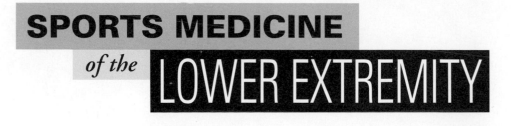

SPORTS MEDICINE
of the LOWER EXTREMITY

EDITION 2

SPORTS MEDICINE
of the LOWER EXTREMITY

EDITION 2

STEVEN I. SUBOTNICK, D.P.M., N.D., D.C.

Clinical Professor
Departments of Biomechanics and Surgery
California College of Podiatric Medicine
San Francisco, California
Adjunct Professor
Department of Kinesiology
California State University
Hayward, California

CHURCHILL LIVINGSTONE

A Division of Harcourt Brace & Company
New York, Edinburgh, London, Madrid, Melbourne, San Francisco, Tokyo

CHURCHILL LIVINGSTONE
A Division of Harcourt Brace & Company

The Curtis Center
Independence Square West
Philadelphia, Pennsylvania 19106

Library of Congress Cataloging-in-Publication Data

Sports medicine of the lower extremity / edited by Steven
  I. Subotnick. — 2nd ed.
      p.   cm.
    Includes bibliographical references and index.
    ISBN 0–443–08999–X
    1. Sports medicine.   2. Leg—Wounds and injuries.   3. Human
  mechanics.   I. Subotnick, Steven I.
    RC1236.L43S66   1999
  617-5'8044—DC21
  DLC   98–21519

SPORTS MEDICINE OF THE LOWER EXTREMITY   ISBN 0-443-08999-X

Copyright © 1999, 1989 by Churchill Livingstone

Churchill Livingstone® is a registered trademark of Harcourt Brace & Company

℗ is a trademark of Harcourt Brace & Company.

Printed in the United States of America.

Last digit is the print number: 9   8   7   6   5   4   3   2   1

In loving memory of my father, Leonard Subotnick
May 19, 1988.
To my mother, Ruth Subotnick; my wonderfully supportive wife, Janice;
and my marvelous children, Mark, Ali, and Kari.

Contributors

David R. Allen, MD
Founder-President, Integrative Medicine, Los Angeles, California
Chinese Medicine and the Treatment of Lower Extremity Problems

Barry T. Bates, BSE, PhD
Professor Emeritus, Biomechanics, Department of Exercise and Movement Science, University of Oregon, Eugene, Oregon
Normal Patterns of Walking and Running; Forces Acting on the Lower Extremity

Richard T. Bouché, DPM
Podiatric Surgical Residency Training Committee, Providence-Seattle Medical Center; Chief, Podiatric Medicine and Surgical Services, Virginia Mason Clinic, Seattle, Washington
Exercise-Induced Leg Pain

Donald A. Chu, RPT, PhD
Ather Sports Clinic, Castro Valley, California
Physical Therapy

Drew Collins, ND
South West Naturopathic Medical Center, Scottsdale, Arizona
Naturopathic Sports Medicine

Jan M. Corwin, DC, CCSP
Oak Bay Chiropractic, Oakland, California
Sports Chiropractic

Howard J. Dananberg, DPM
Staff, Catholic Medical Center, Elliott Hospital, Bedford, New Hampshire
Sagittal Plane Biomechanics

George J. Davies, MED, PT, ATC
Professor, University of Wisconsin; Lacrosse Graduate Program in Physical Therapy; Director, Clinical and Research Services, Gunderson-Lutheran Sports Medicine, La Crosse, Wisconsin
Physical Therapy

Don G. Davis, DC
Private practice, Hayward, California
Manipulation

Patrick A. DeHeer, DPM
Private practice, Winona Foot and Ankle Centers, Muncie, Indiana; Extern Director, Assistant Residency Director, Winona Memorial Hospital; Editorial Board, *Podiatry Today*; Co-Chairman of Continuing Education Committee, Indiana Podiatric Medical Association, Indianapolis, Indiana
Arthroscopy and Endoscopy

Harvey N. Dulberg, PhD
Private practice, Brookline, Massachusetts
The Adult Athlete; Children and Sports

Harry D. Friedman, DO
Assistant Professor, San Francisco College of Osteopathic Medicine; Staff Physician, St. Mary's Spine Center, San Francisco, California
Osteopathic Approach to the Athlete

Ayne Furman, DPM
Courtesy Staff, Alexandria Hospital, Alexandria, Virginia
Golf Injuries

Gary Gordon, DPM
Adjunct Assistant Professor of Podiatric Medicine, Department of Orthopedic Surgery, University of Pennsylvania School of Medicine; Assistant Professor, Department of Community Health, Pennsylvania College of Podiatric Medicine, Philadelphia, Pennsylvania
Basketball Injuries

Elson M. Haas, MD
Private practice, San Rafael, California
Proper Nutrition for Athletes: Maintaining a Balance

Gary Jarvis, OPA-C, ATC
Rehabilitation Consultant, Dallas, Texas
Knee and Thigh Injuries; Hip, Pelvis, and Low Back Injuries

Donald Johnson, MD
Associate Professor of Orthopaedic Surgery, Department of Surgery, University of Ottawa School of Medicine; Director, Sports Medicine Clinic, Carleton University; Orthopaedic Surgeon, Ottawa Civic Hospital, Ottawa, Ontario, Canada
Knee and Thigh Injuries; Hip, Pelvis, and Low Back Injuries

James D. Key, MD, JD, MBA
Regional Teaching Faculty, Kansas City School of Medicine, Kansas City, Kansas; Visiting Lecturer, Uniformed Services University of the Health Sciences, Bethesda Naval Hospital, Bethesda, Maryland; Previously, Chief of Orthopedics, Lutheran Medical Systems Hospital, Dallas, Texas; Clinical Faculty, Southwestern Medical Center (Parkland), Dallas, Texas
Knee and Thigh Injuries; Hip, Pelvis, and Low Back Injuries

Steven R. Kravitz, DPM, FACFAS

Assistant Professor, Department of Orthopedics, Pennsylvania College of Podiatric Medicine; Adjunct Faculty, Department of Surgery, Pennsylvania College of Podiatric Medicine, Philadelphia, Pennsylvania; Surgical Podiatric Residency Director, Allegheny University Hospital, Bucks County, Warminster, Pennsylvania; Faculty, Baja Project for Crippled Children, Los Angeles, California
The Mechanics of Dance and Dance-Related Injuries

Dana J. Lawrence, DC

Director, Department of Publication and Editorial Review; Professor, Department of Chiropractic Practice, National College of Chiropractic, Lombard, Illinois
Manipulation of the Lower Extremity: Chiropractic

Buck Levin, PhD, RD

Associate Professor of Nutrition, Bastyr University, Bothell, Washington
Selected Aspects of Nutrition and Physical Performance

Michael K. Lowe, DPM

Private practice, East Salt Lake City, Utah
Basketball Injuries

Richard O. Lundeen, DPM

Auxiliary Clinical Associate Professor, Ohio College of Podiatric Medicine, Cleveland, Ohio; Private practice, Lundeen Regional Foot and Ankle Center, PC, Indianapolis, Indiana
Arthroscopy and Endoscopy

John E. McNerney, DPM

Adjunct Professor, New York College of Podiatric Medicine, Barry University of Podiatry, Scholl's College of Podiatry, Westwood, New Jersey; Chief of Podiatric Surgery, Pascack Valley Hospital; Consultant Podiatrist, New York Giants, New Jersey MetroStars; New Jersey Devils
Football Injuries

Lyle J. Micheli, MD

Associate Clinical Professor of Orthopaedic Surgery, Harvard Medical School; Director, Division of Sports Medicine, Children's Hospital, Boston, Massachusetts
Lower Extremity Sports Injuries in Children

Carla J. Murgia, PhD

Assistant Professor, Biomechanics and Kinesiology, Dance, Department of Physical Education, Kean University, Union, New Jersey
The Mechanics of Dance and Dance-Related Injuries

C. Michael Neuwelt, MD

Clinical Professor of Medicine, Stanford University, Palo Alto, California; and University of California, San Francisco; Chief of Rheumatology, Alameda County Medical Center, Oakland, California
Anti-inflammatory Medications, Analgesics, and Anesthetics

Robert M. Parks, DPM

Staff Physician, Lovelace Medical Center, Albuquerque, New Mexico
Skiing Injuries/Cross-Country Skiing

David Ponsonby, MEd

Faculty, Research Department, Parker Chiropractice College, Dallas, Texas
Knee and Thigh Injuries; Hip, Pelvis, and Low Back Injuries

John Queally, DPM

Private practice, Brookline, Massachusetts
The Adult Athlete

Nicholas M. Romansky, DPM

Private practice, Philadelphia, Media, and Phoenixville, Pennsylvania; Consultant podiatrist, US Soccer World Cup National and Olympic Men's and Women's soccer teams
Soccer Injuries

Jeffrey A. Ross, DPM, FACFAS

Assistant Clinical Professor, Baylor College of Medicine; Chief, Diabetic Foot Clinic, Ben Taub Hospital, Houston, Texas
Step/Bench Aerobic Dance and Its Potential for Injuries of the Lower Extremity; In Alpine Skiing; A Comparison of Alpine and Cross-Country Skiing; Snowboarding; Tennis Injuries

Allan J. Ryan, MD

University of Wisconsin-Madison, Madison, Wisconsin-Retired; American College of Sports Medicine Fellow
The Sports Medicine Specialist

Michael A. Schmidt, DC, CCN, CNS

Visiting Professor, Applied Biochemistry and Clinical Nutrition, Northwestern College, Bloomington, Minnesota
Selected Aspects of Nutrition and Physical Performance

Pamela Sisney, DPM

Instructor, University of Cincinnati, Cincinnati, Ohio
General Concepts of Injury; Cross-Training and Associated Injuries

Kristin Smith, PT

Candidate, Master of Science in Nutrition, Bastyr University, Bothell, Washington
Selected Aspects of Nutrition and Physical Performance

Nicholas Stergiou, PhD

Assistant Professor of Biomechanics, Department HPER, University of Nebraska at Omaha, Omaha, Nebraska
Normal Patterns of Walking and Running; Forces Acting on the Lower Extremity

Steven I. Subotnick, DPM, ND, DC

Clinical Professor, Departments of Biomechanics and Surgery, California College of Podiatric Medicine, San Francisco, California; Adjunct Professor, Department of Kinesiology, California State University, Hayward, California
The Sports Medicine Specialist of the Lower Extremity, The Podiatrist; The Four Phases of Running; Athletic Training and Conditioning; Injury Prevention; Normal Anatomy, Functional Anatomy; Biomechanics of the Foot and Ankle; Sports-Specific Biomechanics; General Concepts of Injury; Foot Injuries, Ankle Injuries; History and Physical Examination; Diagnostic Imaging; Orthoses; Surgical Intervention in the Foot and Ankle; In Alpine Skiing; Complementary Approaches Introduction; Homeopathic Medicine

Yvonne Sun, MD
Tricity Imaging, Fremont, California
Diagnostic Imaging

Paul M. Taylor, DPM
Clinical Instructor, Department of Orthopedics (Podiatry), Georgetown University School of
Medicine, Washington, DC; Past President, American Academy of Podiatric Sports Medicine
Basketball Injuries

Ronald Valmassey, DPM
Professor, Department of Podiatric Biomechanics, California College of Podiatric Medicine; Staff
Podiatrist, Center for Sports Medicine, St. Francis Hospital, San Francisco, California
Orthoses

William L. Van Pelt, DPM
Visiting Lecturer, Ricci University; Harris County Podiatric Medical Residency Program; Chief of
Podiatry, Memorial City Medical Center, Houston, Texas
Accommodation, Strapping, and Bracing

Harold W. Vogler, DPM
Visiting Professor, Orthopaedics, Malmö University Hospital, Malmö, Sweden; Adjunct Professor of
Surgery, Pennsylvania College of Podiatric Medicine, Philadelphia, Pennsylvania; Research Fellow in
Biomechanics and Functional Anatomy, Panum Institute, University of Copenhagen, Copenhagen,
Denmark; Chairman, Section of Foot Surgery, University Community Hospital, Tampa, Florida
Surgical Intervention in the Foot and Ankle

Roger F. Widmann, MD
Instructor in Surgery (Orthopaedics), Cornell University Medical College; Assistant Attending
Orthopaedic Surgeon, Hospital for Special Surgery, New York, New York
Lower Extremity Sports Injuries in Children

Robert J. Wysocki, DPM*
Private practice, Central Podiatry Associates, Inc., Toledo, Ohio; Diplomate, American Board of
Podiatric Surgery (Ambulatory)
Bowling Injuries

Jeffrey F. Yale, DPM
Adjunct Professor, California College of Podiatric Medicine; Illinois College of Podiatric Medicine,
Chicago, Illinois; Chairman, Podiatry Division, Department of Surgery, Griffin Hospital,
Derby, Connecticut
Baseball Injuries

---

*Deceased

Preface

This revision of Sports Medicine of the Lower Extremity represents an integrated approach to treating the athlete, as evidenced by the number of specialists from various disciplines who have contributed to the revision. It also represents a broadening of the field of sports medicine as it enters a new millennium with new, ever-changing patient expectations, and a generation of athlete-physicians and their patients who are entering middle age and beyond, becoming senior citizens. Sports medicine of the past focused on the younger athlete on high-school, college, and professional teams. Then, with the fitness and running revolution of the early 1970s, the 30-something recreational athletes became the majority of many of our practices. As we and our athletes became older, the emphasis began to shift to preventative medicine and wellness as well as longevity. Suddenly cholesterol, blood pressure, stress reduction, and maintenance of health became more important.

This revision also reflects my evolution as a physician and healer. I entered podiatry school to become a healer, yet somewhere during the process of my education—4 years of podiatric medical school, my internship at Highland General Hospital, and my surgical residency—I lost touch with that initial calling and became hardened. My healing tools were scalpels, cortisone injections, prescription drugs, and other invasive forms of intervention. At times my successes were gratifying, yet the failures were dismal. The "first do no harm" doctrine began to haunt me. As did most of the contributors in this text, I used the tools I had available and thought little of what existed beyond, viewing any other methods of treatment as being remotely beneficial to the health or recovery of my injured patients.

At this time in my life, I had taken up running as a recreational and fitness activity, and I eventually became a marathoner. My intellectual and professional interest in running helped me to develop the principles of a biomechanical approach to treating the athlete. I now had another tool that helped and did no harm. I began to see the athlete, as well as myself, as more than just a bunch of parts. The idea of an integrated whole far more complex and infinitely more meaningful than the sum of the parts began to emerge. The healer in me, never dead, re-emerged, and my journey into wholeness opened me up to new worlds.

Personal circumstances led me to homeopathic medicine. I completed 3 years of extensive training in classical homeopathy at the Hahnemann College of Homeopathy from a faculty of physicians who inspired me and taught by example the meaning of being a healer. They were all superbly grounded in conventional medicine, yet relied upon homeopathic medicine to treat a variety of acute as well as chronic diseases that often had failed to respond to orthodox medicine.

Yet despite its elegance and ability to heal the whole person deeply on all levels, classical homeopathy wasn't the answer for every patient or all conditions. I needed a system that integrated all of the various healing techniques that I had been taught were valuable to the athlete—sometimes by the athletes themselves, who had always been in favor of exercise, nutrition, and natural modalities over drugs or surgery, whenever possible, to improve performance or heal an injury. I found that system in naturopathic medicine. The naturopathic physician goes through 4 years of medical school, with the same emphasis on medical sciences that all disciplines share during their first 2 years, followed by study of natural therapeutics such as diet and nutritional therapies, physiotherapy, manual therapies, herbal and homeopathic remedies, and psychotherapy. The naturopath treats the whole person, appreciating that health or disease comes from a complex interaction of physical, emotional, dietary, genetic, environmental, life-style, and other factors.

I then furthered my studies in manipulative medicine by becoming a chiropractor. I gained a greater appreciation of the innate healing process that we all possess, and learned new methods to unlock this force when it becomes slowed down or suppressed by subluxations or nerve impingement. The meaning of biomechanical efficiency took on new proportions as I integrated chiropractic into my holistic sports medicine practice. Most importantly, I gained a healthy respect for the education and skills that chiropractors possess, and the importance of chiropractors integrated into the health care system as entry-level caregivers.

I now, after 25 years of practice, have tools to treat a wide variety of injuries and illness, I can advise about and help to prevent disease, and I have methods and modalities to reverse or cure chronic disease. I have answers for those patients who have exhausted what orthodox medicine has to offer. I rely heavily on my allopathic background, I operate when I have tried all else and believe surgery is the only option left, use antibiotics when indicated, order imaging studies, and refer to my medical colleagues for consultation and treatment.

I know the territory, the "lay of the land," and can individualize a treatment plan for wellness, life enhancement, and recovery that suits each individual according to his or her own unique constitution. I, like my brethren sports medicine specialists, am becoming the healer I have always dreamed of being, a generalist with specialist skills.

This revision, and especially the chapter on complementary approaches to medicine, reflects this wholeness transformation that is so essential for the future of sports medicine, and medicine in general, as they enter the next century.

Preface to the First Edition

This text assembles and synthesizes a diverse body of knowledge essential to podiatrists and other health professionals involved in sports medicine. A basic knowledge of podiatric and/or orthopedic medicine is not enough to qualify one as a sports medicine specialist; in addition, it is necessary to understand both the principles of athletic medicine as a whole and the biomechanical peculiarities and associated injuries of specific sports. The sports medicine specialist must also be familiar with the functional changes in anatomy and biomechanics characteristic of athletes participating in various sports.

This book includes chapters on fitness, exercise physiology, training methods, and the podiatric considerations of various sports. The normal anatomy, functional anatomy, and biomechanics of the lower extremity are presented in detail. The mechanisms and biodynamics of injury are discussed, as are the tools of diagnosis and the differential diagnoses of athletic injuries. Initial and subsequent treatments, including physical therapy, manipulation, orthoses, strapping, surgery, and arthroscopy, are covered thoroughly, with a chapter devoted to each treatment modality. The psychological aspects of sports and sports injury in the adult and child are discussed.

This comprehensive text is intended for podiatric physicians and sports medicine specialists who wish to give individualized, well-considered treatment to their patients. To win in sports, the team must work together; likewise, in sports medicine, a team approach is often best. This text draws on the experience of each contributor in his or her field and, like sports medicine itself, is the result of a well-integrated team effort.

I wish to give special thanks to Podiatric Sports Medicine fellows Pamela Sisney, D.P.M., Walter E. Roth III, D.P.M., Lawrence M. Horn, D.P.M., and Richard Jones, D.P.M., for their editing, writing, proofreading, and tremendous support; and a very grateful thanks to Stanley Newell, D.P.M., for his illustrations. I am also grateful to Kim Loretucci and Leslie Burgess of Churchill Livingstone for their support and encouragement.

Finally, thank you to Barbara Howard, my secretary. Without her help, this project could never have been completed.

Contents

I

Sports Medicine
and Athletics

1

The Expanding Sports Medicine Specialty

The Sports Medicine Specialist

ALLAN J. RYAN

HISTORICAL REVIEW

The first attempt in recent history to bring together physicians with a special interest in sports and exercise appears to have been the establishment of a separate section on "Hygiene of Physical Exercise" at the World Hygiene Exposition held in Dresden in 1911. Physicians meeting during the second winter Olympic Games in St. Moritz in February 1928, and again in August of the same year, at the games of the Ninth Olympiad in Amsterdam, established the Association Internationale Medico-Sportive; this group subsequently became known as the International Federation of Sports Medicine. As a result of this, teaching and research in this field developed in many European countries, and in some a specialty certification was established. The first publications dealing with this subject in England and the United States appeared in 1927, and medical services of this type were offered chiefly to college and university athletes. There was no organized interest in the United States until the 1950s.

DEFINITION

Although interest on the part of physicians has grown steadily since then (many are devoting a major portion of their time to sports medicine), there has been no initiative to establish sports medicine as a formal medical specialty.

This puzzles some people, especially those regularly and vigorously involved in physical exercise and sports, because they are looking for expert advice and treatment and have become accustomed to increasing specialization in other fields of medicine. To understand why this is not happening in sports medicine, it is necessary to understand how the field is defined today.

Sports medicine is currently understood to include (1) the medical supervision and care of the competitive and recreational athlete, (2) the provision of appropriate physical exercise and sports for persons who are handicapped in any way, (3) advice about the conduct and supervision of activities that develop and maintain physical fitness, and (4) the organization and provision of exercise and sports activities for people being rehabilitated from illness or injury. Physicians are active in all four phases of this field; however, the extent and variety of the planning, research, and activities involved go beyond those ordinarily considered medical practice, and often involve the participation of people with different educational backgrounds, training, and occupations.

This fact alone, however, is not a barrier to the designation of the physicians involved as members of a medical specialty group. Standards appropriate for training in such a specialty could be developed, and examinations (both oral and written, as well as of a practical nature) could be prepared to establish qualification. Practitioners who demonstrated their qualifications by virtue of their specific training and by examination could then be certified as specialists and required to limit their practice to this field. One result of this approach would be the exclusion of physicians not so qualified or those holding certification in other specialties from practicing in this field.

The central problem with establishing sports medicine as a separate and distinct specialty is that the medical activities involved in the field, taken as a whole, cut across many established medical specialties: much of the care involved in treatment of the injured athlete requires the special skills of the orthopedic surgeon; the examination and qualification of the very young athlete requires the special knowledge and experience of the pediatrician or family practitioner. For example, testing of and recommending exercise to the person with heart disease requires the judgment and abilities of the cardiologist or general internist; management of injuries to the central nervous system requires the services of a neurologist or neurosurgeon; and the special problems involved in the correct identification and treatment of problems in the lower extremities demands the knowledge and skills of the orthopedist or podiatrist. The relationships of all these problems to the sports medicine situation in which they are encountered may require special knowledge and preparation, but the basic aspects require the standard preparation for each of these specialties.

Another consideration is the willingness of physicians qualified in these other specialties to give up their practices in those fields and devote themselves entirely to sports medicine; how desirable this is for society must be considered also.

ESTABLISHING THE SPECIALITY

Since sports medicine practice cuts across many established medical specialties, a decision to establish it as another specialty must be based on three basic requirements. The first of these is whether a distinct body of knowledge defining it as a field separate from other specialties can be established. The second is to determine whether a sufficient body of knowledge exists to allow practitioners to establish practices independent of other specialties. The third is whether specific training programs can be identified that would produce physicians qualified in, and with the necessary skills to apply, this body of knowledge correctly.

An already vast and still growing collection of literature in the field of sports medicine indicates that a distinct body of knowledge does exist. This has been further confirmed by a group of interested and involved physicians by their development of a database outline delineating the scope and

specific topics that compose this body of knowledge. This database draws from many different fields of basic science and medical specialities, integrating this information in ways unique to the purposes that have been defined for this field. For example, the diagnosis and management of acute brain injury fall within the field of knowledge that is part of the medical specialties of neurology and neurosurgery; however, the question of when a person who has suffered a concussion is able, with a reasonable degree of caution, to return to sports and competition requires the additional knowledge and experience of the sports physician.

The practice of sports medicine in the United States today does not engage most physicians full time, since they also see and treat patients who come to them for their special qualifications as internists, pediatricians, orthopedic surgeons, or podiatrists. If a physician trained in family practice, for example, decided to devote himself to a full-time sports medicine practice—that is, to the medical supervision of recreational and competitive athletes, to examination and counseling handicapped persons for participation in modified or adapted exercises and sports, to developing and supervising programs for the development and maintenance of physical fitness, and to advising and supervising for programs of therapeutic exercise—there would certainly be sufficient work to maintain an independent practice. Practices of this type would also provide abundant opportunities for research and teaching to advance the sports medicine field.

None of the academic degree programs in the United States is devoted in its entirety to turning out specialists in sports medicine. Limited sections of residency training programs in family practice and orthopedic surgery are devoted to sports medicine. Fellowships in sports medicine are offered by some departments of orthopedics for a school term for those students who have already satisfied their training requirements in that specialty. Podiatric sports medicine fellowships running for 6 months to 1 year have been in existence since 1977. However, in general, today's practicing physicians and podiatrists learn about and become involved in sports medicine by attending conferences, seminars, and special courses in the field; reading the literature; and learning from practical experience, individually or as an apprentice to someone already established in the field.

THE SPORTS MEDICINE PRACTITIONER TODAY

Those who practice sports medicine as a part of their regular occupation include not only physicians—especially family and general practitioners, general surgeons, orthopedic surgeons, pediatricians, and podiatrists—but also dentists, physiologists, physical educators, coaches, physical therapists, and psychologists. These people work both independently and in teams, teamwork being characteristic of sports medicine as it is of sports. They share their special knowledges and skills for the purpose of providing the best possible advice and management to the exercising person.

The multidisciplinary character of this field of practice is demonstrated by the number of different professional organizations to which its practitioners may belong. Although each group may have its origin and primary support within a special field, all of them welcome the membership of interested and involved persons from other professional backgrounds. These organizations include the American College of Sports Medicine (ACSM); the American Orthopedic Society for Sports Medicine; the American Osteopathic of Podiatric Sports Medicine; the Academy of Sports Dentistry; the American Alliance for Health, Physical Education, Recreation and Dance; the Sports Medicine Section of the American Physical Therapy Association; the National Athletic Trainers Association; and the North American Society for Sports Psychology.

Further possibilities for special training and qualification in the field include the expansion of existing programs and the development of new ones. Opportunities for expanding existing programs are limited by the objectives of the organizations now operating them, and the need to engage more qualified instructors and find additional funds to do this. Most programs currently operate at or beyond their financial limits. Their expenses continue to increase while their overall operating funds have not increased proportionately. Government support in this field has been virtually nonexistent, and private support has been limited by the fact that there has been little appreciation of these programs' overall contribution to the general welfare and economy.

CERTIFICATION IN SPORTS MEDICINE FOR PHYSICIANS

After years of consideration and discussion concerning the qualification of physicians who examine, supervise, and care for athletes, physician members of the ACSM opened discussions about how this would and should be done with other medical associations and organizations who were catering to the interests and activities of physicians providing advice and services in the general field of sports medicine. A preliminary step was the establishment in 1987 of a clinical conference of the College in the midwinter to allow

more opportunities for medically oriented presentations for physician members and fellows of the College and other interested persons, since the annual meeting had become so congested with papers describing research findings in exercise physiology, nutrition, biomechanics, psychology, and rehabilitation that were health, rather than sports, related.

On March 19 to 24, 1989, the ACSM inaugurated the Team Physician Course in Orlando, Florida, in collaboration with the American Orthopedic Society for Sports Medicine, the American Osteopathic Academy, the Canadian Academy of Sports Medicine, the American College of Surgeons, the American Academy of Pediatrics, the American College of Obstetrics and Gynecology, the American Academy of Neurological Surgeons, the American Academy of Ophthalmology, and the American College of Emergency Physicians. The course is directed to the individual possessing an M.D. or D.O. degree, which the ACSM and the cooperating organizations feel is the minimum background necessary to benefit from the course.

The 54-hour curriculum is designed to disseminate the information necessary for a physician to cover comfortably an educational institution's athletic problems or an athletic event. The term *team physician* recognizes the tradition in the United States that was established by the appointment of the first football team physician for the Harvard Athletic Association, Dr. William M. Conant, in 1890. Football at that time was the leading college, and later high school, sport and produced the greatest number of injury problems among all organized sports, but the team physicians came gradually to accept similar responsibilities for athletes engaged in other sports as well.

The Team Physician Course was originally organized in three parts, each to be given in successive winter seasons, and the three parts were presented in 1989, 1990, and 1991. As one result of the great demand for admission to this course, Part I was presented again in 1992, and Parts II and III were presented concurrently in March 1993 at Lake Buena Vista in Florida. The original three-part course was then redesigned so that it could be completed in 2 years by adding aspects of Parts II and III to Part I and designated the remainder as Part II. The new Part I was offered in Dallas, Texas, in 1994. Parts I and II have been offered annually at different locations. Beginning in 1998 they will be combined at a conference preceding the annual ACSM meeting offering 57 hours of experience.

The program goal for the Team Physician Course was stated as follows:

Upon completion of the three parts of the American

College of Sports Medicine Team Physician Course, a physician will have been presented the information to perform the duties of a team physician. These include

1. Organization of medical care for athletic teams and events.
2. Delivery of medical care for the athletes:
   a. Preparticipation evaluation
   b. Treatment of illness and injuries
   c. Identification of proper management of nutritional, psychological, and drug problems
3. Assisting in the development of conditioning and training programs.
4. Providing coverage for games and other athletic events, including mass participation events.
5. Hands-on experience.

Completion of each part entitles the physician to credit hours in Category I of the Physicians Recognition Award of the American Medical Association, and the program is acceptable for Prescribed Hours by the American Academy of Family Physicians.

The establishment of the Team Physicians Course was accompanied by the production of a series of five 20-minute tapes: ACSM's Guidelines for the Team Physician.[1]

This series is not a part of the course but is meant to supplement it as well as to inform physicians who have not taken but may wish to take the course.

Certificates indicating completion of Parts I and II of the course are issued by the ACSM on behalf of all the cooperating Colleges, academies, and societies with the date of completion.

The establishment of a certification for physicians in sports medicine provides all interested parties with a reasonable means of identifying persons who are qualified to serve as team physicians at all levels. It does not exclude any physician who does not have this certification from serving as a team physician from practicing what is generally regarded as sports medicine in general in the promotion, establishment, and maintenance of physical fitness and good health. Medical clinics, both public and private, and hospitals that operate inpatient and outpatient services for both general and special populations, will probably welcome physicians as members and consultants to answer the needs they are specially qualified to serve.

The American Medical Society for Sports Medicine was formed in 1991 to fill an apparent need to foster a collegial relationship among sports medicine physicians who offer primary nonsurgical care in this field. It has cooperated with the American Orthopedic Society for Sports Medicine to present courses on Current Concepts for the Team Physician.

The Sports Medicine Specialist of the Lower Extremity, the Podiatrist
STEVEN I. SUBOTNICK

As the specialty of sports medicine continues to grow, the body of knowledge required to adequately diagnose, treat, refer for a team approach, and finally return an injured athlete to activity or competition, grows exponentially. When the first edition of *Sports Medicine of the Lower Extremity* was written, well-defined lines existed between the respective professions involved in the treatment of the athlete. Now, as of the second edition, those distinctions are less apparent. All of us in sports medicine have our specific fields of expertise; the podiatrist is the specialist of the foot and ankle, as well as biomechanics of the lower extremity. The orthopedist is the "knee doctor." The osteopath or chiropractor is the "back doctor." In practice, however, all must know the foot, ankle, leg, knee, thigh, hip, and back; nutrition; training; general medicine; sports psychology; and so on. The sports medicine specialist is in reality the sports medicine *generalist*. There is so much overlap that degrees and artificial boundaries have no place in sports medicine. What counts is a broad base of knowledge, experience, and a desire to help the athlete, whatever caliber—recreational, fitness, or professional—enjoy a healthy, fulfilling life with sports as part of an overall balanced life-style. The relationship between physical activity and health-related quality of life is well documented.[2] Physical activity and physical fitness avert premature mortality while promoting health and favoring longevity.[3] The importance of an eclectic "bag of tricks" borrowing from many disciplines becomes obvious when faced with the responsibility of keeping our patients active and exercising, enjoying pain-free sports and fitness participation.

Within this field, sports medicine of the lower extremity is particularly important, since most sports depend on proper foot function for maximum performance and to avoid overuse or traumatic injuries to other parts of the body. Variations in the angle of gait in different sports must be considered when treating lower extremity athletic injuries.[4–6] Similarly, these variations must be considered when attempting to decrease the likelihood of injury while coaching athletes or helping them improve their performance.[7,8] The sports medicine podiatrist is a valuable and indispensible member of the sports medicine team.

DEFINITION

The application of podiatric medical, biomechanical, palliative, surgical, and diagnostic methods to the athlete defines the scope of podiatric sports medicine. Knowledge of functional biomechanics; orthopedics; training, coaching, and conditioning methods; exercise physiology; and sports psychology, nutrition, physical therapy, and rehabilitation must be integrated into the discipline of podiatric medicine.

Podiatric sports medicine also assumes a basic working knowledge of the unique demands placed on athletes. Their emotional needs must be addressed, as must physiologic, biomechanical, and metabolic needs. It goes without saying that sports medicine podiatrists must be well versed in sport-specific biomechanics and kinetics, injury patterns, and rehabilitative exercises that are unique to different sports or positions in team sports. Furthermore, age-related injuries and preventative measures must be appreciated, as well as those general medical factors related to gender. It is the goal of the podiatric sports medicine specialist to return athletes to sports competition in better condition than they were in before injury. This means improving strength, flexibility, balance, power, and biomechanical function. This also includes imparting to the athlete an increased awareness of the mechanism of injury and of what can be done to prevent injury in the future.

The sports medicine podiatrist should approach each injured athlete with the following general and specific questions in mind:

1. Who am I treating? A professional, college, or high school athlete? A recreational athlete? An addicted, phase III, marathoner or triathelete? A senior citizen fitness walker or jogger? An occasional athlete, the "weekend warrior"?

2. How important is it for my patient to get back to competition?

3. What are the inherent risks involved in the sport, and what can be done to minimize them?

4. How will treatment affect the ability of the athlete to return to safe participation or competition?

5. Is treatment more likely to fail because of the biodynamics and/or biomechanics of the sport?

6. Are the biodynamics of the sport such that no form of interventive treatment is appropriate (e.g., surgery in a ballet dancer)?

7. How can exercise withdrawal be handled in the "addicted" athlete? What types of alternate aerobic exercises are available?

When dealing with fitness athletes:

8. How much aerobic exercise is enough for basic health and fitness? What are the benefits of aerobic versus anaerobic exercise?

9. What are the characteristics of an overuse injury? What are the pros and cons of exercise and/or sports as a way of life?

10. What is the effect of the sport on the complaint or injury?

And finally:

11. When is it time to tell an athlete to change sports, *to hang up their shoes*?

These questions take into account the scope of sports medicine and the specific needs of each athlete. Their answers will point the sports medicine podiatrist toward the appropriate form of treatment, rehabilitation, and conditioning for the injured athletic patient.

PROFILE OF PODIATRIC SPORTS MEDICINE PATIENTS

The athletes who see a sports medicine practitioner are of a broad spectrum in fitness levels, commitment to sports, body types, and age. Even within the same sport, genetic polymorphism produces uniquely individual athletes who have personalities of their own. Factors that lend themselves to predicting performance or injury predilection are broad and generalized at best.[9] In an effort to identify the types of athletes and specific injury patterns, data have been obtained in an ongoing retrospective study from a profile of the various sports medicine patients seen in a podiatric sports medicine practice, averaging 1,000 patients per year, between 1971 and 1996. This created a database of 25,000 to 26,000 athletes. The age group ranged from 5 to 94 years. Originally, in the 1970s, most of the patients were joggers, recreational athletes, and long-distance runners; during the 1980s, interest among women in aerobic dance and jazzercise paralleled the growing women's rights movement, and these activities continue in popularity in the late 1990s, and hopefully into the next millenium. Fitness walking became more prevalent in the late 1980s and is growing ever stronger in the late 1990s. Fitness and recreational walkers have overtaken both runners and aerobic exercise participants as the most commonly injured fitness enthusiasts. As the "baby boomers" begin to enter their late 40s and early 50s, those who were once runners and joggers become walkers, and for good reason—walking is safe and excellent aerobic exercise.[10]

It is estimated that in the late 1970s long-distance running had about 35 million participants in the United States. In May 1996, in San Francisco, 78,000 people participated in the Bay-to-Breakers race-carnival through the streets of San Francisco, between 7 and 8 miles. As of 1987, aerobics could claim 25 million participants; walking as of 1996 has well over 75 million fitness and recreational enthusiasts. As the population ages, one can assume that walking will continue to be a major fitness activity.[11] Golf and bowling continue to grow in popularity and, as their participants age, more foot-related injuries are presenting to foot specialists and general practioners. There is virtually an epidemic of heel injuries endemic to an active, although aging, population. These "athletes" need the treatment and biomechanical expertise of the sports podiatrist; they simply will not recover, despite all the good intentions of the primary care "gatekeeper" without this specialized knowledge and approach.

Youth league soccer contributes a considerable number of aches and strains in youngsters with problems associated with rapid growth spurts, such as apophysitis. Summer league softball, gymnastics, skiing, field hockey, tennis, basketball, race walking, and football all are popular and have their own host of associated injuries.

It is of particular interest that most athletes seen have few problems during everyday activities.[12] They might occasionally complain of problems secondary to improper shoe fit or postural fatigue due to biomechanical imbalances; the sports merely aggravated the deformity. Those who had bony or retrocalcaneal exostoses were previously asymptomatic in everyday foot gear; those who had plantar fasciitis and/or heel-spur syndrome were generally asymptomatic before the athletic endeavor. Those who had leg complaints, such as chronic periostitis or medial shin syndrome, were invariably asymptomatic before engaging in sports; the same is true of those with generalized overuse injury about the knee. Similarly, athletes with neuroma-type pain were usually asymptomatic prior to athletic endeavor and increased stress under the forefoot.

A TREATMENT APPROACH

It is vital for all those in sports medicine to realize the importance of the function of the foot and the interdependence of the entire kinetic chain above the foot to proper foot functioning. During most sports that include running, approximately three times the body weight is borne on the support foot. Thus biomechanical abnormalities of the lower extremity must be multiplied by 3 to realize their true importance. For example, a 3-degree forefoot varus imbalance allowing for abnormal pronation, which normally would cause few symptoms in everyday activities, is as important in the athlete as would be a 9-degree deformity in the nonathlete. This 3-degree forefoot varus deformity would be enough to cause abnormal pronation and delayed resupination in the athlete, which could affect the foot, ankle, leg, knee, thigh, hip, or even the back.[13] Conversely, variations in the functioning of the back, pelvis, hip, knee, leg, or ankle can also affect the foot. The entire kinetic chain must be evaluated to see which part is causing the abnormal effect on the other members.[14]

Many lower extremity overuse or traumatic injuries will respond to a combined approach of improving foot function and providing for symptom relief and total rehabilitation. An approach that has worked well for me is the use of temporary foot orthotics, made out of soft materials, on the initial visit. This improves foot function and aids the evaluation of its effect on the presenting complaint. For example, an athlete may enter my office with a complaint of chondralgia patella secondary to increased mileage in long-distance running. This athlete may have been jogging 30 miles each week with no pain, but upon increasing mileage to 40 miles a week began to experience stiffness that gradually became pain and then disability in the peripatellar area. Abnormal footwear on the symptomatic side may also be noted. My approach would be a complete biomechanical examination of the lower extremity to rule out serious abnormalities in the knee joint itself. Soft temporary orthotics are fabricated on the initial visit, and the patient is evaluated running on a treadmill. The orthotics are adjusted until biomechanical functional foot control is nearly restored. The athlete is then put on a rehabilitation program to strengthen the quadriceps muscles. If within 3 to 4 weeks the symptoms decrease and foot function is improved, a more permanent functional orthosis is made. Orthotic foot control is only part of the total rehabilitation of this athlete, but a very important part.

It is also possible that the complaint is not due to a biomechanical foot imbalance. The chondralgia patella could have been caused by an improper foot function secondary to a short leg, to an imbalance within the anatomic structure of the foot itself, or to an abnormality within the knee. In these cases, it is important for the sports medicine practitioner to recognize the cause and refer the patient to an orthopedist.

SUMMARY

It is imperative for the entire sports medicine team to realize the importance of lower extremity function, as well as the role of the sports medicine podiatrist. It is equally important for the sports medicine podiatrist to recognize those problems that will not respond to functional biome-chanical treatment and to be prepared to refer the patient to the appropriate specialists on the sports medicine team (or elsewhere) when the need arises.

REFERENCES

The Sports Medicine Specialist

1. Cantu RC, Kibler B, Micheli L et al: ACSM's Guidelines for the Team Physician. Five-tape set. Williams & Wilkins, Baltimore, 1992

The Sports Medicine Specialist of the Lower Extremity, the Podiatrist

2. Rejeski WJ, Brawley LR, Schumaker SA: Physical activity in health-related quality of life. Exercise Sport Sci Rev 24: 71, 1996
3. Lee IM, Paffenbarger RS: Physical activity and physical fitness avert premature mortality. Exercise Sport Sci Rev 24: 135, 1996
4. Marti B, Vadar JP, Minder CE et al: On the epidemiology of running injuries: the 1984 Bern Grand-Prix study. Am J Sports Med 16:265, 1988
5. Subotnick SI: Variations in angles of gait in running. Physician Sports Med 7:110, 1979
6. Macera CA, Pate RR, Powell KE et al: Predicting lower extremity injuries among habitual runners. Arch Intern Med 149:2565, 1989
7. Brill PA, Macera CA: The influence of running patterns on running injuries. Sports Med 20:365, 1995
8. Mero A, Komi PV, Gregor RJ: Biomechanics of sprint running: a review. Sports Med 13:376, 1992
9. Bouchard C, Dionne FT: Genetics of aerobic and anaerobic performance. Exercise Sport Sci Rev 20:27, 1992
10. Davison RC, Grant S: Is walking sufficient exercise for health? [editorial] Sports Med 16:369, 1993
11. Kallinen M, Markku A: Aging, physical activity and sports injuries: an overview of common sports injuries in the elderly. Sports Med 80:41, 1995
12. Kibler WB, Chandler TJ, Stracener ES: Musculoskeletal adaptations and injuries due to overtraining. Exercise Sport Sci Rev 20:99, 1992
13. Subotnick SI: Orthotic foot control and the overuse syndrome. Physician Sports Med 3:61, 1975
14. Plowman SA: Physical activity, physical fitness, and low back pain. Exercise Sport Sci Rev 20:221, 1992

2

Psychological Considerations

The Adult Athlete

HARVEY N. DULBERG
JOHN QUEALLY

For many years, our society has considered the pursuit of sport and exercise as an activity that should be dominated by our youth. Except for the professional adult athlete, researchers have geared their studies toward the physical and psychological benefits that children and adolescents take away from sports. Accordingly, parents have focused so much of their attention on their child's progress that they have rarely had time to consider their own needs as "athletes." But along with the health-conscious 1980s came the well-justified belief that people of all ages, child through senior citizen, can improve their physical as well as psychological well-being through sports and exercise. In other words, each and every person should consider him- or herself an athlete to some degree. Thus, in conjunction with this athletic enlightenment, researchers have begun to look at the psychological needs and problems facing young and middle-aged adults, as well as senior citizens. This chapter highlights some of the more recent findings dealing with the psychological issues of motivation, injuries, overtraining, and burnout as applied to the non-professional adult athlete.

MOTIVATING FACTORS

The most fundamental reason one can give for participating in sports or some exercise program is the physical benefits these activities provide. Whether it be decreasing the heart rate through aerobic workouts or lifting weights to increase strength and muscle mass, the goal of an improved body for increased longevity of life is quite common. But by no means is this the single goal of participation. As Clough, Shepherd, and Maughan[1] have demonstrated, psychological factors play a significant role in motivating an athlete into action. In their study, Clough et al. presented a list of 70 reasons for running to 521 runners, asking them to rate the salience of each reason as it applied to them. The format of the list allowed the researchers to determine the importance of six basic motivating factors in the lives of runners: challenge, health/fitness, mental well-being, addiction, status, and social factors. What the findings revealed was that two of the three top motivating factors, including the most salient motive, were psychologically based. The most powerful motivator runners cited was the self-esteem created by meeting the athletic challenge of running. After health and fitness came the third top answer, the mental well-being that running provides. Participants feel a reduction in stress, an elevation of mood, and a general feeling of control over one's life after engaging in this activity.[1] Although the desire for better physical health is a more worthwhile goal of sport and exercise, we cannot emphasize enough what these activities do for the mind and spirit of the athlete.

In accordance with the psychological motives presented by Clough et al.,[1] Ewart[2] discovered that athletes may also be motivated by the process through which they can release anger that has been building inside of them. In a similarly constructed study of mountain climbers, Ewart found that the experience of a catharsis can be very important to an athlete. For example, the athlete who is under an enormous amount of stress and is carrying strong aggressive and negative emotions may channel or sublimate these emotions into a positive activity, such as sport. The athletic arena usually provides a safe and socially acceptable environment in which to release these emotions. The entire process, which then results in a more positive mood, is commonly known as a catharsis. Without an outlet such as sports, the anger and stress produced by the everyday lives of the average adult may be overwhelming. Only now is our society beginning to fully understand the impact athletic activity can have on our lives.

As we have seen, a number of people are seeking to escape the effects of their day-to-day lives. There are also adults who are trying to escape something else: the myths that accompany old age. Society's impression of seniors has never been one of the successful athlete, but instead a frail and dependent being. But as O'Brien and Vertinsky[3] describe, "obtaining the knowledge and power to be more in control of one's body in late life are liberating forces that more and more aging adults seek." To be able to shed such a popular misconception must do wonders for the self-esteem of these elder athletes. From these seniors, the adult population as a whole can take away the knowledge that it is never too late to start playing.

THE PROVEN BENEFITS OF EXERCISE

The relationship between sports or exercise and one's psychological well-being is more than just an abstract idea. Countless studies have empirically examined the positive effects of these activities on the psyches of recognized athletes and nonathletes alike. According to Hughes,[4] by 1984 alone, more than 1,000 studies had dealt with the topic, and most of the results were in agreement as to the power of exercise. In fact, one of the few points of debate seems to be over which types of exercise are more effective psychologically. In a study done by Steptoe et al.,[5] results indicated that moderate aerobic workouts, in this case consisting of jogging, alleviated psychological tension in both normal psychologically healthy people, as well as those who suffer from moderate anxiety. Nonaerobic exercise such as weight or flexibility training produced no such effect in either group.

More recent studies in the area, however, such as those conducted by Ossip-Klien and colleagues[6] and then by Stein and Motta,[7] contradict the notion of nonaerobic ex-

ercise as being psychologically useless. Ossip-Klien et al. discovered that, compared to an aerobic group, those participating in a nonaerobic program showed slightly better results in a test of their self-concept. In addition, Stein and Motta cited in their study that, "while only the aerobic group improved cardiovascularly, both the aerobic and non-aerobic exercise groups experienced a reduction in depression relative to that of the control group." As the studies mount up, the proof that sports and exercise create psychological benefits cannot be denied. The goal that we now face is to target the activities that provide the most positive impact.

WHO IS NOT MOTIVATED?

Still, in the face of all this evidence, national participation in sports in not what it should be. In 1986, less than 20% of adults 18 to 65 years old exercised at sufficient levels. By 1992, the level had increased to only 25%.[8] Thus researchers have been left wondering exactly who is not motivated and why more than half of the people who start exercise programs do not finish them.

With so many people not motivated to exercise, it is hard to pinpoint one trait or characteristic that is common to all of them, but tendencies do exist. There are some qualities to the nonparticipant that can be seen more often than not. For example, as LeUnes and Nation[8] explain, numerous studies have found that smokers are notorious for having poor adherence rates in exercise programs. In addition, researchers have found just as strong a tendency for nonsmokers to be adamant followers of their own program. Type A personalities also have difficulty in maintaining the will to continue an exercise program. The belief is that the aggressive, time-pressured characteristics of the type A personality are in conflict with the sometimes slow pace and progression of a program.

As the wide range of reasons that adults produce for not participating in sports or exercise programs piles up, one that is common to many, yet rarely mentioned, is the protection of one's ego. For many, the fear of failure, according to O'Brien and Vertinsky,[3] can create considerable anxiety and distress, so much so that the fear becomes insurmountable and participation becomes out of the question. Former athletes, specifically, are prone to this problem. They feel they must live up to standards set in their youth, standards to which their bodies just cannot accommodate. Therefore, instead of accepting what they can do, these adults unfortunately leave the activity altogether. The challenge that lies ahead for the nation is to help adults understand what exercise and sport really are, and what these activities can do for them. Adults must see that these things are not a vehicle for social status, but an essential element to all-around health, no matter the level at which they are practiced.

INJURIES

For many athletes, participation in sports and exercise not only presents the fear of damage to one's self-concept, but also the fear of physical injury. Even in athletes who were once active, the overwhelming fear of injury may have caused diminished concentration and muscle tension to such a degree that performance considerably deteriorated,[9] and thus, the athlete was driven out of the activity altogether. Of course, people cannot be led into sports under the impression that they will never get hurt. An estimated 17 million sports-related injuries occur yearly among American athletes.[9] The job of those trained in sports and exercise, therefore, is to help people understand that the physical and psychological benefits of activity far outweigh any risks to the body.

Obviously, as the numbers indicate, injuries do happen, and when they do they must be dealt with not only on the physical but also the psychological level. Once an athlete becomes injured, it is crucial to understand what emotions will follow and how the athlete will deal with them. Presently, two quite similar theories dominate thinking on the subject. The first was based on Kubler-Ross' work done on those grieving from the death of a loved one. Like a grieving friend or relative, the athlete progresses through a series of five stages immediately following the injury and into rehabilitation.[9] At first, the athlete experiences denial and disbelief over what has happened. Anger then sets in, followed by downplaying the severity of the injury, leading to the next stage, depression. Finally, the athlete comes to accept the true extent of the injury, and hopefully a committed effort at rehabilitation will begin.

The variation of this theory proposed by Steadman[10] consists of only three stages: denial, distress, and determined coping. Basically, it is a condensed form of the process as proposed by Rotella.[11] The difference is that, as opposed to the Rotella process, which cycles only once, the Steadman theory states that the process can cycle several times, often being sparked by an event in rehabilitation. For example, an athlete who has progressed through denial and distress, and who is now in determined coping,

may experience a setback in recovery that delays return to competition. Denial over this relatively minor event will follow, thus initiating the cycle again.

But even when the body is fully recovered from injury, that does not mean that the mind has followed. Many times, "fear or anxiety manifests itself when a rehabilitated athlete encounters situations resembling those in which the injury occurred."[9] This problem is known as a phobic response to injury and has the ability to interfere with performance and increase the risk of reinjury. Ironically, players so conscious of reinjury will tend to play tentatively, which only increases the chances of their worst fear. Like other phobias, however, this can be treated with stress inoculation or systematic desensitization.

OVERTRAINING

We now move from those who believe that the risk of injury is too great for them to participate, to those who participate so much that they create and then ignore their own injuries. As defined by Lehmann et al.,[12] overtraining is an imbalance between training and recovery, exercise and exercise capacity, stress and stress tolerance. There are two recognized forms of overtraining: the short-term overreaching, from which one can recover in a matter of days, and the long-term overtraining syndrome, which requires a much longer recovery period. The two are distinguished by the number and intensity of the workouts. Therefore, an overzealous athlete will first experience overreaching followed by full-blown overtraining. The long-term form of the disorder is then subdivided into the common parasympathetic type, produced mostly by aerobic sports, and the quite rare sympathetic type, brought on by nonaerobic sports.

Although the research findings on the psychological factors contributing to overtraining are not very extensive, Heil[9] has provided a few possible reasons for the overtraining phenomenon. The first suggestion is that, as opposed to unmotivated athletes who drop out of a program if they cannot keep up with peers, athletes who suffer from the overtraining syndrome feel the need to push themselves to meet self-expectations, as well as the expectations of others. The fear of failure is so great that it drives the athlete to participate at unhealthy levels. A second psychological factor may involve the amount of stress that the athlete is under. Exercising may be the only way an athlete knows how to cope with stress; therefore, times of great stress can bring great physical punishment to the athlete.[9] Now that the dedicated athlete trains 12 months a year and "two-a-days" seem to be the rule not the exception, it becomes more important than ever for coaches and trainers to recognize the signs and symptoms of overtraining so that irreversible damage to the athlete is prevented.

BURNOUT

If the long-term overtraining syndrome is left unchecked and untreated, it will eventually lead to its logical conclusion, burnout. As defined by Henschen,[13] burnout is specifically the state of mental, emotional, and physical exhaustion brought on by persistent devotion to a goal. But those who burn out should not be confused with those who drop out. As we have seen, many athletes withdraw from activities because they become disenchanted. Their performance may not be up to par, or they may dislike the leader or the coach and decide that leaving is the easiest answer. Burnouts, on the other hand, almost work until they drop. In most cases, they are perfectionists who set unrealistic standards for themselves, and who are too hard on themselves once failure strikes.

Like many psychological problems involved in both sports and other facets of life, burnout can be detected through the Profile of Mood States (POMS) test. In 1977, Morgan and Johnson[14] used this test to psychologically define the successful athlete as one who is high in vigor and low in tension, depression, anger, fatigue, and confusion. Athletes who possess these traits were described as having the "iceberg profile."[14] Ten years later, in a study of swimmers and wrestlers, Morgan and co-workers[15] found that the profile of the unsuccessful or burned out athlete was exactly the opposite of the iceberg profile. According to Morgan et al., as the season wore on, there was a stepwise increase in the mood disturbance of the athletes, indicating that burnout had become a factor by the end of the season.[15]

Unfortunately, once an athlete reaches the burnout stage, many of the signs and symptoms indicating its onset have already been ignored. But there are actions that can possibly remotivate the athlete into competition. The first would be to completely remove the athlete from the situation. The monotony of practice and the stagnation of performance are prime contributors to the affect of the athlete. To be able to get away and relax is a necessity in this situation. In addition, coaches or exercise program leaders may want to reestablish the goals the athlete is trying to attain. A fresh new approach with salient and manageable goals may be just what an athlete needs to get back on track.

Children and Sports
HARVEY N. DULBERG

Involving children in sports is a rite of passage that almost all families will experience. Sports are said to build character and strength as well as to teach the child about life and competition. These small athletes are, however, being increasingly thought of and treated as miniature adult athletes. More emphasis is placed on winning than on the simple enjoyment of the sport. Extrinsic rewards are being used rather than teaching the values of sports. In order to ensure a good sports experience for their child, parents must examine the needs of the child rather than fulfilling their own needs.

All adults involved in youth sports can influence a child, but the parental role is perhaps the most important. The child will look to the parent for support, approval, and guidance. If parents place emphasis on the wrong aspect of sports, their child could become discouraged and leave sports forever. Confidence and self-esteem could falter. The parents should keep in mind that the goal of youth sports is not winning, but becoming a better, stronger, more skilled and capable person—and to have fun.

BECOMING INVOLVED

There are many things to think about when a child becomes involved in youth sports. The focus of the program should be keeping children in an environment that will develop and nurture them as people as well as athletes. Young children are very much influenced by their involvement in sports. Here, they will learn lessons that they will carry with them throughout life. There are a variety of determining factors when deciding if a child is ready for organized youth sports. If they are not ready, children could have a negative rather than a positive experience.

There are two aspects to a child's readiness: motivational readiness and maturity or cognitive readiness. Children are socially ready to participate in organized group sports before they are intellectually ready. In social development, a child first begins to master individual physical skills. At age 5 or 6 children begin to compare their abilities to others their age. By 6 or 7, all social interactions are turned into a competition. It is at this age that competition becomes an isolated event and is separated from everyday situations. It is also at this age that children are motivationally ready to enter the world of competitive sports, wishing to compare themselves against peers.

However, the child may not be intellectually ready to do so. The child may know that winning is good and losing is bad, but does not really understand the essence of competition. It is only when children can begin to see others' points of view and relate to team, not individual goals, that they can begin to understand true competition. The ability to role play, to take on another's perspective, does not occur until ages 8 to 10. The ability to take on a group perspective is not learned until 10 to 12. This is when the team goal can be understood and when playing to win should ideally begin. It is at this age that concepts such as sacrificing one's own goals for the good of the team are understood. Now the child can understand that everyone needs to work together for the good of the team to bring about a winning effort.

Determining the right time to participate in team sports may be a tough decision. The child must be ready to learn the necessary skills of the game as well as understand it. During a child's younger years, emphasis should be on teaching, developing, and refining physical skills. At these ages, fun and social activities should be the focus, not winning the World Cup or World Series. When the child is older, about 10 or 12, competition can become more of a focus, but the emphasis should still be on skills training. The program should take into account both the child's ability and the program goal when deciding which children are ready to participate.

WHAT ARE YOUTH SPORTS FOR?

Why do children want to participate in sports? What keeps them interested in sports? In determining the goal of youth sports, these questions need to be answered. In

a survey done by the Athletic Footware Association on American Youth and Sports Participation, children stated that the most important reason they play sports is to have fun. They stop playing when they lose interest or when the fun stops. When asked reasons for joining sports, children responded with fun, learning skills, staying in shape, being good at something, and competition. Winning placed 10th out of 10. This shows that for children, fun is developing skills and self-knowledge.

PARENTING YOUTH IN SPORTS

Parents play a critical role in shaping a child's sports experience. For children to have a positive experience, parents must act as role models and guides. Children are very impressionable and they are led by actions, not just by words. Parents need to set good examples for their children. The focus should be on skill development rather than winning. Parents also need to be sensitive to the child's needs. Children should play at their own individual skill levels and in a sport they want to play. Forcing children to play at a higher level or in a sport they do not want to play will lead to failure and possibly injury. Asking a child to live out a parent's fantasy is also unhealthy emotionally.

Parents need to be sensitive to the child's feelings. Children should be asked if they want vocal encouragement during the game or just quiet viewing, or whether they want extra coaching from mom and dad or to figure it out for themselves. Parents need to ask their children about their feelings, especially when it comes to coaching. Many children would love to have mom or dad coach them, but many would not. It may be embarrassing to have their parents directing them and their friends. It is important to keep sports in perspective. Parents should always find something positive to say to their child, and should remember that very few become superstars. This is youth sports; parents should not expect their child to remember every play and to concentrate for long periods of time. Sometimes butterflies flying by or a pattern of clouds is more interesting than the game. Children are children, and they will always do the unexpected. These are games, not chances to prove their innate worth. Parents can get involved by watching the games, helping to run practices, driving, or making team dinners. The more the child sees that the parents care, the happier and healthier the child's experience will be.

Children progress at their own pace. They need to be

given the opportunity to play and to learn under game conditions. Playing only against the best players turns a lot of children off to sports. Doing the same activity day after day is no fun either, and interest levels will drop accordingly. Parents should never let their first question be, "Did you win?" Also, the child should not be asked, "How many points did you score?" The focus is fun, not winning. If performance is the parents' focus, children will equate self-worth with how many points they score. A better question to ask children is whether or not they had fun, or what they learned today, or who played with them. "Did you do your best?" is also a good question. The score will eventually be brought up but in its own time.

There are so many things that sports can teach children about life. Sports helps self-confidence and physical skill development, and it provides role models and friends. Functioning well in a sports situation can generalize to functioning as a productive member of society in the future. Important skills such as teamwork are learned, and children learn to set goals and to work to achieve them.

YOUTH SPORTS AND LIFE

Children can learn much about life through their sports experiences. The way people behave in sports often generalizes to the way they will behave in a nonsports situation. Learning to win or lose graciously preserves self-respect and mutual admiration both on and off the playing field. Being able to perform well in a sporting situation will bring confidence in sports as well as other aspects of life. The confidence learned on the field will bring a general feeling of accomplishment that will always stay with the child.

Learning values is a big part of sports. The "win at all costs" attitude must be discouraged. Good sportsmanship is crucial. Cheating is not to be tolerated. When the sports world is functioning at its best, everyone is having fun. Competitors push each other, and winning is much sweeter when athletes know that they have won playing within the rules. Even the losers come away from the competition knowing that they played their best and that the competition itself was a winning experience. The same applies to the world outside of sports.

Improving a skill or learning a new one will be a boost to one's self-esteem. Skill mastery provides a sense of accomplishment and self-worth.

Handling success and failure in sports is perhaps the most important lesson for sports, and also for life. Everyone makes mistakes, so one must learn to move on. Mistakes can never be taken away, but they can be used as a learning tool. Whether a child has just made a terrible play or a terrific one, there is still the rest of the game to think about. When the game is over, that moment can be relived, but now is the time to stay in the game and not let one mistake turn into another. Other great lessons include refocusing on the goal ("Just do it!"), always staying in the present, concentrating on the task at hand, and giving it your best shot. No child is like any other, and each is to be treasured as an individual. Once the right level of competition has been found, the child will thrive. When children are matched against others at their own level, skill mastery becomes easier. There are so many good things that sport can teach us about life. The earlier our children learn those lessons, the better off they will be.

The Four Phases of Running
STEVEN I. SUBOTNICK

Understanding the four phases that most runners pass through helps the health practitioner to more easily evaluate the status of the patient, as well as the patient's needs. The conceptual origin of these four phases is derived from my experience as a runner and clinician.

PHASE I

Phase I describes casual, beginning runners. They may be a bit overweight and out of shape and are entering the sport of running after having had a period of time away from sports. A background in sports is usually present, although these athletes were almost never full-fledged runners in the past.

The phase I runner is a consistent, yet casual, runner, usually going 3 miles 4 or 5 days a week. The total mileage run in a week is 12 to 15, fitting well within the guidelines for sensible aerobic fitness. The phase I runner soon notices a gradual firming of the body, along with a loss of weight. Most approach 80 percent of their ideal racing weight. Most phase I runners find that they have much more energy during the day, have a better attitude, and generally accomplish more with greater ease than they did before they started exercising. Their thoughts are clearer, and they look forward to a relaxing run at anywhere from 8 to $9\frac{1}{2}$ min/mile. These athletes seldom run far enough to experience a "runner's high" and/or to become dependent on the sport of running from the influence of endorphins and enkephalins. They are, however, habituated to feeling good and to the positive results of their aerobic fitness program. They are often involved in other sports, such as golf, bowling, tennis, skiing, racquetball, or an occasional game of softball or basketball.

PHASE II

Phase II runners are the occasional racers who are serious but not obsessed about running. They average about 30 miles a week and tend to go 5 to 7 miles a day, 5 days a week. Phase II runners occasionally will be involved in a 5- or 10-km race. Once in awhile, they will consider a half-marathon or, very rarely, will train for a marathon. They enjoy their occasional races and thoroughly enjoy the benefits of aerobic exercise. They are putting in enough mileage to benefit from the psychological aspects of running and may use running for stress reduction. These runners have realized, through trial and error, that after running for about 25 to 30 minutes they experience a "runner's high" or "second wind." This occurs when the metabolism changes from glycogen metabolism to free fatty acid metabolism.[16] This normally takes 25 to 30 minutes to occur and is associated with increased endogenous endorphins and enkephalins, referred to by the layman as endogenous morphine-type substances, that make the runner feel good or "high." There is also more free association in runners after running for more than 30 minutes, and this has considerable positive psychological and stress-reduction effects.

Thus the phase II runner is benefiting from increased aerobic fitness and psychological well-being. Running may very well be a safety valve for the runner, but the phase II runner is not truly addicted to running and has a healthy sense of proportion. This runner realizes that 2 days of rest each week reduces injuries and the aches and pains associated with running. There are no qualms about taking a vacation or missing a week or two of running. They will follow instructions and cut down on their mileage when necessary, and are very cooperative in rehabilitative programs.

PHASE III

Phase III runners tend to be obsessive-compulsive in behavior. They are psychologically and physiologically dependent on the "runner's high" and on the increased endorphins and enkephalins created by the run. They may use running as an escape from other problems. They often feel guilty when they miss workouts or have poor performances, and will choose their running workout over business or personal appointments, or both. They devote at least 90 minutes a day to their workout. These phase III runners can be young, gifted athletes, aiming toward careers in sports or the Olympics; however, they can also be men or women going through a divorce, trying to lose weight, or changing their way of looking at the world, who are using running as an escape.

The sports health practitioner must realize that phase III runners believe that they are invincible. They feel that they have put in their time training and thus should avoid injury. They do not take responsibility for their injuries, and may blame family members or their physician when they do not rapidly recover from an injury. They become depressed, angry, and litigious, and may exhibit hysterical personality traits, praising the doctor for improvements one moment and blaming the doctor for a prolonged recovery or poor performance the next.

The withdrawal that phase III runners go through when injured is both psychological and physiologic. To ease their anguish somewhat, the physician can prescribe an alternative aerobic exercise that will enhance rehabilitation of injured parts while providing the benefits of aerobic fitness. Running in a swimming pool with a support vest, biking, swimming, and race walking are good aerobic substitutes to jogging and enable the injured part to rest while exercising the noninjured parts.

These injured athletes usually report to the physician with severe dynamic and functional imbalance. They may have very tight, weak muscles. Common injuries include myositis, periostitis, tendinitis, or stress fractures. A legitimate medical diagnosis is often requested by these athletes; otherwise, they feel that their colleagues and friends may "make fun" of them or consider them quitters or failures. In these patients, the use of cast brace immobilization or splints is helpful. This allows for motion when appropriate and rest when indicated. The splints may be removed to permit exercise of the injured part within physiologic tolerance and under supervision. For phase III athletes, sport is a safety valve, as well as a major focus of life. Their perceptions of themselves and others may be skewed. They are often overly talkative and may be poor listeners. When working with these patients, interventive therapy such as surgery should be avoided, if at all possible. Rehabilitation, reassurance, and help with redefining goals is the treatment of choice.

PHASE IV

Phase IV runners are those who have gone through the phase III stage of their running careers. They usually exercise at 70 to 75 percent of their maximum cardiac output;

when they were phase III runners, they often went higher by doing intervals, fartlek, and running under 8 min/mile. At phase IV they are satisfied with an 8- to 8½-minute mile. They are seldom interested in other than casual competition.

These runners have mellowed out and are wiser than they were when they were phase III runners. As patients, they are a pleasure to treat and will follow instructions and respond well to rehabilitative measures.

REFERENCES

The Adult Athlete

1. Clough P, Shepherd J, Maughan R: Motives for participation in recreational running. J Leisure Res 21:297, 1989
2. Ewart A: Why people climb: the relationship of participant motives and experience level to mountaineering. J Leisure Res 17:241, 1985
3. O'Brien S, Vertinsky A: Perspectives on older adults in physical activity and sports. Educ Gerontol 18:461, 1992
4. Hughes JR: Psychological effects of habitual aerobic exercise: a critical review. Prev Med 13:148, 1984
5. Steptoe A, Edwards S, Moses J, Mathews A: The effects of exercise training on mood and perceived coping ability in anxious adults from the general population. J Psychosom 33:537, 1989
6. Ossip-Klien DJ, Doyne EJ, Bowman KM et al: Effects of running or weight training on self-concept in clinically depressed women. J Consult Clin Psychol 57:158, 1989
7. Stein PN, Motta RW: Effects of aerobic and nonaerobic exercise on depression and self-concept. Percept Motor Skills 74:79, 1992
8. LeUnes AD, Nation J: Sports Psychology: An Introduction. Nelson-Hall Publishers, Chicago, 1989
9. Heil J: Psychology of Sport Injury. Human Kinetics Publishers, Champaign, IL, 1993
10. Steadman R: A psychologist's view of the personal challenge of injury p. 35. In Heil J (ed): Psychology of Sports Injury, Human Kinetics Publishers, Champaign, IL, 1993
11. Rotella R: A psychologist's view of the personal challenge of injury p. 35. In Heil J (ed): Psychology of Sports Injury. Human Kinetics Publishers, Champaign, IL, 1993
12. Lehmann M, Foster C, Keul J: Overtraining in endurance athletes: a critical review. Med Sci Sports Exerc 25:854, 1993
13. Henschen KP: Athletic staleness and burnout: diagnosis, prevention and treatment p. 328. In Williams JM (ed): Applied Sport Psychology. Mayfield Publishing Company, Mountain View, CA, 1993

14. Morgan WP, Johnson RW: Psychological characterization of the elite wrestler: a mental health model. Med Sci Sports 9:55, 1977

15. Morgan WP, Brown DR, Raglin JS et al: Psychological monitoring of overtraining and staleness. Br J Sports Med 21:107, 1987

The Four Phases of Running

16. Costill D: Physiologic basis for training Track Field News, Palo Alto, CA, 1976

SUGGESTED READINGS

The Four Phases of Running

King AC: Community intervention for promotion of physical activity and fitness. Exerc Sport Sci Rev 19:221, 1991

North CT, McCullagh P: Effects of exercise on depression. Exerc Sport Sci Rev 18:379, 1990

Weiss MR, Brenemier BJ: Moral development in sports. Exerc Sport Sci Rev 18:307, 1990

Wojtek J, Moore MS: Physical fitness and cognitive functioning in aging. Exerc Sport Sci Rev 22:121, 1994

3

Lower Extremity Sports Injuries in Children

ROGER F. WIDMANN
LYLE J. MICHELI

As ever-increasing numbers of children participate in organized athletic activities, the numbers of pediatric sports injuries presenting for medical care will continue to rise. Both intrinsic and extrinsic factors play a role in a child's risk of musculoskeletal injury. Extrinsic factors include the environment, equipment, and training program, while intrinsic factors include musculoskeletal strength, flexibility and bulk, associated disease states, and potential for growth.[1] This potential for growth makes children's anatomy and physiology uniquely different from that of adults.

Although the child's musculoskeletal system has the ability to heal and remodel injuries faster than adults, the open growth plates and the rapid growth of the musculotendinous units and the bones present a unique set of musculoskeletal injuries. While a young child can completely remodel a poorly reduced long bone metaphyseal fracture in the plane of a joint, severe growth plate injuries in a young child can result in complete cessation of growth and major deformity and disability.

Sports-related injuries can be broadly classified into the two categories of high-energy macrotrauma and repetitive microtrauma injuries. Macrotrauma includes acute fractures, dislocations, sprains, and ligament tears. Repetitive microtrauma is responsible for such injuries as stress fractures and apophysitis. Rapid growth and relative inflexibility may both predispose the adolescent athlete to overuse injuries.[1]

An understanding of the unique anatomy and physiology of the pediatric athlete as well as the extrinsic factors contributing to the potential for musculoskeletal injury will assist in rapid diagnosis and appropriate treatment of sports injuries of the lower extremity in children. In addition, the aim is to use this knowledge to prevent injury. This chapter reviews the diagnosis and treatment of some of the common pediatric sports injuries of the lower extremity.

INJURIES TO THE HIP AND PELVIS

Acute pelvis and hip fractures are rare in children. When these fractures occur, they usually result from high-energy trauma. A review of pediatric pelvic fractures requiring hospital admission revealed that only 3.5 percent of pelvic fractures occurred during athletics.[2] Most pelvic fractures in this study resulted from motor vehicle accidents or falls. The pediatric pelvis is more elastic and flexible than the adult pelvis and, therefore, can tolerate greater deformation prior to acute fracture. Thus, pelvis fractures in children can be associated with significant injuries to the viscera, major blood vessels, and nerves. Rapid evaluation and treatment may decrease the high rate of associated morbidity and mortality.[3]

Hip fractures are likewise quite rare in children, comprising less than 1 percent of all fractures.[4] These fractures also are often associated with other injuries that may require urgent treatment. Rapid evaluation, diagnosis, and treatment of acute physeal fractures as well as femoral neck fractures will decrease the incidence of late complications such as avascular necrosis, growth arrest, nonunion and progressive deformity, and degenerative changes (Fig. 3-1).

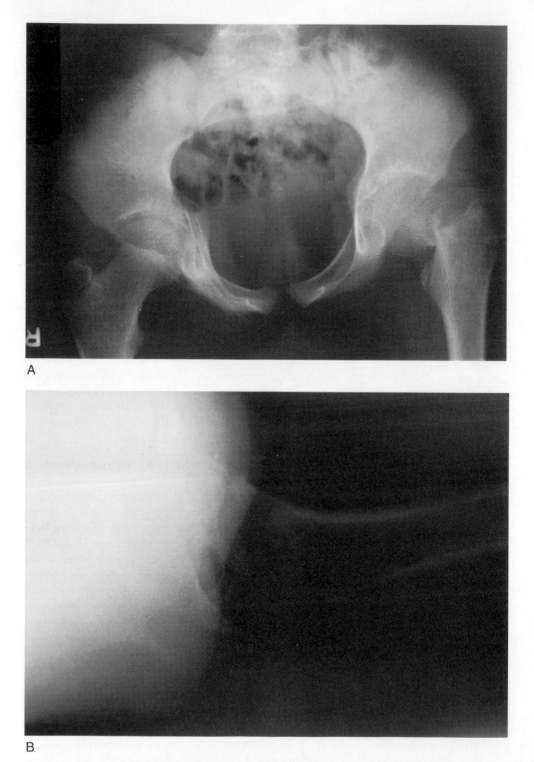

Figure 3-1 Anteroposterior (AP) (**A**) and lateral (**B**) radiographs demonstrating a displaced femoral neck fracture in a 10-year-old girl. (*Figure continues.*)

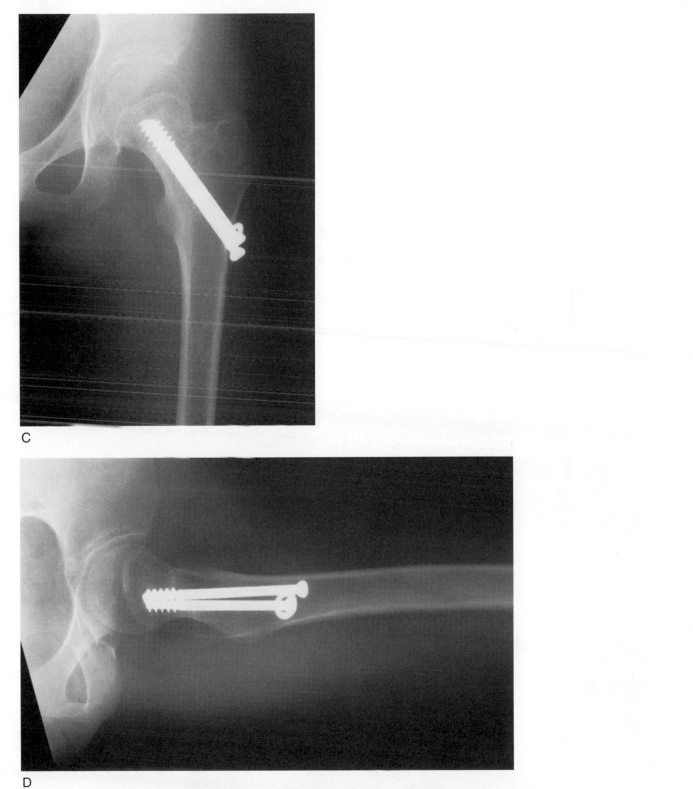

C

D

Figure 3-1 *(Continued)* This injury was treated with immediate closed reduction, internal fixation, and capsular decompression (**C & D**).

Avulsion Fractures of the Pelvis and Hip

Avulsion fractures of the pelvis and proximal femur result from vigorous muscle contractions or stretch across an open apophysis.[5] These injuries include avulsion of the hamstrings from the ischial tuberosity, the iliopsoas from the lesser trochanter, the rectus femoris from the anterior inferior iliac spine, the sartorius from the anterior superior iliac spine, and the abdominal muscles from the iliac crest. Avulsion fractures typically occur in children between the ages of 13 and 17 after the appearance, but prior to the fusion, of the secondary center of ossification.[6-8] This developmental stage corresponds to a period of rapid growth and relative inflexibility.[1] Although historically boys have been affected far more often than girls, reports suggest that the incidence of avulsion fractures is increasing significantly in girls.[7]

Avulsion injuries typically occur in association with kicking, sprinting, or jumping activities, with immediate onset of localized pain and swelling. Physical exam reveals local tenderness, guarding, and decreased muscle excursion secondary to pain. Radiographs confirm the diagnosis (Fig. 3-2).[9] Ischial tuberosity avulsions appear to be the most common.[5,7]

Three stages of apophyseal avulsion have been noted. The first stage consists of nondisplaced apophyseal injuries termed apophysiolysis. The second stage consists of acute avulsion fractures, and the third stage is chronic nonunion.[10] Patients with nondisplaced apophyseal injuries respond well to rest and partial weight bearing. Most displaced avulsion fractures with nonunion are asymptomatic. Some will continue to cause pain with activity or with sitting, and these may require excision.

Most authors concur that conservative nonoperative treatment with rest, partial weight bearing, and extremity positioning to minimize muscle stretch is indicated in the treatment of acute avulsion fractures. Metzmaker and Pappas[11] outlined a five-step rehabilitation plan consisting of (1) protected gait, (2) protected gait and guided exercise, (3) progressive resistance training, (4) gradual return to athletics, and (5) return to competition. These authors reported that 24 of 27 athletes with acute avulsion fractures of the pelvis returned to their preinjury level of function within 4 months of injury.[11] Other authors have suggested that conservative nonoperative treatment is associated with a significantly higher incidence of functional disability and inability to return to competitive athletic activity.[7,12] Specifically, these authors have noted that functional disability

Figure 3-2 A displaced anterior inferior iliac spine avulsion fracture is easily seen on the AP pelvis radiograph.

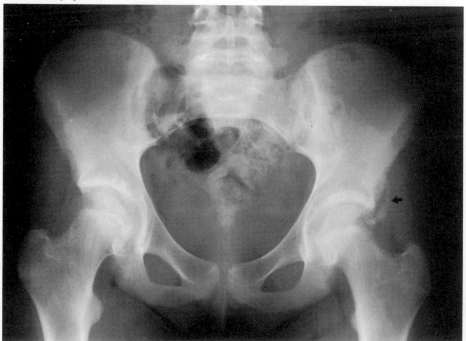

is primarily associated with displaced ischial tuberosity fractures.

Iliac Apophysitis

Iliac crest apophysitis is an unusual traction apophysitis that originally was described in adolescent distance runners between the ages of 14 and 17 years.[13,14] Clancy and Foltz[13] described mostly nondisplaced cases of apophysitis and a few case of discrete avulsion fractures that they called stress fractures. All patients in this study were involved in active track running programs, and all presented with gradual onset of localized tenderness to palpation and localized pain with resisted abduction of the hip. Both anterior and posterior iliac crest apophysitis syndromes have been described. Anterior iliac crest apophysitis has been attributed to overpull of the tensor fascia lata, the gluteus medius, and the oblique abdominal muscles, whereas posterior iliac crest apophysitis has been attributed to overpull of the latissimus dorsi or gluteus maximus. Most patients responded well to 3 to 4 weeks of rest, with complete resolution of symptoms and resumption of training.

Hip Dislocation

Although hip dislocations are rare injuries in children, when this injury occurs, it is commonly caused by mild to moderate trauma during athletic activities.[15,16] Hip dislocations occur in all age groups, with an average age between 7 and 10 years.[17] Most dislocations are posterior, and physical exam is quite helpful in differentiating between anterior and posterior displacement. The posteriorly dislocated hip will be shortened, flexed, adducted, and internally rotated, whereas the anteriorly dislocated hip will be abducted, flexed, and externally rotated.[9] Complete neurologic exam is mandatory prior to reduction since sciatic nerve injury may occur in association with hip dislocation.

In older children, hip dislocation is associated with more severe trauma and associated other injuries.[16] In addition, higher energy trauma is correlated with late degenerative changes and radiographic abnormalities.[15] Management of the pediatric hip dislocation includes rapid diagnosis with complete physical exam and plain radiographs, emergent gentle closed reduction or open reduction if needed, follow-up computed tomography (CT) scan, and protected weight bearing for 4 to 6 weeks.[9,18] Complications include soft tissue interposition, nerve injury, avascular necrosis,

premature closure of the triradiate cartilage, recurrent dislocation, and osteoarthritis.

Slipped Capital Femoral Epiphysis and Perthes' Disease

Although slipped capital femoral epiphysis and Perthes' disease are not sports injuries, the pediatric sports medicine practitioner must consider both of these conditions in the differential diagnosis of any skeletally immature patient with hip or knee pain and limp.

Slipped capital femoral epiphysis is a very common problem in adolescents between ages 11 and 15, and it affects between 0.7 and 3.4 children per 100,000.[19] The disorder consists of a chronic or acute disruption of the proximal femoral growth plate with a clinical presentation of pain, limp, and limited hip internal rotation.[20] Standard radiographs include anteroposterior (AP) pelvis, including both hips, and frog lateral of both hips (Fig. 3-3). Both hips are included on the initial and subsequent radiographs because of the high incidence of bilateral disease, which approaches 40 percent.[21,22] The hips are classified as stable or unstable based on the patient's ability to ambulate.[23]

Standard treatment of both groups consists of single-pin fixation as expeditiously as possible.[24,25] The major complications of slipped capital femoral epiphysis are avascular necrosis and chondrolysis. Both avascular necrosis and chondrolysis are associated with increasing severity of the slip and with reduction of the slip.[20]

Perthes' disease is a poorly understood pathologic process of avascular necrosis of the proximal femoral epiphysis. The diagnosis of Perthes' disease must be considered in the management of children with limp and restricted hip range of motion between the ages of 3 and 12, and most commonly between the ages of 5 and 7.[26] The disease affects boys approximately three to five times as frequently as girls. The etiology is unknown, but the pathophysiology is consistent with avascular necrosis. Clinical exam will demonstrate restricted hip internal rotation and abduction, Trendelenburg gait, and hip pain or referred thigh or knee pain. The history will be consistent with activity-related symptoms.[26,27]

Both surgical and nonsurgical treatment options have been advocated for Perthes' disease, depending on the calendar or bone age of the patient and the stage of the disease; however, no consensus has been achieved on ideal treatment.[28] Herring[28] outlined the basic goals of treatment as relief of symptoms, containment of the femoral head, and

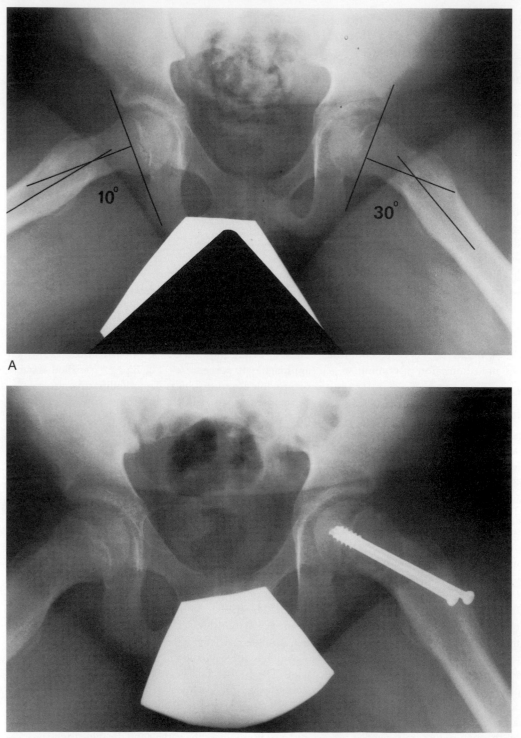

A

B

Figure 3-3 (**A**) Slipped capital femoral epiphysis is best seen on the frog lateral radiographic view. Note the slip angle of 30 degrees on the involved left side, versus the 10-degree slip angle on the uninvolved right side. (**B**) Stabilization was performed via percutaneous screw fixation.

restoration of range of motion. Return to athletic activities is restricted during the active phase of Perthes' disease until the patient is well into the healing phase, in order to protect the revascularized epiphysis.[9]

QUADRICEPS CONTUSION AND MYOSITIS OSSIFICANS

Muscle contusions are frequent injuries in the pediatric athlete, comprising up to 38 percent of injuries in large studies of pediatric athletes.[29,30] The mechanism of injury is most commonly direct contact of an opponent's knee with the patient's quadriceps muscle.[31] Although quadriceps contusions occur in many athletic activities, the greatest number occurred as a result of tackle football injuries in Jackson and Feagin's landmark study.[31]

Jackson and Feagin classified injuries into mild, moderate, and severe depending on knee motion of 90 degrees or greater, less than 90 degrees, and less than 45 degrees, respectively, at 2 days after injury. He described a rational three-phase approach to treatment and rehabilitation: phase I consists of rest, ice, elevation, and compression; phase II involves restoration of active knee range of motion with full extension and over 90 degrees of flexion; and phase III concerns progressive resistance training and gradual return to athletics once full strength and range of motion are achieved.

Myositis ossificans is an unusual complication of quadriceps contusion in young athletes sustaining moderate and severe injuries.[32] Reinjury of the quadriceps in the recovery phase is associated with the development of subsequent myositis, as is the severity of the original injury.[31] It is essential to differentiate between heterotopic ossification resulting from trauma and the heterotopic ossification of malignancy. An appropriate history of trauma with corresponding radiographic findings is most helpful (Fig. 3-4). A positive bone scan is helpful in the early diagnosis of heterotopic ossification, and CT scan may assist in defining the mass, should surgical intervention be necessary.[33,34] Magnetic resonance imaging (MRI) findings are often nonspecific.[35,36] Conservative management is the mainstay of treatment in myositis ossificans. Protection of the patient from reinjury is essential in preventing myositis. Most patients achieve normal function despite the appearance of heterotopic bone.[31] In addition, surgical intervention prior to maturation of the myositis ossificans lesion may result in an increased rate of recurrence compared with late surgery. Persistent symptoms after at least 1 year of observation and radiographic maturation of the lesion may warrant surgical excision in a small percentage of patients.[37]

KNEE INJURIES

Patellofemoral Stress Syndrome

Anterior knee pain in the child and adolescent can be difficult to classify based on physical examination. A system of classification based on etiology, including primarily trauma, malalignment, or a combination of both, appears to be a very reasonable approach.[38]

The patellofemoral stress syndrome is an overuse injury of the extensor mechanism that results from repetitive microtrauma in susceptible individuals during the period of most active growth.[1] The syndrome results from a complex interplay of mild soft tissue imbalance without overt bony malalignment. With rapid growth the tight lateral structures, including the fascia lata and vastus lateralis, exert lateral forces on the patella that are countered by the relatively weak vastus medialis. Patients typically present with pain with activity, difficulty with prolonged sitting, and a history of the knee giving way. Acute symptoms may follow abrupt increases in training programs. Physical examination reveals lateral patellar tightness without overt bony malalignment.

Initial treatment of patellofemoral stress syndrome in the young athlete consists of training modification, strengthening of the medial quadriceps, and stretching of the fascia lata and hamstrings.[1] Bilateral progressive straight leg raises with a goal of 12 pounds achieves pain relief in most patients. Over a 27-month study period, 93 percent of patients responded well to conservative therapy.[39] Patients who fail conservative treatment are offered lateral patellar retinacular release, with a 76.7 percent rate of good or excellent results. The best results from lateral release have been achieved in patients who are without evidence of hypermobility of the patella and who have normal alignment clinically.[40]

Osgood-Schlatter Disease and Sinding-Larsen-Johansson Disease

Osgood-Schlatter disease and Sinding-Larsen-Johansson disease are two common overuse injuries of the extensor mechanism about the knee. Osgood-Schlatter disease results from repetitive microtrauma at the level of the skeletally immature tibial tubercle.[41] It occurs more commonly

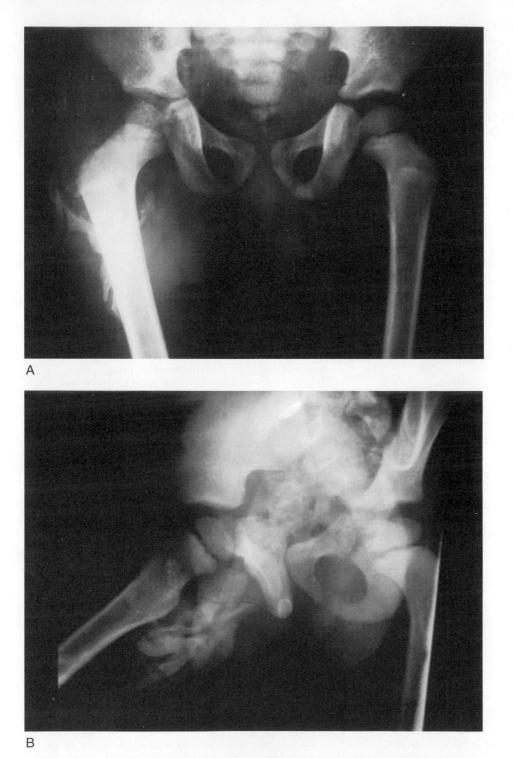

A

B

Figure 3-4 Mature myositis ossificans resulting from proximal thigh trauma as seen on AP (**A**) and lateral (**B**) views.

in boys, and more commonly in athletes participating in sports involving kicking, jumping, and squatting.[42] Patients typically present with pain to palpation over the tibial tubercle with associated swelling and exacerbation of symptoms with resisted extension of the knee. Histologic studies support the theory that this condition results from avulsion of the developing ossification center of the tibial tubercle.[43] Plain radiographs will demonstrate fragmentation of the tibial tubercle, as well as patella alta.[44]

A report from Japan supports the strong role of developmental factors in the etiology of this condition.[45] This longitudinal study found that the onset of Osgood-Schlatter disease is related to the start of the second growth spurt. Clinical symptoms were usually manifest 4 to 6 months after peak growth velocity.

Conservative treatment of Osgood-Schlatter disease consists of pain relief with anti-inflammatory medication and modality therapy as needed, as well as a quadriceps stretching and strengthening program.[1,42] Brief periods of immobilization may be necessary in rare cases resistant to usual measures. About 12 percent of patients develop a distinct, symptomatic, mobile ossicle and will fail to respond to conservative treatment. Early surgical intervention to excise the ossicle may be indicated in this small group.[41]

Sinding-Larsen-Johansson disease is a closely related overuse injury of the extensor mechanism resulting from traction tendinitis of the proximal attachment of the patellar tendon at the inferior pole of the patella.[46] This syndrome represents a subset of the broader classification of patients with "jumper's knee," which includes adults who may or may not have distinctive radiographic findings.[47] Boys are affected more often than girls, and the typical age group is between 10 and 13 years. Clinical presentation is quite similar to Osgood-Schlatter disease, with pain and swelling over the inferior pole of the patella and pain with resisted knee extension. Radiographs demonstrate calcification of the inferior pole of the patella that may over time coalesce and fuse to the patella or form a separate ossicle.

Most patients do well with conservative treatment as described for Osgood-Schlatter disease, with full return of function between 3 and 13 months from initial presentation.[46] These uniformly excellent results in children contrast sharply with the results of both conservative treatment and surgery in the older athletic population with jumper's knee.[47]

Plica

Synovial plicae of the knee are a common cause of anterior knee pain in adolescent athletes.[48] Plicae have been described anatomically as folds of synovium located in the infrapatellar, suprapatellar, medial patellar, and lateral patellar regions of the knee.[49] Patel's review of the literature reveals a reported incidence of medial patellar plica between 18.5 and 55 percent based on arthroscopic and cadaver studies.[49] The incidence of symptomatic plicae is far lower, but difficult to quantify.

Clinical presentation typically follows either an acute blunt injury to the knee or a sudden increase in exercise.[50] In addition, a relative growth spurt, with resultant proximal and lateral deviation of the patella, and tension on the medial retinaculum may be a factor. Patients complain of pain, swelling, and pseudolocking of the knee that may be confused with acute internal derangement.[48] Physical examination reveals a palpable shelf above the joint line and sometimes an audible snap.[49,50]

Since this pathologic process most commonly represents an overuse injury, conservative treatment is indicated initially, with modification of activities and symptomatic treatment. A prospective, randomized study of patients with symptomatic synovial plicae demonstrated 83 percent good and excellent results with arthroscopic plicae division in patients who had initially failed 3 months of conservative treatment.[48]

Bipartite Patella

Bipartite patella is an unusual anatomic variant that occurs in 2 to 3 percent of the population.[51] Although most bipartite patellae are asymptomatic, both acute and overuse injuries have been described. Ogden et al.'s studies suggest that the bipartite nature of the patella results from an unfused secondary center of ossification.[51] Adolescent male athletes typically present with anterior knee pain and localized tenderness (Fig. 3-5).[52] Conservative treatment with modification of activities is successful in chronic cases. Acute injuries that fail to respond to activity modification may be successfully treated by excision, internal fixation, or release of the vastus lateralis tendon insertion from the fragment.[51,53,54]

Meniscal Tears

Although meniscal injuries were thought to be rare, especially in children under age 10, studies have demonstrated significant numbers of meniscal injuries in children and adolescents.[55] A study of acute hemarthroses in children and adolescents demonstrated that 45 percent of children and 47 percent of adolescents had acute meniscal tears

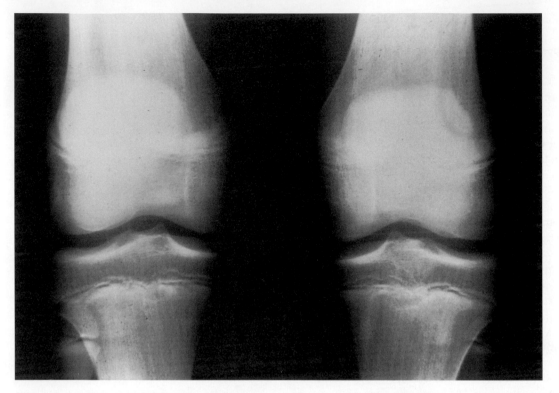

Figure 3-5 Symptomatic left bipartite patella as seen on AP radiograph of both knees.

either alone or in combination with anterior cruciate ligament injuries. Thus the incidence of meniscal tears in the presence of acute hemarthrosis was similar in the preadolescent and adolescent age groups.[56]

History and physical examination have been shown to be less reliable in the diagnosis of meniscal injury in younger children, and this may have contributed to hesitancy on the part of orthopedists to diagnose and treat these injuries in the past.[57] The use of arthroscopy as a diagnostic tool has significantly increased the accuracy of diagnosis of acute traumatic knee injuries in children and adolescents.[58]

Routine evaluation, including history and physical examination, may provide useful information, particularly in the older patient. Physical examination must include observation for abnormal gait, thigh atrophy, or knee effusion; palpation for tenderness, especially along the joint lines; and examination for range of motion and stability.[55]

Basic trends in treatment of meniscal lesions are toward preservation of the meniscus whenever possible.[59] Long-term follow-up studies in children and adolescents who underwent meniscectomy have clearly demonstrated un-

satisfactory results in upward of 40 percent of patients.[60,61] Nonoperative treatment is indicated in patients with stable vertical longitudinal tears in the periphery of the menisci because these tears have a propensity toward spontaneous healing.[62] Meniscal repair should be attempted on traumatic tears over 7 mm in length, which occur in the vascular zone of the meniscus, within 3 to 5 mm of the periphery.[59] Menisci with more central tears or major structural damage are best treated with partial meniscectomy. Postoperative supervised rehabilitation is a prerequisite for return to athletics.

Anterior Cruciate Ligament

Anterior cruciate ligament injuries are being reported with increased frequency in children and adolescents. This apparent increased incidence is due to greater participation by children in organized athletics, improved diagnostic techniques, and increased awareness of these injuries.[63] Review of a large series of children with acute hemarthrosis who underwent arthroscopy revealed a 47 percent incidence of anterior cruciate ligament tears in children ages 7 to 12 years and a 65 percent incidence in adolescents ages 13 to 18 years.[56] These injuries often occur in association with other ligamentous and meniscal injuries. Anterior cruciate ligament tears in children and adolescents should no longer be considered an unusual diagnosis.

Rapid diagnosis depends on an accurate history and physical exam, as well as appropriate imaging studies as in the adult population (Fig. 3-6). Rehabilitation, bracing, and activity modification have been the basic tenets of treatment until recently. Two groups of patients, all under age 14, with anterior cruciate ligament tears were followed for over 2 years on average, with successful return to athletic competition in over 90 percent of patients undergoing either extra-articular or intra-articular ligament reconstruction.[64] Only 44 percent of patients treated nonoperatively returned to sports, and all suffered repeat episodes of giving way, effusions, and pain.

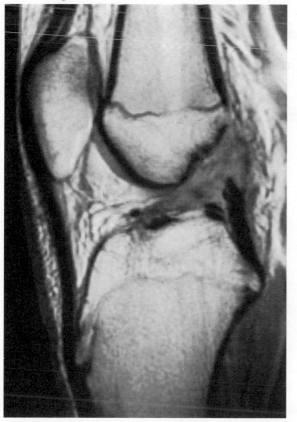

Figure 3-6 Anterior cruciate ligament tear is easily seen on sagittal MRI image of this 16-year-old boy's knee, which was injured in a soccer game.

Different techniques for reconstruction have been advocated depending on the patient's skeletal maturity. Techniques that violate the open physis can result in growth arrest, with resultant limb length inequality and angular deformity. Various techniques, including extra-articular and intra-articular reconstruction, have been utilized successfully. Brace treatment and observation until skeletal maturity is an option. Only one significant leg length discrepancy of 2 cm was observed in one series of 24 patients ages 12 to 15 who underwent hamstring tendon anterior cruciate ligament reconstruction with the graft crossing the proximal tibial physis.[65] It is quite clear that midsubstance repair of the anterior cruciate ligament fails in children as it does in adults.[66]

Anterior Cruciate Ligament Avulsions

Avulsion fractures of the tibial eminence are the most common type of anterior cruciate ligament injury in the skeletally immature individual.[67] Most fractures result from athletic injuries. Falling from a bicycle was the mechanism in approximately 50 percent of children in two large studies.[68,69] Myers and McKeever[69] proposed a classification system that remains useful: grade I avulsions are minimally displaced, grade II avulsions are hinged open anteriorly but remain attached posteriorly, and grade III avulsions are completely detached and may be rotated or comminuted.[70]

Closed treatment with cast immobilization remains the gold standard for grade I and II injuries that can be reduced anatomically. Controversy exists as to the optimal position of knee immobilization, either in full extension or in 30 degrees of flexion. Displaced grade II and most grade III avulsions merit arthroscopic or open reduction and internal fixation (Fig. 3-7). No matter what the form of treatment, a high incidence of residual knee laxity has been noted in long-term follow-up studies.[71,72]

Medial Collateral Ligament Injury

Medial collateral ligament injuries commonly result from valgus and external rotation forces on the knee, which are most commonly encountered in contact sports such as football and rugby.[73] Clinical exam remains diagnostic, with valgus instability noted with the knee in 30 degrees of flexion. Hemarthrosis or instability in full extension are clues to other internal derangements of the knee.[73] Nonoperative treatment has been demonstrated to be as good as operative repair in prospective studies of isolated

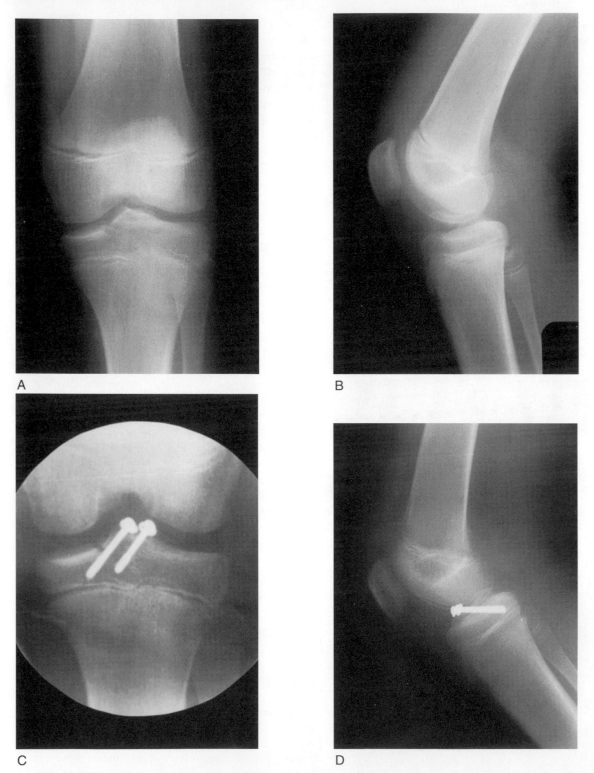

A

B

C

D

Figure 3-7 Grade II avulsion of the tibial eminence is seen on AP (**A**) and lateral (**B**) radiographs. Note the posterior hinge. This fracture was not reducible with closed reduction, and was treated with arthroscopically assisted reduction and internal fixation (**C & D**).

complete grade III medial collateral ligament tears in college athletes.[74] Similar findings have been noted in high school athletes.[75] Treatment protocols stress rapid return of function with full weight bearing as soon as possible and early range-of-motion exercises.

FOOT AND ANKLE

Children and adolescents are subject to a variety of acute and overuse injuries of the foot and ankle. Acute injuries include sprains and dislocations. Anatomic considerations explain the significantly higher incidence of physeal ankle fractures compared to sprains in skeletally immature individuals. The ligaments insert below the physes, and the open physis is weaker than the adjacent bone and ligaments.[76]

Physeal fractures of the ankle in children can be classified both by the mechanism of injury and by the Salter-Harris system. Several fracture types deserve special attention because of the high incidence of complications, including growth arrest with shortening of the extremity and angular deformity, as well as joint incongruity. These high-risk fractures include Salter-Harris type III and IV fractures as well as juvenile Tillaux fractures, triplane fractures, and comminuted epiphyseal fractures. In a retrospective review of these high-risk fractures, the overall complication rate was 32 percent.[77]

Juvenile Tillaux fractures are intra-articular Salter-Harris III fractures involving the lateral portion of the distal tibial epiphysis (Fig. 3-8).[78] These fractures occur toward the end of skeletal growth after the medial portion of the growth plate has already closed. The mechanism of injury

Figure 3-8 (**A**) Juvenile Tillaux fracture with intra-articular incongruity is best seen on mortice view. (**B**) This fracture was treated successfully with open reduction and internal fixation.

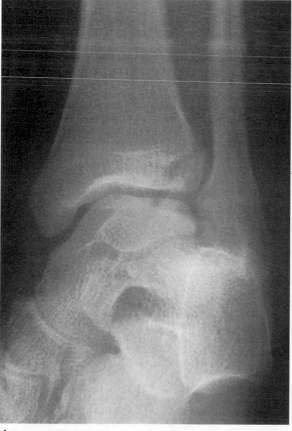

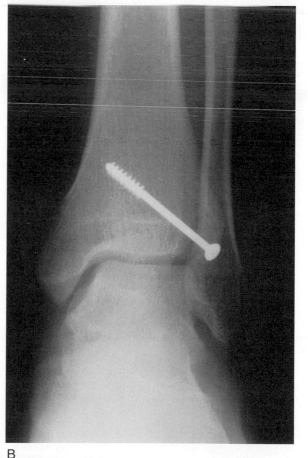

A

B

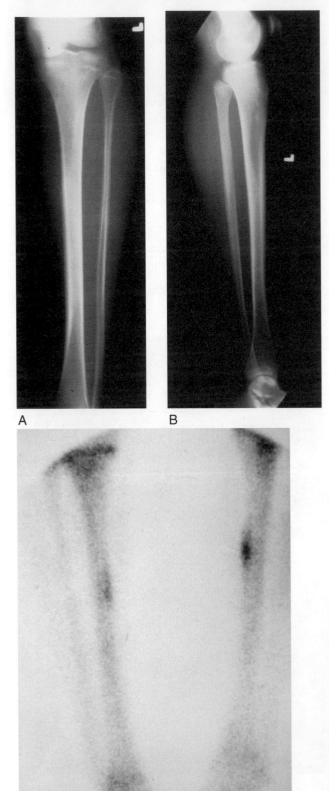

A   B

Figure 3-9 The plain radiographs (**A & B**) of a 14-year-old girl with left tibia pain are negative after 1 week of symptoms. The bone scan (**C**) and MRI (**D**) are positive at this time, however. Note the presence of bilateral proximal tibia diaphyseal stress fractures as seen on bone scan and MRI. The patient subsequently complained of bilateral symptoms.

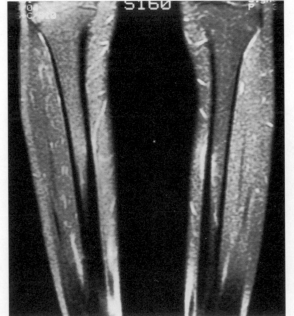

C   D

is an external rotation force applied to the supinated foot. Management of this intra-articular fracture involves precise realignment of the joint surface. CT or plain tomograms can help in the assessment of appropriate reduction. Open reduction and internal fixation is indicated for articular incongruities of more than 3 mm.[79]

Other less common acute injuries include sprains and osteochondral lesions. The overuse injuries include Sever's apophysitis, plantar fasciitis, and stress fractures. Stress fractures of the lower extremity are discussed below.

STRESS FRACTURES

Stress fractures in skeletally immature athletes are a common type of overuse injury. Almost every bone in the lower extremity and pelvis is susceptible to stress fracture. The mechanism of injury is thought to be excessive, repetitive forces acting across the bone.[80] An association between certain sports and specific types of stress fractures has been demonstrated.[81] The typical clinical presentation includes a history of gradual onset of localized pain that is relieved by rest. Patients may also have localized tenderness and swelling. Continued activity may increase the severity of the pain, and in unfortunate circumstances the affected bone may go on to complete fracture.

Early diagnosis of suspected stress fractures is simplified with the use of bone scans (Fig. 3-9). Bone scans will often reveal multiple foci of increased uptake correlating with abnormal stress.[82] Plain radiographs will subsequently demonstrate periosteal reaction and may demonstrate complete fractures if progression occurs. The major diagnostic dilemma is differentiating stress fractures from osteomyelitis and osteogenic sarcoma.[83] The history will provide the most valuable information in this regard.

Initial management of stress fractures includes activity modification, non-weight bearing, and at times cast treatment. Tibial diaphyseal stress fractures exhibit a unique tendency to go on to nonunion and complete fracture despite conservative treatment. Surgical excision and bone grafting of the tibial diaphysis has been successful in treating this condition.[84]

REFERENCES

1. Micheli LJ: Overuse injuries in children's sports: the growth factor. Orthop Clin North Am 14:337, 1983
2. Torode I, Zeig D: Pelvic fractures in children. J Pediatr Orthop 5:76, 1985
3. Garvin KL, McCarthy RE, Barnes CL, Dodge BM: Pediatric pelvic ring fractures. J Pediatr Orthop 10:577, 1990
4. Swiontkowski MF: Fractures and dislocations about the hip and pelvis. p. 307. In Green NE, Swiontkowski MF (eds): Skeletal Trauma in Children. Vol. 3. WB Saunders, Philadelphia, 1994
5. Fernbach SK, Wilkinson RH: Avulsion injuries of the pelvis and proximal femur. Am J Radiol 137:581, 1981
6. Hamada G, Rida A: Ischial apophysiolysis: report of a case and review of the literature. Clin Orthop 31:117, 1969
7. Sundar M, Carty H: Avulsion fractures of the pelvis in children: a report of 32 fractures and their outcome. Skel Radiol 23:85, 1994
8. Heinrich SD: Pediatric pelvic fractures. p. 247. In MacEwen GD, Kasser JR, Heinrich SD (eds): Pediatric Fractures. Williams & Wilkins, Baltimore, 1993
9. Waters PM, Millis MB: Hip and pelvic injuries in the young athlete. p. 279. In Stanitski CL, DeLee JC, Drez DD (eds): Pediatric and Adolescent Sports Medicine. WB Saunders, Philadelphia, 1994
10. Martin TA, Pipkin G: Treatment of avulsion of the ischial tuberosity. Clin Orthop 10:108, 1957
11. Metzmaker JN, Pappas AM: Avulsion fractures of the pelvis. Am J Sports Med 13:349, 1985
12. Schlonsky J, Olix ML: Functional disability following avulsion fracture of the ischial epiphysis. J Bone Joint Surg [Am] 54:641, 1972
13. Clancy WG, Foltz AS: Iliac apophysitis and stress fractures in adolescent runners. Am J Sports Med 4:214, 1976
14. Fox IM: Iliac apophysitis in teenage distance runners. J Am Podiatr Assoc 76:294, 1986
15. Gartland JJ, Benner JH: Traumatic dislocations in the lower extremity in children. Orthop Clin North Am 7:687, 1976
16. Offierski CM: Traumatic dislocation of the hip in children. J Bone Joint Surg [Br] 63:194, 1981
17. Heinrich SD: Proximal femur fractures: hip dislocations. p. 263. In MacEwen GD, Kasser JR, Heinrich SD (eds): Pediatric Fractures. Williams & Wilkins, Baltimore, 1993
18. Barquet A: Traumatic hip dislocation in childhood. Acta Orthop Scand 50:549, 1979
19. Stanitski CL: Acute slipped capital femoral epiphysis: treatment alternatives. J Am Acad Orthop Surg 2:96, 1994
20. Carney BT, Weinstein SL, Noble J: Long-term follow-up of slipped capital femoral epiphysis. J Bone Joint Surg [Am] 73:667, 1991
21. Jerre R, Billing L, Hansson G, Wallin J: The contralateral hip in patients primarily treated for unilateral slipped upper femoral epiphysis. J Bone Joint Surg [Br] 76:563, 1994
22. Loder RT, Aronson DD, Greenfield ML: The epidemiology of bilateral slipped capital femoral epiphysis. J Bone Joint Surg [Am] 75:1141, 1993
23. Loder RT, Richards BS, Shapiro PS et al: Acute slipped capital femoral epiphysis: the importance of physeal stability. J Bone Joint Surg [Am] 75:1134, 1993

24. Aronson DD, Carlson WE: Slipped capital femoral epiphysis. J Bone Joint Surg [Am] 74:810, 1992

25. Ward WT, Stefko J, Wood KB, Stanitski CL: Fixation with a single screw for slipped capital femoral epiphysis. J Bone Joint Surg [Am] 74:799, 1992

26. Wenger DR, Ward WT, Herring JA: Current concepts review: Legg-Calve-Perthes disease. J Bone Joint Surg [Am] 73:778, 1991

27. Weinstein SL: Legg-Calve-Perthes disease. p. 851. In Morrissy RT (ed): Lovell and Winter's Pediatric Orthopaedics. 3rd ed. JB Lippincott, New York, 1990

28. Herring JA: Current concepts review: the treatment of Legg-Calve-Perthes disease. J Bone Joint Surg [Am] 76:448, 1994

29. Sullivan JA, Gross RH, Grana WA, Garcia-Moral CA: Evaluation of injuries in youth soccer. Am J Sports Med 8:325, 1980

30. Watson AWS: Sports injuries during one academic year in 6799 Irish school children. Am J Sports Med 12:65, 1984

31. Jackson DW, Feagin JA: Quadriceps contusions in young athletes. J Bone Joint Surg [Am] 55:95, 1973

32. Rothwell AG: Quadriceps hematoma: a prospective study. Clin Orthop 171:97, 1982

33. Tyler JL, Derbekyan V, Lisbona R: Early diagnosis of myositis ossificans with Tc-99m diphosphonate imaging. Clin Nucl Med 9:256, 1984

34. Zeanah WR, Hudson TM: Myositis ossificans. Clin Orthop 168:187, 1982

35. Kransdorf MJ, Meis JM, Jelinek JS: Myositis ossificans: MR appearance with radiologic-pathologic correlation. Am J Radiol 157:1243, 1991

36. De Smet AA, Norris MA, Fisher DR: Magnetic resonance imaging of myositis ossificans: analysis of seven cases. Skel Radiol 21:503, 1992

37. Thorndike A: Myositis ossificans traumatica. J Bone Joint Surg [Am] 22:315, 1940

38. Yates CK, Grana WA: Patellofemoral pain in children. Clin Orthop 255:36, 1990

39. Micheli LJ, Stanitski CL: Lateral patellar retinacular release. Am J Sports Med 9:330, 1981

40. Kolowich PA, Paulos LE, Rosenberg TD, Farnsworth S: Lateral release of the patella: indications and contraindications. Am J Sports Med 18:359, 1990

41. Mital MA, Matza RA, Cohen J: The so-called unresolved Osgood-Schlatter lesion. J Bone Joint Surg [Am] 62:732, 1980

42. Kujala UM, Kvist M, Heinonen O: Osgood-Schlatter's disease in adolescent athletes. Am J Sports Med 13:236, 1985

43. Ogden JA, Southwick WO: Osgood-Schlatter's disease and tibial tuberosity development. Clin Orthop 116:180, 1976

44. Jakob RP, Von Gumppenberg S, Engelhardt P: Does Osgood-Schlatter disease influence the position of the patella? J Bone Joint Surg [Br] 63:579, 1981

45. Sekiguchi H, Koga Y, Ushiyama Y: Skeletal maturation growth velocity curve and the onset of Osgood disease. Abstract presented at 2nd Combined Meeting of AAOSM/ JOSSM, Maui, Hawaii, March 23, 1993

46. Medlar RC, Lyne ED: Sinding-Larsen-Johansson disease. J Bone Joint Surg [Am] 60:1113, 1978

47. Blazina ME, Kerlan RK, Jobe FW et al: Jumper's knee. Orthop Clin North Am 4:665, 1973

48. Johnson DP, Eastwood DM, Witherow PJ: Symptomatic synovial plicae of the knee. J Bone Joint Surg [Am] 75:1485, 1993

49. Patel D: Plica as a cause of anterior knee pain. Orthop Clin North Am 17:273, 1986

50. Hardaker WT, Whipple TL, Bassett FH: Diagnosis and treatment of the plica syndrome of the knee. J Bone Joint Surg [Am] 62:221, 1980

51. Ogden JA, McCarthy SM, Jabl P: The painful bipartite patella. J Pediatr Orthop 2:263, 1982

52. Weaver JK: Bipartite patella as a cause of disability in the athlete. Am J Sports Med 5:137, 1977

53. Ishikawa H, Sakurai A, Hirata S et al: Painful bipartite patella in young athletes. Clin Orthop 305:223, 1994

54. Ogata K: Painful bipartite patella. J Bone Joint Surg [Am] 76:573, 1994

55. Stanitski CL: Meniscal lesions. p. 371. In Stanitski CL, DeLee JC, Drez D (eds): Pediatric and Adolescent Sports Medicine. Vol. 3. WB Saunders, Philadelphia, 1994

56. Stanitski CL, Harvell JC, Fu F: Observations on acute knee hemarthrosis in children and adolescents. J Pediatr Orthop 13:506, 1993

57. King AG: Meniscal lesions in children and adolescents: a review of the pathology and clinical presentation. Injury 15: 105, 1983

58. Harvell JC, Fu FH, Stanitski CL: Diagnostic arthroscopy of the knee in children and adolescents. Orthopedics 12:1555, 1989

59. DeHaven KE: Decision-making factors in the treatment of meniscus lesions. Clin Orthop 252:49, 1990

60. Wroble RR, Henderson RC, Campion ER et al: Meniscectomy in children and adolescents: a long-term follow-up study. Clin Orthop 279:180, 1992

61. Manzione M, Pizzutillo PD, Peoples AB, Schweizer PA: Meniscectomy in children: a long-term follow-up study. Am J Sports Med 11:111, 1983

62. Weiss CB, Lundberg M, Hamberg P et al: Non-operative treatment of meniscal tears. J Bone Joint Surg [Am] 71:811, 1989

63. DeLee JC: Ligamentous injury of the knee. p. 406. In Stanitski CL, DeLee JC, Drez D (eds): Pediatric and Adolescent Sports Medicine. Vol. 3. WB Saunders, Philadelphia, 1994

64. McCarroll JR, Rettig AC, Shelbourne KD: Anterior cruciate ligament injuries in the young athlete with open physes. Am J Sports Med 16:44, 1988

65. Lipscomb AB, Anderson AF: Tears of the anterior cruciate ligament in adolescents. J Bone Joint Surg [Am] 68:19, 1986

66. DeLee JC, Curtis R: Anterior cruciate ligament insufficiency in children. Clin Orthop 172:112, 1983
67. Sullivan JA: Ligamentous injuries of the knee in children. Clin Orthop 255:44, 1990
68. Meyers MH, McKeever FM: Fracture of the intercondylar eminence of the tibia. J Bone Joint Surg [Am] 41:209, 1959
69. Meyers MH, McKeever FM: Fracture of the intercondylar eminence of the tibia. J Bone Joint Surg [Am] 52:1677, 1970
70. Zaricznyj B: Avulsion fracture of the tibial eminence: treatment by open reduction and pinning. J Bone Joint Surg [Am] 59:1111, 1977
71. Baxter MP, Wiley JJ: Fractures of the tibial spine in children. J Bone Joint Surg [Br] 70:228, 1988
72. Wiley JJ, Baxter MP: Tibial spine fractures in children. Clin Orthop 255:54, 1990
73. Indelicato PA: Isolated medial collateral ligament injuries in the knee. J Am Acad Orthop Surg 3:9, 1995
74. Indelicato PA, Hermansdorfer J, Huegel M: Nonoperative management of complete tears of the medial collateral ligament of the knee in intercollegiate football players. Clin Orthop 256:174, 1990
75. Jones RI, Henley MB, Francis P: Nonoperative management of isolated grade III collateral ligament injuries in high school football players. Clin Orthop 213:137, 1986
76. Sullivan JA: Ankle and foot injuries in the pediatric athlete. p. 441. In Stanitski CL, DeLee JC, Drez D (eds): Pediatric and Adolescent Sports Medicine. Vol. 3. WB Saunders, Philadelphia, 1994
77. Speigel PG, Cooperman DR, Laros GS: Epiphyseal fractures of the distal ends of the tibia and fibula. J Bone Joint Surg [Am] 60:1046, 1978
78. Kleiger B, Mankin HJ: Fracture of the lateral portion of the distal tibial epiphysis. J Bone Joint Surg [Am] 46:25, 1964
79. Crawford AH: Fractures and dislocations of the foot and ankle. p. 449. In Green NE, Swiontkowski MF (eds): Skeletal Trauma in Children. Vol. 3. WB Saunders, Philadelphia, 1994
80. Stanitski CL, McMaster JH, Scranton PE: On the nature of stress fractures. Am J Sports Med 6:391, 1978
81. Walter NE, Wolf MD: Stress fractures in young athletes. Am J Sports Med 5:165, 1977
82. Rosen PR, Micheli LJ, Treves S: Early scintigraphic diagnosis of bone stress and fractures in athletic adolescents. Pediatrics 70:11, 1982
83. Levin DC, Blazina ME, Levine E: Fatigue fractures of the shaft of the femur: simulation of malignant tumor. Radiology 89:883, 1967
84. Green NE, Rogers RA, Lipscomb AB: Nonunions of stress fractures of the tibia. Am J Sports Med 13:171, 1985

4

Athletic Training and Conditioning

STEVEN I. SUBOTNICK

THE EFFECT OF TRAINING ON THE BODY

Physical fitness is an essential part of any wellness prescription. The Centers for Disease Control and Prevention estimates that 70 to 80 percent of chronic disease is preventable. Americans who are not involved in a regular fitness program or acrobics program would benefit from an evaluation of their life-style. Are they truly healthy enough to ignore the multitude of benefits of regular moderate-intensity aerobic exercise? Previously sedentary patients can experience improvement in health with exercise intensity as low as 50 percent of their VO_{2max}. Stress reduction, aerobic exercise, stretching, and diet modification had been shown to reverse cardiovascular disease by Dean Ornish, M.D. at U.C.S.F. Medical School in San Francisco. He is currently a White House adviser to President and Mrs. Clinton.[1]

An awareness of the increased health risks associated with sedentary jobs, sedentary life-style, and improper diet or social habits has many people of all ages looking toward aerobic exercise as a way to reduce the risk factors associated with cardiovascular disease and stress, improve the quality of their lives, and lose weight.[2-4] Along with this increased desire for fitness has come an increased number of athletic injuries. There is literally an epidemic of heel-spur syndrome with plantar fasciitis occurring in middle-aged to senior citizen fitness walkers. The "baby boomer" marathoners of the early 1970s have become the fitness walkers of today, with over 70 million of us walking 2 to 6 miles 5 days a week. We have learned that fitness is no longer just recreation, it is a presription for life. Every patient a physician sees must be given a fitness prescription in terms of intensity, frequency, duration, and progression. Exercise and nutrition are the medicines! Yet injuries occur. As in the case of heel-spur syndrome, why?

Most of these injuries are due primarily to training errors, accentuated by biomechanical imbalances. Gear is a primary factor, and even nutritional deficiencies can be involved. The sports medicine physician must be able to prescribe a sensible and reasonable fitness program for both the entry-level and the established athlete.

The U.S. population embarked on a fitness and aerobics renaissance during the early 1970s: for example, the New York Marathon had 120 contestants in 1970, compared with 25,000 in 1987. Three million people regularly run for aerobic fitness in the United States, and it is not unusual to have 20,000 to 25,000 entrants in a marathon in the United States, Europe, or the Orient. Also experiencing a resurgence during the late 1970s was exercise walking. There are now an estimated 65 million to 70 million people involved in regular active walking for aerobic fitness and exercise. In addition to the popularity of running and walking is the aerobics revolution, which began mainly as a woman's sport. In the United States 15 million to 20 million women are currently involved in regular aerobic dance or high- or low-impact aerobics for fitness.[5,6]

Other examples of an increased desire for fitness can be found in the increased membership in the YMCA over the past 15 years, and an increase in the memberships of swimming and biking clubs. In addition, hundreds of companies have hired fitness directors for their employees, and hotels have installed exercise facilities. Golf is growing at phenomenal rates and especially attracting retired senior citizens. Bowling remains ever-popular.

In spite of all this participation, there is a generalized unawareness among the public about how to begin an appropriate fitness program or how to prevent or treat associated injuries; the sports medicine physician is then referred to for advice.[7]

There is a misconception among the public that all exercise leads to fitness. Exercise may lead to fitness, but not necessarily *total* fitness. Often, exercise is not even aerobic and does little for the cardiovascular system.[2,8]

The necessary elements of total fitness include a dynamic balance of the physical, emotional, mental, and spiritual dimensions of the person. Physical fitness includes

1. Cardiovascular exercise
2. Proper eating habits and nutrition
3. Weight control
4. Elimination of smoking
5. Elimination of excessive alcohol consumption
6. Stress management
7. Establishment and maintenance of flexibility, strength, endurance, and power.

The American Heart Association has estimated that 1 million Americans die each year from cardiovascular disease. This accounts for 55 percent of all deaths.[3] There has been an alarming increase in cardiovascular disease among young adults in the age group of 24 to 40 years, and women in high-stress occupations are also suffering from cardiovascular disease. The advantage of total fitness is that it decreases the likelihood of cardiovascular attack while increasing the chance for recovery if one does suffer such an attack.[3,8] In addition, there are many other positive by-products of total fitness, some of which are listed here:

1. Greater strength, stamina, and suppleness, with corresponding reduction of minor aches and pains, stiffness, and soreness
2. Better posture and fewer back problems
3. Renewed energy and vitality
4. Improved digestion

5. More restful sleep
6. Enhanced ability to control tension, anxiety, and stress
7. Increased coordination, ease, and grace of movement
8. Improved appearance
9. Better self-image, including self-confidence and improved disposition
10. Increased efficiency, clear thinking, and better decision-making skills
11. Greater sexual enjoyment

Health care is at a crossroads; chronic disease, despite the advances in medicine, is growing at alarming rates. Sports medicine and fitness medicine are a big part of the solution.

COMPONENTS OF A CARDIOVASCULAR FITNESS PROGRAM

The amount of time necessary for an appropriate fitness program is 30 to 40 minutes every other day. The most important part of a fitness program is compliance. Studies have shown that people who have never been involved in an aerobics program before and who start a program on their own have about an 80 percent failure rate after 2 to 4 weeks. When these same people are placed within a supervised program with a knowledgeable exercise leader, the survival rate at the end of 4 weeks is at least 80 percent (Dr. Michael Pollock, personal communication, 1987). Appropriate instruction, encouragement, and group motivation are all important. This is especially true for endomorphic people, who tend to be obese and rather self-conscious, and who prefer the company of groups. Mesomorphs are more muscular people who respond to the challenges of the program. Ectomorphs are rather slender people who take naturally to running and aerobic exercise and have little trouble with compliance.[2,9]

Several components should be incorporated into an exercise program that is regularly scheduled, personally tailored, and initially recorded in a fitness improvement log: warmup, aerobic exercise, cooldown, and conditioning.

The Warmup

The warmup enables the muscles to stretch to their physiologic length. Maximum muscle function is achieved when the muscles have been stretched to 110 percent of their physiologic length. This must be done slowly and nonballistically. The stretch should be held for approximately 30 seconds. Five such stretches suffice for the various body parts. Stretching is often enhanced by yoga-type breathing. The athlete should gently inhale first, then exhale while doing a slow, steady stretch.[7,10] Tight posterior muscles, such as the hamstrings and calf muscles, must be stretched before engaging in aerobic exercise. The same holds true for the anterior muscle groups. Rotational exercise of the various joints of the lower extremity, including the ankle, subtalar, and midtarsal joints, is also recommended. Bouncing up and down gently on the ball of the foot, with the feet not leaving the ground, tones and stretches the intrinsic foot muscles. As a supplement to the warmup, a mini-yoga program or tai chi are most helpful in improving and maintaining flexibility. These type of activities may be carried out two to three times a week.

A brief upper extremity warmup with forward and backward arm rolls is helpful. A fast-walking session speeds up the heart rate and lung action and marks the termination of the warmup session. The warmup is crucial to helping prevent injuries and to avoid overtaxing the cardiovascular system.[7]

In colder weather or for athletes who tend to be stiff, such as senior citizens, warming up on an exercise bike can be beneficial. Ten to 15 minutes of gentle biking before running tones the cardiovascular system as it warms up the lower extremities, decreasing the likelihood of injuries. Brisk walking is also an excellent warmup exercise. This should be done for at least 5 minutes before, as well as 5 minutes after, athletic participation. The longer or harder a workout is, the more time should be spent in preparing for the event. Many athletes hedge by cutting down on the warmup as well as the cooldown to increase the amount of time they spend actually training. Since cutting back on the warmup can lead to injury, an important part of any sports-related history-taking should include questioning athletes about warmup and cooldown routines. Since most injuries are caused in part by training errors, suggestions as to improved warmup and cooldown by the sports physician are of considerable importance. Cooldown is discussed following the section on aerobics.

Figure 4-1 depicts various warmup exercises. These exercises are suggested prior to running, and are also a good warmup for overall general conditioning and other sports.

Aerobic Exercise

Aerobic training is an essential part of any successful fitness program. It entails a steady, continuous activity using major muscles, increasing blood flow and the pumping action of the heart. Associated with aerobic exercises are improved functioning of the heart, lungs, and blood vessels.[11]

Aerobic exercises were popularized by Dr. Kenneth Cooper. In his publications on aerobics, he stated that aerobic exercise is exercise that roughly doubles the resting pulse rate, maintained for 20 to 30 minutes per workout, 3 to 4 days a week.[5,6] This doubled pulse is approximately 80 percent of maximum cardiac output. The maximum benefit range (MBR) is 70 to 85 percent of maximum pulse rate. When aerobic exercise is being carried out at this level, athletes are able to talk with ease; as the aerobic threshold is approached, talking becomes uncomfortable. When an athlete becomes "out of breath," it is time to switch from aerobic to anaerobic exercise.

Aerobic exercise uses oxygen that is stored in the body. Any exercise that uses the larger muscles in the body, mostly the leg muscles, is helpful in maintaining aerobic fitness. Many beginning athletes undertake aerobic programs in an effort to lose weight. A total of 3,500 calories must be burned off to lose 1 pound. Since 250 to 300 calories are metabolized per mile when running 8 to 9 min/mile, running 35 miles/wk would theoretically lead to the loss of 1 pound/wk, provided caloric intake is not increased. Most effective weight reduction programs include aerobic exercise as a key component.

One metabolic benefit of aerobic exercise is increased growth of mitochondria in the muscles. Mitochondria are increased threefold in major muscle groups and up to sevenfold in the calf muscles, according to Costill.[12] As the mitochondria content increases, the body's efficiency at metabolizing food increases, and the muscles are more capable of storing glycogen. Free fatty acids are more readily metabolized and used for fuel.

Work done by Costil[12] demonstrates that between 25 and 30 minutes into an aerobic workout, there is a crossover from metabolizing stored glycogen in the muscles to metabolizing free fatty acids. This condition is colloquially referred to as a "runner's high" or "second wind." The free fatty acids and glycogen metabolism graphs cross at about 30 minutes and, for the next 30 minutes, the athlete metabolizes increasing amounts of free fatty acid while decreasing the amount of stored glycogen being metabolized. At about 1 hour, very little glycogen is metabolized and, instead, the free fatty acids are used. In addition, there is an increase in the amount of neurotransmitters in the body that parallels increased free fatty acid metabolism and increases endorphins and enkephalins, which improves stress

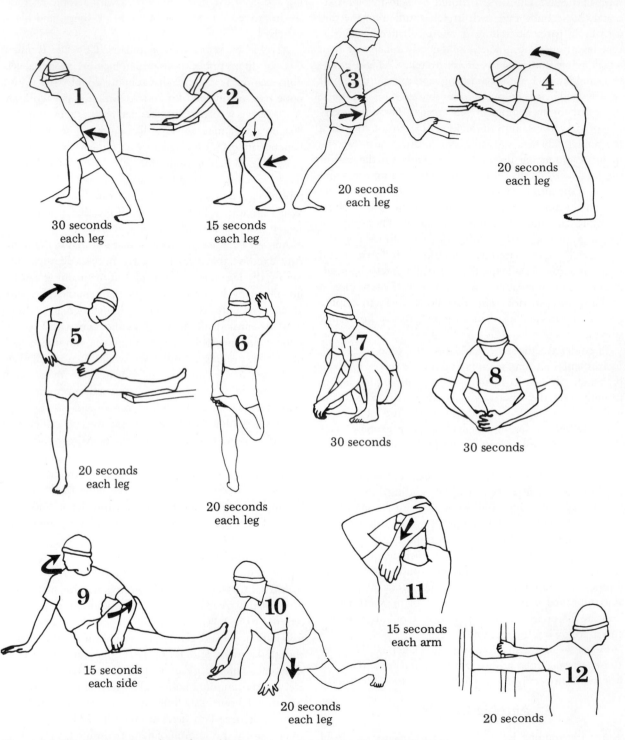

Figure 4–1 Warmup exercises to be performed before running (takes approximately 9 minutes).

reduction. The increased level of neurotransmitters appears to reach a peak after 45 to 50 minutes of aerobic activity.

Aerobic exercise also has an effect on cholesterol. Low-density lipoproteins (LDLs) are decreased and a corresponding increase in high-density lipoproteins (HDLs) occurs. A positive correlation between decreased atherosclerosis and increased HDLs has been demonstrated. In addition, total body fat decreases with an aerobic exercise program. These factors help decrease the risk factors associated with cardiovascular disease.[12]

Aerobic exercise uses slow-twitch muscle fibers, which metabolize more slowly and are more prevalent in endurance-type activity. Anaerobic exercise uses fast-twitch fibers as well as stored glycogen. Long-distance running increases endurance but does not improve speed; intervals or fartlek (speed play) increase quickness and speed; and calisthenics and conditioning exercises improve balance and proprioception. All three are necessary for maximum conditioning and fitness.

The physiologic changes associated with aerobic exercise are listed in Table 4-1. There are several protective

PROTECTIVE BENEFITS OF REGULAR AEROBIC EXERCISE

Decreased cardiovascular disease

Decrease in degenerative disease with increased longevity

Shift toward increased HDL

Decrease and lowering of the triglycerides

Increased rapid fat metabolism

Dietary changes with a trend away from simple carbohydrates toward more complex carbohydrates

benefits of regular aerobic exercise (see Box).[3] The overall effects are increased longevity, increased endurance, and greater ability to withstand or recover from disease.

AEROBIC EXERCISE: DEFINITION

In order for aerobic exercise to be successful in a fitness program, it must accomplish a number of things. The resting heart rate must be increased to a training level or MBR. This is the rate that is 70 to 85 percent of the maximum pulse rate—the maximum number of beats that the heart can beat in 1 minute. The maximum pulse rate is affected primarily by age: the older the patient, the lower the maximum. To determine maximum pulse rate, the person's age is subtracted from 220. The result is that person's maximum pulse rate. A person's target aerobic workout pulse rate is the maximum pulse rate times the desired intensity of exercise, or MBR. For example, if a man of 40 years of age has a maximum pulse rate of 180, his MBR is 70 to 85 percent of 180, or 126 to 153 beats/min.[2,9]

To qualify as an aerobic activity, exercise must succeed in raising the pulse rate to this level for a minimum of 12 to 15 continuous minutes. Exercise should last for 20 to 30 minutes and be done 4 to 5 days a week to maintain baseline aerobic fitness. In order to obtain the psychological benefits of exercise, this pulse rate must be maintained for at least 30 minutes, with the maximum benefit taking place at between 45 minutes and 1 hour.

Energy expenditure during exercise is measured in metabolic equivalents (mets). One met represents an oxygen consumption rate of 3.5 ml/kg/min, the approximate resting rate of a 70-kg (154-pound) adult. The expenditure in various types of exercise are as follows:

Table 4-1 Physiologic Changes Associated with Regular Aerobic Exercise

Organ/System	Physiologic Changes
Heart	Increased efficiency; increased stroke volume; decreased diastolic pressure
Lungs	Increased vital oxygen capacity; increased oxygen diffusion
Cardiovascular system	Increased red cell mass; increase in the collateral circulatory tree; increase in the plasma volume
Muscles	Increase in the slow-twitch fibers; increase in mitochondria; $3\frac{1}{4}$ times more oxidative capacity in most muscles; up to 7 times increased efficiency and capacity for gastrocnemius–soleus muscles, with concomitant increase in mitochondria and associated fat-burning capacity
Gastrointestinal system	Increased digestive function and peristalsis
Musculoskeletal system	Increased lubrication and nutrition of joints, provided abuse is avoided
Metabolism	Increased metabolic efficiency with a decrease in dysmenorrhea; decrease in total body fat; increase in HDL and decrease in LDL; increase in oxygen utilization, transportation, and consumption

Walking at 3 miles/hr	3.3 mets
Walking at 4 miles/hr	4.5 mets
Doubles tennis	6 mets
Speed walking	6 mets
Slow jogging	6 mets
Fast biking	6 mets
Cross-country skiing	6 mets
Jogging a 10-minute mile	10 mets
Running	12–14 mets

SAFETY IN AN AEROBIC FITNESS PROGRAM

Patients of all abilities ask their physicians for guidelines in beginning or accelerating an aerobic fitness program; what follows are some basic guidelines. The beginning athlete should be told to train and not strain. It should be emphasized to athletes of all levels that conditioning and training involve *gradual* adaptation to stress. Excessive stress leads to overstress injuries. The hard–easy rule applies to all athletes: a hard workout one day should be followed by an easy one. Two hard days in a row do not permit the soft tissue to recover to a level that will accept rigorous activity. Recreational athletes or those involved for fitness should have at least 2 days per week when they are not involved in their primary activity. Thus runners should run only 5 days a week and may hike or swim on the two nonrunning days. Runners are well advised not to go more than 3 days in a row without a break or rest with a substitute alternate aerobic activity. Running more than 5 days per week is clinically associated with 50 percent more injuries.

At the beginning of an aerobic program, a person should exercise at the low end of the MBR (70 percent of maximum pulse rate). This is particularly true if the potential athlete is overweight, has been inactive for more than 2 to 3 years, or is over 35 years of age. The risk of a myocardial infarction in a 50-year-old engaging in 1 hour of moderate to heavy exercise (target pulse 70 to 75 percent of maximum) equals 1 in 1 million; for a sedentary 50-year-old the risk is 1 in 10,000. Trained athletes in the intermediate stages of their program can be advised to exercise at 75 percent of their maximum pulse rate (mid-range MBR). Only top competitive athletes should be exercising at 85 percent of their maximum pulse rate (upper range MBR).

A clinical tool helpful to athletes is to suggest to them that, if they are able to talk during their workouts but prefer not to, they are close to 80 to 85 percent of their maximum pulse rate. If talking is impossible, they are beyond 85 percent. This "talk test" is important for beginning athletes, who should be advised to exercise only at levels at which talking is comfortable.[14]

Fitness walkers or runners need not go more than 15 miles/wk. Competitive/recreational runners need not run more than 35 miles/wk. Marathoners may put in 50 to 65 miles/wk beginning 4 months before the actual competition. Needless to say, there is a high risk of injury with this high mileage.[12]

When creating a successful exercise program, it is important for the physician to have patients record the following data that may be transferred to a log for the physician's review:

1. Maximum pulse rate (220 minus age)
2. Seventy percent maximum pulse rate (lower range aerobic threshold)
3. Seventy-five percent maximum pulse rate (mid-range MBR)
4. Eighty percent maximum pulse rate (upper range MBR)
5. Eighty-five percent maximum pulse rate (aerobic threshold, for competitive athletes only)

In addition to these data, it is helpful to note the type of footwear used; the time of day when the athletic program is undertaken; a brief explanation as to warmup, stretching exercises, and cooldown; and some information as to lifestyle, stresses, and diet.

The exercise physician should suggest or prescribe alternative aerobic exercise to the injured athlete; for example, a cross-country ski machine may be used by an injured runner who has sustained a stress fracture, permitting maintenance of muscle tone and aerobic fitness while decreasing impact. Various aerobic exercises can be selected for a fitness program in order of their relative merit (see Box).

Walking is an excellent alternative or primary aerobic activity. Although walking is listed last in relative merit (see Box), fitness or exercise walking can deliver benefits similar to those achieved with jogging or running. Since the knee is extended upon contact, athletes who would otherwise have knee pain with running, jumping, or cutting sports may be able to exercise or pace walk without pain. The same holds true for race walking, which has aerobic benefits that may exceed those of running. Exercise walking at about 14 min/mile uses approximately 6 mets. For each additional pound added with hand weights, 1

ORDER OF BENEFITS TO PATIENT OF VARIOUS AEROBIC EXERCISES

1. Cross-country skiing
2. Jogging and running
3. Skipping rope
4. Aerobic dance or jazzercise
5. Swimming
6. Bicyling—indoor or outdoor
7. Skating—roller or ice
8. Jumping jacks
9. Running in place
10. Stair stepping
11. Walking

met is gained; thus fitness walking with 3 pounds in each hand, vigorously pumping the arms rhythmically in pace with the leg swing, can accomplish an aerobic workout at a level of 12 mets, equivalent to running at 8 to 9 min/mile.[2] Thus walking is an excellent alternative for the patient who is out of shape and overweight.

The exercise physician should remember that each patient has 633 muscles in the body. There is a tendency toward overspecialization in sports, which overdevelops some muscles at the expense of others. This leads to stiffness as well as dynamic imbalance. Encouraging patients to participate in activities that use both the upper and lower extremities increases their fitness and decreases the likelihood of injury. Thus the inclusion of alternative aerobic exercise in the workout program is recommended.

VALUE OF RECREATIONAL SPORTS

Recreational sports, such as tennis, squash, racquetball, handball, and volleyball, have little aerobic exercise value. They are fun and relaxing and have great social merit. They do not, however, raise the pulse to the appropriate MBR. Good aerobic fitness, however, enables one to enjoy these sports with more vigor and less fatigue.

The Cooldown

A successful fitness program includes gradual cooldown for at least 5 minutes following the workout, be it aerobic or anaerobic. It must be stressed to athletes that the cool-down period prevents soreness, cramps, nausea, and dizziness, as well as circulatory problems. During the aerobic exercise, the athlete's heart, lungs, and blood vessels work at an increased rate to supply the muscles with extra oxygen. This need for increased oxygen consumption continues for a few minutes after the aerobic exercise stops, hence the importance of maintaining the pumping action of the heart and major veins and the aerobic capacity of the lungs during the cooldown. Athletes can be instructed simply to walk rapidly while pumping or swinging the arms forward and backward.[12,15]

The physician should urge the athlete not to sit down immediately after any workout, but instead to keep moving for at least 5 minutes. This guards against circulatory collapse. Athletes are advised not to rush into a hot or cold shower, hot tub, sauna, or steam room until they have cooled down. This guards against excessive vasodilation and/or syncope.

Athletes are advised to stretch after the cooldown period, since their muscles are warm and supple, providing added gain in length of these tight structures. A period of 5 to 10 minutes of stretching is suggested as a post-aerobic workout session.

Figure 4-2 illustrates appropriate cooldown stretching exercises for running and other similar activities. These exercises help maintain general conditioning of the musculoskeletal system.

CONDITIONING

Specific conditioning advice is often asked of the sports physician. Conditioning involves the use of exercise to tone, firm, and strengthen the body; however, it does not produce aerobic fitness. Conditioning exercises are done in addition to aerobics to increase the efficiency of the body and improve muscle tone. Range of motion of the joints is improved as well. Athletes involved in an aerobic training program tend to ignore general conditioning, since they do not appreciate its benefits. The physician must remind athletes that conditioning both improves their ability to perform and decreases the likelihood of injury.

Conditioning may be done on alternative days of aerobic workout. Traditional exercises include the use of Nautilus-type equipment, free weights, slant boards, and calisthenics. Light repetitive weights are useful in developing strength and speed. Conventional situps, pushups, pullups, jumping jacks, and a mini–yoga program are all advisable.

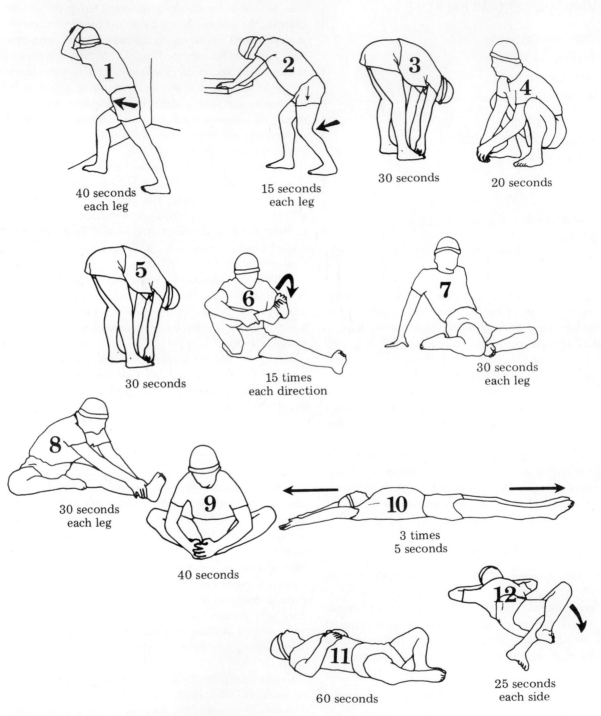

40 seconds
each leg

15 seconds
each leg

30 seconds

20 seconds

30 seconds

15 times
each direction

30 seconds
each leg

30 seconds
each leg

40 seconds

3 times
5 seconds

60 seconds

25 seconds
each side

Figure 4–2 Cooldown exercises to be performed after running (takes approximately 9 minutes).

In addition, conditioning involves improved balance and kinesthetic tone. Proprioception is enhanced. Athletes are advised to stand on one foot with their eyes closed and arms extended, like a stork, practicing balancing on one foot. Reflexes are improved as they hop from foot to foot. Proprioception and balance exercises prevent ankle injuries and are essential following rehabilitation of the athlete who has injured any joint. Athletes must be reminded that total fitness involves strength, flexibility, balance, and endurance.

Overall Conditioning Methods

STRENGTH

Strength requires some form of weight training. If an injury is present, Cybex testing is usually suggested to ascertain the amount of weakness. Appropriate rehabilitation through Cybex and other weight machines with an exercise physical therapist is essential. Overall strength is maintained and improved through weight training. As muscular strength is improved, so is power and endurance. Light weights with increased repetitions improve strength and endurance, yet do not contribute to muscular hypertrophy. High weight–low repetition results in improved strength and endurance as well as muscular hypertrophy. Appropriate strength training includes concentric, eccentric, and isometric exercise. Injured athletes should receive specific exercise testing via Cybex, as well as rehabilitation from an exercise physical therapist. The sports physician should be familiar with existing facilities to which to refer patients who need additional instruction or overall conditioning from trained exercise and strength coaches.

FLEXIBILITY

Flexibility is often overlooked in overall conditioning. Appropriate flexibility is as important as appropriate strength. Flexibility exercises, such as the exercises illustrated in Figures 4-1 and 4-2, may be carried out both before and after the specific exercise event. Major muscle groups should be slowly stretched over a period of 20 to 25 seconds. Nonballistic stretching is preferred. Ballistic stretching may actually pull a muscle, causing injury. Rapid jerking movements evoke the reflex arc, causing contraction of the muscle, which should be relaxed for the gentle stretch. This reverse myostatic reflex is avoided by gentle breathing and relaxed slow stretching. It is important to inform athletes to hold the stretch to at least a count of

20. Progressively stretching the same muscle group gently results in improved flexibility as well as increased length. Athletes who are usually tight may benefit from enrolling in a yoga class. Flexibility and yoga classes for athletes are often offered through the YMCA or similar facilities.

BALANCE

Balance and proprioception decrease the likelihood of injury. Specific exercises to improve and maintain proprioception are part of an overall conditioning program. Exercise physicians instruct their athletes in balancing on one foot with their eyes closed. Athletes are then instructed to hop from foot to foot rapidly with their eyes closed. Improved proprioception and balance may also be achieved by balance boards or working out on a mini-trampoline. Balance boards are most helpful following rehabilitation from a sprained ankle. In testing athletes, the exercise physician should have the athlete demonstrate proprioception by standing on one foot and balancing and then comparing this with the opposite foot. Often, when an injury has been incompletely rehabilitated, there will be some functional limitation of proprioception on the injured side, which should be corrected.

ENDURANCE

Fatigue leads to injury. Athletes lose their ability to concentrate when fatigued, making injury more likely. Fatigued muscles lose their ability to absorb shock or provide dynamic stability for joints. Thus, bone and joints are at greater risk when the athlete is fatigued. Increased endurance is the goal of most athletes and is improved by gradually increasing exercise or workout time. Endurance is also improved by weight training, which improves the power and strength of muscles. Cross-training using swimming, biking, or running allows for increased workout time with decreased strain to the body. This method is preferable to running alone as a means of increasing endurance. Endurance is accomplished by exercising at approximately 70 to 75 percent of maximum pulse rate. Speed is improved by exercising beyond 85 percent of maximum pulse rate. This is accomplished by doing interval training with repeat short bursts of speed from 100 to 440 yards, once or twice a week. In another form of speed play, called fartlek, an athlete focuses on an object in the distance and then runs close to maximum speed to this object. Hill running is another popular way to increase speed and endurance. Running uphill has less impact and allows harder workouts with decreased stress; running downhill has the opposite effect.[13]

THE VALUE OF BIOFEEDBACK

Biofeedback and positive imaging are also important for a total fitness program. The physician should instruct athletes to observe themselves periodically when standing in front of a mirror. If they have a dropped shoulder or curvature of the spine, one hip low, or one hip high, they may have dynamic imbalances that need to be corrected with specific exercises. There also may be biomechanical imbalances. Running on a treadmill with a mirror is a good way to teach athletes how to run with appropriate form. Biodynamic foot orthotics (a biofeedback device) encourage athletes to have appropriate foot function. Videotaping athletes undergoing various movements that are components of their sports helps the physician pick up errors and prescribe appropriate rehabilitative exercises. Consultation with a coach is often helpful in correcting errors that decrease efficiency and increase the likelihood of injury.

TRAINING TOWARD A SPECIFIC EVENT

The sports physician is often asked for appropriate advice about training toward a certain event. These questions usually come from runners. They want to know how to increase their mileage safely while improving speed. The "rule of three" is applicable here and can be explained to the patient (see Ch. 6). Most runners can compete at about three times their average daily mileage. Cyclic, rather than progressive, training is associated with fewer overuse injuries.

In cyclic training, a plateau is reached every 3 weeks. Thus a runner exercising at 3 miles/day 5 days a week, or 15 miles/wk, who is interested in running a half-marathon, would be advised to increase total weekly mileage by 5 miles every 3 weeks. After 3 weeks of running 15 miles per week, the athlete would then run 20 miles per week for 3 weeks. The first week would be a relatively easy week, the second week one of intermediate intensity, and the third week easy again, in preparation for the next increase to 25 miles per week. If stiffness, soreness, or pain is encountered, the mileage is reduced back to the original level and maintained there for an additional 3 weeks; persistent discomfort or discomfort that becomes pain should be evaluated by the sports physician.

Athletes seeking improved speed can do interval training. Quarter-mile fast runs at 70 to 80 percent maximum speed can be carried out once or twice a week. Six to eight of these intervals usually suffice. Half-mile or mile intervals are helpful in preparing for a marathon. Marathon preparation also requires long runs once a week. These runs are in the range of 15 to 20 miles at a time. Marathon preparation requires a base of 50 to 60 miles for 2 months prior to the marathon. Two weeks before the marathon, mileage is decreased by about 60 percent. Most athletes rest 2 days before a marathon, doing only flexibility exercises or perhaps light jogging for up to 3 miles.

Athletes are advised to eat complex carbohydrates when preparing for endurance events. Food should not be eaten within 3 hours of an endurance event. In general, the most appropriate fluid for endurance events is water.

Athletes who have been injured or operated on need specific advice on how to get back to their specific sport. Return to training is easier, provided some substitute form of aerobic activity has been used during the rehabilitative period. Athletes are not allowed to run until they can demonstrate the ability to walk for 3 miles at a pace of 15 min/mile. Appropriate flexibility, proprioception, and strength must be demonstrated. Once 45 minutes of rapid walking without pain or discomfort is achieved, the athletes are put on a 5–10 program: they walk for 5 minutes, then run easily for 10 minutes. They continue doing this for 3 miles. This program is maintained for 5 days. Alternative aerobics are then prescribed for the next 2 days. The new week is started with a 5–10 program. Every week, 20 minutes more of running is added to the program, as long as there is no pain or prolonged stiffness. Once the athlete can run for 30 minutes without pain at about an 8-minute pace, he or she is put in a cyclic training program, increasing mileage by 5 miles/wk every 3 weeks as described above.

SUMMARY

The sports medicine physician must be prepared to prescribe a safe fitness program. In addition, suggestions for improving an established program are imperative. A successful fitness program is done regularly at least four times per week. Strenuous exercise should only be done every other day; for example, running 5 days a week increases the risk for injury. The importance of a warmup and cooldown cannot be overstressed. Aerobic fitness is achieved by exercising at 70 to 80 percent of MBR. Sedentary individuals can benefit from exercises at as little as 50% of MBR. Everyone is capable of some form of regular aerobic exercise program; patients must be educated and empowered to share the responsibility for their fitness, health, and wellness with their wellness advocate, their physician.

Since running is such a popular aerobic exercise, the exercise physician should suggest or prescribe alternative aerobic exercise to permit increased workout time with decreased strain to the musculoskeletal system and to provide for rehabilitative exercise while decreasing strain to an injured part. Alternative aerobic exercises (cross-training) include biking, exercise walking, exerstriding, swimming, rowing, cross-country ski machines, or jazzercise.

Suggesting that the athlete keep an exercise journal is a good way to discover training errors. The log should include duration and intensity of workout; pulse rate before, during, and after a workout; and general observations about attitude, body form, diet, and sleep patterns. Notations about any discomfort or pain that occurs in body parts may be valuable.

The sports medicine physician should advise athletic patients that exercising with discomfort may be allowable, but that exercising with pain is not. Athletes are advised to "listen" to their bodies and are instructed to stop exercising if any unusual discomfort, tightness or pain in the chest, shortness of breath, dizziness, light-headedness, or loss of muscle control occurs.

A sports physician must keep a positive attitude and encourage patients to keep fit. The two main reasons for relinquishing an exercise program are overexercise and unsuitable exercise; other factors include inappropriate gear and training errors. All these factors must be taken into consideration when a successful exercise program is designed, or an unsuccessful one evaluated for causes of failure or injury.

The sports physician must always remember that injured athletes detrain three times as fast as they train. All injured athletes should be given alternative aerobic exercises within the limits of their injury. Often the exercise prescription is the most important one a sports physician can give.

REFERENCES

1. Ornish D: Alternative Ther Health Med 1:84, 1995
2. Wilmer J: Sensible Fitness. Leisure Press, Champaign, IL, 1986
3. Kiel P, Fritinghuessen J: Keep Your Heart Running. Winchester Press, New York, 1976
4. Hastings A, Fadaman J, Gordon J: Health for the Whole Person: Institute of Noetic Sciences. Westview Press, Boulder, CO, 1980
5. Cooper K: The Aerobics Way. Bantam Books, New York, 1977
6. Cooper K: Aerobics for Women. Bantam Books, New York, 1973
7. Lawrence N, Rajla J, Sciutto C: Total Fitness for the Working Person. Corporate Fitness, 1980
8. Bailey C: Fit or Fat. Houghton-Mifflin, Boston, 1978
9. Haycock C: Sportsmedicine for the Athletic Female. Medical Economics, Oradell, NJ, 1980
10. Anderson RA: Stretching. Shelter Publications, 1980
11. Library of Health: Exercising for Fitness. Time-Life Books, New York, 1981
12. Costill D: A scientific approach to distance running. Track Field News, Palo Alto, CA, 1979
13. Henderson J: The Complete Marathoner. World Publications, Mountain View, CA, 1978
14. Sheehan G: Running and Being. Simon & Schuster, New York, 1978
15. Williams JP, Sperryn PN: Sports Medicine. 2nd Ed. Butler and Tanner, London, 1976

5

Sports Nutrition

Proper Nutrition for Athletes: Maintaining a Balance

ELSON M. HAAS

Regular exercise is one of my four key components for staying healthy, along with proper nutrition that is, eating a balanced diet appropriate to our individual needs, managing stress, and keeping a positive attitude toward life that motivates us to treat our bodies healthily because we want to experience health, vitality, and longevity. As we know from both naturopathic and oriental philosophies of medicine, circulation and proper function must be maintained to continually generate health. This proper circulation applies to all body systems: energy (or Qi), blood, lymph, emotions, ideas, and the like. For adequate function, we must maintain circulation and the acquisition of all the right essential nutrients—vitamins, minerals, amino acids, and fatty acids.

Functional medicine practice applies to an underlying systematic approach within health care delivery that both assesses adequate function in such areas as digestion and assimilation, subtle endocrinology, detoxification pathways, and oxidative stress, and measures essential nutrients in body tissues. The therapies utilized to regain and sustain adequate function involve multiple disciplines: manual modalities (manipulation and massage) for structural function; medical prescriptions for normalization of hormones and eradicating unwanted microbes, especially in the gastrointestinal tract; nutritional support for making sure adequate nutrients are available to our tissues and cells 24 hours a day; herbal treatments for strengthening, balancing, and detoxifying as needed individually; and energetic and emotional support through such therapies as acupuncture, counseling, and stress management education.

Athletes, especially competitive athletes, must maintain finely tuned machines, their bodies. To do this, each athlete must eat a diet that is right for him or her, whether that is a high-fiber, carbohydrate-based diet or a high-protein, low-carbohydrate diet. Clearly, any athlete's diet should be wholesome, incorporating a variety of natural foods that include some fruits and whole grains, lots of fresh vegetables, and appropriate proteins and oil-based foods, such as legumes, nuts, and seeds; low-fat dairy products if tolerated; and animal proteins if desired. The body can be supported adequately on both vegetarian and omnivorian diets. To sustain long-term health, an athlete should avoid wasted-calorie foods such as refined sugars and flours as well as the persistent use of the generally accepted toxins of society—caffeine, alcohol, and nicotine—that undermine the quality of health.

There are several additional areas that relate to athletes and nutritional medicine. First, athletes need nutritional supplementation to support optimum function. This is in addition to a balanced and healthful diet. Drinking an adequate amount of water is also crucial to maintaining tissue health and hydration. Appropriate intake of the essential fatty acids, while avoiding "junky" fats such as hydrogenated oils, excessive saturated fats, and trans-fatty acids, allows proper lubrication and health of the tissues, protecting them from damage. Secondarily, exercise generates oxidative stress via free radical toxins that can inflame and irritate tissues and may increase potential for injury. As a consequence, athletes may require additional antioxidant nutrients to protect their cells and tissues and to manage oxidative stress. Antioxidant supplementation would include the regular use of vitamins C and E, β-carotene, zinc, and selenium.

The use of individual nutritional and functional assessments for competitive athletes is state-of-the-art medicine. Designing specific dietary and nutrient programs can make the difference between health and injury, as well as enhancing performance and general well-being.

Remember, balance in life is important; balance in terms of our exercise is also crucial to performance and overall function. An exercise program, then, should provide the following balance: daily stretching to maintain flexibility and prevent injury, weight training to build and sustain muscle tone and strength, aerobic activity to support circulation and endurance, and relaxation to prevent tensions and injuries. Our attitude regarding exercise is best kept playful and geared toward organization of personal performance, which can enhance team performance. We should have fun, take care of ourselves, and be aware of our bodies and our health as it enhances our athletic potential.

Selected Aspects of Nutrition and Physical Performance

BUCK LEVIN
KRISTIN SMITH
MICHAEL A. SCHMIDT

NUTRITIONAL CONSIDERATIONS IN OPTIMAL PERFORMANCE

Athletes represent a unique population in nutritional practice. As a group, they are often highly motivated to make dietary modifications that might benefit performance. Nutritional "ergogenic aids" have become commonplace items on store shelves, and numerous popular publications advocate specialized dietary practices to enhance performance. Research on nutritional practices of athletes, however, has called into question the validity of many such practices, including such basic components as percentage carbohydrate intake.[1] In addition, numerous controversies exist in the research literature regarding the effectiveness of dietary modification or nutritional supplementation.

Macronutrients in Optimal Performance

PROTEIN

Both intensity of exercise[2] and duration of exercise[3] have been shown to affect protein metabolism. By comparing urinary urea output with maximal and submaximal oxygen consumption, researchers have been able to quantify net increased protein needs. Amino acid availability over time has also been evaluated in the context of diminishing glycogen stores. Numerous studies have shown protein intake in the 1.5 to 2.0 g/kg/day range to be required for maintenance of positive nitrogen balance,[4] and actual intake of trained athletes has also been estimated to fall into this range.[5] For a 175-pound individual, this requirement would amount to approximately 120 to 160 g of protein per day.

Equally or more important than quantity of protein intake may be quality of protein intake in terms of constitutive fatty acids. Researchers working out of the Department of Sports and Performance Medicine at the University Medical Hospital in Freiburg, Germany, have examined the balance of branched-chain amino acids (BCAAs: leucine, isoleucine, and valine) versus aromatic amino acids (tyrosine, tryptophan, and phenylalanine) in ultra triathletes, and determined strong decreases reflecting a catabolic state.[6] While total serum amino acid levels were determined to fall by 18 percent as a result of the endurance activity, specific amino acid decreases varied from 9 to 56 percent. Unique patterns were observed for sulfur-containing amino acids (cystine and methionine). Because of the unique relationship between sulfur metabolism and oxidative stress involving activity of the tripeptide glutathione, adequacy of sulfur-containing amino acids may be of special importance in prevention of exercise-induced injury. Nuts and seeds (e.g., sesame seeds), grain germs (e.g., wheat germ or rice germ), egg yolk, and soft cheeses (e.g., ricotta or cottage cheese) are rich sources of the sulfur-containing amino acids. In addition, since BCAAs are preferentially metabolized by mitochondria in production of aerobic energy, maintenance of BCAA body pools would also be an important consideration for all athletes. Rich dietary sources of the BCAAs include most beans (especially black and lima beans), brewer's yeast, herring, sardines, and most cheeses.

CARBOHYDRATE

Both size and oxidative capacity of muscle fibers undergo change as a result of training. Depending upon intensity and duration of activity, the muscle fibers in an athlete's body undergo differential recruitment and place differential demands upon fuel supply. When athletes are performing at 50 to 60 percent of maximal oxygen consumption and have been consuming diets with a macronutrient balance of approximately 60:20:20 (60 percent of total calories from carbohydrate, 20 percent from protein, and 20 percent from fat), about half of their metabolic energy is derived from carbohydrate. As 100 percent oxygen capacity is reached, this percentage contribution by carbohydrate rises sharply. In addition, at the onset of any exercise, carbohydrate plays a critical role in performance, since muscle and liver glycogen stores serve as the exclusive metabolic fuel source.

Since the early 1960s, "carbohydrate loading" has been a widely practiced method for increasing muscle glycogen stores for improved performance. More recent research has demonstrated that complex carbohydrates (starches obtained from whole, unprocessed foods) are a superior source of muscle glycogen to refined, simple sugars.[7] In its 1960s debut, carbohydrate loading involved an initial low-carbohydrate phase in which the diet was depleted of all high-carbohydrate foods. This phase was believed to stimulate increased muscle glycogen synthesis once dietary carbohydrate was restored through a negative feedback mechanism. Because the enzyme glycogen synthetase appears to respond primarily to training itself, it is now recognized that low-carbohydrate feeding alone cannot help stimulate subsequent glycogen synthesis, and that an athlete must allow the training itself to deplete glycogen stores. In addition, the glycogen-depleting training must involve the same muscle groups that the athlete will be utilizing during performance.

Numerous studies have documented the beneficial effect of carbohydrate intake during performance. In cyclists, fatigue has been postponed by an average of 26 percent through intermittent carbohydrate feedings.[8] For endurance events, a research-based recommendation has been made for consumption of approximately 25 to 30 g of carbohydrate every half-hour.[9] In the sports nutrition marketplace, "sports gels"—typically combining about 17 to 25 g of simple sugars, long-chain carbohydrates, and glucose polymers in a liquid-filled, palm-sized foil packet—have been developed for this application.[10]

FAT

In the popular press—and to a much lesser extent the research literature—a 1990s equivalent to the 1960s carbohydrate-loading practice has emerged, referred to by some researchers as "fat loading."[11] A carbohydrate-sparing effect of increased fat intake has been proposed, along with increased availability of fatty acids as fuel sources for aerobic metabolism in endurance events. Several researchers have gone so far as to investigate the effects of an 85 percent fat diet on exercise in men, revealing a neutral effect upon performance.[12] Medium-chain triglyceride feeding has also failed to elevate serum fatty acids or improved endurance following increased consumption.[13]

Caffeine has been proposed as an ergogenic aid capable of elevating free fatty acid pools pre-exercise because of its inhibitory effect on the phosphodiesterase enzyme. Several international competitions have in fact prohibited pre-event consumption of caffeine for this reason. However, research in this area has been mixed and has suggested that, although caffeine may in fact be beneficial in untrained individuals, training may largely negate its effect, as may consumption of high-carbohydrate foods along with caffeine. In several studies, the amount of caffeine investigated was similar to that contained two 8-ounce cups of coffee, or approximately 100 to 150 mg.[14]

Discussed later in this chapter is the key importance of essential fatty acid intake—and fatty acid balance—in avoiding oxidative stress and chronic inflammatory events that can be associated with aerobic exercise. This aspect of fat intake is absolutely essential in dietary planning for all athletes. The Ratio of ω-3 to ω-6 fatty acids appears to be a critical determinant in inhibiting proinflammatory eicosanoid synthesis from arachidonic acid.[15] In the United States, ω-3:ω-6 ratios have been estimated to fall somewhere between a 1:10 and 1:25 range, as compared with a worldwide average of 1:2. Virtually all dietary recommendations from public health agencies have indirectly placed the ratio in further jeopardy, either by focusing on intake of ω-9 fatty acids (e.g., recommendations of increased olive oil in the diet) or by encouraging use of plant oils extremely high in ω-6 fatty acids (e.g., canola, safflower, sunflower). ω-3 Fatty acids are difficult to obtain from animal products, where they are essentially limited to cold-water fish such as salmon and halibut. From plant sources they are less rare but also limited. Especially rich sources include seeds (and their oils) such as flax, borage, and black currant. Ability of the body to convert ω-3 fatty acids into anti-inflammatory regulatory molecules such as series 3 prostaglandins and thromboxanes depends upon enzyme activity. Because ω-6 fatty acids use the same elongase and desaturase enzymes for conversion into their prostaglandin and thromboxane equivalents, excessive intake of ω-6 relative to ω-3 fatty acids can saturate enzyme activity and prevent manufacture of anti-inflammatory substances even when ω-3 fatty acids are available.

Micronutrients in Optimal Performance

VITAMINS

In comparison to the general population, athletes have clearly increased vitamin needs and benefit from increased vitamin nutriture.[16] These increased needs are related to a variety of physiologic events, including increased lean body mass, increased enzymatic activity, increased nutrient transport, increased anabolism/catabolism, and increased fluid loss from perspiration. Biochemical profiles of endurance athletes have repeatedly shown alterations in vitamin biochemistry.[17,18] While these effects have not generally been interpreted as either negative or health compromising, the uniqueness of vitamin nutrition in athletes has repeatedly been confirmed.

Vitamin supplementation has not consistently been shown to enhance performance in physically active individuals, except in instances where deficiency has been previously confirmed. For example, even marginal vitamin C status has been shown to impair performance,[19] while supplementation in vitamin C–sufficient athletes has demonstrated no beneficial performance effects.[20]

van der Beek and colleagues,[21] working out of the Toxicology and Nutrition Institute in the Netherlands, have examined functional performance in healthy male subjects and determined that, within 8 weeks, a diet of "normal food products" can deplete body stores of vitamins B_1, B_2, B_6, and C as measured by decreased red blood cell enzyme activities and excretion of urinary metabolites. Subjects undergoing depletion were also found to have significantly decreased VO_{2max} and nonsignificantly decreased maximal workload.[21] Nonsignificant, yet measurable, differences in VO_{2max} and training distance were determined by Weight et al. after examination of male runners undergoing multivitamin-mineral supplementation, even though those authors summarized the results of the study as failing to confirm a performance effect.[22]

Supplementation of vitamin E appears to be an exception to the previous rule, consistently resulting in improved performance and decreased risk of oxidative stress and inflammation. Cannon et al.[23] found that supplementation of d-α-tocopherol at 800 IU allowed postexercise elevations of creatine kinase to return to baseline much more quickly than levels in control subjects and, in addition, brought plasma levels in older subjects down to levels similar to those in younger subjects. While a more recent review by Tiidus and Houston[24] has noted mixed results in the intervention literature, close examination reveals consistently positive results in the methodologically more sophisticated studies.

MINERALS

While minerals and vitamins share a common role as enzymatic cofactors, the unique role of minerals in bone health, and their potential for loss in perspiration, require them to be treated uniquely in nutritional support of performance. However, like vitamins, most of the intervention studies on minerals suggest a clear benefit to supplementation only when deficiency has been previously established.

Human perspiration contains approximately 40 to 60 mEq/L of sodium, 3 to 5 mEq/L of potassium, 25 mEq/L of calcium, and 10 mEq/L of magnesium. As the sweat rate increases, loss of sodium increases, loss of calcium decreases, and losses of potassium and magnesium stay approximately the same. The potential for zinc loss in perspiration has been estimated at 8 to 14 μmol/day in healthy nonexercising men consuming zinc diets at about 50 percent of the recommended dietary allowance (RDA),[25] and would be expected to be higher in exercising individuals. Taken as a whole, these observations point to the necessity of individualizing nutritional support for athletes who may vary greatly (both interindividually and intraindividually) in their surface loss of minerals.

Zinc

Oxidative stress and inflammatory response can trigger significant drops in plasma zinc levels.[26] Because both of these risks are prominent for the endurance athlete (and are discussed at length in the final segments of this chapter), attention to zinc status may be of special importance in sports nutrition.

Researchers working out of the University of Padua in Italy have shown that physical exertion causes a significant redistribution of the trace minerals zinc and copper between target tissues, body stores, and the blood, posing a risk of copper and zinc deficiency even when total body pools appear normal.[27] Their research further confirms the necessity of utilizing highly sensitive, functional measurements of zinc (and other mineral) status rather than static, momentary, and potentially misleading quantifications in the blood. In a study of swimmers, dietary intake of zinc (as well as the minerals copper, magnesium, and iron) has also been found to be predictive of 100-yard freestyle performance.[28] Debates over the optimal delivery form for zinc remained unresolved, but most research favors a monomethionine, picolinate, or gluconate delivery form, and points away from an oxide version.

Electrolytes and Water

Normal hydration status has been shown to be critical for performance of any kind, and closely related to the question of electrolyte balance. A 145-pound person, without exercising, will lose approximately 2.5 quarts of water per day. Approximately 1.5 quarts will be lost rhough urination, and the remaining quart through perspiration and insentient loss. Thermoregulation is the primary factor in perspiration rate. Intense exercise can result in as much as 3.5 L/hr of sweat loss. Losses increase at approximately 7 percent per each degree Fahrenheit increase in temperature. When water loss exceeds 3 percent of body weight, endurance time for muscle contractions is reduced. For example, a 4 percent loss of body weight from dehydration can result in a 31 percent shorter muscle endurance time.

Glucose-electrolyte replacement drinks have been shown to increase the rate at which fluid is absorbed from the gastrointestinal tract.[29] Dilute solutions of sodium (e.g., 0.45 g of sodium chloride per 100 ml of water) have been shown to improve rehydration following performance.[30] As in general dietary intake, a sodium/potassium ratio of approximately 1 : 1 is recommended for electrolyte replenishment.

Interestingly, hydration status and plasma osmolality also appear to have significant regulatory impact upon immune function. Greenleaf and colleagues, reporting from the Laboratory for Human Environmental Physiology at the Ames Research Center in California, have noted regression of mean $CD4^+/CD8^+$ T-lymphocyte ratios in dehydrated men who had just completed 70 minutes of submaximal lower extremity cycle exercise.[31]

Selenium

Exercise that involves aerobic production of energy places a special focus on selenium, because four atoms of the mineral are required for proper function of each glutathione peroxidase enzyme, a key component in oxidative metabolism. This enzyme—and much of the body's glutathione—are especially active in the body's mitochondria. Training induces increased numbers of mitochondria in the working muscle as well as increased intracellular surface area occupied by these subcellular organelles. Selenium supplementation has been shown to help regulate short-term plasticity of the mitochondria in ways that reduce risk of oxidative stress.[32] Researchers have hypothesized higher efficiency of glutathione peroxidase enzyme activity as a possible mechanism for this effect. Tessier et al. have also shown selenium supplementation to have no direct effect upon performance in presumably selenium-adequate subjects.[33]

NUTRITIONAL SUPPORT IN EXERCISE-RELATED FATIGUE

Fatigue is commonly associated with altered physiologic function, reduced immune vigilance, and increased risk of injury. Therefore, attention to the biologic factors that contribute to fatigue may be important in training and therapeutic considerations. This section provides a brief discussion of factors that may give rise to fatigue in athletes and nutritional support considerations.

Fatigue and Immunosuppression

There appears to be a variable immune response to exercise. Moderate physical activity has been shown to stimulate immune function.[34] However, a growing body of literature suggests that heavy training may cause suppression of several markers of immune function.[35] This has been associated with increased incidence of infection.[36–39] In fact, it has been observed that athletes such as endurance runners lose more training days to infection than to injury. Although the solution to the immunosuppressive effects of intense exercise is undoubtedly complex, there is evidence suggesting that antioxidant nutrient support may reduce some of the adverse immune consequences.[40]

Inadequate Fluid Intake

As body temperature rises during training, the body perspires in an effort to cool itself. This phenomenon may lead to substantial fluid loss. In a 2-hour period of intense physical activity, for example, an individual may lose as much as five to eight pounds of fluid. This fluid loss may also be accompanied by loss of electrolytes (described elsewhere in this chapter). Dehydration, therefore, is one important cause of fatigue in athletes. Attention to water and electrolyte needs before, during, and after training sessions must be a priority in order to maintain fluid balance.

Poorly Balanced Diets

Athletes commonly employ diets aimed at improving performance. While there are many potential benefits to be gained by well-designed programs, many such diets are not well conceived and may lead to metabolic consequences that result in fatigue. For example, wrestlers commonly cut calories in order to attain a specific weight. This may lead to dehydration and poor nutrient intake. Wrestlers have been found to be low in protein; vitamins A, B_1, and B_6; and iron, zinc, and magnesium.[41] Gymnasts commonly restrict calories in an effort to remain lean and small for competition. Dancers and gymnasts have been

found to consume less than the RDA for vitamin B_6, folic acid, calcium, zinc, and magnesium.[42]

Many athletes emphasize protein or carbohydrate intake and de-emphasize fat in their training regimens. Such choices may lead to metabolic alterations that contribute to fatigue. Athletes must be observed for their food and nutrient intake. In many cases, specific supplementation strategies can be tailored to the unique demand of individual sports.

Sleep and Rest

Athletic training places considerable demands on the body, which must be met with adequate sleep and rest. When training intensity is increased, the need for additional rest commonly increases as well.[43] Athletes who do not obtain rest commensurate with the physical demands of their sport may be at increased risk of injury, immune suppression, poor performance, and generalized fatigue.

Exposure to Environmental Pollutants

Athletes in certain sports are more likely to be exposed to environmental pollutants that may affect physiology and performance. For example, swimmers who suffer inordinately from asthma have been observed to have higher levels of chloroform measurable in their blood. This is presumably a result of chlorinated compounds added to disinfect swimming pools.[44] Runners who train in city environments have been found to have elevated carboxyhemoglobin, a marker of carbon monoxide binding. Motor vehicle exhaust is the likely pollutant source in these individuals.[45] Such exposure may adversely impact energy metabolism, affecting both stamina and performance. Athletes who compete in areas in which pollutant exposure is likely must modify training to minimize exposure. They may further benefit from nutritional support that targets antioxidants and nutrients that support detoxification.

Overall Nutrient Needs in Fatigue

The demands of physical training may increase the requirement for certain nutrients. Moreover, insufficiency of specific nutrients may contribute to symptoms of fatigue in the nonathlete and should be considered in the athlete as well. These have been reviewed by Schmidt, and include selected amino acids, carnitine, coenzyme Q10, essential fatty acids, folic acid, glutathione, iron, magnesium, molybdenum, pantothenic acid, thiamine, pyridoxine, cobalamin, ascorbate, and zinc.[46] In addition to micronutrients, caloric intake must be commensurate with the physiologic demands of each sport.[47]

NUTRITIONAL SUPPORT OF POSTINJURY HEALING AND RECOVERY

Tissue Damage in Athletic Injury

Statistically, every athlete has a 50 percent chance of sustaining injury. Once injured, the athlete is faced with the challenge of completing healing in minimal recovery time and with minimal loss of performance. Premature re-entry into competition can put the athlete into great jeopardy. However, many athletes are unaware of the diverse ways in which nutrition can enhance healing, shorten recovery time, and minimize loss of performance.

Musculoskeletal tissue is the most commonly damaged tissue in athletic injury, and accounts for over 90 percent of all sports injury.[48] During physical activity, stress and force are placed on muscle, bone, and connective tissue. Even in the absence of injury, delayed onset muscle soreness is often reported at the muscle–tendon junction, as well as throughout the muscle.[49]

Because movement of the body is potentiated by the joints, tissues involved in maintenance of joint stability, flexion, rotation, and the like are of special importance when there is disruption of movement as a result of athletic injury. Heading the list of tissue types involved in joint health is connective tissue. This type of tissue includes the tendons, ligaments, and fasciae. While not considered connective tissue proper, cartilage, bone, and blood are also classified as connective tissue given their developmental origin in the embryonic mesenchyme.

Unique Structure of Connective Tissue

Nutritional support of postinjury healing must be adapted to fit the unique structure of the connective tissue. This tissue type is somewhat unique in its composition because, unlike other primary tissues composed predominantly of cells, connective tissue is noncellular and composed predominantly of extracellular matrix (ECM). In the ECM are found three basic components: ground substance, fibers, and fluid.

GLYCOSAMINOGLYCANS AND GLYCOPROTEINS

Two major families of molecules are found in the ground substance of connective tissue, and both have been investigated for their role in nutritional support of postinjury healing. The first family, or glycosaminoglycans (GAGs), are the best researched and most widely used substances in nutritional support of damaged connective tissue. The GAG molecules, also traditionally referred to as mucopolysaccharides, can themselves be linked together to form proteoglycans. Except for hyaluronic acid, all GAGs are sulfated, linear polysaccharides containing a repeating disaccharide unit, which is usually composed of a uronic acid and a hexosamine. Sulfation of the GAGs takes place in the Golgi apparatus of the osteoblast cells.

Glucosamine and galactosamine are the most common of the hexosamines found in GAGs. Glucuronic acid is the most common uronic acid. While the half-life of all GAGs is fairly short, hyaluronic acid's 2- to 4-day half-life is significantly shorter than the average half-life of the sulfated GAGs (7 to 10 days). Glucosamine has clearly emerged as a central player in the GAG literature. Availability of glucosamine appears to be the rate-limiting step in synthesis of most GAGs.[50,51] In addition, n-acetylglucosamine (along with n-acetylgalactosamine) has been shown to inhibit release of superoxide anion radicals in certain cells.[52]

Along with their structural role in the formation of ground substance within connective tissue, GAGs play important metabolic roles as well. Ion transport, diffusion of nutrients, water retention, collagen fibrogenesis, growth factor binding, cell signaling, and other aspects of cell regulation also depend on proper GAG functioning.[53] Cytokine growth factors widely studied in molecular medicine for their role in cell signaling, angiogenesis, and carcinogenesis, including platelet-derived endothelial cell growth factor, transforming growth factor β, and basic fibroblast growth factor, have been shown to stimulate synthesis of at least one GAG (hyaluronic acid).[54] In addition, fibroblasts have been shown to routinely produce hyaluronic acid during the early stages of wound healing.[55]

Glycoproteins constitute the second family of molecules found in the ground substance of connective tissue. They are less well researched and not commonly available in supplemental form. The carbohydrate portion of these molecules typically consists of a branching structure and is represented by the structure found in fibronectin, laminin, and chondronectin.

GLYCOSAMINOGLYCAN INTERVENTION STUDIES

Many hexosamines, uronic acids, and GAGs are widely available as oral supplements, including glucosamine sulfate, galactosamine sulfate, d-glucuronic acid, chondroitin sulfates, heparan sulfates, keratan sulfates, and dermatan sulfates. However, the best researched of the GAG supplements is clearly glucosamine sulfate. Oral glucosamine sulfate in a daily dose range of 750 to 1,500 mg (usually in three to six divided doses) has been examined in numerous studies of osteoarthritis, arthrosis, and other chronic degenerative articular disorders, with repeated success. In a double-blind study comparing glucosamine sulfate to ibuprofen in treatment of osteoarthritis of the knees, glucosamine sulfate was found to be slower in alleviating symptoms but more effective over an 8-week period.[56] A large, multicenter trial in Portugal involving 252 physicians and 1,208 subjects found oral supplementation to be more effective than all previous treatments (except glucosamine injection) in reducing pain from exercise and decreasing limitations on active and passive movement after 6 to 12 weeks.[57] Double-blind comparisons to piperazine/chlorbutanol[58] and placebo[59] have also yielded strong positive results. While none of these studies was focused specifically on the nature of athletic injury, the parameters studied have substantial overlap with postinjury healing in the recovering athlete.

OXIDATIVE STRESS IN ATHLETIC PERFORMANCE

Oxidative stress is defined as a physiologic condition in which an increased concentration of reactive oxygen species (ROS) is not properly counterbalanced by an increased presence of oxygen metabolite–processing enzymes and free radical–quenching molecules. At a molecular level, oxidative stress is related to electrochemical redox potential. Because biologic oxidations are electron transfer reactions, the activities of reducing agents (electron donors) and oxidizing agents (electron acceptors) are required to bring about redox reactions. When molecules are left with single, unpaired electrons as a result of electron transfer processes, the molecules become "free radicals"—the most reactive type of all ROS.

Athletic activity is typically accompanied by a significant increase in oxygen uptake. Strenuous exercise can increase oxygen consumption as much as 10 to 15 times over resting levels.[60] This increased oxygen uptake occurs at a whole-body level, but is of particular importance in the skeletal muscle. The ability of mitochondria within the muscle

to regenerate adenosine triphosphate (ATP) for muscular energetics depends upon the availability of oxygen. During mitochondrial regeneration of ATP, however, about 2 to 5 percent of available oxygen becomes converted into ROS, including hydrogen peroxide, superoxide anion radical, and hydroxyl radical.[61] It is the increased presence of ROS that places high demands on the body's capacity to scavenge free radicals with molecular redox agents and maintain proper activity of enzymes reducing oxidative stress. Key redox agents studied in the oxidative stress literature include ascorbic acid (vitamin C), tocopherol (vitamin E), glutathione (GSH, a tripeptide consisting of glycine, cysteine, and glutamic acid), lipoic acid, and cysteine. Key oxidative enzymes include superoxide dismutase (SOD), which is needed to convert superoxide anion radical into hydrogen peroxide; glutathione peroxidase (GPO), which is able to convert hydrogen peroxide into water; and catalase, which is also able in the presence of molecular oxygen to produce water from hydrogen peroxide. Each of these oxidative enzymes requires at least one nutrient cofactor. For intracellular SOD, specific ratios of zinc to copper are required; for mitochondrial SOD, the required cofactor is the mineral manganese; for catalase, enzymatic activity changes in relationship to its mineral cofactor, iron.

Ji[62] has reviewed the relationship of oxidative stress to exercise, with several key observations. First, he notes clearly identified electron paramagnetic resonance–based free radical signaling from contracting muscle.[63] This increased free radical signaling—which may be as high as 70 percent—can be accompanied by increased lipid peroxidation and by other markers of oxidative stress. Second, he details the nature of oxidative-based changes to the muscle cell membrane and other cellular components. These changes include ROS-based modification of membrane phospholipids, intracellular enzymes, and nuclear material, including DNA. Using urinary 8-hydroxy-deoxyguanosine as a biochemical marker, Alessio has determined DNA damage to be significantly increased following marathon-level activity.[64] Poulsen et al.[65] have made similar observations on endurance athletes in Denmark. Finally, Ji[62] reviews changes in intracellular redox balance, noting depletion of reduced glutathione, induction of antioxidant enzymes, and supportive effects of antioxidant supplementation in training athletes.

Exercise and the Glutathione System

The tripeptide GSH (L-γ-glutamyl-L-cysteinylglycine) is a redox agent whose oxidized and reduced forms play a key role in oxidative metabolism. The known functions of GSH in cellular metabolism continue to expand, almost exponentially, with increasing research on the molecule. These functions presently include regulation of redox balance, free radical scavenging, regulation of prostaglandin metabolism, deoxyribonucleotide synthesis, cell proliferation, and immune messaging.[66] Shuffling of glutathione between its reduced (GSH) and oxidized (glutathione disulfide, or GSSG) forms is accomplished by the glutathione reductase and GPO enzymes. The reductase is a vitamin B_2–requiring enzyme that also needs the reducing factor NADPH as generated by the hexose monophosphate shunt metabolic pathway. GPO is a selenium-requiring enzyme.

In both animals and humans, exercise has been shown to induce activity of the oxidative enzymes SOD, GPO, and catalase.[67] Although results have been mixed, the ratio of reduced to oxidized glutathione (GSH:GSSG) appears to be decreased in many tissue in response to strenuous activity, but these decreases appear dependent upon dietary intake, nutritional supplementation, and endocrine balance.[67–69]

Selenium, n-acetylcysteine (NAC), and GSH supplementation have all been investigated in relationship to oxidative stress, with significant results only consistently observed for selenium and cysteine supplementation. Significant effects of selenium supplementation at 240 μg/day on GPO activity have been demonstrated by Tessier et al. in their studies of young healthy men and treadmill performance.[70] In an animal model, decreased levels of GSH following exhaustive running have been shown to take 96 hours to be replenished.[71] Further confirmation of an oxidative stress mechanism in the study was found in the ability of allopurinol, an inhibitor of the xanthine oxidase enzyme, to cut recovery time in half. Repair of oxidatively damaged tissue in lung disease has been shown to benefit from oral supplementation with NAC.[72] This type of damage has frequently been demonstrated to occur in ultramarathon-type events, along with severe depletion of liver GSH.[73] Doses of NAC in oxidative-stress studies have ranged from 1,000 mg to 100 mg/kg body weight (or approximately 7,000 mg) per day.[74]

ANTIOXIDANT SUPPLEMENTATION AS A MODIFIER OF EXERCISE-RELATED OXIDATIVE STRESS

Physical performance that involves a high workload and participation of many muscle groups can place the athlete in a situation in which oxygen requirement exceeds maximal oxygen intake. Although maximal oxygen uptake can be increased with training, heavy workloads can cause 98 percent maximal oxygen uptake within minutes regardless of maximal capacity.

Any exercise that increases oxygen uptake can increase formation of ROS and pose a risk of cellular damage. Nuclear and mitochondrial DNA[75]; lipids within the cell membrane, mitochondrial membrane, and bloodstream[76]; and other cellular proteins[62] may all be exposed to oxidative insult when oxygen uptake is increased. Ironically, reduced blood flow causing transient ischemia can pose an even greater risk of oxidative tissue damage than increased oxygen uptake. When low-oxygen tissues can no longer maintain aerobic generation of ATP through oxidative phosphorylation, the ATP molecule is enzymatically converted into hypoxanthine. Low oxygen conditions induce further transformation of hypoxanthine into xanthine through activity of xanthine oxidase, but the activity of this enzyme also generates the superoxide anion radical and potentiates free radical damage to cell components.

Vitamin E

Antioxidant status has been shown to play a key role in prevention of tissue damage from oxidative stress during strenuous exercise. While studies of vitamin E and performance have repeatedly shown little or no benefit from supplementation except at altitude,[77] studies have shown effectiveness of vitamin E supplementation in reducing oxidative damage to muscle as measured by reduced serum creatine kinase activity.[78] A double-blind, placebo controlled study of young (22 to 29 years of age) and older (55 to 74 years) adult men doing eccentric treadmill running at 75 percent maximum heart rate after 48 days of supplementation at 800 IU/day of d-α-tocopherol found numerous indicators of protective effect.[23] These indicators included alterations in fatty acid composition, vitamin E concentration, and lipid-conjugated dienes in muscle together with changes in urine lipid peroxides. The authors viewed all changes as consistent with a protective effect of vitamin E against oxidative injury produced by strenuous exercise.

Supplemental doses of vitamin E in clinical studies have ranged widely, from 400 to 1,600 IU, but most interventions have targeted a 400 to 800–IU range. The ability of vitamin E to protect phospholipid bilayers[79] of cell membranes and to scavenge free radicals[80,81] has been clearly demonstrated in all areas of medicine, and lends strong support to the smaller quantity of work that has been done in sports nutrition.

Vitamin C

Vitamin C has long been identified as a free radical scavenger and key component in oxidative metabolism. Dietary deficiency of vitamin C has been shown to reduce oxidative capacity during exercise in an animal model.[82] The vitamin has also been shown to be involved in carnitine synthesis, which is upregulated during endurance exercise in order to shuffle substrate into the mitochondria.[83]

In humans, supplementation of vitamin C at the 1-g/day level has been shown to reduce exercise-induced oxidative stress as measured by the thiobarbituric acid–reactive substances test of blood plasma.[84] Contractile function in the triceps muscle of healthy, physically active adults has been shown to be improved by supplementation of ascorbic acid at the 400 mg/day level, with less decrement being observed in the 20/50 Hz ratio of tetanic tension both postexercise (60 minutes of box stepping) and during recovery.[85] At the other end of the vitamin C spectrum, deficient intake has repeatedly been shown to reduce work capacity,[86] and even marginal intake of vitamin C can compromise performance.[87]

Coenzyme Q

Use of ubiquinone—the benzoquinone with a conjugated isoprenoid side chain, commonly referred to as coenzyme Q—has reached almost legendary status in the treatment of cardiovascular disease, with over 300 indexed journal studies to support its clinical efficacy with conditions such as arrhythmia, atherosclerosis, cardiomyopathy, and congestive heart failure. The literature should not be surprising, since cardiac muscle is one of the few tissues in the body to be continuously aerobic, and coenzyme Q occupies a totally unique and central spot in aerobic metabolism. Stationed near the center of the mitochondrial electron transport chain, it is the only nonprotein component of the chain, as well as the only component with a capability for moving two electrons simultaneously along the chain. Both heart and red muscle cells of endurance-trained animals have shown significantly increased concentrations of coenzyme Q.[88,89] Supplementation at 60 mg/day for 8 weeks has been shown to significantly improve aerobic performance in healthy young men,[90] and at 90 mg coenzyme Q has improved exercise capacity in

older subjects with a history of chronic obstructive pulmonary disease.[91] Exercise tolerance in chronic stable angina pectoris has also been shown to be significantly improved by supplementation of coenzyme Q at 150 mg/day (divided into three 50-mg doses).[92]

Zinc

In the United States, high-carbohydrate diets based upon commonly chosen supermarket foods have been shown to be zinc deficient.[93] Since many athletes practice preperformance carbohydrate loading and consume overall diets high in carbohydrate, risk of zinc deficiency may be particularly high in this population. Further confirming this risk has been the finding, in both male and female athletes, that loss of zinc in sweat and urine can potentiate zinc deficiency.[94] In male runners, zinc supplementation at 50 mg/day over a 6-day period significantly reduced production of ROS following treadmill running at 75 percent maximal oxygen uptake until exhaustion.[95] Researchers used tritiated thymidine incorporation by mitogen-treated mononuclear cell cultures and respiratory burst activity of neutrophils as markers for oxidative and immune changes.

Antioxidant Synergism

Coenzyme Q, vitamin E, and vitamin C synergisms are well documented in the research literature. In its reduced form, coenzyme Q helps reduce oxidized forms of vitamin E.[96] Redox potentials of vitamins C and E have been shown to be interlinked, and the vitamins have been shown to interact synergistically in scavenging free radicals[97] and reducing lipid peroxides in human subjects.[98]

NUTRIENT MODULATION OF EXERCISE-INDUCED INFLAMMATION

Inflammation is a time-honored concept in medicine, dating back at least as far as 1650 BC.[99] The four major types of symptoms (heat, swelling, redness, and pain) that we associate with inflammation were first identified at that time. Acute inflammation is widely recognized as a natural component in the body's healing processes and, when well regulated, performs essential tasks in wound healing and recovery from injury. A wide variety of risks with which athletes are routinely confronted—including toxic exposures, inhaled particulates, cuts, bruises, abrasions, and trauma—are known triggers for inflammation.

During inflammation, vasodilation and increased blood pressure allow for rapid delivery of nutrients to the injured site. Complement—a group of approximately 20 proteins that are delivered to the injured site—is an extensively studied feature of the inflammatory process, and some of the complement proteins are regarded as excellent markers of inflammatory conditions. One such protein is C-reactive protein (CRP). Training is believed to have a dampening effect on the release of CRP during potentially inflammatory athletic activity, and attempts are currently being made to establish CRP standards for endurance events such as long-distance running to monitor inflammation-related health risk.[100] Release of heat-shock proteins and stress proteins is another parameter undergoing similar investigation.[101]

Ligaments and tendons, once injured, have been shown to heal in the following sequence: hemorrhage, inflammation, proliferation, and remodeling. The timing of these events is critical to full recovery. Underactivation and overactivation of inflammatory processes both serve as detriments to healing. Overexpression of T cells in an immune response, for example, can lead to a triggering event in adhesion formation and result in increased scarring and fibrosis. Adhesion formation has been shown to be the most common complication associated with tendon healing.[102] By binding tendons to surrounding tissue and putting increased pressure on blood vessels and nerves, adhesions decrease the supply of oxygen and nutrients to healing tissue.[103] Also, once anchored to surrounding sites, connective tissue components lack the fluidity to function normally.

Increased appearance of inflammatory cells in the synovial sheath and epitenon is known to precede increased production of fibronectin by tendon cells.[104] Excess fibronectin produced at the site of injury may also promote excessive formation of fibrotic tissue during wound healing. Because fibronectin synthesis is under partial regulation by immune cytokines and growth factors, any factors that might upregulate synthesis of proinflammatory cytokines might also compromise the healing process by overactivating synthesis of fibronectin. Also playing a potentially key role in fibrosis is the influence of oxidative stress. As discussed earlier, formation of ROS is a phenomenon intrinsic to oxidative metabolism, but one that must be balanced by sufficient enzyme and antioxidant activity. Unsupported oxidative metabolism resulting in the forma-

tion of excess ROS has been shown to contribute to fibrosis and prevent proper healing.[105]

The cytokine immune messaging system is also critical in postinjury healing because of its ability to regulate collagen synthesis. Collagen is the primary structural macromolecule in all tissues whose primary functions are weight bearing, transmission of force, protection, compartmentalization, transmission of light, or distribution of fluid. Collagen in the most abundant protein in the body (constituting approximately 30 percent of all body protein by weight) and is of critical importance in recovery from injury. About 90 percent of total body collagen is classified as type I, in which protein fibers are aligned parallel to the direction of force and provide optimal tissue strength. During the healing process, a second, more pliable type of collagen—referred to as type III—is initially laid down at the site of injury to provide for more rapid formation of crosslinks and to stabilize the repair site efficiently. The flexibility of this type III collagen originates in the random alignment of its fibers, which are more flexible yet less able to resist tensile forces. As healing progresses, type III collagen gets remodeled into type I. However, this natural healing sequence can be interrupted by cytokine activity, such that excessive immune response and proinflammatory activity can result in destabilization of repaired connective tissue and incomplete recovery.[106]

The inflammatory process places high demands on nutrient adequacy and availability. Bioavailability of fatty acids, amino acids, saccharides, vitamins, and minerals plays a key role in healthy inflammatory response. In addition, whether occurring in bone, muscle, connective tissue, or skin, healthy inflammatory response requires maintenance of at least two basic underlying balances in the body: oxidant/antioxidant, or redox balance; and glycemic balance. The role of nutrients in support and regulation of these balances is discussed next.

Oxidant/Antioxidant Balance in Inflammation

Oxidant/antioxidant balance comes into play during all episodes of inflammation because of the key role played by fatty acid metabolism in regulation of inflammatory events, and because of the actual use of oxygen-based free radicals in killing of microorganisms that pose a risk of infection. The critical role of fatty acid metabolism in inflammation focuses on the eicosanoids, a class of fatty acid molecules each containing 20 carbon atoms. The eicosanoids include highly potent regulatory molecules in the prostaglandin, leukotriene, and thromboxane families. During several metabolic steps that occur in inflammation, oxidative enzymes are required to produce proper eicosanoid balance and maintain healthy response.

Phospholipase A_2, located on the cell membrane, is initially responsible for mobilizing arachidonic acid $(20:4\omega6)$ to be used as the substrate for eicosanoid synthesis. Activity of this enzyme is inhibited by numerous dietary antioxidants, including vitamin E, quercitin, and licorice. The prescription drug cortisone also works through this mechanism. Synthesis of the series 2 prostaglandins and series 2 thromboxanes requires transformation of arachidonic acid by the cyclo-oxygenase (COX) enzyme. This enzyme is found in two isoforms—COX-1 and COX-2—and, because the COX-2 form is highly inducible, its excessive conversion of arachidonic acid into series 2 prostaglandins can be a key factor in excessive inflammatory response. Production of hydrogen peroxide by the enzyme is also a potential source of increased ROS. Nonsteroidal anti-inflammatory drugs target COX but are unable to selectively inhibited the COX-2 form.[107] Ginger and turmeric are dietary inhibitors of the enzyme. Production of leukotrienes from arachidonic acid requires activity of the lipoxygenase enzyme, which generates epoxide and peroxide metabolites. These metabolites may help regulate leukotriene production, but they may also pose oxidative risk. Dietary inhibitors of the lipoxygenase enzyme include onion, garlic, turmeric, and vitamin E.

Glycemic Balance in Inflammation

Maintenance of proper blood sugar levels, and overall glycemic regulation, are long-established goals in sports nutrition. The popularity of glucose-based sports drinks, and the evaluation of these drinks in research, have both focused on the issues of absorption and availability to working muscle. In general, pre-exercise intake of glucose (and starch) has been shown to increase glucose availability and to improve performance.

An important aspect of glycemic balance not typically addressed in the sports nutrition literature is its relationship to inflammation. Chronic insulin resistance (the inability of insulin to stimulate glucose uptake by the cells) can result from many factors, including diet, life-style, and genetic inheritance.[108] Athletic activity typically has an inverse relationship with insulin resistance, and exercise training has become an important component of diabetes treatment for

precisely this reason.[109] While trained athletes are less likely to become insulin resistant than untrained individuals,[110] even trained individuals must pursue a diet that promotes glycemic balance.

A key link between inflammatory risk and glycemic balance involves the previously discussed area of eicosanoid metabolism. Any glycemic imbalance leading to overstimulation of the pancreatic cells with glucose is known to result in release of arachidonic acid from membrane phospholipids and, through the activity of COX-2 (as previously discussed), the release of series 2 prostaglandins. These eicosanoid molecules have a proinflammatory effect in the body and are overproduced in chronic inflammation. When dietary intake fails to support glycemic balance and/or eicosanoid balance, risk of inflammation is increased.

In the popular press, and to a lesser extent in the professional literature, macronutrient balance, eicosanoid metabolism, and glycemic control have been issues of debate. This debate is of interest in relation to sports nutrition, since athletes in the United States have generally chosen high-carbohydrate, low-fat, moderate protein diets for maximization of performance. The carbohydrate/protein/fat ratio in such diets has typically approximated $60:20:20$, When deviating from this balance, most athletes have upped carbohydrate or protein at the expense of fat, moving in the direction of a $70:15:15$ balance. Seldom have athletes increased either protein or fat at the expense of carbohydrate. This practice has been questioned, however, and many writers in the popular press have begun to advocate a $40:30:30$ macronutrient ratio for promoting glycemic balance, eicosanoid balance, and minimized risk of inflammation.

Researchers at the University Hospital in London, Ontario, have performed a "protein-for-carbohydrate switch" in which normocholesterolemic and hypercholesterolemic subjects randomly assigned to high- or low-protein diets crossed over after 4 to 5 weeks onto experimental diets in which varying percentages of protein calories were substituted for carbohydrate calories. At all levels of substitution, the substitution of protein for carbohydrate was found to lower cardiovascular risk as estimated by standard lipid profiles.[111]

A fascinating inverse correlation between the protein/carbohydrate ratio and blood testosterone levels has been found by Volek et al.[112] in a study of endocrine response to exercise. In their research, pre-exercise levels of testosterone were found to be significantly and inversely related to the pre-exercise protein/carbohydrate ratio. In other words, as dietary percentage protein increased, pre-exercise levels of this key androgenic hormone decreased. In their studies of weight training, Chandler et al.[113] have also determined that carbohydrate supplementation causes a significant decline in testosterone level, but that this decline may not necessarily have a negative impact upon training since it is accompanied by a simultaneous rise in insulin and growth hormone levels, which could favor muscle growth.

The ability of a dietary parameter to modulate hormone levels—in this case, testosterone—is important, since the testosterone/cortisol ratio is often selected as a monitoring device in management of athletic training. A decreased testosterone/cortisol ratio is often viewed as an indicator of metabolic disturbance foreshadowing a drop-off in performance. This drop-off is hypothesized to involve the role of testosterone as a myotrophic hormone that directly binds to receptor sites on muscle cells and enhances anabolic events.[114] Similarly, the role of increased cortisol has been interpreted as a catabolic one, throwing the athlete's metabolism into anabolic-catabolic imbalance. In studies of competitive swimmers, total testosterone/cortisol ratio has been shown to significantly correlate with performance ($r = .86$, $p < .01$).[115]

The dietary modulation of this ratio is important for a second reason involving the impact of hypercortisolemia on inflammation. Studies of physical and emotional stress have revealed that stress-induced elevations of cortisol are often associated with depression of dehydroepiandrosterone and insulin insensitivity.[116] This combination of events may greatly enhance production of proinflammatory cytokines in the body's immune system,[117] thereby increasing the risk of inflammatory response.

SUMMARY

Nutritional support of athletic performance has shifted in emphasis over the past few decades from a focus on quantitative supply of macronutrients and body "fuels" to a focus on qualitative aspects of micronutrition. Ratios of dietary fatty acids, amino acids, and saccharides have replaced absolute amounts of fat, protein, and carbohydrate as critical research issues. These ratios include ω-3 : ω-6 fatty acids, branched-chain/aromatic amino acids, processed/unprocessed carbohydrate, sodium/potassium, and zinc/copper. Functional measurement of nutrient status in athletes, involving enzyme challenge and intracellular concentration, has been found to be far more sensitive

to performance-related issues than static quantification in the blood. The issues of oxidative stress and inflammation have become critical areas for consideration in nutritional support of optimal performance and postinjury recovery.

REFERENCES

1. Hawley JA, Denis SC, Lindsay FH et al: Nutritional practices of athletes: are they suboptimal? J Sports Sci 13:S75, 1995
2. Lemon PWR, Dolny DG, Yarasheski KE: Effect of intensity on protein utilization during prolonged exercise [Abstract]. Med Sci Sports Exerc 16:151, 1984
3. Haralanbie G, Berg A: Serum urea and amino nitrogen changes with exercise duration. Eur J Appl Physiol Occup Physiol 36:39, 1976
4. Marable NL, Hickson JK, Korslund MK et al: Urinary nitrogen excretion as influenced by muscle building exercise program and protein intake variation. Nutr Rep Int 19: 795, 1979
5. Burke LM, Read RSD: Diet patterns of elite Australian male triathletes. Physician Sports Med 15:140, 1987
6. Lehmann M, Huonker M, Dimeo F et al: Serum amino acid concentrations in nine athletes before and after the 1993 Colmar ultra triathlon. Int J Sports Med 16:155, 1995
7. Costill DL, Sherman WM, Fink WJ et al: The role of dietary carbohydrates in muscle glycogen resynthesis after strenuous running. Am J Clin Nutr 34:1831, 1981
8. Coyle EF, Hagberg JM, Hurley BF et al: Carbohydrate feeding during prolonged strenuous exercise can delay fatigue. J Appl Physiol 55:230, 1983
9. Coyle EF, Coggan AR, Hemmert MK et al: Muscle glycogen utilization during prolonged strenuous exercise when fed carbohydrate. J Appl Physiol 61:165, 1986
10. Costill D, Hargraves M: Carbohydrate nutrition and fatigue. Sports Med 13:86, 1992
11. Sherman WM, Leenders N: Fat loading: the next magic bullet? Int J Sports Nutr 5(suppl)S1, 1995
12. Phinney SD, Bistrian BR, Wolfe RR et al: The human metabolic response to chronic ketosis without caloric restriction: physical and biochemical adaptation. Metabolism 32:757, 1983
13. Decombaz J, Arnaud MJ, Milon H et al: Energy metabolism of medium-chain triglycerides versus carbohydrates during exercise. Eur J Appl Physiol 52:9, 1983
14. O'Neil FT, Hynak-Hankinson MT, Gorman J: Research and application of current topics in sports nutrition. JADA 86:1007, 1986
15. Boudreau MD, Chanmugam S, Hart SB et al: Lack of dose response by dietary n-3 fatty acids at a constant ratio of n-3 to n-6 fatty acids in suppressing eicosanoid biosynthesis from arachidonic acid. Am J Clin Nutr 54:111, 1991

16. Grandjean AC, Ruud JS: Nutrition for cyclists. Clin Sports Med 13:235, 1994

17. Singh A, Evans P, Gallagher KL et al: Dietary intakes and biochemical profiles of nutritional status of ultra-marathoners. Med Sci Sports Exerc 25:329, 1993

18. Fogelholm GM, Himberg JJ, Alopaeus K et al: Dietary and biochemical indices of nutritional status in male athletes and controls. J Am Coll Nutr 11:181, 1992

19. Howald H, Segesser B: Ascorbic acid and athletic performance. Ann NY Acad Sci 258:458, 1975

20. Keren G: The effect of high dosage vitamin C on aerobic and anaerobic capacity. J Sports Med Phys Fitness 20:145, 1980

21. van der Beek EJ, van Dokkum W, Schrijver J et al: Thiamin, riboflavin, and vitamins B-6 and C: impact of combined restricted intake on functional performance in man. Am J Clin Nutr 48:1451, 1988

22. Weight LM, Myburgh KH, Noakes TD: Vitamin and mineral supplementation: effect on the running performance of trained athletes. Am J Clin Nutr 47:192, 1988

23. Cannon JG, Orencole SF, Fielding RA et al: Acute phase response in exercise: interaction of age and vitamin E on neutrophils and muscle enzyme release. Am J Physiol 259: R12114, 1990

24. Tiidus PM, Houston ME: Vitamin E status and response to exercise training. Sports Med 20:12, 1995

25. Johnson PE, Hunt CD, Milne DB et al: Homeostatic control of zinc metabolism in men: zinc excretion and balance in men fed diets low in zinc. Am J Clin Nutr 57:557, 1993

26. Thurnham DI: Micronutrients and immune function: some recent developments. J Clin Pathol 50:887, 1997

27. Bordin D, Sartorelli L, Bonani G et al: High intensity physical exercise induced effects on plasma levels of copper and zinc. Biol Trace Elem Res 36:129, 1993

28. Lukaski HC, Siders WA, Hoverson BS et al: Iron, copper, magnesium, and zinc status as predictors of swimming performance. Int J Sports Med 17:535, 1996

29. Murray R: The effects of consuming carbohydrate-electrolyte beverages on gastric emptying and fluid absorption during and following exercise. Sports Med 4:322, 1987

30. Nose H, Mack GW, Shi X et al: Role of osmolality and plasma volume during rehydration in humans. J Appl Physiol 65:325, 1988

31. Greenleaf JE, Jackson CG, Lawless D: CD4+/CD8+ T-lymphocyte ratio: effects of rehydration before exercise in dehydrated men. Med Sci Sports Exerc 27:194, 1995

32. Zamora AJ, Tessier F, Marconnet P et al: Mitochondrial changes in human muscle after prolonged exercise, endurance training, and selenium supplementation. Eur J Appl Physiol 71:505, 1995

33. Tessier F, Margaritis I, Richard MJ et al: Selenium and training effects on the glutathione system and aerobic performance. Med Sci Sports Exerc 27:390, 1995

34. Neiman DC, Nehlsen-Canarella SL: The effects of moderate training on natural killer cells and acute upper respiratory tract infections. Int J Sports Med 11:467, 1990

35. Mackinnon LT: Current challenges and future expectations in exercise immunology: back to the future. Med Sci Sports Exerc 26:191, 1994

36. Surikina ID: Stress and immunity among athletes. Soviet Sports Rev 17:198, 1987

37. Asgiersson G, Bellanti JA: Exercise immunity and infection. Semin Adolescent Med 3:199, 1987

38. Heath GW: Exercise and the incidence of upper respiratory tract infections. Med Sci Sports Exerc 23:152, 1991

39. Peters EM, Bateman ED: Ultramarathon running and upper respiratory tract infections: an epidemiologic survey. S Afr Med J 64:582, 1983

40. Peters EM: Vitamin C supplementation reduces the incidence of post-race symptoms of upper respiratory tract infection in ultramarathon runners. Am J Clin Nutr 57:170, 1993

41. Steen SN, McKinney S. Physician Sports Med 14:100, 1986

42. Moffat RJ: Dietary status of elite female high school gymnasts: inadequacy of vitamin and mineral intake. J Am Diet Assoc 84:136, 1984

43. Fitzgerald L: Exercise and the immune system. Immunol Today 9:337, 1989

44. Aggozzoti G: Plasma chloroform concentrations in swimmers using indoor swimming pools. Arch Environ Health 45:175, 1990

45. Nicholson JP, Case DB: Carboxyhemoglobin levels in New York City runners. Physician Sports Med 11:135, 1983

46. Schmidt MA: Tired of Being Tired. p. 39. North Atlantic Books, Berkeley, CA, 1995

47. Budgett R: The post-viral fatigue syndrome in athletes. p. 345. In Jenkins R, Mowbray JF (eds): Post-Viral Fatigue Syndrome. John Wiley & Sons, New York, 1991

48. Arnheim DD: Principles of Athletic Training, 6th ed. Times Mirror/Mosby, St. Louis, 1985

49. MacIntyre DL, Reid WD, McKenzie DC: Delayed muscle soreness: the inflammatory response to muscle injury and its clinical implications. Sports Med 20:24, 1995

50. McCarty MF: Glucosamine for wound healing. Med Hypotheses 47:273, 1996

51. Karzel K, Domenjoz R: Effects of hexosamine derivatives and uronic acid derivatives on glycosaminoglycan metabolism of fibroblast cultures. Pharm 5:337, 1971

52. Kamel M, Alnahdi M: Inhibition of superoxide anion release from human polymorphonuclear leukocytes by n-acetyl galactosamine and n-acetyl glucosamine. Clin Rheumatol 11:254, 1992

53. Leadbetter WB: Cell matrix response in tendon injury. Clin Sports Med 11:533, 1992

54. Shyjan AM, Heldin P, Butcher EC et al: Functional cloning of the cDNA for a human hyaluronan synthase. J Biol Chem 271:23395, 1996

55. McCarty MF: Glucosamine for wound healing. Med Hypotheses 47:273, 1996
56. Vaz AL: Double-blind clinical evaluation of the relative efficacy of ibuprofen and glucosamine sulfate in the management of osteoarthrosis of the knee in out-patients. Curr Med Res Opin 8:145, 1982
57. Tapadinhas MJ, Rivera IC, Bigamini AA: Oral glucosamine sulphate in the management of arthrosis: report on a multicentre open investigation in Portugal. Pharmatherapeutica 3:157, 1982
58. D-Ambrosio E, Casa B, Bompani R et al: Glucosamine sulphate: a controlled clinical investigation in arthrosis. Pharmatherapeutica 2:504, 1981
59. Pujalte JM, Llavore EP, Ylescupidez FR: Double-blind clinical evaluation of oral glucosamine sulfate in the basic treatment of osetoarthritis. Curr Med Res Opin 7:110, 1980
60. Clarkson PM: Antioxidants and physical performance. Crit Rev Food Sci Nutr 35:131, 1995
61. Chance B, Sies H, Boveris A: Hydroperoxide metabolism in mammalian organs. Physiol Rev 59:527, 1979
62. Ji LL: Oxidative stress during exercise: implication of antioxidant nutrients. Free Radic Biol Med 18:1079, 1995
63. Jackson M, Edwards RHT, Symons MCR: Electron spin resonance studies from intact mammalian skeletal muscle. Biochim Biophys Acta 847:185, 1985
64. Alessio HM: Exercise-induced oxidative stress. Med Sci Sports Exerc 25:218, 1993
65. Poulsen HE, Loft S, Vistisen K: Extreme exercise and oxidative DNA modification. J Sports Sci 14:343, 1996
66. Bray TM, Taylor CG: Tissue glutathione, nutrition, and oxidative stress. Can J Physiol Pharmacol 71:746, 1993
67. Reddy VK, Kumar CT, Prasad M et al: Exercise-induced oxidant stress in the lung tissue: role of dietary supplementation of vitamin E and selenium. Biochem Int 26:863, 1992
68. Rokitzki L, Logemann E, Sagredos AN et al: Lipid peroxidation and antioxidative vitamins under extreme endurance stress. Acta Physiol Scand 151:149, 1994
69. Sen CK, Atalay M, Hanninen O: Exercise-induced oxidative stress: glutathione supplementation and deficiency. J Appl Physiol 77:2177, 1994
70. Tessier F, Hida H, Favier A et al: Muscle GSH-Px activity after prolonged exercise, training, and selenium supplementation. Biol Trace Elem Res 47:279, 1995
71. Duarte JA, Appell HJ, Carvalho F et al: Endothelium-derived oxidative stress may contribute to exercise-induced muscle damage. Int J Sports Med 14:440, 1993
72. Suter PM, Domenghetti G, Schaller MD et al: N-acetylcysteine enhances recovery from acute lung injury in man: a randomized, double-blind, placebo-controlled clinical study. Chest 105:190, 1994
73. Pyke S, Lew H, Quintanilha A: Severe depletion in liver glutathione during physical exercise. Biochem Biophys Res Commun 139:926, 1986
74. Sochman J, Vrbska J, Musilova B et al: Infarct size limitation: acute n-acetylcysteine defense (ISLAND trial): preliminary analysis and report after the first 30 patients. Clin Cardiol 19:94, 1996
75. Poulsen HE, Loft S, Vistien K: Extreme exercise and oxidative DNA modification. J Sports Sci 14:343, 1996
76. Rokitzki L, Logemann E, Sagredos AN et al: Lipid peroxidation and antioxidative vitamins under extreme endurance stress. Acta Physiol Scand 151:149, 1994
77. Tiidus PM, Houston ME: Vitamin E status and response to exercise training. Sports Med 20:12, 1995
78. Rokitzki L, Logemann E, Huber G et al: α-Tocopherol supplementation in racing cyclists during extreme endurance training. Int J Sports Nutr 4:253, 1994
79. Liebler DC, Kling DS, Reed DL: Antioxidant protection of phospholipid bilayers by α-tocopherol. J Biol Chem 15:12114, 1996
80. Burton GW, Joyce A, Ingold KU: First proof that vitamin E is a major lipid-soluble, chain-breaking antioxidant in human blood plasma. Lancet 2:327, 1982
81. Kamal-Eldin A, Appelqvist L-A: The chemistry and antioxidant properties of tocopherols and tocotrienols. Lipids 31:671, 1996
82. Packer L, Gohil K, DeLumen B et al: A comparative study on the effects of ascorbic acid deficiency and supplementation on endurance and mitochondrial oxidative capacities in various tissues of the guinea pig. Comp Biochem Physiol 83B:235, 1986
83. Johnston CS: Supplemental vitamin C, carnitine, and endurance performance [Abstract]. J Am Coll Nutr 12:615, 1993
84. Alessio HM, Goldfarb AH, Cao G: Exercise-induced oxidative stress before and after vitamin C supplementation. Int J Sports Nutr 7:1, 1997
85. Jakeman P, Maxwell S: Effect of antioxidant vitamin supplementation on muscle function after eccentric exercise. Eur J Appl Physiol 67:426, 1993
86. Buzina R, Grgic Z, Jusic M et al: Nutritional status and physical working capacity. Hum Nutr Clin Nutr 36C:429, 1982
87. Gerster H: The role of vitamin C in athletic performance. J Am Coll Nutr 8:636, 1989
88. Beyer RE: Elevation of coenzyme Q and cytochrome c concentration by endurance exercise in the rat. Arch Biochem Biophys 234:323, 1984
89. Gohill K: Effect of exercise training on tissue E and ubiquinone content. J Appl Physiol 63:1638, 1987
90. Folkers K: Biomedical and Clinical Aspects of Coenzyme Q, Vol 3. Elsevier, Amsterdam, 1981
91. Fujimoto S: Effects of coenzyme Q administration on pulmonary function and exercise performance in patients with chronic lung diseases. Clin Invest 71:S162, 1993
92. Kamikawa T, Kobayashi A, Yamashita T et al: Effects of

coenzyme Q10 on exercise tolerance in chronic stable angina pectoris. Am J Cardiol 56:247, 1985

93. Lane HW: Some trace elements related to physical activity: zinc, copper, selenium, chromium, and iodine. p. 301. In Wolinsky I, Hickson JF (eds): Nutrition in Exercise and Sport. CRC Press, Boca Raton, FL, 1989

94. Clarkson PM: Minerals: exercise performance and supplementation in athletes. J Sports Sci 9(spec issue):91, 1991

95. Singh A, Failla ML, Deuster PA: Exercise-induced changes in immune function: effects of zinc supplementation. J Appl Physiol 76:2298, 1994

96. McGuire JJ, Kagan V, Ackrell BAC et al: Succinate-ubiquinone reductase linked recycling of alpha-tocopherol in reconstituted systems and mitochondria: requirement for reduced ubiquinol. Arch Biochem Biophys 292:47, 1992

97. Lambelet P, Saucy F, Loliger J: Chemical evidence for interactions between vitamins E and C. Experientia 41:1384, 1985

98. Kunert KJ, Tappel AL: The effect of vitamin C on in vivo lipid peroxidation in guinea pigs as measured by pentane and ethane production. Lipids 18:271, 1983

99. Ryan GB, Majno G: Inflammation. p. 6. Upjohn Company, Kalamazoo, MI, 1977

100. Strachan AF, Noakes TD, Kotzenberg G et al: C reactive protein concentrations during long distance running. Br Med J 289:1249, 1984

101. Locke M, Noble EG: Stress proteins: the exercise response. Can J Appl Physiol 20:155, 1995

102. Taras JS, Gray RM, Culp RW: Complications of flexor tendon injuries. Hand Clin 10:103, 1994

103. Leadbetter WB: Cell matrix response in tendon injury. Clin Sports Med 11:533, 1992

104. Brigman BE, Hu P, Yin H et al: Fibronectin in the tendon-sinovial complex: quantitation in vivo and in vitro by ELISA and relative mRNA levels by polymerase chain reaction and Northern blot. J Orthop Res 12:253, 1994

105. Panasyuk A, Frati E, Ribault D et al: Effect of reactive oxygen species on the biosynthesis and structure of newly synthesized proteoglycans. Free Radic Biol Med 16:157, 1994

106. Oryan A: Role of collagen in soft connective tissue wound healing. Transplant Proc 27:2759, 1995

107. Masferrer JL, Kulkarni PS: Cyclooxygenase-2 inhibitors: a new approach to the therapy of ocular inflammation. Surv Ophthalmol 41(suppl 2)S35, 1997

108. Reaven GM: Pathophysiology of insulin resistance in human disease. Physiol Rep 75:473, 1995

109. Richter EA, Turcotte L, Hespel P et al: Metabolic responses to exercise: effects of endurance training and implications for diabetes. Diabetes Care 15:1767, 1992

110. Tremblay A, Pinsard D, Coveney S et al: Counterregulatory response to insulin-induced hypoglycemia in trained and nontrained humans. Metabolism 39:1138, 1990

111. Wolfe BM: Potential role of raising dietary protein intake for reducing risk of atherosclerosis. Can J Cardiol 11(suppl G)127G, 1995

112. Volek JS, Kraemer WJ, Bush JA et al: Testosterone and cortisol in relationship to dietary nutrients and resistance exercise. J Appl Physiol 82:49, 1997

113. Chandler RM, Byrne HK, Patterson JG et al: Dietary supplements affect the anabolic hormones after weight-training exercise. J Appl Physiol 76:839, 1994

114. Michel G, Baulieu E-E: Androgen receptor in rat skeletal muscle: characterization and physiological variations. Endocrinology 107:2088, 1980

115. Mujika I, Chatard JC, Padilla S et al: Hormonal responses to training and its tapering off in competitive swimmers: relationships with performance. Eur J Appl Physiol 74:361, 1996

116. Bernton E, Hoover D, Galloway R et al: Adaptation to chronic stress in military trainees. Ann NY Acad Sci 774: 217, 1995

117. Kutten WH, Raney WE, Carr BR: Regulation of interleukin-6 production in human fetal Kupffer cells. Scand J Immunol 33:607, 1991

6

Injury Prevention

STEVEN I. SUBOTNICK

Injury prevention is enhanced by appropriate conditioning, including strength, flexibility, balance, and endurance. The sports physician must remain mindful of these factors when counseling patients.

THE RULE OF THREE

A good thing to keep in mind when giving advice to athletes about avoiding injury is the Rule of Three, which was obtained from information on running but is adaptable to almost all sports. There are many ways that the Rule of Three can be applied. For example, when an individual is standing, half of the body weight goes through each foot; when standing on one foot, the full body weight goes through that foot. In easy walking, 1 to 1.5 times the body weight goes through the foot. In running, however, the amount of force going through the lower extremity is at least three times greater; this is the Rule of Three. The rule demonstrates to the athlete why even a slight imbalance needs correction. Minor imbalances of the lower extremity are three times more important for the runner than for the nonathlete; thus, a one-eighth inch limb length discrepancy has a relative importance of a three-eighths-inch limb length discrepancy in a nonathlete. An imbalance of 3 degrees in the forefoot of the athlete has a relative importance of a 9-degree imbalance in the nonathlete.

Athletes must be advised that injury results in the loss of 3 weeks of training for every week away from competition. Athletes detrain as fast as they train; the need for substitute aerobic activity when an injury is being treated cannot be overemphasized.

The Rule of Three also applies to workouts: athletes can increase the duration and intensity of their workout every 3 weeks in a cyclic method; the duration of a competitive event may be three times greater than the average daily workout. The Rule of Three can also be used to explain to athletes that they have three times more mitochondria in their muscles than untrained individuals, and thus are three times more efficient at metabolizing the food they eat. They also have three times greater endurance.

The Rule of Three is used to remind the athlete that triple training is safer than concentrating on a single activity. I suggest to my athletes that they combine biking, swimming, and running. Other aerobic sports may be combined as well. The important point is to decrease the likelihood of injury secondary to chronic repetitive stress and overspecification of various muscles.

INTERNAL FACTORS

Importance of Warmup

Injury prevention is enhanced by giving good commonsense advice to athletic patients. In preparing for a workout or competition, movement should be initiated in larger muscles during the warmup period, since this has a greater warming effect. The athlete should walk or jog easily for at least 5 minutes, perspiring gently but avoiding a state of breathlessness.

Lack of appropriate warmup on cold mornings is associated with increased frequency of injury. The colder the weather or the longer the period of inactivity prior to exercise, the longer and more careful the warmup should be. Similarly, it is difficult to stretch cold, stiff muscles. A brisk walk or gentle jog for 5 to 7 minutes before stretching is helpful. Once a general warmup with flexibility exercises has terminated, athletes can do calisthenics as preparation for team sports, such as football.

Stretching

The axiom "Train, don't strain" is good advice for the athletic patient. It applies to stretching as well as the athletic event. Stretching should be done slowly and gently to avoid invoking the myostatic reflex, whereby the muscle contracts to prevent being overstretched. Athletes who are particularly stiff and inflexible should be referred to a sports physical therapist for proprioceptive neuromuscular facilitation (PNF) (see Ch. 21). With PNF, an isometric contraction is held at the initial boundary of the range of motion, followed by relaxation and, usually, a greater range of motion.

Biofeedback

It is helpful to inform athletic running patients that the skills of walking, as well as running, are learned and not inherited. A treadmill with a video camera and mirrors that enable patients to analyze their own running form is valuable when teaching technique and encouraging appropriate biofeedback. Some basic rules about form are helpful. Walkers are shown how to land gently on the heel with the foot in front of the knee, and then to roll onto the ball of the foot, finally toeing off through the first and second toes. They are taught to keep their feet pointing straight ahead on parallel tracks. With walking, the left arm goes forward when the right leg does. Faster walking is accompanied by greater circumduction at the hips.

Running has a zero base of gait, with the feet pointing straight ahead. One foot lands where the other foot was. Runners may land on the heel, flat-footed, or on the ball of the foot, depending on their foot type or preferred running style. The recreational and distance runner, however, uses a heel–foot–toe form. In running, the foot should land under the knee and, correspondingly, under the center of gravity of the body. Athletes should be told to keep the foot on the ground as long as possible, and not lift it off prematurely. The center of gravity should be lowered, and attempts should be made to stop it from going up and down abruptly. Proper arm swing is accompanied by proper leg swing. In general, a short, comfortable stride is preferred.

Through biofeedback, foot technique can be taught to runners, and they can be shown how to contact gently on the outside of the heel in a somewhat supinated position, then proceed to a foot-flat position with the calcaneus gently everted. The runner is then shown how to resupinate the foot as the heel leaves the ground, and the foot proceeds to toe-off through the first and second (and, at times, third) toes. A neutral position is explained and demonstrated by establishing congruency of the talonavicular joint. The athlete is taught to stand with both feet in a neutral position, and then on one foot alone, which simulates the middle of mid-stance when neutral position is desirable.

Runners are encouraged to land gently on their feet. The audio portion of a videotape setup is used to record the foot plant. With this audio aid, the sports physician and athlete can correct foot slap or asymmetric contact.

Patients involved in dance or similar activities are shown how to align the foot with the knee. The second toe is aligned with the middle of the kneecap. This, in general, keeps the foot in neutral while the dancer rotates the leg internally or externally from the hip. Turnout from the foot, with associated pronation, is demonstrated to the athlete as an error in form, and the importance of correcting this is stressed.

Fatigue

The importance of fatigue should be explained to the athletic patient. Fatigue undermines resistance to injury in a number of ways. The proprioceptive system, so important in preventing joint laxity, is part of the reflex nervous system, which is unable to respond autonomously to situations when muscle function is impaired secondary to fatigue. Fatigue compromises skills as well as muscle metabolism. The incidence of both noncollision and collision injuries is higher in the fatigued athlete. Fatigue may be present after one specific event or workout, or it may be chronic, as is seen in the overuse syndrome. Chronic overuse and fatigue have systemic signs and symptoms. Often an influenza-like flatness is the first sign of overstress. The athlete should be warned to watch for sleep difficulty, increased irritability, or increased resting pulse in the morning. If the pulse is 10 beats/min faster than normal in the morning, the athlete is overstressed and overfatigued. Athletes must be advised to decrease their workouts and rest until this condition reverses.

EXTERNAL FACTORS

Gear

Injuries can often be avoided with appropriate advice about gear. Athletes' shoes should be carefully examined for deformities secondary to abnormal forces. A fractured or broken counter of a shoe, either lateral or medial, correlates with excessive lateral or medial forces. An athlete with lateral instability of the rearfoot or ankle and lateral override of the rearfoot counter needs appropriate shoes with a lateral buildup or reinforcement of the counter. The athlete with excessive pronation and associated symptoms, with medial breakdown of the counter of the shoe, needs a firmer shoe with a reinforced counter. The mid-sole of a shoe may fatigue after 350 to 750 miles if it is made out of ethyl vinyl acetate (EVA) or polyurethane. Injury can be prevented by replacing shoes at appropriate intervals. Shoes should be inspected for excessive compression and fatigue of the mid-sole material. Decreased recovery and shock attenuation of the shoe are felt in the muscles as increased soreness and stiffness. Even shoes that look sound may have mid-sole material oxidation and failure. Treadmill analysis often shows that runners have better form going barefooted than in their running shoes. This is due to the softness of shoes, which promotes excessive motion. Selecting shoes with firmer mid-soles and reinforced counters and using some form of foot orthosis improve foot function during running. Most athletes need a running shoe one size larger than their street shoes. Often their street shoes are too small anyways! Our feet get larger as we age, or postpartum. Improper-fitting shoes cause multiple foot and lower extremity problems.

The athletic patient who is involved in recreational or serious competition may wish to have a pair of shoes specifically made for the competitive event. Although this is understandable for an intermediate- or high-caliber competitor, it is unnecessary, and often harmful, for the beginner or novice. Competitive road-running shoes are usually lighter and more flexible and offer less impact protection. Competition shoes are usually made on an in-toed last. In contradistinction, training shoes may be made on a straight last for the pronator, or on a slightly curved last for the stable foot. An excessively in-toed, curved last competitive shoe for a novice runner with a pronated straight foot leads to serious problems. As a runner goes from heel–foot–toe to ball-of-the-foot contact, the foot supinates, which is the rationale for a more in-toed competitive running shoe.

The shape of the foot should correspond to the shape of the shoe. If the foot is held in a neutral position and traced on a piece of paper, the shoe can be superimposed on this tracing. A correct last should be prescribed for the patient, depending on the foot type. In general, a pronator does better with a straight-last shoe. A high-arch cavus foot does better with a C-shaped or mildly adducted last. Athletes with lateral instability of the ankle or a tendency toward ankle instability may do better with a high-top athletic shoe, since these increase proprioception about the ankle and thereby reduce injury. The total amount of strength afforded by a high-top shoe is estimated to be only 10 to 15 percent beyond that of a low-top shoe.

Many athletic shoes, especially those designed for aerobics, walking, or running, have a removable innersole or sock liner. Once these fatigue, there may be increased pain at the plantar aspect of the heel or under the ball of the foot. The sports physician should remove these portions from the shoe and inspect them to see whether they need replacement. If so, they may be replaced with a similar type of innersole, a full-length viscoelastic innersole if shock attenuation is desirable, or some form of biodynamic orthosis for specific imbalance problems.

Weather Conditions

Injury can be prevented or avoided with appropriate advice from the exercise physician on topics concerning weather and humidity. Weather and humidity are important, and athletes must be aware of the signs of heat prostration. Heat prostration is associated with cold sweats, dizziness, and excessive fatigue on otherwise warm days. Athletes living in colder areas may be training for an event to be held in a warmer areas, such as the Hawaii Marathon, held in December. They should be cautioned about heat prostration and the effects of excessive humidity. Runners are advised to take it easy, running at least 1 minute slower than their normal pace in hot and humid weather.

The absence of hot, humid weather does not preclude heat prostration, fluid depletion, or electrolyte imbalance. I have observed cases of heat prostration with rectal temperatures above 105°F during Olympic Marathon tryouts in cool weather (65°F). Treatment for these cases consists of immediate fluid replacement, rest, and cardiovascular monitoring.

Running in cold weather with an excessive wind chill factor can subject toes, fingers, or nose to frostbite. Wet weather may cause the shoes and socks to get soaking wet, predisposing the foot to blistering. This can also occur on a day on which one is competing in a race in which by-standers are using hoses to cool down the participants.

Altitude

It takes at least 2 weeks to acclimate to large changes in altitude. Athletes must be advised to run slower with less intensity when going to higher altitudes. This same advice holds when athletes are competing in areas with higher humidity or higher heat than they are accustomed to.

THE OVERUSE SYNDROME

Both the sports physician and the athletic patient should be well aware of the overuse syndrome. *Overuse* is a term applied to those injuries that have a gradual onset. They usually start off as a tightness or ache that is present 1 or 2 hours after exercise. If the training error is ignored, or biomechanical imbalances are not corrected, this tightness or ache will progress and be present at the beginning of the athletic event. It then goes away as the athlete warms up, only to reoccur 1 or 2 hours following the event. The athlete will wake up in the morning very stiff and achy and will have soreness in one or two major portions of the body. When the athlete continues to train or run through this injury, eventually there is pain during the entire event to such an extent that the intensity, duration, or speed of the workout must be drastically reduced. Finally, the injury progresses to a point at which there is pain during walking, and athletic endeavors are impossible. Unfortunately, this is usually when the athlete presents to the sports practitioner for help. Invariably, when the overuse syndrome is present, training errors have been compounded by biomechanical imbalances, as well as dynamic imbalances of muscle. There may be sleep disturbance, increased irritability, generalized feeling of malaise with influenza-like symptoms, or systemic complaints similar to that of mononucleosis. Eating patterns may be disrupted. The morning resting pulse is usually elevated by 10 to 15 beats/min. Fever blisters are prevalent, and there is a general achiness in muscles and joints. There are many common examples of overuse injuries (see Box).

Biomechanical imbalances are accompanied by dynamic imbalances. Characteristically, in a runner, there will be tight posterior structures and relatively weak anterior–anti-gravity structures. When overuse syndrome is present, the first and most immediate treatment is that of rest. Biomechanical imbalances must be corrected with appropriate

---

COMMON EXAMPLES OF OVERUSE INJURIES

Plantar fasciitis

Morton's interdigital neuroma

Subungual hematoma

Heel-spur syndrome

Retrocalcaneal bursitis or exostosis

Subluxed cuboid

Midtarsal joint strain or sprain

Achilles tenosynovitis or paratenonitis

Sinus tarsi syndrome

Ankle synovitis or strain

Anterior enthesitis or shin-splint syndrome

Posterior musculature, enthesitis, or shin-splint syndrome.

Runner's knee—chondralgia patella, including peripatellar pain, pes anserinus bursitis, iliotibial band friction syndrome, intra-articular damage, and posterior knee pain

Thigh strains

Hamstring strains

Greater trochanteric bursitis

Hip and/or low back strain

---

gear and a temporary full-length running orthosis. Once appropriate shoes and foot function have been accounted for, dynamic imbalances must be corrected with appropriate flexibility and strengthening exercises. Running form is checked, and corrections are made as deemed necessary. When pain and inflammation are present, anti-inflammatory measures are prudent to prevent chronic fibrosis, with subsequent painful or reduced range of motion. Physical therapy, manipulations, homeopathic remedies, herbs, nonsteroidal anti-inflammatory medications, or pain medications may be necessary at times. Exercise participation must be monitored by the sports physician whenever artificial measures are used to reduce pain or inflammation. As with any injury, appropriate diagnostic tests, including radiography or laboratory tests, may be indicated.

Further injury is prevented by appropriate instruction and education from the sports physician. If a true injury prevents involvement in a high-impact sport, substitute aerobic exercises within the tolerance of the injured part are prescribed.

As can be seen from the previous list (see Box, p. 70) the overuse syndromes of the lower extremity involve almost all parts of the soft tissue, skeleton, or joint anatomy. They are all attributed to training errors, accumulated microtrauma, biomechanical imbalances, improper foot gear, and "too much, too soon." These topics are covered in greater depth in the section on injuries (see Ch. 13 through 18).

OVERTRAINING SYNDROME

The overtraining syndrome is similar to the overuse syndrome. With overtraining, there is greater emphasis on the physiologic response. Athletes who overtrain become irritable. They have a tendency to lose touch with reality. Overtraining also leads to poor sleep patterns and to disturbances in eating patterns, such as anorexia. These athletes normally notice an increased pulse rate in the morning when they awake, as with the overuse syndrome, of 10 to 15 beats/min above normal. They have a generalized feeling of being stale and a fear of their ability to perform. Most present with a myriad of overuse injuries, all of which seem minor to the examining physician but are considered critical by the athlete. Upon reviewing the training records of these athletes, it becomes obvious that they are pushing themselves too hard.

The sports practitioner can help these athletes by pointing out to them that they are overtraining. The systemic effects of overtraining are explained. Sports physicians can counsel their competitive athletic patients who are pushing themselves too hard to realize that the quality of a workout is more important than the quantity. Single-activity athletes are encouraged to cross-train. Runners are advised to add swimming and biking to their workout schedule. The addicted competitive athlete with systemic overtraining symptoms may benefit from psychological counseling.

FIRST AID FOR ACUTE AND OVERUSE INJURIES

When one is acting in a medical capacity at a track and field athletic event, total preparation is essential. Immediate first aid equipment includes ice, Ace bandages, splints, airway, rescusitation bag, and fluid replacements for intravenous administration. Rectal thermometers should be on hand, as should appropriate means to rest the athlete and to treat shock. Blood pressure and pulse must be monitored if an athlete is injured. A well-planned evacuation system will facilitate triage to an appropriate medical facility. Cardiac support medications and units are helpful.

For simple soft tissue injuries, the use of ice packs and/ or ethyl chloride sprays for contracted or spastic muscles is helpful. The acronym RICE (rest, ice, compression, and elevation) is a useful mnemonic device. An athlete with a sore foot or leg is suspected of having sustained a stress fracture until proved otherwise.

When acting in the capacity of a medical director at field events, if a sprained ankle occurs, the general rule is that the athlete must be able to hop up and down on the involved side before returning to competition. Often, a grade II sprain can be reduced to a grade I sprain by appropriate icing and compression followed by supportive taping. With head injuries, return to competition is discouraged until after a complete medical clearance.

DIET AND FLUIDS

Diet and nutrition have always been a controversial subject. By and large, most athletes do well with a diet composed of complex carbohydrates, moderate protein, and abundant fluid. The best fluid is water, but athletes also do well with juices. No carbohydrates should be taken within 3 hours of any event, although water intake is advisable.

Fad diets are to be discouraged. A common example is carbohydrate loading—the athlete begins to deplete carbohydrates by consuming only protein for 3 days while rigorously working out. This crash regimen is followed by 3 days of gentle workout or rest accompanied by increased carbohydrate intake before the event. Costill and coworkers (personal communication) suggest that this regimen does nothing to improve the glycogen stores in the mitochondria. The problem with carbohydrate loading is that it increases the risk of injury to the athlete, who is working out while fatigued during the carbohydrate-sparing, protein-rich, workout-intensity phase. Many an athlete has shown up at the starting line of a marathon following carbohydrate loading with an upset stomach, as well as a bloated feeling.

The purpose of carbohydrate loading is to increase glycogen storage in the mitochondria. The same objective can be achieved, without the side effects, by having the athlete decrease the intensity and duration of a workout beginning 1 week before an endurance event. During this time, the athlete is encouraged to consume more complex carbohydrates and to avoid heavy protein intake. Then, no food is taken within 3 hours of the athletic endurance event, in order to prevent the problem of initial hyperglycemia followed by hypoglycemia.

VITAMINS

Multiple vitamins are also commonly used, and there is little clinical evidence of harm in doing so. In fact, evidence supports the use of multiple vitamins for all athletes. Apparently the modern mass farming techniques used today, although responsible for abundant crops, are producing crops seriously deficient in trace minerals and vitamins so necessary for our metabolic functions. Vitamins, minerals, and trace elements are beneficial to aid in metabolic well-being, especially in those athletes who are interested in losing weight or in modifying their diet or caloric intake to maintain a low weight. Many doctors discourage their patients from taking vitamins, yet take vitamins themselves, as do members of their families. Apparently the peace of mind that vitamins afford is worth the price.

Iron-deficiency anemia among women with low total body fat is well recognized. For female as well as male athletes complaining of staleness or overuse syndrome, appropriate laboratory tests should be ordered to rule out iron-deficiency anemia. Dr. Joan Ullyot, a prominent sports physician, recommends that all female endurance athletes take some form of iron supplementation. Gerontologists suggest that elderly athletes, especially postmeno-pausal women, increase their calcium and magnesium along with the trace minerals boron, vanadium, molybdenum, and selenium. Chromium and pyridoxine (vitamin B_6) are essential for diabetics.[1] Zinc and vitamin C are essential for collagen well-being, and decrease the risk of the common cold.[2]

Summary

Injury prevention is a joint effort between the sports physician, knowledgeable of the simple measures that may be taken to prevent injuries or overuse, and the athlete and coach/trainer.

Vitamins, once a controversial topic, are now becoming part of mainstream preventative and treatment medical prescriptions. Most athletes take at least 2g of vitamin C a day. All of them in my practice are anxious for advice as to vitamins, trace elements, nutritional supplements, and diet. They all are trying something on their own without adequate guidance. The need for iron in women, as well as calcium and magnesium in postmenopausal women, is well documented, as is the use of folic acid in pregnant women. Vitamins and supplements are here to stay, and it behooves all physicians to become well versed in their indications and uses.

REFERENCES

1. Marion JE: Diabetes—New Therapies, 1995 (available from author at Route 4, Box 1647, Mt. Pleasant, Texas 75455)
2. Gaby AR: Townsend Letter, issue 148 (Nov.):26, 1995 (Fax 360–385–6021)

II

Anatomy and
Biomechanics of the
Lower Extremity

7

Normal Anatomy

STEVEN I. SUBOTNICK

OSTEOLOGY

The foot consists of 26 bones and 55 articulations, conveniently divided into three regions: forefoot, midfoot, and rearfoot. The forefoot is represented by the 14 bones of the toes and five metatarsals. The midfoot consists of the three cuneiform bones, the cuboid, and the navicular. Finally, the rearfoot, or greater tarsus, is composed of the talus and the calcaneus. The foot contains two arches, the longitudinal or mid-part and the transverse or forepart (Fig. 7-1). The transverse arch forms the convexity of the dorsum of the foot (Fig. 7-2). The tarsal and tarsometatarsal articulations constitute the longitudinal arch, maintained primarily by the plantar ligaments and aponeurosis. People's feet are as individual as people are, and there are many variations to the illustrations presented here. Often, it is these variations that alter the mechanics and cause subsequent sequelae. The bones of the foot, ossification schedule, and architectural relationships are illustrated in Figures 7-1 through 7-6.

The phalanges of the foot are similar in number and distribution to those of the hand, although they are somewhat shorter and broader than their counterparts. The hallux contains two phalanges, and each of the four lateral toes consists of three phalanges. The concave bases of the proximal phalanges articulate with the convex heads of the metatarsals. The saddle-shaped articular fossa of the head of the proximal phalanx receives the base of the intermediate phalanx. This, in turn, articulates with the smaller and flatter distal phalanx.

Proximally, the five metatarsals articulate with the lesser tarsus and with themselves through broad concavities. The first metatarsal is the shortest and strongest and contains plantar articulations near its heads for the two sesamoid bones (tibial and fibular) located in the tendon of the flexor hallucis brevis. The second metatarsal is the longest and the least mobile of the metatarsals and serves as the anatomic touchstone for abduction and adduction of the foot. The fifth metatarsal is noted for the lateral prominence (styloid processes) at its base, which serves as the insertion site for the tendon of the peroneus brevis. The styloid area is often avulsed during acute inversion injuries of the foot (Fig. 7-4B).

Lesser Tarsus

Distally, the three cuneiform bones (medial, intermediate, and lateral) articulate with the first three metatarsal bones; proximally, they articulate with the navicular. Their wedge shape assists in the formation of the transverse arch, with the middle cuneiform serving as the keystone. Laterally, the cuboid bone articulates with the fourth and fifth metatarsal distally and with the calcaneus proximally. Medially, the cuboid has a fossa for the navicular and lateral cuneiform bones. On its plantar distal suface, there is a small groove for the peroneus longus tendon. The cuneiforms, together with articulations with the metatarsal bones, form Lisfranc's joint. The navicular bone articulates with the cuneiforms distally and with the talus proximally. The navicular tuberosity present on the medial plantar suface is the insertion point of the tibialis posterior tendon.

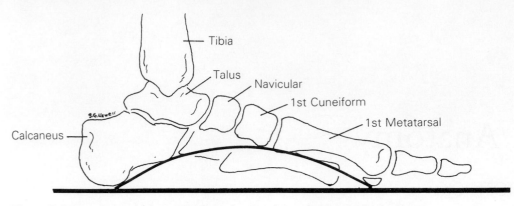

Figure 7-1 Lateral view of the medial foot, showing the medial longitudinal arch.

The midtarsal joint is formed by the articulations between the navicular and talus, and between the cuboid and calcaneus (Fig. 7-4A).

Greater Tarsus

The largest tarsal bone, the calcaneus (os calcis) (Fig. 7-5), serves four basic functions. One-half the body's weight, which is transmitted through the talus, is borne by the calcaneus. The remaining weight is shared by the five metatarsal heads. Posteriorly, the calcaneus completes the longitudinal arch. The calcaneus, through its articulation with the talus, joins the foot to the leg. Finally, the posterior third of the calcaneus serves as the insertion point for the tendo Achillis, providing an effective lever for the calf muscle. Anteriorly, one-third of the calcaneus articulates with the cuboid bone. The superior surface of the calcaneus consists of a series of convexities for the articulation of the talus. It contains three facets for this articulation: the anterior, middle, and posterior facets. A canal or groove runs across the middle facet that, with a corresponding groove on the plantar surface of the talus, forms the sinus

Figure 7-2 Cross section of the forefoot, showing the transverse metatarsal arch.

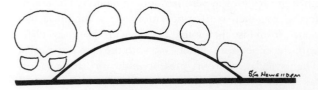

tarsi. The plantar posterior surface of the calcaneus contains a medial and a lateral tuberosity. From the medial calcaneal tuberosity, much of the foot's intrinsic musculature and the plantar aponeurosis take origin (Fig. 7-5). It is important to note that compression fractures most commonly occur in the calcaneus because it contains a high percentage of cancellous bone, and, because of its structure and location, it is subjected to much of the body's transferred weight.

The attachment of the foot to the leg occurs through the talus (astragalus) (Fig. 7-4). Medially and laterally, the talus articulates with the tibial and fibular malleoli and the talar trochlea, forming the ankle joint. The anterior portion of the talar trochlea is wider than the posterior portion and curves slightly, which provides inherent stability during dorsiflexion as it wedges upward (Fig. 7-6). The principal motions of the ankle joint are dorsiflexion and plantar flexion. The plantar surface of the talus articulates with the dorsal surface of the calcaneus in the subtalar joint. The talus has no muscular attachments and, combined with the high surface pressures it bears, this means it is susceptible to vascular damage during trauma. Fractures of the talus are therefore frequently associated with avascular necrosis, as all blood supply is derived from the capsule. Talar fractures also occur at the posterior process or os trigonum. In addition to fracture, bones of the ankle may be involved with arthritis, osteochondral fractures, or osteochondritis dissecans.

Accessory Bones

A number of sesamoids and accessory bones are variably present in the foot (Fig. 7-7). The sesamoids are usually present within tendons juxtaposed to articulations and are

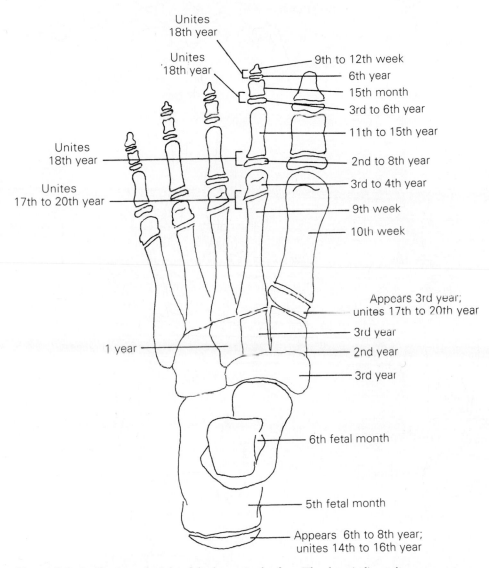

Unites
18th year

Unites
18th year

9th to 12th week

6th year

15th month

3rd to 6th year

11th to 15th year

Unites
18th year

2nd to 8th year

3rd to 4th year

Unites
17th to 20th year

9th week

10th week

Appears 3rd year;
unites 17th to 20th year

3rd year

1 year

2nd year

3rd year

6th fetal month

5th fetal month

Appears 6th to 8th year;
unites 14th to 16th year

Figure 7-3 Ossification schedule of the bones in the foot. The dates indicate the appearance of ossification centers.

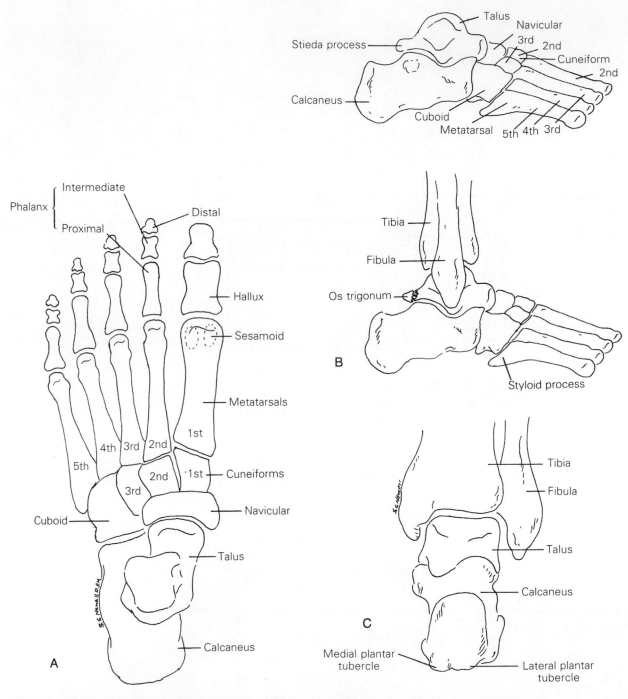

Figure 7-4 Bones of the foot and ankle. **(A)** Dorsal, **(B)** lateral, and **(C)** posterior views.

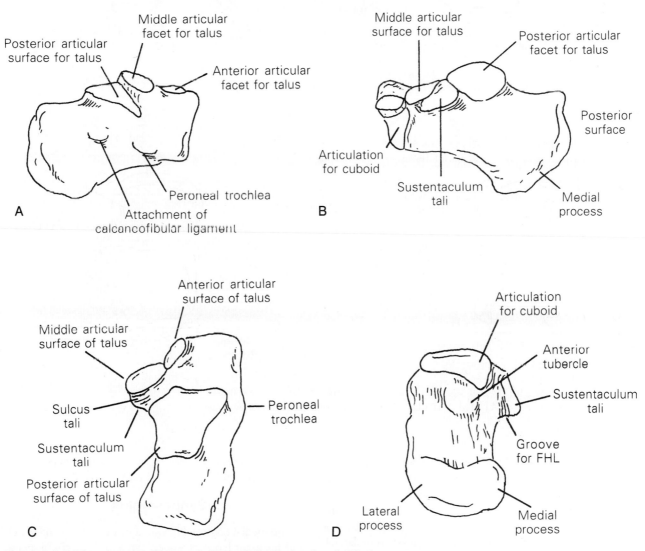

Figure 7-5 Right calcaneus. **(A)** Lateral, **(B)** medial, **(C)** dorsal, and **(D)** plantar views.

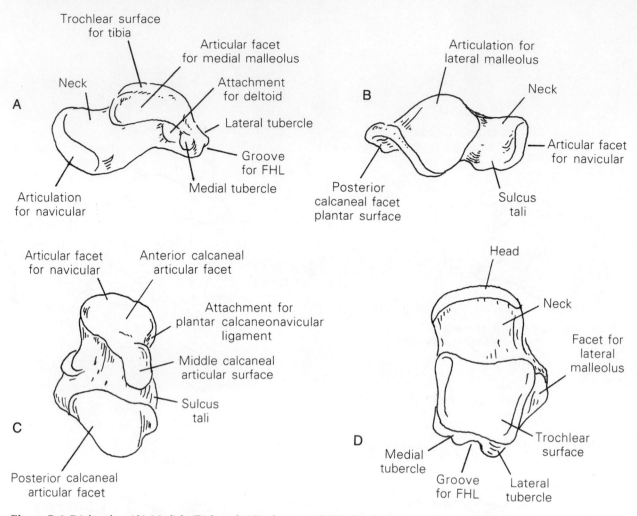

Figure 7-6 Right talus. **(A)** Medial, **(B)** lateral, **(C)** plantar, and **(D)** dorsal views.

frequently incompletely ossified (e.g., contain cartilage, fibrous tissue, and bone). The tibial (medial) and fibular (lateral) sesamoids of the flexor hallucis brevis are always present plantar to the first metatarsal head. The lateral one is usually single, but the medial one may be bi-, tri-, or quadripartite. Usually multipartite sesamoids are bilateral. Other locations where sesamoids may be found are under the heads of the four lateral metatarsals or in the tendons of the tibialis anterior, tibialis posterior, or peroneus longus. Accessory bones appear in the foot between the ages of 10 and 20. Common examples include an os trigonum at the posterior plantar surface of the talus, an accessory of the navicular bone (os tibiale externum) located at the medial border, and ossicles at the base of the fifth metatarsal

(os vesalianum pedis) (Fig. 7-7). Accessory bones can become sources of irritation and require excision.

Syndesmology

The medial collateral ligament of the ankle joint or deltoid ligament has both superficial and deep components. Superficially, the ligament consists of the tibionavicular, tibiocalcaneal, and posterior tibiotalar components. The anterior middle component also stabilizes the subtalar joint. The deep portion of the deltoid ligament is the anterior tibiotalar ligament, which is responsible for stabilizing the medial malleolus and talus. Together, these ligaments form an exceptionally strong band, which is not easily disrupted (Fig. 7-8A).

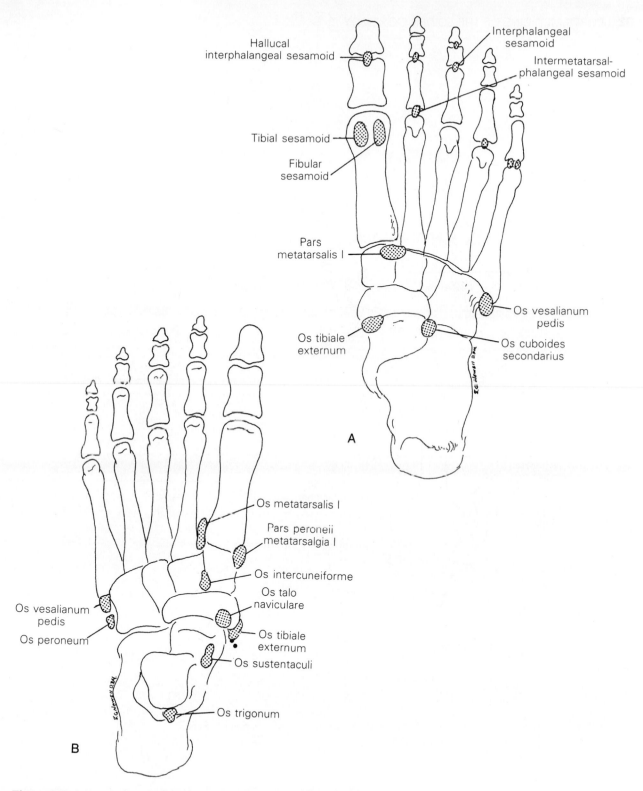

Figure 7-7 Accessory bones of the foot. **(A)** Plantar view. **(B)** Dorsal view.

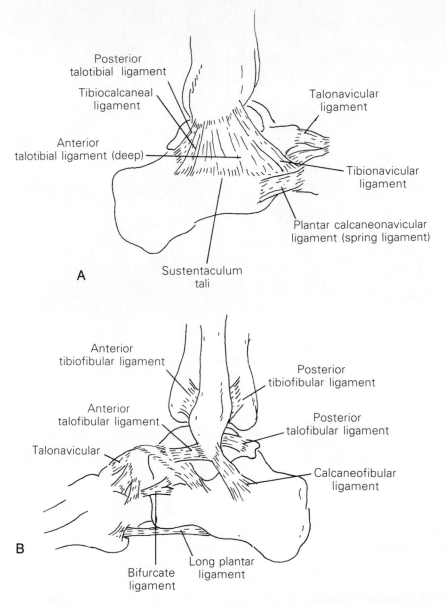

A

B

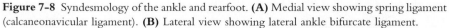

Figure 7–8 Syndesmology of the ankle and rearfoot. **(A)** Medial view showing spring ligament (calcaneonavicular ligament). **(B)** Lateral view showing lateral ankle bifurcate ligament.

Laterally, the ligamentous structure is not as sturdy, consisting of three ligaments, the anterior talofibular, the calcaneofibular, and the posterior talofibular ligaments. In concert, they constitute the lateral collateral ligament. These are commonly torn with inversion sprains, whereas the deltoid is rarely torn (Fig. 7-8B).

The subtalar (talocalcaneal) joint is surrounded by a thin, nonsupportive joint capsule. Stability in the joint is essentially maintained by four sturdy ligaments: the medial collateral, interosseous, calcaneal, and cervical ligaments. The first three prevent excessive eversion while the cervical ligament inhibits inversion along with the lateral collateral ligaments (Fig. 7-8).

The spring ligament (inferior calcaneonavicular ligament) firmly connects the navicular bone to the sustentaculum tali on the calcaneus. The ligaments of the calcaneocuboid joint include the plantar ligament and a portion of the bifurcate ligament dorsally. The long plantar ligament joins the cuboid to the base of the third, fourth, and occasionally fifth metatarsal. Its origin is the calcaneus, and it forms a tunnel for the peroneus longus muscle. The short plantar ligament also binds the cuboid to the calcaneus and, together with the long plantar ligament, helps maintain a longitudinal arch (Fig. 7-8, and see Fig. 7-13).

There are numerous small ligamentous attachments between each bone of the foot and its neighbor, anchoring and creating inherent stability within the foot. Without this internal structure, the foot would simply be a bag of bones (Fig. 7-9). Of the ligaments between the metatarsals and midtarsus, the ligament of Lisfranc between the first cuneiform and second metatarsal base is of prime importance. Traumatic injuries that disrupt this ligament lead to disastrous dislocation of the medial aspect of the foot as the first metatarsal and first cuneiform separate from the second metatarsal and second cuneiform. The arrangements of the ligaments between the metatarsals and midtarsals are illustrated in Figure 7-9. Figure 7-10 shows the complexity of the ligamentous structures about the first metatarsophalangeal joint. The delicate balance of this joint is appreciated by looking at the plantar view with the flexor hallucis brevis inserting proximally into both sesamoids and distal attachments from the sesamoids into the base of the first metatarsal. The intersesamoidal ligament is important in maintaining a proper relationship between both sesamoids, which act as lever pulley systems in increasing the mechanical advantage of the first metatarsophalangeal joint. Figure 7-11 illustrates the delicate balances and the extensor apparatus of the lesser metatarsophalangeal joints. One can appreciate the contribution made by the lumbricales and interossei to the exten-

sor foot apparatus. Figure 7-11 shows the deep transverse metatarsal ligaments.

The plantar aponeurosis (Fig. 7-12) consists of a strong fibrous central portion and small thinner medial and lateral sections. Each is oriented longitudinally on the plantar aspect of the foot. The central portion runs from the medial calcaneal tuberosity and inserts distally, with the superficial portion attaching the skin to the pads of the toes and a deeper portion blending with flexor tendon sheaths. The medial and lateral components of the plantar aponeurosis provide vertical intermuscular septa for the plantar musculature. This aponeurosis is analogous to the one in the hand. As the toes are dorsiflexed, this band tightens up and raises the longitudinal arch while it inverts the foot. The superficial and deep plantar ligaments of the foot are illustrated in Figure 7-13.

Beneath the plantar aponeurosis–plantar fascia are the four muscular layers of the plantar intrinsic foot muscles, as well as the plantar ligaments of the rearfoot and midfoot. The plantar superficial and deep ligaments help maintain the architectural arrangement of the foot. The long plantar and short plantar ligaments have their origins at the calcaneal plantar tubercles. The long plantar ligament is superficial to the short plantar ligament and extends into the metatarsal bases (Fig. 7-13).

There are four important ankle retinacula (Fig. 7-14), which bind the leg tendons as they enter the foot. The extensor retinaculum consists of two portions: superior and inferior. Continuous with the deep leg fascia, the superior extensor retinaculum serves to contain the tendons of the extensor digitorum longus, extensor hallucis longus, tibialis anterior, and peroneus tertius. The Y-shaped inferior retinaculum consists of an upper and a lower band that run from the lateral calcaneus to the medial malleolus and plantar aponeurosis, preventing "bowstringing" of the dorsal tendons.

Coursing between the distal fibula and the lateral calcaneus are the peroneal retinacula, which firmly secure the peroneus longus and brevis tendons behind the fibular malleolus (Figs. 7-14 and 7-15). Medially, the flexor retinaculum extends from the calcaneus to the tibial malleolus and provides a firm support structure for the neurovascular bundle, flexor digitorum longus, flexor hallucis longus, and tibialis posterior (Fig. 7-16).

MYOLOGY

Extrinsic Musculature of the Foot

The muscles of the foot can be divided into extrinsic and intrinsic compartments (Figs. 7-17 through 7-27). Extrinsic muscles consist of the anterior (pretibial) compart-

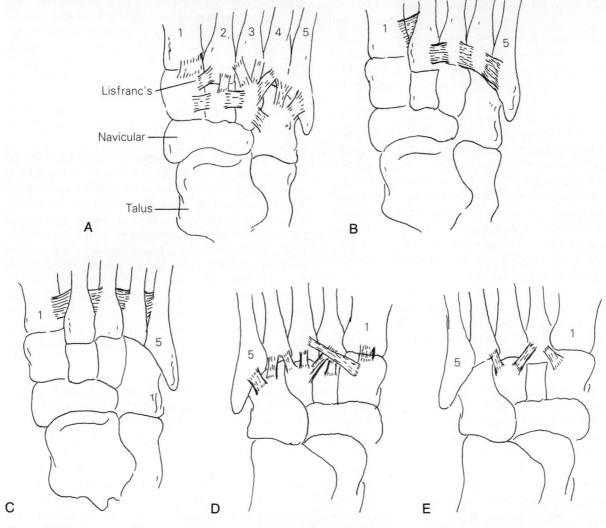

Figure 7-9 Tarsometatarsal ligaments. **(A)** Dorsal tarsometatarsal ligaments. **(B)** Dorsal intermetatarsal ligaments. **(C)** Intermetatarsal ligaments. **(D)** Plantar tarsometatarsal ligaments. **(E)** Interosseous tarsometatarsal ligaments.

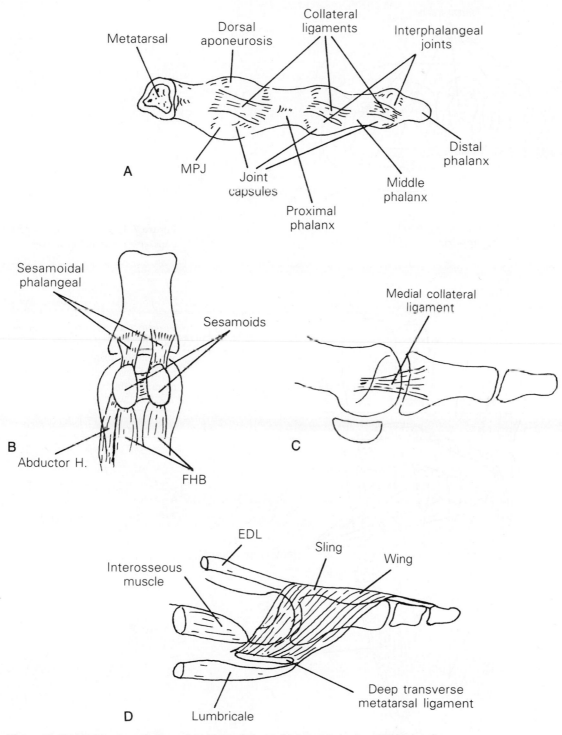

Figure 7-10 **(A)** Metatarsophalangeal and interphalangeal joint organization. **(B)** Plantar ligaments of the metatarsophalangeal joint. **(C)** Medial ligaments of the metatarsophalangeal joint. **(D)** Phalangeal apparatus.

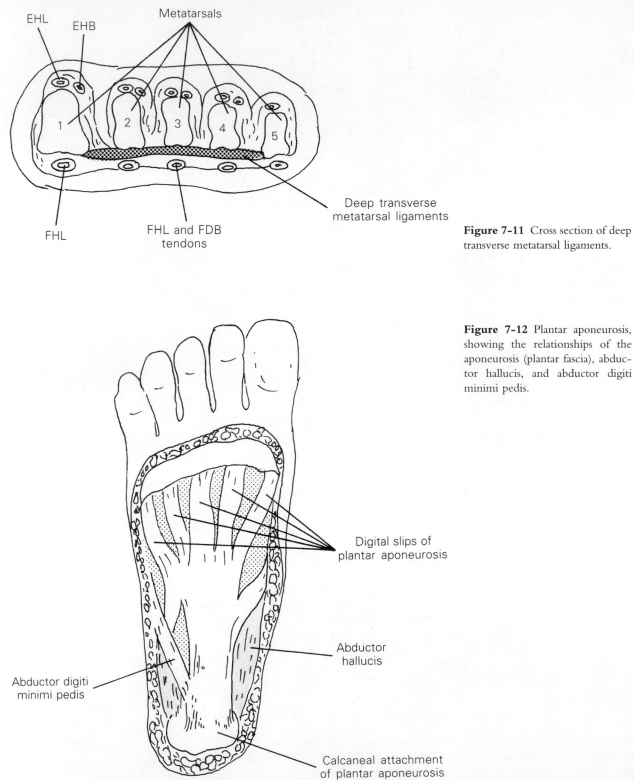

Figure 7–11 Cross section of deep transverse metatarsal ligaments.

Figure 7–12 Plantar aponeurosis, showing the relationships of the aponeurosis (plantar fascia), abductor hallucis, and abductor digiti minimi pedis.

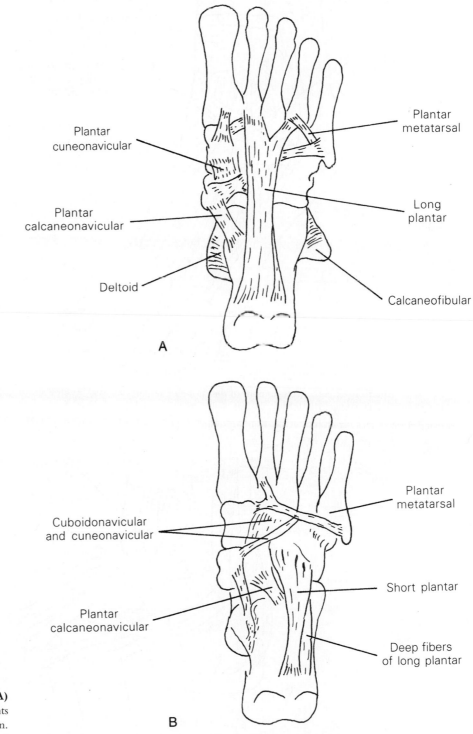

Figure 7-13 Plantar ligaments. **(A)** Superficial and **(B)** deep ligaments of the plantar midtarsal joint region.

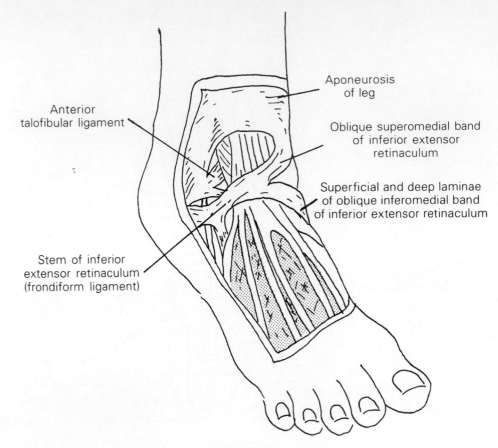

Figure 7-14 Anterior (extensor) retinaculum of the foot and ankle.

Figure 7-15 Lateral retinaculum of the foot and ankle.

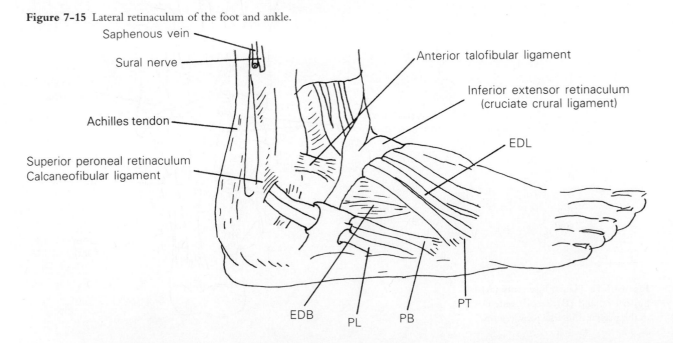

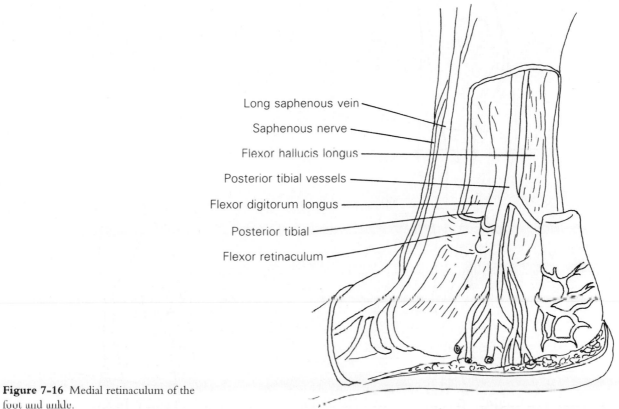

Long saphenous vein

Saphenous nerve

Flexor hallucis longus

Posterior tibial vessels

Flexor digitorum longus

Posterior tibial

Flexor retinaculum

Figure 7-16 Medial retinaculum of the foot and ankle.

Figure 7-17 Cross section of leg showing extrinsic muscles of the foot.

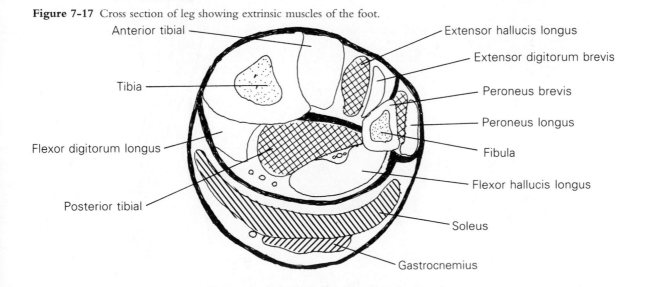

Anterior tibial

Extensor hallucis longus

Extensor digitorum brevis

Tibia

Peroneus brevis

Peroneus longus

Flexor digitorum longus

Fibula

Flexor hallucis longus

Posterior tibial

Soleus

Gastrocnemius

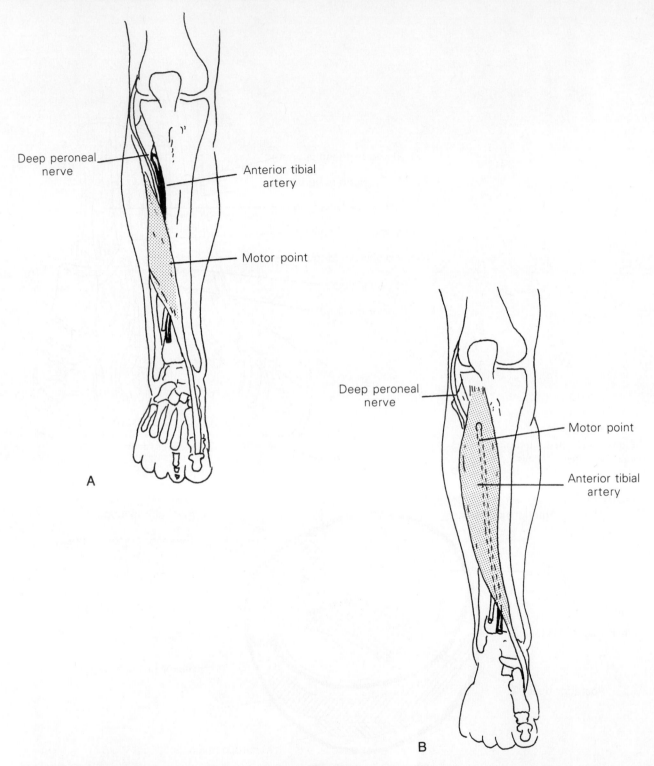

Figure 7-18 Anterior muscle group. **(A)** Extensor hallucis. **(B)** Tibialis anterior. (*Figure continues.*)

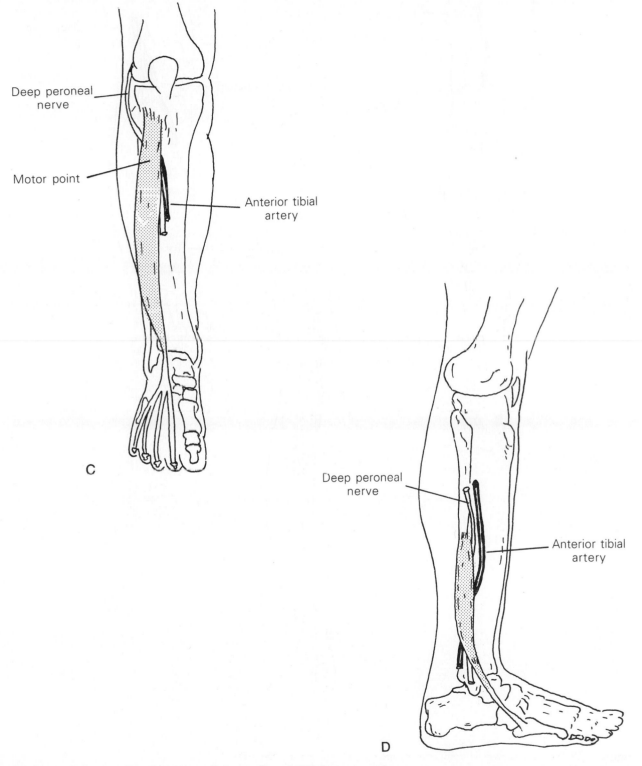

Deep peroneal
nerve

Motor point

Anterior tibial
artery

C

Deep peroneal
nerve

Anterior tibial
artery

D

Figure 7-18 (*Continued*). **(C)** Extensor digitorum longus. **(D)** Peroneus tertius.

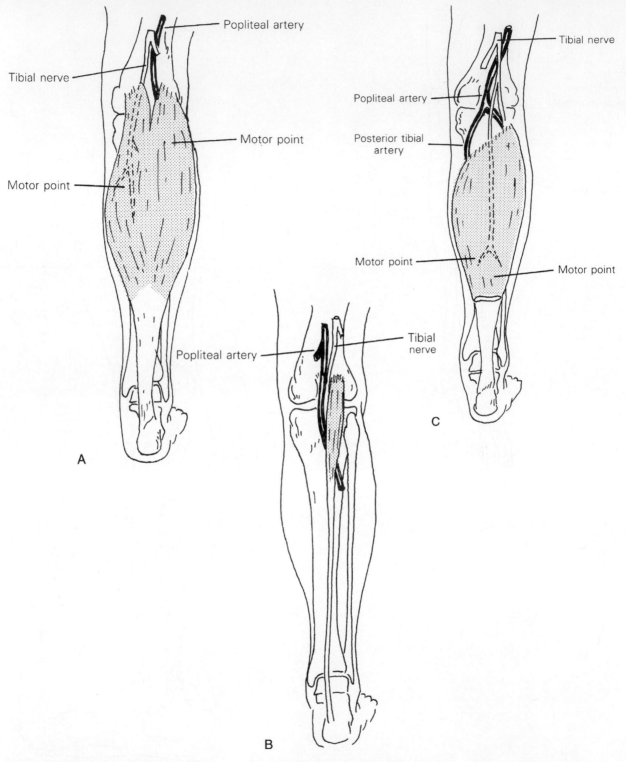

Figure 7-19 Posterior superficial compartment muscles. **(A)** Gastrocnemius. **(B)** Plantaris **(C)** soleus.

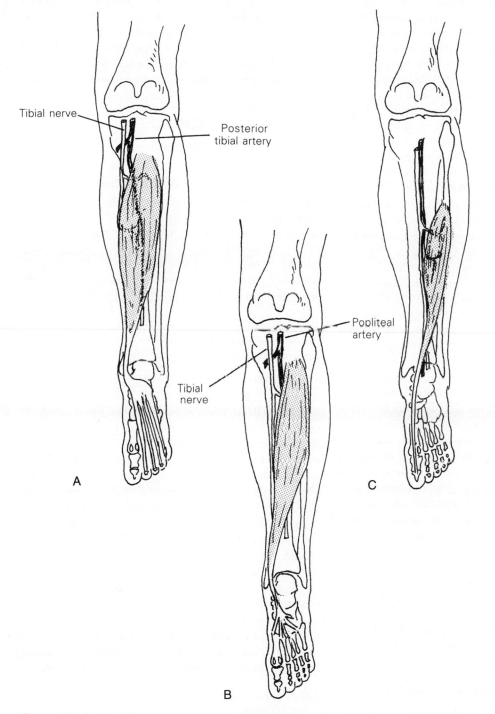

Figure 7-20 Posterior deep compartment muscles. **(A)** Flexor digitorum longus. **(B)** Tibialis posterior. **(C)** Flexor hallucis longus.

ment, the posterior superficial compartment, posterior deep compartment (flexors), and the lateral musculature.

The anterior compartment of the leg contains the dorsiflexors or extensors of the foot. They are the tibialis anterior, extensor digitorum longus, extensor hallucis longus, and peroneus tertius. The muscles of the pretibial group, along with their major artery and nerve, are seen in Figure 7-18.

The posterior superficial muscle group consists of the calf muscles. These flexors of the foot are located posterior to the interosseous membrane and consist of the gastrocnemius, plantaris, and soleus. The gastrocnemius and plantaris arise from the femur, whereas the soleus originates from the posterior surface of the proximal fibula and tibia. The three muscles collectively constitute the triceps surae and are innervated by a branch of the tibial nerve. Collectively, they form the tendo Achillis as they merge to insert into the posterior surface of the calcaneus. The Achilles is the largest and strongest tendon in the human body. The posterior superficial muscle group, along with its innervation, main artery, and motor point, is shown in Figure 7-19.

The posterior deep muscle group (the flexors) courses behind the medial malleolus. They make up the bulk of the leg at the medial posterior aspect. This compartment includes the tibialis posterior, flexor digitorum longus, and flexor hallucis longus. The tibialis posterior inserts into the navicular bone and medial and intermediate cuneiforms and into the base of the second, third, and fourth metatarsals. It is important in maintaining the medial longitudinal arch, as well as in providing foot inversion and decelerating rapid internal rotation associated with pronation. The tibialis posterior is a major inhibitor to pronation. The flexor hallucis longus and flexor digitorum longus join the posterior tibial tendon through the tarsal tunnel. These three muscles, with their respective artery, nerve, and motor points, are shown in Figure 7-20. The lateral compartment contains the peroneals, both longus and brevis. The peroneus longus plantar flexes the base of the first metatarsal. It passes down the lateral aspect of the leg underneath the cuboid in the peroneal groove to the plantar aspect of the first metatarsal and first cuneiform. The peroneus brevis inserts into the styloid process of the fifth metatarsal and is an abductor of the foot. These two muscles, with their respective arteries, nerves, and motor points, are seen in Figure 7-21.

Intrinsic Musculature of the Foot

DORSAL INTRINSIC MUSCLES

The dorsal intrinsic muscles of the foot are the extensor digitorum brevis and extensor hallucis brevis. These muscles run from the anterior region of the superior lateral aspect of the calcaneus to the dorsum of the first four toes. The extensor hallucis brevis inserts into the base of the proximal phalanx of the great toe, and the extensor digitorum brevis inserts into the base of the second, third, and fourth proximal phalanges. The lateral terminal branch of the deep peroneal nerve innervates these muscles (Fig. 7-22).

PLANTAR INTRINSIC MUSCLES

Layer 1 of Plantar Intrinsic Foot Muscles

There are four layers to the plantar intrinsic muscles of the foot, all of which are innervated by the medial or lateral plantar nerves. The first layer is the most plantar and consists of the following from medial to lateral: the abductor hallucis, flexor digitorum brevis, and abductor digiti minimi pedis. These muscles arise from the calcaneal tuberosity and insert into the toes. They are important in providing dynamic stability to the longitudinal arch (Figs. 7-23 and 7-24).

Layer 2 of Plantar Intrinsic Foot Muscles

The quadratus plantae and lumbricales make up the second layer, along with the tendons of the flexor digitorum longus and flexor hallucis longus as they pass through this region on their way to their respective insertions (Fig. 7-25). The quadratus plantae and lumbricales are in the central aspect of the second layer. The flexor hallucis longus tendon is medial. The flexor digitorum longus tendon begins medially and is then central, with a portion being lateral. The quadratus plantae arises from the two heads on the medial and lateral calcaneal tuberosity and terminates in the tendinous slips, joining the long flexor tendons to the second, third, fourth, and, occasionally, fifth toes. The lumbricales arise from the tendon of the flexor digitorum longus and insert into the dorsal aspect of the proximal phalanges as part of the extensor hood apparatus. Their function is to flex the metatarsophalangeal joint and extend the proximal interphalangeal joint. Paralysis or absence of the lumbricales results in claw toes. Inadvertent sectioning during neuroma surgery results in digital contracture.

Layer 3 of Plantar Intrinsic Foot Muscles

The third layer consists of the adductor hallucis, flexor hallucis brevis, and flexor digiti minimi brevis (Fig. 7-26). The adductor hallucis is in the central and medial portion

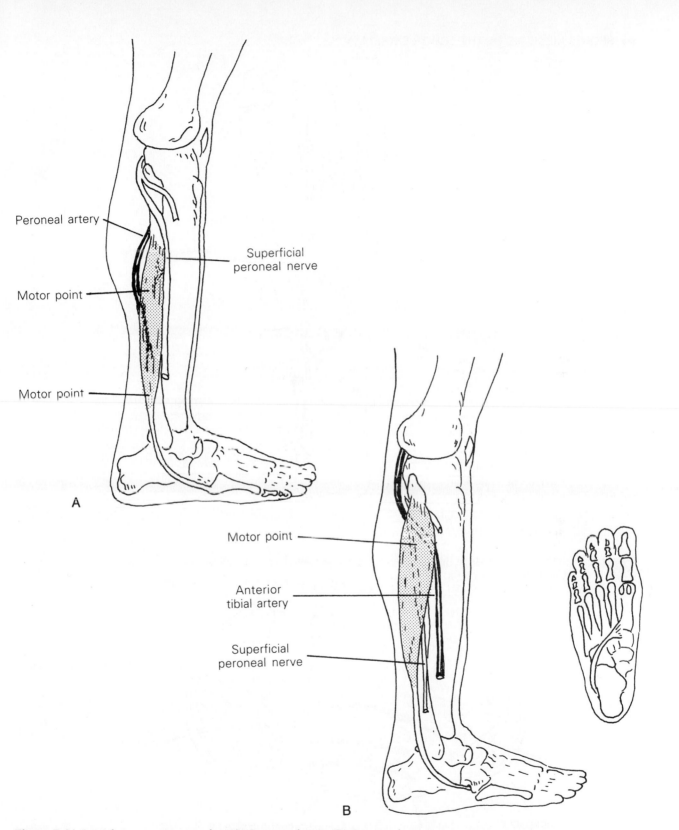

Figure 7-21 Lateral compartment muscles. **(A)** Peroneus brevis. **(B)** Peroneus longus.

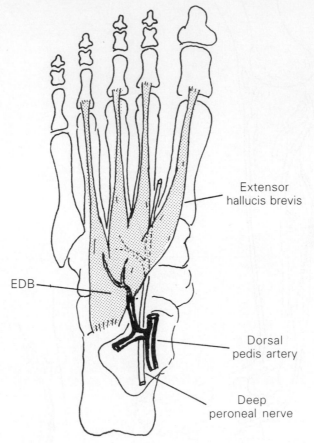

Figure 7-22 Dorsal intrinsic musculature of the foot, showing extensor hallucis brevis and extensor digitorum brevis (EDB).

Figure 7-23 Intrinsic musculature of the foot. Cross-sectional diagram of the relationships of plantar forefoot muscles.

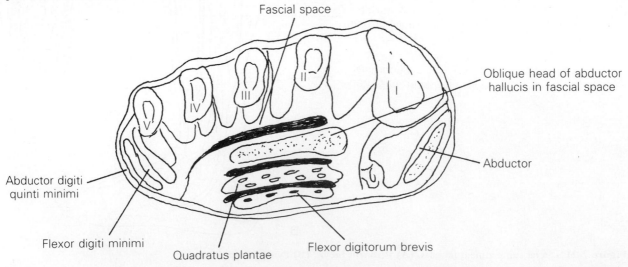

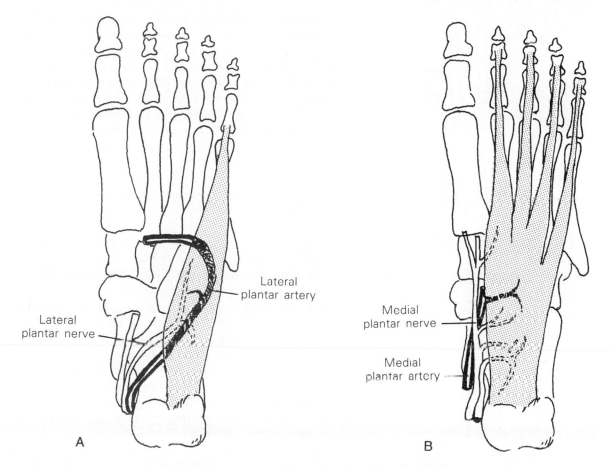

Figure 7-24 Plantar intrinsic muscles, layer 1. **(A)** Abductor digiti minimi pedis. **(B)** Flexor digitorum brevis. (*Figure continues.*)

of the foot; the flexor hallucis brevis is also in the central medial portion, with the flexor digiti minimi brevis at the lateral aspect.

The flexor hallucis brevis arises from the cuboid and lateral cuneiform. It divides into the medial and lateral components before its insertion into the corresponding aspects of the base of the proximal phalanx of the first toe. A sesamoid is present in each of its tendons, the tibial and fibular, respectively, from medial to lateral. This muscle stabilizes the hallux during propulsion. Loss of the medial aspect of the flexor hallucis brevis may result in hallux valgus, whereas absence of function of the lateral head may predispose to hallux varus.

The oblique and transverse heads of the adductor hallucis insert into the lateral border of the flexor hallucis brevis and fibular sesamoid. The bases of the second, third, and fourth metatarsal heads give rise to the oblique head of

the adductor hallucis, while the deep transverse metatarsal ligament between the third, fourth, and fifth metatarsals provides the site of origin for the smaller transverse head.

The abductor digiti minimi pedis inserts into the lateral side of the base of the proximal phalanx of the fifth toe from an origin at the base of the fifth metatarsal (Figs. 7-23 and 7-26).

Layer 4 of Intrinsic Foot Muscles

The fourth layer of intrinsic muscles is made up of the plantar and dorsal interossei. Found also in this layer are the tendons of the peroneus longus and tibialis posterior. The four dorsal interossei are bipennate and are in the intermetatarsal areas. Their function is to abduct the second, third, and fourth toes from an axis through the second metatarsal ray. The three plantar interossei are unipennate

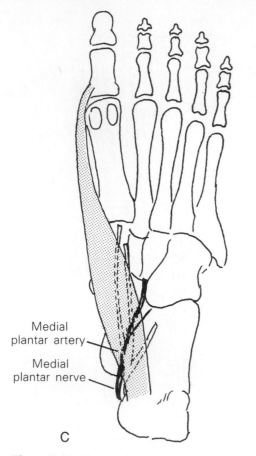

Medial
plantar artery

Medial
plantar nerve

C

Figure 7-24 (*Continued*). **(C)** Abductor hallucis.

and function to adduct the three lateral toes by inserting into the medial sides of the bases of the proximal phalanges of the third, fourth, and fifth toes. Inadvertent sectioning of these tendons while dissecting metatarsophalangeal joints or interspace may lead to digital imbalance (Fig. 7-27).

NERVES

The sciatic nerve (Fig. 7-28) provides the motor and sensory innervation of the foot. It divides into the common peroneal and tibial nerves, both of which are derived from L4 to S3 and lie within a common sheath. The smaller branch, the common peroneal nerve, divides into superficial and deep components. The superficial peroneal nerve (musculocutaneous) provides the cutaneous sensory distri-

bution to the dorsum of the foot, the medial portion of the hallux, the lateral side of the second toe, and the medial surface of the third toe and adjacent sides of the third, fourth, and fifth toes, as well as the lateral portion of the ankle (Figs. 7-29 and 7-30). The motor portion of the superficial peroneal nerve innervates the peroneus longus and brevis muscles. The deep peroneal nerve (anterior tibial nerve) supplies the extensor hallucis longus, tibialis anterior, extensor digitorum longus and brevis, and peroneus tertius, and provides sensory innervation of the first web space (Fig. 7-30B). The third component of the common peroneal nerve is the sural nerve, which provides sensory distribution to the skin of the lateral malleoli of the foot (Fig. 7-29).

The tibial nerve (Fig. 7-31) (posterior tibial or medial popliteal) supplies the medial heel and sole of the foot, as well as the posterior compartments of the leg. It divides into the medial and lateral plantar nerves at the level of the arch, serving the intrinsic muscles of the foot with the exception of the extensor digitorum brevis (Fig. 7-32). The nerve and its branch provide cutaneous innervation to most of the plantar aspect of the foot. The saphenous, the largest cutaneous branch of the femoral nerve (L2 to L4), provides cutaneous innervation to the medial aspect of the foot, often extending as far as the metatarsophalangeal joint of the hallux (Fig. 7-29). It is the only nerve to the foot that is of nonsciatic origin.

ARTERIES

The anterior and posterior tibial arteries and the two terminal branches of the popliteal arteries constitute the main blood supply to the foot (Fig. 7-33). The anterior tibial artery, in concert with the associated deep veins, passes beneath the superior and inferior extensor retinacula to the dorsum of the foot as the dorsalis pedis artery. The anterior tibial artery also gives rise to the anterior medial and lateral malleolar arteries. The origin of the anastomotic network is formed by the anterior malleolar arteries. The medial and lateral tarsal branches are derived from the dorsalis pedis. The dorsalis pedis gives rise to the arcuate artery and the first dorsal and plantar metatarsal artery (Fig. 7-33).

The larger posterior tibial artery, in accompanying the deep veins, courses behind the medial malleolus, just medial to the tendo Achillis, and divides into the medial and lateral plantar arteries after passing underneath the flexor retinaculum. The smaller medial plantar artery supplies the medial aspect of the first ray. The larger lateral plantar artery anastomoses with the dorsalis pedis to create the

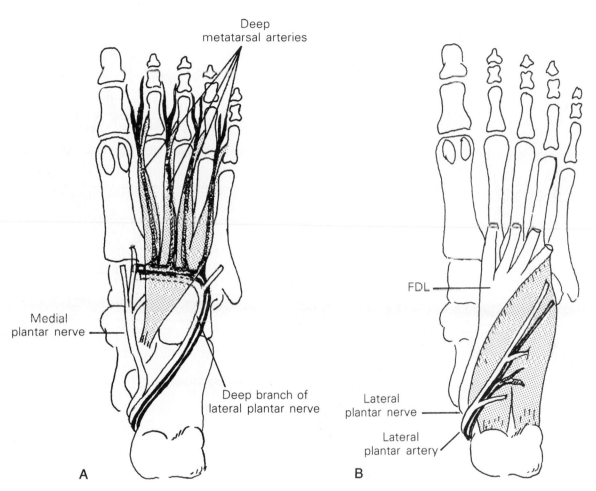

Figure 7-25 Plantar intrinsic muscles, layer 2. **(A)** Lumbricales. **(B)** Flexor accessorius (quadratus plantar).

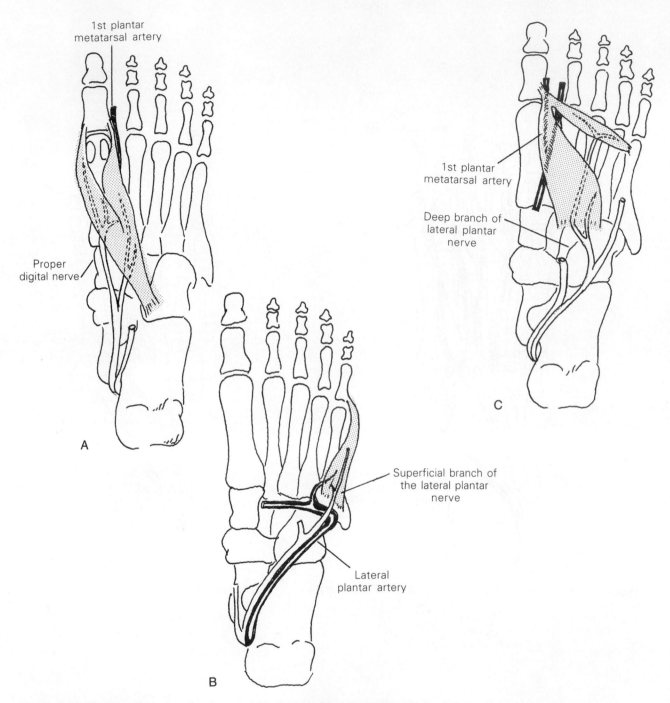

Figure 7-26 Plantar intrinsic muscles, layer 3. **(A)** Flexor hallucis brevis. **(B)** Flexor digiti minimi brevis. **(C)** Adductor hallucis.

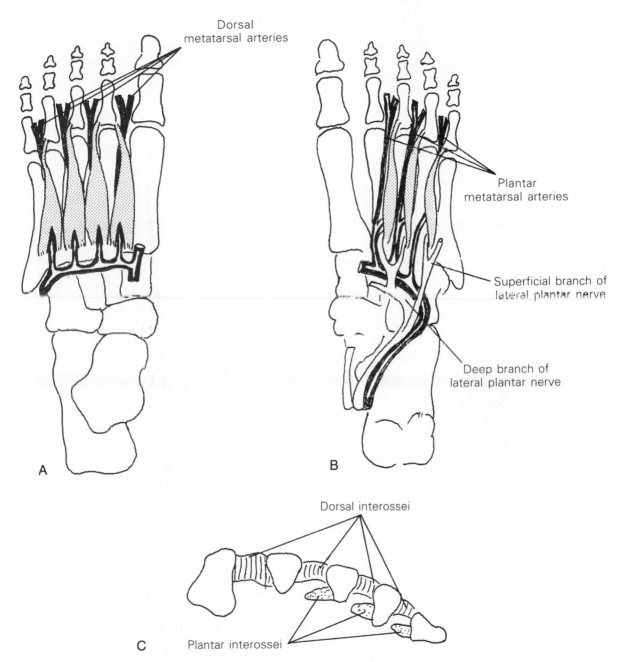

Figure 7-27 Plantar intrinsic muscles, layer 4. **(A)** Dorsal interossei. **(B)** Plantar interossei. **(C)** Relationships of interosseus muscles.

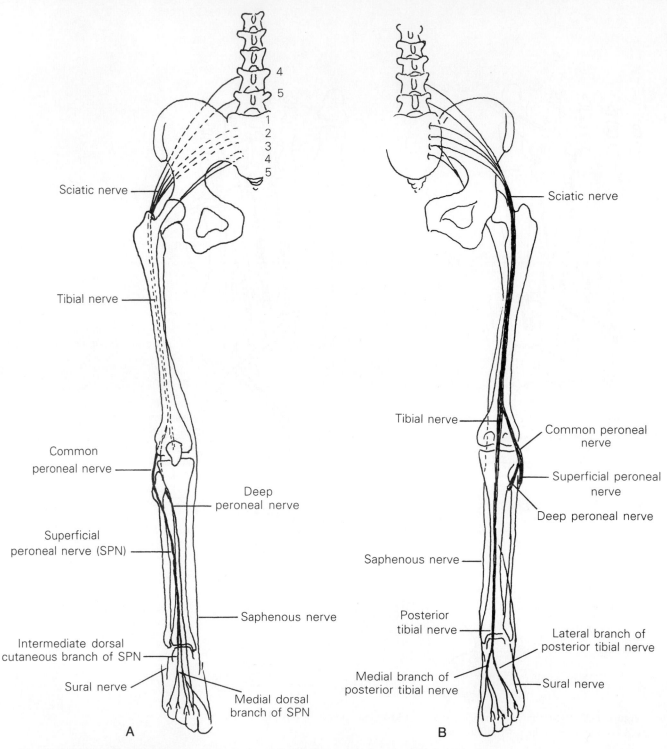

Figure 7-28 Neurology of the leg. **(A)** Anterior view. **(B)** Posterior view. (Adapted from Turek S: Orthopaedics: Principles and Their Applications. 4th Ed. JB Lippincott, Philadelphia, 1983, with permission.)

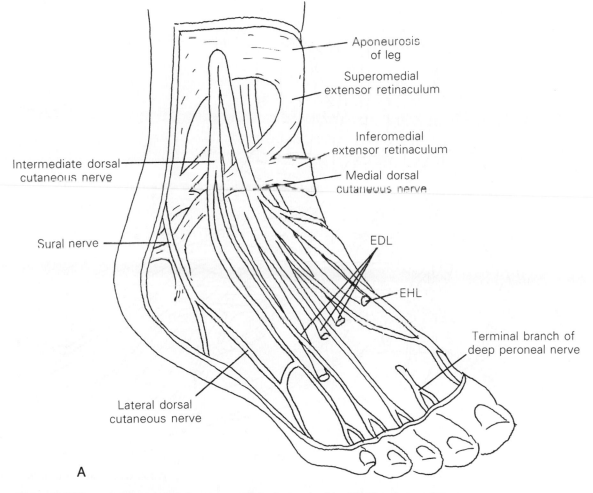

Aponeurosis
of leg

Superomedial
extensor retinaculum

Inferomedial
extensor retinaculum

Intermediate dorsal
cutaneous nerve

Medial dorsal
cutaneous nerve

Sural nerve

EDL

EHL

Terminal branch of
deep peroneal nerve

Lateral dorsal
cutaneous nerve

A

Figure 7-29 Lateral nerves and vital structures of the foot and ankle. **(A)** Dorsal view. (*Figure continues.*)

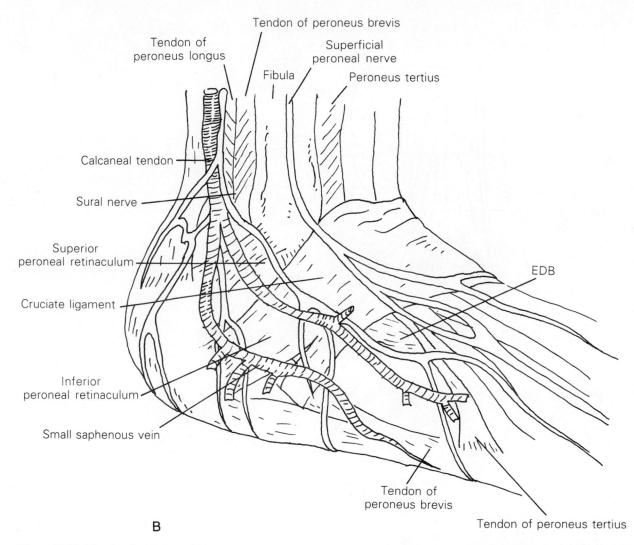

B

Figure 7-29 (*Continued*). **(B)** Lateral view.

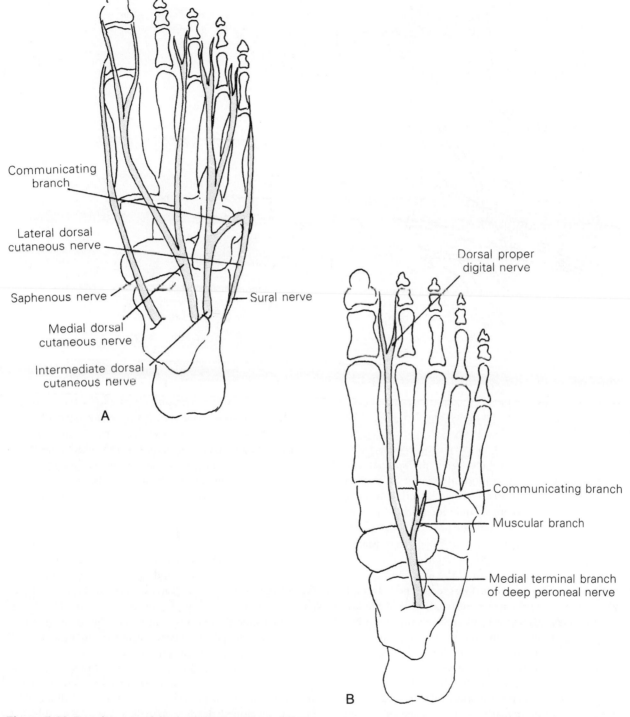

Communicating branch

Lateral dorsal cutaneous nerve

Saphenous nerve

Medial dorsal cutaneous nerve

Intermediate dorsal cutaneous nerve

Sural nerve

A

Dorsal proper digital nerve

Communicating branch

Muscular branch

Medial terminal branch of deep peroneal nerve

B

Figure 7-30 Dorsal nerves of the foot. **(A)** Superficial. **(B)** Deep.

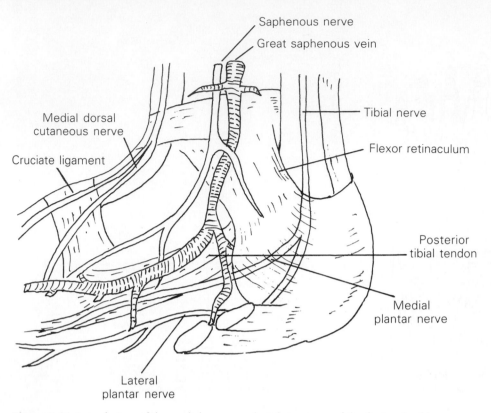

Saphenous nerve
Great saphenous vein
Medial dorsal cutaneous nerve
Cruciate ligament
Tibial nerve
Flexor retinaculum
Posterior tibial tendon
Medial plantar nerve
Lateral plantar nerve

Figure 7-31 Lateral view of the medial nerves and vital structures of the foot and ankle.

plantar vascular arch, which provides the arterial supply to the intermetatarsal spaces and digits (Fig. 7-33). The largest branch of the posterior tibial artery is the perforating peroneal artery, which supplies the lateral and posterior aspects of the calcaneus to anastomosis with the anterior lateral malleolar branches. It is important to bear in mind that there is a wide variation in arterial architecture in the foot and leg. Up to 15 percent of individuals may be missing a dorsalis pedis artery, although the posterior tibial is almost always present. When the anterior tibial artery is absent, a dorsal peroneal artery may be present.

The venous drainage system of the foot consists of both superficial and deep branches. The greater and lesser saphenous veins are the principal superficial veins of the lower leg, with a deep plantar venous arch serving as a primary deep drainage system. This arch system empties into the venae comitantes, uniting in the region of the interosseous membrane to form the popliteal vein, which eventually empties into the femoral vein. It is important to note that the superficial and deep networks of the veins communicate extensively, particularly near the edge of the ankle and the distal and medial portion of the leg. The valvular

arrangement in the perforating veins allows for blood to flow from the superficial veins to the deep network, but not in the opposite direction under normal conditions.

There are no lymphatic nodes found within the foot. The dorsal aspect of the foot receives the lymphatic plexus of the digits within the lymphatic vessels, following the course of the saphenous vein to the inguinal or popliteal nodes.

SUMMARY

Knowledge of normal anatomy serves as a common reference point for evaluation and treatment of various maladies of the human body. Variations from the normal are commonplace. For example, an accessory branch of the extensor hallucis brevis may cross over the medial branch of the superficial peroneal nerve, causing entrapment neuropathy. The gastrocnemius muscle belly may extend distally into the ankle, predisposing to chronic posterior compartment syndrome. A tibial sesamoid may be congenitally absent, leading to hallux valgus. The abductor hallucis may be overdeveloped, leading to hallux varus. Examples of anatomic variation are numerous. A strong basis in normal

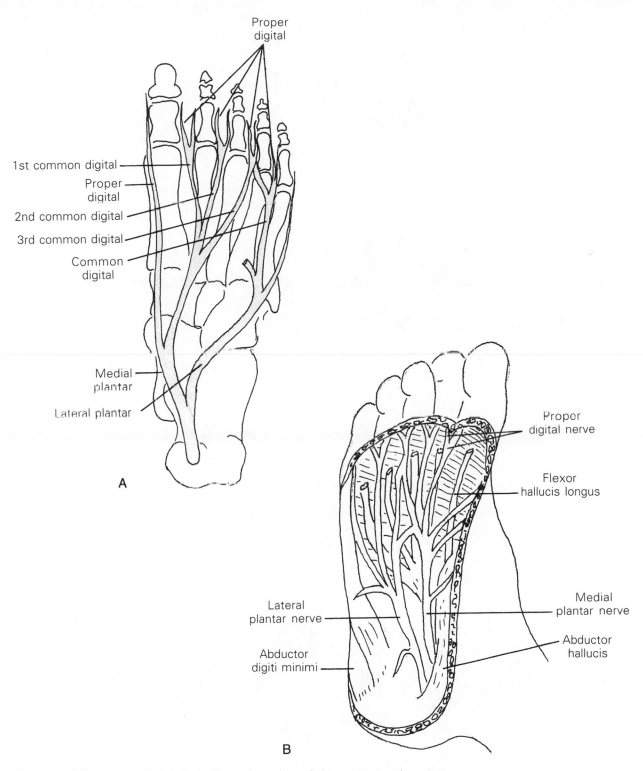

Proper
digital

1st common digital
Proper
digital
2nd common digital
3rd common digital
Common
digital

Medial
plantar

Lateral plantar

A

Proper
digital nerve

Flexor
hallucis longus

Lateral
plantar nerve

Medial
plantar nerve

Abductor
digiti minimi

Abductor
hallucis

B

Figure 7-32 Plantar nerves of the foot. **(A)** Relationships of plantar nerves and contiguous structures. **(B)** Diagram of plantar nerves.

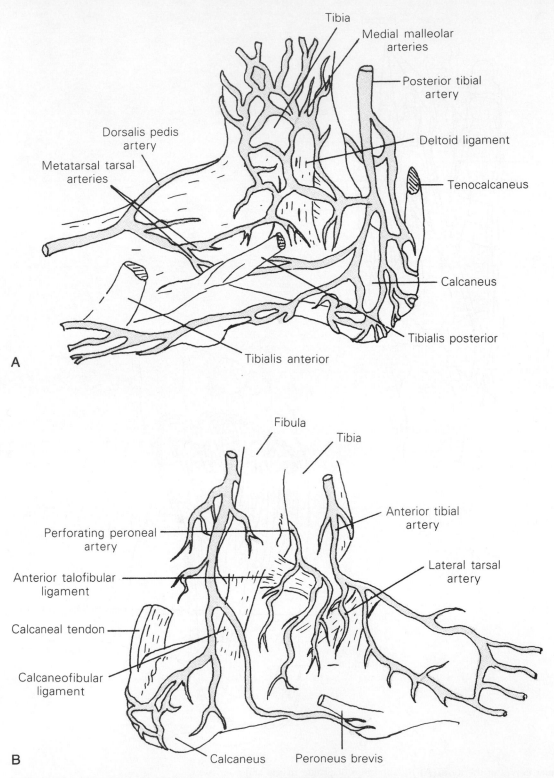

Figure 7-33 Arteries and veins of the foot and ankle. **(A)** Medial. **(B)** Lateral. (*Figure continues.*)

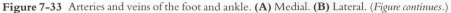

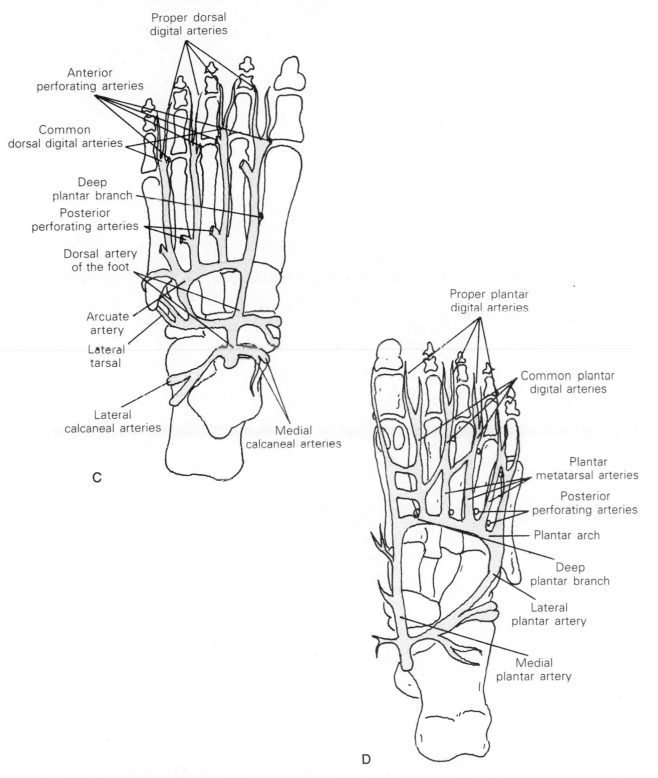

Figure 7-33 (*Continued*). **(C)** Dorsal. **(D)** Plantar. (*Figure continues.*)

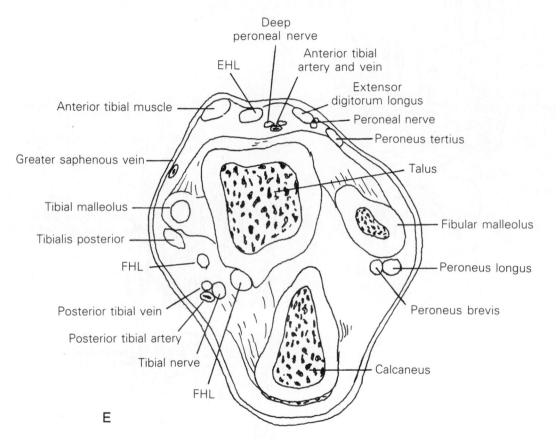

E

Figure 7-33 (*Continued*). (**E**) Cross section of ankle at joint level.

anatomy is the foundation for understanding function as well as pathology.

SUGGESTED READINGS

Draves DJ: Anatomy of the Lower Extremity. Williams & Wilkins, Baltimore, 1986

Evans EG: Biomechanical Studies of the Musculoskeletal System. Charles C Thomas, Springfield, IL, 1961

Helfet AJ, Gruebel Lee DM: Disorders of the Foot. JB Lippincott, Philadelphia, 1980

Inman VT: Surgery of the Foot. 3rd Ed. CV Mosby, St. Louis, 1973

Inman VT: The Joints of the Ankle. Williams & Wilkins, Baltimore, 1976

Inman VT, Ralston HJ, Todd F: Human Walking. Williams & Wilkins, Baltimore, 1984

Kapandji IA: The Physiology of the Joints. Vol. 2. The Lower Limb. 5th Ed. Churchill Livingstone, Edinburgh, 1988

Mack RP: The Foot and Leg in Running Sports. CV Mosby, St. Louis, 1982

McGlamry ED, Banks AS, Downey MS: Comprehensive Textbook of Foot Surgery. p. 3. Williams & Wilkins, Baltimore, 1992

McMinn RMH, Hutchings RT, Logan BM: Color Atlas of Foot and Ankle Anatomy. 2nd Ed. CV Mosby, St. Louis, 1996

Moore KL: Clinically Oriented Anatomy. Williams & Wilkins, Baltimore, 1980

Nordin M, Frankel VH: Basic Biomechanics of the Musculoskeletal System. 2nd Ed. Williams & Wilkins, Baltimore, 1989

Root ML, Orien WP, Weed JH: Normal and Abnormal Function of the Foot. Clinical Biomechanics, Los Angeles, 1977

Sarrafian SK: Anatomy of the Foot and Ankle. 2nd Ed. JB Lippincott, Philadelphia, 1993

Steindler A: Kinesiology of the Human Body Under Normal and Pathological Conditions. Charles C Thomas, Springfield, IL, 1970

Travell JG, Simons DG: Myofascial Pain and Dysfunction: The Trigger Point Manual. Vol. 2 The Lower Extremity. Williams & Wilkins, Baltimore, 1992

Williams PL (ed): Gray's Anatomy. 38th Ed. Churchill Livingstone, Edinburgh, 1995

8

Functional Anatomy

STEVEN I. SUBOTNICK

Phasic activity of the muscles in various activities, as well as muscle function relative to joint position and axis and activity, are important considerations in sports medicine. A considerable amount is known about the phasic activity of muscles during normal ambulation on various surfaces, as well as walking uphill and downhill.[1-9] Burns et al.[10] have broken the gait cycle down into phases, and muscular activity is described in reference to these phases rather than in precise percentages. The phasic activities that they recorded are a compilation of reports of many investigators. These results are shown in Figure 8-1. This graphic representation shows that various muscles belonging to associated muscle groups have similar phasic activity. The groups also have similar function in that their anatomic location allows for similar function as the muscles and tendons cross the various axes of the joints of the foot. Figure 8-1 demonstrates that the stance phase is 60 percent of the total gait cycle, whereas the swing phase constitutes 40 percent.

The posterior superficial muscle group consists of the gastrocnemius, soleus, and plantaris. The deep posterior muscle group consists of the posterior tibial, flexor digitorum longus, and flexor hallucis longus. The lateral muscle group consists of the peroneus longus and peroneus brevis. The anterior muscle group (pretibial group) consists of the anterior tibial, extensor hallucis longus, extensor digitorum longus, and peroneus tertius.

The intrinsic musculature dorsally contains the extensor digitorum brevis and the extensor hallucis brevis. The medial plantar intrinsic musculature includes the abductor hallucis and the flexor digitorum brevis. Other deep plantar

intrinsic muscles include the quadratus plantae, the lumbricales, the flexor hallucis brevis, and the adductor hallucis.

Phasic activity can generally be divided into swing phase and stance phase. The posterior superficial muscle group is active throughout most of the stance phase of gait, ceasing its activity after heel-off just before toe-off.

The deep posterior musculature includes the posterior tibial muscle. It is active from contact until push-off. The flexor muscle group, consisting of the flexor digitorum longus and flexor hallucis longus, becomes active from 10 percent of the stance phase of gait, at the end of contact, throughout midstance, until toe-off. This group takes over at the final stages of propulsion after the posterior superficial muscle group has ceased its activity. The lateral muscle group is active during both midstance and propulsion. The posterior superficial, posterior deep, and lateral musculature are therefore primarily active during stance phase and are called the gravity muscle group.

The antigravity muscle group is active during the swing phase. The anterior tibial, extensor hallucis longus, and extensor digitorum longus are biphasic. They function during the end of the stance phase as well as during the early portion of the swing phase. There is also function during the late swing and early contact phases.

The dorsal intrinsic musculature is active during midstance and propulsion. The plantar intrinsic musculature is active from midstance to liftoff. With walking, then, it can be seen that those muscles active during the first 15 percent of the entire gait cycle are assisting in decelerating the rapid plantar flexion of the forefoot as it approaches the support surface. These muscles also stabilize the rearfoot at initial heel strike, as well as decelerating the internal rota-

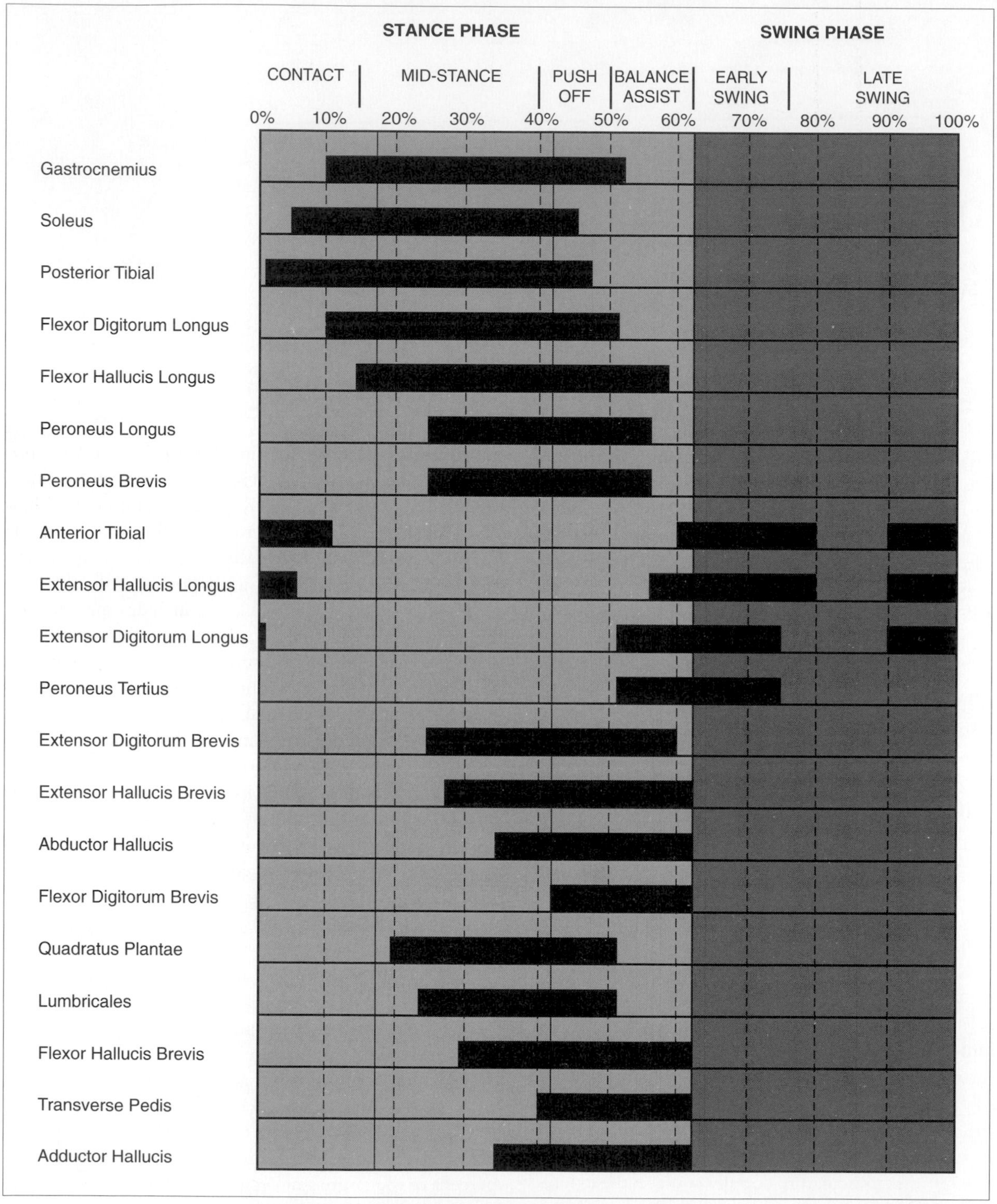

Figure 8-1 Phasic muscular activity during normal ambulation. (From McGlamry, JE: Fundamentals of Foot Surgery. Williams & Wilkins, Baltimore, 1987, with permission.)

tion of the tibia and concomitant closed kinetic chain pronation of the foot. Those muscles that are active during the midstance portion of gait are involved in resupination from the maximally pronated position at the beginning of midstance, to a neutral position at the middle of midstance, to a supinated position at heel-off and toe-off. Those muscles that are active during propulsion stabilize the metatarsophalangeal joint, flexing the metatarsophalangeal joints, plantar-flexing the first ray, and supinating the forefoot. Thus, at the end of propulsion into early swing, the muscles dorsiflex the foot, preparing it to clear the ground. Those muscles that are active at the later portions of the swing phase function to stabilize the forefoot and decrease foot slap.

COMPARISON OF WALKING AND RUNNING PHASIC ACTIVITY

During normal walking at a rate of 120 steps/min, each walking cycle (from heel strike to heel strike of the same foot) consumes 1 second. The stance portion of this cycle is approximately 60 percent or, in real time, 0.6 second. Given a runner proceeding at a pace of 6 min/mile, the total cycle time is 0.6 second, and the stance phase is approximately 0.2 second. By increasing speed, the runner has decreased the time the foot is on the ground from 0.6 second (600 msec) to 0.2 second (200 msec). That being the case, all events occurring during the stance phase must occur three times faster as the speed of gait is increased. The period of time between initial ground contact and maximum pronation is 150 msec during walking but 30 msec during running.

In running, the subtalar joint reaches its maximum angular velocity within 15 msec. The heel contacts the support surface in a more inverted position. Each of these events requires that all the extrinsic muscles acting on the foot become active simultaneously at foot contact during running (Subotnick SI, Chu D: Unpublished clinical data, California State University, Department of Kinesiology, 1973). Furthermore, the electromyographic muscle activity can be increased or decreased, depending on biomechanical stability or instability of the foot or speed (Subotnick SI, Chu D: Unpublished clinical data, California State University, Department of Kinesiology, 1973; Subotnick SI, Aston J, Carrollo J: Unpublished research, Texas Scottish Rite Hospital for Crippled Children, Department of Biomechanics, Dallas, 1982).

Knowledge of the phasic activity of the various muscles and muscle groups in walking helps explain the function of these muscle groups during running and other sport activities. It must be understood as well that, as the speed of running increases, the impact force and the amount of energy absorbed by the muscles progressively increase as well. The four major extrinsic muscle groups affecting the function of the foot, as well as their individual muscle components, are discussed below.

EXTRINSIC MUSCLES OF THE FOOT

Posterior Superficial Muscle Group

The posterior calf muscle group, the gastrocnemius–soleus group and the peroneal muscles, appear to function as a unit. During walking, this group is active during the midstance phase, when it resists the progressive dorsiflexion of the ankle joint through an eccentric contraction.[4,11] After this group initiates plantar flexion of the ankle joint, activity ceases. In running, however, this muscle group becomes active late in the swing phase and remains active for approximately 70 percent of the stance phase. The late swing phase and initial stance phase activity most likely provide stability to the ankle and subtalar joints while controlling the forward movement of the tibia over the fixed foot. This eccentric contraction lasts for approximately 50 percent of the plantar flexion of the foot.

Recalling that the triceps surae has its origins from the femoral condyles and inserts into the posterior one-third of the calcaneus, it becomes obvious that this muscle group acts on three joints: the knee, ankle, and subtalar. In open kinetic chain action, the triceps surae is a flexor of the knee, plantar flexor of the ankle, and supinator of the subtalar joint. During closed kinetic chain activity, the triceps surae has a considerable stabilizing role as it undergoes eccentric rather than concentric contraction. The function of the triceps after heel contact is to decelerate knee extension. This is done by decreasing the forward progression of the tibia while undergoing an eccentric contraction. As the soleus plantar-flexes the foot, the lateral column is stabilized. This eccentric contraction is approximately six times more effective than a similar concentric contraction would be in producing force and stability (Fig. 8-2A).

The next function of the triceps surae is to simultaneously flex the knee and plantar-flex the ankle. During final propulsion, plantar flexion of the ankle has reached its peak, and the activity of the gastrocnemius is ceasing. During midstance, the triceps contraction helps convert the

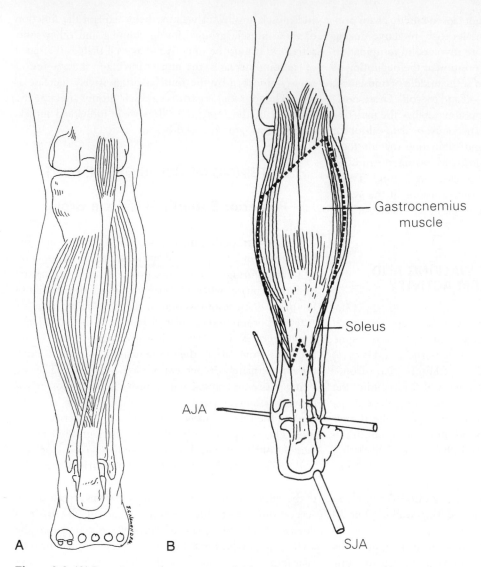

Figure 8-2 (**A**) Posterior muscle group, superficial, with gastrocnemius removed. (**B**) Posterior muscle group, superficial; also subtalar and ankle joint axes. SJA, subtalar joint axis; AJA, ankle joint axis.

foot from a mobile adaptor to a rigid lever. It stabilizes the lateral column of the foot while the peroneus longus plantar-flexes the first ray in preparation of propulsion. The foot thus becomes a rigid lever, ensuring forefoot stability.

There is controversy regarding the amount of push-off accomplished by the posterior superficial muscle group during normal walking. Some investigators who have studied the triceps surae believe that the main function of this group during walking is restraint of the forward movement of the tibia over the ankle rather than active plantar flexion of the forefoot against the support surface, producing active push-off. This same concept may hold true for unidirectional running on relatively level surfaces at a constant speed. This is not the case with acceleration, deceleration, jumping, or rapid turns. During these activities, the triceps surae is active, and active forces are generated during propulsion. The triceps may also be assisted by the long flexors of the great toe and lesser toes during running and, especially, jumping sports. Because this muscle group crosses three joints, it has enormous influence on the function of biomechanics of the lower extremity. Tightness or contracture of this muscle group can cause improper function of the knee, ankle, or subtalar joints (Fig. 8-2B). The muscle undergoes concentric, eccentric, and isometric contraction. It can therefore be easily injured, as can the Achilles tendon, from sudden rapid excessive motion at any one of these joints. An example of rapid dorsiflexion of the foot at the ankle when the triceps surae is acting as a stabilizer for the knee, ankle, and subtalar joint is skiing downhill and then suddenly hitting an uphill object. Another example would be during rebounding (landing on another player's foot), which can cause a rapid, forceful, unexpected dorsiflexion of the foot when the muscles are prepared for contact on the ball of the foot (Fig. 8-2B).

Posterior Deep Muscle Group

The posterior deep muscle group has been called the flexor muscle group. It includes the posterior tibial, flexor digitorum longus, and flexor hallucis longus. The long flexors act together as a unit, whereas the posterior tibial has some unique functions and activity.

POSTERIOR TIBIAL MUSCLE

The posterior tibial muscle originates from the lateral posterior aspect of the body of the tibia and the medial aspect of the body of the fibula, as well as the interosseous membrane of the proximal two-thirds of the leg. It passes over the deltoid ligament in the flexor canal and inserts into the navicular, giving off branches into the cuneiforms as well as the metatarsal bases. In an open kinetic chain, it is a weak plantar flexor of the ankle, yet a substantial supinator of the subtalar and midtarsal joints. During walking, the posterior tibial muscle is a decelerator of initial rapid pronation that takes place at the subtalar joint until 50 percent of the gait cycle. It then functions as a stabilizer of the midtarsal joint and helps reverse leg rotation through subtalar joint resupination. This takes place primarily around the midtarsal joint oblique axis. The importance of this muscle is readily appreciated when observing the patient with weakness or a rupture of the posterior tibial tendon. There is a progressive eversion of the calcaneus with lowering of the medial longitudinal arch, as the foot pronates and loses its ability to function (Fig. 8-3A and B). During running, there is rapid internal rotation of the tibia as the calcaneus goes from an inverted to an everted position. This inversion is secondary to the functional

varus of running, with its narrow base of gait, as well as the activity of the anterior tibial muscle, which acts actively during the late portion of the swing phase of gait to produce dorsiflexion and inversion of the foot.[12] In Cavanagh's series, the average subject contacted in a position of 4 to 6 degrees of inversion and then actively pronated to about 10 degrees calcaneal eversion. Some subjects landed in 30-degree inversion and pronated to a 5-degree inverted position. Others landed in 5 to 6 degrees of inversion and pronated to 25 degrees of eversion.

Subotnick found that those runners with calcaneal varus or cavus foot landed in a high degree of inversion, yet had more transverse plane rotation of the tibia than calcaneal eversion going from initial heel strike to the foot-flat position (unpublished data from clinical observations, 1986). Those patients with a normal foot landed in about 10 to 12 degrees of varus and then rapidly pronated to 6 or 8 degrees of valgus. Those with a weaker or more pronated foot landed in 6 to 8 degrees of calcaneal inversion and pronated up to 15 or 16 degrees of calcaneal eversion. The addition of a running shoe increased the amount of pronation due to the softness of the midsole material and the ability of the foot and counter to pronate through the midsole at the medial aspect of the shoe. There was considerably more pronation during running than during walking, especially in those athletes who had more "normal feet." They might walk with a minimal amount of pronation yet, during running, would have excessive pronation due to a combination of factors, including functional varus, impact or contact forces, and accentuated biomechanical abnormalities (e.g., forefoot varus or supinatus, or both). All these movements place a considerable load on the posterior tibial tendon in an attempt to decrease the rapid internal rotation of the tibia while decelerating concurrent lowering of the medial longitudinal arch (Fig. 8-3).

LONG FLEXOR GROUP

The long flexors have similar action, which occurs nearly simultaneously. The flexor digitorum longus arises from the posterior aspect of the tibia and inserts into the base of the distal phalanx of the four lesser toes. It produces open kinetic chain supination of the subtalar as well as the midtarsal oblique joint. This weak plantar flexor of the ankle functions during an open kinetic chain to plantarflex the digits at the metatarsophalangeal joints. In a closed kinetic chain situation in which the digits are stable, the effects of the flexor digitorum longus are to stabilize the metatarsophalangeal joints as momentum carries the foot

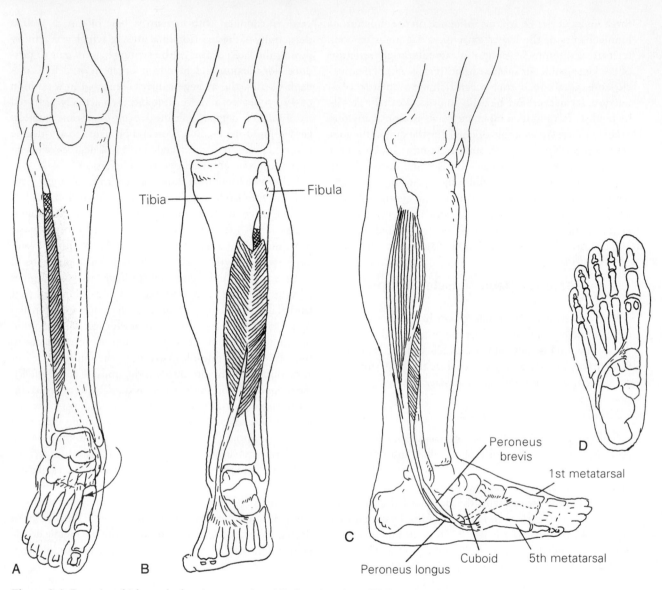

Figure 8–3 Posterior tibial muscle showing pronation. **(A)** Anterior view. **(B)** Posterior view. **(C)** Lateral view. **(D)** Plantar view.

over these joints during propulsion. The flexor hallucis longus originates from the distal two-thirds of the posterior surface of the fibula, inserting into the plantar aspect of the base of the distal phalanx of the hallux. It follows the same course as the flexor digitorum longus, just medial to the os trigonum, and passes through the tarsal tunnel. The flexor hallucis longus has a function similar to that of the flexor digitorum longus at the ankle, subtalar, and midtarsal joints. Its primary action at the midtarsal joint is about the

oblique axis. It produces open kinetic chain supination at the subtalar and oblique midtarsal joints and, depending on the longitudinal axis of the midtarsal joint location, can produce midtarsal joint inversion. Its effect on the hallux is similar to that of the digitorum longus on the lesser digits. During normal ambulation, it produces translatory stabilization. During jumping, cutting, and running sports with changes of velocity, as well as diving or working out on a trampoline, active plantar flexion takes place just before toe-off or liftoff. The flexor digitorum longus becomes active sooner than the flexor hallucis longus, which remains active longer. Both are active during the latter stages of contact, throughout midstance, and during the initial and later stages of the propulsive stage of normal ambulation. Interestingly enough, there is no activity during the latter stages of propulsion during normal ambulation, suggesting that the final phases of propulsion are liftoff rather than active propulsion. The flexors remain active throughout the propulsive phase of running sports and, in fact, are active throughout the stance phase.

When the toes are stable, the long flexors assist the posterior tibial muscles in stabilizing the subtalar and midtarsal joints during closed kinetic chain function. When the digits are unstable, such as with hammertoe deformity, the long flexors produce progressive instability and deformity at the interphalangeal and metatarsophalangeal joints. A weak posterior tibial tendon may be surgically reinforced with the long flexors.

Lateral Muscle Group

The lateral extrinsic muscle group consists of the peroneus longus and peroneus brevis.

PERONEUS LONGUS

The peroneus longus originates from the head and lateral aspect of the proximal two-thirds of the fibula (Fig. 8-4). It passes posterior to the lateral malleolus and inferior to it in a groove shared with the peroneus brevis. It continues out along the calcaneus to the lateral side of the cuboid, where it then passes plantarly in the peroneal cuboid groove, as it goes obliquely distally and inserts into the lateral aspect of the base of the first metatarsal and medial cuneiform. During normal ambulation, it has a weak potential for plantar flexion at the ankle joint. It has open kinetic chain potential to pronate the subtalar joint. It likewise has the potential to pronate the oblique axis of the midtarsal joint while everting about the longitudinal axis in an open kinetic chain situation. It inserts into the base of the first metatarsal nearly perpendicular to the axis of motion of the first ray. In an open kinetic chain, it produces plantar flexion as well as eversion of the first ray.

In a closed kinetic chain, the peroneus longus resists plantar flexion of the foot by plantar-flexing the first ray. In normal ambulation, the peroneus longus is active during the latter three-fourths of midstance into the early and middle stages of propulsion. As it plantar-flexes the first

ray, inversion occurs at the forefoot, resulting in supination at the subtalar joint. A hyperactive or strong peroneus longus with a weak antagonistic anterior tibial muscle, therefore, produces a cavus foot with plantar flexion of the first ray and supination of the forefoot as well as subtalar joint (Fig. 8-5).

The activity of the peroneus longus during normal ambulation is to stabilize the lateral column of the foot (the calcaneocuboid joint) while also providing for stability of the medial column of the foot (the first ray). The cuboid

Figure 8-4 **(A)** Lateral muscle group. **(B)** Plantar view, showing insertion of the peroneus longus into the medial cuneiform and first metatarsal.

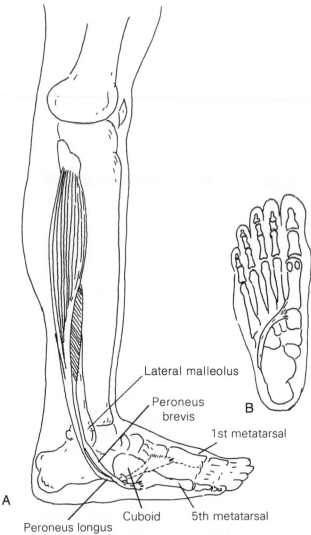

Lateral malleolus

Peroneus brevis

1st metatarsal

B

A

Peroneus longus

Cuboid

5th metatarsal

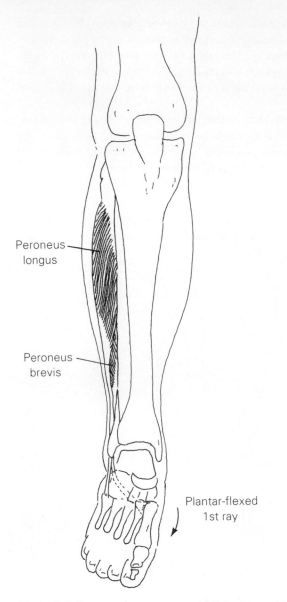

Peroneus
longus

Peroneus
brevis

Plantar-flexed
1st ray

Figure 8-5 Peroneus longus spasm and tightness resulting in a plantar-flexed first ray.

umn of the foot. The peroneus longus is assisted by the posterior tibial and long plantar musculature, as well as the plantar fascia and the locking mechanism in the midtarsal joint, in stabilizing the medial column of the foot. A weak peroneus longus muscle, secondary to neuromuscular causes, or an unstable calcaneocuboid joint, leads to metatarsus primus elevatus and a dorsal bunion.

In running, the peroneus longus may be used as an adjunctory plantar flexor. Faster, more talented long-distance runners tend to have a greater range of plantar flexion at the ankle joint. They plantar-flex actively just before contact when landing on the ball of the foot. The peroneus longus is used for this active plantar flexion and to stabilize the foot during impact. It creates a functional cavus when it is overdeveloped. Athletes with 3 to 4 degrees of forefoot varus may function mildly pronated during normal ambulation yet function with a relatively plantar-flexed first ray and cavus foot during fast running. Obviously, orthoses with medial buildup, although useful for walking, would be damaging for running in these athletes. When functional forefoot valgus is present, a lateral forefoot wedge is helpful to control excessive supinatory forces with lateral instability of the foot and ankle. A functional forefoot valgus may also be present during jumping and rebound sports as the athlete actively plantar-flexes the first ray in preparation for touchdown following jumping maneuvers. A forefoot lateral wedge likewise may be useful in preventing sprains or strain in these athletes.

PERONEUS BREVIS

The peroneus brevis originates from the distal two-thirds of the fibula and is deep to the peroneus longus. As with all the brevis muscles, the muscle extends more distal than the corresponding longus muscle. It passes in a groove similar to that of the peroneus longus and then attaches to the lateral aspect of the styloid process of the base of the fifth metatarsal. In an open kinetic chain, it exerts a weak plantar-flexory force at the ankle joint. Its primary action is about the fifth metatarsal cuboid and calcaneocuboid articulations (Fig. 8-5).

It has activity similar to the peroneus longus muscle, but with slightly longer duration. It becomes active about midway through midstance and continues in its activity until just before toe-off.

In a closed kinetic chain, little motion is accomplished. The chief purpose is that of stabilization of the lateral column of the foot, especially at the calcaneocuboid joint. In doing so, it assists the peroneus longus in its function of plantar-flexing the first ray and providing for medial column stability during ambulation and propulsion.

must be stable for the peroneus longus to produce plantar flexion of the first ray. The stability of the calcaneocuboid joint is dependent on subtalar joint functioning around a neutral or supinated position. The midtarsal joint must be fully pronated about the oblique axis, and the peroneus brevis and triceps surae actively stabilize the lateral column of the foot relative to the support surface. With this stable fulcrum, the peroneus longus can stabilize the medial col-

Pathology of the subtalar or midtarsal joints, such as a coalition, fracture, or arthritis, causes the peroneus brevis to act as a splinter, abducting the forefoot. A spastic peroneus brevis muscle is a tipoff to pathology in the subtalar or midtarsal joints.

Both the peroneus longus and peroneus brevis muscles must be strengthened and rehabilitated following lateral ankle sprains. Appropriate kinesthetic strength and flexibility of these muscles are important in preventing recurrent lateral ankle sprains.

The peroneus brevis is opposed by the posterior tibial muscle. It abducts the forefoot, whereas the posterior tibial adducts the forefoot. When the peroneus brevis tendon, in part or in whole, is used for lateral stabilization of the ankle, little functional loss occurs in the foot.

Anterior Muscle Group

The anterior muscle group has been called the pretibial group or the antigravity group. All three muscles act in concert. In normal ambulation, they are active just before toe-off, and their activity continues throughout the swing

Figure 8-6 Function of anterior muscle group (shaded) during gait.

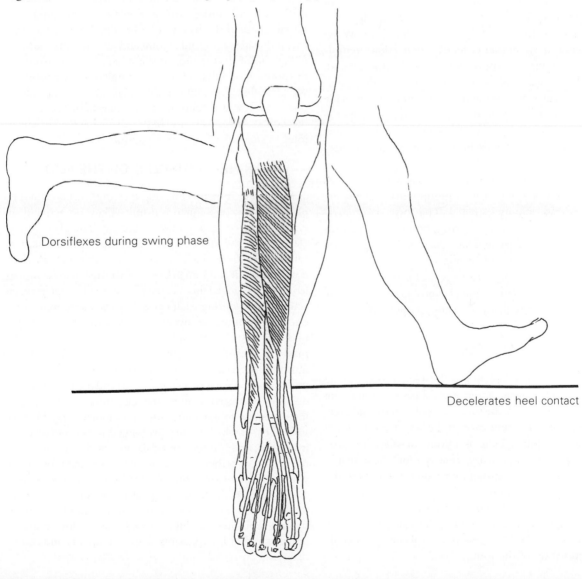

Dorsiflexes during swing phase

Decelerates heel contact

phase, when activity ceases at the midway portion of contact. The muscles function throughout the swing phase; however, they are biphasic. Stance phase activity takes place when there is limited weight stress passing through the foot.

The activity of the anterior muscles, as a group, during the late swing and early contact phase is to decelerate plantar flexion of the forefoot against the support surface, in effect reducing foot slap. During propulsion, this group functions in the stability of the metatarsophalangeal joint, as well as in dorsiflexion of the toes and forefoot to clear the toes of the support surface during propulsion and early swing (Fig. 8-6).

The anterior muscle group undergoes an eccentric or lengthening contraction at the end of the stance phase and a concentric or shortening contraction during the swing phase, followed by another eccentric contraction after initial ground contact, until the foot is flat on the ground. During the late stance phase, just before toe-off, they function in stabilizing the foot and ankle. They then provide dorsiflexion at the ankle joint to provide for adequate toe clearance during swing. These muscles are active in controlling initial plantar flexion of the forefoot until the foot-flat position.

As the speed of ambulation increases, swing phase activity of the anterior compartment group remains the same, but stance phase activity increases. The anterior compartment muscles remain active during the initial 50 percent of the stance phase of gait and then decrease in their activity after the ankle joint begins plantar-flexing. During running, this group functions to provide for stability of the ankle during initial contact and also provides for acceleration of the tibia over the foot during propulsion.

ANTERIOR TIBIAL MUSCLE

The anterior tibial muscle is a dorsiflexor of the ankle joint. The tendon of the anterior tibial passes through the subtalar joint axis when the subtalar joint is in neutral position. It functions as a supinator of the subtalar joint when the subtalar is supinated and as a pronator when it is pronated. It has a slight supinatory capacity about the midtarsal joint oblique axis and a strong inversion activity about the longitudinal axis (Fig. 8-6).

A strong or tight anterior tibial muscle might create a functional supinatus during running. A weak anterior tibial muscle is associated with excessive medial column instability and pronation of the foot.

EXTENSORS

The extensor digitorum longus dorsiflexes the ankle. It is lateral to the subtalar joint axis and therefore has a pronatory force arm. It also pronates the oblique axis of the midtarsal joint. Its primary function is extension of the toes at the metatarsophalangeal joints.

The peroneus tertius is part of the antigravity muscle group, functioning with the extensor digitorum longus. Its action is similar to that of the extensor digitorum longus at the ankle, subtalar, and oblique axis of the midtarsal. It inserts into the fifth ray at the dorsal aspect of the base of the fifth metatarsal and has a potential pronatory force at this axis.

The extensor hallucis longus arises from the middle half of the anterior surface of the fibula and inserts into the dorsal aspect of the base of the distal phalanx of the great toe. It dorsiflexes the ankle joint and pronates the midtarsal oblique joint. Its function at the subtalar joint depends on the position of the subtalar joint. It will pronate a pronated subtalar while supinating a supinated subtalar. It produces dorsiflexion and extension of the interphalangeal joint of the hallux, and dorsiflexion of the first metatarsophalangeal joint through the extensor expansion.

INTRINSIC MUSCLES OF THE FOOT

Mann and Inman[7] conclude that the intrinsic muscles of the foot act as a functional unit. They are active from early midstance until just before toe-off. The plantar muscles crossing the midtarsal joint become important supinators around the oblique midtarsal joint axis once the heel is raised. Mann and Inman believe that the intrinsic musculature in a pronated foot becomes active earlier and remains active longer during each cycle. This is an attempt to reduce the amount of hypermobility around the oblique midtarsal as well as the subtalar joint axis. The lumbricales may fire with the long extensors during swing.[13] These intrinsic foot muscles help stabilize the midtarsal joint as well as the metatarsophalangeal joints and digits, depending on their respective origins and insertions. This accounts for excessive foot fatigue with a compensating forefoot varus foot, in which there is prolonged and excessive activity of the intrinsic foot musculature. It also accounts for the success of orthotic foot control in relieving foot fatigue when forefoot varus is present. Intrinsic foot muscles delicately balance the metatarsophalangeal joints; when fatigue, neuromuscular disease, or dysfunction of the intrinsic muscles is present, this delicate balance is lost, resulting in metatarsal or interphalangeal joint instability and abnormality.

The flexor hallucis brevis muscle inserts into the respective tibial and fibular sesamoids. It then inserts into the base of the proximal phalanx of the hallux. Loss of the effect of the medial portion of the flexor hallucis brevis may result in hallux valgus, whereas loss of the lateral portion may lead to hallux varus. When both portions of the muscles are rendered ineffectual, such as when both sesamoids are removed, a hallux hammertoe may be the end result due to loss of stability of the plantar aspect of the first metatarsophalangeal joint, hence the philosophy of preserving the function of the sesamoids and those muscles and tendons attaching to them whenever possible.

MUSCLE FUNCTION AT HIP AND KNEE JOINT DURING RUNNING
Hip Joint

Mack,[14] in his American Association of Orthopaedic Surgeons section on biomechanics of running, has studied muscle function during running at the hip, knee, and ankle. This study was carried out at the Gait Analysis Laboratory at Shriner's Hospital in San Francisco. Mack studied the gluteus maximus, hamstrings, hip abductors, and hip adductors. The study noted that, during walking, the gluteus maximus is active from the end of swing phase until the foot is flat on the ground at approximately 10 percent of the walking cycle. The hamstring muscles demonstrate a similar period of activity. These two muscle groups probably function to decelerate the swinging thigh and initiate extension of the hip joint.

During jogging and running, the gluteus maximus continues to have late swing phase activity, and the period of activity during stance phase increases to approximately 30 percent of stance phase during jogging and nearly 50 percent during running. The gluteus maximus plays a role in hip extension during the stance phase of running.

The gluteals are more active when walking or running uphill or climbing stairs. The hamstrings demonstrate a longer period of swing and stance phase activity during both jogging and running. The hamstrings are active during the last 50 percent of swing phase during jogging and the last 25 percent of swing phase during running. The hamstrings are active for the first 50 percent of the stance phase of running and jogging. Mack[14] believes that they function synergistically with the gluteus maximus to bring about rapid hip extension during the running gait.

The hip abductors demonstrate essentially the same period of activity at all speeds of gait. The abductors become active late in the swing phase and remain active during approximately the first 50 percent of the stance phase. The abductors function to stabilize the stance leg and hemipelvis at the time of initial ground contact, thereby preventing excessive sagging of the swing leg hemipelvis.[15]

During walking, the hip adductors are active in the last third of the stance phase. During jogging and running, their period of activity extends throughout the entire stance and swing phase.

Knee Joint

During walking, the quadriceps muscles become active late in the swing phase and remain active during the stance phase, until the initial period of knee flexion has been completed and extension of the knee joint once again begins (15 percent of the gait cycle). The quadriceps group acts to stabilize the knee at initial ground contact until foot flat has been accomplished. During jogging, the same phasic activity is noted during walking. During running, however, quadriceps activity during swing phase increases considerably. Mack[14] postulated that the quadriceps activity increase probably helps bring about knee extension, which passes through a much greater arc of motion during running than during walking. The stance phase activity, although consuming nearly 50 percent of the stance phase, is briefer in real time than during walking.

S.I. Subotnick, J. Aston, and J. Carollo (unpublished research, 1982) measured the activity of the vastus medialis during walking and running with and without orthotics and neutral foot control. These workers found electrical activity of the vastus medialis to decrease with neutral foot control and to increase with excessive pronation at contact. They postulated that a functional valgus at the knee associated with excessive contact and midstance pronation accounted for excessive activity of the vastus medialis.

Clinically, a weak vastus medialis is associated with patellofemoral pathology and lateral maltracking of the patella in runners (Fig. 8-7).

The hamstrings influence both the hip and knee joints. The hamstring probably helps stabilize the knee joint at the time of initial contact. It participates actively in extension of the hip. The flexion at the knee during the period of hamstring activity is brought about by the weight of the body against the knee, rather than by active hamstring contraction. During late swing, the hamstrings function to modulate speed of knee extension and participate in hip extension. Tight hamstrings are characteristic of long-distance runners. When the hamstrings become too short, they limit hip and knee extension, thereby shortening the stride length. This may predispose to inefficient stride or injury, or both.

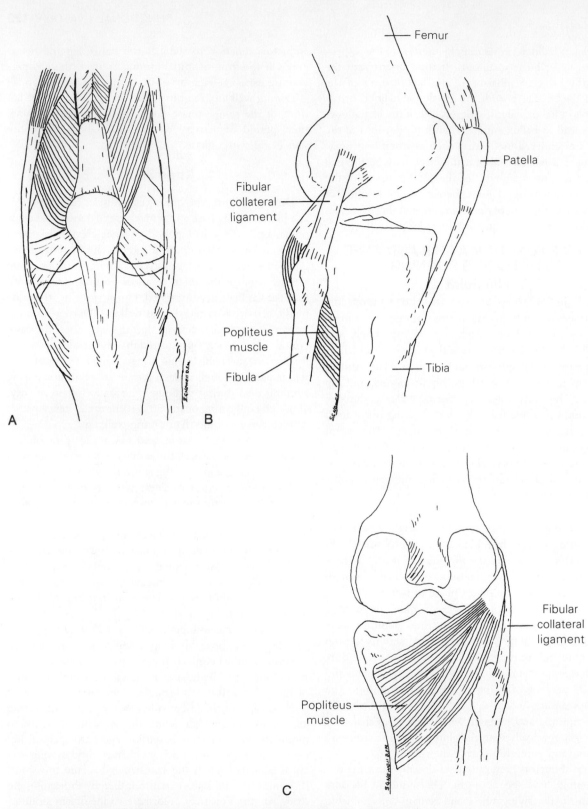

Figure 8–7 Anatomy of right knee. **(A)** Anterior view. **(B)** Lateral view. **(C)** Posterior view.

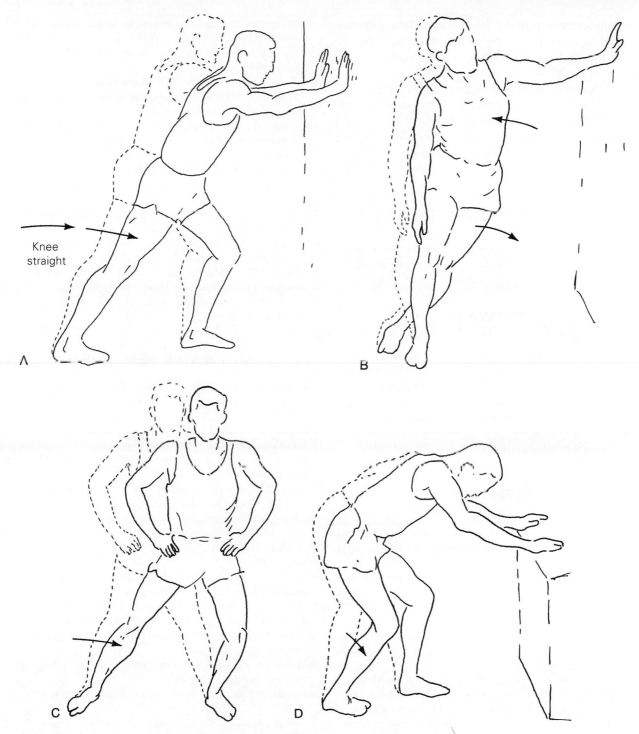

Figure 8-8 Simple diagrams of muscle stretches. **(A)** Adductor stretch. **(B)** Abductor and iliotibial tract stretch. **(C)** Stretch for hamstring, plantar fascia, Achilles tendon, and gastrocnemius. **(D)** Bent knee, posterior leg stretch, isolating structures that originate below the knee joint: soleus, posterior tibial muscles, and plantar fascia.

Contracture or tightness of the muscles affecting the medial aspect of the knee—the pes anserinus, including the medial hamstrings and sartorius—can cause tendinitis or pes anserinus bursitis about the knee. This can also be precipitated by excessive functional valgus at the knee (Fig. 8-7A).

Weakness or tightness of the tensor fascia lata and associated iliotibial band may create iliotibial band (friction rub) syndrome. This muscle may become weak during endurance events (Fig. 8-7 A and B). Excessive rotatory instability of the knee may cause a popliteus tendinitis (Fig. 8-7). Balance between the quadriceps and hamstrings is important in the athlete. The hamstrings should be at least 60 percent, and preferably 80 percent, as strong as their antagonistic counterparts, the quadriceps. Tight hamstrings are often thought to be strong, whereas this is usually not the case. Tightness is most often an indication of dynamic imbalance and improper stretching rather than of actual strength.

SUMMARY

Appropriate stretching and strengthening of all the muscles of the lower extremity provide for a more efficient, biomechanically sound gait. Dynamic imbalance leads to joint position abnormalities and to secondary compensatory mechanisms that invariably lead to fatigue and injury. A series of stretching exercises for the leg and foot muscles is illustrated in Figure 8-8.

REFERENCES

1. Root ML, Orien WP, Weed JH: Normal and Abnormal Functions of the Foot. Clinical Biomechanics Corporation, Los Angeles, 1977
2. Perry J: The mechanics of walking, a clinical interpretation. Phys Ther 47:778, 1967
3. Inman VT: Human locomotion. Can Med Assoc J 9:1047, 1966
4. Sutherland DH: An electromyographic study of the posterior flexors of the ankle in normal walking on a level. J Bone Joint Surg [Am] 48:66, 1966
5. Murray MP, Drought AB, Korry RC: Walking patterns of normal men. J Bone Joint Surg [Am] 46:335, 1964
6. Hautz SJ, Walsh FP: Electromyographic analysis of the function of the muscles acting on the ankle during weightbearing with special reference to the triceps surae. J Bone Joint Surg [Am] 41:1469, 1959
7. Mann R, Inman VT: Phasic activity of intrinsic muscles of the foot. J Bone Joint Surg [Am] 46:469, 1964
8. Elftman H: The function of muscles in locomotion. Am J Physiol 125:357, 1939
9. Mann RA: Surgery of the Foot. 5th Ed. CV Mosby, St. Louis, 1986
10. Burns MJ, McGlamry ED: Biomechanics. p. 111. In McGlamry ED (ed): Fundamentals of Foot Surgery. Williams & Wilkins, Baltimore, 1987
11. Simon SR, Mann RA, Hagy JL, Larsen LJ: Role of the posterior calf muscles in normal gait. J Bone Joint Surg [Am] 60:465, 1978
12. Cavanagh RR: The shoe-ground interface in running. In Mack RP (ed): AAOS Symposium on the Foot and Leg in Running Sports. CV Mosby, St. Louis, 1982
13. Jarrett BA, Manzi JA, Green DR: Interossei and lumbricales muscles of the foot. J Am Podiatry Assoc 70:1, 1980
14. Mack RP: AAOS Symposium on the Foot and Leg in Running Sports. CV Mosby, St. Louis, 1982
15. Inman VT: Functional aspects of the abductor muscles of the hip. J Bone Joint Surg [Am] 29:607, 1947
16. McGlamry JE: Fundamentals of Foot Surgery. Williams & Wilkins, Baltimore, 1987

SUGGESTED READINGS

Adrian M, Deutsch H: Biomechanics: 1984 Olympic Scientific Congress Proceedings, Microform Publications, University of Oregon, Eugene, 1984
Cavanagh PR: The Running Shoe Book. Anderson World, Mountain View, CA, 1980
Ducroquet R: Walking and Limping. JB Lippincott, Philadelphia, 1965
Frederick EC: Sports Shoes and Playing Surfaces: Human Kinetics. Nike Human Kinetics Publishers, Champaign, IL, 1984
Gottlieb LL: Muscle compliance: implications for the control of movement. Exerc Sport Sci Rev 24:1, 1996
Inman VT: The Joints of the Ankle: Williams & Wilkins, Baltimore, 1976
McCarthy DJ: Anatomy. p. 3. In McGlamry ED (ed): Fundamentals of Foot Surgery. Williams & Wilkins, Baltimore, 1987
Nicholas JA, Hershman EB: The Lower Extremity and Spine in Sports Medicine. 2nd Ed. CV Mosby, St. Louis, 1995
Sarrafian SK: Anatomy of the Foot and Ankle. 2nd Ed. JB Lippincott, Philadelphia, 1993
Steindler A: Kinesiology of the Human Body. Charles C Thomas, Springfield, IL, 1955
Subotnick SI: Podiatric Sports Medicine. Futura, Mt. Kisco, NY, 1975
Travell JG, Simons, DG: Myofascial Pain and Dysfunction: The Trigger Point Manual. Vol. 2. The Lower Extremity. Williams & Wilkins, Baltimore, 1992
Williams PL: Gray's Anatomy. 38th Ed. Churchill Livingstone, Edinburgh, 1995

9

Clinical Biomechanics

Biomechanics of the Foot and Ankle

STEVEN I. SUBOTNICK

CLASSIFICATION OF FOOT TYPES

The classification of foot types—cavus, normal, or flat—has been presented in Chapter 7. Foot types have also been classified as to their neutral position at the ankle, subtalar, and midtarsal joints. Furthermore, they may be classified as to their relative laxity or stiffness. These classifications are useful in making clinical decisions as to diagnosis, treatment, and rehabilitation and are most helpful in making decisions relating to orthotic requirements and shoes. In addition, correlation of the predisposition to various overuse and acute injuries with the generalized foot types is relatively accurate and useful.

All these foot types are variants of the "ideal" neutral foot. However, this neutral functional position at the middle of midstance is *not* a normal functional position for most athletes because of the unique genetic and individual characteristics of each person. It is merely a theoretical functional neutral position that seems to improve overall function once achieved. The neutral foot is used as a baseline that clinicians strive to reproduce functionally with biodynamic functional foot orthotics and musculoskeletal techniques such as stretching, manipulation, strength training, and good coaching.

The Normal Foot

A hypothetical ideal working-model foot has a subtalar joint range of motion of about 21 to 30 degrees; give or take 3 to 5 degrees, the forefoot is perpendicular to the rearfoot with no obvious forefoot varus or valgus. In the sagittal plane, the plantar aspect of the ball of the foot is parallel and level with the plantar surface of the heel. There is no forefoot equinus or hypermobility of the first ray. In the transverse plane, the forefoot-to-rearfoot angle is approximately 10 to 12 degrees adducted. The medial lateral columns of the foot are respectively balanced to each other and to the posterior column. In essence, there are perpendicular relationships at the ankle, rearfoot, and forefoot. The foot is perpendicular to the leg at the ankle joint. The subtalar joint is neutral, neither pronated nor supinated (Fig. 9-1); the midtarsal joint is maximally pronated; and the metatarsophalangeal and interphalangeal joints are neutral.

The Pronated Foot

The pronated foot has been called a "weak foot," "Morton's foot," or "hypermobile flatfoot." Idiopathic unilateral flatfoot had been associated with posterior tibial tendon insufficiency or rupture. Moderate pronation and hypermobility is best termed *weak foot*. Severe hypermobility with flattening of the foot is termed *hypermobile flatfoot*. It may be associated with a congenital or ligamentous laxity. There is a general increase in the range of motion at the subtalar and midtarsal joints as the degree of laxity and

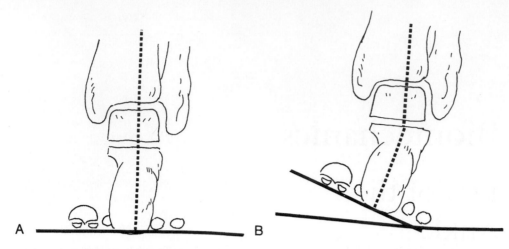

Figure 9-1 (A) Neutral subtalar joint with perpendicular calcaneus. **(B)** Calcaneal varus (C-shaped heel) with neutral subtalar joint and forefoot inverted to the floor, although perpendicular and neutral to the subtalar.

deformity increases (e.g., Morton's foot; Figs. 9-2 and 9-3). This increases the parallel arrangement on the midtarsal axis, permitting greater range of motion.

The weak foot or hypermobile flatfoot may cause symptoms in everyday walking and activity, such as postural fatigue with aching at the plantar foot and posteromedial aspects of the leg. The physician examining the patient can usually readily tell when there is excessive pronation. The heel will be in valgus and the medial arch dropped, the forefoot is externally positioned on the rearfoot, and the foot is usually toed out, with the second toe lateral to the middle of the patella. This position further forces the foot to pronate because the center of gravity and force is lateral to the long axis of the foot, which roughly bisects the rearfoot and exits out the second toe.

Excessive pronation of the foot can also be caused by subtalar varus, equinus at the ankle, or a plantar-flexed lateral column. Thus the foot may appear relatively normal with no weight on it, or even when walking, but pronates excessively during running. This type of foot may give few symptoms during everyday activity but considerable symptoms in sports. Rearfoot varus or functional varus of unilateral running creates excessive pronation at heel contact. This rearfoot pronation is often associated with excessive forefoot pronation and delayed resupination. Ankle equinus secondary to bony or soft tissue limitation results in increased dorsiflexion of the forefoot at the rearfoot around the midtarsal joint oblique axis. This creates pronation of the forefoot and rearfoot, based on the unique relationship between the subtalar and midtarsal joints. A plantar-flexed lateral column produces pronation by virtue of the fact that the fourth and fifth metatarsals are lower than the adjacent third metatarsal. When they contact the surface, pronatory force is generated, which causes prona-

Figure 9-2 Morton's foot pronation. Short hypermobile first metatarsal and increased midtarsal joint pronation are typical.

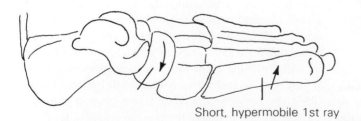

Short, hypermobile 1st ray

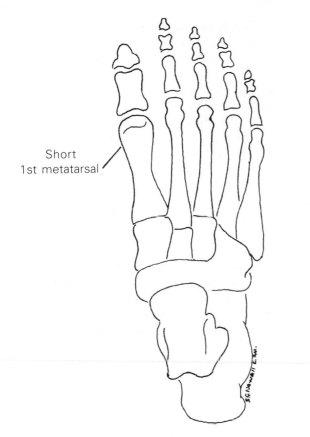

Figure 9-3 Morton's foot. Characteristics include short first metatarsal and a hypermobile first ray.

tion at the distal medial aspect of the forefoot. This is usually associated with an increase of the calcaneal inclination angle.

Foot deformity may be static or dynamic. A dynamic weak foot or flatfoot is relatively neutral or normal during non-weight bearing and excessively pronated with weight bearing. A static deformity is present with or without weight bearing. A functional or dynamic situation is present when the athlete has pronation only while performing a sport and has a relatively normal foot when standing and walking.

With the pronated foot, in running, the key factor is for the foot to be neutral in the middle of midstance. When there is no sequential phasic resupination, torque and countertorque result, causing injury. Fatigue results when muscles work overtime against unstable fulcrums and when joints that should be stable and locked are unlocked and hypermobile.

In some sports, a pronated foot is essential. Pronation is necessary for the uneven surfaces of a golf course, and is an essential part of the golf swing and stance. Pronation is also essential when setting the inside edge in sports such as skiing. In these situations, limited pronation can be as detrimental as excessive pronation.

The Cavus Foot

At the opposite end of the spectrum is the high-arched cavus foot with decreased or limited pronation. Whereas a normal amount of pronation dissipates stress and helps protect bone and soft tissue supporting structures, lack of normal pronation is associated with excessive shock to bone and supporting structures. The high-arched cavus foot has decreased range of motion, increased stiffness, and decreased pronatory compensation. The cavus foot usually has increased rearfoot varus, as well as a higher incidence of lateral instability of the foot and ankle. The forefoot equinus component of the cavus foot is associated with hammertoes or claw toes and with anterior migration of the plantar forefoot fat pad, leaving the metatarsal heads unprotected and predisposing to sesamoiditis, metatarsalgia, neuromas, and keratomas.

PERFORMANCE BASED ON FOOT TYPE

Performance is decreased with excessive supination or pronation in most sports. The pronated foot has increased recruitment of motor units during stance in the attempt to stabilize the foot. This leads to fatigue and inefficiency. The cavus foot has increased kinetic energy in the musculature of the lower extremity as a result of decreased stress dissipation from normal joint motion. However, gross generalizations as to foot type and success in various sporting events can be made.

Sports in which the feet are externally rotated and wide apart, with a lower center of gravity, require excessive pronation. Thus the lineman on a football team would need to have normal to excessive pronation at the subtalar and midtarsal joints. The lineman's forward lean demands ankle dorsiflexion and often leads to anterior compression ankle spurs. Hiking or running on irregular surfaces with abrupt changes of the terrain requires normal to excessive pronation. Limitations of pronation lead to lateral instability and may predispose to strains or sprains. Golf requires pronation and supination for the stance and swing. Short sprint events require pronation as the athlete takes off out of the blocks with the feet externally rotated and pronated.[1]

A relatively normal neutral foot with forward ankle lean and mobility is required for skiing. Excessive hypermobility decreases the amount of pronation available to set the inside control edge. Excessive tibial varum or rearfoot varus may cause boot cuff abnormal fit pressure, predisposing to lateral edge overriding. A decrease in the amount of pronation available for inside edge control occurs with compensation. Long-distance running requires a neutral foot; whereas excessive pronation results in an overuse syndrome, excessive supination results in overstress. Neutral foot function is also preferable for jumping and rebound sports. Track and field events such as the javelin throw require a crossover step and relative freedom of the rearfoot to supinate and pronate.[2]

It has been observed that halfbacks on a football or soccer team do well with a semirigid cavus foot. This foot type permits quick cutting and maneuverability. It has been long observed by coaches that the pigeon-toed athlete is faster and more responsive. In middle- and long-distance running, athletes with greater plantar flexion at the ankle joints are more efficient and faster. Long-distance runners develop functional limitations, such as tight hamstrings and limited range of motion in the subtalar as well as midtarsal joints. In effect, they develop mild functional cavus feet with excessive rearfoot varus of a soft tissue nature if they do not stretch appropriately. Tight hamstrings and calf muscles affect stride length by reducing knee extension and creating a functional equinus by reducing dorsiflexion at the ankle. Eventually, the efficiency of the runner is decreased, predisposing to inefficient stride with a predictable increase in overuse injuries.

The high-arched cavus foot, although well suited for quick cutting, pivoting, and speed, is poorly adapted to jumping. This foot tends to be plantar flexed in a position of forefoot valgus during rebounding, which predisposes to lateral instability. Limited range of motion in the subtalar and midtarsal joints creates greater stress in the bones of the foot and leg. The anterior equinus associated with cavus foot produces greater stress under the ball of the foot, while straining the plantar fascia and posterior structures that insert into the calcaneus. These limitations and strains decrease efficiency of performance.

INJURY PREVENTION BASED ON FOOT TYPE

Realizing the characteristics of the basic foot types, one can make predictions as to injury predilections on the basis of foot type (see next section). These injuries can be de-

creased with appropriate individualized training schedules, foot gear, orthoses, shock-absorbing and attenuating materials, and conditioning exercises that concentrate on strength, balance, flexibility, and endurance. Thus the athlete with a high-arched cavus foot requiring more flexibility might do yoga in conjunction with swimming pool workouts. Full workouts with a flotation vest would allow speed work for running to be carried out with little risk of stress-related injuries (Fig. 9-4). The water movements increase the range of motion of the various joints in the lower extremity. Yoga would also increase the range of motion.[3]

The athlete with a hypermobile flatfoot requiring more neutral function could be given appropriate shoes with increased medial stability and orthoses, and exercises to strengthen the muscles that resist pronation and support the medial longitudinal arch, specifically the intrinsics and extrinsics, tibialis posterior, tibialis anterior, and long flexors. Athletes with forefoot valgus and increased subtalar joint motion predisposed to lateral instability of the foot would be given appropriate balance and kinesthetic exercises to decrease the likelihood of sprain as well as supportive measures, such as orthoses and shoes with lateral wedges. The athlete with the miserable malalignment syn-

Figure 9-4 Running in water using a flotation device is an excellent workout for those with a high-arched cavus foot. It is also a useful rehabilitation technique.

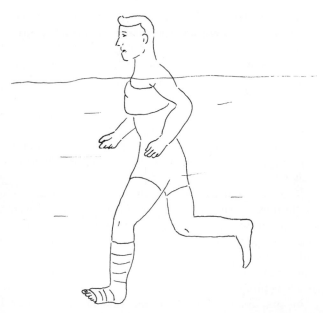

drome (anteversion, knee valgus, and excessive pronation of the feet) would be encouraged toward sports other than long-distance running. If long-distance running is desired, appropriate shoes, orthoses, and exercises are necessary.

The relative height and integrity of the medial and lateral longitudinal, as well as transverse metatarsal, arches are also factors to be considered in planning treatment modalities, as well as the orthosis prescription. For instance, plantar flexed lateral column, wherein the fourth and fifth metatarsals hang lower, closer to the weight-bearing surface, than the bottom of the heel and the adjacent third metatarsal, is often associated with lateral subtalar and ankle sprain with rebounding or jumping and landing on the outside of the forefoot. Knowing this foot type ahead of time allows for preventative intervention with a lateral accommodation and valgus wedge forefoot extension to prevent the lateral instability and subsequent increased risk of injury.

INJURY PREDILECTION BASED ON FOOT TYPE

Injury predilection may be based on foot type in regard to the relaxed stance position of the foot or on the amount of calcaneal varus or valgus present during function. Injury may also be predicted by evaluating the individual joints, including the ankle, subtalar, midtarsal, and metatarsal–tarsal articulations. The former type of injury predilection is discussed here; that based on joint evaluation is discussed in a later section.

Relaxed Calcaneal Stance Position

As relaxed stance position of the foot or amount of calcaneal valgus or varus varies from the ideal situation with the bisection of the posterior surface of the calcaneus parallel to the bisection of the posterior aspect of the lower one-third of the leg, more symptoms appear to be prevalent in the athlete. Predictably, as the degree of pronation or calcaneal valgus increases, there is concomitant increase in predilection for medial overuse injuries. Thus, as the foot pronates and the forefoot abducts on the rearfoot, there is a greater incidence of abductor hallucis longus strains, as well as medial plantar fasciitis. There is also a greater likelihood for medial shin syndrome. A functional valgus is present at the knee secondary to excessive pronation, and there appears to be an increase in overuse injuries about the knee, with patellofemoral symptoms, with excessive pronation.[4]

By contrast, as the amount of calcaneal varus increases,

one progresses from a neutral foot to a semiflexible or inflexible cavus foot. There is a greater lateral instability and higher incidence of lateral sprains of the ankle.[5] There are also more impact-related injuries. The amount of subtalar joint pronation and supination decreases as the arch raises and the stiffness of the foot increases. Subtalar joint limited range of motion is associated with midtarsal joint axis obliquity and decreased range of motion, as previously explained. Thus semiflexible and inflexible cavus feet become more rigid and have less pronatory motion to help dissipate and absorb impact shock. Decreased range of motion is associated with poor adaptability to irregular surfaces. An extreme example is the athlete who has had a triple arthrodesis or who has subtalar and midtarsal joint arthritis with no range of motion. Although the foot may function adequately in unidirectional walking or jogging, it does poorly on irregular surfaces because of lack of adaptability of these major joints.

Hypermobile Flatfoot

As the stability of the foot decreases, as seen in the weak foot or hypermobile flatfoot, demands are placed on the extrinsic and intrinsic dynamic stabilizers. Thus muscles try to stabilize the foot, which should have its own intrinsic stability but does not; these muscles become fatigued, and overuse injuries secondary to loss of shock absorbance of the soft tissue structures and malpositioning of the joints, as well as oblique pull of the muscles, is the end result. At the end of the range of motion of maximum pronation, if the foot contacts maximally pronated during gait, the normal pronatory dissipation of stress is also lost. The foot becomes a poor shock absorber. The weak or hypermobile flatfoot responds well to orthosis treatment combined with muscular rehabilitation when treated early in life.[6]

Cavus Foot

Retardation of progression of cavus foot deformity is less successful even when treated early with appropriate physical therapy, exercises, and orthosis and shoe therapy. With cavus foot, orthoses and shoes that increase the range of motion of the subtalar joint and provide for a stable foot-to-floor relationship are helpful. Plantar fascia and intrinsic foot muscle stretching are beneficial. When the first ray is plantar flexed, the peroneus longus should be stretched and antagonistic muscles strengthened. Occult or detectable neuromuscular disease must be considered when cavus foot is progressive.

STRESS FRACTURES AND FOOT TYPE

Pronated Foot

The pronated foot has increased calcaneal valgus with secondary excessive stress upon the fibular malleolus. Thus there is an increased tendency toward fibular malleolar stress fractures in the weak hypermobile foot. There are also distal medial stress fractures at the tibia secondary to posteromedial shin syndrome. This syndrome is produced by rapid excessive pronation and oblique pulling of the posterior tibial muscle away from the tibia. There is, first, periostitis, then stress reaction of bone. The end result may be single or multiple stress fractures.[7–9]

With excessive prolonged pronation in the pronated foot, there is dorsiflexion and inversion of the first ray, exposing the tibial sesamoid to more stress. As the first ray dorsiflexes, the second metatarsal becomes vulnerable to stress reaction of bone or stress fractures, or both. Stress fractures of the second ray are more prevalent with a hypermobile short first ray. With the pronated foot, if the first metatarsal is hypermobile and the second metatarsal is short, there may be a stress fracture of the third metatarsal. Excessive pronation during jumping in the pronated foot may pull the navicular tuberosity away from the main body, producing either an avulsion or stress fracture. As the pronated foot contacts everted, there is more stress on the medial tubercle of the calcaneus, predisposing it to excessive trauma. There may be a stress fracture. In the younger athlete, plantar calcaneal apophysitis is prevalent with excessive pronation.

Cavus Foot

The cavus foot has reduced range of motion in the joints and limited pronatory shock attenuation. There is usually an anterior equinus. The anterior equinus predisposes the plantar aspect of the first metatarsal to more stress, and there are more stress fractures of the tibial and fibular sesamoids. Stress fractures at the base of the first metatarsal may occur. With anterior equinus, any metatarsal that is relatively long or plantar flexed is subjected to more stress. Forefoot valgus and adductus of the forefoot with cavus foot predisposes the styloid process of the fifth metatarsal to more fractures. The same is true at the base of the fifth metatarsal with so-called Jones fractures. Limited subtalar joint motion produces more stress in the calcaneous with a higher incidence of calcaneal stress fractures. This rigid foot puts more stress on the midtarsal bones, and there may be a stress fracture of the navicular, cuneiforms, or cuboid. Tibial stress fractures in the cavus foot are more proximal. Femoral stress fractures may be distal or proximal (at the neck) with this foot type. Pelvis stress fractures may also occur with decreased shock attenuation.

SOFT TISSUE INJURIES AND FOOT TYPE

Pronated Foot

Soft tissue injuries in the pronated foot are secondary to increased mobility, along with abduction of the forefoot on the rearfoot. In the foot, there is increased medial plantar fasciitis and abductor myositis. The pronated foot has a higher incidence of hallux valgus with bunion deformity. Shear keratomas or callosities may occur secondary to excessive pronation and motion of the metatarsal over the underlying ball of the foot. There is a higher incidence of posterior and anterior tibial tendinitis and associated anterior and medial shin syndrome. Medial strain of the Achilles tendon is prevalent. The pronated foot produces a functional valgus at the knee during running with increased strain along the medial aspect of the knee. Thus there is patellofemoral compression with mild lateral instability and maltracking of the patella. There is medial retinaculitis with pes anserinus bursitis. The medial quadriceps may be strained or overworked. Excessive rotation at the hips may aggravate the muscles about the groin or pelvis.

Cavus Foot

The cavus foot with anterior equinus also has a higher incidence of plantar fascial strain or tears. With claw toe deformity, there are increased callosities under the ball of the foot. Hallux limitus or rigidus is more common, especially if the first ray is longer than the second. There is a higher incidence of peroneus longus and brevis tendinitis, and peroneal cuboid syndrome is present with pain under the cuboid in the peroneal groove. Increased rearfoot varus with the cavus foot produces retrocalcaneal bursitis, exostosis, or both. There may be strains about the central or lateral aspect of the Achilles tendon. The anterior equinus produces more load at the plantar aspect of the calcaneus, thus stretching the intrinsic foot muscles, plantar fascia, and gastrocnemius–soleus complex. This produces overload and pathology of all these structures.

The lateral instability associated with forefoot valgus and cavus foot predisposes the foot and ankle to more sprains. Thus there may be sprains of the midtarsal, subtalar, or ankle joint at the lateral aspect. At the knee, there is a higher incidence of iliotibial band syndrome. Greater trochanteric bursitis is prevalent. Whereas the pronated foot causes anterior shin syndrome secondary to excessive pulling of the anterior tibial muscle, the cavus foot produces anterior compartment or shin syndrome secondary to increased kinetic energy absorption by this muscle group.

Implication for Orthotics

As an overgeneralization, it might be said that the pronated foot has more medial symptomatology, whereas the supinated foot has more lateral symptomatology. This characterization has direct clinical applications to orthosis treatment. An orthosis that overcorrects in regard to medial control might produce the same symptomatology as a cavus foot. The same holds true for an orthosis designed to treat a cavus foot, which pronates the foot excessively, creating a functional medial imbalance and associated symptomatology.

FOREFOOT-TO-REARFOOT RELATIONSHIP

It is helpful to understand the relationship of the forefoot to rearfoot in all three planes. For example, there may be forefoot rectus, abductus, or adductus. There may be anterior equinus or a metatarsus primus elevatus. Forefoot varus, the true fixed joint positional variation from the ideal, or supinatus, a soft tissue compensatory and reducible malposition, can be contrasted to the more common forefoot valgus, with a plantar-flexed first ray, which may be flexible, semiflexible, or rigid.

Transverse Plane Relationships

RECTUS FOOT

A rectus foot exists when there is a straight relationship between the forefoot and the rearfoot. This foot has relatively few problems unless it is forced into a shoe with a C-shaped last. A straight last is preferable.

ADDUCTED FOREFOOT

A metatarsus adductus or forefoot adductus exists when the forefoot or metatarsals are adducted on the rearfoot. Angulation above 25 to 30 degrees may produce pathol-

ogy. This foot is supinated and tends to have lateral stability. Shoe fit is an important problem. With excessive adduction of the forefoot on the rearfoot, there is usually external rotation and pronatory compensation to provide for a more straighthead gait. This pronatory compensation creates medial instability in the foot if there is enough motion available. Thus, depending on the range of motion and stiffness of the joints, there may be supination, relatively neutral function, or pronation with a metatarsus adductus or forefoot adductus.

FOREFOOT ABDUCTUS

Forefoot abductus is associated with a hypermobile forefoot or excessive pronation at the midtarsal joint. It may also be secondary to arthritic changes in the midtarsal joint or a spastic peroneus brevis secondary to damage of the midtarsal, subtalar, or ankle joint. Appropriate diagnosis and etiology are important. Lower extremity injury is dependent on the etiology of the abductus condition.

JOINT FUNCTION AND INJURY PREDILECTION

Congenital or static joint limitations must be dealt with through the use of appropriate orthoses and shoes. Acquired dynamic hyper- or hypomobility is aided greatly by muscle re-education and flexibility exercises. It is helpful to discuss the ankle and foot joints individually and consider the effect they have on compensated function or injury.

Ankle Joint

Ankle equinus, or limited dorsiflexion at the ankle, causes pathology in the lower extremity. Ten degrees of dorsiflexion of the neutral foot at the ankle joint is necessary for normal ambulation. An equinus deformity is present when there is less than 10 degrees of dorsiflexion at the ankle. This may be compensated for by a mobile transverse axis at the midtarsal joint.[10]

It is important to differentiate between bony and soft tissue limitations at the ankle. Dorsiflexion at the ankle should be checked with the knee both extended and flexed. To differentiate between bony and soft tissue limitation, the knee should be flexed with the patient in a prone position. As the knee is then extended and the foot rapidly plantar-flexes into an equinus position, there is a soft tissue contracture of the posterior superficial muscle group. This usually occurs during the last 20 degrees going from flexion to full extension at the knee. In limited dorsiflexion with both the extended and flexed knee position and a firm endpoint to the range of motion, there is usually a bony block. This is termed *anterior impingement exostosis* of the ankle. With a less definitive end of the range of motion, there may be a soleus contracture. A lateral stress radiograph of the ankle helps differentiate the two and definitively makes the diagnosis of anterior impingement exostosis (see Fig. 20-14).[11]

Soft tissue equinus in runners and athletes is usually secondary to dynamic imbalance with tight gravity muscles and relatively weak antigravity muscles. They respond well to a physical therapy program designed to reverse this condition. Osseous limitation may require surgical excision.

Soft tissue equinus at the ankle joint creates excessive pronation of the foot. The dorsiflexion that should have been taking place at the ankle joint is now made up for around the oblique axis of the midtarsal joint. For this joint to function adequately, the subtalar joint must be pronated to unlock the midtarsal joint. Thus the gastrocnemius–soleus contracture creates excessive pronation in the foot as it compensates at the midtarsal joint.

During gait, an early heel-off is seen. This is usually associated with a bouncy gait that aggravates the medial head of the gastrocnemius, as well as the Achilles tendon. This bounciness also overloads the plantar fascia. Runners with a functional equinus tend to land on the balls of their feet, have the heel sag to the ground, and spring off the ball, using the style of the middle-distance runner.

The pronatory injuries related to the functional or anatomic equinus are the same as those seen with other conditions that cause excessive pronation in addition to unique problems of the calf muscles. Ankle bony limitations create pain at the anterior aspect of the ankle. The foot plant depends on the location of the anterior bone blocks. An antero lateral exostosis creates a supinated foot plant; an antero medial, a pronated foot plant. There is a higher incidence of Achilles tendon pathology with anterior impingement exostosis at the ankle. Bony limitation of ankle joint dorsiflexion is associated with pathology of the Achilles tendon and gastrocnemius–soleus complex, which is trying to dorsiflex the foot despite the fact that there is a bony limitation.[12,13]

Subtalar Joint

The most common positional abnormality of the subtalar joint is subtalar varus. This causes increased lateral heel contact and excessive pronation from this position to either a perpendicular calcaneal position or beyond, to a valgus position. Rapid pronation from this varus contact position predisposes to retrocalcaneal exostosis (Figs. 9-5 and 9-6). Increased lateral heel contact with excessive compression of the lateral aspect of the shoe may lead to instability of the shoe and a tendency toward lateral instability with sprains.

In walking, rearfoot varus leads to postural fatigue. In running, it leads to instability of the subtalar joint with overuse of the posterior tibial muscle. In edge control sports, compensatory pronation is necessary to bring the

Figure 9-5 Retrocalcaneal bursa.

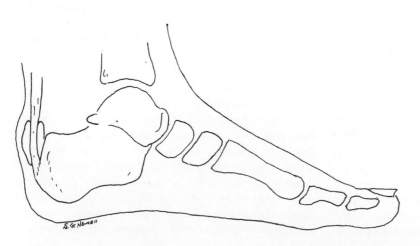

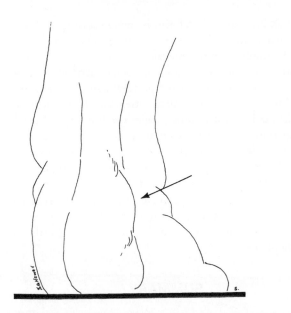

Figure 9-6 Retrocalcaneal exostosis and irritation of the Achilles tendon. Note lateral compression of the ankle and subtalar joints, which results from excessive pronation.

Midtarsal Joint

FOREFOOT VARUS

Forefoot varus is associated with increased strain to the medial plantar aspect of the foot. There is a higher incidence of medial plantar fasciitis, abductor myositis, or both. Medial heel-spur syndrome and postural fatigue of the intrinsic muscles of the foot are prevalent. There is medial imbalance of the foot with hallux valgus and bunion deformity. Abduction of the forefoot on the rearfoot during gait may produce shear calluses, keratomas, or neuromas. Abduction of the forefoot on the rearfoot predisposes the fifth toe to pressure from the shoe, and a fifth-digit hammertoe may be the end result, along with tailor's bunionette. Forefoot varus is part of the miserable malalignment syndrome, with external rotation of the foot and valgus at the ankle. There is a functional valgus at the knee with excessive internal rotation of the tibia and femur. Thus there is increased medial symptomatology in the foot,

ankle, leg, knee, and thigh. There is increased lumbar lordosis with excessive pronation, and low back pain may be the end result. Forefoot varus has increased incidence of stress fractures about the fibular malleolus and, in the forefoot, about the second or third metatarsal.

Forefoot Varus with Plantar-Flexed Lateral Column

Forefoot varus with plantar-flexed lateral column differs from forefoot varus inasmuch as the fourth and fifth metatarsal are plantar to the plane of the posterior aspect of the

Figure 9-7 Forefoot varus and compensation. **(A)** Non-weight-bearing neutral foot showing plantar-flexed lateral column. **(B)** Compensatory pronation.

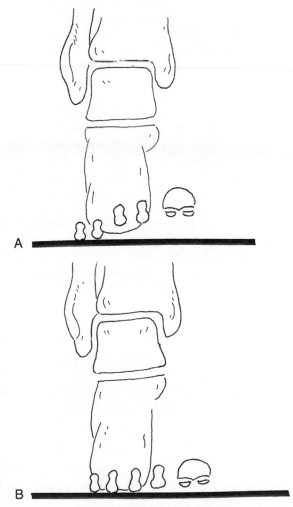

foot to a flat position. This uses up the pronation necessary for edge control and greatly hampers the ability of the athlete to perform turning maneuvers safely.

rearfoot. There is excessive pronation of the forefoot with concomitant increase of the calcaneal inclination angle as the lateral column of the foot is raised during compensation. This foot nonetheless causes pronatory compensation and symptomatology. There may be medial shin splint syndrome in the leg or imbalance about the knee. There is also a higher incidence of imbalance of the forefoot with hallux valgus and bunion deformity (Fig. 9-7).

FOREFOOT VALGUS

Forefoot valgus is associated with increased pressure beneath the first metatarsal and lateral instability of the foot and ankle. There are increased stress fractures in the sesamoids of the first metatarsal and at the base of the first metatarsal. Rapid supination places stress at the lateral aspect of the foot, and there are increased fractures at the base of the fifth metatarsal and the styloid process of the fifth metatarsal. There is a higher incidence of peroneal cuboid syndrome and lateral sprains of the midtarsal, subtalar, and ankle joints. Peroneal tendinitis is prevalent.

ANTERIOR EQUINUS

An anteromedial local equinus is a plantar-flexed first ray or local forefoot valgus. The first metatarsal is plantar to the adjacent second metatarsal and causes supinatory compensation. The same injuries as seen with forefoot valgus are present. There is also a component of anterior equinus that places more stress on the posterior musculature. With anterior equinus, the whole forefoot is plantar to the plantar surface of the calcaneus. This causes increased strain on the plantar fascia, as well as on the posterior structures about the subtalar and ankle joint—in particular, strains to the gastrocnemius, soleus, and Achilles tendon. Excessive shearing at the ball of the foot must be dealt with. Often, claw toe deformities are associated with the anterior equinus. The metatarsals are plantar flexed, and stress fractures are more prevalent.

Functional hallux limitus has been described by Dananberg as a cause of chronic postural pain.[14] This common biomechanical imbalance is treated with an orthosis with a kinetic hallux limitus wedge as well an applied kinesiology muscle-balancing technique focusing especially on strengthening the peroneals, which have been weakened by the lateral column instability and subsequent hypermobility of the first ray with resultant functional hallux limitus. In Dananberg's series, 70 percent of his patients reported 50 to 70 percent improved of myriad types of body chronic postural pain when surveyed 2 years following orthosis treatment.

SUMMARY

In closing, it should be emphasized that many factors may alter the function or range of motion of joints. These include functional adaptation and dynamic imbalance, systemic conditions such as arthritis, post-traumatic conditions, and congenital problems such as coalitions. These changes in foot mechanics have far-ranging impact upon bodily function and have been implicated as an etiology of chronic postural pain, as well as acute and overuse injuries in the lower extremity of the athlete. Certainly, the relationship between back pain and foot mechanics is well appreciated. Radiographs are helpful in ruling out congenital blocks, as are specific diagnostic tests such as magnetic resonance imaging and computed tomography. Despite the etiology of the joint malfunction and secondary ramifications, treatment centered around sound biomechanics, rehabilitative medicine, and shoe therapy is often quite rewarding.

Sagittal Plane Biomechanics
HOWARD J. DANANBERG

The focus of most sporting events is getting from point A to point B in the fastest, most efficient manner. This may involve running bases or catching a diving fly ball in baseball or being a wide receiver in a football game. It may mean reaching the finish line in the 100-m dash with an all-out effort, or in the marathon by carefully balancing speed with endurance. In all cases, the movement can be simplified to the concept of efficient forward advancement. It involves moving the body's center over the weight-bearing limb, first over one side, then over the other. This basic viewpoint is true in both running and walking. How this happens involves some of the most intriguing biomechanical interactions of the human body.

Over the last 1.8 million years, our species has gradually achieved an erect posture while relying on a bipedal style for ambulation. This has involved changes in the structures of the pelvis and spine; muscular balance alteration between gluteals, hamstrings, and quadriceps; and reorientation of the hips, knees, and ankles. The foot, in particular, has achieved a remarkable ability to support body weight while permitting forward motion above it. Through a complex interaction between its various components, the foot is able to endure the crushing loads applied over thousands of cycles per day while simultaneously being sufficiently mobile to serve as the central site about which movement must occur. This is no small task; it requires an elegant coordination of abilities and movements.

This portion of this chapter is divided into four main sections in order to describe the significance of sagittal plane movement on athletics. The first section demonstrates how power is generated for movement, how the foot serves as a sagittal plane pivot, and how these coordinate to create a supportive structure. The second section describes how blockages to sagittal plane movement can develop at various sites in the foot and ankle. The third section demonstrates methods of clinical evaluation for sagittal plane blockages, and the fourth section describes treatment with both foot orthotic devices and techniques in manual manipulation.

SAGITTAL PLANE PERSPECTIVE OF THE FOOT

Power of Motion

In order to understand sagittal plane biomechanics, it is essential to first grasp the nature of how the body creates the power to move itself forward. To simply think of walking or running as being the result of concentric contractions of the weight-bearing calf, thigh, and hip musculature causing powerful joint movements is to miss the elegance of the efficiency in the various styles of human ambulation. The literature supporting a different type of motion-creating power source is quite extensive. Mann et al.[15] concluded that

It would appear, based upon this data, as though little or no push-off per se is occurring from the posterior calf musculature. It should be noted, however, that during this same period of time the swinging limb, and in particular the hip, is undergoing rapid flexion that reaches its peak just after plantar flexion of the ankle joint begins. It is therefore postulated that the majority of the forward propulsion during jogging, running, and sprinting is brought about by the rapid hip flexion of the swing limb, rather than the push-off of the stance limb.

Claeys wrote, in regard to the motion of the swinging arms and legs, "This 'pull phase', is . . . the major cause of the forward propulsion."[16] Dorman has written of the elastic energy that is stored in the fascia and ligaments by reciprocal arm and leg swing motion and how it plays a significant role in providing energy for movement.[17] Grecovetsky published a textbook dedicated to reviewing the ability of the spine to store and return energy for all tasks, including walking and running.[18] In detailed anatomic dissections, Vleeming et al.[19] have shown previously undescribed anatomic connections that support the interactions of various postural and lower extremity segments reported by Grecovetsky and Dorman. The movements and interactions chronicled by these authors form the basis for understanding the storage and return mechanisms for the power of movement.

The primary aim is to use the entire body to facilitate motion of the center of body mass (COM) over either of the planted feet during the single-support phase of the step. (For the purpose of this discussion, walking is specifically addressed. Similar mechanisms exist for other methods of ambulating, including running.) At heel strike, impact forces are resisted at the various joints from the foot/ankle, knee, and hip. This activity can be thought of as a loading of these components as the surrounding musculature fires eccentrically (resisting collapse), storing elastic energy in the process. As heel strike occurs on one side, a preswing motion is taking place on the other. This trailing hip and knee initiate a rapid flexion motion from their fully extending position, which occurred just prior to opposite heel strike. This coincides with the continuation of ankle joint plantar flexion.

Figure 9-8 (A) Posteriorly, the latissimus dorsi and guteals align from ipsilateral superior to contralateral inferior almost as an "X" pattern via the boxed area containing the fascia thoracolumbocalis. **(B)** The fibers of the superior right can be seen interconnecting with the fibers from the inferior left in the darkened area. These structures can therefore work as a unit, storing and returning energy as the shoulder and pelvic girdle reciprocally rotate during gait. (From Vleeming A: A new light on low back pain. p. 147. In The Integrated Function of the Lumbar Spine and Pelvis. Vleeming A, Mooney V, Dorman, T, Snijders C [eds]: Proceedings of the 2nd Interdisciplinary Congress on Low Back Pain, San Diego, CA, November 9–11, 1995, with permission.)

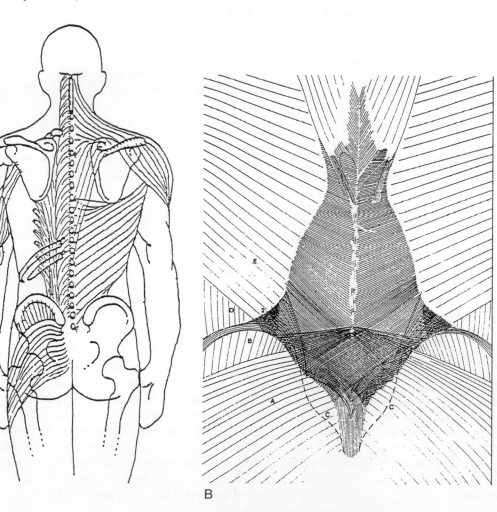

A   B

This preswing motion is critical to normal, efficient ambulation and is a result of the following intercoordinations.

The lumbar spine acts as a gear-like system to direct transverse, rotary force to the pelvis.[18] The elastic components that drive this "gear box" relate to a cross-linkage from top left (or right) to bottom right (or left). This anatomic interconnection results from the ipsilateral latissimus dorsi attachment to the contralateral gluteus maximus via the fascia thoracolumbocalis[20] (Fig. 9-8). Therefore, as the arms and legs swing reciprocally, energy is stored within this cross-linked mechanism, preparing it for the next step. As one steps ends and the other begins, the pelvis is redirected via a release in the sacroiliac joint. This release causes a forward-directed acceleration of the pelvis and is matched with the preswing limb's acceleration and serves

as a preparatory mechanism for toe-off. These intercoordinations permit adequate forward speed to develop within the preswing limb with minimal muscular assistance. Therefore, toe-off can occur with only a brief burst of activity of the iliopsoas muscle to perpetuate hip flexion (Fig. 9-9). As this limb now kicks off the ground and accelerates forward, the COM of the body will be pulled up and forward, over the now single-support, weight-bearing side. Once the COM has advanced over the support limb, gravity will continue to act on it, pulling it toward the ground. Body weight therefore becomes the final "thruster" for propulsion. As the trailing limb reaches the fully extended position during this period, advancement is perpetuated by the lever effect of the limb against the ground. Newton's third law of motion dictates that, with this thrust of body weight against the limb, which in turn

Figure 9-9 (A) At the end of the right single-support phase, the trailing limb reaches its fully extended position on the hip joint. **(B)** As single support transitions to double support, the trailing limb begins its preswing motion. From the fully extended position, it accelerates forward via hip and knee flexion to a point where the thigh is directly below the hip. At toe-off, the iliopsoas fires, perpetuating the hip flexion, and swing phase begins.

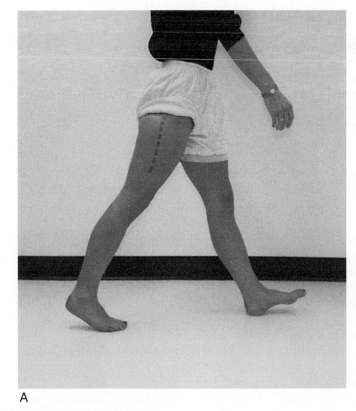

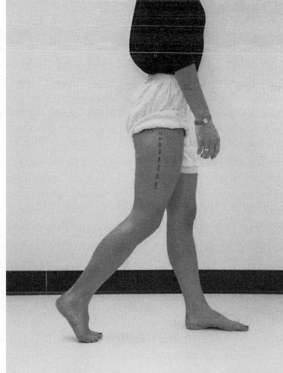

A

B

acts against the ground, forward motion occurs. The pendular effects of the arms and legs feed energy to each other, recycling step by step.

The Foot as a Sagittal Plane Pivot

As the power to move the COM over the foot is created, the foot must respond by simultaneously allowing the COM this range of motion. To perform this task, it functions as a sagittal plane pivot. This requires that movement be permitted as the power to create it develops, in addition to being able to achieve adequate stability required for managing the increasing force levels that are applied to the foot. This section describes the mechanics of the pivotal role, while support mechanics are detailed in the next. It is important to recognize that, while described separately, these actions occur simultaneously.

The foot, by its arch-like shape, would at first not appear to be well suited as a sagittal pivot. The curved foot-piece of a rocking chair would initially seem to be the ideal form, but that would only be true if the foot were to be considered a rigid body. The normally hypermobile, rocker-bottom foot is well known as a pathologic entity; therefore, the pivotal action must be accomplished via a different mechanism. In fact it is accomplished through an intricate interaction with three sites serving as sequential rotational locations. These are, in order, the round underside of the calcaneus, the dorsiflexion motion of the ankle, and the dorsiflexion of the metatarsophalangeal joints.[21] As one component reaches its end range capacity, the next begins to provide motion. This occurs as follows.

During heel strike, the initial rotational site is the plantar surface of the calcaneus (Fig. 9-10A). It permits the COM to move from behind the planted foot to directly over it. (This occurs simultaneously with loading of the heel and ends at the point of peak loading.) With essentially no moving parts, this is a very standard motion and appears quite similar in most subjects. Once the COM has moved to a point directly over the foot, the inferior calcaneus can no longer provide for forward rotation because the forefoot is now in firm ground contact. This blocks any further progression while the heel remains loaded on the support surface. For continued advancement, the site of rotation must now switch to the ankle (Fig. 9-10B). The leg normally is capable of moving 10 degrees over the talus, as the calcaneus is gradually unweighted from its peak load bearing by this "leg-over-foot" movement at the ankle.

During this ankle dorsiflexion motion, the fibula component of the ankle translates in a cranial-lateral direction, opening the ankle mortise and allowing it to receive the wider anterior talar dome. This movement permits the simultaneous COM movement as the calcaneus unweights. Once unweighted, heel lift becomes visible, and ankle dorsiflexion ends with reversal to plantar flexion. The final rotational site is now at the metatarsophalangeal joints. With the raising of the heel from the ground, the forefoot must commit to sagittal motion through the end of the single-support phase. Approximately 25 to 30 degrees of range of motion (ROM), is necessary prior to the opposite side's impact against the ground (Fig. 9-10C). By the conclusion of single support, the previously described foot motion occurs simultaneously with the knee and hip moving to their fully extended positions.[22] (Fig. 9-11).

The Coordination of Sagittal Plane Movement with Autosupport

The advancement of the COM over the support foot causes loads to be applied at the ground level that exceed body weight by 125 percent in walking. In running, these loads can reach 300 to 400 percent of body weight. To function normally, the foot and proximal structures must achieve a strengthened posture to appropriately manage these high-force loads. The coordination of specific, timely joint movements with the changing position of the COM creates such a supported structure. In addition, rotational changes from internal to external within the leg and pelvis must be accommodated at the foot/ground level. The method by which the foot becomes both supportive to loads and accommodative to rotational motions involves the ability to function as a tension–compression system. This method is not unlike that of a child's kite; the balsa wood framework and plastic cover require tension to be applied via the string, which bows the frame, creating a stable, united structure capable of withstanding the forces of the wind. Without the tension provided by the string, the kite, with all its other components, would be unable to resist the forces applied to it. The balsa wood is more of a compression strut than a beam support column, and a plastic cover in combination with the string provides the necessary tension banding. This permits a lightweight structure to function with remarkable strength. Buckminster Fuller has described this as "tensegity" and has demonstrated its prevalence throughout all of nature.[23]

In 1979, Bosjen-Möller described the interrelationship

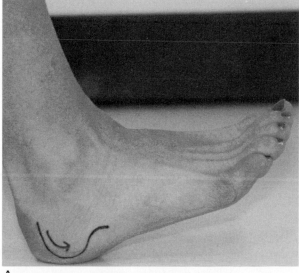

A

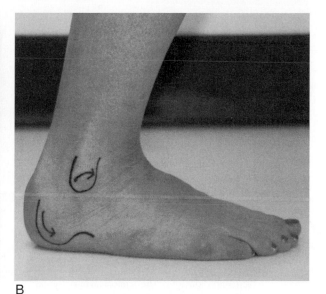

B

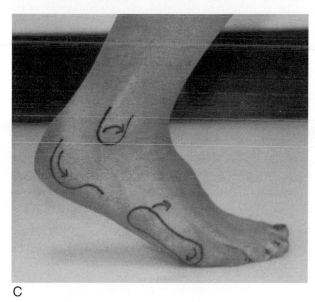

C

Figure 9-10 **(A)** At heel strike, the round underside of the calcaneus serves as the initial pivotal site, permitting the foot to move to the foot flat position **(B)** Once in complete ground contact, the next pivotal site becomes the ankle. This permits the body to travel over the planted foot. Approximately 10 degrees of ankle joint dorsiflexion is required for this motion to occur. **(C)** At heel-off, ankle motion reverses to plantar flexion while the pivotal site transitions to the metatarsophalangeal joints. During the single-support phase, approximately 25 degrees of flexion is required at the metatarsophalangeal joints for efficient function.

between the plantar fascia and the compression of the calcanocuboid joint. He was able to demonstrate that when, via a successful weight transfer during the midstance phase, the plantar fascia is tightened, calcaneocuboid joint becomes subject to compression from both the distal and proximal aspects. This effect, referred to as "closed packed," creates a stabilization of both the tarsus and midtarsus in the second half of the single-support phase of the step.[24]

The anatomy of the plantar fascia and its relationship to the osseous structures is critical to understanding how it

can create the closed-packed alignment. The fascia originates from the inferior calcaneus and inserts in the plantar aspect of the proximal phalangeal bases as well as the fat pad under the metatarsal heads. When tightened by digital dorsiflexion, the fat pad becomes "fixed" beneath the metatarsal heads, providing a slippery surface about which they can rotate the bases about the heads. The alignment of the fascia also is affected by the metatarsal's parabolic shape, and, when subject to increasing loads during the second half of single support, can cause increased fascial tension as weight shifts to a point between the first and second

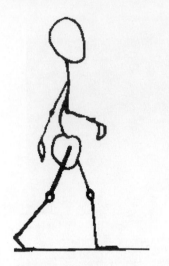

Figure 9–11 By the end of single-support phase, the thigh extends on the hip approximately 15 degrees while the knee achieves a fully extended and rectus position.

metatarsal heads. This effect is due to the longer perpendicular bisection of the axis formed by the first and second metatarsals heads versus the shorter axis formed by oblique relationship of metatarsal heads two through five. The timing of this shift must occur prior to the heel-off phase of the step. When coupled with this increased tension created by weight shift across this longer axis, the shift causes compression of the cuboid from both distal and proximal, and thus intrinsic foot stability just prior to the higher loads applied to the foot at heel lift[24] (Fig. 9-12).

Once the heel lifts from the ground, two simultaneous actions occur that continue to promote this reactive autosupport posture. As the metatarsal bases rotate about the heads, the metatarsals achieve a more perpendicular alignment to the support surface. This permits enhanced weight transfer from distal to proximal. This transfer is a response of ground reaction force relative to the Parallelogram of Forces Axiom:

If two forces whose lines of action intersect are acting on a body, their action is equivalent to the action of a single force whose vector representation is the diagonal of the parallelogram of which the two original force vectors are sides. With respect to any horizontal support surface, the diagonal vector formed by this design is greatest when the two lines of action are parallel (vertical) to the diagonal, and least (equal to zero) when they are directly perpendicular (horizontal) to it.[25]

This, when combined with the tension of the fascia, permits increased compression across the osseous structures and intrinsic support.[26]

As the metatarsal heads pivot, the digits, particularly the hallux, tighten the fascia by wrapping them around the metatarsal heads. This has been described by Hicks as the windlass effect.[27] The effect is to supinate the foot and externally rotate the lower leg as the wrapping of the fascia shortens the distance between the heel and forefoot. Hicks referred to this motion as "irresistable"; once the toes hinge, the supinatory motion becomes part and parcel to digital dorsiflexion.

In summary, the appropriate timing of weight transfer creates a combination tension–compression effect between the plantar fascia and the ligamentous, and osseous structures. Immediately following the weight transfer, heel-off, permitted by metatarsal head pivotal motion, occurs. This empowers the foot with the positional strategy by which it resists greater compressive loads while supinating the foot via the windlass action. All told, the foot is adequately stabilized to forces applied to it in terms of both vertical load and rotational reorientation (internal-to-external limb rotation).

SAGITTAL PLANE BLOCKADE

In broad terms, to think of the foot as an axis of a wheel about which the entire body advances is to create an image of the sagittal plane motion it provides. If, for some reason, the ability to permit this ROM is unavailable, a consequence to the entire ambulation sequence must develop. It is this senario in which sagittal plane blockade should be considered.

To understand sagittal plane motion blockade, each site about which the sagittal plane motion develops must be appreciated. These include the plantar surface of the calcaneus, the ankle joint, and the metatarsophalangeal joints. It is important to keep in mind that more than one site may be involved in any particular patient. Blockade may also occur unilaterally and therefore be responsible for postural motions and rotations that take place more to one side than the other. In this section, the restriction of motion at each site is described separately and then the overall effect of sagittal plane blockage is characterized.

Plantar Calcaneus

The plantar calcaneus has a round underside to permit the foot to roll over it during the contact phase of the step. This site has, relatively speaking, no moving parts, so disruption of motion is unusual. Disruption is most often

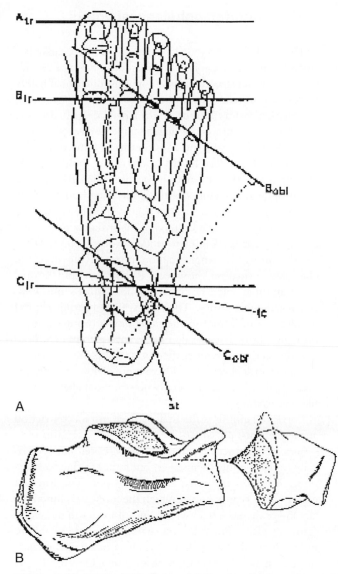

A

B

Figure 9-12 (A) In 1979, Bosjen-Möller described a two-part, high- and low-gear system used by the parabolic shape of the metatarsal heads to permit efficient propulsion. Line B_{tr} is formed by the axis of metatarsal heads one and two. Line B_{obl} is formed by metatarsal heads two through five. In this system, the perpendicular bisection of the oblique axis (B_{obl}) is far shorter than the transverse axis (B_{tr}). This shorter radius arm permits an efficient use of leverage about which heel lift can begin. Once the heel unweights sufficiently for liftoff, weight can shift to the longer radius for efficient use of the power created to pull the body forward. **(B)** As the weight shift from the oblique to the transverse axis occurs, the plantar aponeurosis tightens as a result of the longer radius arm associated with the transverse axis. The effect of this is to "close pack" the calcaneocuboid joint and thus stabilize the tarsus and midtarsus as the body load is beginning to increase across the forefoot. Without this mechanism, the osseous structures of the foot would not be able to resist the increasing loads applied, and this task would then fall to the soft tissues, with implications for overuse phenomena becoming more prevalent. (From Bosjen-Möller F: Calcaneocuboid joint and stability of the longitudinal arch of the foot at high and low gear push off. J Anat 129:165, 1979, with permission.)

present following severe injury to the heel, such as calcaneal fracture comminuting to the subtalar joint. Effectively, the loss of the rotation causes heel strike to become a "foot flat" contact, with the forefoot contacting simultaneously with the heel. This creates a significant reduction in the momentum created by the normal "rolling" heel strike motion, and affects the movement of the COM during the initial portion of the step. While thankfully not common, blockage here does present a difficult obstacle to forward progression.

Ankle Joint

Once the calcaneus permits motion to the foot flat stage, motion of the leg and all superior structures is dependent on ankle joint dorsiflexion for continued advancement until heel lift occurs. This accounts for approximately 40 percent of the single-support sagittal plane pivot. Restriction of ROM of the ankle to dorsiflexion therefore presents a significant obstruction to normal forward progression. There are essentially two types of restriction, structural and functional.

A structural restriction to ankle ROM can involve either degenerative or traumatic destruction of the ankle. Osseous lipping along the anterior tibia can also create a restriction to normal progression. True triceps surae (Achilles) tendon shortness, while more rare than generally believed, can restrict proper ankle joint dorsiflexion. Prior surgical intervention with fusion may be present, but in all cases ROM is either absent or very limited.

A functional restriction describes an equinus condition in which the normal 10 degrees of dorsiflexion is not available. This condition has often been attributed to congenital or acquired tightness in the triceps surae or Achilles tendon. While this has been the accepted wisdom regarding equinus, mechanical dysfunction of the fibula may restrict normal ankle ROM and mimic the tight heel cord condition. In this "fibula-related equinus," a fixation (temporary immobility) of the fibula prevents its normal translation motion from occurring. This blocks the ability of the ankle to broaden and accept the wider, anterior dome of the talus into the joint space as dorsiflexion occurs. While otherwise identical to the structural equinus, this condition will usually respond immediately to manipulation and spontaneously demonstrate normal dorsiflexion capacity. (The examination and manipulation for this are covered in the treatment section.)

Metatarsophalangeal Joints

The final site of pivotal motion is the metatarsophalangeal joints. These joints exhibit several types of restrictions, including structural hallux limitus, functional hallux limitus, and forefoot equinus.

Structural hallux limitus (SHL) is well described in the literature.[28] It represents a degenerative disease of the first metatarsophalangeal joint. Motion can be limited on both clinical and functional ROM examination. Pain is usually present at this site and may be accompanied by swelling and proliferative changes in the underlying bone.

Functional hallux limitus (FHL) has also been described in the literature.[29] It is defined as the inability of the first metatarsophalangeal joint to undergo dorsiflexion ROM strictly during the single-support phase of the step. On clinical examination, however, ROM is within normal limits and may even be hypermobile. In this sense, FHL is a paradoxical entity. The non-weight-bearing clinical findings are unrelated to the functional attributes present during walking. Patients do not describe pain in or around this joint and cannot relate their other symptoms to the first metatarsophalangeal joint. There is no edema or erythema present, and there are generally no structural changes visible within the joint.

Forefoot equinus is the final form of motion restriction at the metatarsophalangeal joints (Fig. 9-13). In this case, however, the absence of movement is related not specifically to these joints themselves, but rather to their relative position versus the remainder of the foot. The forefoot equinus foot type is one in which the forefoot is functionally lower than the heel when viewed from the transverse (ground) plane. Since the metatarsal bones are unable to move "beneath the ground," the effect of a forefoot equinus is to make the heel tip backward to achieve both heel and forefoot contact. In essence, having this foot shape causes the subject to walk uphill. Each time the metatarsophalangeal joints are required to provide motion, it is like climbing a small mound.

Compensations for Sagittal Plane Motion Blockade

The body, through its intricate design, efficiently creates the power to move the COM over the weight-bearing foot. The entire weight-bearing limb can therefore be viewed as passive, with the remainder of the body being involved in powering itself forward. The

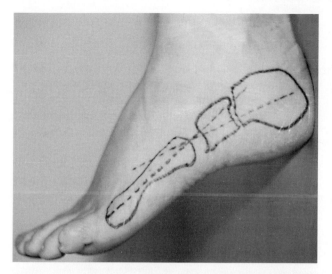

Figure 9-13 Forefoot equinus. Even when loaded, this foot (typically high arched) demonstrates a high sagittal declination angle of the forefoot on the rearfoot. During weight bearing, for heel and forefoot contact to occur, this foot must shift backward, causing an "uphill" position to be assumed. Despite full ROM of the metatarsophalangeal joints, sagittal plane blockade exists based on the shape of the foot structure.

role of the weight-bearing side is therefore to (1) efficiently transmit the power to the support surface, where a reactive longitudinal ground thrust develops, and (2) support the COM as it moves over that side. Since both the advancement of the COM and autosupport depend on the ability of the foot to provide specifically directed sagittal plane motion, a failure to perform correctly will result in a breakdown in either or both of the required actions. Recognizing the lower extremity and postural motions that result from sagittal plane motion blockade is the focus of this section.

As a general rule, the appropriate utilization of the power created for walking, when viewed in the second half of the single-support phase, causes joint motions in the direction of extension (first metatarsophalangeal joint dorsiflexion, medial longitudinal arch raising, ankle plantar flexion, knee extension, hip extension, erect torso [lumbar lordosis], erect head position [cervical lordosis]). This is consistent with efficient mechanical activity. Conversely, joint motion in the second half of single support, when viewed as flexion movements (failure of first metatarsophalangeal joint dorsiflexion, lowering of the medial longitudinal arch, prolonged ankle dorsiflexion, failure to reach full knee extension, failure to reach full hip

extension, flexed posture [straight lumbar spine], and forward head posture, can be indicative of compensatory accommodations to sagittal plane blockade. While these flexion motions have classically been viewed as single joint problems, looking at the entire picture of walking reveals their interrelationships. Each joint movement should be considered integrally related to the others. In the presence of sagittal plane blockade, flexion collapse of the knee and hip, for instance, should be considered as a single motion, rather than two completely separate ones. As an example, when a 10-car pileup occurs on a highway, the barrier created by the first two cars involved stops all movement along this path. The momentum of the cars behind them then causes a series of collisions to develop. This cause-and-effect activity creates a chain of events in which the cars further down the road are affected by the blockage directly in front of them. So too can the flexion joint collapse be viewed as the foot failing to provide the correct motion at the correct time. Since each joint is dependent on the motions adjacent to it, failure of the pivotal site with the ground, in the presence of the power designed to move the joints, leads to compensatory maneuvers as described previously.[30]

Conceptually, the flexion response is related to the power creation aspect of walking. The direction in which this power creates motion must be accommodated when failure to sagittally advance is not available. This is often quite subtle and may not immediately be related to sagittal plane blockade. For instance, in the classic pronated foot, the medial longitudinal arch can often be seen progressively lowering during the step. Considering that FHL is invariably present in this foot type, the accommodation in the sagittal plane direction is visible as this collapsing arch. As the heel is raised from the ground by the advancement of the COM over the foot, a failure to pivot at the first metatarsophalangeal joint results in the need to accommodate heel lift in the more proximal foot joints. The medial longitudinal arch, at the oblique midtarsal joint axis, is capable of allowing some amount of sagittal plane motion. This accommodation becomes visible as medial longitudinal arch collapse and, unfortunately, occurs during the period in which arch raising should occur. This motion reversal, coupled with the loss of autosupport related to the failure of the first metatarsophalangeal joint to dorsiflex, results in a pronated foot. This is not to say the FHL is the only cause of a pronated foot; however, it provides a recognition of the powerful influence of sagittal plane blockade and subsequent accommodation of various joints and motion segments (Fig. 9-14).

More proximally, the compensatory accommodation of sagittal plane blockade is visible as limitations to full ROM. For instance, in normal walking, the extension of the thigh on the hip should reach between 15 and 20 degrees by the end of the single-support phase. When sagittal plane blockade is present, the ability of the hip joint to undergo full-range extension is lost. Limitation is visible with 5 to 10 degrees of extension at the hip.[30] In addition, there may be addition accommodation with flexion of the torso as an adjustment to the loss of hip ROM. The classic flexed-posture geriatric patient is an example of the end result of this process. Systematic, gradual flexion accommodation to failed sagittal plane extension mechanics results in a form that has over time

followed a functional adaptation. Julius Wolffe described this "Form follows Function" axiom in the mid 1800s, and D'Arcy Thompson expanded on these principles in the early 1900s. Understanding the accommodation mechanisms as related to sagittal plane blockade provides a detailed understanding of the process of postural decay following the Wolffe axiom. Common sports injuries, such as plantar fasciitis and Achilles tendinitis, particularly when chronic, can relate to long-term, subtle sagittal plane blockade. Overload of these structures as a result of the negative implications of segment length and loss of autosupportive mechanisms will, over time, result in their becoming symptomatic. Specifically addressing the appropriate sagittal plane blockade site rather than the apparent symptomatic location can result in rapid and long-term cure. Readers are directed to other publica-

Figure 9-14 (A) This diagram is designed to demonstrate the alignment of the foot joints when viewed sagittally just prior to the onset of heel lift. Note the medial longitudinal arch form created by the osseous structures. **(B)** In the presence of FHL, as the heel is pulled from the ground by the advancing body above it, the midfoot must accommodate the failure of sagittal plane motion to develop at the metatarsophalangeal joints. This is visible as collapse of the medial longitudinal arch.

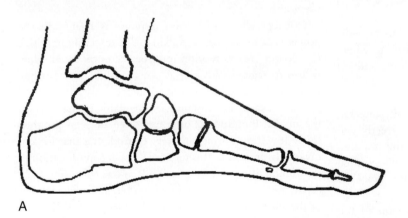

A

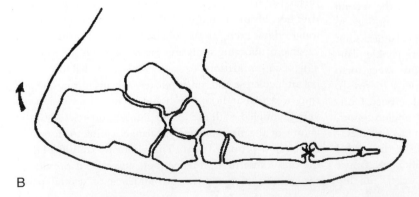

B

tions by this author that describe in detail the pathomechanics of this process and how they relate to various symptoms in the foot, ankle, and lower back.[31]

METHODS OF EVALUATION

In the examination for sagittal plane blockade, several basic factors must be considered. First, the patients exhibiting this phenomenon will complain of symptoms rather than motion restrictions. Second, these symptoms may be remote to the restricted motion site. It therefore becomes the clinical responsibility of the sports medicine practitioner to understand the relationship between the motion inhibitions and secondary symptoms.

Ankle Joint Sagittal Plane Clinical Examination

The examination of the ankle for the wide range of pathomechanical problems that may exist is beyond the scope of this chapter. Instead, dorsiflexion ROM with specific attention to fibula translation is addressed. However, determining total dorsiflexion ROM of the ankle is important in the overall evaluation. Should this motion be restricted (or absent) as a result of traumatic or degenerative arthritis or even prior fusion surgery, it is essential to keep this in mind and relate it to other sites where ROM losses can be accommodated. For instance, should ankle motion be restricted and FHL be simultaneously present, then virtually all the sagittal plane motion sites available during single support are blocked. Significant pain syndromes can develop under these circumstances, and the examiner must aware of the consequences. Establishing ROM at the functionally restricted side can go a long way toward establishing an improved patient outcome.

With the subtalar joint held in the neutral position and the subject's knee fully extended, ROM of the ankle can be evaluated. Normally, 10 degrees of dorsiflexion should be available. Limitations can exist to a point at which no or even negative dorsiflexion is present. Once existing ROM of the ankle is established, this examination repeated with the examiner palpating the head of the fibula just lateral and distal to the knee. The fibula head should be felt moving both laterally and cranially. Comparison of the left and right legs should be performed to judge relative differences of both in terms of fibula translation and total ankle joint motion. Restrictions in this palpable ROM of the fibula head can indicate restriction based on fibula fixation (temporary motion restriction, which responds to manual manipulative therapy). Patients may involuntarily flex the knee during attempts to dorsiflex the ankle, and care should be taken to prevent this from occurring. In addition, tightness in the triceps surae and Achilles tendon and/or tightness and pain in the popliteal fossa may also be indicative of fibula-related equinus. Although equinus deformity (lack of normal ankle joint dorsiflexion ROM) has been associated with short Achilles tendons, triceps surae complex, and subsequent need for surgical lengthening, fibula fixation can mimic this situation. Appropriate manual manipulative treatment (covered in the final section of this chapter) can immediately resolve this situation.

Symptoms that can be related to fibula-related equinus include Achilles tendinitis, plantar fasciitis, acute (or chronic) forefoot bursitis or vague metatarsalgia, chronic or acute posterior calf pain, and pain in the medial or posterior knee. Some cases of chronic sacroiliac joint pain may also relate to a fibula equinus. Anatomic connections between the fibula and sacrum via the biceps femoris and sacrotuberous ligament have been established. Limited ROM of the fibula can therefore affect motion of the sacrum, and chronic symptoms can result. Detailed explanation of this phenomenon is beyond the scope of the chapter, and readers are referred elsewhere for more complete descriptions.[32]

Functional Hallux Limitus

As described earlier, FHL is a paradox. On standard clinical examination, ROM of the first metatarsophalangeal joint can be normal or even hypermobile. Effective clinical evaluation involves partial reproduction of weight bearing so that motion can be studied with the joints under load. Several methods can be employed to assess for FHL.

With the patient seated or lying supine and the examiner seated at the foot of the patient, ROM of the first metatarsophalangeal joint in the dorsiflexion direction is evaluated. Then the examiner's opposite thumb is used to load the plantar surface of the first metatarsal head just between the sesamoids. Moderate, not excessive, upward pressure is all that is necessary. Hallux dorsiflexion is then repeated while the load is maintained on the first metatarsal head. Normally, 15 to 20 degrees of dorsiflexion should be available with the first metatarsal head loaded. Failure to obtain

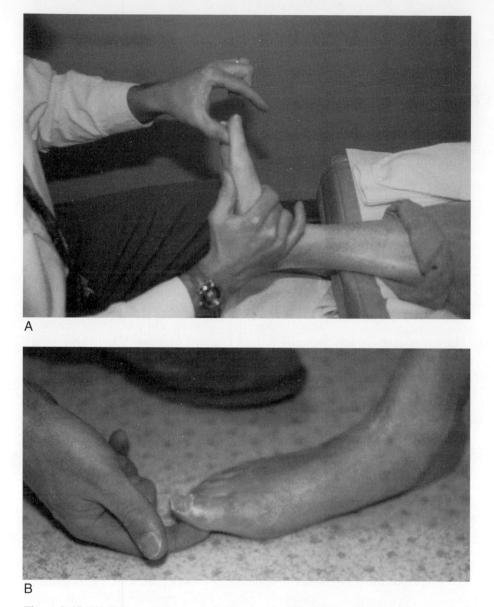

Figure 9-15 (A) FHL test (patient seated). The thumb of the right hand loads the first metatarsal head while the thumb of the left hand examines for metatarsophalangeal joint range of motion. Failure to achieve 15 to 20 degrees of metatarsophalangeal joint dorsiflexion is positive for FHL. **(B)** FHL test (patient standing). Using the examiner's index finger, dorsiflexion ROM of the hallux is attempted. Less than 15 to 20 degrees of first metatarsophalangeal joint ROM is positive for FHL.

this amount of motion indicates a positive test for FHL (Fig. 9-15A).

In an alternative approach, ROM can be evaluated with the patient standing (Fig. 9-15B). The subject is instructed to stand on one foot. The examiner then attempts to dor-

siflex the hallux. Failure to achieve 15 to 20 degrees of hallux dorsiflexion is again positive for FHL.

Symptoms of FHL can be wide ranging. Since sagittal plane blockade can be either accommodated or avoided, a large array of chronic problems can be associated with this entity. These can include the entire list associated with fibula-related equinus and can additionally include interdigital neuromas and chronic lateral foot pain. Chronic postural symptoms, including lower back pain, patello femoral syndrome, greater trochanteric bursitis, and iliotibial band syndrome, have also been linked to FHL.[33] Of particular interest, long-term cure of chronic lower back pain has been reported when FHL is addressed, despite that fact that FHL, in and of itself, remains asymptomatic. Careful examination for FHL should be undertaken in all patients with these symptoms.

Structural Hallux Limitus

Structural hallux limitus has been extensively described in the literature. ROM of the joint will be less than the required 65 degrees. Often, total ROM is one-half or less of normal amounts. SHL has been described as being preceded by FHL.[28] In some cases SHL will eventually result, whereas in others ROM remains apparently normal yet is restricted during gait (FHL). In either case, the examination technique described for FHL can be employed for SHL. Should the available ROM with the joint loaded be less than that of the nonloaded joint, then at least some component of FHL can exist within this structural deformity. Treatment concepts are addressed in the final section.

Forefoot Equinus

This type of blockade is easily detectable via clinical examination. With the subject either supine or seated, the foot is viewed in a nonloaded condition. Examination is directed to the lateral aspect of the foot. From the base of the fifth metatarsal, there will be a plantar declination of the structures distalward. With the rearfoot then stabilized with one hand, the entire forefoot, via pressure across the metatarsal heads, is dorsiflexed. If the level of declination cannot be reduced so that the plantar-flexed attitude is no longer visible, then a positive identification of forefoot equinus can be made.

Symptoms of forefoot equinus are typically plantar fasciitis, lateral foot pain at the cuboid and/or lateral ankle, and an array of forefoot symptoms from bursitis to metatarsalgia.

TREATMENT: MANIPULATIVE CARE AND ORTHOTIC MANAGEMENT

Manipulative Care

The concept of manipulation dates back to Hippocrates. Skilled, rapid movement of joints has been shown to increase ROM and reduce pain sensation. The relationship between pain and motion is one that has been extensively explored in the neuroscience literature.[34–37] The primary pain receptor in all vertebrates, the primary afferent nociceptor, is a C-fiber, nonmyelinated structure that transmits signals to the spinal cord in a relatively slow fashion. The sensitivity of this nociceptor has also been shown to be modulable. Changes in nerve compression, joint motion, and/or muscle hypertonicity can alter the threshold at which a nociceptor signals a pain response to the central nervous system. While there are dedicated nociceptor synaptic sites in the spinal cord, there are also locations in which proprioceptive-type motion signals synapse with nociceptive input. These are known as wide dynamic range cells. When the motion signals are improper, particularly if range is limited and present over an extended period of time, the nociceptive input can be "misinterpreted." The pain level is then perceived as far greater than would otherwise be the case. In other words, a signal that would not normally relay a painful experience is sensed as severe pain. When rapid, specific manipulation is performed, the effect is not only local but systemic. The intense stimulation of the rapid-firing proprioceptive receptors causes the wide dynamic range cells to be "reset," and nociceptive input is again sensed as normal. Thresholds return to typical levels and pain perception decreases. This effect, in combination with the biomechanical aspects of normal ROM, is the one that is sought in manipulative therapy.

MANIPULATIONS FOR FIBULA-RELATED EQUINUS

After careful examination of fibula translation, absence of motion can be significant as a primary pathomechanical entity causing ankle equinus. Manipulation of the fibula can be performed with immediate return to normal ankle ROM. There are three basic techniques for fibula manipulation, two direct at the proximal fibula and one indirect at the ankle joint.

Fibula Manipulation: Patient Supine

With the patient either seated in the examination chair or supine on an examination table, the knee is flexed and the foot is placed flat on the chair or table. Standing in

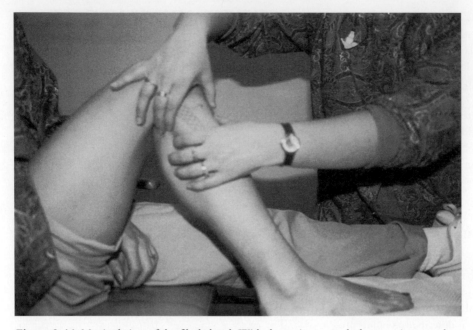

Figure 9-16 Manipulation of the fibula head. With the patient seated, the examiner stands at the foot end of the table. Grasping the fibula head above and below the peroneal nerve, the manipulation is performed by "pulling" the head forward (posterior to anterior). The thumbs are used as an anchor over the tibia. There is no audible sensation with the maneuver and, until ankle joint ROM is re-examined and increased range demonstrated, it may appear as though little to no result is achieved.

front of the affected side, the examiner grasps the fibula head with both hands, using the middle and index fingers (Fig. 9-16). The top hand is placed at the superior surface of the fibula head, and the bottom hand is placed below the peroneal notch on the fibula. (Care must be taken to avoid compression of the peroneal nerve during the manipulation process.) Once the fingers are in place on the fibula, the examiner's thumbs are then used to grasp the anteromedial portion of the tibia. Using the thumbs as an anchor, the fibula is then manipulated with a rapid "squeeze" action of the fingers, pulling the fibula head forward relative to the tibia. There is no audible sound associated with this maneuver, and there is often no sense that movement of the fibula has occurred. Effectiveness of this maneuver is evaluated by change in ankle joint ROM, which is immediately assessed following manipulation.

Fibula Manipulation: Patient Prone

This technique is useful in patients with large legs or where there is extreme tenderness over the anterior aspect of the tibia. With the supine technique, grasping the tibia

can be acutely painful and therefore should be avoided where a history of tibial tenderness exists.

With the patient in the prone position, the fibula can first be loosened using a muscle energy technique. The leg is flexed to 90 degrees to the thigh. Standing in front of the leg, the examiner grasps the ankle and tries to extend the knee while the patient is asked to resist this movement. This is performed to an 8-second count and is a relatively gentle maneuver. It is not necessary to provide excessive extension force; rather, the examiner should match the patient's strength. Once this maneuver is completed, the knee is then extended so that the entire limb is flat on the table. The examiner then places his or her palm on the posterior fibula head and a manipulation from posterior to anterior is performed (Fig. 9-17). Only moderate force need be applied. Ankle joint ROM is then used to measure success of this manipulation.

Manipulation of the Talus

In cases of longstanding fibula-related equinus, it is often necessary to free both the proximal and the distal fibula. The distal fibula is mobilized using the wedge shape of the talus.

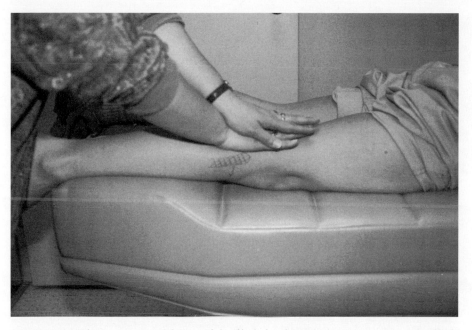

Figure 9-17 Alternative manipulation of the fibula head. With the patient prone, the fibula head is palpated. With the palm placed directly over the fibula head, a gentle downward thrust is imparted. Again, there is no audible sensation with the maneuver and, until ankle joint ROM is re-examined and increased range demonstrated, it may appear as though little to no result is achieved.

With the patient in the seated position, the affected limb is placed in a fully extended position. The examiner stands at the foot of the patient, and the foot is grasped with thumbs over the dorsum of the talus and middle and long fingers over the posterior calcaneus. Longitudinal traction is then applied for at least 30 to 45 seconds in an effort to relax the ankle. Without releasing the traction, the manipulation is performed (Fig. 9-18). The thrust is performed in an anterior-to-posterior direction, moving the talus between the fibula and tibia. There can be an audible "pop" associated with this maneuver. ROM of the ankle is then examined as a method of evaluation of this procedure.

Orthotic Care

The approach to orthotic management of pedal pathology has been one for which the standard has been "motion control." It was believed that overpronation of the subtalar joint during the contact phase was responsible for an "unlocking" of the midfoot and rearfoot complex. This would render the foot incapable of becoming an effective "rigid lever" at propulsion. It was therefore a logical conclusion

that controlling this impact pronation would be an effective therapy. As the concept of sagittal plane motion blockade has come into prominence, a new method of orthotic management has developed. This is the philosophy of "motion enhancement." Rather than limiting pronation at heel contact, the conceptual change is to positively influence the mechanics by enhancing sagittal plane motion. For instance, preventing the development of FHL thereby permits the normal autosupportive mechanisms to operate at the appropriate time in the gait cycle. Creating a device that places the foot in a position in which it is capable of supporting itself becomes the challenge. It is this approach that is discussed in this section.

FABRICATION STRATEGY

The orthotics fabricated for sagittal plane motion enhancement depend on the functional examination findings described earlier in this chapter. Essentially, there are three type of devices that can be designed depending on the specific site or sites of sagittal blockade. Each is discussed here based on foot type, with general suggestions as to

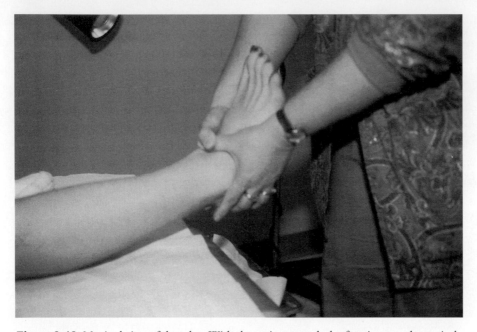

Figure 9–18 Manipulation of the talus. With the patient seated, the foot is grasped superiorly over the talus and posteriorly over the calcaneus. Long traction is then applied for 20 to 30 seconds. The thrust is then performed from anterior to posterior, manipulating the talus between the ankle bones. There may be an audible sensation associated with this maneuver. ROM of the ankle in dorsiflexion should be immediately attempted following the manipulation.

posting and extension modifications. Some other specifics regarding materials are also described.

The need for rigid materials for motion enhancement devices is not as critical as in motion control devices. When the foot has a moderate or high arch, rigid materials tend to be contraindicated. Flexible shell materials such as Toprel or 2 to 3-mm subortholene provide considerable comfort and proper alignment.

The Kinetic Wedge (KW) extension is used for specific foot types. This is a patented extension whereby the area under the first metatarsal head is both softer than the remaining extension material and wider medially than laterally (Fig. 9-19). It is specifically used when FHL is present. It can be fabricated in several styles, including a firm material under metatarsals two through five when lateral balance is important. When FHL is present and the forefoot is sensitive, then materials such as PPT or medical-grade Poron can be utilized. In the latter case, the second through fifth metatarsal area is made of 1/8–inch-thick material while the sub–first metatarsal material is 1/16 inch thick. This effect is to promote first metatarsal plantar flexion/eversion while dorsiflexing the base of the proximal phalanx of the hallux relative the first metatarsal head. The following labs are currently licensed to fabricate this device: Langer Biomechanics Lab (Deer Park, NY), Applied Orthotic Lab (Londonderry, NH), and Ruch Orthotic Lab (Pekin, IL).

In addition to the KW itself, a digital platform can be used to enhance hallux dorsiflexion relative to first ray plantar flexion (Fig. 9-20). The platform can be fabricated from firm material and extends from the sulcus to the ends of the digits. In cases where excessive hallux dorsiflexion is necessary, this digital platform can be fabricated thicker distally than proximally to ensure proper great toe positioning. If this is the case, care must be taken to have the patient purchase shoes with an adequate toebox to prevent hallux jamming.

The KW is designed to be fabricated with an orthotic shell incorporating a first ray cutout. While the standard orthotics cutout has been used in the past, with this type of material the amount removed from under the first ray is far more extensive. There are three basic cutout designs: standard (small), bidirectional, and long (Fig. 9-21).

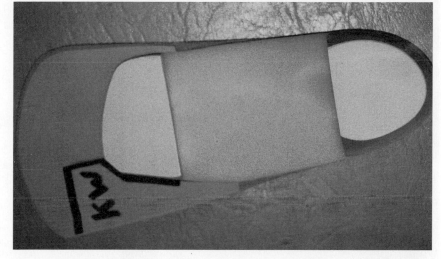

Figure 9-19 An orthotic with a Kinetic Wedge extension (KW). The distal aspect is configured to the transverse axis as described by Bosjen-Möller. It is wider medially than laterally to permit both plantar flexion and eversion of the first metatarsal head.

Standard: This involves removing a small amount of material from under the very tip of the medial-distal aspect of the orthotic. This is useful when limited amounts of first ray plantar flexion are desired.

Bidirectional: By far the most commonly used, this involves using the orthotic shell to rotate (evert) as well as plantar-flex the first metatarsal. This is the ideal cutout to be used with FHL.

Long: This is useful when first ray plantar flexion is very difficult and loading of the plantar surface of the metatarsal is minimal. This is very helpful in cases of structural hallux limitus/rigidus when 15 degrees of motion or more is available. If less than 15 degrees' motion exists, the concept of motion enhancement is not a successful model for treatment of this condition without surgical intervention[38]

SAMPLE ORTHOTIC DESIGNS

Forefoot Equinus

In this foot, the plantar-flexed position of the forefoot relative to the heel creates a situation in which the patient is essentially walking uphill. The goal of the orthotic is to neutralize this effect and permit ease of heel lift.

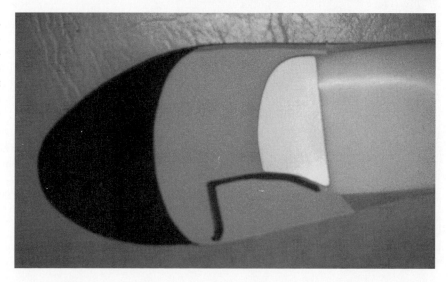

Figure 9-20 A KW extension incorporating a digital platform. The black-colored material distal to the KW extension is fabricated from a firmer material so as to create a dorsiflexed hallux relative to a plantar-flexed metatarsal. This is very effective in difficult-to-treat FHL.

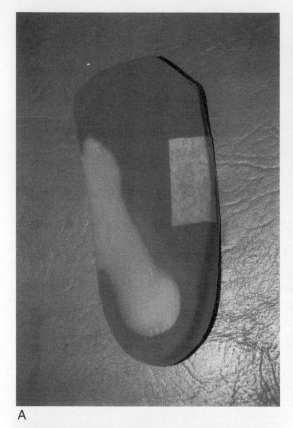

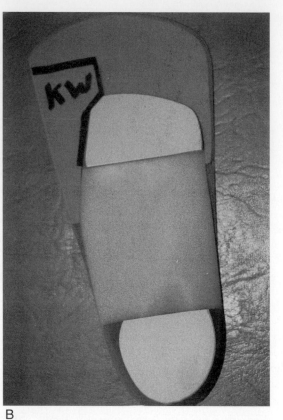

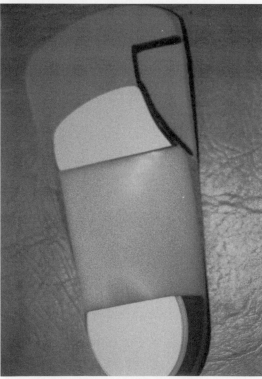

Figure 9–21 (A) Standard first ray cutout in a right foot orthotic without a KW. The smaller size cutout is indicated when FHL is minimally present. **(B)** Bidirectional first ray cutout in a left foot orthotic with a KW. Note the two-directional cutout. This permits plantar flexion while creating an environment for eversion of the first metatarsal. It is indicated in cases of FHL and early SHL with ROM greater than 30 degrees. **(C)** Long first cutout in a right foot device, and the largest cutout used. It is indicated in resistant FHL or SHL where ROM is less than 30 degrees.

Shell material: 2- or 3-mm subortholene or cork/leather

Rearfoot post: neutral (0 degrees)

Heel lift: 1/8 inch + amount of limb shortness

Forefoot post: none to 2 degrees of valgus

First ray cutout: small (none if first ray rigidly plantar flexed)

Extension: none

An interesting note involves the complaint of forefoot metatarsalgia-type symptoms that this foot type tends to develop. The use of padding is actually contraindicated for this foot because the ability of the metatarsal head to "drop off" accomodating the metatarsal heads to drop, promotes far better function and will usually eliminate symptoms that exist. Padding this type of foot seems to prevent proper loading and often leads to continued pain and disability.

Pronating Flatfoot

Care must be taken with this foot to ensure that any fibula-related equinus is adequately addressed by manipulation and stretching. Once this is done, then the following type of prescription is often helpful.

Shell material: 4-mm subortholene or other suitable rigid material

Rearfoot post: 0 to 4 degrees (use only up to 2 degrees in most cases)

Forefoot post: 1 to 3 degrees depending on forefoot position

First ray: cutout in bidirectional style

Extension: KW-type extension (soft or firm)

Digital platform: firm

Flexible Forefoot Valgus

Shell material: 2- to 3-mm subortholene

Rearfoot post: 0 degrees

Forefoot post: 1 to 3 degrees of valgus

First ray: bidirectional cutout

Extension: KW (firm under second through fifth metatarsals)

Digital platform: optional

CONCLUSION

The ability to identify pathologic motions within the sagittal plane extends the sports practitioner's scope of understanding a wide range of chronic disorders that plague athletes. Using skills that combine diagnostic ability with manipulative and orthotic fabrication, long-term cures can be obtained. Utilizing an approach that reflects the new concept of motion enhancement permits the clinician to view overuse problems in a different light, and thus represents another tool for patient management.

REFERENCES

Biomechanics of the Foot and Ankle

1. Mero A, Komi PV, Gregar RJ: Biomechanics of sprint running: a review. Sports Med 13:376, 1992
2. Morris C, Bartlett R: Biomechanical factors critical for performance in the men's javelin throw. Sports Med 21:438, 1996
3. Wilder RP, Brennan DK: Physiological responses to deep water running in athletes. Sport Med 16:374, 1993
4. LaBrier K, O'Neill DB: Patellofemoral stress syndrome. Sports Med 16:449, 1993
5. Barrett J, Bilisko T: The role of shoes in the prevention of ankle sprains. Sports Med 20:227, 1995
6. Subotnick SI: The flexible flatfoot. Arch Podiatr Med Foot Surg 1:7, 1973
7. Walz D, Craig BM et al: Bone imaging showing shin splints and stress fractures. Clin Nucl Med 12:92, 1987
8. Detmer DE: Chronic shin spints: classification and management of medial tibial stress syndrome. Sports Med 3:436, 1986
9. Aspegren DD et al: Detection of stress fractures in athletes and non athletes. J Manipulative and Physiol Ther 12:298, 1989
10. Root M, Weed J, Orien W: Normal and Abnormal Function of the Foot, Vol. 2. Clinical Biomechanics, Los Angeles, 1977
11. Ferkel RD: Ankle arthroscopic treatment of anterolateral impingement of the ankle. Presented at the 15th annual meeting of the American Orthopedic Society for Sports Medicine, Traverse City, MI, June 1989
12. Kvist M et al: Chronic Achilles paratenenitis on athletes. Pathology 19:1, 1987
13. Laine HR et al: Ultrasonography as a differential diagnostic aid in achilodynia. J Ultrasound Med 6:351, 1992
14. Dananberg HJ: Functional hallux limitus. J Am Podiatr Med Assoc 83:433, 1993

Sagittal Plane-Biomechanics

15. Mann RA, Moran GT, Dougherty S: Comparative electromyography of the lower extremity in jogging, running, and sprinting. Am J Sports Med 14:501, 1986
16. Claeys R: The analysis of ground reaction forces in pathologic gait. Int Orthop Spring:113, 1983
17. Dorman T: Elastic energy of the pelvis. p. 365. In Dorman T (ed): Spine: State of the Art Reviews, Vol. 9. Hanley and Belfus, Philadelphia, 1995
18. Gracovetsky S: The Spinal Engine. Springer-Verlag, Heidelberg, 1987
19. Vleeming A, Pool-Goiudzwaard A, Stoeckart R et al: The posterior layer of the thoracolumbar fascia. Spine 20:753, 1995
20. Vleeming A: The posterior layer of the thoracolumbar fascia. p. 139. In Vleeming A, Mooney V, Dorman T, Snijders C (eds): The Integrated Function of the Lumbar Spine and Sacroiliac Joint, Part 1. Proceedings of the 2nd Congress on Lower Back Pain, San Diego, CA, November 9–11, 1995
21. Perry J: Gait Analysis: Normal and Pathologic Function. Slack Inc, Thorofare, NJ, 1992
22. Dananberg HJ: Gait style as an etiology to chronic postural pain, Part I. Functional hallux limitus. J Am Podiatr Med Assoc 83:433, 1993
23. Fuller B: Synergetics. Collier Books, New York, 1975
24. Bosjen-Möller F: Calcaneocuboid joint and stability of the longitudinal arch of the foot at high and low gear push off. J Anat 129:165, 1979
25. Mechanics: energy, forces and their effects. p. 805. In Encyclopedia Brittanica, 15th ed. Encyclopedia Britannica, Chicago, 1987
26. Root M et al: Abnormal and Normal Function of the Foot. Clinical Biomechanics Corp, Los Angeles, 1977
27. Hicks JH: The mechanics of the foot II: The plantar aponeurosis and the arch. J Anat 000:25, 1954
28. Drago JJ, Oloff L, Jacobs AM: Comprehensive review of hallux limitus. J Foot Surg 23:213, 1984
29. Dananberg HJ: Functional hallux limitus and its relationship to gait efficiency. J Am Podiatr Med Assoc 76:648, 1986
30. Dananberg HJ: Lower extremity pathomechanics and its effect on sacroiliac function. p. 389. In Dorman T (ed): Spine: State of the Art Reviews, Vol. 9. Belfus and Hanley, Philadelphia, 1995
31. Dananberg HJ: Lower back pain as a gait related repetitive motion injury. p. 253. In Vleeming A, Mooney V, Dorman T et al. (eds): Movement: The Pelvis and Low Back Pain—An Interdisciplinary Approach. Churchill Livingstone, Edinburgh, 1997
32. Vleeming A: A new light on low back pain. p. 147. In Vleeming A, Mooney V, Dorman T, Snijders C (eds): The Integrated Function of the Lumbar Spine and Sacroiliac Joint, Part 1. Proceedings of the 2nd Congress on Lower Back Pain, San Diego, CA, November 9–11, 1995
33. Dananberg HJ: Gait style as an etiology to chronic postural pain, Part II. The postural compensatory process. J Am Podiatr Med Assoc 83:11615, 1993
34. Zimmermann M: Pain mechanisms and mediators in osteoarthritis. Semin Arthritis Rheum 18 (suppl):22, 1989
35. Levine J, Fields HL, Basbaum AI: Peptides and the primary afferent nociceptor. J Neurosci 13:2273, 1993
36. Cornefjord M, Olmarker K, Farley DB et al: Neuropeptide changes in compressed spinal nerve roots. Spine 20:670, 1995
37. Levine JD, Moskowitz MA, Basbaum AI: The contribution of neurogenic inflammation in experimental arthritis. J Immunol 135:843, 1995
38. Dananberg HJ, Phillips AJ, Blaakman H: A rational approach to the nonsurgical treatment of hallux limitus. p. 67. In Richard J (ed): Advances in Podiatric Medicine and Surgery II. CV Mosby, St. Louis, MO, 1996

SUGGESTED READINGS

Biomechanics of the Foot and Ankle

Chessler SM, Grumbine NA: An examination procedure for cavo-adducto-varus. J Foot Surg 18:1, 1978

Evans D: Calcaneal valgus deformity. J Bone Joint Surg [Br] 57:270, 1975

Grumbine NA, Chessler SM: An evaluation for compensated anterior cavus. J Foot Surg 19:142, 1980

Subotnick SI: Biomechanical approach to running injuries. Ann N Y Acad Sci 301:888, 1977

10

Normal Patterns of Walking and Running*

BARRY BATES
NICHOLAS STERGIOU

Normal human locomotion is the translation of the body from one point to another using a series of rhythmical, alternating movements of the limbs and trunk. The repetitive events that occur during walking or running constitute the gait cycle. The gait cycle begins when the foot contacts the ground and ends with the following ground contact of the same foot. The two major components of the gait cycle are stance phase and swing phase. A limb is in stance phase when it is in contact with the ground, and it is in swing phase when it is not in contact. The period when only one limb is in contact with the ground is referred to as single support, while double support occurs when both limbs are in contact with the ground simultaneously. The approximate amounts of time spent in each phase of the gait cycle during walking are stance phase, 60 percent of the cycle; swing phase, 40 percent of the cycle; and double support, 20 percent of the cycle (Fig. 10-1). With increased walking speed there is an increase in time spent in the swing phase, and at slower speed there is a decrease. The duration of double support decreases as walking speed increases and eventually is eliminated with the transition to running. The running cycle consists of a support phase and an airborne phase, with each limb moving through a support and a swing phase. The support phases vary from about 60 to 40 percent for

slow to fast running, respectively, with corresponding relative nonsupport periods of 40 to 60 percent for both limbs. The relationship between the support and swing phases for each limb varies between 20 to 30 percent and 80 to 70 percent, respectively. These support and swing phases can be further divided as indicated in Figure 10-1. The completion of a single step occurs when the opposite limb makes contact with the ground about midway through the forward swing subphase at about 70 to 80 percent of the limb cycle.

WALKING VERSUS RUNNING

A theoretical model of locomotion should be considered as a starting point to describe and understand the gait patterns of walking and running. The major observation is that in walking the body is always in contact with the ground, whereas in running there is a flight phase. Thus, from a purely mechanical perspective, the body's center of gravity (COG) must travel more in the vertical direction during running than in walking. Mathematically, the vertical displacement in locomotion can be described as a sinusoidal function. The simple pendulum-like motion associated with this function is known as harmonic motion. The differential equation for harmonic motion is

$$\theta'' + \omega^2\theta = 0$$

where θ = angle of the oscillation and ω = angular

---

* This chapter is adapted from the chapter by James W. Aston, Jr., and James J. Carollo that appeared in the first edition.

157

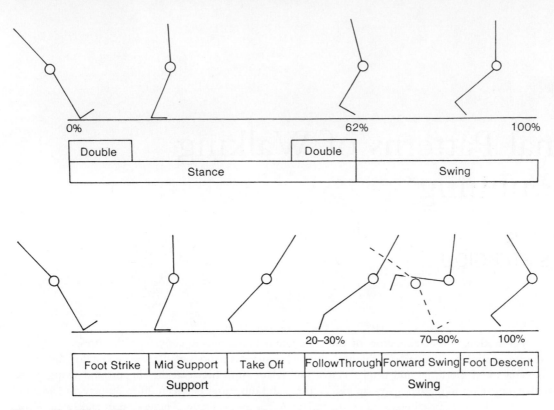

Figure 10-1 The walk cycle (top) and run cycle (bottom). (Redrawn from Slocum, DB: Overuse syndromes of the lower leg and foot in athletes. American Academy of Orthopedic Surgeons Instructional Course Lectures, Vol. 17. CV Mosby, St Louis, 1960, with permission.)

frequency. The sinusoidal wave function will be elongated or shortened by changes in frequency and will be increased or decreased in magnitude by changes in angle of oscillation. Therefore, stride length (angle of oscillation) and stride frequency, and their product, the resultant speed, are extremely important components of locomotion.

Changes in frequency and stride length will be mirrored in energy transfer. Plotting the energy expenditure versus speed in walking will result in a parabola.[2] Increases in speed result in increased frequency, and lower or higher speeds require greater energy per step compared to an intermediate speed. The parabolic function indicates that there is an optimal minimum at which walking is more efficient that is associated with an individual's preferred speed. If speed is further increased, a transition to running will eventually occur. In running, increases in speed result in increases first in stride length and then in stride frequency. The energy expenditure curve is also a parabolic function.[3] Shortly after the transition from walking to running, energy expenditure will drop to an optimal minimum where frequency and stride length work together to the body's best advantage.

Basically, the sinusoidal curve of the vertical displacement of the COG reflects the transitions between potential and kinetic energy (Fig. 10-2). At the lower points the kinetic energy is maximal, whereas at the higher points the potential energy is maximal. The transfer of energy back and forth from kinetic to potential is occurring in both running and walking,[4] and as a result energy is conserved within the body. Thus the work of the muscular system is minimized. However, Inman[5] pointed out that the system in locomotion is not perfect. He estimated that the transfer of energy is about 50 percent efficient and the remaining energy must be supplied by muscle action. The higher the potential energy that is generated from the greater vertical deviations of the body's COG while moving from walking to running (and introducing flight phases), the more kinetic energy needs to be generated. The generation of the kinetic energy occurs on the ground, where Newton's action–reaction law and friction are crucial. The harder the push against the ground, the larger the propulsion will be. Subsequently, the increase in stride length is not a result of reaching but of the greater push-off power generated by the lower extremity. The generation of larger amounts of kinetic energy will result in increased energy expenditure as described above. Williams and Cavanagh[6] showed that, in running at 3.6 m/s, an increase of 0.5 cm of vertical displacement of the COG resulted in significant increases in VO_2.

The horizontal component of the COG reflects the task of the movement, which is to move the body forward. Thus the horizontal component can be represented as a linear equation ($y = ax + b$). Increases in speed will affect the slope of this function and it will become steeper. However, a comparison with data from the literature reveals that what actually happens is not exactly what has been hypothesized. The reason is that the body experiences de-

celeration every time it contacts the ground. The body's inertia must be controlled; otherwise, the body will fall forward. Following contact, the velocity decreases during the braking phase of the movement. This phase is more critical in running, where the COG has been raised higher and accumulated more potential energy, resulting in greater vertical velocity at contact, with greater kinetic energy ($K = 1/2mv^2$, where m is a constant). This results not only in a braking action but also an impact phenomenon due to the collision of the body with the ground. Therefore, in running the action of the lower extremities is not only to maintain forward motion and accelerate the COG against external and internal resistances but also to support the body's weight and absorb the impact at contact. Subsequently, when speed increases, energy expenditure increases not only due to the propulsion phase but additionally because the muscu-

Figure 10-2 The transitions between kinetic and potential energy.

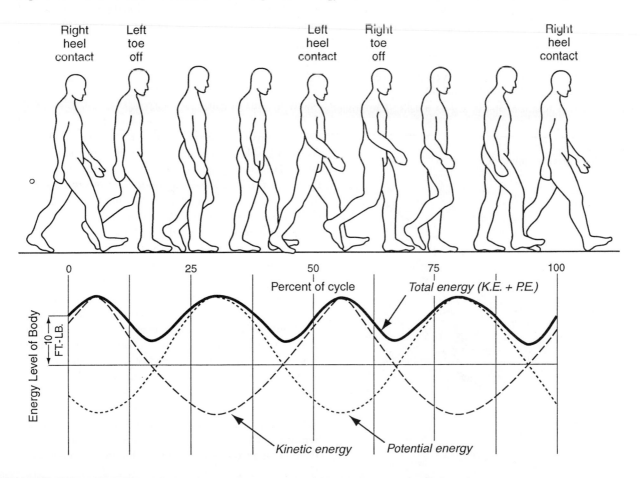

Right heel contact   Left toe off   Left heel contact   Right toe off   Right heel contact

Percent of cycle

Total energy (K.E. + P.E.)

Energy Level of Body — 10 — FT.-LB.

Kinetic energy   Potential energy

loskeletal system must dissipate impact forces and decelerate the body.

IMPACT

During the impact stage, maximum force is generated, although the joints undergo minimal motion. Joints are stable at the end of their range and unstable in between these extremes (Fig. 10-3). This inherent stability is afforded both by the bony architecture and by the ligaments spanning the joint. For instance, the hip owes much of its stability to its tight ball-and-socket fit, whereas the knee must depend primarily on ligaments for support. All joints have an endpoint stability if allowed to collapse. Were it not for muscles, all joints would collapse completely at impact. During impact, the hip extensors check excessive hip flexion as the quadriceps muscles prevent the knee from buckling into extreme flexion. At the same time, ankle dorsiflexors resist the foot slap that would otherwise occur as the ankle quickly plantar-flexes.

As the limb is vertically loaded, the head of the talus falls over the calcaneus medially, lowering the arch, pushing the heel laterally, and pronating the foot. The posterior tibial muscle contracts to prevent excessive talar descent. Because the talus is mortised within the ankle joint, it causes passive internal rotation of the leg as it falls. The ankle

Figure 10-3 Status of joints during impact.

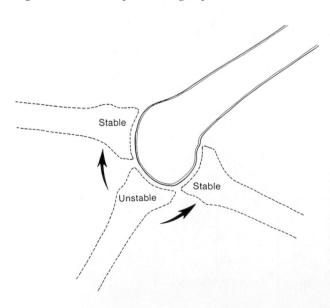

is thereby oriented to operate in the line of progression, even though the foot is positioned in external rotation (Fig. 10-4).

TRANSFER

During transfer, force diminishes while motion is maximal. Internal rotation of the limb is obligatory at foot contact as a part of talar descent and begins at the ankle and foot level. By contrast, unloading in external rotation begins at the hip level. The swing limb rotates the pelvis, causing external rotation of the stance limb, unwinding the rotation from the hip downward. The femur imparts its external rotation to the tibia via the knee joint. This rotational effort must increase if the tibia is excessively internally rotated, as is common in foot pronation. The result is a varus stress to the knee and lateral patellar compression, both contributory to the pain of runner's knee. The rotational reversal that occurs during transfer unlocks the joints from a relatively stable to an unstable midrange position. It is in this free range that the joints, while more vulnerable to injury, are most efficient at converting an otherwise stiff-legged vaulting gait into a motion that is both smooth and energy efficient. During transfer, the COG is moved alternately from side to side over the supporting foot (Fig. 10-5). Acting in this way, the joints have been called the "determinants of gait."[5]

As external rotation reaches the ankle, the talus is twisted back on the calcaneus and the subtalar and midtarsal joints are now stable in the opposite (inversion) end of their range. The soleus muscle contracts, preventing ankle dorsiflexion as the heel leaves the floor. Because the joints of the foot have now been made stable, the foot can act as a single rigid lever. Takeoff can occur properly at the toes instead of merely straining the midfoot.

Impact, transfer, and recovery are appropriate terms for slow running as well as walking. Long-distance runners commonly show a heel–foot–toe ground contact pattern, whereas mid-distance runners contact foot–toe. Sprinters try to avoid rearfoot contact altogether but often do make total foot contact following a forefoot contact. The force at impact is much greater in running, reaching two to three times body weight. As the speed of running increases, the muscles and joints make adaptive changes. Balance, a part of normal bipedal walking, is less important in running, and the base of support narrows. While the COG moves over the support limb in walking, it is the limbs that move beneath the COG in running, eliminating transfer (Fig. 10-6). This accommodative hip adduction and knee varus

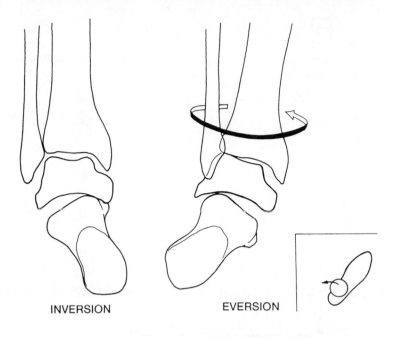

Figure 10-4 Inversion and eversion.

INVERSION   EVERSION

can so tighten the iliotibial band that the inflammatory iliotibial band syndrome results. Conditions that exaggerate the varus attitude include the uphill limb in incline running, excessive internal rotation of the foot on contact, worn lateral heels of the shoes, and the cavus foot.

The joints exhibit more flexion at the hip and knee during running, presumably for better absorption of the increased force and accommodation of the lowered COG. While exaggerated in range of motion, the joints generally act similarly in walking and running. Muscles, too, generally contract phasically in running as well as walking. Mann and Hagy[7] showed that, with increased speed, muscles increase their time of contraction, beginning earlier and lasting longer.

Figure 10-5 Line of progression: walking.

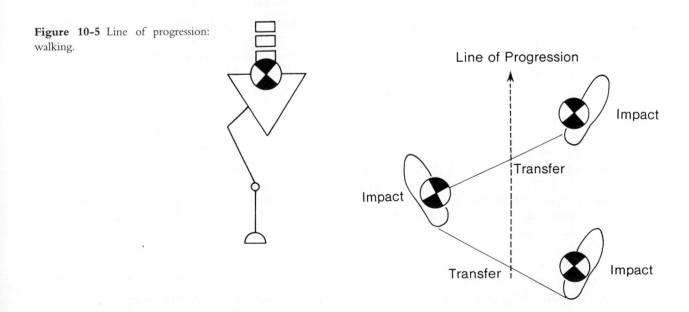

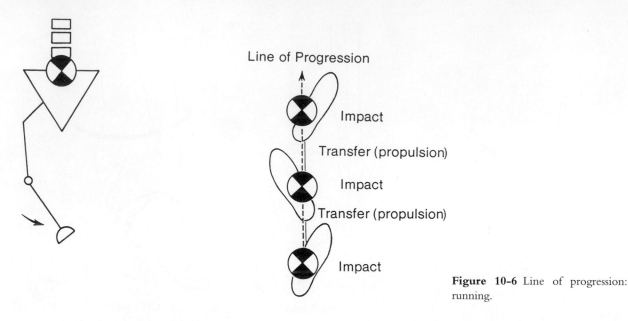

Figure 10-6 Line of progression: running.

DETERMINANTS OF GAIT

As previously indicated, walking is clearly separated from running by the existence of a double support period; thus, before one leg finishes its support phase, the other comes in contact with the ground. The system, within the same support phase, must account for the other leg's contact. From an energy perspective, besides push-off, the trailing leg also must "climb the hill"[5] over the opposite extended leg following contact. These actions result in a rise and fall of the COG of approximately 2 inches during walking. However, the mechanical model described by Fenn[8] rises and falls 3 inches. Most of this discrepancy can be accounted for by the determinants of gait identified by Inman.[5] These include

1. *Transverse pelvic rotation.* While both feet rest on the ground after a step, the pelvis is at its lowest point. Therefore, the COG has made a drop across an arc and the pelvis is perpendicular to the line of progression. Rotation of the body forward with the swinging leg will elevate the COG and rotate it forward. This rotation cuts the angle of the femur with the floor. If the vertical component of the femur is lengthened toward its lowest point by increasing the segment angle relative to the ground, that can save the COG drop at its lowest point. Thus three-eighths of an inch of the COG drop has been saved at its lowest point.

2. *Pelvic tilt.* The pelvis drops on the side of the swinging leg. This leads to a depression of the COG apex at the highest point by lowering the swinging leg, which saves a COG elevation of three-sixteenths of an inch at the highest point.

3. *Knee flexion.* The knee flexes about 15 degrees during the support phase. Using a rigid leg would result in the COG rising to its highest point at the middle of stance. With knee flexion, the COG drops and its apex will be depressed. This results in seven-sixteenths of an inch less elevation of the COG.

These first three determinants total 1 inch of elevation, accounting for the difference between 2 and 3 inches mentioned earlier and resulting in less energy expenditure. The remaining three determinants of gait are responsible for modifications in the shape of the COG curve.

4. *Lateral motion of the pelvis.* The COG must be directly above the support point on the ground for a person to balance on one leg. If the leg segments are parallel, the COG would have to shift from 8 to 12 inches; however, the femurs are adducted and the tibias are in slight valgus, which narrows the base of support, narrowing the necessary maximum displacement by several inches. Also, because of the dynamic nature of gait, transfer from one limb to the other does not have to be complete, with the reduction in lateral movement being dependent upon speed of progression (Fig. 10-5).

5. *Foot and ankle motion.* At heel strike the foot is dor-

siflexed. The ankle's center of rotation rises and then falls at foot flat. During foot flat there is no rise or fall of the center of rotation. When heel-off starts, the center of rotation starts rising and keeps rising until toe-off. As the COG is dropping and the leg flexes, this center of rotation rise might slow the drop a slight amount, smoothing the path of the COG. Additionally, the actions of the ankle, foot, and knee smooth the COG by acting as a cushion during heel strike. Thus the combination of the foot and ankle motions along with the knee motion smooths the potentially abrupt changes of the COG path.

6. *Knee motion.* During the gait cycle the knee flexes, extends, and flexes again in conjunction with foot and ankle motion during stance. These actions help smooth out the gait cycle. Knee flexion occurs as the COG approaches its apex, reducing the height of the rise. It also occurs in conjunction with the rise of the center of rotation of the ankle joint (Fig. 10-2).

As in walking, during running the knee joint (and the entire lower extremity) is acting as a cushion or shock absorber. However, due to the greater impact, this cushioning effect is increased with additional knee flexion and ankle dorsiflexion. The added flexion activity (knee, ankle) places the muscles under stretch, and now the muscular system is ready to work. The simultaneous extension of the hip and knee will give 10 more degrees at the hip to operate and provide a good follow-through. After that, the leg reverses its action to swing over the opposite leg, which now is on the ground.[9] In walking, the swing starts within the stance phase to bring the body over the opposite leg. The swinging leg, with the assistance of the hip flexors, gains kinetic energy and moves forward. As Inman[5] observed, this kinetic energy will be transmitted to the torso as the leg decelerates by hamstring activity. This deceleration will further help in the forward motion of the body. Inman identified the stance phase in walking as the high-energy phase since (1) the leg is decelerated at heel strike, (2) the shock is absorbed at time of heel strike, (3) the torso is balanced at midstance, and (4) push-off is initiated. Conversely, the swing phase is the low-energy phase: (1) hip flexion is initiated, (2) the quads damp excess heel rise, (3) the ankle is dorsiflexed in midswing, and (4) the hamstrings are decelerating the swinging leg.

In running, the lower extremity's inertia and the power available to accelerate and decelerate are crucial. During early swing, the knee flexes passively due to the rapid forward acceleration of the thigh. Newton's third law is applied by the two segments in the air. Additionally, flexion of the knee will result in a change of inertia and an increase in velocity, a desirable result, almost like figure skaters using their hands during an axel. Furthermore, the biarticular nature of the hamstrings plays an important role. The hamstrings not only extend the hip but also flex the knee. When the hip is flexing, the distance between the origins and insertions of the hamstrings increases. Knee flexion reduces this distance to help the hamstrings operate within a larger range of motion. Kapandji[10] reported 30 more degrees of hip flexion with the knee flexed. The forward swing is also assisted by the hip flexors. Eventually, this movement will be arrested by the hamstrings and the knee will start to extend in preparation for the heel strike.

ASSESSMENT OF ABNORMALITIES

Any physical examination designed to identify the nature of a particular abnormality must include observing the patient walk and run. To increase objectivity, measurement of important parameters may also be included. But what should be measured? Obviously, if one were to quantify all the important features associated with walking and running, a fairly sophisticated and expensive measurement system would be required. Even if such a system were accessible, however, the measurements themselves often do little more than document the subtle differences between the subject and some statistically determined "normal" pattern. Just as in walking, each runner possesses a unique style of running that arises from morphologic constraints (size, weight, limb segment length, etc.), as well as from different experiences. Comparison with "normal" values without considering the individualistic nature of running leads to error. Judgment must be used both in selecting appropriate measurements and in using these measurements to assess running conditions. In this context, it is important to distinguish between the terms *measurement* and *assessment*. Measurements yield facts that describe the characteristics of a system or individual, whereas assessments are context-specific conclusions made after consideration of many facts.[11] For example, suppose a runner's best time in the 100-m dash is measured and found to be 13.5 seconds; this fact can be used by a coach or trainer to make the assessment that the athlete is too slow to be a sprinter. If other measurements, such as 1,000-m time and aerobic capacity, are considered, the runner's ability to be a long-distance runner can be assessed instead. Measurements, then, are the tools of assessment. However, such tools are only as good as the person using them and are no substitute for a comprehensive knowledge of running or walking mechanics or both.

Types of Measurement Tools

To assess abnormalities properly, the clinician should select those measurement tools that provide information considered most useful in distinguishing pathologic from normal gait. These measurements can be categorized into five groups: temporal measurements, kinematic measurements, kinetic measurements, energy consumption, and measures of muscle activity.[12]

Temporal measurements are concerned with simple measurements of stride rate and timed events. In conjunction with distance measures, stride length and average velocity can be computed. Simple and inexpensive systems have been developed to measure these parameters. In addition, they can be obtained from any system capable of making kinematic measurements. These measurements are most useful in assessing walking and are particularly helpful in documenting pre- and post-treatment changes in gait.

Kinematic measurements describe the geometry of limb movement as well as the translation of the body as a whole. Angular displacements, velocities, and accelerations of either the joints of the lower limb or the limb segments themselves can be obtained using these tools. The information can be presented both qualitatively, in the form of sequentially recorded images on film or video, and quantitatively, by calculating segment trajectories and joint angles from marker position data.

Kinetic measurements are concerned with the forces that give rise to, or result from, limb movements. The forces associated with muscular contractions responsible for limb segment movements cannot be measured directly. However, measurement of the forces imparted to the ground by the stance limb, the so-called ground reaction forces, can be easily measured. Combining this information with kinematic data permits the calculation of joint torques, which represent the sum of all muscle activity about the joint. The primary kinetic measurement device is the force platform, which measures the three components of the ground reaction force vector and the moments about each axis. Center of pressure measurements can be obtained from force platform data as well as various pressure transducers that conform to or are attached to the sole of the foot to show the pressure profiles under the foot during contact.[13]

Methods employed for energy analysis during walking or running are concerned with either direct measurement of the rate of metabolic oxygen consumption or approximation of this rate using a combination of walking speed, heart rate, and/or mechanical energies associated with each limb segment. Oxygen consumption can be measured directly using the same apparatus commonly used in administering a cardiac stress test, but, unfortunately, this requires that the subject run on a treadmill with bulky equipment. However, telemetric equipment is also available to measure oxygen consumption, permitting the subject to walk or run without being directly connected to the recording machinery.

Electromyography is the only realistic method for evaluating the phasic activity of the muscles during walking or running.[14] In this technique, electrodes are positioned either within (intramuscular electrodes) or directly over (surface electrodes) the belly of the muscle to be monitored. The electrochemical potential generated during the muscle contraction is received by the electrodes, and after appropriate signal conditioning can be displayed on any device that produces a voltage-versus-time display. Preamplification and telemetry can be used to permit the subject to run without being directly connected to the final display and recording equipment.

A Simple Clinical Gait Assessment System

Although comprehensive analyses of walking and running require system components from each of the five categories, most of the running problems that are encountered can be identified using a simple videotaping system and manual calculation of stride parameters. Using any of the current generation of high-quality video cameras or slow-motion videocassette recorders (VCRs) designed for the home or commercial market, video records of the subject can be easily obtained. Of particular merit are the so-called digital VCRs, which incorporate a video-frame store (video-frame memory) for capturing frames of interest, which allow slow motion and freeze-frame analysis. Most of the moderately priced cameras available today give good-quality pictures, but the best choice is a solid-state (closed-circuit device, or CCD) camera that uses a chip as the image sensor rather than a conventional video tube.

Reasonable approximations of all stride parameters can also be made from the videotape record. First, the length of the walkway should be measured and the beginning and end of the walkway marked with high-contrast tape. A camera is then placed perpendicular to the walkway at a distance that permits the start and stop markers to be clearly visible in the frame. Next, the subject is recorded running down the walkway, making sure that the speed at which the subject crosses the starting line is maintained over the entire walkway. By playing the video record back one frame at a time, the number of frames is counted from the instant the subject crosses the starting line to each event in the cycle (e.g., left foot contact, left foot toe-off). The frame count for the entire time that the subject is on the walkway is determined. Finally, a determination is made of the duration of each event, noting that each frame of the video equals 1/30th of a second (33.33 ms). Average velocity is equal to the length of the walkway divided by the time from start to finish, and each step length is equal to the average velocity multiplied by each relative step time.

SUMMARY

Except for the obvious incapacitating injury discovered on table examination, which would preclude running, the physician should observe the patient running. Often this means asking patients to run on a runway or treadmill until they begin to experience the discomfort they complain of. Observing from the side, the examiner should look for any overstriding, a possible explanation for hamstring pull. Excessive lordosis of the lumbar spine, especially evident in downhill running, may contribute to back pain. The rear view shows the attitude of the heel at impact as well as the degree of pronation during this stage. Exaggerated trunk rotation and arm motion as well as excessive rotational and angular displacement of the knee are best seen from the front.

In summary, prescribing appropriate treatment requires an understanding of the biomechanics of running as well as the pathophysiology of those conditions common to the runner. The assessment should be made on the basis of information gathered from the running history and physical examination, it should also include measurements collected during observation of the running gait.

REFERENCES

1. Slocum DB: Overuse syndromes of the lower leg and foot in athletes. American Academy of Orthopedic Surgeons Instructional Course Lectures, Vol. 17. CV Mosby, St. Louis, 1960
2. Ralston HJ: Energetics of human walking. In Herman RM, Grillner S, Stein PSG, Stuart DG (eds): Neural Control of Locomotion. Plenum, New York, 1976
3. Hreljac A: Preferred and energetically optimal gait transition speeds in human locomotion. Med Sci Sports Exerc 25:1158, 1993
4. Alexander RMcN, Jayes AS: Vertical movements in walking and running. J Zool (Lond) 185:27, 1978
5. Inman VT: Human locomotion. Can Med Assoc J 9:1047, 1966
6. Williams KR, Cavanagh PR: Relationship between distance running mechanics, running economy, and performance. J Appl Physiol 63:1235, 1987
7. Mann RA, Hagy J: Biomechanics of walking, running and sprinting. Am J Sports Med 8:345, 1980
8. Fenn WO: Work against gravity and work due to velocity changes in running. Am J Physiol 93:433, 1931
9. Bates BT, Haven BH: An analysis of the mechanics of highly skilled female runners. p. 237. In Bluestein JL (ed): Mechanics and Sport. Vol. 4. AMSE, New York, 1973
10. Kapandji IA: The Physiology of the Joints. Churchill Livingstone, New York, 1985
11. Kondraske GV: Looking at the study of human performance. Soma 7:50, 1987
12. Inman VT, Ralston HJ, Todd F: Human Walking. Williams & Wilkins, Baltimore, 1981
13. Cheskin MP, Sherkin KJ, Bates BT: The Complete Handbook of Athletic Footwear. Fairchild Publishers, New York, 1987
14. Vaughan CL: Biomechanics of running gait. Crit Rev Biomed Eng 12:1, 1984

11

Forces Acting on the Lower Extremity

BARRY BATES
NICHOLAS STERGIOU

Athletes encounter a variety of surfaces during a workout. The pitch or terrain may vary. The effect of acceleration, ground reaction force (GRF), and surfaces on the various tissues of the body have important clinical ramifications. Running surfaces are usually grass, dirt, asphalt, or concrete. The effects of these surfaces on performance, injury/shock-attenuating mechanisms of the body, and range of motion of the joints are important. Artificial surfaces are encountered in dance, basketball, football, aerobics, and various court sports, to mention just a few. Many athletes involved in multiple sports are subjected to various surfaces with changes in elasticity, terrain, and slope, all of which have an effect on the body.

Various ways to assess, quantify, and qualify motion and shock are helpful when evaluating the athlete, planning appropriate training and rehabilitative schedules, and designing protective foot gear. Forces acting on the lower extremity are related to the various activities in sports. In general, as one progresses from walking to running and, finally, jumping, the impact forces increase as a function of body mass and velocity at contact. Normally, a walker goes about one-third as fast as a runner. The GRF, measured by a force platform, as well as the acceleration, measured by accelerometers, are about two-thirds less in a walker than those of a runner (Fig. 11-1). When the walker increases speed to one-half that of the runner, however, the forces increase to about one-half of those found in running.

During ambulation, high forces of short duration are repetitively transmitted through the lower extremity of the skeleton to the low back and up through the spine to the head. At heel strike during normal walking, peak forces at the tibia and skull have been recorded at 5 and 0.5 gravities (g), respectively.[1] These data indicate that, as the forces travel from the foot through the body to the skull, they can be attenuated by a factor as great as 10. Corresponding forces of 7 to 12 and 2 to 3 g have been reported for the tibia and the skull during running. Forces during landing of four to nine times body weight are not uncommon, with maximum values reaching 15 times body weight.[2] Attenuation up through the body has not been reported for landing.

MEASURING FORCES AND MOVEMENT

Forces acting on the lower extremity can be measured using force platforms, accelerometers, and foot sensor systems. Each of these measuring devices has its own applicability to the individual or athlete. In addition, videography and cinematography can be used independently or in conjunction with these devices to evaluate the effects of the forces on the body.

Force Platform

Ground reaction forces are the main external forces acting on the human body during running. They occur when the runner is in contact with the ground. These forces can be measured using a force platform. The platforms commonly used are piezoelectric or strain-gauge technologies, which typically have resonance frequencies above 300

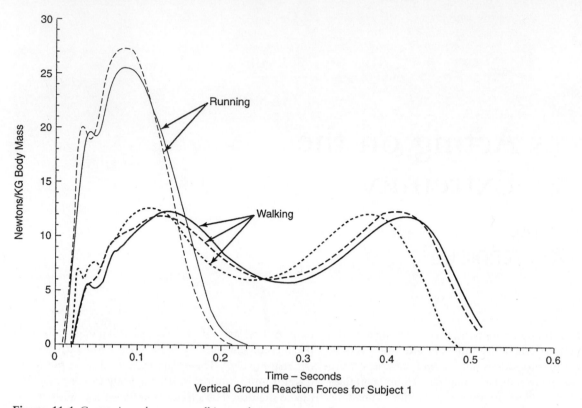

Figure 11-1 Comparisons between walking and running ground reaction force curves for different shoe conditions.

Hz. Force platforms permit quantification of the GRF and its components (F_x, F_y, and F_z); the point of application of the force, which can be mapped onto the foot; and the free moment of rotation around the vertical axis, M_z, with respect to the point of application.

The resultant force is a vector, which has three conventional components: F_z, vertical force; F_y, anteroposterior force; and F_x, mediolateral force (Fig. 11-2). The vertical force is the component of the GRF in the vertical direction and is always positive. F_y is negative during the braking phase of stance and positive during the propulsive phase. The mediolateral force, F_x, is associated with foot stability and the actions of pronation/supination. In terms of absolute impulse, the vertical force comprises approximately 85 percent of the GRF, with the anteroposterior and mediolateral forces contributing about 12 to 15 percent and 2 to 5 percent, respectively.

Bates and colleagues[4] developed a model made up of a minimum but complete set of unique parameters that adequately describe the three components of the GRF.

Based on data from 12 subjects running in six different shoe conditions, they identified a set of 23 parameters describing temporal and kinetic characteristics of the three conventional GRF components.

The GRF can also be separated into two functional components: (1) a high-frequency impact or passive force and (2) a lower frequency loading or active force. In the vertical component of the GRF, the impact force produces the first maximum force while the loading force produces the second maximum force. The impact force, especially in the vertical direction, initiates a shock wave that propagates through the musculoskeletal system and must be attenuated by the various elastic components of the system. The loading force has a similar effect except that the rate of force application is much slower. Both forces must be absorbed by various internal and external components of the system. The external components consist of the shoe and the surface, while the internal components include the bones, muscles, tendons/ligaments, cartilage, and other soft tissue (heel fat pad).

Accelerometers

Accelerometers can be used to quantify the shock transmitted through the body following heel strike. Various accelerometer designs include piezoelectric, piezoresistive, and strain-gauge components. Light and McLellan[5] used accelerometers mounted to Kirschner wires, placed within the tibia below the knee, and a metallic bite bar held in the mouth to measure the effects of impact forces. The results were compared with those from skin-mounted accelerometers. Results were comparable, with only a slight delay noted between the bone-mounted and the skin-mounted accelerometers. In a later study different shock waves were observed at heel strike during normal walking in different footwear[1] using the same experimental setup. The use of the skin-mounted and bone-mounted accelerometers again produced similar results in magnitude, but a slight time lag was observed for the skin-mounted device. Accelerations of 5 g with hard shoes and only 2.5 g with a more compliant heel were measured at the tibia. The rise time to the peak was about 50 percent longer for the more compliant shoes. Although the transient shock wave was greatly attenuated as it passed up the skeleton, the acceleration and displacement were still 0.5 g and 0.5 mm, respectively, at the head. Light and co-workers concluded that the shock wave at heel strike is initially moderated by the viscoelastic tissue of the heel pad and is then further attenuated and delayed about 10 ms as it passes to the head. Because its speed of propagation exceeds that of afferent nerve conduction velocities, this rapid transmission of shock may serve as a signal for the body to react to the variety of surfaces at heel strike.

Hennig and Lafortune[6] examined the relationship between GRF and tibial bone acceleration values during running. The peak values for the two measurement devices were only moderately correlated ($r = 0.76$), with GRF peak forces occurring 5.2 ms later. Average accelerometer values of 5.39 were observed compared to force platform values of 2.2 times body weight. In a later study, Hennig et al.[7] used a similar procedure to evaluate runners' perceptions of footwear midsole construction.

Figure 11-2 Graphs of the three force–time components: F_x, F_y, and F_z. (**Left**) One subject with one shoe graphed over 10 trials. (**Right**) Same subject tested with 10 different shoes. A high degree of reliability is found when one subject is tested many times with one shoe; variance is expected when the shoes are changed. (From Nigg BM: Biomechanics of Running Shoes. Human Kinetic Publishers, Champaign, IL, 1980 with permission.)

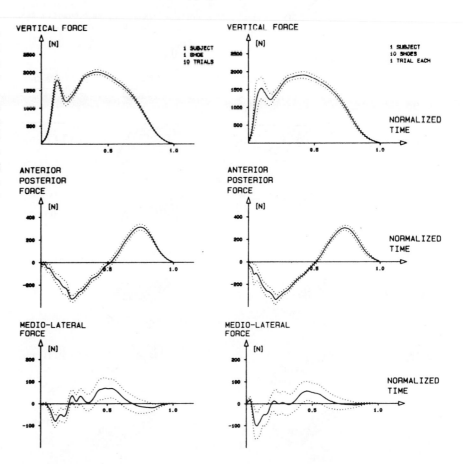

Foot Sensor Systems

Foot sensor systems can be used to measure the distribution of pressures at discrete locations beneath the foot. Figure 11-3 shows the position and relative amounts of pressure distributions during running barefooted and with running shoes.[8] The effect of running shoes on impact loading is illustrated. The system used was a pressure platform with piezoceramic transducer elements.

More recently, Henning and Milani[9] used a discrete pressure sensor system in conjunction with a force platform to examine the effects of shoes on GRFs. The pressure sensor system consisted of eight discrete piezoceramic transducers (4×4 mm) less than 2 mm thick that were positioned at specific anatomic locations on the bottom of the foot using adhesive tape. Differences in plantar foot pressures among shoe models indicated that shoes do make a difference and that foot function can be evaluated using the sensor system. The researchers were also able to estimate the GRF from the pressure data.

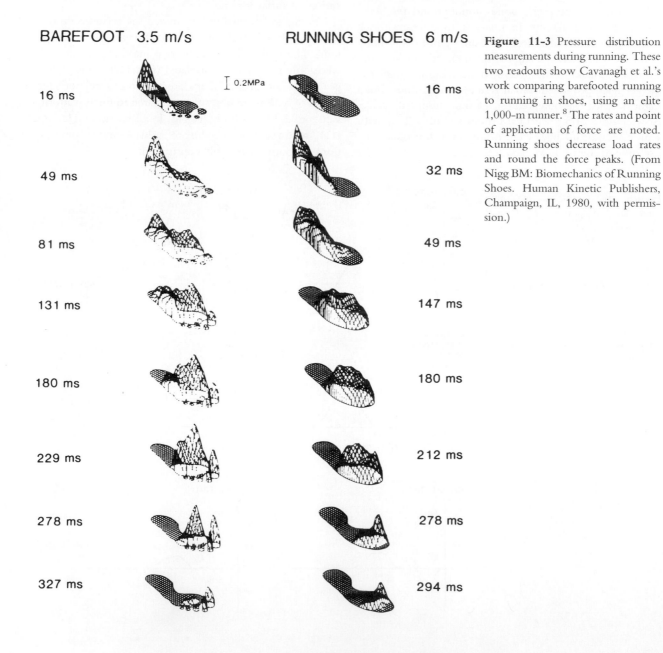

BAREFOOT 3.5 m/s

16 ms
49 ms
81 ms
131 ms
180 ms
229 ms
278 ms
327 ms

0.2MPa

RUNNING SHOES 6 m/s

16 ms
32 ms
49 ms
147 ms
180 ms
212 ms
278 ms
294 ms

Figure 11-3 Pressure distribution measurements during running. These two readouts show Cavanagh et al.'s work comparing barefooted running to running in shoes, using an elite 1,000-m runner.[8] The rates and point of application of force are noted. Running shoes decrease load rates and round the force peaks. (From Nigg BM: Biomechanics of Running Shoes. Human Kinetic Publishers, Champaign, IL, 1980, with permission.)

Figure 11-4 Heel contact and early heel-off, illustrating excessive pronation. (**A**) First contact. (**B**) during the Maximum pronation.

Several positive features are associated with these systems. First, the clinician can evaluate the patient in virtually any environment. Second, data can be produced quickly indicating the times at which each point of the foot on which a sensor is located is actively involved in support or shock absorbency. Third, since such systems can be placed in the shoe, data relative to the foot, shoe, or foot–orthosis interface can be collected.

Video

Video is very practical and helpful in a clinical setting. It allows the practitioner to observe the effects of various forces in terms of motion and to assess the effectiveness of components such as orthoses and shoes. Appropriately mounted mirrors around a treadmill can be helpful in teaching proper running form and in giving the athlete positive feedback. Video and cinematography also lend themselves to slow-motion playback for more in-depth study of various gait phases in evaluating qualitative biomechanics.

As an example, video or cinematography can be used to study the amount of relative pronation by measuring the angle of the Achilles tendon and rearfoot during ground contact in heel–toe running. They can also be used to measure stride length, contact position of the foot, angle of gait, base of gait, and position of the foot during toe-off. The difference in pronation at heel contact and early heel-off is illustrated in Figure 11-4.

OVERVIEW OF RUNNING

Running is a cyclic activity consisting of a series of support and airborne phases, with each leg going through a support and a swing phase (Fig. 11-5). (These phases were previously defined in Chapter 10.) Ground contact following the airborne phase results in an external GRF being applied to the body. The specific characteristics of the force vary as a result of factors such as running style, speed, footwear, and surfaces. The GRF is typically separated into three orthogonal components. Some representative curves are given in Figure 11-2. The focus of this brief overview is on the support phase of running, since most injuries are the result of events during this portion of the gait cycle.

Figure 11-5 Running stride phases for (**a**) both legs, (**b**) right leg only, and (**c**) left leg only. RS/LS, right/left support; RNS/LNS, right/left nonsupport; RR/LR, right/left recovery.

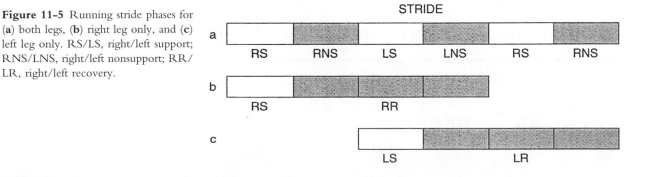

Table 11-1 Support Phase Events

Body Position[a]	Event[b]	Relative Time During Support Phase	
		Individual (%)	Mean (%)
1	Touch down (TD)	0.0	0.0
1a[c]	Begin pronation (BP)	5.0–20.0	6.8–14.8
	Impact (MI)	5.0–16.2	9.0–12.1
2	Min. force (MF)	7.8–24.7	11.8–21.4
	Max. brake (MB)	13.0–25.5	17.5–23.4
3	Max. pronation (MP)	24.0–62.8	30.9–48.6
	Max. knee (MK)	33.0–46.2	32.6–43.2
	Max. load (ML)	31.5–52.5	35.3–48.9
	Brake-propulsion (BP)	26.3–55.7	38.7–53.4
4	Max. ankle (MA)	48.0–57.7	49.4–54.3
5	Max. propulsion (MP)	63.6–74.5	66.1–74.4
	End pronation (EP)	60.0–88.0	68.3–86.2
6	Toe-off (TO)	100.0	100.0

[a] See Figure 11-7 for body positions corresponding to numbers.

[b] See Figure 11-6 for kinematic depiction.

[c] Not shown.

Research has identified a number of phases and events that are important for understanding support-phase activities and their possible relationship to running injuries. The critical events are identified in Table 11-1. Also given are the relative times for the occurrence of these events for individuals as well as groups of individuals. The individual results are more variable than the group results, as should be expected, but considerable variability still exists among the group mean values. In spite of these variations, the events have been grouped to form what we believe can be used as a representative model when evaluating the support phase of the gait cycle. The kinematic body positions for these grouped events are shown in Figure 11-7, and a graphic representation is given in Figure 11-6. The relationship of these events to lower extremity joint actions are given in Figure 11-8 and Table 11-2, as are movements of the center of gravity (COG) in the vertical and horizontal (anteroposterior) directions and the corresponding GRFs. Understanding the relationships among these events and actions is critical to the evaluation of performance and injury mechanisms. More detailed explanations of some of these relationships are given in the following sections.

MECHANISMS ASSOCIATED WITH RUNNING INJURIES

The majority of runners land on the lateral heel with the COG trailing the action. The foot at this point is slightly supinated, which is an inherent structural movement of the lower extremity[10] (Fig. 11-9). The foot is slightly adducted, inverted, and plantar flexed. Thus the forefoot is closer to the ground and the foot can go through a greater

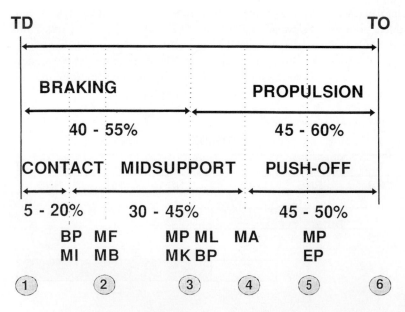

Figure 11-6 Support-phase phases and events. See Table 11-1 for definition of symbols and Figure 11-7 for body positions corresponding to numbers.

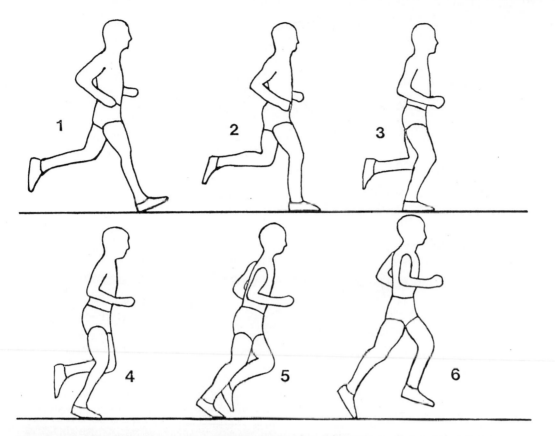

Figure 11-7 Selected body positions during the support phase of running.

range of motion during the upcoming stance phase to absorb the impact forces. The knee is also extended since this position gives it greater stability. However, it is not fully extended (only to about 170 degrees), since landing on a stiff leg can result in problems. At heel strike, the impact forces result in the transmission of a vertical shock through the body that carries the potential for injury.[11] This shock wave is attenuated by various internal (muscles, tendons, etc.) and external (shoe, surface) elastic components. The heel pad[12] and knee joint flexion (acting like a soft spring) have been identified as major components in the attenuation of the traveling shock wave.

The vertical shock will generate mostly compressive forces at the knee, which have the potential to produce osteoarthritis, as found by Radin and colleagues[13] in their animal experiments. The menisci play an important role as an elastic coupling (a "washer" between the bones) that transmits these compressive forces between the femur and tibia. Damage to the menisci can induce premature development of osteoarthritis.

Another interesting point deals with the part of the foot that first comes in contact with the ground. Three types of runners have been identified: heel strikers, midfoot strikers, and forefoot strikers. The foot strike pattern is the result of strategy (performance), structure, or both. It is interesting to observe that the first maximum or impact force is not always present in the GRF for forefoot strikers. Traditionally, forefoot running at slower and even moderate speeds has been approached as a system deficiency and has been associated with increased stress in the region of the Achilles tendon.[14] However, it seems that, since the system's structure defines its function, a forefoot strike may be the natural outcome of a system adaptation to eliminate the deleterious effects of impact. In a study of skilled runners, most followed the progression from heel to forefoot contact as speed increased, but there were some individuals who maintained their contact pattern independent of speed.[15] For example, a forefoot striker might lack adequate heel pad thickness; however, the lack of research in this area only allows for speculation. Furthermore, the

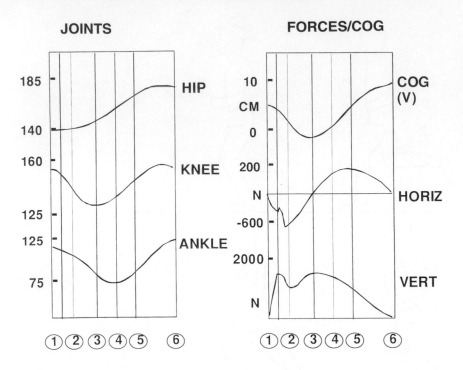

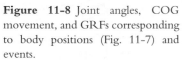

Figure 11-8 Joint angles, COG movement, and GRFs corresponding to body positions (Fig. 11-7) and events.

function of the lower extremity and its role as a shock absorber must be evaluated from an individual performance approach. As impact forces increase, some individuals respond mechanically (with an increase in the measured impact force) while others respond neurologically (by increasing knee flexion) to reduce the forces. Bates and co-workers[16] suggested that differential response patterns seem perfectly reasonable since it is unlikely that individuals will have the same experiences and the same perceptions of the environment that are necessary to produce the same performance adjustments.

At contact, the foot will be in a slightly supinated position, although the action will be pronation. Within the first 5 to 20 percent of the stance phase the foot will pass through the neutral position into a pronated position. With increased pronation the foot unlocks at the midtarsal joint and becomes flexible to achieve surface adaptation and force absorption. The loading forces are directed toward the musculoskeletal system and must be absorbed by the elastic components of the system. The subtalar joint function facilitates the talus as a load distributor over the entire foot. The load is transmitted (1) posteriorly to the heel via the posterior subtalar joint, (2) anteriorly and laterally to the lateral arch via the anterior subtalar joint, and (3) anteriorly and medially to the medial arch via the talonavicular joint. The talus lies at the top of the plantar vault, which is another important functional component. Besides load distribution over the foot, the plantar vault itself contributes as a shock-absorbing mechanism by flattening during the loading phase. The flattening of the plantar vault is checked by the contraction of the plantar tighteners. At the end of the propulsive phase, these tighteners will also contribute to the propulsive thrust by releasing their stored energy and shortening the plantar vault. The function of

Table 11-2 Joint Actions and COG Movements

Body Position and Relative Time During Support Phase[a]					
1 0%	2 10–25%	3 30–50%	4 50–55%	5 65–80%	6 100%
Hip	F or E	E	E	E	E
Knee	F	F	E	E	F or E
Ankle	DF	DF	DF	PF	PF
Pronation/ supination	PR	PR	S	S	S
COG (V)	D	D	U	U	U
COG (H)	B	B	P	P	P

Abbreviations: B, braking; D, down; DF, dorsiflexion; E, extension; F, flexion; P, propulsion; PF, plantar flexion; PR, pronation; S, supination; U, up.

[a] Numbers refer to body positions as illustrated in Figure 11-7.

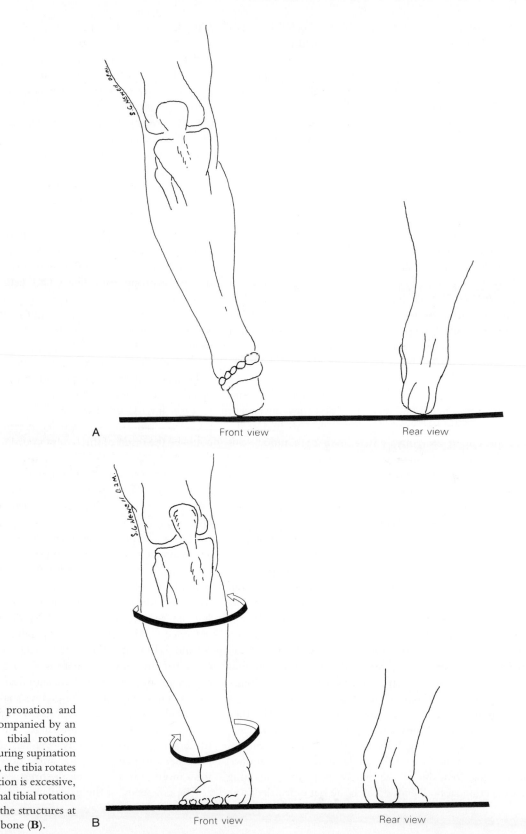

A   Front view   Rear view

Figure 11-9 Foot pronation and knee flexion is accompanied by an obligatory internal tibial rotation (**A**). Conversely, during supination and knee extension, the tibia rotates externally. If pronation is excessive, the obligatory internal tibial rotation increases, straining the structures at the two ends of the bone (**B**).

B   Front view   Rear view the plantar vault can be pathologically affected by a pes planus (flatfoot) or a pes cavus (high-arched foot). However, a lack of significant relationship between pronation and foot type has been reported in the literature, and thus it has been suggested that static measures are not always reflective of dynamic function.[17,18]

The most prevalent site of running injuries is the knee joint.[19,20] The knee is typically recognized as part of the impact-absorbing mechanism during running.[21–24] McMahon et al.[23] investigated the mechanics of running to determine the effect of vertical stiffness of the body. They concluded that stiffness increased with running speed and that at any given speed the stiffness could be reduced in a controlled fashion by running with greater knee flexion than normal. In addition, they found that the transmission of the mechanical shock due to impact was very sensitive to the degree of knee flexion. Running with flexed knees ($\theta = 60$ degrees) diminished the ratio of the acceleration peak from the foot to the skull by 80 percent but required an increase in oxygen consumption of as much as 50 percent. Furthermore, Kim et al.[24] developed a mathematical model that describes the dissipation and attenuation of the impulsive shock loads produced during impact that can be used to analyze the effect of various components. They found that an 80 percent reduction of peak shock amplitude could be achieved between the tibia and the rest of the body. Based upon their model, this attenuation was attributed to the knee joint. A similar attenuation value (70 percent) was observed by Wosk and Voloshin[22] that was also credited to the knee joint.

Maximum pronation occurs about 35 to 45 percent into the support phase along with maximum knee flexion. At this point the body's COG passes over the base of support and the braking/absorbing force period ends (Table 11-1; Figs. 11-6 to 11-8). Active hip extension and the body's inertia help the body advance over the foot. At maximum flexion, the knee has its greatest degree of mobility. Mobility is essential because it allows axial rotation of the tibia so the foot can perform pronation/supination. However, mobility also means instability. Therefore, ligaments and menisci are susceptible to injury in this position. Both foot pronation and knee flexion are accompanied by an obligatory internal tibial rotation. Conversely, as propulsion begins, supination and knee extension occur and the tibia rotates externally. If pronation is excessive or prolonged, the ankle then sags medially and the obligatory internal tibial rotation increases at the ankle joint but is restrained at the knee joint due to the extension, possibly straining the structures at both ends of the bone but especially those

at the knee joint (Fig. 11-9). Research has shown that the asynchronous function of pronation and flexion can be initiated by increases in the GRF.[25–27] This will result in the generation of opposite moments at the two ends of the tibia along with increases in shear force. These events combined with femoral rotation might be the reason for the observed increase in knee injuries over the last 10 years.[20] Furthermore, these problems can be enhanced with genu varum (bowlegs) or genu valgum (knock-knees).

As the propulsion phase begins, the knee extends, the ankle continues to dorsiflex, and the foot stays in a relatively maximally pronated position. The ankle reaches maximum dorsiflexion at about 55 percent of the support phase. This added ankle dorsiflexion results in additional stretch to the gastrocnemius, which is now ready to contribute to propulsion. The COG velocity increases and eventually the foot moves from a pronated to a supinated position at about 65 to 85 percent of the support phase. Supination locks the foot and makes it a rigid lever to propel the body forward. Propulsion is also assisted by the extension of the great toe and the plantar vault.

However, if excessive pronation occurs, the foot may be prevented from returning to the more stable, supinated position for toe-off. Bates et al.[10] showed that excessive pronation can be facilitated by running barefoot. That could be the result of the system's need to protect the body from the increased GRF, since the shoe is not there to help with cushioning. In addition, shoe or surface hardness or both can affect pronation. A softer midsole or surface can give greater mobility to the rearfoot and result in increased pronation.

During the propulsion phase, knee extension results in a more stable joint, which is important since the knee now is subjected to stresses resulting from lengthening lever arms. The simultaneous knee and hip extensions allow for more effective use of the powerful muscles of the hip. The hip can be extended 10 more degrees when the knee is extended.[28] That gives more operational room for push-off and follow-through. Additionally, with the two joints extended the gluteus maximus has a greater mechanical advantage and can contribute significantly to propulsion. This is important since the gluteus maximus is the most powerful muscle in the body and can produce forces 50 percent greater than the hamstrings.[28] Furthermore, during the braking phase the body stretches the extensors with knee flexion, pelvic tilt, and ankle dorsiflexion, allowing for a more powerful extensor thrust.

The efficiency of the gastrocnemius, a biarticular muscle, strongly depends on the degree of flexion at the knee. As the knee is fully flexed or fully extended, the displacement of the origin of the muscle produces a relative lengthening or shortening of the muscle, which is equal to or exceeds its length of contraction. Thus, when the knee is extended, the gastrocnemius is passively stretched and works at its best advantage, which allows some of the power of the quadriceps to be transferred to the ankle. In contrast, when the knee is flexed, the gastrocnemius loosens and looses most of its efficiency. Then only the soleus is active; its power would be inadequate in running unless knee extension was an essential part of the process. A simultaneous extension of the ankle and the knee joint enhances the action of the gastrocnemius.

The coupling of ankle plantar flexion and foot supination can be further explained by an additional functional point that has to do with the biarticularity of the triceps surae. The triceps surae acts on the ankle joint through the subtalar joint; thus it moves these joints in sequence. First it extends the ankle and then it tilts the calcaneus, which results in supination. The way the triceps surae functions explains why decreased pronation results in reduced ankle dorsiflexion.[10] This helps explain why individuals who lack flexibility of the triceps surae often try to compensate with increased knee flexion and pronation.

Finally, as mentioned above, individuality is a critical aspect of foot function. Bates and co-workers[2] compared the fastest and the slowest runners of a 4×400 relay race and showed similarities and differences that they attributed to the runners' previous training. The fastest runner had as her primary event the 400-m run, while the slowest runner was primarily a 1,500-m runner. Running is a skill, and like all skills depends upon an individual's genetic (structural) makeup, development, and experiences. These latter factors are practice driven where the notion of specificity is critical.

BODY MECHANISMS FOR SHOCK ABSORPTION AND ATTENUATION

Body Tissues

Active attenuation of skeletal shock forces takes place with proprioception, joint position, and muscle tone. Passive attenuation takes place with the elasticity of bone, cartilage, and soft tissues such as the heel pad. Intervertebral discs as well as the menisci aid in passive shock attenuation.

Although it is readily understood that muscles produce energy, it is less appreciated that muscles absorb kinetic energy. Muscles that absorb abnormal, prolonged amounts of kinetic energy become fatigued, and postural fatigue is the end result. The rate and amount of loading are also important factors. Rapid application of high force is damaging to the elastic properties of soft tissue and bone. Chronic repetitive stress or overstress leads to fatigue of dynamic movers and stabilizers, which exposes muscle as well as bone and soft tissue to additional stress. When muscles lose their ability to absorb energy, more energy is transmitted to the skeletal system. This accounts for the higher number of stress-related bone problems (stress fractures or stress reaction of bone) during the later parts of a marathon, when muscles are presumably fatigued.

Calcaneal Fat Pad

Of the body's natural shock absorbers, the calcaneal fat pad is one of the most effective in the lower extremity. The fat pad has a columnar arrangement that allows for attenuation of impact load; at the same time, it has near-perfect memory as it accepts shear and torsional forces without deforming. It therefore has the ability to attenuate shock and deform, followed by rapid recovery, so that it may repeat the same function at the next heel strike.

Aging and system conditions may decrease the effect of the calcaneal fat pad. Kinoshita and associates[30,31] observed decreases in the shock-absorbing capability of the fat pad with age that were also a function of loading rate. At lower rates there was a mean reduction of 11.8 percent for the oldest group (ages 71 to 86) compared to a mean reduction of 16.0 percent for the higher loading rate for the same group. There was also less energy absorbed by the fat pad for these older individuals. Notable among systemic conditions are the collagen diseases. Higher incidences of calcaneodynia in heavier patients, who presumably place more stress on their calcaneal fat pads, with secondary degeneration of the columnar arrangements, have been observed. This same phenomenon has been noted in athletes with very low total body fat, who appear to have an atrophic fat pad of the calcaneus. Shoes with a heel cup (an anatomic rearfoot last), rounded to fit the contour of the plantar surface of the heel, can help hold the calcaneal fat pad in place and decrease spreading.

De Clerq and colleagues[32] studied the compressive properties of the heel pad during heel strike using cinematography (150 Hz) and a force platform. An average maximum deformation of 60.5 percent was observed for barefoot running compared to only 35.5 percent for the shod condition, without a significant change in contact forces.

The authors suggested that in barefoot running the heel pad was compromised in its role of local protection of the heel bone, and that a well-fitted shoe actually increases the effective stiffness of the heel pad. In a previous study, Paul et al.[33] did observe degeneration in the knee even though the heel pad reduced the shock wave applied to the tibial shafts of rabbits by 25 percent during rapid, cyclic loading.

Foot Type

The high-arched cavus foot with limited range of motion attenuates shock poorly compared with a normal foot. The hypermobile flatfoot or weak foot also often does poorly in shock attenuation when it functions near the end of the range of motion. Pronation is a necessary component of shock attenuation. In running, the normal foot contacts in a slightly supinated position and then rapidly pronates, continuing its pronation through about 30 to 45 percent of the support phase. However, although this is generally true, it is important to remember that foot function during running is dynamic and a static assessment can be misleading. Several studies[17,18] have failed to show a relationship between foot type and dynamic function.

Conditions that limit joint motion place additional stress on proximal and distal joints, as well as soft tissue structures. Thus, a midtarsal joint coalition with peroneal spasm places excessive stress on the medial structures of the foot and ankle. A subtalar joint coalition, with no pronatory compensation, places undue stress about the hip and knee joints. Hallux rigidus places excessive stress on the plantar fascia as well as on the Achilles tendon. Ligamentous laxity with excessive pronation places undue stress on the posterior tibial muscle and tendon. Limited ankle dorsiflexion overloads the plantar fascia and intrinsic musculature of the foot, as well as the gastrocnemius–soleus muscles and Achilles tendon. Tight posterior structures of the knee decrease knee extension and alter foot plant. Variations from ideal biomechanical phasic sequences decrease the body's shock-attenuating mechanisms, predisposing to overuse injuries. Furthermore, fatigue decreases the athlete's ability to respond rapidly to changing situations, increasing the risk of acute injuries.

EXTERNAL FACTORS RELATED TO RUNNING INJURIES

The Effect of Slope

The slope or variability of the terrain affects foot contact as well as toe-off position. The bank of the road may pronate or supinate the foot. The irregular terrain of a golf course requires supinatory or pronatory changes in foot plant. Running on a banked track may create excessive pronation or supination. The same is true when rounding a curve on a traditional track[34]: the inside foot pronates more than the outside foot. There is also asymmetry of swing length when rounding a curve. These variations influence the system's ability to attenuate kinetic energy.

Ground reaction forces of 3 g at impact during normal running were reported by Subotnick[35] compared to uphill values of only 2 g. Downhill running exhibits an increased impact spike along with increased braking as the athlete typically lands with the foot considerably in front of the body's center of gravity due to overstriding. Decreased GRF values are seen in uphill running as a result of less landing energy. The impact force is often absent since the runner typically lands on the ball of the foot. This landing style is brought about by a combination of forward body lean and a shortened stride length due to earlier contact with the surface on the upward slope. Thus it can clearly be seen that downhill running generates greater GRFs as compared with level or uphill running, which can result in a higher incidence of stress fractures and stress-related injuries with continued downhill running. Uphill and downhill running also affect pelvic tilt, as shown in Figure 11-10.

The Effect of Surfaces

Unold and co-workers[36,37] investigated the effects of walking and running on different surfaces by placing accelerometers on the shin, hip, and head. The test surfaces included grass, asphalt, and synthetic track. They found that the acceleration measured at the tibia varied significantly, being the least on grass and relatively equal on asphalt and synthetic track. Hip and head measurements remained almost constant, showing that the body protects the trunk and the head from large shock waves by dampening the applied load in the lower extremities. For each surface, the acceleration at the tibia was 5 to 10 times greater than that in the trunk.

McMahon and Greene[21] developed a mathematical model to determine the effect of surface stiffness on running speed. They hypothesized that a compliant surface acts as a spring and that, if the stiffness of the spring is closely tuned to the mechanical properties of the runner, the runner's speed can be increased. Their model showed that the ground contact time was the most important factor in predicting the effect of track stiffness on running speed.

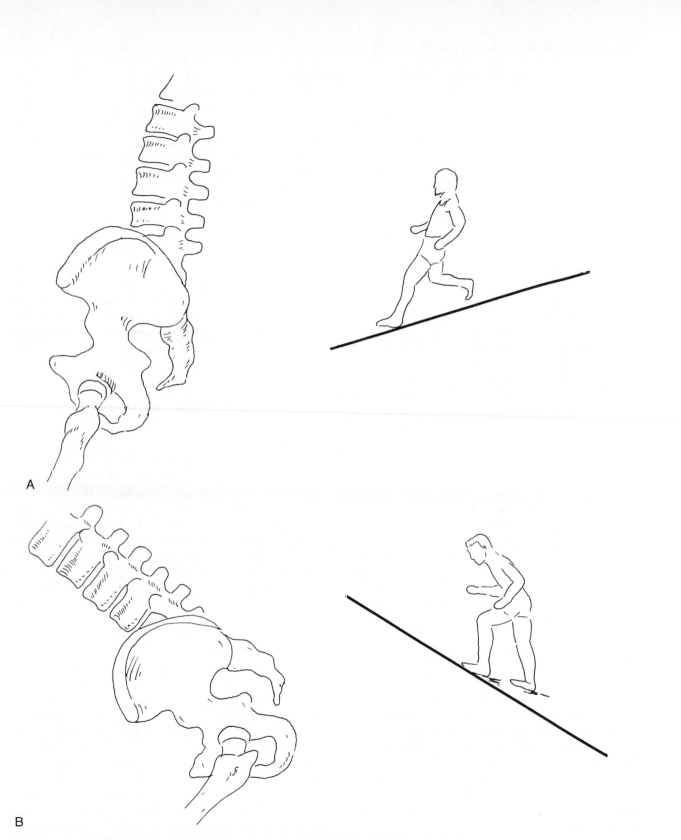

Figure 11-10 Effect of (**A**) downhill and (**B**) uphill running on pelvic tilt. Uphill running accentuates anterior tilt. Downhill running increases posterior tilt and hyperextends the spine (lordosis).

A

B

As expected, the ground contact time on soft surfaces was longer. It might be expected that ground contact time decreases as surface hardness increases, suggesting that a surface such as concrete would be the fastest. The results were not as would be expected, however; the ground contact time did not decrease over the entire range of compliances. The damping effect in the spring of human muscle affects the ground contact time such that it reaches a minimum at intermediate compliance, where the stiffness is two to four times greater than the runner's stiffness. At this optimum compliance, the runner stores elastic energy in the surface, much as a pole vaulter stores elastic energy while bending a fiberglass pole, and the energy is recovered as the runner springs forward. The model was used to design a six-lane 200-yard track at Harvard University, featuring banked turns, a polyurethane top surface, and a substructure made primarily of wood. Times run on the Harvard track averaged 2.9 percent faster than at other facilities during the first year of use.

Feehery[38] attempted to determine the influence of three different surfaces (asphalt, concrete, and grass) on the GRF at the foot and the acceleration of the head during distance running. The head measurement was included to assess the magnitude of shock transmitted through the body and to determine whether differences between surfaces measured at the foot are reflected at the head. Different test surfaces were laid on a Kistler force platform on which GRFs were obtained. The vertical acceleration of the head was measured with a uniaxial accelerometer mounted on a Plexiglas bite bar, as previously described by Light and McLellan.[1] Research determined that the overall shape of the force and acceleration curves for the three surfaces showed only small variations between surfaces, in agreement with the results of Holden and Muncey.[39] The GRF time records were similar in shape to those reported by Cavanagh and La Fortune.[40] The largest differences attributable to the surfaces were seen in the vertical force component and in the acceleration at the head. Contrary to what was expected, Feehery[38] found slightly lesser peak forces when the athlete was running on concrete. He postulated that the athletes were altering their running mechanisms (strategy) in preparation for landing on what they perceived to be a harder surface. The existence of strategies has been confirmed for both running and landing by Dufek and colleagues.[41] Hennig et al.[7] also reported altered loading patterns on the plantar surfaces of the feet when midsole hardness was changed, indicating adaptation or a change in strategy.

Subotnick[35] observed fewer shock attenuation-related injuries due to running on softer surfaces, such as grass. By contrast, increased motion problems were associated with very soft surfaces, such as sand, especially among runners unaccustomed to these soft, poorly tuned surfaces. Nigg[42] reported fewer injuries for tennis players playing on natural surfaces compared to a composition surface.

Variable changes of the slope, pitch, and terrain can be beneficial to the body, given average biomechanical stability. Induced variability results in greater range of motion of the joints and distribution of forces, with a decreased likelihood of chronic repetitive stress and fatigue. The need for precise biomechanical control at midstance is far less on natural, varying surfaces than on hard, flat, unyielding surfaces such as roads. Also, uneven surfaces require less protection from the functional varus seen in unidirectional sports. Some runners actually run in different shoes to create functional variability and modify the force distribution on a daily basis to avoid repetitive stress injuries.

The Effect of Shoes

The anatomic structure and anthropometric relationships within a runner's foot are usually inherent and cannot be changed, as pointed out by Nigg.[42] He noted, however, that what can be changed is the anatomy of the running shoe. Certain features of the shoe can influence the lines of action of forces by changing lever arm lengths. The shape of a shoe midsole can increase or decrease the amount of pronation. The shape or last of the shoe as it corresponds to the shape of the foot can increase or decrease foot stability, predisposing the runner to excessive pronation. For example, a low-arched rectus foot put in a C-shaped shoe will pronate through the shoe and have no support under the medial longitudinal arch, accentuating the instability of this already pronated foot. Nigg[42] observed that rearfoot movements during barefoot running show a minimal amount of initial and maximal pronation compared to such movements in a shod foot. Nigg reported that the excessive lateral flare of the running shoe, as well as the excessive posterior flare (the so-called heel spoiler), increase pronation and foot slap. The effect of increasing the lever arm on shoes is illustrated in Figure 11-11. The effect of a biomechanically sound shoe with dual-density midsole material and a slightly rounded heel is shown in Figure 11-12, which demonstrates a decrease in excessive pronation. This can further be enhanced with the use of an orthosis within the shoe.[43]

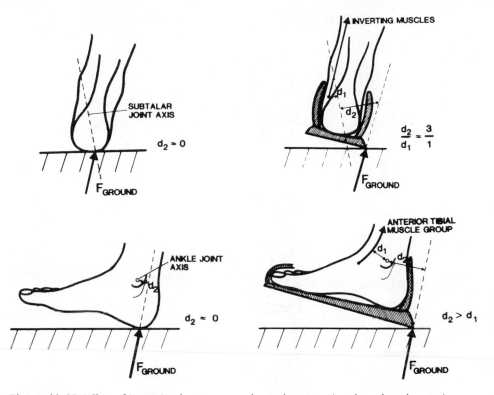

Figure 11-11 Effect of increasing lever arm on shoes, demonstrating that a lateral posterior lever arm in shoes increases pronation and foot slap. (From Nigg BM: Biomechanics of Running Shoes. Human Kinetic Publishers, Champaign, IL, 1980, with permission.)

There is a delicate balance between the ability of a shoe to decrease excessive pronation and its ability to also attenuate shock. In extreme cases, soft midsoles are good for cushioning while firmer midsoles create a stable base that allows for less pronation. Bates and colleagues[44] examined the effects of several shoes, including one with a dual-density midsole, using dynamic tests—runners running across a force platform. Although their results generally supported the functional differences of midsole construction on foot function, the authors concluded that there is no "best" design because each person's feet are anatomically and functionally different. Bates[45,46] further elaborated upon the importance of the individual and the related issues of performer variability and research methodology when evaluating footwear and performance.

There are many factors involved in the shoe's ability to perform all of its functions. Among these are shoe mechanical factors, such as the durometer of the midsole material, interface between the counter and the midsole, fatigue of midsole material, shape and lasting of the shoe, and components of the outsole. Also included are the geometry and fabrication of the heel counter; the presence or absence of innersoles, soft support systems, or orthotics; and biomechanical factors, such as surface, touchdown velocity, and foot pronation. Further biomechanical factors include foot type as well as laxity or stiffness of ligaments. An anatomically lasted shoe increases the shoe's ability to attenuate shock but also improves the stability of the foot within the shoe and decreases excessive pronation. When additional control is necessary, orthotics are helpful. Orthotics must be contoured to fit the inside of the shoe by grinding along the interior surfaces.

Based upon clinical evidence, Subotnick (personal communication) has suggested that the closed-cell midsole material ethylvinyl acetate (EVA) fatigues within 500 to 750 miles of running on hard surfaces. Hamill and Bates[47] reported losses in cushioning of 7.3 percent after 250 miles. These values are considerably less than the 27.0 and 40.4 percent for 50 and 250 miles, respectively, reported by Cook and co-workers[48] based upon impact testing. They also reported in vivo results of 20 and 30 percent for 150 and 500 miles, respectively. Temperature can also have a

SUBJECT A　　　　　**SUBJECT B**

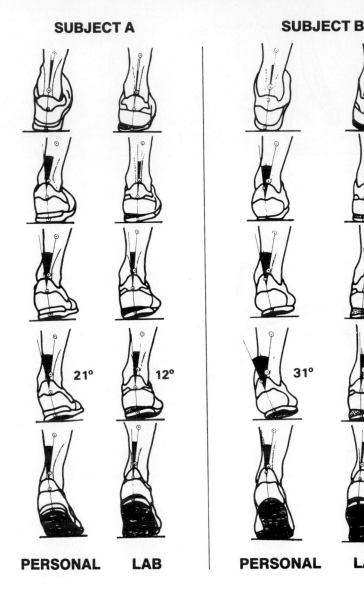

21°　　12°　　　31°　　12°

PERSONAL　　**LAB**　　　**PERSONAL**　　**LAB**

Figure 11-12 Effect of dual-density midsole in two subjects running at 4 m/s. Decrease in pronation while increasing the biomechanical effectiveness of shoes is the difference between subject A and subject B. A decrease in lateral and posterior flare improves the efficiency of the shoe and decreases unwanted abnormal pronation. (From Nigg BM: Biomechanics of Running Shoes. Human Kinetic Publishers, Champaign, IL, 1980, with permission.)

dramatic effect on EVA function. Kinoshita and Bates[30] reported losses in cushioning properties of up to 50 percent over temperature ranges from −5 to 55°C. These factors suggest that runners should be sensitive to the condition of their shoes and also consider choosing different shoes, in terms of hardness, for different environmental conditions.

Artificial Shock Attenuation

Light and colleagues[1] conducted research to evaluate the effect of artificial shock attenuation. They found that different shock waves pass up the skeleton following heel strike with normal walking in different footwear. They used three accelerometers, two on the leg and one supported by a bite bar held between the teeth. One of the leg accelerometers was placed invasively into the tibia, while the other was secured externally to the skin for the purpose of determining how accurately the externally mounted accelerometer recorded actual shock in the tibia. The use of the skin-mounted accelerometers was quite accurate, although there was a slight lag time when compared with the accelerometer mounted on a Kirschner wire implanted in the tibia. Accelerations of 5 g with hard shoes and of only 2.5 g with more compliant heels were found at the tibia. The rise time to this peak was about 50 percent longer in the more compliant shoes. Although the transient shock wave was greatly attenuated in its passage up the skeleton, the acceleration and displacement were still 0.5 g and 0.5 mm, respectively, at the head. Therefore, about 90 percent of the shock registered at the tibia was attenuated during the 10-ms travel time to the head. The investigators concluded that the shock wave at heel strike is initially moderated by the viscoelastic tissue at the heel pad and is then further attenuated and delayed about 10 ms as it passes to the head. Because its speed of propagation exceeds that of the afferent nerve conduction velocity, this rapid transmission of shock may serve as a signal for the body to react to the variety of surfaces at heel strike.

Wosk and Veloshin[22] did further research using accelerometers to study the effect of vibrational pathology on the development of joint degeneration. Fredrich[49] reported that the initial deceleration at heel strike can produce a shock of up to 30 g on the heel that then passes through the body at more than 200 mph. Fredrich discussed the role that viscoelastic polymers can play in decreasing both the frequency and magnitude of the shock wave. Studies have shown that viscoelastic polymers can assist the viscoelastic properties of the calcaneal fat pad in decreasing the vibration and frequency of shock waves to the tibia by approximately 40 percent.

McLellan reported results achieved using modified polyurethane with a high hysteresis as an insert in the posterior one-third of the heel.[35] A 6-mm-thick insert mounted in an otherwise hard heel construction produced a slightly greater reduction in heel strike transient than did the 18-mm-thick soft crepe rubber used in his research with Light et al.[1] Most impressive, however, was the attenuation–reverberation phenomenon seen with the crepe rubber construction. By using the viscoelastic polymer, about half the amplitudes during rebound were avoided. It was suggested that rebound transients propagated as waves traveling up the skeleton, producing nonuniform, nonsynchronous accelerations to various parts of the body, could possibly lead to osteoarthritis, musculoskeletal symptoms, or both. It was further suggested that the use of viscoelastic polymers to attenuate heel strike transients might be helpful in preventing or treating musculoskeletal periosteal tissue inflammation and associated pathology. Results of the utilization of the viscoelastic polymer heel insert are shown in Figure 11-13. Most notable is the 50 percent reduction in force with marked decrease in reverberation. Viscoelastic materials have also been used to reduce forefoot impact transient shock and reverberation.

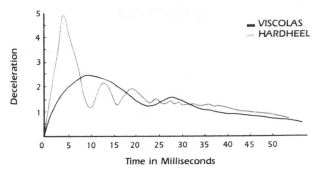

Figure 11-13 Decrease in impact and rebound when Viscolas polymer heel is compared with a hard heel. (Graph courtesy of Chattanooga Corporation, Chattanooga, TN.)

The Effect of Orthoses

Orthoses are discussed in detail in Chapter 24. It is generally appreciated that an orthosis that decreases abnormal pronation also reduces the need for eccentric contracture of muscles that reduce the rate of impact loading. This includes the posterior and anterior tibial muscles. When excessive impact pronation is decreased, the likelihood of posteromedial or anterolateral shin syndrome is decreased, as is the subsequent stress reaction of bone. Orthoses theoretically improve the efficiency of an athlete, decreasing fatigue and theoretically improving the ability of the body to attenuate impact shock. Orthoses can be made with semiflexible materials that encompass shock-attenuating fillers. Thus the added biodynamic control as well as shock-attenuating properties of foot orthoses afford additional protection against injury. The combination of orthoses with viscoelastic polymer components in a well-constructed shoe appears to enhance the body's ability to attenuate shock.

In a study of 180 running patients, James and associates[19] reported that 83 individuals (46 percent) were prescribed orthotic devices and that 65 of these runners (78 percent) were able to return to their previous running program. Six of these runners were later evaluated while running barefooted in regular running shoes and while wearing their orthoses using high-speed (200-Hz) cinematography.[43] Both the period of pronation and maximum pronation were reduced for the shoe condition compared to the barefooted condition, with even further reductions as a result of the orthotic condition, thus confirming the positive influence these devices can have on controlling pronation.

REFERENCES

1. Light LH, McLellan GE, Klenerman K: Skeletal transients on heel strike in normal walking with different foot wear. J Biomech 13:477, 1980
2. Dufek JS, Bates BT: Biomechanical factors associated with injury during landing in jump sports. Sports Med 12:326, 1991
3. Nigg BM: Biomechanics of Running Shoes. Human Kinetic Publishers, Champaign, IL, 1980
4. Bates BT, Ostering LR, Sawhill JA, Hamill J: Identification of critical variables describing ground reaction forces during running. p. 635. In Matsui H, Kobayashi K (eds): Biomechanics VIII-B. Human Kinetic Publishers, Champaign, IL, 1983
5. Light LH, McLellan GE: Skeletal transients associated with heel strike. J Physiol 272:9, 1977
6. Hennig EM, Lafortune MA: Relationship between ground reaction force and tibial bone acceleration parameter. Int J Sport Biomech 7:303, 1991
7. Henning EM, Valiant GA, Lui Q: Biomechanical variables and the perception of cushioning for running in various types of footwear. J Appl Biomech 12:143, 1996
8. Cavanagh PR, Hennig EM, Bunch RP, Macmillan NH: A new device for the measurement of pressure distribution inside the shoe. p. 1089. In Matsui H, Kobayashi K (eds): Biomechanics VIII-B. Human Kinetics Publishers, Champaign, IL, 1983
9. Hennig EM, Milani TL: In-shoe pressure distribution for running in various types of footwear. J Appl Biomech 11:299, 1995
10. Bates BT, James SL, Osternig LR: Foot function during the support phase of running. Running 4:19, 1978
11. Voloshin AS, Wosk J: An in vivo study of low back pain and shock absorption in the human locomotor system. J Biomech 15:21, 1981
12. Jorgensen V: Achillodynia and loss of heel pad shock absorbency. Am J Sports Med 16:185, 1985
13. Radin EL, Paul IL, Rose RM: Role of mechanical factors in pathogenesis of primary osteoarthritis. Lancet 1:519, 1972
14. Brody DM: Running injuries. Clin Symp 32:2, 1980
15. Mason BR: A kinematic and kinetic analysis of selected parameters during the support phase of running. Unpublished doctoral dissertation, University of Oregon, Eugene, 1980
16. Bates BT, Hamill J, Devita P: The evaluation of strategies to accommodate additional loads during running. p. 40. In: Proceedings of the Biennial Conference of the Canadian Society of Biomechanics: Human Locomotion V, Vol. 5. Kingston, Ontario, Canadian Society of Biomechanics, 1988
17. Bates BT, Francis PR, Kinoshita H: Functional capabilities of runners having extreme foot types. p. 98. In Proceedings of the Second Biannual Conference of the Canadian Society of Biomechanics. Kingston, Ontario, Canadian Society of Biomechanics, 1982
18. Hamill J, Bates BT, Knutzen KM, Kirkpatrick GM: Relationship between selected static and dynamic lower extremity measures. Clin Biomech 4:217, 1989
19. James SL, Bates BT, Osternig LR: Injuries to runners. Am J Sports Med 6(2):40, 1978
20. Van Mechelen W: Running injuries: a review of the epidemiological literature. Sports Med 14:320, 1992
21. McMahon TA, Greene PR: The influence of track compliance on running. J Biomech 12:893, 1979
22. Wosk J, Voloshin A: Wave attenuation in skeletons in young healthy persons. J Biomech 14:261, 1981
23. McMahon TA, Valiant G, Frederick ED: Groucho running. J Appl Physiol 87:2326, 1987
24. Kim W, Voloshin AS, Johnson SH: Modelling of heel strike transients during running. Hum Movement Sci 13:221, 1994
25. Hamill J, Bates BT, Holt KG: Timing of lower extremity joint actions during treadmill running. Med Sci Sports Exerc 24:807, 1992
26. Stergiou N: Mechanisms associated with running injuries. Unpublished doctoral dissertation, University of Oregon, Eugene, 1995
27. Stergiou N, Bates BT: Relationship between subtalar and knee joint function during running on different surfaces. Gait Posture 6:177, 1997
28. Kapandji IA: The Physiology of the Joints. Churchill Livingstone, New York, 1985
29. Bates BT, Osternig LR, Mason BR, James SL: Functional variability of the lower extremity during the support phase of running. Med Sci Sports 11:328, 1979
30. Kinoshita H, Bates BT: The effect of environmental temperature on the properties of running shoes. J Appl Biomech 12:258, 1996
31. Kinoshita H, Francis PR, Murase T et al: The mechanical properties of the heel pad in elderly adults. Eur J Appl Physiol 73:404, 1996
32. De Clercq D, Aerts P, Kunnen M: The mechanical characteristics of the human heel pad during foot strike in running: an in vivo cineradiographic study. J Biomech 27:1213, 1994
33. Paul JL, Munro MB, Abernathy SR et al: Musculoskeletal shock absorption: relative contribution of bone and soft tissue at various frequencies. J Biomech 2:237, 1978
34. Hamill J, Murphy M, Sussman D: The effects of track turns on lower extremity function. Int J Sport Biomech 3:276, 1987
35. Subotnick SI: The Running Foot Doctor. Mountain View, CA, World Publications, 1975
36. Unold EM: Acceleration on different surfaces. Track Technique 69:211, 1977
37. Unold EM, Neukonum PN, Nigg B: Continuous acceleration measurements in humans during locomotion on different surfaces. Biotelemetry II: Second International Symposium, 1974

38. Feehery RV: Biomechanics of running on different surfaces. Clin Pediatr Med Surg 3:4, 1986
39. Holden TS, Muncey RW: Pressures on the human foot during walking. Aust J Appl Sci 4:405, 1953
40. Cavanagh PR, Lafortune MA: Ground reactive forces in distance running. J Biomech 13:397, 1980
41. Dufek JS, Bates BT, Stergiou N, James CR: Interactive effects between group and single-subject response patterns. Hum Movement Sci 14:301, 1995
42. Nigg BN: External force measurements with sport shoes and playing surfaces. p. 11 In Nigg BN, Kerr BA (eds): Biomechanical Aspects of Sport Shoes and Playing Surfaces, Calgary, Alberta, University Printing, 1983
43. Bates BT, Osternig LR, Mason BR, James SL: Foot orthotic devices to modify selected aspects of lower extremity mechanics. Am J Sports Med 7:338, 1979
44. Bates BT, Osternig LR, Sawhill JA, James SL: An assessment of subject variability, subject-shoe interaction, and the evaluation of running shoes using ground reaction force data. J Biomech 16:181, 1983
45. Bates BT: Comment on "The influence of running velocity and midsole hardness on external impact forces in heel-toe running." J Biomech 22:963, 1989
46. Bates BT: Single-subject methodology: an alternative approach. Med Sci Sports Exerc 28:631, 1996
47. Hamill J, Bates BT: A kinetic evaluation of the effects of in vivo loading on running shoes. J Orthop Sports Phys Ther 10:47, 1988
48. Cook SD, Kester MS, Brunet ME: Shock absorption characteristics of running shoes. Am J Sports Med 9:47, 1985
49. Fredrich EC (ed): Sport Shoes and Playing Surfaces. Human Kinetics Publishers, Champaign, IL, 1984

12

Sports–Specific Biomechanics

STEVEN I. SUBOTNICK

UNIDIRECTIONAL VERSUS MULTIDIRECTIONAL SPORTS

Sports may include such activities as jumping, pivoting, cutting, sprinting, backpedaling, jogging, balancing, hurdling, or edging. One might be called upon to treat an athlete involved in field events, such as the pole vault, shot put, discus, or javelin. High jumping has different requirements than does the jumping seen in basketball or aerobics. Differences as well as similarities of various activities aid in making the appropriate diagnosis and planning for meaningful treatment.[1-3]

Different sports require various movement styles because each style serves a different purpose. One might compare the backpedaling of the basketball guard with that of the broken-field running of a football halfback. The rebounding and pivoting of a basketball player could be compared with the tennis player going from a stance position to a backhand or forehand position. The rebounding basketball player could be compared with the spiking volleyball player. It is essential for a volleyball player to have a wide base of gait with flexed knees in preparation for returning a serve with underhand fist contact. It is also essential for a lineman on a football team to have a wide base of gait with a low center of gravity in preparation for rapid cutting, blocking, or collision. In long-distance running, however, this wide base of gait with excessive flexion at the knee would give an inefficient gait and clumsy running style.

There are several factors to consider when comparing unidirectional with multidirectional sports. Among them are the angle of gait, base of gait, center of gravity, and direction of gait, as well as the likelihood of collision or contact.

Angle of gait: The angle of gait is determined from the angle that forms between the long axis of the foot as it compares with the line of progression (Fig. 12-1).

Base of gait: The base of gait is that distance between the inner aspects of both feet at the level of the medial malleolus (Fig. 12-1).

Direction of motion: The direction of motion may be unidirectional, multidirectional, or a combination of the two with cutting, pivoting, twisting, jumping, or kicking.

Speed: The speed of running or walking influences biomechanics. In general, as speed increases, the angle of gait and base of gait decrease and the impact increases. Some sports require constant speed, such as sprinting, middle-distance running, and long-distance running. Other sports demand rapid changes in acceleration and deceleration. The foot may change from a pronated attitude to a supinated attitude as the athlete moves from slow running with a wide base of gait to sprinting.

Characteristics of Unidirectional Sports

Unidirectional activities, such as walking, exercise walking, race walking, and running, in general have a higher center of gravity than is present with multidirectional sports, such as broken-field running. In unidirectional activity, the feet point relatively straight ahead. The angle of gait is mildly externally rotated with leisure walking, whereas it is more commonly straight ahead with running.[4]

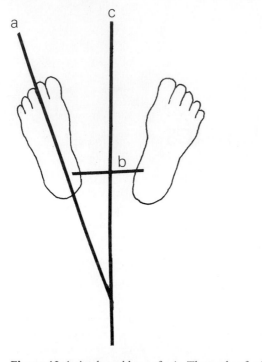

Figure 12-1 Angle and base of gait. The angle of gait (*a*) is the long axis of the foot compared to the forward line of progression (*c*). The base of gait (*b*) is the distance between the feet at the level of the medial malleolus when they are in a position of function.

The base of gait becomes narrower as the speed increases.[5,6]

The direction of gait in walking is straight ahead, and the feet travel on parallel tracks. In race walking as well as running, one foot lands where the other foot was on the line of progression directly beneath the center of gravity. Therefore, a 0 base of gait is used in race walking and running compared with a base of gait 6 to 10 inches apart during leisure walking. In general, as the base of gait increases, the feet become externally rotated. Increased angle of gait is associated with increased base of gait[4] (Fig. 12-2).

A wide base of gait is necessary for stability. With the feet far apart, the center of gravity is lower and the feet are externally rotated. This allows for a quick response in any direction, as seen in the set position of tennis or shortstop position in baseball. A narrow base of gait, with its associated narrow angle of gait, is necessary for fast-forward progression, as is seen in running. It allows for longer stride length with greater speed and running efficiency.

Characteristics of Multidirectional Sports

In multidirectional sports, the center of gravity is lowered as the base of gait and angle of gait are increased. This position is essential for collision sports, including rugby, football, and, at times, basketball and soccer. Normal variations of the angle of gait can be sports specific, while pathologic variations of the angle of gait can be caused by or lead to biomechanical imbalance.

Variations of the Angle and Base of Gait

The angle of gait and base of gait change with the demands of the sport. In sports with frequent changes of direction and acceleration, the foot is usually externally rotated with a relative wide base. The athlete usually cuts away from the support foot. In pivot sports, the foot is anchored on the surface and the body rotates above the support foot. In contact and collision sports, there may be backpedaling (backward running) with the athlete on the balls of the feet initially, then going backward with a relatively wide base and angle of gait. Pivoting can take place on the heel, forefoot, or whole foot. A wide base of gait is necessary for stability. A pronated foot position is necessary for adaptability to varying surfaces and to allow for bipedal stability. A supinated foot position is necessary for liftoff in rebounding or jumping.

Thus in contact or collision sports, in which balance may be precarious, a player tries to keep the center of gravity low and to use a wide base of gait with externally rotated feet. As the athlete (e.g., football player) breaks away from any would-be opponent, a more upright position is assumed; as speed increases, the base of gait gets narrower and narrower until the angle of gait is almost 0, as is the base. When rapid changes of direction are necessary or when there is a chance for collision and upset balance, the athlete again lowers the center of gravity and assumes a wide stance.[7]

Variations in functional capacity might lead to decreased performance or injury in multidirectional or unidirectional sports. Conditions such as hypermobility, hypomobility, loss of dynamic stability, or asymmetry in variations of neutral position are such examples. These can be secondary to injury, genetic factors, or dynamic imbalance with functional abnormalities. Sports-specific overspecialization may lead to functional imbalance. Previous injury with

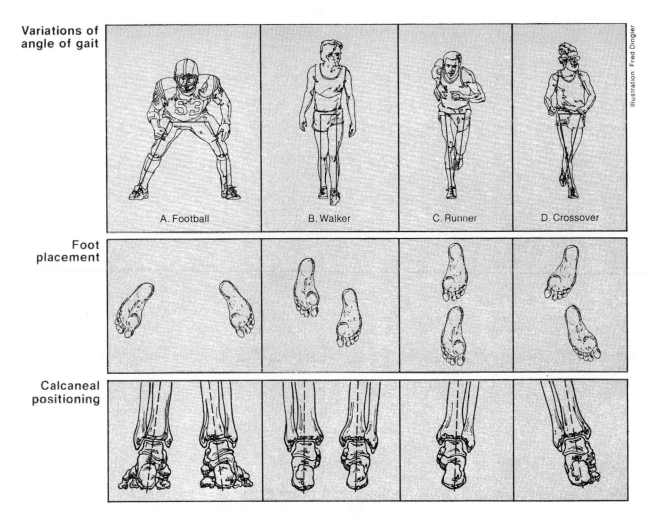

Figure 12-2 Comparison of the angle and base of gait. **(A)** Football players, with a low center of gravity, have a wide angle and base of gait and a pronated rearfoot. **(B)** Exercise walkers, with a narrow base of gait, have a parallel angle of gait and a neutral rearfoot. **(C)** Runners, with a high center of gravity, have a 0 base and angle of gait and a varus rearfoot. **(D)** Joggers usually have crossover and functional varus. (From Subotnick SI: Variations in angles of gait in running. Physician Sports Med 7:205, 1979, with permission.)

inadequate rehabilitation results in functional limitations. There may be acquired or developed limits in joint motion predisposing to imbalance in proximal or distal joints. Such an example is functional valgus at the knee secondary to increased internal rotation of the hips.[7]

BIOMECHANICS OF RUNNING

Comparison of Walking to Running

Problems resulting from variations in the angle of gait or contact position of the foot can be further appreciated when one compares walking to running (Fig. 12-2). In walking, there is a period of bipedal stance at contact followed by unipedal support during midstance and again followed by bipedal stance during toe-off (Fig. 12-3). There is a wider base of gait than in running, and the foot assumes a neutral position in the middle of midstance just prior to heel-off. Because there is a wide base of gait, the feet move along parallel lines of progression, which are not directly along the line of progression.

During running, there is a float phase (levitation) when neither foot is on the ground, followed by unipedal support (Fig. 12-4; see Fig. 12-6). In ideal running form, the angle of gait is 0 and the foot lands on the line of progression. Variations from this ideal may be seen in athletes who do not have a normal biomechanical structure or perfect running form (Fig. 12-5). Athletes with limited rotation in the hips or who have a leg length variation may find it more comfortable or natural to toe out for greater stability. This is not ideal running form for those with more normal biomechanical structure or requirements. In the absence of ideal intrinsic stability, the body is supported by excessive muscular activity instead of being balanced by efficient positioning. The result is rapid fatigue. In running, as in walking, the foot should be neutral at midstance (Figs. 12-3B and 12-6), in order to balance the body above the support foot. In running, as in walking, there is single support during midstance.

Figure 12-3 Gait cycle in walking. Stance phase compared with swing phase. The stance phase is balance support, midstance, and finally propulson. The gait cycle involves limb rotation. Internal rotation occurs during the first 25 percent of the stance phase of gait. External rotation takes place from foot flat to toe-off; internal rotation occurs during the swing phase. (From Subotnick SI (ed): p. 14. Podiatric Sports Medicine. Futura, Mt. Kisco, NY, 1975, with permission.)

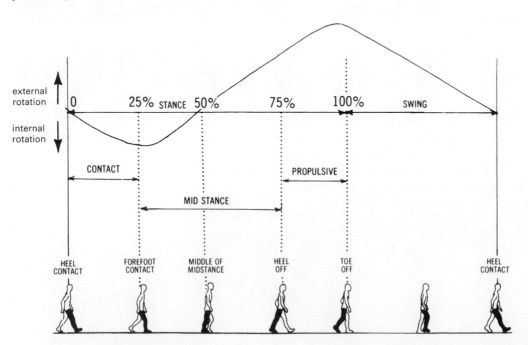

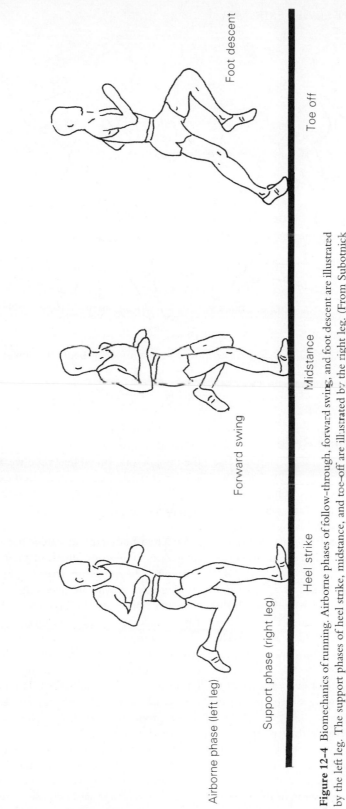

Figure 12–4 Biomechanics of running. Airborne phases of follow-through, forward swing, and foot descent are illustrated by the left leg. The support phases of heel strike, midstance, and toe-off are illustrated by the right leg. (From Subotnick SI (ed): p. 18. Podiatric Sports Medicine. Futura, Mt. Kisco. NY, 1975, with permission.)

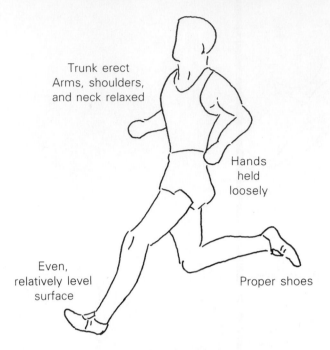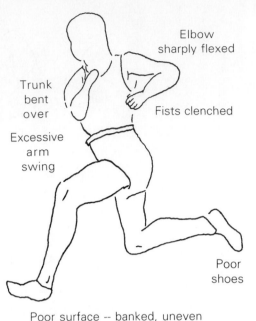

Figure 12-5 Comparison of good and bad running form.

Analysis of Running Style

Several investigations have been made of the characteristics of walking and running styles.[5,6,8–11] Of prime importance is the increase in functional varus seen as one progresses from leisure walking to race walking to running, and finally to sprinting.[4,12,13] This functional varus increases the speed and amount of pronation when one compares walking to running (Fig. 12-7).

The difference between bipedal stance in walking and unipedal stance in running varies markedly. The athlete may have pronated feet in stance yet run with supinated feet. This might be due to plantar flexing at the ankle during running, using the peroneus longus and producing a functional forefoot valgus. This athlete might need orthoses with varus control for walking or everyday activity, compared with running orthoses with a forefoot valgus post.

Many athletes believe that, because they wear down the lateral aspects of the heels of their shoes, they are not pronating excessively. They conclude that, if pronation were a problem, they would be landing on the inner aspects of their heels. Excessive lateral wear of the shoe is secondary to abrasion during contact. Contact is followed by rapid pronation, which may be excessive. That being the case, despite lateral heel shoe wear, functional varus is usually associated with rapid, often excessive, pronation.

BODY TYPES

Different body types dictate variance in individual running styles. The stride length of a tall, long-legged athlete is certainly different from that of a short, squatty one. Beginning runners who are overweight have excessive fat on the inner aspects of their thighs. They will characteristically have a wide base of gait and increased angle of gait. They may circumduct at the hips to decrease the medial rub at the inner aspects of the thighs. Circumduction is also necessary to allow for forward swing of the foot without hitting the opposite stance foot. This excessive circumduction creates crossover, with excessive abduction and accentuated pronation[4,8] (Fig. 12-2) (S. I. Subotnick, unpublished data). As the beginning jogger or runner loses weight, the body changes. Running style and biomechanical function also change. Thus the shoe and orthotic requirements of runners vary as their running style and body types change. Shoe and orthosis requirements change as runners learn to run more efficiently, with improved bio-

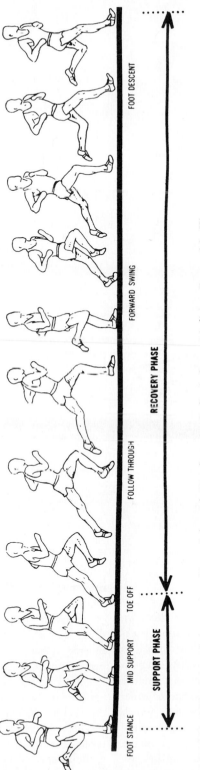
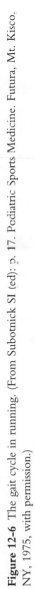

Figure 12-6 The gait cycle in running. (From Subotnick SI (ed): p. 17. Pediatric Sports Medicine. Futura, Mt. Kisco, NY, 1975, with permission.)

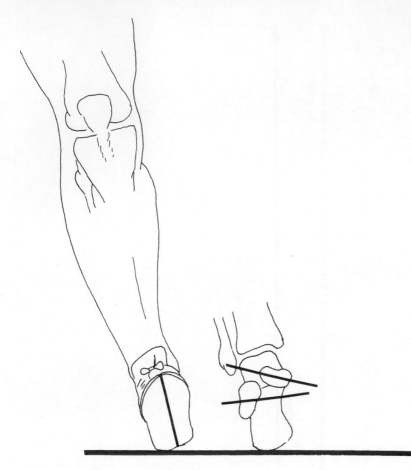

Figure 12-7 Functional varus in running.

mechanics. This accompanies the physical changes that occur as the athlete progresses from the fitness to the competitive level.

LIMB LENGTH DISCREPANCIES

Variations in the angles of gait in running are caused by limb length discrepancies. Most often, the short leg externally rotates for increased stability. The short leg is often associated with a posteroinferior pelvis imbalance on the involved side. There is usually overstriding on the short side. The foot on the short side is therefore subjected to greater force over a shorter period of time. This is compounded by the external position, which increases the pronatory force on the foot as well as the knee. Overstriding produces contact at the rear of the shoe as the foot lands in front of the center of gravity. This braking, in fact, increases contact load and acceler-

ates foot slap, placing excessive strain on the antigravity anterior muscle group of the leg as braking occurs. Anterior shin splints (enthesitis) might occur (S. I. Subotnick, unpublished data).

Discrepancies as little as 1/8 inch are corrected in the runner. If the difference in limb length is less than 5/8 inch, an intrinsic heel lift may be used. This is usually made of ethyl vinyl acetate (EVA) or Korex and applied to the rearfoot post of the orthosis. With heel lift the calcaneus inverts; thus a perpendicular rearfoot post is preferred to prevent lateral ankle instability.

Discrepancies greater than 6/8 inch are corrected with extrinsic midsole shoe partial correction of about one-half the heel lift, increase modification, in running sports.[7]

These differences in limb length can also affect skiing proficiency, and correction is advised, usually extrinsic with full-correction lifts under the heel and forefoot of the boot bindings.

CONSIDERATIONS FOR ORTHOTIC TREATMENT

Activity influences biomechanical treatment or control for various sports. In jumping sports, such as aerobics and basketball, shoes and orthoses allow for shock attenuation of both the forefoot and rearfoot. A perpendicular heel position is preferred, and a semiflexible device works best (Fig. 12-8). The device should be full length.

In pivoting sports, such as tennis, basketball, golf, racquetball, or handball, full-length semiflexible orthoses with perpendicular rearfoot control are used. The rearfoot post should be compressible to allow for pronation. The same compressible rearfoot post is used in jumping sports. If additional shock attenuation is desired, the orthoses may be filled with a shock-attenuating material, such as Viscolas (Chattanooga Corp., Chattanooga, TN) or Poron (Stein Podiatry Supplies, Hackensack, NJ). If additional shock attenuation or accommodation under metatarsal heads is desirable, as is often the case in pivoting or jumping sports, EVA, Poron, or Viscolas may be used under the metatarsal heads with a compressible forefoot wedge. These wedges may be drilled out to accommodate metatarsal heads that

are plantarly positioned and that have associated lesions or bursitis, or both.

Cutting sports, such as football, basketball, or soccer, have biomechanical requirements similar to those of pivoting. The orthosis is semiflexible and may have perpendicular compressible rearfoot control or no rearfoot control, depending upon the foot type. The cavus foot might require perpendicular rearfoot control to prevent lateral instability; a 1/8-inch heel lift may be necessary for anterior equinus. A perpendicular-to-valgus forefoot extension might be necessary to prevent sprains in rebounding during basketball. Since soccer shoes are rather snug, an in-shoe cast may be preferable.

Unidirectional running, such as sprinting, middle-distance running, or long-distance running, requires orthoses with varying degrees of rearfoot and forefoot control. Sprinting requires a flexible orthosis with compressible forefoot control. The orthosis must be full length to provide for forefoot control. Since contact is on the ball of the foot, rearfoot control is unnecessary. A flexible soft orthosis with forefoot wedging is preferred. In middle-distance running, there is forefoot followed by rearfoot contact. Some rearfoot control is desirable and may be

Figure 12-8 Soft orthoses used in sports. Left to right: Custom-molded leather; custom-made semirigid, with or without post; "off-the-shelf" soft plastic.

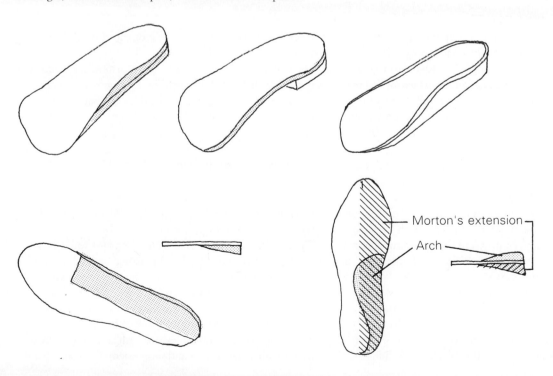

Morton's extension

Arch

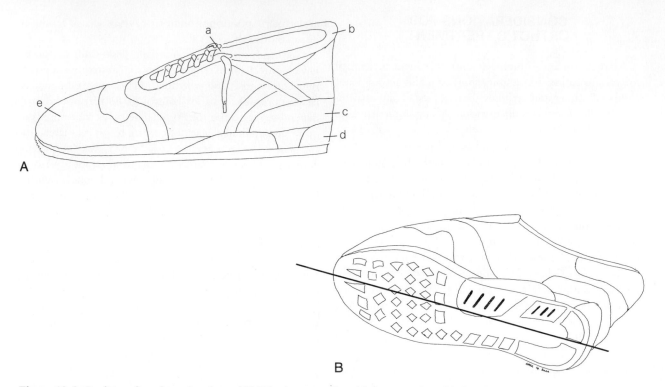

Figure 12-9 Qualities of good running shoes. **(A)** Side view. *a*, well-padded tongue; *b*, molded Achilles pad; *c*, firm heel counter; *d*, flared and beveled heel; *e*, high, rounded toebox. **(B)** Bottom view. Straight last and studded sole.

anywhere from 3 to 5 degrees, depending on the foot type and contact position. Additional varus control of the forefoot is desirable to prevent propulsive pronation. In long-distance running there is a functional varus, and rearfoot control with semicompressible material in from 3 to 5 degrees of varus is needed. The forefoot is posted with a wedge from behind the metatarsal heads to the sulcus to prevent any motion between the forefoot and rearfoot. This prevents excessive propulsive pronation and stabilizes the forefoot during takeoff. Figure 12-9 shows the basic features of good running shoes.

In multidirectional running sports, such as baseball, racquetball, or tennis, a semiflexible orthosis with perpendicular compressible rearfoot post and shock-attenuating material under the forefoot is preferred. Sometimes no rearfoot control works best.

Edge sports, such as hockey, skiing, roller skating, or ice skating, often require an in-boot cast. Perpendicular to 3- to 4-degree varus rearfoot control may be used, depending on the foot type and biomechanics. The forefoot is balanced perpendicular to the rearfoot. A full-length

device is desired to pad the ball of the foot and increase proprioception under the toes.

Balancing sports, such as dancing or fencing, require a soft to flexible full-length orthosis with no rearfoot control and shock-attenuating material under the ball of the foot. Field events in track require full-length soft or flexible orthoses with no rearfoot control and padding under the ball of the foot. Hurdling requires a full-length flexible orthosis with 3- to 5-degree compressible rearfoot varus control and shock-attenuating material under the ball of the foot. A forefoot wedge may be desired. If additional medial forefoot stability is required, a Morton's extension may be added (see Fig. 12-8).

In all orthoses, functional hallux limitus should be corrected with a Kinetic Wedge. I personally grind out under the first metatarsal head on the forefoot wedge extension, and then, if needed add a Vylyte (Stein Podiatry, Trenton, NJ) Morton's extension. With any varus forefoot running wedge, the first metatarsal head should be plantar flexed to prevent metatarsus primus elevatus with jamming of the first metatarsophalangeal joint and subsequent functional hallux limitus, which over the long term leads to permanent joint changes with bony hallux limitus.

SHOE MODIFICATIONS

Shoes may be modified depending on the needs of the athlete and the biomechanical foot type (Fig. 12-10). In unidirectional sports, the lateral flare at the rearfoot oftentimes acts as a lever arm and accentuates pronation. The posterior projection on running shoes may increase foot slap. Shoes are routinely modified by grinding the lateral and posterior flare. This decreases excessive pronation and

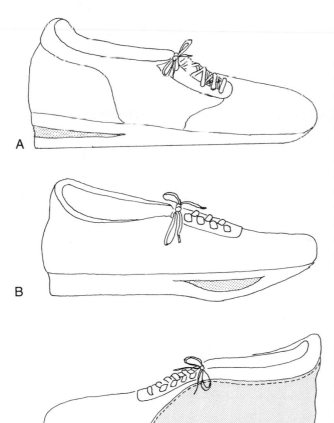

Figure 12-10 Examples of compensatory shoe correction. **(A)** Schuster heel wedge for Achilles tendinitis. **(B)** Rubber rocker bottom inserted in sole for metatarsal pain. **(C)** Leather-reinforced upper on medial side prevents hyperpronation and recurrent lateral ankle syndrome.

foot slap. Shoes that are stiff at the metatarsophalangeal joint are given additional flexibility by cutting transverse grooves in the outsole and midsole, decreasing strain on the posterior musculature. This is especially helpful in young athletes who have tendencies toward posterior apophysitis. Pain under the ball of the foot can be alleviated with a rocker sole built into the shoe. Athletes with excessive pronation in standard shoes can be given additional medial rearfoot support with leather reinforcement. Weak counters can also be reinforced with leather.

Conditions such as Haglund's deformity, retrocalcaneal exostosis, and pump bumps are best treated by removing the plastic counter from the back of the shoe and replacing it with soft leather or elastic. All pressure is thereby removed from the posterior heel, allowing the bursae and osteitis to heal. One can also smash the counter with a hammer to relieve pressure. Similarly, ski boots are heat-punched out with a ball-and-ring stretcher and a heat gun. (It is always easier to operate on the shoes than the feet!) Shoes with excessive medial compression can be built up with firmer durometer EVA or polyurethane medial wedges in the midsole of the shoe.

A toebox that is causing dorsal pressure on toes can be modified by cutting through the shoe, creating space for the toes. Tailor's bunion could be alleviated by a lateral cut in the shoe, whereas hallux valgus and bunion can be helped by a medial cut in the shoe. Retrocalcaneal exostosis is aided by softening the counter of the shoe with a hammer. Variations in foot size are treated by fitting the largest foot. The smaller foot is aided by placing 1/8-inch felt under the tongue of the shoe to prevent forward sliding of the foot. Running shoes may be modified for race walkers by grinding down the posterior flare. Whereas the weak or pronated foot requires additional medial control, the cavus foot requires a narrow width at the rearfoot. Thus medial and lateral grinding of the flare of the running shoe increases motion in the cavus foot.

SUMMARY

The various biomechanical characteristics of each sport must be understood and correlated with the biomechanical foot type. With this knowledge, appropriate shoes, or orthoses when indicated, may be prescribed. Shoe modifications, or brand or style changes, can often solve an athlete's problem. Sports specialists dealing with feet must also be shoe specialists. A referral to a certified pedorthotist for shoe modifications can be remarkably effective in relieving foot pain and improving function.

REFERENCES

1. Maffulli N, Baxter, Jones AD: Common skeletal injuries in young athletes. Sports Med 19:137, 1995
2. Brill PA, Macera CA: The influence of running patterns on running injuries. Sports Med 20:365, 1995
3. Van den Bogert AJ: Analysis and simulation of mechanical loads on the human musculoskeletal system: a methodological overview. Exerc Sport Sci Rev 22:23, 1994
4. Subotnick SI: Variations in angles of gait in running. Physician Sports Med 7:110, 1979
5. Andriacchi TP, Ogle JA, Galante JO: Walking speed as a basis for normal and abnormal gait measurements. Biomechanics 10:261, 1977
6. Cairns MA, Burdett RG, Pisciotta JC, Simon SR: A biomechanical analysis of race walking gait. Med Sci Sport Exerc 18:446, 1986
7. Subotnick SI: Orthotic foot control and the overuse syndrome. Physician Sports Med 3:61, 1975
8. Subotnick SI (ed): Podiatric Sports Medicine. pp 21–56. Futura, Mt. Kisco, NY, 1975
9. Cavanagh PR, Pollack ML, Landa J: A biomechanical comparison of elite and good distance runners. p. 328. In Milvy P (ed): The Marathon: Physiological, Medical Epidemiological and Psychological Studies, Vol. 3. New York Academy of Sciences, New York, 1977
10. Subotnick SI: A biomechanical approach to running injuries. In Milvy P (ed): The Marathon: Physiological, Medical, Epidemiological, and Psychological Studies, Vol. 3. New York Academy of Sciences, New York, 1977
11. Nelson RC, Brooks CM, Pike NL: Biomechanical comparison of male and female distance runners. p. 793. In Milvy P (ed): The Marathon: Physiological, Medical, Epidemiological, and Psychological Studies, Vol. 3. New York Academy of Sciences, New York, 1977
12. Mero A, Cromi PV, Gregor, RJ: Biomechanics of sprint running: a review. Sports Medicine 13:376, 1992
13. Högberg P: Length of stride; stride frequency, slight period, and maximum distance between the feet during running with different speeds. Arbeitsphysiologie 14:431, 1952

SUGGESTED READINGS

James ST, Brubaker CD: Biomechanics of running. Orthop Clin North Am 4:604, 1973
Sgarlato TE: A Compendium of Podiatric Biomechanics. California College of Podiatric Medicine, San Francisco, 1971
Subotnick SI: The abuses of orthotic devices. J Am Podiatry Assoc 63:1025, 1975
Subotnick SI: The Running Foot Doctor. World Publications, Mountain View, CA, 1977
Subotnick SI: Sports and Exercise Injuries. North Atlantic Press, Berkeley, CA, 1992

III

Injuries of the Lower Extremity

13

General Concepts of Injury

STEVEN I. SUBOTNICK
PAMELA SISNEY

Injuries of the lower extremity may be acute, chronic but improving (overuse), or chronic and not improving. An understanding of the basic concepts of tissue response to trauma is helpful when creating an appropriate treatment plan and anticipating the eventual outcome.[1] Aging may even play a role in physical activity and sports injuries.[2] In addition, when evaluating sport injuries, as stressed in the sports psychology discussions in Chapter 2, exercise dependency syndrome is always a factor in etiology and treatment.[3] Finally, exercise itself has inherent risks depending upon the particular program engaged in by the athlete.[4]

ACUTE INJURY

Acute injury or trauma occurs when a sudden episode stresses tissue beyond its normal physiologic limits. Thus a ligament ruptures when the normal range of motion of a joint is exceeded. A tendon ruptures when its tensile strength is exceeded. Acute trauma is followed by a predictable sequence of events centered around the inflammatory process. The acute inflammatory process lasts 24 hours and is characterized by vasodilation, local necrosis of tissue, and release of inflammatory cellular elements, including prostaglandin, serotonin, and histamine. This initial inflammatory phase is best treated by using components of the mnemonic RICE: rest, ice, compression, and elevation. This treatment decreases the undesirable effects of the acute inflammatory phase. Icing and compression can be accomplished with a cold moist Ace bandage or with

ice packs secured with Ace wraps. Icing decreases inflammation and pain, which allows early range of motion. Eventually, secondary vasodilation from the ice, and the combination of motion, decrease of pain, and splinting, increases the clearing away of the inflammatory cellular elements and decreases local necrosis. Nonsteroidal antiinflammatory medications decrease the prostaglandin release and allow pain-free range of motion, with eventual recovery.[5–8]

Once the initial 24-hour acute inflammatory process has passed, chronic inflammatory changes persist. The waste products of injury are cleared away by the body, and healing takes place over a period of 3 to 4 weeks. Use of physical therapy, including early gentle range of motion within the tolerances of discomfort, increases circulation and the clearing away of inflammation waste products, and decreases atrophy. This accelerates healing and decreases the disability the athlete experiences. Acute injuries may require splinting with a posterior fiberglass splint, which can be removed four to five times a day to allow for protected range-of-motion exercises. Complete immobilization in a cast causes considerable atrophy, and there is evidence that prolonged cast immobilization increases the likelihood of decreased range of motion in joints, as well as osteophytic and arthritic changes. A loss of conditioning occurs rapidly when the athlete is immobilized, and should be counteracted by using safe forms of aerobic activity, such as swimming or riding an exercise bike.

These same principles apply to surgical trauma. A stable repair of a ligamentous rupture of the ankle best responds to early range-of-motion exercise, which is within the tolerance of the repaired structures. This hastens the healing of ligamentous structures and helps prevent atrophy of surrounding muscular tissue; it also decreases the possibility that limited joint motion will result. Postoperative physical therapy decreases inflammation, aids healing, and allows for a more functional outcome from the surgical repairs. A treatment consisting of rigid internal fixation for osteotomies or fractures, followed by early passive and active range of motion, is prudent when possible with the athlete.[9–11] The use of abrasion arthroplasties of osteochondritic lesions, followed by early range of motion with non-weight-bearing activity for 6 weeks, permits the formation of healthy fibrocartilage, and more functional results are obtained.

OVERUSE INJURY

Overuse injuries are chronic injuries. They occur secondary to microtrauma and microinflammatory processes that accompany the trauma and are sometimes called subclinical changes. There is evidence to suggest that microtrauma, which follows excessive training, causes inflammation and damage that follow the same, although less severe, sequence as that found in acute injuries. If one ignores the signs of overuse injury, which include stiffness and soreness but not the gross signs of inflammation, and continues to push in spite of the injury, a more acute condition may ensue. Enzyme studies done on runners after marathons reveal that considerable muscular damage can occur.[9–15] This will best respond to an initial treatment of ice, rest, and elevation, followed by training and physical therapy modalities to decrease inflammation and increase range of motion and function without re-injuring the injured structures. Recovery from a rigorous endurance event takes at least 4 weeks.

Athletes must be taught that conditioning consists of training the body to accept stress. Rushing this training creates too much stress, which leads to overuse injury and its associated microinflammatory changes and trauma. When overuse injuries are present, a dynamic imbalance may exist. The examining physician may find that injuries that occurred some time ago were never fully rehabilitated; thus the athlete's performance is compromised and other structures are injured. Complete rehabilitation of all structures is necessary after an acute or overuse injury occurs. Strength, flexibility, balance, and functional biomechanics are the goals of appropriate rehabilitation.

CHRONIC STATIC INJURY

A third category of injuries are the chronic static conditions. These are situations that persist beyond 1 to 2 years after acute trauma or overuse injury. In spite of appropriate conservative therapy, the conditions do not get better and, in fact, may get worse. An example of this type of injury is anterior impingement arthropathy of the ankle: limited dorsiflexion exists; osteophytes or spurs may be present; and certain activities, such as jumping or running fast on hills, result in pain and capsulitis. The athlete living within the confines of this disability must consider surgery, such as an anterior arthroplasty of the ankle, for resolution. Chronic tenosynovitis of the Achilles tendon that persists 1 to 2 years after injury and does not respond to physical therapy and appropriate biomechanical control of the lower extremity is another example. The athlete may always experience pain when running more than 3 to 4 miles. Surgery is the treatment of choice unless the athlete chooses to live within the confines of the injury. Repeated bouts of inflammation and pain that occur secondary to exceeding the limits of the paratenon of the Achilles tendon may lead to central necrosis of the tendon and eventual partial or complete rupture.[16,17]

There are, however, chronic injuries that resolve with time. An example is a hamstring strain, which lingers for 1 to 2 years and then finally goes away. Another example is chronic chondralgia patella about the right knee, which gradually goes away over a period of 1 to 2 years, only to be replaced with chondralgia patella of the left knee. Often, these injuries persist because of continued training errors. Once the training errors are corrected, the problems tend to go away. At other times, the reason for recovery is more obscure.

DEGREES OF INJURY

Injuries are generally classified as first, second, or third degree. First-degree injury is mild. There is initial pain, which goes away with rest, ice, compression, and elevation. Stability of the joints and the surrounding soft tissue structures are intact, and the athlete can generally return to competition after a careful evaluation and a short period of rest. Supportive therapy, such as taping or an Ace wrap, may be necessary. Before going back into competition, the athlete will need to demonstrate the ability to jump up and down on the affected lower extremity without pain and to run without pain. In the case of a sprained ankle, there may be some discomfort when jumping up and down on the ankle or doing figure eights. Once this subsides completely with appropriate treatment of the ankle, the athlete can return to competition.

In a second-degree injury, a moderate degree of damage occurs. There may be more extensive tearing of soft tissue structures about a joint or a strain of the muscle–tendon unit. Inflammation exists, and a moderate acute inflammatory process occurs. Although the athlete can walk on the lower extremity, there may be a slight limp. Running is uncomfortable; jumping up and down on the ball of the foot is difficult or impossible. An evaluation is done to rule out more serious damage, such as a fracture or complete rupture; rest, ice, compression, and elevation are used. After this the athlete is evaluated again, and, if able to walk, is then asked to run; if able to run, he or she is asked to jump up and down on the ball of the foot. In the case of an inversion sprain of the ankle, taping may be done, and, if the athlete can perform satisfactorily, return to competition is allowed. In this case, the tape transforms a second-degree injury into a first-degree injury.

Third-degree injuries involve complete disruption of tissue. Examples include a third-degree sprain or complete rupture of the ligament, or a third-degree strain with complete rupture of a muscle–tendon unit. In these cases, walking will be most difficult; the athlete will limp or be unable to bear weight on the involved lower extremity. Initial evaluation will reveal instability of the joint. Radiographic studies are done to rule out fracture, and appropriate supportive therapy (rest, ice, compression, elevation, and analgesics) is instituted. Immobilization with a posterior cast is helpful. Return to competition is not allowed until the patient is fully recovered, which may take anywhere from 3 to 6 weeks.

STRAINS

A strain is a tear of a tendon or muscle–tendon complex. Strains are generally graded as *first degree* if they are mild to minimal, *second degree* if moderate, and *third degree* if there is complete rupture in the muscle–tendon unit. Unless there is a complete rupture of the myotendinous unit, it is difficult to accurately assess the severity of the strain. Initial palpation, if done at the time of injury, may reveal a void or rift when a rupture has occurred. Complete rupture of the tendo Achillis is associated with a positive Thompson's test (squeezing of the calf is not associated with plantar flexion of the foot); however, other muscle–tendon units are more difficult to evaluate. The amount of pain, swelling, and spasm helps in classifying first-, second-, and third-degree deformity. The manner in which the athlete responds to RICE treatment will also give an indication of the severity of the injury.

First-degree injuries are associated with less tissue injury and a decreased inflammatory response. They tend to heal more readily, thus allowing an early return to full training. A second-degree injury must be treated more cautiously, inasmuch as it may progress to a third-degree strain if treated inappropriately. Protected weight bearing and range of motion are preferred. A second-degree sprain, if allowed to go untreated, results in excessive scar tissue formation, with delayed healing and compromised function.

Rifts of the myotendinous unit heal by fibrosis. Initially, the crisscrossed collagen that fills in the void is very inelastic and needs constant physical therapy, consisting of flexibility and stretching exercises, to encourage a more parallel arrangement of collagen bundles and increased functional results. Failure to use appropriate rehabilitative and physical therapy modalities will lead to chronic disability and pain.

SPRAINS

Sprains are disruptions of the ligamentous structures about joints. The primary function of ligaments is to limit excessive normal range of motion. Ligaments do not function well when forced to limit abnormal motion occurring around a joint.

The most common sprain is the first- or second-degree sprain of the anterior talofibular ligament of the ankle. This injury occurs during plantar flexion and inversion. This motion places excessive strain on the anterior lateral collateral ligament, which is mildly torn with a first-degree injury and more considerably torn and stretched with a second-degree injury. A complete disruption occurs with a third-degree rupture. The mechanism that causes the sprain puts excessive force on the ligamentous tissue, which is stretched beyond its physiologic tolerance until it fails with incomplete or complete rupture. Although it is possible for the ruptured ligament to heal without surgical intervention, some degree of instability may persist due to initial stretching of the ligaments. In children, recovery of ruptured ligaments is more complete than in adults; thus, surgical intervention is seldom necessary in the pediatric age group. Intervention may be appropriate in the athlete in the postadolescent to young adult age groups.

During the first hour after an acute injury has occurred, the degree of instability or damage can be more easily assessed. By the day following injury, enough inflammatory change has taken place that appropriate clinical evaluation of the severity of damage is more difficult. In the case of a ruptured ligament, an arthrogram may be helpful because the leakage of dye into the extracapsular tissue spaces indicates a disruption of capsule and ligamentous tissue.[18] This is especially true of the ankle joint.

First-degree sprains will show mild to moderate pain or inflammation initially. This responds rapidly to rest, ice, compression, and elevation. The athlete gains full ability to cut and jump up and down on the foot after a short period of rest. Supportive taping decreases the chance of re-injury, and the athlete may return to competition.

Second-degree sprains will have more excessive pain and swelling. The athlete will be limping. Attempts to cut or jump up and down on the foot are met with pain, and taping of the foot, although it provides for stability, will not completely eliminate the pain. If the pain is minimal with a supportive taping, the athlete may return to competition; however, if the athlete cannot jump up and down on the foot or cut, even with the taping, then return to competition is not advised. This type of injury is best treated with supportive therapy for the initial inflammatory process and then physical therapy and rehabilitation. When the athlete returns to competition, tape or bracing should be used to support the joint and permit complete healing of the injured ligament; otherwise, a second-degree sprain can progress to a third-degree sprain and complete rupture.

Sprains are accompanied by decreased kinesthetic responses, and appropriate proprioceptive rehabilitation is necessary.[19] Supportive taping or bracing should be used for 2 months following a second-degree sprain. Crutches are used until comfortable weight bearing is possible without external support. A posterior cast may initially be helpful, holding the foot in dorsiflexion and eversion to approximate the ruptured ligaments and allow healing with ligament lengthening with subsequent laxity.

A third-degree sprain is a complete disruption of a ligament. Considerable capsular damage with a partial tear and secondary inflammation are almost always present. Ecchymosis occurs as blood vessels in the capsule are torn. There may be associated tendon damage. Severe injuries may result in osteochondral defects or osteochondritis. These lesions are not always seen on plain radiograms and may need special studies, such as a computed tomography (CT) scan, for identification. Chronic pain following a grade III sprain is an indication for special radiographic studies to rule out bony damage, such as osteochondritis or impingement accompanied by meniscoid degeneration of the joint. Meniscoid lesions are best seen with magnetic resonance imaging (MRI) or via arthroscopic evaluation.

Initial evaluation of a third-degree sprain will reveal instability. In the ankle joint, there is a positive anterior drawer test; the calcaneus is pulled forward and the tibia pushed posteriorly. This indicates complete disruption of the anterior lateral collateral ligament. In the knee, a rupture of the medial collateral ligament, when evaluated initially after trauma, is accompanied by instability and a palpable rift where the ligament has been ruptured.

A third-degree sprain in a serious athlete is appropriately treated by primary surgical repair. The recreational athlete may choose conservative treatment, initially using a posterior cast and physical therapy three times a week. However, if chronic instability with repeated sprains is the end result, surgery is the treatment of choice. If complete disruption has occurred, optimal results are obtained with anatomic reapproximation of injured tissue.

Arthrograms and stress tests are most helpful in evaluating the severity of sprains, especially during the acute inflammatory phase when there is considerble ecchymosis, edema, and splinting. MRI evaluation is useful for older injuries to demonstrate fluid in tendons or ligaments, as well as fibrosis. CT scans help demonstrate transchondral and osteochondral fractures that often accompany grade III ankle sprains but are occult on plain radiographs.

ENTHESITIS

Enthesitis is defined as an inflammation of the attachments of muscles to bone. Medial shin syndrome (deep flexor compartment shin splints) results from a pulling of the soft tissue from the medial aspect of the tibia; this is an enthesitis. With enthesitis, there is pain with palpation at the junction of the soft tissue and bone, and pain with activity also occurs. When only soft tissue damage is present, enthesitis is the primary diagnosis. However, there may also be inflammation and a stress reaction of bone present. Chronic repetitive damage to bone with increased stress may lead to a stress fracture, and repeated trauma to a stress fracture may lead to a complete fracture. Thus it is important when making a diagnosis to differentiate enthesitis from stress reaction of bone and from stress fracture.[20–23] Radiographic studies and bone scans help differentiate these entities.

Enthesitis will respond to physical therapy and anti-inflammatory measures. At times, surgery is necessary to free the inflamed soft tissue from its attachments to bone, such as when the chronic shin-splint or heel-spur syndromes occur. Stress reaction of bone requires rest and then appropriate rehabilitation. Stress fractures also require rest and rehabilitation.

REFERENCES

1. Fredickson M: Common injuries in runners: diagnosis, rehabilitation and prevention. Sports Med 21:49, 1996
2. Kallinen M, Markku A: Aging, physical activity and sports injuries: an overview of common sports injuries in the elderly. Sports Med 80:41, 1995
3. Pierce EF: Exercise dependency syndrome in runners. Sports Med 18:149, 1994
4. Jones BH, Cowan DN, Knapik JJ: Exercise, training and injuries. Sports Med 18:202, 1994
5. Obel AO: Practical therapeutics: The newer non-steroidal anti-inflammatory drugs. East Afr Med J 59:366, 1982
6. Aronoff GM: The use of non-narcotic drugs and other alternatives for analgesia as part of a comprehensive pain management program. J Med 13:191, 1982
7. Non-steroidal anti-inflammatory drugs (editorial). Del Med J 53:486, 1981
8. Weissman G: The biochemistry of inflammation. J Miss State Med Assoc 23(3):66, 1982
9. Knudsen HA, et al: Ankle fracture classification with approaches to surgical repair by AO-ASIF technique. J Foot Surg 22:145, 1983
10. Rand JA, et al: Biomechanical factors in fracture treatment. Minn Med 65:558, 1982
11. Mulltier ME, Allgowier M, Schneidier A, Willizneggier H: Manual of Internal Fixation: Springer-Verlag, Berlin, 1979
12. Bouleau RA, et al: Physiological characteristics of elite middle, and long distance runners. Can J Appl Sport Sci 7:167, 1982
13. Keul J, et al: Biochemical changes in a 100 km run. Eur J Appl Physiol 47:181, 1981
14. Ali M, Brown E, Fayemi AO: Elevated CK-MB levels in marathon runners (letter). JAMA 274:2368, 1982
15. White R, et al: Hematological and chemical profile in long distance runners. Ann NY Acad Sci 7:346, 1977
16. Thompson TC: Spontaneous rupture of tendon Achilles: a new clinical diagnostic test. J Trauma 2:126, 1962
17. Bruce RK, et al: Ultrasonography evaluation for ruptured Achilles tendon. J Am Podiatry Assoc 72:15, 1982
18. Olson RW: Ankle arthrography. Radiol Clin North Am 19:255, 1981
19. Newton RA: Joint receptor contributions to reflexive and kinesthetic responses. Phys Ther 62:22, 1982
20. Dugan RC, et al: Fibular stress fractures in runners. J Fam Pract 17:415, 1983
21. Moss A, et al: Ultrasonic assessment of stress fractures. Br Med J 286:1479, 1983
22. Daffner RH, et al: Stress fractures in runners. JAMA 247:1039, 1982
23. Belin SC: Stress fractures in athletes. Orthop Clin North Am 11:735, 1980

SUGGESTED READINGS

Colson JC, Armour WJ: Sports Injuries and Their Treatment. Paul, London, 1975

Dolan JP: Treatment and Prevention of Athletic Injuries. Interstate, Danville, IL, 1967

Dominguez RH: The Complete Book of Sports Medicine. Scribner, New York, 1979

Kulund DN: The Injured Athlete. JB Lippincott, Philadelphia, 1982

Mack RP: AAOS Symposium on the Foot and Leg in Running Sports. CV Mosby, St. Louis, 1982

Nafpliotis H: Soccer Injuries. Vantage Press, New York, 1981

O'Donoghue DH: Treatment of Injuries to Athletes. WB Saunders, Philadelphia, 1962

Reynolds FC: AAOS Symposium on Sports Medicine. CV Mosby, St. Louis, 1962

Sheehan GC: An Encyclopedia of Athletic Medicine. Runner's World Magazine, Mountain View, CA, 1972

14

Foot Injuries

STEVEN I. SUBOTNICK

The foot is composed of 26 bones making up the forefoot, midfoot, and rearfoot. Athletic injuries of the foot are similarly classified by these three regions. The similarity of their functions lends itself readily to this classification. An excellent updated review of the literature of common injuries by Fredericson chronicles the literature from the early 1970s to the present,[1] and includes the knee, leg, Achilles, ankle, and foot.

THE FOREFOOT

The forefoot is the part of the foot distal to the metatarsal cuneiform–cuboid articulations. It includes the five long metatarsals and the associated phalanges of the toes. The metatarsal–cuneiform and metatarsophalangeal joints are of prime importance. Injuries may likewise occur to the interphalangeal joints. The ball of the foot takes considerable stress during sports, and frequent acute, as well as chronic, injuries occur in this area.[2-4]

The soft tissue of the foot consists of the thin dorsal skin as well as the thicker plantar skin. Plantar cutaneous lesions under metatarsal heads—keratomas—may be secondary to increased friction or shearing forces. Thick subcutaneous tissue under metatarsal heads helps decrease the shock transmitted to the bones of the forefoot. Proprioceptive nerve endings are present in the foot and aid the athlete in balance. Toenails are dermal appendages; they may be involved in a myriad of pathologic conditions or injuries.

Nail Pathology

Nails are horny curved structures or plates found on the anterior dorsal surfaces of the distal phalanges of the toes (Fig. 14-1). They function to protect the tender tips of the toes from abnormal pressure. Both macrotrauma and microtrauma may give rise to changes in the shape and appearance of nails. When a damaged nail plate is treated immediately and there is no damage to the nail bed or matrix, it is possible to have a normal nail continue to grow. When the nail bed or matrix has been damaged, when there is a long delay in the treatment of the macrotrauma, or when microtrauma is the cause of the abnormality, the new nail will usually be deformed.

SUBUNGUAL HEMATOMA

A subungual hematoma is a benign tumorlike mass containing effused blood. It is called "black toenails" or "runner's toe." Runners and athletes frequently develop bleeding under the toenails from chronic friction, from rubbing or bumping the nail against the end of an improperly fitting shoe, or from a direct blow to the dorsal aspect of the toe itself. Running downhill with the foot sliding forward in the shoe or hitting an object and stubbing the toe often causes a subungual hematoma. Considerable pain is usually associated with this problem due to the extreme sensitivity of the nail bed, and bleeding into a closed space; it is seldom confused with other pathology, such as subungual pigmented nevi. The acute problem occurs suddenly and is most often accompanied by severe pain. The chronic problem tends to become more painful toward the final stages.

In most cases, there is pressure in the space between the nail and the nail bed, and there is exquisite pain and tenderness upon palpation. The painful toenail turns partially or completely black or red, and the hallux throbs.

Treatment of the acute problem consists of decom-

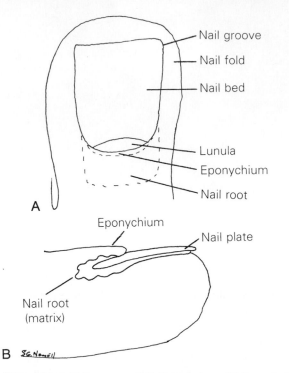

A

B SG.Newell

Figure 14–1 Nail anatomy. **(A)** Dorsal view. **(B)** Lateral view.

pressing the hematoma by using a paper clip heated in an alcohol burner. The clip is heated until it is red hot and used to burn a hole through the nail, decompressing the hematoma.

Chronic hemorrhage under a nail will cause the nail plate to loosen from the bed. A compressive dressing is necessary to prevent further bleeding and to maintain pressure on the nail bed to decrease the likelihood of deformity of the new nail that will form. Homeopathic remedies include *hypericum* 30c for pain, or *Arnica* 200c for hematoma (three pellets sublingually every 2 to 3 hours until better). Traumeel (Biological Homeopathic Industries, Inc., Albuquerque, NM), 10 drops sublingually every hour until better, is often very helpful.

A dystrophic nail may be the end result of a subungual hematoma. This is especially true when the pathology is secondary to chronic repetitive microtrauma. In these cases, the nails may be thick and unsightly. The thickness of the nail may cause chronic pain due to impingement on the dorsal aspect of the toebox of the shoe. At times, the thick, deformed nails grow into the distal aspect of the hallux soft tissue. Chronic ingrowing on the medial or lateral border may be secondary to dystrophic changes.

These nails may need constant care, such as mechanical grinding down and curettage of nail borders. If chronic pain persists and conservative treatment fails to yield a manageable nail, a total matricectomy may be necessary. For those patients desirous of preserving the toenail, avulsion of the nail and thinning of the matrix with a laser may give satisfactory cosmetic results. Partial matricectomies may be necessary for chronic ingrowing of the tibial or fibular nail border. Radiographs should be taken to rule out subungual exostosis, which may be the end result of chronic dorsal subungual pressure.[5]

Nail pathology may be avoided by using shoes that fit properly. An athletic shoe should be one size longer than a street shoe in most cases. Most street shoes are a size too small anyway! Feet get larger with age, or after childbirth, yet people persist in wearing the same size. Tight-fitting shoes that predispose to nail damage should be avoided. Protecting the nails with properly fitting socks is important. Wrinkled or tight socks can cause nail pathology.

SUBUNGUAL EXOSTOSIS

A subungual exostosis is hypertrophic bone at the dorsal distal aspect of the phalanx, usually of the great toe. It may begin as an osteochondroma, which is a bony growth of the cartilaginous cap. Excessive pressure causes reactive hypertrophic bone.

The subungual exostosis may cause chronic pain at the distal aspect of the hallux and may likewise cause the nail to grow deformed and excessively convex. The subungual exostosis itself should be differentiated from a hypertrophic dorsal distal tuft. The hypertrophic tuft is usually acquired in nature and involves a greater area of the dorsal distal aspect of the phalanx. Dystrophic nails may grow into the soft tissue just proximal to the tuft, causing considerable discomfort.

The diagnosis of subungual exostosis or hypertrophic tuft is made with a radiograph of the propped-up hallux. The dorsal slope of the distal phalanx itself should be appreciated in the radiograph, since it may be contributing to subungual pain and impingement.

Conservative treatment for subungual exostosis consists of decreasing the width of hypertrophic nails and using foot gear with a deep toebox. Chronic discomfort or pain, despite conservative therapy, is treated with an open excision of the subungual exostosis or of the hypertrophic dorsal distal tuft, or both. This minor surgical procedure is well worth the comfort it affords.

ONYCHOCRYPTOSIS

Onychocryptosis, or ingrown toenails, is a common malady of the hallux in the athlete. It may be secondary to abnormal pressure of the shoe over the tibial or fibular nail borders or secondary to improper cutting of the nail. The cryptosis is frequently accompanied by secondary pyogenic infection, or paronychia (Fig. 14-2). Strictly speaking, onychocryptosis should be differentiated from unguis incurvatum. Onychocryptosis is a condition whereby the nail is growing into the flesh, with a hook of nail embedded in the skin. Onychocryptosis without paronychia is treated conservatively by removing the portion of the nail that is offending the soft tissue. This may be done with a nail splitter; the nail border is then smoothed with a curette. If chronic deep involvement fails to respond to conservative therapy, local anesthesia may be necessary and a partial matricectomy may be the treatment of choice. Such treatments as wedging of the toenail distally or excising the spicula and applying a piece of cotton in the nail groove are conservative and may yield satisfactory results. When inflammation of the skin is present following removal of onychocryptosis, moist dressings with Epsom salt and water or Burow's solution are helpful. Antibiotics may be necessary if paronychia and lymphangitis are present.

Figure 14-2 Onychocryptosis of the fibular border of the hallux nail. Paronychia is present.

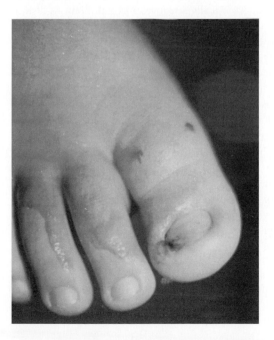

When the skin is dry, the application of a lubricant as the nail grows back ensures a smoother, more comfortable nail groove. Chronic onychocryptosis is treated by a partial matricectomy. I prefer a phenol procedure whereby the matrix under the offending portion of the nail, be it a tibial or fibular border, is eradicated with three applications of full-strength phenol for 90 seconds.[5] This procedure is easily carried out under local anesthesia on an outpatient basis, and there is very little postoperative discomfort or pain. Usually, athletic activities need not be interrupted.

ONYCHIA

Onychia is an infection of one or both sides of the nail and nail plate. This most commonly occurs on the hallux nail but may be present on lesser digital nails. Chronic pressure on the nail plate as well as allergy, nail polish, or certain soaps may lead to onychia. Suppurative onychia is usually caused by *Staphylococcus*. Occasionally, a mixed infection is present. Nonsuppurative onychia may be caused by *Candida albicans*. Trauma from improperly cutting the nails is the most frequent cause of onychia.[6] If the skin is nicked when the nail is cut, this becomes the basis for infection. If the matrix is not damaged, the prognosis is good for a healthy nail following appropriate treatment of the ingrown toenail. If the matrix is damaged, the nail plate becomes discolored, and it will become disturbed and cracked. Chronic onychodystrophy will be the end result. Recurrent onychia may lead to a hypertrophic nail plate. Paronychia is an infection of both sides, as well as the base, of the nail.

Onychia involving one border of the nail is treated by partial avulsion of the offending border. This is done under local anesthesia. At times, a partial wedge resection of the nail can be carried out without anesthesia. The patient is placed on supportive therapy for infection, such as Betadine (povidone-iodine) soaks with 1 tablespoon of Betadine per pan of lukewarm water, with soaks carried out for 15 minutes three times a day. Antibiotic topical therapy is given with triple antibiotic cream or Neosporin G. If there is significant cellulitis or lymphangitis, systemic antibiotics should be administered. A semisynthetic penicillin, such as dicloxacillin, 500 mg qid, will usually suffice. At times an oral cephalosporin is necessary. High-risk patients, such as diabetics prone to mixed infections, usually respond to ciprofloxacin 500 to 750 mg bid for 7 to 10 days.

Pyrogenium 30c is a homeopathic remedy that may be given 3 pellets tid to those patients who prefer not to take antibiotics if at all possible (e.g., nursing women). The remedies are safe and often as effective as antibiotics, once the offending nail border is removed. In these cases the temperature and local wound condition must be carefully monitored and, when indicated, antibiotics given. In most instances, simply removing the ingrown nail, which is acting as a foreign body, will permit rapid resolution of the infection without the aid of systemic antibiotics. A phenol partial matricectomy may be carried out, even when there is infection and inflammation. Phenol is bactericidal. Surgical partial matricectomy should be done once infection has been ablated, if preferred over the phenol technique.

ONYCHAUXIS

Onychauxis is an overgrowth of the nail that may be due to trauma, peripheral neuritis, old age, or decreased circulation. The nail may become thickened, long, and hard and grayish or yellow in discoloration. Secondary fungal infection with chronic onychomycosis may occur. Digital deformity or contractures may predispose to abnormal pressure on nails and onychauxis.

Women often complain of onychauxis secondary to tight-fitting sport shoes. These nails look unsightly in open-toed shoes. At times, they are associated with subungual exostosis or hypertrophic bone and discomfort and pain.

Treatment consists of electric debridement of the nails. Appropriate cleansing of the nails with an old toothbrush and soap and water is helpful. The use of shoes with wide toeboxes is encouraged to decrease repeated trauma to the nail bed.

ONYCHOMYCOSIS

Chronic fungal conditions of the nail (onychomycosis) are treated with regular debridement and topical applications of antifungal medication and a salicylic–lactic acid preparation. Fifteen percent salicylic acid with 15 percent lactic acid in a flexible collodion base softens the nail and allows for penetration of a topical antifungal agent. Lamasil Cream 1% (Sandoz) (terbinafine HCl) is combined with the acid solution to effect appropriate topical antifungal therapy. Although systemic antifungal preparations, such as griseofulvin and ketoconazole, may be used, I prefer not. This, to me, appears to be a case of "treatment worse than the disease." I have found that it takes 3 to 6 months of griseofulvin preparations to eradicate chronic fungal infections. Liver function must be monitored and, as soon as the systemic antifungals are discontinued, the onychomycosis returns. In the meantime the antifungals often cause bowel flora disruption leading to dysbiosis and the *leaky gut syndrome.*

Vigorous treatment of the nails and nail beds, as well as topical antifungal medications, may bring about a cure. I have had success with electric grinding followed by laser perforation of the remaining nail plate with numerous laser holes. This is done with the CO_2 laser at a setting of 5 to 6 watts, pulse width 25, and literally hundreds of very small holes are scored upon the nail plate. Local anesthesia is unnecessary. The perforations allow for the penetration of topical antifungals such as Mycocide NS (benzalkonium chloride; Woodward Labs) nail solution or Fungoid Tincture (miconazole nitrate 2 percent). The holes are kept open by having the patient scrub the nail plate with a toothbrush. It may be necessary to repeat the laser partial nail ablation every 2 months until the plate is clear. At the same time the patient is detoxified and drained and bowel flora are rebalanced with natural measures. This method has given good overall results, and, should small areas of recurrence be present in the months to come, they are easily eradicated painlessly with relasing.

I have also had success with complete removal of a fungal nail followed by treatment of the hypertrophic nail bed with laser thinning and sterilization. The remaining nail bed is then treated with Lamasil.

There is, however, at least 20 percent recurrence of onychomycosis with any therapy other than total nail avulsion and matricectomy. Following this, once healing has taken place, the nail is composed of firm cornified epithelium that is cosmetically adequate and is difficult to distinguish from a healthy nail, once nail polish is applied. The high rate of recurrence exists because the real problem with onychomycosis is in the *ecology* of the foot and nail itself. The circumstances are right for the fungus to invade and live off the dead keratin. To really cure onychomycosis, complex homeopathic (homotoxicologic) drainage and detoxification, followed by a constitutional homeopathic remedy, is necessary. This changes the *biological terrain* so the fungus no longer finds the environment conducive to colonization. The cause has been eliminated rather than just the symptom. Simply using enteric antifungals is like using chlorine to sterilize water contaminated by raw sewage, rather than stopping the contamination. It is a matter of ecology and getting to the cause.

SUBUNGUAL AND PERIUNGUAL CLAVUS

A subungual or periungual clavus is a corn located under the nail or in the nail groove, respectively. Because any sort of pressure may cause keratotic tissue to become a clavus, such a lesion may be found on almost any part of the body. A subungual or periungual clavus may be caused by inverted or thickened nails or merely by pressure due to shortness, narrowness, or shallowness of the toebox of the shoe. On the smaller toes, these clavi usually develop under the immediate free edge of the nail. On the fifth toe, they occur most often at the lateral dorsal aspect of the toe secondary to pressure from the shoe. The dorsolateral fifth toe clavi often overlie a hypertrophic osteophyte arising from the lateral base of the distal phalanx. The toes are usually rotated into valgus, predisposing to excessive lateral pressure. The clavi may grow to such a size as to elevate the nail, resembling a subungual exostosis. The pain is usually constant. The clavus is usually visible through the nail. Pressure from a bed sheet is enough to cause pain. Palliative treatment consists of debridement of the clavus. Surgical wedge resection may be necessary, along with removal of underlying hypertrophic bone. With significant toe malalignment or rotation, correctional realignment or derotational arthroplastic correction is indicated.

Toes

Toes are important for balance, proprioception, and propulsion. They are traumatized by shoes and stubbing; they are involved in cleat injuries and can be strained, sprained, or fractured. The skin of the toes may be afflicted with blisters, bursae, or corns and calluses (Fig. 14-3). Trauma to toes may result in tendinitis, neuritis, or synovitis. Occasionally dislocations occur, after stubbing toes. Treatment is symptomatic and may include anti-inflammatory drugs, splinting, padding, or surgical correction for painful fixed deformities, hammertoes, trigger toes, or mallet toes.

BLISTERS

Blisters occur secondary to friction and shearing. Lysis occurs between layers of the skin. A narrow toebox may cause blisters at the medial aspect of the hallux and fifth toe. A shallow toebox may cause blisters on the dorsal aspect of the toes. Loose-fitting shoes may result in blisters of the distal plantar aspect of the toes as they grasp the shoe to decrease excessive motion. Obviously, a properly fitting shoe is crucial in preventing blisters. Friction-decreasing insoles, such as Spenco, PPT, or Viscolas, are very helpful. When blisters are caused by excessive motion, such as pronation or supination, an orthosis is usually helpful. A common example is with blisters under a plantar-

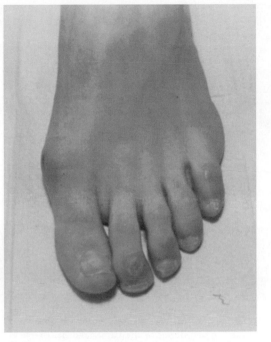

Figure 14-3 Claw toe of the second digit with associated lesion.

flexed first metatarsal. An orthotic with a long compressive extrinsic post to bring the heel to perpendicular while accommodating the first metatarsal head will remedy the blister problem. Blisters may be associated with or complicated by hyperhidrosis. Foot powders to dry the skin and foot soaking in astringents, such as one-half cup of vinegar per pan of water, can help. Simply spraying the foot with deodorant may solve the problem. Socks knit of a combination of natural and synthetic fibers are of primary importance. These socks will pad the toes and wick fluid away from the feet. When selecting shoes, it is a good idea to allow for the width of the thumb at the end of the longest toe in the end of the shoe. Feet get larger with age, and athletic shoes are often a size larger than street shoes!

Acute blisters may be treated by decompression through a puncture hole followed by the application of an antibiotic topical preparation and then compressive dressings. The skin may be left intact and will act as a biologic graft. The feet should be kept clean and may be soaked with appropriate antibacterial solutions, such as Hibiclens or Betadine and water. The toes may then be taped with one-quarter-inch adhesive tape prior to runs to decrease friction on the toes. Tube foam or gel pads are often helpful. Chronic problems may be treated with moleskin applied over tincture of benzoin placed on the area in which blis-

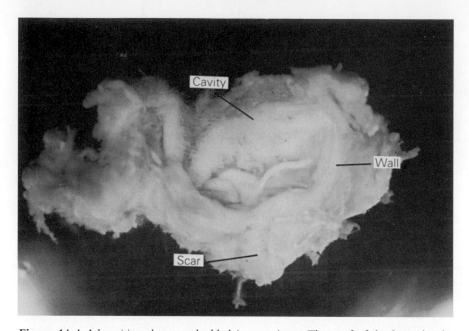

Figure 14-4 Adventitious bursa embedded in scar tissue. The roof of the bursa has been removed, and the folded lining of the cavity and hairlike projections into the lumen can be seen.

ters occur. As a general rule, dry skin may be lubricated with 10 percent urea cream, aloe vera gel or lotion, calendula oil, or other skin preparations; moist skin should be dried with foot powder and appropriate soaks.

BURSAE

A bursa is a blister deep in the body (Fig. 14-4). Bursae in toes occur underneath clavi, between the clavi and the underlying bony protuberances. A clavus is a corn that occurs over a bony pressure point on a toe. Simple paring of the clavus will usually release the pressure on significant bursitis, an intrabursal injection of a small amount of a long- and slow-acting corticosteroid preparation and local anesthetic may be indicated. In those patients preferring no cortisone, injection with Traumeel or *Ruta graveolens* gives excellent results. These remedies are also effective orally. Persistent clavi and bursae usually indicate a hammertoe condition or exostosis that may require minor surgical correction. In most instances, conservative therapy with accommodative felt or moleskin padding will suffice.

CLAVI

Clavi are areas of thickened skin overlying bony prominences in toes. A soft corn is called a heloma molle. A hard corn is a heloma durum (Fig. 14-5). Soft corns occur

Figure 14-5 Heloma durum secondary to hammertoe of the fifth digit.

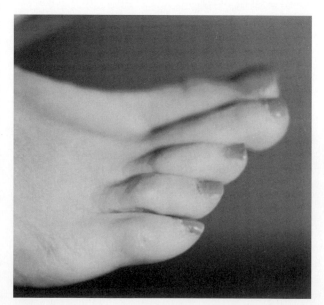

most commonly between the fourth and fifth toes and are caused by pressure between the head of the proximal phalanx of the fifth toe and the base of the proximal phalanx of the fourth toe in the fourth interspace. Maceration may occur, and a secondary sinus tract or infection may be the end result. These soft corns are secondary to pressure from tight toeboxes of shoes. They are quite common in women who wear high-heeled shoes. They may occur in athletes wearing bike shoes or various forms of boots.

Conservative treatment involves debriding the clavus and using padding between the fourth and fifth toes. When extreme pain is present, I prefer to inject a local anesthetic and cortisone or Traumeel into the interspace under the adjacent soft corns. Then deep debridement with tissue nippers is possible. Foam rubber pads or cotton is placed between the toes. Wider foot gear is usually mandatory. The injection, deep debridement, padding, and foot gear change often take care of the problem, although regular preventative debridement is usually required. Chronic persistent soft corns that do not respond to conservative therapy will respond to minor surgical procedures to excise the hypertrophic bone or correct a hammertoe deformity. Deep-seated chronic soft corns in the fifth interspace respond well to hammertoe correction along with syndactylism of the fourth to fifth toes. This is easily accomplished under local anesthesia.

With rotated hammertoe fifth toe deformity, the head of the proximal phalanx of the fifth toe may be excised and a derotational arthroplasty carried out to remedy a clavus at the dorsolateral aspect of the proximal interphalangeal joint with a coexistent soft corn in the fourth interspace. If there is a soft corn deformity only, partial ostectomy may suffice if overall toe deformity is not severe.

Soft corns may occur between any toes and commonly are found between the second and third toes or the hallux and second toe. Appropriate sponge rubber padding or felt padding is the treatment of choice, following paring down of the lesions. Occasionally, partial ostectomy is indicated for chronic persistent problems.

Hard corns (heloma durum) are most common at the dorsal aspect of toes or at the dorsolateral aspect of the fifth toe. They are accompanied by hammertoe contracture of the toes and are secondary to impingement of soft tissue between the bone and shoe (Fig. 14-5). Conservative treatment consists of paring down of the hypertrophic tissue and injecting the inflamed subclaval bursa with corticosteroid and local anesthetic preparations, or local anesthetic, Wydase (hyaluronidase), and Traumeel. Appropriate accommodative padding with one-eighth-inch

adherent felt is quite helpful. Persistent annoying problems that fail to respond to conservative therapy may be treated with partial ostectomy, arthroplasty, or arthrodesis of the involved toes.

TINEA PEDIS

Tinea pedis may occur in the interspaces of toes or on the tissue of the toes themselves. The moist interspaces of the toes may be infected with *Candida albicans*. The drier tissue of the toes may be infected with dermatophytes. Mixed yeast and dermatophyte infections may occur in the interspaces. Acute or chronic tinea pedis should be treated with appropriate local therapy using soaks with one-half cup of vinegar per pan of water, three times a day. Following this, a topical antifungal preparation, such as Lamasil, may be used. Antifungal powder should be placed in socks and shoes. Shoes and socks should be changed regularly. Dilute vinegar and water soaks or compresses are helpful. As with onychomycosis, homeopathic detoxification and drainage along with appropriate specific remedies for the skin are preferred over oral antifungals due to their untoward effects, including liver toxicity, bowel dysbiosis, and the usual recurrence of symptoms and lesions once the medications are stopped. Tinea pedis is an internal problem associated with a change in the body *ecology* favoring fungal invasion. The ecology must therefore be changed.

TENDINITIS

Tendinitis is an inflammation of a tendon. The flexor tendons in the toes may be strained or sprained secondary to stubbing of the toes or hyperextension injuries. Chronic overuse injury in the plantar surfaces of the toes may predispose to flexor tendinitis.

The tendons on the plantar aspect of the toes are palpated as the toes are taken through a range of motion, both actively and passively. If there is pain upon utilization of the tendons, one may presume that tendinitis is present.

Treatment consists of resting the toes and using anti-inflammatory physical therapy modalities, such as ultrasound, interferential stimulation, or electrogalvanic therapy. The involved toe may be splinted to an adjacent uninvolved toe with one-quarter-inch tape, Coban, or Elastikon. Biomechanical factors, such as clawing of the toes secondary to intrinsic muscle weakness and instability with a hyperpronated foot, should be corrected with a biodynamic neutral orthosis. A crest pad may be helpful in decreasing the load on the flexor tendons to the toes.

The extensor tendons of the toes may become inflamed secondary to tight, ill-fitting shoes. They respond to local anti-inflammatory therapy, such as cool soaks or various physical therapy modalities, interferential stimulation being one of the most versatile and effective. Appropriate adjustment of foot gear is essential.

TOE SPRAINS AND TURF TOE

Toe sprains may result from the stubbing of a foot. Toes could be traumatized when the athlete steps in a hole or bangs the toes on a hard running surface. Sprains of the first metatarsophalangeal joint can be quite debilitating. They may occur secondary to a fall, abnormal biomechanics, or running form.

Turf toe, a sprain of the interphalangeal joint of the great toe in the direction of hyperextension, may be secondary to running on artificial turf. This injury can be quite debilitating if plantar capsular tissue is torn. Treatment consists of splinting, physical therapy, anti-inflammatory medications, a firm-soled shoe limiting motion of the great toe for 6 weeks, and trigger point injection therapy, in later stages, if adhesions persist.

Athletes with sprained toes complain of pain and swelling at the metatarsophalangeal or interphalangeal joints. There is pain with motion, and effusion may be present in the joint. Capsulitis, synovitis, or both will be apparent.

Nonspecific capsulitis of the second metatarsophalangeal joint may occur insidiously, or after an identifiable traumatic hyperextension injury. The plantar capsule is stretched or ruptured and may progress to hyperextension of the second toe with chronic instability. A claw toe can develop with associated plantar flexion of the second metatarsal head. This, in turn, causes metatarsalgia under the second metatarsal head. Early recognition and splinting, as well as the precautions outlined for turf toe, may prevent the otherwise predictable degenerative changes and deformity. Otherwise, with progressive deformity, surgery is required to stabilize the second toe and plantar second metatarsophalangeal joint capsule. With chronic instability and claw toe formation, the joints are usually subluxed with subsequent arthritic changes. Surgery, in these cases, consists of resection of either the base of the proximal phalanx or the head of the metatarsal. If arthritis is minimal, an osteotomy of the second metatarsal, with surgical correction of the second toe, may suffice.

NEURITIS

The digits of the feet may be painful secondary to irritation of a nerve. Friction or traction neuritis may be present. At times, there may be a digital neuroma (Figs. 14-6 and 14-7). An example of this is *Joplin's neuroma* at the medial aspect of the hallux plantarly. This is an inflammation of the medial plantar nerve to the great toe secondary to abnormal pressure, which may be due to excessive pronation during toe-off. The diagnosis is made by palpation of the area at the junction of the thin and thick skin near the first metatarsophalangeal joint and proximal and distal to this. A clicking mass may be felt, associated with pain radiating distally to the medial plantar aspect of the hallux, and may be confused with tibial sesamoiditis. Injection along the nerve with a small amount of local anesthetic and long- and slow-acting cortisone will decrease the inflammation

Figure 14-6 Traumatic neuroma, stained to enhance features. The nerve is paler than scar tissue and can be traced across the specimen. Nodular mass of scar below the nerve, containing several bursa clefts, stands out clearly.

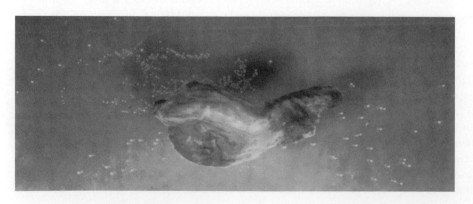

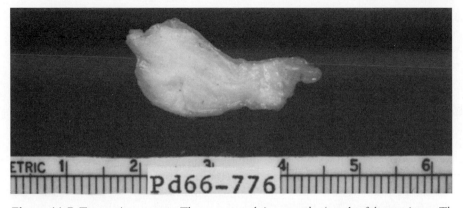

Figure 14-7 Traumatic neuroma. The nerve trunk is seen at both ends of the specimen. The course of the nerve along the upper portion of the scar tissue mass is faintly visible. The greater bulk of scar tissue below the nerve contains a vertical cleft, representing adventitious bursa. (Courtesy of John McNeal.)

and, along with treating the problem, help establish the diagnosis. Corrective orthotics with accommodation usually allow the traumatic neuroma to heal. Surgery may be required for resistent Joplin's neuromas. When resecting the nerve, the free distal end must be transferred under the abductor hallucis muscle belly to guard against postoperative amputation neuromas, which are otherwise, unfortunately, not uncommon following surgery of peripheral nerves. Quite commonly, the nerve is associated with an inflamed bursa that goes under one or both of the sesamoids and may be misdiagnosed as sesamoiditis.

The fifth toe may have an entrapment neuropathy of a superficial nerve secondary to pressure from the shoe at the dorsolateral aspect. This is treated by appropriate change in foot gear and local anti-inflammatory physical therapy modalities. Occasionally, injection therapy is indicated. I have also seen digital neuromas at the plantar medial branch of the fifth toe secondary to varus rotation deformity and abnormal nerve pressure. Any toe may have an isolated digital neuroma; in fact, at the time of hammertoe surgery, it is common to see a digital neuoma under the ellipsed hypertrophic corn (heloma durum).

HAMMERTOES

Hammertoes or claw toes (see Fig. 14-3) are contractures. There may be contractures of the toes themselves at the interphalangeal joints or contractures involving the metatarsophalangeal and interphalangeal joints (Fig. 14-8). Severity ranges from hammertoe to mallet toe to claw toe. A *hammertoe* is usually defined as a contracture at the proxi-

mal interphalangeal joint plantarly with a mild dorsal contracture at the metatarsophalangeal joint. A *mallet toe* is a plantar contracture at the distal interphalangeal joint, and a *claw toe* is an advanced contracture dorsally at the metatarsophalangeal joint and a plantar contracture at the proximal

Figure 14-8 Hallux valgus, with an overriding second toe, with hammertoe of the fifth digit and ingrown tibial border of the hallux.

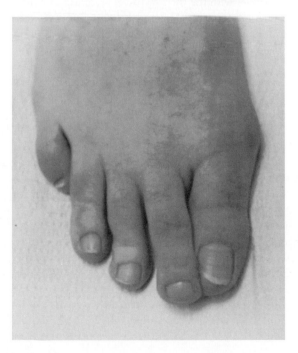

interphalangeal and distal interphalangeal joints. When digital deformities exist, unless present from birth, they usually develop from intrinsic muscle fatigue and overpowering by the long extrinsic muscles, the flexors and extensors. The intrinsic foot muscles stabilize the toes at the metatarsophalangeal joints as well as the proximal interphalangeal joints. They become fatigued, and finally atrophic, secondary to chronic pronation. They also become overpowered with cavus feet or the dropped forefoot (anterior equinus). Hammertoes may also develop from high-heeled shoes, which by their nature cause shortening of the flexors and elongation of the extensors, resulting in secondary hammertoe and finally claw toe deformity. As the toes contract, they pull the plantar fat pads distally from their anatomic functional position under the metatarsal heads. Calluses and deep-seated keratomas develop as the metatarsal heads are driven plantarly by the retrograde digital force. With time, flexible deformity becomes semireducible, and finally fixed and ankylosed in position. Pointed-toe shoes cause obvious digital deformity. I will often trace patients' feet on paper while they are standing and then place their dress shoes on the foot tracings; most often the foot is far larger than the shoe! To further illustrate, I radiograph the foot while in the dress shoe.

The solution to hammertoe is foot orthotics to re-establish biomechanically stable lever systems, sensible shoes, and intrinsic muscle strengthening exercises, such as picking up marbles with the toes, or towel toe grasp exercises. Tight extrinsic foot muscles must be stretched and weak muscles strengthened to overcome dynamic imbalance. Finally, I encourage fashion-conscious patients to wear sensible shoes whenever possible, while carrying their dress shoes and wearing them only when indicated by social circumstances. Fixed contractures of toes require surgical correction.

A claw toe usually has a distal plantar lesion or clavus secondary to abnormal pressure at the distal pulp of the toe, and a painful callus over the proximal interphalangeal joints dorsally (Fig. 14-3). Often there is an associated plantar keratoma under the metatarsal head, plantar flexed secondary to retrograde pressure from the claw toe.

The mallet toe has a distal lesion at the tip of the toe due to abnormal pressure, and there is usually an associated dorsal lesion at the distal interphalangeal joint. The hammertoe has a lesion over the proximal interphalangeal joint. The most common hammertoe is perhaps the hammertoe fifth toe, with a callus at the dorsolateral aspect of the toe.

Hammertoes are treated conservatively by paring and debridement of keratomas and by the use of crest pads, as well as accommodative dressings with moleskin or tape. Recalcitrant hammertoes are treated surgically. Hard and soft corns between toes without severe contracture are treated with partial ostectomy. Contracted toes are treated with arthroplasties or arthrodesis of the proximal interphalangeal joints for hammertoes and the distal interphalangeal joints for mallet toes. Thomas Sgarlato (Sgarlato Labs, San Jose, California, personal communication) reports good results using Silastic digital implants to maintain flexibility while providing stability with hammertoe contracture. Hammertoe second toe, with associated hallux valgus, is often best treated with arthrodesis to stabilize against the hallux. Contracted metatarsophalangeal joints must be released to reposition the plantar fat pad and balance the dorsal toe extensor hood apparatus.

Claw toes are treated with release of the metatarsophalangeal and interphalangeal joints and arthrodesis of the interphalangeal joints. Hammertoe second toe or claw toe second toe often needs an arthrodesis at unstable joints. Flexible clawing of toes may be treated effectively with flexor tendon transfers, which often also release painful keratomas under plantar-flexed metatarsal heads. Long-standing fixed deformity requires bony resection and arthrodesis stabilization for lasting results. These procedures are generally well tolerated by athletes. Short-term symptomatic relief during the competitive season can be achieved with sublesional cortisone [Celestone (betamethasone)] or homeopathic (Traumeel) injections, padding, and strapping. Anterior heel or rocker-bottom bars can be placed on running, tennis, or everyday shoes to relieve metatarsal pain associated with digital contractures. Athletic shoes can be modified by placing elastic material over painful toes in the shoe toebox, or simply making longitudinal slits through the shoe toebox to take pressure off of painful contracted toes. It often is easier to operate on the shoes than the patient!

The digital bones of athletes may be symptomatic secondary to exostoses. Exostoses form secondary to abnormal pressure on the bone, which responds with reactive hyperostosis. These painful bumps respond to padding, moleskin, or gels. When exostoses are chronic and painful, simple exostectomy is well tolerated with good results.

DIGITAL FRACTURES

Toe fractures in athletes occur secondary to running barefooted, stepping on rocks or in potholes, or trauma from spikes or the foot gear of other athletes. Most commonly, the fifth toe is broken while walking barefooted, catching against some object and bending sideways.

Broken toes usually cause severe pain and swelling. There may also be bleeding into the soft tissue and a crunching sensation. Athletes are most often aware of the trauma that led to the fracture. Radiographs will confirm the diagnosis.

Fractures of lesser toes most often will respond to splinting of the injured toe to adjacent uninjured toes. The homeopathic remedy *Symphytum caucasicum* (bone knit) often speeds up the healing of these fractures. *Arnica* or *Ruta graveolens* reduces pain and swelling. Fractures of the hallux may be more serious. Intra-articular fractures of the interphalangeal joint of the great toe are most often treated conservatively. At times, internal fixation is indicated to prevent postinjury arthritis. Intra-articular fractures may result in permanent disability and necessitate excision of nonunion or malunion of fragments within the joint. Fusion or an implant may be necessary. The usual treatment of choice, however, is arthroplastic procedures and early range-of-motion exercises.

Fractures of the first metatarsophalangeal joint may be quite serious when intra-articular. They can lead to permanent disability and arthritis and may necessitate secondary surgical procedures. Whereas the athlete can resume participation in competition with a fracture of a lesser toe, a fracture of the hallux or first metatarsophalangeal joint may necessitate immobilization and rest.

Soft Tissue of the Forefoot

PLANTAR KERATOMAS

Plantar keratomas range from friction calluses, which are a mere annoyance, to intractable plantar keratomas, which are debilitating. Shearing or friction superficial keratomas usually still have the skin lines running through them. Intractable plantar keratomas are discrete, well-circumscribed keratotic lesions. The skin lines cease at their margins. They may be keratotic and involved with vascular or nerve lesions at their base, and are usually caused by excessive impingement of the soft tissue between the metatarsal plantar condyles and the opposing surfaces, such as the shoe.[7–9] Long metatarsals and plantar-flexed metatarsals predispose to keratomas. Abnormal biomechanics with excessive pronation and motion predispose to friction calluses or superficial keratomas. The severe nucleated intractable keratoma has a fibrotic scarred base, which may cause extreme symptoms (Fig. 14-9).

Treatment consists of sublesion local anesthesia, Wydase and a steroid or Traumeel, and deep debridement. In the

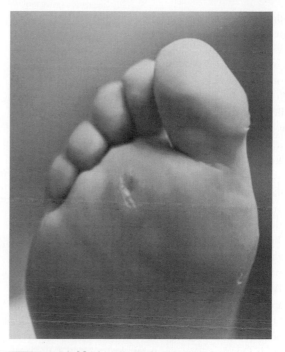

Figure 14-9 Nucleated plantar keratoma.

less intractable lesion, simple paring will suffice. Accommodative felt or sponge padding; Poron, Spenco, Sorbothane, or Viscolas intersoles; accommodative orthoses; and shoe modification (metatarsal bars) are all very helpful. Surgery consists of correction of digital fixed deformity, often with dorsal displacement osteotomy of the plantar-flexed metatarsal. Rheumatoid patients do surprisingly well with panmetatarsal head resection and manipulation of toes under anesthesia, followed by Kirschner wire stabilization for 4 to 6 weeks to allow for functional position reankylosis.

VERRUCA

Verruca is a viral lesion secondary to papillomavirus. A benign verrucous tumor on the plantar aspect of the foot causes considerable pain when underneath bony prominences or weight-bearing surfaces. Verrucae are treated conservatively by debridement and chemocautery with a combination of 15 percent lactic acid and 15 percent salicylic acid in a flexible collodion base. This preparation is available commercially under the brand name of Duofilm (Schering-Plough, Memphis, TN). Patients are given a bottle of Duofilm to be applied every evening to the verruca. It is helpful if the Duofilm is jabbed into the verruca. This may be associated with some discomfort. The goal of chemocautery is to form a mild sterile abscess, which then permits sloughing of the verrucous lesion. Stronger acids will more readily facilitate the sterile abscess but cause more pain and disability when eradicating the verruca; therefore, the weaker acid solution is preferred, even though it takes longer to treat the lesion. The homeopathic remedies *Thuja* and *antimonium crudum* are often suprisingly effective in eliminating warty lesions. Topical *Thuja* may be applied bid, and is supplemented with *Thuja* oral pellets 12c taken bid.

Excision of verrucae on the plantar aspect of the foot may lead to painful scarring and should be reserved for only recalcitrant problems.[10] I prefer laser surgery for verrucae due to its precise nature and decreased likelihood of painful postoperative scars. Laser ablation of verrucae may lead to rapid resolution of the problem, but one must take care not to pierce the dermal layer, which will lead to scar tissue. Verrucae are also found on the toes or periungually; these are treated in a manner similar to that described for the plantar aspect of the foot. For digital verrucae, the homeopathic remedy nitric acid 12c bid is often effective, along with Duofilm chemocautery or by itself. Repeated trauma to the plantar aspect may predispose to recurrent verruca; therefore, appropriate biomechanics and accommodations are necessary.

TYLOMAS

A tyloma is a thick callus at the plantar aspect of the foot that usually occurs at the medial plantar aspect of the great toe. In this case it is termed a *pinch callus*. It may occur at the interphalangeal or metatarsophalangeal joint and is secondary to abnormal propulsive sequences and weight bearing. Excessive propulsion will lead to shearing and friction and secondary hyperkeratotic tissue formation. Hallux limitus (decreased dorsal range of motion in the first metatarsophalangeal joint) leads to hyperextension of the distal interphalangeal joint; often there will be a plantar tyloma. A tyloma may likewise be present over the lateral aspect of the foot near the fifth metatarsophalangeal joint, secondary to abnormal shoe pressure or propulsive sequences. Treatment consists of debridement of hyperkeratotic tissue, protective padding, shoe modification, and rebalancing of the foot with an orthosis, including appropriate accommodations. Occasionally, there may be an instance in which a plantar tyloma under the medial aspect of the hallux is associated with hypertrophic bone; when this occurs, partial ostectomy is indicated. Central hallux tylomas are associated with bony or cartilagenous

interphalangeal sesamoids in the hallux interphalangeal joint. They may require excision.

MORTON'S NEUROMA

Interdigital (Morton's) neuroma is common in the second or third interspace of athletes. In my experience, it is equally prevalent in the second and third interspaces. It is less common in the first interspace and is rarely, although occasionally, found in the fourth interspace. A neuroma is a benign neoplasm of the nerve secondary to abnormal pressure. The nerve is squeezed between the transverse metatarsal ligament and adjacent bone. The athlete will complain of pain in tight shoes that compress the metatarsal heads and put pressure on the nerve. Some athletes state that it feels like the sock is wadded up in the shoe, causing them to take the shoe off and rub the foot so that the burning, numbing pain will go away. A denervation supersensitivity with pain and numbness result as the nerve loses its normal blood supply from abnormal pressure.

Upon physical examination, the examining physician should apply a lubricant to the plantar aspect of the foot to facilitate palpation. The fingers are moved from interspace to interspace. A clicking mass will be felt in the symptomatic interspace consistent with a plantar mass. This is the Morton's neuroma (Fig. 14-10). The neuroma may be manually impinged on adjacent bone to confirm the diagnosis. Pain will be elicited with palpation. Plantar digital nerves are palpated in a similar manner to rule out digital neuromas. A cotton applicator stick may be used to evaluate digital nerves.

More than one neuroma may be present; for example, there may be pain and pathology in the second and third interspaces. Neuromas may be associated with bursitis, tendinitis, or both; therefore, interspace pain is not always a neuroma. The treatment, however, is the same. Conservative treatment consists of injection therapy using a combination of a small amount of a long- and slow-acting corticosteroid (Celestone), Wydase, vitamin B_{12}, and local anesthetic. I use 4 mg prednisolone acetate and 4 mg dexamethasone phosphate with 1 ml of 1 percent Xylocaine (lidocaine) plain, 1 ml of 0.5 percent Marcaine (bupivacaine) plain, 0.5 ml Wydase, and 0.5 ml vitamin B_{12}. This is injected through a 27- or 30-gauge needle from dorsal to plantar, and the needle is moved back and forth to effect a local neurolysis between the transverse metatarsal ligament and the neuroma. More recently, I have begun injecting into the interspace, between spread toes, aiming for the space between the nerve and the transverse metatarsal

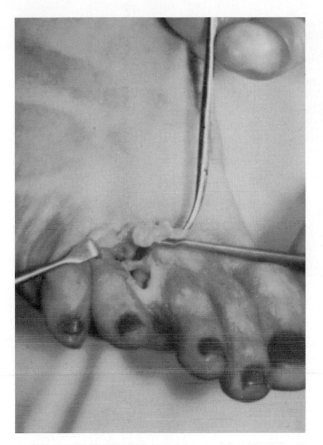

Figure 14-10 Morton's neuroma.

homeopathic injection cocktails. In the 30 percent of cases that have recurrent neuromas or are recalcitrant to injection therapy, excision under local anesthesia is carried out. This is an outpatient procedure.

There may be as high as 7 percent recurrence of neuromas, even with the most careful surgical procedures, using loupe magnification and proximal resection under the metatarsal neck. The athlete should be informed that there is a 7 percent recurrence rate and that there may be permanent loss of sensation on the plantar aspect of the foot in regard to the adjacent aspects of the toes. I have found that, in most cases, regrowth of superficial nerves may be expected in 8 to 12 months, and sensation likewise recurs. The athlete must be warned that there could be a stump neuroma, which would present a particular problem. Fibrosis in the interspaces is bothersome to some athletes. Despite these objections, neuroma surgery usually has a high degree of success. More recently, I have performed neurolysis with transection of the transverse metatarsal ligament when the nerve appears more compressed than involved with neuromatous changes. These procedures are done endoscopically by some, but statistics are not yet available for adequate evaluation of long-term results. At this time I prefer visualizing all structures with open surgical technique and loupe magnification.

Joints of the Forefoot

PATHOLOGY OF THE FIRST METATARSOPHALANGEAL JOINT

The most common pathology of the first metatarsophalangeal joint is hallux valgus. Conditions may range from hallux limitus to hallux rigidus. Hallus valgus is the lateral deviation of the hallux and medial deviation of the first metatarsal. Hallux valgus is often accompanied by an axial rotation of the great toe as it goes into valgus. Mechanical instability of the forefoot predisposes to hallux valgus and bunion formation. The long flexors, which previously stabilized the first metatarsophalangeal joint, become deforming factors when there is excessive pronation and splaying of the first metatarsal. The first metatarsal moves medially, and the sesamoids are relatively subluxed in a lateral displacement. As the sesamoids sublux, they erode the plantar aspect of the first metatarsal head and the crista; chondromalacia of the sesamoids may be the end result. This causes considerable plantar pain, which hinders the athlete's performance, and eventually leads to chronic irreversible arthritis. With sesamoid glide dysfunction, de-

ligament. A fluid neurolysis is the desired result. In selected patients, I inject a mixture of 1 ml Traumeel or *Hypericum* (instead of the cortisone mixture) along with the remainder of my injection "cocktail." Three to five of the cortisone cocktail mixtures are given at weekly or 2-week intervals. At least three injections must be given to prevent recurrence. The homeopathic cocktail may be given weekly for 6 to 8 weeks, or longer if results are favorable, without ill effect. Cortisone repeat injections may lead to unwanted fat and soft tissue necrosis. A thinning of the plantar fat pad from excessive use of cortisone is to be avoided.

Following the injection, ultrasound is used to enhance the effectiveness of the injection; gentle massage and mobilization of the metatarsal heads are then carried out. A soft temporary orthotic is made for the athlete, and a metatarsal pad is used to elevate depressed metatarsal heads and to spread the heads where neuromas are present. Wide appropriate foot gear is recommended. The success rate with this treatment is 70 percent with both the cortisone and

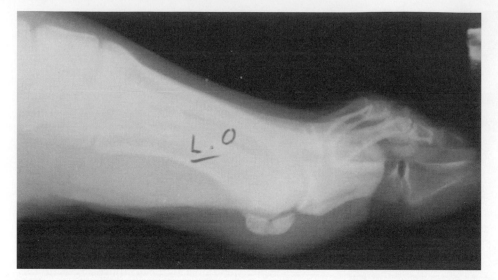

Figure 14-11 Fractured tibial sesamoid.

creased hallus dorsiflexion is the end result, with additional strain on joints proximal and distal to the first metatarsophalangeal joint. Faulty biomechanics, or a congenitally long first metatarsal, may lead to limited dorsiflexion of the first metatarsophalangeal joint (hallux limitus). Intraarticular pathology, arthritis, or fracture may lead to hallux rigidus. A long first metatarsal appears to be associated with more incidents of hallux limitus and hallux rigidus.[11,12] A hypermobile first metatarsal in the pronated foot is associated with a higher frequency of hallux abductovalgus with bunion formation.

Certain sports predispose to pathology of the first metatarsophalangeal joint. Ballet, when done on point, often leads to dorsal bunion, hallux valgus with dorsomedial bunion, or hallux limitus. With improper dismount, gymnastics can cause injury to the first metatarsophalangeal joint. Running, jumping, or hurdling may injure the sesamoid–first metatarsal articulation with stress fractures or complete fractures (Fig. 14-11). Abnormal pressure from tight ice skating or ski boots may cause bunions. These problems are treated conservatively with orthotics and physical therapy; surgical intervention may be required to increase range of motion. Osteotomies to realign abnormal bony relationships are usually the treatment of choice. Abrasion arthroplasties may be useful for mild to moderate intra-articular pathology, and, when followed by early range-of-motion exercises, often allow for the formation of functional fibrocartilage with subsequent functional range of motion and joint salvage.[13–17] Implants are used

only for those joints that are unsalvageable. Newer articulating metal–plastic composite implant devices may have advantages over the previously used Silastic hinged devices.

For mild to moderate cartilage degeneration I prefer first doing an abrasion arthroplasty with an angular decompression osteotomy of either the first metatarsal head, the proximal phalangeal base, or both. For moderate to advanced degeneration an implant or fusion is required. When arthroplastic salvage procedures fail, an implant or fusion can always be used. Fusions, of course, are more stable and eliminate the long-term eventual implant failure and need for revision. This must be weighed against the advantages of range of motion during athletic competitive years.

PATHOLOGY OF THE LESSER METATARSOPHALANGEAL JOINTS

There may be strains or sprains of the lesser metatarsophalangeal joints. There may also be intra-articular pathology, such as Freiberg's infraction. Freiberg's infraction is an overuse injury of the cartilage of the metatarsal head, which occurs secondary to chronic repetitive stress. It often occurs in a long central metatarsal that mechanically has increased prolonged propulsive stresses during running or jumping. Conservative treatment consists of rest and biodynamic orthoses, following which the metatarsal head may adequately remodel. If not, an abrasion arthroplasty or arthrotomy with or without metatarsal osteotomy may be necessary.

Another problem consists of post-traumatic sprains of

the metatarsophalangeal joints with volar plate disruption. These usually respond to rest, tape splinting in a plantar-flexed position for 6 weeks, a firm-soled shoe to prevent flexion of the toes at propulsion, and physical therapy. With repeated sprains or instability, surgical stabilization is required.

Nonspecific, insidiously occurring capsulitis is treated similarly to a sprain. Intra-articular cortisone injections, although often initially effective, tend to weaken the volar plate and may predispose to plantar ligament failure or rupture. An intra-articular homeopathic cocktail with Traumeel or *Ruta graveolens* may be safely used, often with excellent results. Biomechanical predisposing factors are managed with accommodative biodynamic devices.

TAILOR'S BUNIONS

Splaying of the fifth metatarsal or excessive pressure over the fifth metatarsophalangeal joint from excessive bowing of the metatarsal shaft may give rise to painful pathology with inflamed bursae, called tailor's bunions. More plantar-splayed fifth metatarsals have intractable plantar keratomas associated with painful inflamed tailors bunionettes (Figs. 14-12 and 14-13). In the old days tailors operated their tailor's wheel by pressing with the lateral aspect of the foot, thus developing the hypertrophic "tailor's bunions." These painful fifth metatarsal bunionettes are found in ice skaters, skiers, and other athletes who wear tight boots or shoes, putting excessive pressure over the fifth metatarsal head. Abnormal splaying of the foot with metatarsus quintus abductus leads to tailor's bunion.

Conservative therapy consists of accommodative pads and strapping to decrease the splaying. Tight boots are punched out over the fifth metatarsal head. Shoes are stretched. Anti-inflammatory medications such as ibuprofen, 800 mg, tid with food, give immediate relief. Homeopathic Traumeel or Zeel, topically or 1 tab tid, are often helpful as a natural alternative. Severely inflamed bunionettes and bursae may be injected with a cortisone or homeopathic cocktail.

Persistent cases require surgical osteotomies to decrease the metatarsus quinti varus angle with subsequent abnormal splaying. Moderate deformity will allow for a distal osteotomy; more advanced deformity requires a proximal osteotomy. Partial ostectomy of the fifth metatarsal head often results in long-term failure with recurrence due to persistent splaying deformity and subsequent eventual abnormal excessive pressure.

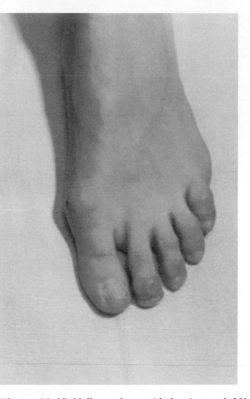

Figure 14-12 Hallux valgus with bunion and fifth metatarsal tailor's bunion.

STRESS FRACTURES

A stress fracture occurs in a metatarsal secondary to chronic repetitive stress. The most commonly fractured bones are the second and third metatarsals. Stress fractures not recognized or treated improperly may convert to complete fractures.

The bone resorptive processes exceed the bone reparative processes. As osteoclastic outstrips osteoblastic activity, weakness develops, and a stress fracture is the end result. Stress fractures in a metatarsal may occur in any location, depending on the forces. They are usually not evident for the first 3 weeks following the incident. They are easily diagnosed by their clinical appearance. There is swelling and redness at the dorsal aspect of the foot over the involved metatarsal. There will be extreme pain in response to digital pressure on the metatarsal. Usually a positive tuning fork test will be present. The vibration of the tuning fork placed upon the bone causes sudden increased pain. This pain is accentuated with motion of the metatarsal during examination. The dorsal swelling is more diffuse than when seen with extensor tendinitis. The general rule

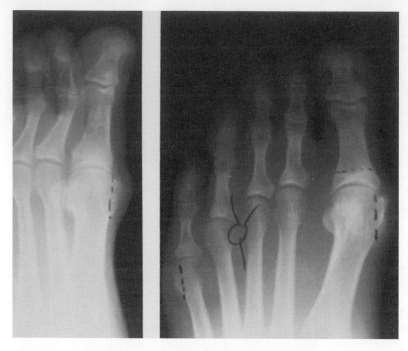

Figure 14-13 Hallux valgus with bunion and tailor's bunion.

is, when in doubt, assume stress fracture until proved otherwise.

Treatment is rest for 3 weeks, using a wooden shoe to eliminate flexion at the metatarsophalangeal joint during push-off. If there is pain with ambulation in the wooden shoe, a foot cast or below-knee (BK) walking cast will suffice. After 3 weeks, a felt large metatarsal or hap pad with tape may be used, and there can be gradual resumption of activity. As with all fractures, homeopathic *Symphytum caucasicum* 12c bid, or calcaria phosphoricum 12c for 3 to 4 weeks bid, may lessen symptoms and hasten healing. At 6 weeks most fractures are healed. When stress fractures are associated with long metatarsals or faulty biomechanics, orthotic correction is understandably indicated.

METATARSAL–CUBOID ARTICULATIONS

Styloid Process and Fifth Metatarsal

The fifth metatarsal styloid process may be involved in trauma, such as avulsion fracture or chronic pressure with secondary bursitis or tendinitis (Fig. 14-14). The peroneus brevis and tertius tendons insert into the base of the fifth metatarsal, and tendinitis may be the end result of abnormal stress or strain or pressure from the shoe. Acute plantar-

flexory supination injuries may lead to avulsion of the base or styloid process of the fifth metatarsal. Avulsion fractures are treated with BK walking cast immoblization for 6 weeks, resting the peroneal tendons. These plantar-flexion inversion injuries can also lead to Jones fractures of the fifth metatarsal base. These fractures have a reportedly high incidence of nonunion and may need internal fixation. Plantar-flexion inversion ankle, subtalar, or midtarsal sprain may result in peroneal–cuboid syndrome with subluxed cuboid. The forced inversion of the foot causes the cuboid to minimally "slip" or "rotate" in the direction of eversion, thus rendering it unstable to the pull of the peroneal tendons. There is pain at the calcaneocuboid or cuboid–fourth/fifth metatarsal articulations as well as pain in the peroneal tunnel under the cuboid where the peroneus longus tendon passes obliquely toward its insertion into the base of the first metatarsal–cuneiform. Pain may be debilitating. In dancers it may more commonly present in the metatarsal–cuboid articulations. A clicking sensation can often be elicited in the involved joint upon careful range-of-motion palpations.

Treatment requires a cuboid or cuboid–metatarsal manipulation (adjustment), followed by a cuboid plantar pad and taping (see Chs. 22 and 25 for technique). With resistant cases, a local anesthetic injection with the Traumeel

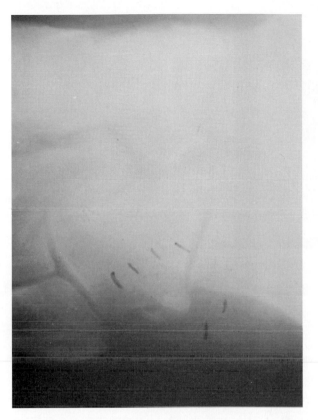

Figure 14-14 Fractured cuboid.

homeopathic cocktail, or cortisone if preferred, is placed in the calcaneocuboid and cuboid–metatarsal joints to facilitate the manipulation correction. When successful, an audible click will be felt and heard as the cuboid is repositoned. Relief will be instantaneous. I have often done this manipulation on the tennis court for foot sprains with subluxed cuboid. The acute subluxation should be treated with icing and manipulation before peroneal muscle spasm sets in. However, fracture should be ruled out first!

Chronic subluxed cuboids are difficult to treat. They may occur secondary to medial heel pain, as in heel-spur syndrome. The patient walks on the outside of the foot to avoid medial pain; this causes the cuboid to rotate and slip into an unstable subluxed position. Correction requires lateral shoe wedging to prevent inversion, injection, and manipulation followed by eversion foot orthotics with a lateral high flange and cuboid stabilizing pad. Persistent cases respond to a BK everted walking cast for 6 to 8 weeks, applied once the cuboid has been repositioned. After final stabilization, a neutral orthotic with high lateral flange and cuboid pad are worn.

I have evaluated patients receiving workers' compensation whose injuries were rated permanent and stationary, with lifetime significant disability awards, who simply had a subluxed cuboid following a foot or ankle sprain. Once corrected, these patients remain symptom free and return to preinjury occupations and athletic participation.

Fractures of the Fifth Metatarsal Base

Fractures of the fifth metatarsal base have been reported to lead to a high degree or percentage of nonunion.[18–20] Although this has not been my experience, the literature shows several cases. I personally find that, if fifth metatarsal fractures are treated with immobilization for 6 weeks, followed by gradual return to activity with taping of the foot, malunion seldom occurs. I also find that those incidents in which malunion is expected usually always heal with time; however, in some cases bone graft and internal fixation are necessary for fifth metatarsal base fractures (socalled Jones fractures).

Dorsal Metatarsal–Cuneiform Pain

The first metatarsal–first cuneiform articulation or the region of the first metatarsal and adjacent cuneiforms can be associated with dorsal hyperostosis and pain. This occurs especially at the first metatarsal–cuneiform articulation due to the unique biomechanics of the first ray (Fig. 14-15). The saddle-shaped joint at the first metatarsal–cuneiform articulation allows for dorsiflexion and plantar flexion of the first metatarsal with some inversion or eversion, respectively. Excessive force going through the first metatarsal head from plantarward causes impingement of the joint and secondary reactive hyperostosis. This dorsal exostosis is often uncomfortable in tight-fitting foot gear (Fig. 14-16). Initially, treatment for the dorsal exostosis is accommodation with felt and appropriate modification of foot gear. If the problem is persistent and there is a large exostosis on radiographs, excision is the treatment of choice. Bone must be removed to create a crater at the dorsal aspect of the first metatarsal–cuneiform joint. If intra-articular pathology is present, an arthrotomy should be carried out.

THE MIDFOOT

The midfoot is that portion of the foot between the tarsal bones and the metatarsals. It is made up of the midtarsus bones: the three cuneiforms, the cuboid, and the navicular.

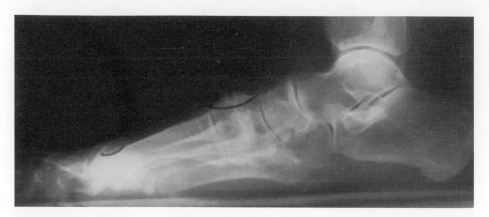

Figure 14-15 First metatarsal–cuneiform exostosis.

Figure 14-16 First metatarsal–cuneiform exostosis, which caused boot irritation in a skier.

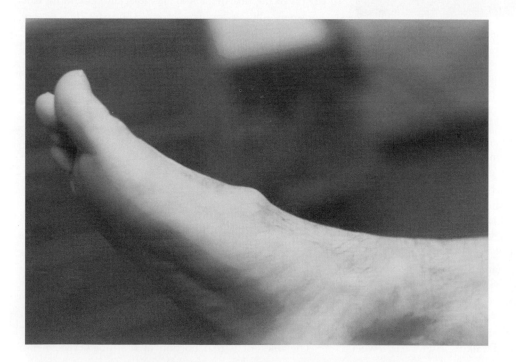

Soft Tissues of the Midfoot

SEED KERATOMAS

The plantar aspect of the skin near the midtarsus or midfoot can be involved with punctate seed keratomas or corns. The etiology of these lesions is speculative.[21] They are diagnosed as a circumscribed seed corn, which is painful at the plantar aspect of the foot at the midtarsus level. They must be differentiated from porokeratosis plantaris discretum, which is a definitive lesion of a plugged sweat duct. These lesions also must be differentiated from verruca plantaris. Seed keratomas are treated by paring and curettage, or laser ablation.

POROKERATOSIS PLANTARIS

Porokeratosis plantaris discretum may be apparent in any aspect of the plantar skin. This apparent plugged sweat duct problem is diagnosed by the appearance of a deep keratotic lesion that has a clear central portion. Upon debridement, the lesion is found to go quite deep, and these are usually not located under pressure points. Treatment consists of injection therapy, using a long- and slow-acting local anesthetic and cortisone, followed by deep paring and curettage. Care must be taken to avoid scarring, which can be as bad as, if not worse than, the original problem. Laser ablation of the lesions is my treatment of choice. With careful technique there is reduced incidence of scarring. Sclerosing the lesions with alcohol injection has met with success in limited cases. No matter what technique is used, even laser ablation, the original or subsequent lesions may recur, disappointing all involved.

Plantar Fasciitis

There has literally been an epidemic of so-called heel-spur syndrome with plantar fasciitis over the past 4 to 5 years. Both conditions are merely anatomic classifications of the same phenomenon. The increased incidence of painful heels and fascia is particularly prevalent among middle-aged walkers, previously inactive, who begin their fitness walking program without adequate preparation. Improper shoes, lack of foot support or shock attenuation, and doing "too much, too soon" are all contributing factors. Since the plantar fascia and deep intrinsic muscles of the foot originate in the medial plantar condyle of the calcaneus, spurs of the heel are merely the result, not the cause, of the problem.

Plantar fasciitis technically is an inflammation of the plantar fascia of the foot. It may be located proximally, at the calcaneal insertion, or more distally (true fasciitis) and usually involves the medial slip of the plantar fascia. There may be chronic repetitive stress leading to chronic irritation of the plantar fascia or an acute injury leading to a partial rupture. Midfoot plantar fasciitis is distinguished from heel-spur syndrome, which is more proximal. Palpation of the plantar fascia at the midfoot level will demonstrate discrete painful areas. When a partial rupture is present, it is palpable; if it is acute, there may be ecchymosis. Chronic partial ruptures have abundant scar tissue, which is palpable. Plantar fibromas may be palpable. Dupuytren's contracture may be present and should be differentiated from plantar fibromas or nodules. Adductor myositis may be present with plantar fasciitis when secondary to excessive pronation, abduction of the forefoot on the rearfoot with subsequent bowing of the soft tissue supportive structures, and abnormal propulsive sequences. Recall that the fascia has a windmill effect that, together with the plantar sesamoids of the first metatarsal, increases the mechanical advantage of the first metatarsophalangeal joint, eccentrically tightening and plantar-flexing the first metatarsal during propulsion. Fast running, rapid acceleration, rebounding, and jumping all can strain the plantar fascia, leading to acute or overuse collagen tissue failure.

TREATMENT

Conservative treatment of plantar fasciitis consists of physical therapy with ultrasound, or interferential stimulation three times a week, for 3 to 4 weeks. The foot is taped, using a hallux lock to prevent dorsiflexion of the hallux, which pulls the abductor hallucis and medial plantar fascia. Various types of plantar fascial rest straps exist and include taping with 2-inch Zonas tape, tape and moleskin strips, and Elastikon (see Ch. 25). A night splint (a posterior BK splint holding the foot at 90 degrees to the leg, and extending the foot itself) prevents contracture of the plantar structures, which otherwise happens with the foot in an exaggerated plantar attitude common during sleep. This is most effective in stopping the morning stiffness and pain so characteristic of plantar fasciitis. If an acute partial rupture has taken place, casting for 4 to 6 weeks is appropriate. With initial swelling, an Unna boot or posterior splint should be used to control edema. Crutches are used based on symptoms.

Oral anti-inflammatory medications are useful, as is the application of topical Traumeel initially for acute conditions, followed by topical Zeel for subacute to chronic fasciitis. Natural anti-inflammatory preparations include *Arnica montana* 12c or 30x, 3 pellets qid until better; Traumeel oral liquid, 10 drops qid for acute fasciitis; and Zeel 10 drops qid for subacute or chronic fasciitis. Single-remedy *Rhus toxicodendron* 12c or 30x is almost specific for the stiffness ("worse initial motion, better continued motion, better heat") of plantar fasciitis. *Ruta graveolens* 12c or 30x, 3 pellets tid to qid, is helpful for fasciitis with associated partial rupture or fibromas. *Hypericum* 12c or 30x may be useful for medial calcaneal neuritis associated with plantar fasciitis and heel-spur syndrome.

CHRONIC PLANTAR FASCIITIS

In a typical case, chronic plantar fasciitis has been present for 3 to 6 weeks. Persistent scar tissue over the plantar fascia may be proximal, near the attachment of the plantar fascia to the plantar tubercle of the calcaneus, or more distal, toward the midaspect of the arch. Usually a palpable rift and pain upon palpation of this trigger point is present. The area is easier to examine if the skin on the plantar aspect of the foot is lubricated. The hallux is taken through a range of motion, which stretches the plantar fascia and permits palpation of the plantar fascia in its entirety. Once areas of scar tissue are isolated, injection therapy is indicated. An injection with a combination cocktail of 4 mg prednisolone acetate, 4 mg dexamethasone phosphate, 1 ml of 0.5 percent Marcaine plain, 0.5 to 1 ml Wydase, and 1 ml of 2 percent Xylocaine plain is most effective. Injection with 1 ml of *Rhus toxicodendron* or Zeel in the cocktail instead of the cortisone is a helpful natural alternative for those patients opposed to cortisone.[22]

Prior to injection, the skin is prepped with Betadine or Hibiclens soap and frozen with ethyl chloride spray as a topical distractor, counterirritant local anesthetic. The initial injection is with a 30-gauge needle. Once anesthesia is obtained, further needling to break up the cross-linked collagen scar with a 27- or 25-gauge needle is useful. Chiropractic manipulation of posterior subluxed calcanei is reported to be helpful in decreasing chronic pulling on plantar structures,[23] and to decrease the pain of the initial thrust of the needle through the superficial tissue. The solution is then carefully deposited in the area of maximum scar tissue formation and the needle moved back and forth, while injecting, to effect a lysis breakup of the excessive collagen tissue. Following the injection, ultrasound is used to increase the penetration of the preparation into the surrounding soft tissue. The foot is then taped using moleskin and tape, incorporating a hallux lock to decrease dorsiflexion and additional strain. The athlete is cautioned to take it easy for the next 3 to 6 weeks, as is the case with any cortisone injection. Injections may be repeated every week or two, for a series of three or four. I prefer to have my patients on either ultrasound or interferential stimulation three times a week with taping for 4 to 6 weeks while healing.

Despite the hazards associated with the injection of cortisone into a joint (e.g., weakening of the cartilage) and the considerable risks attending injection of cortisone into a tendon (e.g., central necrosis and rupture), there is little risk in injecting the plantar fascia. In fact, one of the treatments for chronic plantar fasciitis that does not respond to aggressive conservative therapy is surgical release of the plantar fascia. With resistent cases of plantar fasciitis, especially when associated with heel-spur syndrome, a bone scan should be obtained to rule out calcaneal stress fracture. Resistant cases with or without bony involvement may respond to 6 weeks of cast immobilization. Finally, when conservative measures fail, surgery usually gives good results.

PLANTAR FASCIA SURGERY

The plantar fascia is released from the plantar aspect of the calcaneus, where it attaches to the plantar condyles, through a small medial incision using a meniscotome. If the abductor hallucis is involved, it should be released as well. A heel spur may be rasped smooth using a Maltz rasp. The surgery is performed under local anesthesia, and the patient wears a foot cast or posterior splint for 3 weeks following the surgery in order to stretch the forefoot on the rearfoot and rest the plantar fascia.

Such approaches as Steindler plantar fascial stripping or excision of large portions of the plantar fascia are usually met with some degree of residual deformity. The scar tissue formed and the lack of fascia are often as worrisome as the original problem, which may be a plantar fibroma. Therefore, the plantar fascial release, followed by the use of a well-molded orthotic with a plantar fascial groove, appears a more prudent course. Obviously, the presence of a neoplasm may necessitate wide excision.[1,24]

Muscles of the Midfoot

The muscles of the midfoot are intrinsic to the foot itself, acting as stabilizers. Of prime importance is the abductor hallucis, which is often strained. The strain may occur with sudden pronation in an acute injury and chronic pronation in an overuse injury. Tenderness upon palpation of the abductor hallucis is present. Often, there is associated or accompanying medial plantar fasciitis. The treatment is the same as that for plantar fasciitis. The diagnosis is made by palpating the abductor hallucis and isolating it from surrounding soft tissue. The examining physician must rule out underlying bone damage, such as a sprain of the subtalar or midtarsal joint or os naviculare.

Other muscles of the midfoot include the abductor digiti quinti, the quadratus plantaris, and the lumbricals. These muscles are seldom injured, but they may be involved with chronic aching and stress secondary to abnormal pronation or overuse. The treatment is a biomechanical approach to the foot, eliminating abnormal motions by the use of orthoses. Rehabilitative exercises for weak intrinsic muscles of the foot include curling the toes, picking up marbles with the toes, and walking on the balls of the feet.

The muscle in the dorsal aspect of the midfoot is the extensor digitorum brevis. This muscle has its origin at the lateral anterior aspect of the talus, coursing over the foot into the dorsal aspects of the toes. The extensor digitorum brevis and the extensor hallucis brevis function as stabilizers and extensors of the toes.

Injury may occur secondary to a sprain of the foot. The diagnosis is made upon palpation of the dorsal aspect of the foot, which elicits tenderness over these muscles as the toes are being moved. Underlying trauma, such as stress fracture, complete fracture, or injury to the joints, must be ruled out. Radiographs may be indicated. Acute injuries are treated with appropriate anti-inflammatory local measures and physical therapy, as well as rest of the foot. Oral anti-inflammatory medications may be indicated. Topical Traumeel along with oral Traumeel, one tab qid, is reported to give good results for sports injuries.[25]

Chronic injuries are treated with physical therapy modalities, including ultrasound, interferential stimulation, and deep transverse friction massage. Biomechanical imbalances of the foot are corrected. Taping may be necessary to rest the foot; occasionally, injection therapy is indicated.

Tendons of the Midfoot

The tendons that affect the function of the foot at the midaspect include (dorsomedially to dorsolaterally) the tendons of the anterior tibial, the extensor hallucis longus, the extensor digitorum longus, and the peroneus tertius muscles. These muscles, in conjunction with the triceps surae at the posterior aspect of the foot, constitute the prime movers and stabilizers of the foot and ankle. Situated laterally are the peroneus brevis and the peroneus longus, and, medially, the posterior tibial, flexor hallucis longus, and flexor digitorum longus. These muscles function as prime movers of the foot and as stabilizers with various periods of functional activity, depending on the amount of pronation or supination taking place in the foot.

The phasic activity of walking for the muscles and tendons is different from that for running. Whereas in walking the posterior tibial tendon becomes active at about 12 to 15 percent of the stance phase, in running it is active at contact. Thus the muscles for running function immediately to stabilize the foot, whereas in walking there is a more phasic functional pattern, enabling the muscles to rest at various times during the stance phase of gait. The anterior tibial muscle works as a swing-phase muscle, dorsiflexing the foot, and is helped by the extensors. The peroneals, flexors, and posterior tibial may act as plantar flexors during running. Accomplished runners often will use their peroneus longus as a plantar flexor, creating a functional forefoot valgus. This can cause a strain at the peroneal musculature.

The muscles going into the midfoot have been likened to a stirrup. This is appreciated when one realizes that the peroneus longus runs from the cuboid, under the foot, to the medial aspect of the first metatarsal base; and the posterior tibial courses from medial to lateral. Thus, the peroneus longus and posterior tibial act as a stirrup, supporting the medial and lateral aspects of the foot. They are assisted by the other long muscles.

PERONEAL TENDON INJURY

Peroneal Tendon Trauma/Peroneal Cuboid Syndrome

The peroneus longus muscle plantar flexes, abducts, and everts the foot. It is a plantar flexor of the first ray, causing a functional forefoot valgus. Injuries to the peroneal tendon occur secondary to overuse, poor condition, and acute strain or trauma, such as peroneal tendon dislocation or partial rupture. Overuse may cause a tenosynovitis with inflammation between the tendon and the sheath. Poor biomechanics cause the peroneal to function abnormally and increase the odds for tenosynovitis. Peroneus longus tenosynovitis is diagnosed by palpating the peroneus longus along its course. Tenosynovitis may be present as the peroneal tendon enters the cuboid groove at the lateral plantar aspect of the foot. This could be accompanied by peroneal cuboid syndrome, whereby the cuboid is pulled laterally and dorsally and subluxes minimally. This may be the case following an inversion sprain, which is not uncommon in tennis injuries. The athlete presents with pain over the cuboid and, upon activating the peroneus longus and plantar-flexing the first ray, there is more pain, and crepitation may be palpated beneath the cuboid. Likewise, there may be peroneus longus tenosynovitis proximal to the cuboid. Radiographs are taken to rule out stress fracture or other forms of bony damage.

If crepitation is present, an injection of a cocktail containing a long- and slow-acting local anesthetic, cortisone, and Wydase should be given to decrease the inflammation. This is carried out between the tendon and the sheath but not into the tendon itself, followed by ultrasound, or interferential physical therapy. The previously mentioned Truameel injection cocktail may be substituted when appropriate. The cuboid is then gently manipulated back into place, using a plantar thrust of the thumbs.[21a] Ultrasound or interferential stimulation is then given. A cuboid pad is placed underneath the cuboid with more felt medially than laterally, to help invert it, followed by low-dye strapping using felt and tape, with additional tape placed over the cuboid for stabilization. The athlete's foot is kept in a firm shoe. An exercise bike may be used, but running is decreased or limited for 3 to 6 weeks while healing takes place. A physical therapy program is undertaken three times a week for 3 to 6 weeks. The patient is checked weekly, and additional injections or manipulations may be indicated. Prolotherapy homeopathic sclerosing injections with Zeel or *Ruta graveolens* (or both mixed) help to stabilize previously sprained hypermobile joints.

If biomechanical problems are present, the athlete is eventually fitted for an appropriate orthosis. The orthothosis should have a perpendicular-to-valgus rearfoot control with a high lateral flange and an extended perpendicular-to-valgus long extrinsic forefoot rubber post that tapers distally to the plantar web (junction of the base of the toes and the sole of the foot). A soft temporary orthosis may be used first to validate the necessity of a more permanent orthosis. Partial rupture or intratendinous damage must be ruled out. If the problems persist despite appropriate conservative care, more serious tendon damage such as stenosing tenosynovitis may be present, which may indicate the need for surgical exploration or decompression. Magnetic resonance imaging (MRI) is helpful in evaluating the extent of soft tissue damage.

Peroneus Longus Rupture

Patients with partial rupture of the peroneus longus tendon secondary to inversion sprains with plantar flexion of the ankle and foot were found at clinical examination to have ecchymosis and pain (Fig. 14-17). I have administered conservative therapy to these patients, consisting of cast immobilization and a walking boot for 4 to 6 weeks along with physical therapy. In those cases that were refractory to conservative therapy, surgery was carried out with repair of the rupture. The results have been good. When the peroneus longus tendon is severely degenerated, it can sometimes be reinforced with the peroneus brevis tendon.

Subluxing Peroneal Tendinitis

The peroneus longus tendon may dislocate at the ankle level over the lateral malleolus. This is termed *subluxing peroneal tendon*, also referred to as "trick ankle." The injury occurs secondary to forceful dorsiflexion and eversion, as occurs in downhill skiing injuries. During this motion, when the ski stops suddenly in a snow bank, the skier continues forward and the peroneal tendons move forward on the fibula and avulse the peroneal retinaculum. A "fleck" of bone is often seen on lateral ankle radiographs, indicative of the retinaculum and underlying fibular maleolar avulsion. Chronic snapping of the tendon may follow injury, leading to symptomatic tenosynovitis. Immediate treatment consists of cast immobilization for 4 to 6 weeks. If the instability persists, surgery is the treatment of choice, and a reconstruction of the retinaculum (retinaculoplasty) is carried out.[21,26–28]

The diagnosis is easily made; the examining physician palpates the peroneus longus as the foot is dorsiflexed and everted. The peroneal tendons will anteriorly displace over the fibula. There may be tenosynovitis or tendinitis at the fibular level, usually extending distally to the level of the cuboid. Radiographs will show a fleck of bone from the lateral aspect of the fibula that has been avulsed along with the retinaculum. This is the telltale sign.

PERONEUS TERTIUS INJURY

The peroneus tertius is a small antigravity muscle of the foot, that inserts into the base of the fifth metatarsal dorsally. It is most often injured when there is an inversion plantar-flexion sprain of the foot or ankle. The diagnosis is made by palpating the peroneus tertius as the foot is dorsiflexed and everted against resistance. Radiographs are taken to rule out an avulsion fracture of the base of the fifth metatarsal. Treat-

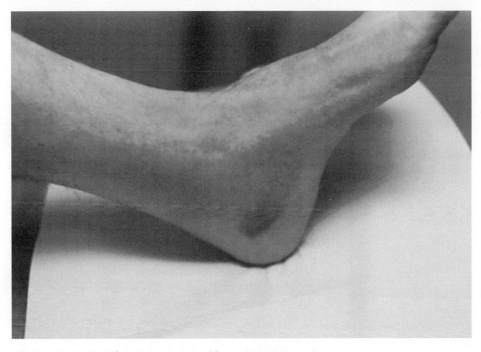

Figure 14-17 Medial ecchymosis caused by an inversion sprain.

ment consists of physical therapy, resting the foot with appropriate taping, and treating biomechanical abnormalities with orthoses. If inflammation is present, anti-inflammatory medications are helpful. These problems respond readily to appropriate conservative therapy.

PERONEUS BREVIS INJURY

The peroneus brevis is an abductor of the foot, opposed by the anterior tibial muscle. The tendon inserts into the styloid process of the fifth metatarsal and is often injured in plantar-flexory inversion sprains. This causes tenosynovitis or partial rupture. An avulsion of the base of the fifth metatarsal may be associated with peroneus brevis tenosynovitis. Radiographs should therefore be taken to rule out fracture in a case of an acute injury along the peroneus brevis. Injury to the peroneus brevis may also be overuse or chronic in nature secondary to chronic repetitive stress in supports or excessive pronation. Both the peroneus longus and brevis tendons may become fatigued or inflamed secondary to attempts at stabilizing the foot. This problem may occur in edge-control sports, such as skiing or ice skating. If there is lateral instability or cavus foot, excessive supination may also predispose the peroneal tendons to strain and injury.

The diagnosis of peroneus brevis tendon pathology is made by active use of the peroneus brevis, moving the foot in the position of abduction and dorsiflexion. This movement is resisted by the examiner's hand. The peroneus brevis tendon is then palpated. If pain is associated with palpation, pathology is present. The peroneus brevis may have a tenosynovitis, which may be sclerosing or chronic in nature. If there is crepitation, the problem is more emergent; injection therapy and rest should be instituted immediately. Failure to respond to conservative therapy would require tenolysis of the sheath. Treatment for tendinitis is similar to that for the peroneus longus: physical therapy, anti-inflammatory medications, and a cuboid pad with taping of the foot. Following the resolution of pain, the athlete's foot is checked for the appropriate biomechanics, and orthoses are used. Rehabilitative exercises designed to strengthen the peroneal tendons and provide for flexibility and balance are prescribed.

EXTENSOR INJURY

The extensor digitorum longus and extensor hallucis longus decelerate the foot at contact (Figs. 8–6 and 14–3). They may become fatigued or injured with running on hard surfaces or downhill. They function as antigravity muscles, decelerating the limb during swing phase and at contact. Their tendons are more susceptible to injury during overstriding, which occurs with downhill running and with such sports as race walking. Overstriding occurs when the foot contacts in front of the knee; the ground pushes the body backward, causing increased shock absorbence in the limb. The shock is absorbed by the soft tissue of the limb as well as by the bone joints. The more overstriding that occurs, the greater the moment of force of acceleration of the forefoot toward the ground, hence the increased need for deceleration by the antigravity muscles. Strengthening exercises for the antigravity muscles with stretching exercises for the gravity muscles decrease this dynamic imbalance and help avoid overstride or deceleration injuries of the anterior soft tissue and musculature.

Extensor Tendinitis

The extensors over the dorsal aspects of the midtarsus may be traumatized secondary to tight laces on shoes or tight foot gear. This is easily treated with local anti-inflammatory measures, changing the patterns of lacing of the shoes, or getting larger shoes. The bruised extensor tendons should be rested and padded with felt or sponge rubber. Analgesics may be helpful. Persistent tendinitis secondary to hypertrophic underlying bony exostosis may require surgery.

ANTERIOR TIBIAL INJURY

The anterior tibial is an antigravity muscle that functions along with the extensors to decrease foot slap at contact. It also works as a dorsiflexor of the foot at toe-off and during swing phase. Anterior tibial as well as extensor tendinitis can occur at the midfoot level from tight shoelaces or eyelets on shoes. Midtarsal joint dorsal hyperostosis may impinge on the tendon and surrounding soft tissue and predispose to tenosynovitis. Excessive pronation elongates the anterior tibial as the medial longitudinal arch drops, causing stress overload with tenosynovitis or partial ruptures. Sudden plantar-flexory eversion injuries may cause partial to complete rupture of the anterior tibial tendon, which may require surgical repair.

Conservative therapy for tenosynovitis of the anterior tibial tendon consists of physical therapy with ultrasound or interferential or electrogalvanic stimulation, as well as the use of oral anti-inflammatory medications or homeopathic remedies such as *Rhus toxicodendron, Ruta graveolens*, or Traumeel. Corticosteroids can be injected judiciously into the peritendinous area, but not intratendinously, since this may cause intratendinous necrosis of the tendon.

Homeopathic cocktail injections are often effective and certainly safer. Initially, resting the foot with Unna boots and tape strapping using a *high-dye* strap incorporating both the foot and ankle is helpful. A soft temporary orthosis is put in place to immediately correct foot imbalances, after which a more permanent orthosis may be indicated. Appropriate rehabilitative exercises are helpful to strengthen the anterior tibial muscle and stretch the peroneals and posterior musculature. Acute partial rupture often necessitates the use of a cast for 4 to 6 weeks, whereas chronic tendinosis requires physical therapy, including transverse friction massage. Ultrasound has been shown to increase the collagen regeneration in damaged tendons.

Chronic tenosynovitis that is not responsive to conservative therapy will respond to surgical tenolysis. If there is intratendinous damage, curettage of necrotic tendon is indicated, with repair of the tendon with a tendon graft if necessary. If the anterior tibial tendon is subjected to repeated impingement secondary to underlying hyperostosis, decompression may be indicated, with excision of hypertrophic dorsal bone at the midtarsus, forming a dell to accommodate the anterior tibial. This is usually carried out in conjunction with partial ostectomy under the extensors.

POSTERIOR TIBIAL TENDINOPATHY

At the midfoot level, the posterior tibial tendon attaches into the talus as well as the navicular. Primary problems occurring with the posterior tibial tendon are tenosynovitis and partial or complete rupture. Posterior tibial tenosynovitis is often associated with a hypertrophic tubercle of the navicular and excessive pronation of the foot, or a separate os naviculare. As the foot pronates excessively, the posterior tibial tendon is subjected to excessive strain as it is eccentrically elongated. With pronation, the forefoot abducts on the rearfoot, effectively elongating and stretching the posterior tibial tendon and muscle, which are eccentrically resisting the pronation. This leads to tendon failure and tenosynovitis, gradual collagen "creep" lengthening (posterior tibial insufficiency), or partial to complete rupture of the tendon with serious posterior tibial insufficiency and secondary progressive unilateral flatfoot. Failure to recognize posterior tibial insufficiency and delayed treatment may lead to progressive subtalar and midtarsal joint subluxatory changes, necessitating subtalar or triple arthrodesis, or both. Early diagnosis and treatment with cast immobilization or tendon repair and reinforcement (modified Cobb or Kidner-Young repairs) may save the athlete from the arthrodesis procedures.

Chronic overloading of the posterior tibial tendon in sports with excessive pronation causes inflammation with tenosynovitis. Repeated trauma may cause partial to complete rupture. The posterior tibial functions to decelerate pronation and internal rotation; thus the forces generated at contact during running sports predispose to injury of this tendon when excessive pronation takes place or when fatigue is present. With mild tenosynovitis, simple backing off of training, slowing down, avoiding hill running and jumping, and resting for 4 to 6 weeks, along with strapping and physical therapy, may allow for complete healing without any tendon creep or persistent deformity.

Acute injury occurs with plantar-flexory eversion stress. These injuries are more common in sports such as soccer and football. Posterior tibial tendinitis must be differentiated from avulsion fracture of the medial navicular tubercle or os naviculare itself, when present as a secondary ossification center.

Acute pathology of the posterior tibial tendon includes tenosynovitis or partial or complete rupture. Tenosynovitis is diagnosed by palpating the posterior tibial tendon and eliciting pain. Swelling is present, yet the strength of the posterior tibial appears intact as the foot is supinated against resistance. Initial treatment consists of rest and anti-inflammatory medications. Acute tenosynovitis will usually respond to taping of the foot and ankle as well as physical therapy with interferential or electrogalvanic stimulation or ultrasound carried out three times a week. Ice massage should be used before and after light workouts. If running causes pain, substituting an alternative aerobic activity, such as biking or swimming, is recommended. It may take 4 to 6 weeks for these problems to respond to conservative therapy. Corticosteroids should not be used for acute problems but may be used judiciously after 3 weeks' duration for chronicity. I prefer injections of the safer Traumeel homeopathic cocktail when injections are required. Repeated cortisone injections are associated with failure of the posterior tibial tendon and subsequent deforming and debilitating posterior tibial insufficiency.

Appropriate orthotic correction of abnormal biomechanics is indicated. Orthoses for posterior tibial tendon pathology often require additional medial wedging at the rearfoot and forefoot with a long extrinsic runner's varus wedge. A deep, 16-mm heel cup is useful along with a high medial clip. Foot gear must be checked and care taken to select shoes that decrease abnormal motion. I have been pleased with the performance of the New Balance 585 model in motion control for runners. A firm counter and midsole are mandatory to control the excessively pronating foot. Because the posterior tibial muscle is the primary decelerator of pronation and internal leg rotation at foot contact, any help from a good supportive shoe is beneficial to the healing of the muscle and tendon. In addition to stable foot gear, rehabilitative muscle and tendon physical therapy is necessary, once the acute phase is over.

Chronic Posterior Tibial Tendinitis

Posterior tibial tendinitis is considered chronic when it persists beyond 3 weeks. In these cases, there is repeated swelling and pain with such sports as running. There may be crepitation along the tenosynovium of the posterior tibial. When this is associated with the os naviculare, avulsion fracture of the os naviculare bone must be ruled out. Treatment includes continuing physical therapy, judicious use of anti-inflammatory agents (oral or injectable), and taping or cast immobilization of the foot. In the event that conservative therapy has been exhausted and pain persists, a tenolysis may be indicated.

Posterior tibial tendinitis may be associated with posterior medial shin syndrome. Periostitis and myositis of the posterior tibial are present in the lower medial posterior portion of the tibia. In these cases I have had gratifying results with trigger point injections using the homeopathic Traumeel and Zeel cocktail. Multiple firm trigger points are palpated and injected with a very small amount (0.5 ml) of a mixture of local anesthetic, Wydase, vitamin B_{12}, Zeel, and Traumeel using a 30-gauge needle. This so-called osteopuncture technique was suggested to me by Ron Lawrence, M.D., President of the American Medical Athletic Association, at one of their meetings (personal communication, 1984). Dr. Lawrence is a long-time Southern California sports medicine physician practicing neurology and medical acupuncture. The trigger point technique has also been advocated by the eminent British orthopedist Sir James Cyriax, and more recently by Dr. Janet Travell.[29,30]

If a symptomatic os naviculare is present, it should be surgically excised. The posterior tibial tendon may be reinforced with the anterior tibial tendon (modified Cobb or Kidner-Young procedures). When these problems are associated with a hypertrophic medial tubercle of the navicular, they should be excised at the time of decompression of the posterior tibial tendon (modified Kidner-Young tenosuspension).

Partial Ruptures of the Posterior Tibial Tendon

Partial ruptures most often will respond to conservative physical therapy, rehabilitation, and initial rest, followed by orthotic control of the foot. In the event that problems persist, surgical decompression of the posterior tibial tendon as well as curettage of intratendinous necrosis are indicated. The posterior tibial tendon may need to be reinforced with a portion of the anterior tibial tendon or the flexors at the time of surgery. The patient is placed in a walking cast for 4 to 6 weeks following this procedure, after which rehabilitation and physical therapy are instituted. The results are uniformly good.

Acute Rupture of the Posterior Tibial Tendon

Acute rupture of the posterior tibial tendon requires immediate surgical repair. Failure to do so will result in prolapse of the medial longitudinal arch. Results of delayed repair of ruptured posterior tibial tendons have been less than satisfactory,[31–33] since the muscle as well as the tendon is weakened. The prolapse of the midtarsal and subtalar joints that occurs with rupture of the posterior tibial tendon is so extensive that triple arthrodesis is often necessary when function of the posterior tibial is lost.

FLEXOR DIGITORUM LONGUS INJURY

The flexor digitorum longus tendon may become inflamed at the plantar aspect medially in the midfoot, secondary to excessive pronation or increased efforts of plantar-flexing the toes during propulsion. Dancing or jumping sports may predispose to excessive strain of the long flexors. The diagnosis is made by palpation over the flexors, at the midaspect of the foot, while the toes are dorsiflexed and plantar flexed. This can be difficult to differentiate from medial plantar fasciitis.

Acute flexor tendinitis is treated with rest and anti-inflammatory medication. Abnormal biomechanics must be corrected. Once the acute phase is over, rehabilitative exercises are instituted with strengthening of the flexors and balancing of the foot. Taping is most helpful and may be necessary for 6 weeks following an acute episode. Crest pads on the toes to decrease overuse of the long flexors during toe-off are helpful. Surgery is rarely indicated for flexor tendon pathology.

FLEXOR HALLUCIS LONGUS INJURY

The flexor hallucis longus is used for push-off. Tenosynovitis may occur secondary to overload, especially in dancing sports. Ballet dancers going on point may have flexor hallucis longus tenosynovitis or tendinitis at the midaspect of the foot. Supporting the foot with tape and rest and using physical therapy and anti-inflammatory medication usually correct this problem.

For acute problems, the foot is rested and the hallux is taped in a plantar-flexory attitude with elastic tape to decrease dorsiflexion. This will rest the long flexor and allow for recovery. Those activities that dispose to injury or pain are eliminated from the athlete's workout, and other aerobic activities are substituted. After 3 to 4 weeks of rest and physical therapy, the athlete usually returns to competition with a hallux lock and low-dye taping of the foot for an additional 3 weeks.

The most common problem is that of tenosynovitis. Partial ruptures may occur; complete ruptures are rare. Complete rupture of the long flexor tendon would require a surgical repair, and partial rupture would require cast immobilization or rest.

The intrinsic musculature of the plantar aspect of the foot includes the flexor brevis and quadratus plantae. These small broad muscles at the plantar aspect of the foot act as stabilizers and may be associated with generalized fatigue of the foot secondary to overuse or excessive pronation. They are usually involved in plantar foot fatigue and pain and will respond to initial taping of the foot, followed by orthotic foot control.

Nerves of the Midfoot

Nerve pathology of the midfoot consists of dorsal compression neuropathy of the superficial nerves or the anterior tibial nerve and distal tarsal tunnel syndrome. In some cases, traction neuropathy of the sural nerve may affect the lateral aspect of the foot. The saphenous nerve may be involved in entrapment neuropathy secondary to tight foot gear at the dorsomedial aspect of the foot.

SUPERFICIAL SENSORY NERVE ENTRAPMENT

The superficial peroneal nerve and musculocutaneous nerves pass from laterodorsal over the midtarsal joints as they course into the dorsal aspects of the toes. These nerves may be damaged secondary to tight foot gear or excessive plantar-flexory sprains; thus a compression or traction neuropathy may be present. The diagnosis is made by palpating individual nerves and tapping them. A positive Tinel's sign implies neuropathy. High-arched cavus-type feet or midtarsal dorsal exostosis may predispose to compression neuropathy of these nerves. Radiographs are helpful. The nerves are readily felt in slender people with thin dorsal skin. They may be more difficult to palpate in muscular, thick feet.

Treatment for compression or traction neuropathy consists of injection therapy with a long- and slow-acting cortisone cocktail or a homeopathic cocktail with *Hypericum* along the nerve, followed by physical therapy with ultrasound, two to three times a week for 3 to 6 weeks, to break up adhesions. Correcting abnormal pressure on the nerve secondary to abnormal foot gear is most helpful. Padding may be necessary between the foot gear and the foot, especially when various forms of boots, such as ski boots, are causing abnormal pressure. I have seen cases of irreversible compression neuropathy of the superficial cutaneous nerve secondary to ski boot pressure. Most cases are reversible, however. Of prime importance is the modification of foot gear by a knowledgeable cobbler. Various expanders and "punch-out" techniques take pressure off the bony prominences that usually underlie compressed nerves.

Treatment for acute problems includes physical therapy, resting the foot, and decreasing abnormal pressure. Anti-inflammatory medications, allopathic or homeopathic, are helpful. *Hypericum* 12c, 3 pellets tid until improvement, is often helpful in promoting nerve repair. Chronic problems respond to injection therapy, physical therapy, balancing of the foot, and padding of the foot. Neurolysis injections with Traumeel or *Hypericum* (1 ml), local anesthetic (1.5 ml), vitamin B_{12} (0.5 ml), and Wydase (0.5 ml) (the homeopathic nerve cocktail), three to five injections, weekly spaced; are often surprisingly effective. Of course, injectable corticosteroids, soluble and insoluble (long and short acting, respectively), can give excellent results.

Chronic resistive problems may require excision of excessive underlying dorsal bone to decompress the nerves. Neurolysis may be carried out but may be unsuccessful in the slender patient with very thin subcutaneous tissue. Transposition of the nerve into healthy fatty tissue is useful. In cases where no substantial fatty layer is available, a neurectomy may be necessary. The neurectomy leaves considerable numbness and is not a desirable procedure unless the patient has intractable pain resistant to all other forms of conservative therapy.[34] Fortunately most pressure neuropathies of nerves in the foot involve only sensory nerves.

SURAL AND SAPHENOUS NERVE PATHOLOGY

Both the saphenous and sural nerves are sensory only in the foot and ankle. The saphenous nerve is at the anteromedial aspect of the midfoot and supplies sensation to the dorsomedial aspect of the foot. It can be involved with an entrapment neuropathy secondary to pressure from ill-fitting boots or shoes.[34–36] This problem usually responds to conservative therapy, such as rest and anti-inflammatory measures, as well as physical therapy. Chronic problems may respond to injection therapy; surgery is rarely indicated.

Sural neuropathy occurs at the lateral aspect of the foot, as the nerve courses behind the lateral malleolus into the foot to serve the lateral aspect of the foot for sensation. It may be involved in traction or other neuropathy secondary to inversion plantar-flexory sprains. Acute conditions usually respond to anti-inflammatory measures, and chronic conditions to injection therapy and physical therapy. Surgery is rarely indicated. As with all neuropathies of the lower extremity, the dermatomal distribution indicates nerve root compression. Generalized neuropathy may be metabolic or systemic in etiology.

ANTERIOR TARSAL TUNNEL SYNDROME

Anterior tarsal tunnel syndrome refers to compression neuropathy of the anterior tibial nerve at the dorsal aspect of the midfoot. The anterior tibial nerve is situated between the anterior tibial tendon and the extensor tendons, and is a mixed sensory and motor nerve. The patient will complain of acute pain radiating over the dorsal aspect of the foot into the first interspace plantarly; thus there may be numbness and pain at the plantar aspects of the hallux and second toes radiating proximally over the dorsal aspect of the foot and extending up the ankle and leg. Diagnosis is made by percussion and palpation of the nerve, which reproduces the symptoms.

The acute problem is treated with physical therapy modalities to decrease inflammation as well as adhesions. Analgesics and anti-inflammatory medications are useful. Traumeel, Lymphomyosot, and vitamin B complex [with 300 mg of pyridoxine (B_6)] help reduce inflammation and adhesion formation while providing nutritional support for nerve repair. The foot is rested and offending foot gear is modified or discarded. Chronic problems may need one or two weekly-spaced homeopathic nerve cocktail or corticosteroid injections with a long- and slow-acting cortisone, followed by appropriate physical therapy to reduce inflammation. When chronicity is present despite conservative therapy, radiographs are taken to rule out underlying hyperostosis or bone problems. When these bone problems are present with excessive dorsal hyperostosis of the midtarsus, a partial ostectomy of the bone is indicated, forming a dell as the neurovascular bundle is decompressed. The extensor retinaculum is sectioned during this surgery and left open during the closure of the surgery to prevent a recurrence of the anterior tarsal tunnel. Electromyography (EMG) and nerve conduction studies may be helpful in confirming the diagnosis[37–39] but, as with posterior tarsal tunnel syndrome, the most important findings are clinical. Therefore, negative neurologic findings in regard to nerve conduction and EMG studies are not in themselves grounds for not performing appropriate surgery.

DISTAL TARSAL TUNNEL SYNDROME

There may be chronic nervelike pain at the medial plantar aspects of the foot from the porta pedis under the abductor hallucis muscle distally. This constitutes a distal tarsal tunnel syndrome or entrapment of the medial or lateral plantar nerve. Medial pain along the long flexor into the hallux indicates medial plantar tarsal tunnel syndrome or entrapment of the medial plantar nerve. That which is lateral is termed lateral distal tarsal tunnel syndrome. Chronic nervelike aching pain, accentuated by activity or pronation, would help confirm this diagnosis. A positive Tinel's sign may be present upon percussion of the nerve distally and plantarly. Neurologic consultation with nerve conduction and EMG studies may be helpful, although lack of neurapraxia does not rule out this form of compression neuropathy.[40–42]

Tarsal tunnel syndrome is more prevalent with excessive pronation, which tends to tighten up the soft tissue at the medial aspect of the foot and close off the porta pedis. Tarsal tunnel syndrome that responds to biomechanical neutral foot control is termed functional tarsal tunnel syndrome, in contradistinction to anatomic tarsal tunnel syndrome, which is symptomatic with or without control of abnormal motion and position. The porta pedis is just above the attachment of the abductor hallucis muscle, and a tight or hypertrophic abductor hallucis may predispose to compression neuropathy or distal tarsal tunnel syndrome.

The acute problem presents with acute pain, numbness, and radiation accentuated by weight bearing. Initial treatment consists of resting the foot, with either taping, an Unna boot, or a BK walking cast for 3 weeks. The use of analgesics and anti-inflammatory medications is recommended. After 3 weeks of rest, if the problem persists and is chronic, injection therapy with long- and slow-acting corticosteroids and anesthetics is helpful. A series of three injections, 1 week apart, may help decrease inflammation around the nerve. The homeopathic nerve cocktail may be substituted for the cortisone in selected cases. The foot is treated with continued supportive therapy, such as ultrasound, transverse friction massage, and rest with taping, splinting, bracing, or casting. Abnormal biomechanics are corrected. This almost universally takes care of the problem. If the problem persists despite appropriate conservative therapy, including casting, resting of the foot with tape, injections, and physical therapy, neurologic consultation is indicated.

When clinical and neurologic findings are consistent with proximal and distal tarsal tunnel syndrome, surgery may be indicated. This consists of a neuroplasty with neurolysis and decompression of the tarsal tunnel proximally under the flexor retinaculum (lacineate ligament) and distally into the arch, including the abductor hallucis muscle and porta pedis. Very careful loupe magnification dissection is necessary, with a bloodless field. At the end of the procedure, the tourniquet is released and the wound closed under a bloody field to ensure that all bleeders are clamped and tied and the vascular components of the neurovascular bundle have not been injured. Compressive dressings are used for 3 weeks following this procedure. Physical therapy is then instituted. Tarsal tunnel surgical procedures usually give a satisfactory result, ranging from 60 to 70 percent success. Re-entrapment following surgical procedures occurs at rates as high as 20 to 30 percent. The athlete must be warned of the possibility of recurrence of entrapment neuropathy following surgery. Distal tarsal tunnel syndrome must be differentiated from more conventional proximal tarsal tunnel syndrome, which occurs under the medial malleolus. This is discussed under the rearfoot section of this chapter.

Joints of the Midfoot

The joints of the midfoot consist of Lisfranc's joint (the articulations of the metatarsals with the three cuneiforms and the cuboid) and the midtarsal joint (the articulations of the calcaneus and the talus with the cuboid and navicular, respectively).

Prolonged pronation causes prolapse of the medial midtarsal joints; synovitis is the end result. Thus, excessive pronation will predispose to chronic capsular spraining of the talonavicular or navicular–cuneiform joints. An acute eversion injury would predispose to acute synovitis and sprain of the medial midtarsal joints. Acute inversion, plantar flexory, or lateral sprains of the foot can result in severe pain over the calcaneocuboid or cuboid–fifth metatarsal joints. There may be sufficient force to the cuboid to cause a dorsiflexory eversion subluxation of the cuboid. This may be accompanied by inflammation of the peroneal tendon, especially in the peroneal groove under the cuboid.

Midtarsal joint sprains may be acute or chronic. Acute sprains are diagnosed by palpating the joints involved and taking the foot through various ranges of motion. Radiographs are taken to rule out fractures. The foot is rested initially for 3 weeks and supported with taping or a cast. Splints are useful inasmuch as they enable the athlete to ambulate, yet can be removed for such sports as swimming, and will also allow for appropriate physical therapy on a daily basis to promote decreased inflammation and increased function. Once the acute phase is over, the foot is treated with a soft temporary support; when significant imbalance is present, a more permanent orthosis is indicated.

A particular problem is sprain of the os naviculare, which may result in permanent instability of the junction of the os naviculare to the main body of the tubercle of the navicular. When this avulsion fracture has taken place, even with conservative therapy such as casting and rest, malunion may be the end result and surgery may be indicated.

Chronic joint pathology may require a single judiciously placed corticosteroid injection.[43] Excessive injections will cause dissolution of the joint cartilage and an iatrogenic pathologic joint.

With sprains of the midtarsal joints, there may be ligamentous damage, treated with rest in the same way as capsular injuries. Recalling that the midtarsal joint is a pronatory–supinatory joint with both an oblique and a longitudinal axis (see Ch. 9), it is possible to appreciate the mechanism of injury, including dorsiflexion forefoot impact (oblique axis), and inversion or eversion longitudinal axis midfoot sprains. Such injuries occur, for example, when the foot steps into a pothole, or lands on a pinecone or rock when running in thin-soled shoes. Often with the classic inversion plantar-flexion ankle sprain, not only is the ankle involved but also the subtalar and midtarsal joints. This helps explain lingering midfoot pain after resolution of the ankle component of the injury. With traumatic episodes, acute or overuse, techniques such as trigger point injection therapy and mobilization with joint-specific adjustments may prove essential in restoring normal joint function. Seldom do injuries involve just one joint; the proximal and distal adjacent joints are also involved, either primarily or secondarily, through compensation and altered function.

As with all trauma, the treating phyician, in partnership with the patient, may choose conventional allopathic medicines and techniques [nonsteroidal anti-inflammatory drugs (NSAIDs), physical therapy, etc.] or less conventional treatments and substances (homeopathic, nutritional, herbal) for treatment. Acupuncture is often of value.

Synovitis about the midtarsal joints may indicate a systemic problem, such as rheumatoid or seronegative arthritis. Gout may be present. Appropriate laboratory tests should be ordered. These problems will respond to the initial acute and chronic care used in the treatment of capsulitis (see previous sections). Resting the foot with splints, taping, an Unna boot, or casting may be helpful. Finally, holding the foot in a neutral functional position facilitates healing of injured joint components under optimal functional conditions, while guarding against re-injury.

Dislocations of bones in the midtarsal joint occur secondary to acute trauma. Such conditions as divergent diastasis between the base of the first and second metatarsal have been reported in football injuries. These subtle Lisfranc's dislocations also occur commonly in motor vehicle accidents, as well as equestrian mishaps as the foot is caught in the stirrup by the falling rider. A forced eversion or twisting of the midfoot causes rupture of the ligaments between the first and second cuneiform dorsally, allowing the lateral four metatarsals to laterally sublux as a unit, creating a gap between the first and second metatarsals and cuneiforms. Lisfranc's ligament is between the second metatarsal base and the medial cuneiform dorsally. It is essential in tethering the second metatarsal, and thus the lateral four metatarsal bases, to the medial cuneiform. Lisfranc's dislocations are particularly disastrous when missed in the initial evaluation. It has been observed by the author that at least 20 percent of these rather rare dislocations are missed. If in doubt as to the presence of subtle Lisfranc's ruptures, a stress test under local or general anesthesia with conventional radiography or C-arm fluoroscopy will be helpful.

Dislocations will require immediate closed reduction and, in resistant cases, open reduction with fixation. Since these injuries are often accompanied by fractures, discrete or obvious, they are reduced and fixed. Chronic cases require fusion procedures, at times with bone graft. Posttraumatic dorsiflexion of the first metatarsal may require fusion with opening wedge osteotomy.

Bursitis may persist about the various joints of the midtarsals. The diagnosis is made upon palpation. Treatment consists initially of using physical therapy, and, for chronic resistant cases, intrabursal corticosteroid or Traumeel injections are useful. Rarely, surgery may be needed for fibrous adherent bursitis with underlying bone spurs.

Persistent strain about the midtarsus with limited motion is an indication of acute or overuse sprain, or a complete or incomplete midtarsal joint coalition. Coalitions, of course, show up as bony growth complexes, and the secondary growth centers close in adolescents. These may be fibrous (syndesmosis), cartilagenous (synchondrosis), or bony (true synostosis). Medial oblique radiographs are indicated. Lateral views often show the telltale dorsal hyperostosis at the talar head, which occurs secondary to limited subtalar or midtarsal motion and altered joint function. Radiography with contrast dye or MRI may be necessary to confirm the diagnosis. Manipulation under general anesthesia with fluoroscopy may be diagnostic as well as therapeutic. Treatment of fibrous coalitions or post-traumatic sprain fibrosis requires injection (corticosteroid, Traumeel, *Ruta graveolens*, or Zeel along with Wydase and a local anesthetic), followed by joint-specific mobilization and manipulation to break up adhesions and restore joint function. Three to five such treatments are often necessary. Synchondrosis may respond to the same treatment. Synostosis requires bony resection and the placement of the extensor hallucis calcaneal origin into the resultant midtarsal void for a myoplasty.

Following joint function restoration, orthotics are most helpful in stabilizing the foot and decreasing abnormal motions, which cause midtarsal joint sprains. Even with synostosis, holding the foot in a semipronated functional position may allow for pain-free function and defer or eliminate surgical intervention. Surgery, however, is met with a high degree of success, unless there has been substantial proximal and distal bony adaptation and altered function.

An acute midtarsal joint sprain presents with pain at the dorsal aspect of the foot radiating through the foot to the plantar aspect, along the plane of the midtarsal joint. These sprains often occur between the calcaneus and navicular at the midtarsal joint level. There may be excessive fibrosis or a synostosis in this area that previously was not a problem, even though motion was limited. Unaccustomed athletic forces that require excessive motion, or acute trauma, may set off the inflammatory cascade of the midtarsal joint.

Acute problems are treated with physical therapy, immobilization of the foot, rest, and support with an Unna boot, or taping and a soft temporary support, to be followed with a permanent orthotic device once edema has resolved. Chronic problems are treated with injection therapy, mobilization, manipulation, and orthotics. Chronic resistant cases are treated with excision of the midtarsal joint coalition by means of extensor brevis arthroplasty (see Ch. 26).

Bones of the Midfoot

The bones of the midfoot consist of the first, second, and third cuneiforms, the cuboid, and the navicular. The midtarsal bones form an archlike structure, termed the proximal transverse arch of the foot. Distally, this arch persists as the metatarsal transverse arch. Loss of the normal architecture of the midfoot occurs with pronation and prolapse of the arches. It may be accompanied by forefoot symptoms, such as central metatarsalgia or keratomas, as the normal transverse arch is reversed. When one examines the foot, there is hypermobility of the fifth and first metatarsals and relative plantar flexion of the second, third, and fourth metatarsals. The excessive force under the central metatarsals may be accompanied by Morton's neuromas, chronic bursitis or metatarsalgia, or both. Large keratomas may be present under metatarsal heads. Prolapse of the midfoot joints and loss of the normal transverse arch at the midtarsal level are accompanied by postural fatigue and plantar strain of the midtarsal joints. This problem is usually reversible with initial taping and strapping of the foot for the acute phase and then using soft supports and finally permanent orthotics to re-establish normal bony architecture of the foot. Strengthening and flexibility exercises are most helpful. The athletes should be taught to walk on their toes and how to strengthen the gravity and antigravity muscles appropriately. Of prime importance is strength of the anterior tibial, posterior tibial, and flexors. A tight gastrocnemius–soleus complex will plantar-flex the foot and predispose to excessive pronation and prolapse of the arch.

FRACTURES OF THE MIDTARSUS

Acute trauma may cause a fracture or fracture-dislocation of the tarsal joints. This requires closed or open reduction with internal fixation. The cuboid may become fractured with inversion plantar-flexory sprains. There may be a stress fracture or complete fracture. Treatment consists of appropriate reduction of the fracture and cast immobilization. The central cuneiforms may be involved with stress fractures. Acute fractures are rare.

The navicular may be involved in stress fractures, which require considerable attention.[44–49] The stress fractures may go undiagnosed despite pain over the navicular, which may result in a complete fracture and malunion. Treatment consists of non-weight-bearing cast immobilization until callus tissue is seen radiographically. An external bone stimulator is helpful when navicular fractures are present. Resistant fractures may require open reduction and a bone graft but, in almost all instances, these fractures will heal with appropriate immobilization and external bone stimulation.

The tubercle of the navicular may be avulsed with acute injuries; likewise, the os naviculare may be avulsed. These fractures are treated acutely, with cast immobilization. After the foot has been in a cast (a walking boot) for 6 weeks, physical therapy is begun. Abnormal pronation is corrected with an orthosis. If malunion occurs, which is not uncommon in both treated and missed cases, especially in case of the os naviculare, surgery (modified Kidner-Young procedure) is indicated (see Figs. 14-19 and 14-24).

THE REARFOOT

The rearfoot consists of the tarsal bones and the soft tissue structures that surround them. The calcaneus is plantar and somewhat lateral, with the talus being dorsal and medial. The tarsal bones are joined to the ankle at the articulation of the talus to the tibia and to the fibular and tibial malleoli. This hinge-type joint allows primarily for plantar flexion and dorsiflexion of the foot, with only a small amount of inversion or eversion. Between the talus and calcaneus is the subtalar joint, a triplane joint allowing for pronation and supination. At the junction of the talus and calcaneus to the midtarsus is the midtarsal joint, which allows for pronation and supination of the forefoot; thus the tarsal bones are involved in the primary motion of the foot. These motions enable the foot and leg to act as an adjustable strut and permit transverse plane rotations to be translated into forward progression motions in the foot.

Any trauma to tarsal bones, such as an intra-articular fracture, results in severe limitation of function to the athlete. An osteochondral fracture of the talus will result in severe limitation of motion with pain at the ankle joint. An intra-articular fracture of the calcaneus into the subtalar joint will result in restricted pronation and supination, and the athlete will be most uncomfortable on uneven surfaces. A subtalar coalition will similarly cause severe restricted motion and limited activity. Trauma affecting the midtarsal joint severely limits the ability of the forefoot to adapt to changing surfaces; it also decreases the ability of the athlete to have normal propulsive sequences.

The tarsal bones form the posterior pillar of the foot, and the talus and the calcaneus help dissipate impact shock at contact during running. This passive shock is registered as ground-resistive force at three times body weight. In reality, 16 to 17 times body weight may be passing through the calcaneus and absorbed by bone and surrounding soft tissue.[50,51] The locking and unlocking of joints and contact pronation helps dissipate this shock. Limited motion or locking mechanisms increase the shock and predispose to considerable injury.

Congenital malpositioning of the tarsal bones leads to permanent and stationary disability. Thus, excessive calcaneal varus with a high-pitched calcaneus leads to cavus foot. Excessive plantar flexion of the talus with calcaneal valgus leads to flatfoot. Overgrowth of the lateral aspect of the foot with an elongated calcaneus and metatarsus adductus leads to forefoot adductus. A long medial column with a short lateral column leads to pronation of the foot with abductus of the forefoot upon the rearfoot. Severe congenital deformities are present with clubfoot. It is estimated that 1 child in 1,000 is born with hypermobile flatfeet with plantar-flexed tali, which may result in disability in later life.

Soft Tissue of the Rearfoot

The skin of the rearfoot consists of the thick plantar fat pad under the calcaneus, extending into the midfoot, and of the thinner skin at the posterior aspect of the calcaneus, extending medially and laterally into the midfoot. The plantar fat pad consists of columnar arrangements of fat beneath the thick plantar skin. This acts as a shock absorber and helps dissipate stress. Atrophy of the fat pad, as occurs in the aging process and with rheumatoid arthritis, predisposes the calcaneus to increased shock and resulting calcaneodynia. Athletes such as long-distance runners, who lose considerable total body fat, tend to have less plantar fat pad protection and may be susceptible to greater plantar heel injury.

The posterior aspect of the heel may form blisters over the retrocalcaneal prominence. Excessive motion of the heel in the counter of the shoe predisposes to blisters. Retrocalcaneal exostosis or excessive posterior calcaneal pitch will impinge soft tissue between the posterior one-third of the calcaneus and the counter of the shoe, predisposing to bursitis or soft tissue injury, such as blisters. Treatment consists of padding the foot with moleskin or with one-eighth-inch foam. The counter of the shoe must be softened or removed by a cobbler; abnormal motion is controlled by taping and soft supports followed by more permanent orthoses. The use of tincture of benzoin over the blister and moleskin is most helpful.

HYPERKERATOSIS

The skin itself can become very painful from plantar fissures of the heel margins, usually posteriorly and laterally. These are associated with dry skin and with wearing sandals or going barefooted. Dietary supplementation with essential fatty acids (3ω, 6ω, and 9ω fatty acids, found in cold-pressed flax seed oil) is often helpful. As with any bony or soft tissue injury or condition, I would be remiss in not considering the nutritional factors (see also Ch. 5). Among them are the bioflavinoids, enzymes, trace minerals, and intermediate catalysts. Herbs, including valerian, are helpful in reducing pain. The skin must be softened and lubricated with topicals [25 percent lactic acid cream, aloe gel, and Kari (Bristol-Myers) lotion are all helpful], and thick stockings must be worn. Initially, padding with moleskin, molefoam, First Skin, or Spenco (Spenco Corp, NJ) decreases symptoms. When fissures are associated with lateral varus heel wear, an orthotic or heel cup is useful. Deep fissures may need debridement with tissue nippers. Seemingly innocuous fissures can cause severe pain and can alter ambulation and athletic function much in the same way as a blister.

PLANTAR FAT PAD SYNDROME

The plantar fat pad syndrome is described as pain at the plantar aspect of the calcaneus proximal to the region where the heel-spur syndrome would occur.[52] Palpation of the heel reveals a thick, painful consolidation of fat. This may be associated with bursitis occurring between the plantar aspect of the calcaneus and the fat pad itself. It also may be associated with medial calcaneal neuritis or neuroma, which may be involved in a fatty bursal mass at the plantar aspect of the heel.

The diagnosis is made by lubricating the tissue to facilitate palpation and by palpating the plantar mass. Palpation of the medial side of the foot may reveal a clicking mass consistent with a medial calcaneal neuroma. At times, a true neuroma is not present; in fact, there is merely an entrapment neuropathy secondary to impingement of the nerve during pronation. The medial and plantar skin impinges upon the nerve at contact during pronation. The pain of plantar fat pad syndrome is present upon contact; rising on the ball of the foot or stretching the plantar fascia does not usually aggravate the pain. With plantar fasciitis or heel-spur syndrome, the opposite is true. Radiographs may be negative or positive for heel spur, but the pain is usually absent distally over the spur and present more proximally. Plantar fat pad syndrome may be present in any foot type, and there does not seem to be a predisposition for it to occur in a more pronated foot. It appears to be secondary to increased contact pressure and to subsequent pathology of the plantar fat pad.

Treatment consists of initially taping the foot to keep the fat under the heel. Heel cups are useful. A well-molded orthotic to decrease abnormal pronation or foot motions and stabilize the calcaneus while holding the fat under the calcaneus is helpful. Appropriate shoes with shock-absorbing midsoles are helpful. Chronic problems will respond to an intrabursal injection. Injection into the fat pad itself with cortisone, however, will cause atrophy of the fat pad and further aggravate the symptoms. Injection with Traumeel, *Ruta graveolens*, or Zeel (homeopathic cocktail) is safe and often effective. These problems usually respond to conservative therapy with physical therapy, nutritional supplementation, herbs, homeopathic remedies (Traumeel, *Ruta graveolens*, Zeel, *Rhus toxicodendron*), analgesics, and anti-inflammatory medications. Viscoelastic heel pads or cups as well as other forms of shock-absorbing material (Poron, Spenco, Violyte) are helpful. Differential diagnosis includes stress fracture of the calcaneus or rheumatoid variants.

Chronic persistent bursitis or retrocalcaneal irritation with radiographic evidence of retrocalcaneal exostosis, retrocalcaneal step, or increased Fowler posterior angulation of the calcaneus may be an indication for surgical correction.[53-55] Procedures involve excision of the retrocalcaneal exostosis with or without osteotomy of the calcaneus (depending on the extent of calcaneal inclination and posterior protuberance) with a dorsal wedge to decompress the posterior aspect and realign the calcaneus. Osteotomies are most helpful when there is an excessive Fowler's angle with no true exostosis, or excessive calcaneal varus predisposing to abnormal pronation at the rearfoot and injury. A biplane osteotomy would be indicated if a two-plane deformity is present (see Ch. 26).

TINEA PEDIS

Tinea pedis may be present anywhere on the skin. Chronic tinea pedis can be on the heel or in the midfoot. It usually presents with redness and itchiness, but may simply appear as dryness and flakiness of the skin. A skin culture for fungus can be taken. Treatment is simple, consisting of soaking the feet in one-half cup of vinegar in a pan of water once a day and applying a topical antifungal agent, such as Lotrimin (clotrimazole) cream. Systemic antifungals are seldom necessary. Antifungal powders are helpful in socks and shoes.

In-depth internal gut function functional tests are essential in treating and reversing the cause of cutaneous fungal infections. These infections are always associated with gut dysbiosis, acquired or iatrogenic (see Ch. 5). Homeopathy and homeotoxicology for drainage and detoxification are an essential part of the global treatment of the whole person (see Ch. 39).

HYPERHIDROSIS OR BROMHIDROSIS

Smelly, sweaty feet are not uncommon in athletes. The more one exercises the greater is one's capacity to dissipate heat by perspiration. Bromhidrosis (smelly feet) is indicative of subtle dysregulation of proper fluid and detoxification pathways. It requires a functional evaluation and finally detoxification, drainage, and correction of any associated gut dysbiosis.

For smelly or sweaty feet, it is necessary to keep the feet dry. I prefer telling the athlete to use soaks or compresses of dilute white vinegar (one-half cup vinegar in a pan of water). Spraying the feet with a deodorant may initially be helpful, but antiperspirants should be avoided. They stop the very reaction the body needs to detoxify and regulate heat, invariably driving the disease deeper into the body, not to mention the potential for antiperspirant-associated aluminum toxicity and concomitant nerve and brain dysfunction. Powders to decrease retention of moisture, such as baby powder or talc (this powder should not be inhaled), are helpful. For resistant cases, utilization of Drysol (aluminum chloride and ethyl alcohol), a commercially available product, is most helpful. It is painted onto the feet in the evening; occlusive dressings, using plastic bags, are applied for the evening. This may be carried out initially every other day and then perhaps once or twice a week for maintenance.

Homeopathic silicea, 6x or 12x, or calcaria carbonica 6x or 12x is helpful for smelly, cool feet. Warmer sweaty, smelly feet often respond to homeopathic sulphur, 6x or 12x, 3 tabs bid.

VERRUCA

Verrucae may be present at the plantar aspect of the foot at any level. These warts are secondary to papillomavirus infection and are best treated conservatively in the athlete, using topical applications of acid. Verrucae are treated in the same manner as described in the forefoot section of this chapter, using Duofilm, which is 15 percent salicylic acid and 15 percent lactic acid in a flexible collodion base. This is applied daily and, once a week, the verrucae are pared down. The verrucae present in the rearfoot, as in the forefoot, as well-circumscribed lesions with white and black dots secondary to perpendicular nerves and capillaries. Chronic resistant verrucae may require punch biopsy followed by laser ablation, avoiding damage to the cutaneous dermal layer, which could result in painful scarification.

SEED CORNS

Seed corns may be found on the plantar aspect of the foot, as either plantar keratomas or porokeratosis plantaris discretum. These well-circumscribed, punctate keratotic lesions may be quite painful. Treatment consists of curettage and debridement. Initial treatment may require a local injection to allow deep debridement. Once controlled, regular follow-up treatment involves only paring and debridement.

Porokeratotic lesions are generally more painful than seed keratomas upon compression, and they appear histologically as a plugged sweat gland syndrome. Treatment of porokeratotic lesions is paring, accommodation, and occasionally injection with a corticosteroid or homeopathic cocktail (injectable silica or graphites are often helpful). These preparations help to dissolve the contents of the plugged sweat gland. Resistant cases do well with laser ablation.

Nerves

The rearfoot nerves are similar to those described for the midfoot. The major problem in these nerves is entrapment, superficial or deep. Thus the patient may have entrapment of the superficial peroneal nerves, musculocutaneous nerves, sural nerve, or saphenous nerve. Peroneal outlet syndrome refers to binding down of the superficial peroneal nerve at the neck of the fibula as it pierces the peroneal fascia to become superficial. It may be associated with proximal peroneal neck entrapment, the so-called double crush syndrome, which renders distal nerves more vulnerable to pressure or entrapment reactions. Both are commonly associated with fibular subluxations, which often respond remarkably to fibular manipulation and adjustment. Biomechanical predisposing factors are, of course, dealt with by means of foot orthotics. These nerve entrapments may be associated with underlying bony prominences. Radiography, MRI, EMG, and nerve conduction studies are all helpful in evaluation.

Tarsal tunnel syndrome, like its counterpart in the wrist carpal tunnel, is a serious problem that occurs under the medial malleolus. The contents of the tarsal tunnel become entrapped under the lacineate ligament (flexor retinaculum).

With all nerve entrapments, supplementation with pyridoxine (vitamin B_6), 300 mg/day, along with vitamin B_{12}, 1-ml subcutaneous injection weekly, helps the nerve recover. Lysis injections with local anesthetic 1 ml vitamin B_{12}, vitamin B_6 Wydase, and Traumeel or *Hypericum*, with or without cortisone (soluble and insoluble), are often effective. These may be given weekly as long as very little or no cortisone is used. Following the injections with ultrasound is often helpful in further breaking up adhesions and preventing postinjection flare-up. Bony underlying spurs, or chronic fibrosis, will require surgical neurolysis with decompression. Peripheral nerve surgery, in the best of hands and with ideal circumstances, is still a crapshoot; the physician should proceed with all due caution and informed consent.

SUPERFICIAL NERVE ENTRAPMENT

Superficial nerves, consisting of the saphenous at the dorsomedial aspect of the ankle, the superficial peroneal with its branches at the dorsolateral aspect of the foot, and the sural at the lateral aspect of the foot, can be a problem. Entrapment of these nerves is usually secondary to tight-fitting foot gear with secondary compression, or it may be secondary to abnormal traction. Treatment is supportive, using physical therapy modalities, resting of the foot, and finally balancing of the foot. Injection therapy or nutritional supplementation as noted in the preceding section may prove fruitful. When all else fails, surgery may be contemplated, but the results are mixed. A decompression of the nerve with neurolysis is suggested if there is enough fatty tissue to cover the nerve following the surgical procedure. Excising underlying bony prominences is helpful. In the very thin patient with loss of subcutaneous fat, a neurectomy may be necessary (see Ch. 26). If so, the free end of the nerve must be buried in muscle to avoid a painful stump neuroma.

Muscles

The muscles in the rearfoot are similar to those of the midfoot. These are the broad flat plantar stabilizers in the foot, the flexor brevis and the quadratus planti. They are occasionally strained with sudden movement or sprained with chronic repetitive stress, such as pronation. They respond to supportive therapy, rest, and orthoses. The same may be said of the dorsal extensor brevis tendon, which has its origin from the lateral dorsal aspect of the calcaneus.

Tendons

The tendons of the rearfoot are the same as those for the midfoot with the exception of the posterior triceps surae. These tendons are stabilizers and prime movers. Their functions, along with their respective muscles, may be concentric, eccentric, or isometric. This must be appreciated and accounted for in passive and active rehabilitation (see Ch. 21).

TENDINOPATHY OF THE TRICEPS SURAE

The gastrocnemius, soleus, and plantaris form the triceps surae, which attaches into the posterior middle one-third of the calcaneus. The soleus has its origin from the fibula and the posterior aspect of the tibia. It then inserts into the Achilles tendon and finally into the posterior surface of the calcaneus. The gastrocnemius is a biarticulate muscle with its origin from the posterior aspect of the femur near the condyles distally. Because of its biarticular nature, it is more susceptible to injury as a stabilizer and mover of both the knee joint and the ankle and subtalar joints. The soleus likewise has its main influence on the ankle and subtalar joints. The plantaris is a small, somewhat insignificant muscle that arises laterally at the posterior aspect of the leg and inserts into the medial aspect of the calcaneus. The gastrocnemius–soleus complex is a major supinator and stabilizer of the rearfoot. It is also responsible for propulsion during gait.

Achilles tendinopathy may be acute or chronic. Chronic problems present as tenosynovitis or partial or complete rupture. Kvist[56] estimates that two-thirds of Achilles tendon injuries in competitive athletes are paratenonitis and one-fifth are insertional complaints (bursitis and insertional tendinitis). The remaining afflictions consist of complaints related to the myotendinous junction and tendinopathies. The sequelae of tenosynovitis or incomplete rupture may be central necrosis of the Achilles tendon, which may present with or without symptoms. Tendinosis or central necrosis of the Achilles tendon, occurring around the posterior aspect of the Achilles, may be asymptomatic if there is no coexistent paratenonitis.

The gastrocnemius–soleus complex comprises four-fifths of the bulk of the leg. This posterior muscle absorbs a considerable amount of shock, as does the Achilles tendon. The age and nutritional status of the patient affect the health and circulation of the Achilles tendon. Generalized atherosclerotic conditions are correlated with degeneration of the Achilles tendon. Circulation to the Achilles tendon decreases after the age of 25, and the fibroblasts of the Achilles tendon in the adult are inactive after 52; thus healing of a partial rupture of the Achilles tendon is dependent on metaplasia from fat cells, which change into fibroblasts and allow for healing.

Acute Achilles tendon tenosynovitis presents as pain over the posterior aspect of the Achilles tendon. The correct term is *paratenonitis*, inasmuch as the Achilles tendon does not have a true sheath, but rather a paratenon, which is loose fatty areolar tissue that moves in concert with the Achilles tendon. Fibrosis of the paratenon secondary to tenosynovitis causes pain upon motion. This has been referred to as adhesive tendinopathy. Essentially a postinflammatory "glue" forms between the tendon and the paratenon. Palpation of the Achilles tendon, when acute tenosynovitis is present, reveals pain over a portion of the Achilles tendon. The examiner usually can feel inflammation in the paratenon. When there has been excessive pronation, the injury is more likely to be at the medial aspect of the tendon. With excessive supination, the injury may be more lateral. The tendon is carefully palpated to rule out a rift or partial rupture. Fusiform swelling may indicate intratendinous damage or partial rupture. Localized palpable swelling in the paratenon is more indicative of tenosynovitis. Soft tissue radiographs may be helpful to delineate this problem, as may xerograms.[57] Newer imaging methods, such as MRI and ultrasound, are very helpful.

Treatment of acute tenosynovitis consists of the supportive anti-inflammatory measures of icing, rest, analgesics and anti-inflammatory medications, and homeopathic, herbal, and nutritional aids. Corticosteroids should not be used in the Achilles tendon, as they predispose to significant central necrosis, degeneration, and partial or complete rupture. A homeopathic cocktail is usually effective, and normally safe. Rest is crucial, as are anti-inflammatory physical therapy measures. Deep transverse friction soft tissue techniques, if they can be tolerated by the patient, will often reverse the condition, especially if complemented with lysis injections. Of course, once the homeopathic medicine and local anesthetic cocktail is administered, deep transverse friction is painlessly carried out as adhesions are palpated, then released. Ultrasound has been shown to actually stimulate collagen synthesis.

Running may have to be stopped for 3 to 6 weeks and replaced by aerobic activities such as biking and swimming. Failure to eliminate the inflammation and repeated insults may lead to repeated adhesive inflammation and eventual degeneration of the tendon from endogenous enzymes, leading to partial and then complete rupture.

Chronic Tenosynovitis

Chronic tenosynovitis is treated with physical therapy (deep transverse friction massage). Ultrasound three times a week, as well as interferential or electrogalvanic stimulation, is most helpful. This is carried out for 3 weeks. Oral anti-inflammatory medications and remedies are used. Ice massage is helpful. Trigger point or lysis injections are valuable. Acupuncture has been helpful for some patients.

The patient should begin an active program of stretching and strengthening. Foot imbalances must be corrected initially with temporary and then with permanent support.

Chronic resistive paratenonitis or tenosynovitis will respond to surgical tenolysis. This has been termed *stripping of the paratenon*. The results have been uniformly satisfactory (see Ch. 26).

Partial Rupture

A partial acute rupture presents with extreme pain and swelling over a portion of the Achilles tendon at the retrocalcaneal area. There is usually more discomfort and pain present than with a paratenonitis. Ecchymosis and bleeding may be present. Treatment consists of ice, anti-inflammatory measures, and rest, using a posterior splint or cast. Immobilization and rest for 3 to 4 weeks are recommended. A posterior splint is helpful because it can be removed and physical therapy instituted immediately, using ultrasound, interferential, or electrogalvanic stimulation. Additionally, a posterior splint permits ambulation without pain and rests the Achilles tendon. Excessive plantar flexion when applying the splint should be avoided, as it leads to calf contracture. I prefer to hold the foot in neutral position. It takes 4 to 6 weeks for partial ruptures to heal, after which an aggressive rehabilitation regimen is instituted to improve balance, flexibility, and strength, while eliminating adhesions. The athlete should not be allowed to run for 6 weeks following this form of injury; a gradual return to activity is then permissible. Substitution of aerobic activity is important during initial rehabilitation. As previously noted, tendon injury healing is facilitated and accelerated with homeopathic and nutritional supplementation.

Chronic partial ruptures are those that persist beyond 6 to 8 weeks. Initially, physical therapy is carried out, especially if no treatment has been rendered in the past. Correcting abnormal biomechanics and instituting balance, strength, and flexibility exercises are most helpful. For chronic resistive cases, a surgical repair is indicated (see Ch. 26).

Complete Rupture—Acute

In an athlete, acute complete rupture is best treated with primary repair. There have been reports in the literature of cast immobilization for 10 to 12 weeks, starting first with an above-knee cast and then gradually proceeding to a walking BK boot.[57,58] However, this prevents full recovery of the strength of the gastrocnemius–soleus complex, so it is therefore preferable to do surgery whenever possible in an athlete to ensure maximal results. Surgery may be an open primary repair or closed percutaneous suturing (see Ch. 26).

Chronic Achilles Tendon Rupture

There have been patients who have had complete rupture of the Achilles tendon who have not sought appropriate treatment. They may present 2 to 3 months following the rupture with significant atrophy of the gastrocnemius–soleus complex and inability to toe off. Despite this, most are ambulatory, although exhibiting a limp with associated pain. The treatment of choice for these patients is surgical repair; I have found it useful to put a tendon graft or synthetic woven Dacron (Meadox) graft in place. The postoperative course is prolonged, but the results are usually good. It may take a year or more for complete recovery from the surgical repair of this injury (see Ch. 26).

POSTERIOR TIBIAL TENDON INJURY

The posterior tibial tendon in the rearfoot is under considerable strain as it functions at heel contact to help decelerate the rapid internal rotation of the lower extremity. Accumulated microtrauma (overuse) can cause tenosynovitis. Acute injury, such as a sprain with excessive pronation, can cause detachment of the posterior tibial from one of its attachments, or tenosynovitis, or partial rupture. A sprain of the midtarsal joint can cause avulsion of the os naviculare and secondary chronic tenosynovitis of the posterior tibial. A rupture of the posterior tibial tendon causes immediate breakdown of the medial longitudinal arch with unrestrained pronation—so-called unilateral idiopathic flatfoot.

Acute Tenosynovitis

Acute tenosynovitis of the posterior tibial tendon in the rearfoot occurs in the area from the medial malleolus to the os naviculare. An acute episode follows prolonged use, such as in a long run, or may occur secondary to an explosive activity or sudden twist of the foot. Acute tenosynovitis can also occur secondary to excessive pressure from foot gear. Inflammation of the synovial sheath of the posterior tibial tendon is obvious. Clinically, there may be a grating sensation or crepitation with motion of the posterior tibial as the foot goes through a range of motion. The classic signs of inflammation are present, with pain on motion, especially when the foot is inverted or when it is averted against resistance. Tenosynovitis may cause increased damage to the tendon and sheath with continued activity. Rest, as well as modalities to decrease inflammation (physical therapy, nutritional, herbal, homeopathic, or allopathic), are required before return to activity. One must rule out intratendinous damage, such as central necrosis or partial rupture. Ultrasound imaging often works well and is far less expensive than conventional MRI. Pain and inflammation that subside following rest and physical therapy but return following activity suggest either chronic tenosynovitis or intratendinous damage. Surgical decompression or repair of the tendon, or both, may be necessary. Metabolic causes of tenosynovitis, such as gout or collagen diseases, should be ruled out. Occasionally, there may be an infectious tenosynovitis. When there is pain along the navicular tubercle, one must rule out avulsion fracture of an os naviculare or stress fracture of the navicular associated with tenosynovitis of the posterior tibial tendon.

When acute tenosynovitis of the posterior tibial tendon is present, rest, ice, compression, and elevation (RICE) are the initial treatments of choice. Short-term, quick-acting analgesics and anti-inflammatory medications are helpful. Traumeel oral along with topical *Arnica* cream or Traumeel cream is useful. The acute episode subsides within 48 to 72 hours; the athlete can then usually start gentle training again. The etiology of the incident must be ascertained and corrected. In the case of training errors, appropriate counseling is necessary. When there is excessive pronation, an orthosis is used. If the area is weakened, it must be rested and protected with bracing or taping methods. A low-dye taping helps re-establish the medial longitudinal arch and decrease pronation, which puts excessive loading on the posterior tibial tendon (level 1 at the navicular insertion, or level 2 between the insertion and the medial maleolus). Proximal posterior or tibial injury at (level 3) or above (level 4) the medial malleolus are better treated with a high-dye Elastikon strapping or an Unna boot. A high-dye strapping adds additional support to the posterior tibial tendon.

When the acute problem is still symptomatic in the

chronic phase, physical therapy is indicated. Ultrasound and electrogalvanic stimulation are helpful initially. If there is no response to this form of therapy, one might consider interferential, ultrasound, Dynawave, or Electroacuscope stimulation. These modalities are generally used three times a week for 3 to 6 weeks, until the athlete is asymptomatic. Then a gradual return to activity is enhanced with soft temporary orthotics or supportive taping of the foot and ankle. The soft supports are replaced with more permanent devices once they are found to be effective. Controlling pronation relaxes tension and stress on the posterior tibial tendon. Taping is used until the patient becomes asymptomatic in workouts, generally for 1 to 2 months. If pain persists and it is difficult to identify whether there is a soft tissue or bony etiology to the pain, radiographs or MRI should be done. Even if these studies are negative, there may be stress reaction of bone or stress fracture; a bone scan is indicated in these difficult cases. For involved cases in which taping does not control symptoms of pain with ambulation, a removable posterior fiberglass splint, or premade adjustable removable cast boot, may offer suitable protection and rest for the lower extremity and yet allow for appropriate rehabilitation, such as swimming and physical therapy.

Acute Sclerosing Tenosynovitis

When there is crepitation, edema, and pain along the posterior tibial tendon, a surgical emergency may be the end result.[21,26–28,59] If these problems fail to subside immediately with RICE, the possibility of a tenolysis must be considered. Most acute and overuse sports injuries do respond to conservative measures. Infectious problems often require open drainage or tenolysis, or both.

Chronic Tenosynovitis

Chronic tenosynovitis is usually an overuse problem but may be the sequela of an acute problem. In the event of an acute problem that then becomes chronic, there is usually discomfort or pain with ambulation, which becomes more severe with the increased activity of running or jumping. This is accompanied by swelling along the medial aspect of the foot along the course of the posterior tibial tendon. There is usually tenderness upon palpation of the sheath and posterior tibial tendon, and pain upon supinating the foot against resistance.

Chronic posterior tibial tenosynovitis usually starts off as discomfort during exercise, progresses to pain during exercise, and persists for 1 or 2 hours after exercise. Ignoring the signs and symptoms of tenosynovitis and continuing to abuse the tendon results in pain during normal ambulation as well as at rest, greatly hindering athletic performance. At times crepitation is present, but more often there is an inflammation and swelling of the synovial sheath of the posterior tibial tendon with pain upon palpation.

The differential diagnosis includes tenosynovitis of the flexor hallucis longus and flexor digitorum longus, as well as tarsal tunnel syndrome. Tarsal tunnel syndrome usually involves a different type of pain. The pain is sharper, and there is a positive Tinel's sign upon percussing the neurovascular bundle beneath the medial malleolus. There is no numbness associated with posterior tibial tenosynovitis, whereas there may be numbness with tarsal tunnel syndrome. It must be noted that posterior tibial tenosynovitis can be coexistent with a tarsal tunnel syndrome. In this instance, there is tenosynovitis of the posterior tibial and, perhaps, the other flexors in the area of the tarsal tunnel, causing swelling and compressing the neurovascular bundle. MRI is very helpful in these cases.

Treatment for tenosynovitis of the posterior tibial initially consists of resting the lower extremity and engaging in physical therapy. Ice massage and transverse friction are of use. Gentle progressive resistive stretching and strengthening exercises are helpful. I use elastic surgical tubing or a bicycle inner tube around the foot to allow for some resistance during inversion of the foot. Homeopathic or anti-inflammatory medications are helpful. Lysis injections with a homeopathic cocktail or a small amount of corticosteroids usually provide relief, but repeated injections with cortisone may lead to rupture. That being the case, they should be used with caution, and the athlete should decrease activity for 3 weeks following an injection. I have also found that ultrasound immediately after an injection enhances its effect.[60]

While the maximum number of cortisone injections is generally three, with each injection combining a small amount of long- and slow-acting corticosteroid, administered at weekly intervals, there are no such limits on the homeopathic injectable cocktail. Following injections the athlete may run lightly, with duration and speed reduced. Biking and swimming as alternative aerobic activities are encouraged.

As with most injuries of the lower extremity, a biomechanical approach is helpful. Thus, when imbalance in the foot is present, a soft temporary support is used. If this is helpful, then a more permanent orthosis is utilized. Because posterior tibial muscle and tendon absorb considerable force during contact and pronation, an orthosis is usually helpful when pathology is present. Even feet that appear to be biomechanically sound may benefit from an orthosis due to the functional varus present in unidirectional sports, such as running. In these instances, an orthotic acts like a cant and decreases the strain on the posterior tibial and other flexors at contact and into midstance. A full-length orthosis with a medial forefoot wedge decreases propulsive pronation and positions the foot in a better attitude for the next contact phase. This also reduces strain on the posterior tibial tendon.

Posterior tibial tenosynovitis that is chronic in nature and not responsive to the usual conservative measures may require surgical exploration. In these instances, a tenolysis is performed and any coexistent pathology of the posterior tibial tendon itself is repaired surgically. A tendon graft or modified Kidner-Young or Cobb tendon reinforcement may be necessary, if there has been central necrosis or a partial rupture of significance.[61-63]

The results of surgery are predictably good when there is pathology of the synovial sheath and the tendon itself is healthy. The extremity is casted in supination for 3 weeks; a posterior splint is then used for an additional 2 to 3 weeks. During this time, physical therapy is carried out at least three times a week, or more if possible, and biking is allowed. Swimming is started as soon as sutures are out and the cast is off, usually within 3 weeks. At the end of 6 weeks, a gradual return to running is instituted.

Posterior Tibial Tendon Rupture

Partial or complete rupture of the posterior tibial tendon creates considerable disability. Running is usually impossible. If a complete rupture has occurred, there is rapid prolapse of the foot. When partial rupture is present, there is still activity of the posterior tibial tendon when the foot is supinated against resistance, but there is considerable pain, and a void is usually palpable.

Treatment for a partial rupture is that of cast immobilization for 4 to 6 weeks with the foot supinated. Physical therapy is then instituted utilizing various modalities, including strengthening and stretching exercises. If the conservative approach is unsuccessful, a surgical repair is indicated.

Complete rupture should be treated immediately with surgical anastomosis. The foot is then immobilized for 4 weeks, followed by physical therapy. Results for repair of acute ruptures are generally good as long as the repair is undertaken within 5 to 7 days of the injury.

Neglected or undiagnosed complete rupture of the posterior tibial tendon can become a considerable problem. Surgical repair should be performed to attempt an end-to-end anastomosis. If balling up has occurred at the ends of the tendons, this excessive collagen tissue must be excised, and the void must be filled with a tendon graft or a graft with a suitable synthetic material, such as woven Dacron. Failure to achieve a strong union results in prolapse of the foot, with excessive pronation and eventually considerable disability. Posterior tibial complete ruptures that have been undiagnosed for 2 to 4 months can be repaired surgically but usually break down over time. In these instances, subtalar or triple arthrodesis may be necessary to restore function to the foot and rid the patient of considerable pain and swelling.

THE LONG FLEXORS

The flexor hallucis longus and flexor digitorum longus have a function similar to that of the posterior tibial tendon: they decrease the rapid internal rotation of the lower extremity at contact. The flexor hallucis longus and flexor digitorum longus also stabilize the metatarsophalangeal joints during toe-off. During jumping sports, these tendons help plantar flex the toes and increase spring from the ground.

Unaccustomed use of the long flexors results in tenosynovitis. Thus running hard and fast on the balls of the feet can produce pain and symptoms. Excessive pronation with propulsion also puts excessive load on the long flexors, producing tenosynovitis and pain.

Flexor Hallucis Longus Tenosynovitis

Tenosynovitis of the flexor hallucis longus is often associated with an os trigonum syndrome.[64,65] The os trigonum is an ossicle at the lateral posterior process of the talus. The posterior talofibular collateral ligament of the ankle attaches here. An avulsion fracture or impaction fracture of the os trigonum or posterolateral process of the talus may occur with an inversion plantar-flexory sprain or with excessive plantar flexion of the foot on the ankle. This causes pain with motion of the flexor hallucis longus, which passes in a tunnel alongside this bony process on the talus. Thus, when the athlete toes off or uses the big toe, there is pain at the posterior aspect of the subtalar joint, somewhat lateral to the Achilles tendon. Radiographs may show an os trigonum or fracture of the posterior process of the talus. Clinically, there is pain upon palpation of the posterior aspect of the subtalar joint, and with moving the big toe up and down.

Crepitation may be present clinically. There is usually some soft tissue swelling. Injection of the os trigonal area with a small amount of lidocaine and Marcaine will stop the pain for 3 to 6 hours. The pain then rapidly recurs. This helps confirm the diagnosis. Radiographs are helpful, as is a bone scan or MRI if an acute fracture is present.

Treatment of flexor hallucis longus tendinopathy associated with os trigonum syndrome is usually surgical. The os trigonum or fractured or dystrophic posterolateral process of the talus must be excised. The prognosis for this surgery is good. The usual postoperative course is that of physical therapy modalities and appropriate rehabilitation.

Flexor Digitorum Longus Tenosynovitis

Tenosynovitis of the flexor digitorum longus is accompanied by pain anteromedial and anterior to the Achilles tendon. This pain progresses into the foot as the flexor digitorum longus dives deep into the plantar aspect of the foot near the porta pedis. The diagnosis is made by flexing the toes and palpating the course of the long flexor tendon. Treatment consists initially of rest and anti-inflammatory medication, as well as physical therapy. Excessive pronation or propulsive pronation is corrected with an orthosis. For some events, taping of the medial longitudinal arch and the use of elastic tape around the toes to prevent excessive dorsiflexion are helpful. This is true in the case of strains at the flexor hallucis longus and the flexor digitorum longus. Crest pads might likewise be helpful to increase the leverage of the toes during propulsion. The crest pad is simply a dental roll at the plantar aspect of the foot at the junction of the toes and the ball of the foot. This may be held in place with elastic tape. Tenosynovitis of these long flexors that is not responsive to the usual conservative therapy may require a surgical decompression. This is rarely indicated, however.

EXTENSOR INJURY

The anterior tibial and the extensors make up the anti-gravity compartment of the leg, ankle, and foot. These tendons function at contact to decrease the impact shock on the ball of the foot. Thus, when contact takes place on the heel, these tendons gently lower the ball of the foot to the ground, resisting the force of gravity. They occupy the anterolateral aspect of the leg.

Anterior Tibial Tendon Tendinopathy

The anterior tibial tendon is involved in tenosynovitis at the rearfoot level secondary to excessive pronation or to compression. The anterior tibial tendon is isolated by dorsiflexing and inverting the foot against resistance. It is palpated until an area of pain and tenosynovitis is found. When tenosynovitis of the anterior tibial is accompanied by excessive pronation, an orthosis is helpful. As the medial longitudinal arch lowers, it puts strain on the anterior tibial tendon, which inserts at the medial plantar aspect of the first metatarsal–cuneiform joint.

Thus treatment for anterior tibial tenosynovitis or tendinopathy is that of resting the tendinous structures by the utilization of an orthosis or taping of the foot. When taping is used, a felt medial longitudinal arch pad is incorporated for additional support. Anti-inflammatory medications, homeopathic remedies, nutritional supplements, and appropriate physical therapy and rehabilitation are instituted. A homeopathic cocktail injection may be helpful.

Anterior Tibial Tendinitis With Underlying Bone Spurs

Tendinopathy of the anterior tibial tendon may be secondary to chronic irritation by underlying bone spurs. Dorsal talar neck impingement exostosis or spurs are often associated with anterior tibial tendinopathy. The spurs are usually palpable, and radiographs confirm the spurs. Radiographs in themselves may not show the extent of the spurring, as the spurs on the dorsal aspect of the talus may be somewhat medial and difficult to demonstrate radiographically. They are, however, readily palpable. Treatment initially is that of utilizing local anti-inflammatory modalities as well as medications, rest, and orthotics. If pain persists, however, then a surgical decompression is necessary. The spurs are easily excised and, when tenosynovitis is present, tenolysis is performed. The postoperative course is rapid, and return to full competition is anticipated within 6 to 8 weeks.

Partial or Complete Rupture of the Anterior Tibial Tendon

Partial or complete ruptures of the anterior tibial tendon are rare in my experience. When they occur, in the acute phase there is usually surrounding inflammation and ecchymosis. Partial ruptures are treated with cast immobilization; complete ruptures are treated with surgical reanastomosis. When the anterior tibial tendon has been completely avulsed from its attachment, then Bunnell pull-out wires are used in the surgical repair.

In some cases, anterior tibial tenosynovitis and underlying talar neck spurs are associated with compression of the neurovascular bundle anteriorly. When this is the case, there will be a positive Tinel's sign, and there may be numbness in the first interspace of the foot. The extensor retinaculum is tight, and there is chronic swelling of the anterior tibial tendon and, at times, of the surrounding extensor tendons. At surgery, the extensor retinaculum is sectioned and the neurovascular bundle inspected. During surgical closure, the retinaculum is not reattached inasmuch as this would create a surgical compression of the neurovascular bundle. This condition has been called anterior tarsal tunnel syndrome.

Extensor Hallucis Longus and Extensor Digitorum Longus Tendinopathy

Tendinopathy of the extensors is diagnosed by extending the hallux, and then the lesser toes, while palpating the extensors. There may be tenosynovitis secondary to compression, such as occurs in a tight ski boot or ice skate boot. Runners who lace their laces too tightly may have compression tendinopathy of the anterior tibial or extensors.

Treatment for compression problems is that of eliminating the compression. Shoes are tied differently, irritated eyelets are removed, and lacing is done in such a way as to avoid areas of irritation. This is especially true when there are underlying spurs that are symptomatic only when the laces cross them. Boots are modified to relieve pressure. Physical therapy and anti-inflammatory remedies or medications may be necessary initially to reduce symptoms. When these problems are chronic and shoe gear has been modified, removal of underlying causes, such as talar neck spurs, must be considered. Tendon adhesions or tenosynovitis is decompressed. However, surgery is usually unnecessary inasmuch as conservative measures most often suffice.

TENDINOPATHY OF THE PERONEALS

The peroneus longus and brevis tendons make up the lateral aspect of the leg and rearfoot. These tendons pass behind the lateral malleolus and then enter the foot. The peroneous tertius, which runs in front of the lateral malleolus, attaches at the dorsal aspect of the styloid process of the fifth metatarsal. The peroneous brevis attaches at the styloid process of the fifth metatarsal. The peroneus longus dives underneath the cuboid in the peroneal tunnel, where it attaches at the plantar aspect of the first metatarsal–cuneiform articulation. The peroneus longus functions in opposition to the posterior tibial. While the posterior tibial plantar-flexes and inverts the foot, the peroneus longus plantar-flexes and everts the foot. The peroneus brevis everts and, to a lesser extent, may plantar-flex the foot, whereas the anterior tibial tendon inverts and dorsiflexes the foot. The peroneus tertius functions along with the extensors. It dorsiflexes and mildly everts the foot.

Tenosynovitis of the Peroneus Longus

The peroneus longus tendon may be associated with tenosynovitis underneath the lateral malleolus or under the cuboid in the peroneal tunnel. A peroneal cuboid syndrome may be present when there is pain beneath the cuboid and tenosynovitis of the peroneus longus. This is diagnosed by everting the foot against resistance while palpating the peroneus longus tendon as it courses deep into the foot under the cuboid.[21a]

Treatment of peroneal cuboid syndrome involves cuboid manipulation followed by stabilizing the foot with a cuboid pad and taping. Resistant cases require trigger point injection therapy with a homeopathic cocktail at the calcanocuboid or cuboid–fifth metatarsal base joint, or both, and then manipulation. An *audible snap* assures that the subluxation is reduced. Peroneus longis tendon tethering or entrapment in the plantar cuboid tunnel often requires a lysis injection. Subsequent palpation reveals improved joint function and a smooth contour to the plantar lateral midfoot surface. With or without injection, with successful manipulation of the cuboid, the relief is dramatic and immediate.

Cavus feet require an orthotic with a lateral wedge and cuboid pad, whereas pronated feet require an orthosis with a medial longitudinal arch as well as a cuboid pad. A cuboid pad is one-quarter-inch felt placed underneath the cuboid, thinner at the lateral border and thicker at the medial border. This cuboid pad tends to invert the cuboid.

The cuboid may become everted or mildly subluxed during supination or inversion injuries of the foot. Manipulation of the cuboid into place and then taping and strapping of the foot is quite helpful. Taping is maintained for 3 to 4 weeks to allow ligament healing and joint stabilization. Eventually even the most stubborn cases resolve. Short-term valgus orthotic wedging may be necessary, along with strapping.

Peroneal tenosynovitis around the lateral malleolus may be secondary to excessive pronation or supination. There is swelling and pain beneath the fibular malleolus. Treatment consists of establishing normal running patterns with the use of orthoses and good shoes. Local anti-inflammatory measures, such as physical therapy, are used. Remedies, supplements, or medications are necessary initially; at times, a homeopathic cocktail or corticosteroid injection is helpful. When pain persists, stress fracture of the fibula must be ruled out.

Peroneus Brevis Tenosynovitis

The peroneus brevis is symptomatic more often at its attachment to the styloid process of the fifth metatarsal. The etiology may be an inversion sprain of the subtalar or midtarsal joint. There is pain upon palpation of the peroneus brevis tendon at its attachment near the fifth metatarsal base. Differential diagnosis includes stress fracture or complete fracture at the base of the fifth metatarsal or the styloid process of the fifth metatarsal. Treatment consists of rest and taping. If a fracture is present, a cast is used. Improper biomechanics are corrected, first with soft temporary supports and then with a more permanent orthosis. Appropriate physical therapy is undertaken; medications may also be helpful. A homeopathic cocktail or corticosteroid injection may be necessary.

Subluxing Peroneal Tendons

The peroneal tendons may sublux anteriorly over the fibular malleolus. When such subluxation is present, there has usually been trauma, such as a ski injury or basketball injury. During these instances, the foot is rapidly dorsiflexed as the leg moves forward. The peroneals move forward with the momentum of the leg and avulse off the peroneal retinaculum from the fibula. Radiographically, there may be a speck of bone present where this avulsion has taken place. Clinically, there is subluxation of the peroneals when the foot is dorsiflexed and everted and the leg moves anteriorly. When subluxation is concurrent with excessive pronation, an orthosis may help stabilize the foot and keep the peroneals behind the fibula. When the problem persists and pain is present, surgical reconstruction of the peroneal retinaculum is easily carried out.[66–68] Even when there is a shallow peroneal groove in the fibula, I have not found it necessary to regroove the fibula. In my experience peroneal retinaculoplasty suffices, and the results are uniformly good. The peroneal retinaculum is re-

constructed from surrounding soft tissue and anchored to the fibula through drill holes.

Peroneus Tertius Tendinopathy

The peroneus tertius may be involved in tenosynovitis near the base of the fifth metatarsal. This is diagnosed by dorsiflexing and everting the foot against resistance while palpating the peroneus tertius tendon. The etiology appears to be that of overuse and improper foot function. Uneven irregular surfaces seem to predispose this tendon to injury. Peroneal tendinitis may also be associated with cuboid subluxations. Treatment consists of local anti-inflammatory physical therapy measures, including cuboid manipulation, or tapping. Medications or an injection may be necessary. The problem usually responds satisfactorily and rapidly to simple treatment.

Joints of the Rearfoot

The joints of the rearfoot are composed of the ankle joint, the subtalar joint, and the midtarsal joint. Specific details as to the ankle joint are covered in Chapter 15. There are multiple ligaments between the joints, such as the spring ligament at the medial aspect of the foot. The spring ligament is the talocalcaneonavicular ligament, which helps support the talus. There is usually a fibrocartilaginous ossicle within the spring ligament at the plantar aspect of the talar head neck. This ligament can be sprained with acute injuries to the midtarsal or subtalar joint, or both. On the lateral side of the foot is the bifurcate ligament, which extends from the anterior lateral beak of the calcaneus to the inferior anterior distal aspect of the talus, and to the dorsal aspect of the cuboid. This ligament may be damaged with inversion injuries to the midtarsal joint. The long plantar ligament from the calcaneus to the cuboid can likewise be sprained, with dorsiflexion injuries to the midtarsal joint.

At the lateral aspect of the subtalar joint is the lateral talocalcaneal ligament, immediately beneath the peroneal ligaments, which may be ruptured with inversion sprains of the subtalar and ankle joint, leading to lateral instability of the subtalar joint.

The lateral collateral ligaments of the ankle include the anterior talofibular ligament; the middle collateral ligament, which is the calcaneofibular ligament; and the posterior talofibular ligament. The posterior talofibular ligament attaches to the os trigonum and may be involved with avulsion fractures of the os trigonum during plantar-flexion inversion injuries of the subtalar and ankle joints. The most commonly injured ligament at the ankle joint level is the anterior talofibular ligament. It is often avulsed from either the talus or the fibula or is ruptured in the central aspect.

At the medial aspect of the rearfoot is the deltoid apparatus. This ligament fans out from the medial malleolus to the sustentaculum tali of the calcaneus. It also attaches to the posteromedial aspect of the talus and calcaneus. Anteriorly, a deep branch, which goes from the medial malleolus to the talus and navicular, is injured with acute external rotatory fractures or with ruptures of the subtalar and ankle joints.

In the sinus tarsi, which is the tunnel between the posterior facet and middle facet of the subtalar joint, is the interosseous talocalcaneal ligament. This ligament is commonly injured with inversion foot and ankle sprain.

PATHOLOGY OF THE SUBTALAR JOINT

Pathology of the subtalar joint is secondary either to acute trauma, such as a fracture, or to a coalition.[69–72] Coalitions are embryonic overgrowths of the joints secondary to congenital causes. They usually become apparent between the ages of 12 and 14. They may be accompanied by peroneal spasm as the foot splints itself in pronation and external rotation. Often, the first symptom of coalition of the subtalar joint is pain when performing on irregular surfaces. The child may be involved in soccer or other sports that require cutting and turning. When these maneuvers are carried out, there is pain at the subtalar joint and the foot goes into peroneal spasm. The peroneus brevis is tight as the foot is externally rotated. Any joint of the subtalar complex can be involved with a coalition; thus there may be a coalition over the middle facet, anterior facet, or posterior facet. The posterior axial view of the subtalar joint facilitates delineation of the posterior facet pathology. Middle and anterior facet coalitions are more easily seen with computed tomography (CT) scan.

Conservative treatment consists of resting the foot in pronation by means of a pronated orthotic or cast immobilization. This approach may calm down the inflammation around the coalition and enable the child to continue to participate in sports, foregoing surgery.

Damage to the posterior facet of the subtalar joint usually necessitates a subtalar or triple arthrodesis following failure of conservative care. Damage to the middle facet may require the use of an excision of the coalition, provided there is no pathology to the posterior facet. I have

had limited experience and some success with the Dow-Corning silicone rubber condylar implant to fill the void of the excised middle facet coalition. This implant is anchored into the talus dorsally. The results of these procedures to date are encouraging, although I have only a small series of a dozen cases in younger (adolescent) patients. In young adults and older active patients, I prefer resecting the middle facet, which still results in limitation of motion, yet often yields a functional result without resorting to a subtalar arthrodesis. Coalitions or pathology of the anterior facet are treated rather easily with excision of the anterior lateral beak of the calcaneus. Results are usually gratifying.

Intra-articular pathology of the subtalar joints may lead to arthritis, which reacts similarly to a coalition—splinting of the foot with peroneal spasm. Ankylosis and fibrous adhesions are the usual post-traumatic sequelae. Finding the most comfortable position (usually one of pronation) of the foot and then maintaining it with an orthosis with a rearfoot post is helpful, as are serial injections followed by manipulation of the foot. Often fibrous adhesions associated with fibrous post-traumatic coalition can be lysed and motion restored. In the event that conservative therapy fails and there is considerable discomfort or pain, an abrasion arthroplasty, open or arthroscopic, or arthrodesis may be necessary. Inflammatory arthritis affecting the subtalar joint leads to chronic subtalar joint pain, especially when walking on irregular surfaces requiring pronation and supination. In these instances, injection, manipulation, a pronated orthosis, or fusion may be necessary. Arthralgia may respond to homeopathy, nutritional intervention (especially inflammatory bowel disease–associated arthritis), manipulation, physical therapy, orthosis, steroids, and/or NSAIDs.

Sinus Tarsi Syndrome

A condition exists over the sinus tarsi at the lateral aspect of the subtalar joint that is called the sinus tarsi fat pad impingement syndrome. This is often the late sequela of an inversion sprain of the ankle and subtalar joint. It may also occur secondary to pronatory sinus tarsi compression. With inversion plantar-flexion sprain there is usually injury to the interosseous talocalcaneal ligament. Chronic fibrosis and subsequent irritation ensue in the later stages of sprain healing, often well after the primary ankle injury has healed. Observation reveals swelling and a bulging mass in the sinus tarsi. Palpation reveals a firm, rubbery mass, and there is appreciable pain upon firm palpation. MRI will help confirm the diagnosis when in doubt. If there is pain with palpation and subtalar motion, a sinus tarsi syndrome may well be present. Treatment consists of homeopathic cocktail or corticosteroid injections followed by joint-specific mobilization and manipulation, and then physical therapy modalities such as interferential stimulation. Orthotics are necessary to maintain the foot in a functional neutral position. Conservative therapy often results in complete recovery from this condition. If the problem persists, especially when advanced fibrosis has set in, it will be necessary to excise the fibrotic contents of the sinus tarsi, with an arthotomy (synovectomy). Results are uniformly successful.

PATHOLOGY OF THE MIDTARSAL JOINT

The midtarsal joint may be involved in coalitions between any of the four bones. The most common coalition is that between the calcaneus and the navicular. The coalition may be a syndesmosis, synchondrosis, or synostosis. Synostosis may be either complete, with bony bridging, or incomplete. A sprain of the midtarsal joint may result in midtarsal pain by rupturing a syndesmosis or synchondrosis. Midtarsal joint coalitions present with pain at the midtarsal joint, usually at the anterior distal aspect of the calcaneus. This joint is found by palpating the origin of the extensor brevis tendon. This origin is at the anterior distal aspect of the calcaneus, somewhat laterally. It covers the lateral superior entrance to the midtarsal joint.

Initial treatment for suspected coalition or sprain, or both, of the midtarsal joint is that of injection with a homeopathic cocktail or corticosteroids to help break up the fibrous adhesions. The foot is then mobilized and manipulated, and physical therapy is instituted. Biomechanical abnormalities are corrected with an orthosis. Oral anti-inflammatory medications may be helpful. In the event that conservative therapy fails and plain radiographs, MRI, or CT scans show evidence of coalition, it may be easily excised with anticipated good results and restoration of functional motion. When the coalition is excised, the origin of the extensor brevis tendon is detached and placed from dorsal to plantar through the void. This is known as an extensor brevis arthroplasty of the midtarsal joint.

Bones of the Rearfoot

The bones of the rearfoot are the talus and the calcaneus. The calcaneus makes up the posterior pillar of the foot. Its weight-bearing surface consists of two plantar condyles, the large medial and the considerably smaller lateral. The medial is most often associated with heel-spur syndrome. On top of the calcaneus is the talus, which fits securely within the mortise of the ankle joint. During closed kinetic chain motions of the lower extremity, when the foot is on the ground, the talus moves with the leg, whereas the calcaneus moves with the foot underneath the talus at the subtalar joint. Thus the talus rotates internally when the foot pronates and rotates externally when the foot supinates. There is plantar flexion of the talus with pronation and dorsiflexion of the talus with supination.

FRACTURES

Fractures of the Calcaneus

Fractures of the calcaneus may be acute or subacute. Acute fractures of the calcaneus include a variety of classifications based on the configuration and mechanism of injury.[73,74] A common sports fracture of the calcaneus is that of the anterior beak. This may be an avulsion fracture secondary to inversion plantar flexion of the midfoot on the rearfoot. There is pain over the anterolateral aspect of the calcaneus, and the avulsion fracture is usually seen on a lateral and medial oblique radiograph. Treatment initially is conservative, with immobilization. If nonunion occurs or there is a loose-floating ossicle that does not respond to conservative therapy, it may be easily excised. This is called the calcaneal anterior beak fracture. Posterior calcaneal process fractures may respond to percutaneous pin fixation, whereas complicated intra-articular crush injuries may required open reduction and internal fixation, which still may necessitate subtalar fusion at a later stage.

Stress Fracture of the Calcaneus

Stress fractures of the calcaneus occur at the junction of the posterior body of the calcaneus with the mid-aspects of the calcaneus. These are overuse injuries secondary to accumulated microtrauma. They may not be present radiographically (Fig. 14-18 shows this in a tibial stress fracture) when the patient presents with pain over the mid-aspect of the calcaneus. There is usually pain with pressure from the mediolateral and lateral aspects of the heel. A bone scan or MRI will confirm the diagnosis.

Treatment consists of rest until healing is complete. Cast immobilization and non-weight bearing may be necessary with advanced stress fracture, especially if there is pain with ambulation. Often MRI will show extensive involvement, especially in postmenopausal or osteporotic women. Bone calcium loss must exceed 60 percent to show up on plain

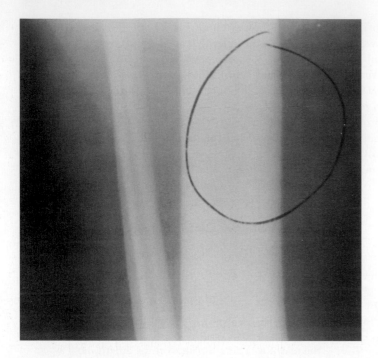

Figure 14-18 Radiograph of tibial stress fracture (in circle) demonstrates how difficult it can be to find a stress fracture on radiographs.

radiographs. Serum calcium levels will always be normal (9 to 11 mg/dl), even with osteoporosis. Bone density photon determinations are reliable evaluations. When in doubt, calcium, magnesium, and supportive trace elements should be supplemented (see Ch. 5). The cause of the overuse accumulated trauma should be investigated. It may be training errors accompanied by improper biomechanics, poor foot gear, and excessive stress to the lower extremity. Heel cups, soft viscoelastic or silicone gel heel pads, or an orthosis will assist the patient in being more comfortable during the convalescence.

Acute Fracture of the Talus

Acute fractures of the talar neck may be disastrous to the athlete. Since the blood supply to the body of the talus comes from the talar neck, there is a high incidence of avascular necrosis of the body of the talus with fractures through the neck. Fractures through the neck occur with sudden forceful dorsiflexion of the foot on the ankle. A similar fracture of the foot is seen in the os naviculare fracture shown in Figure 14-19.

Acute fractures may also occur at the posterior process of the talus, with or without a separate ossicle, the os trigonum. The os trigonum is at the lateral posterior process

of the talus, and may be avulsed with a plantar-flexory or inversion injury, which places tension at the insertion of the posterior fibulotalar ankle ligament into the talus or a separate os trigonum. There may also be a fracture of the posterior process of the talus during acute plantar-flexory injuries of the foot, termed *posterior talar compression*. The posterior process of the talus abuts upon the posteroinferior surface of the tibia, causing a compression fracture (Fig. 14-20). This is usually accompanied by pain of the flexor hallucis longus, which runs along the posterolateral process of the talus. Treatment initially is conservative, with cast immobilization. Despite this, malunion usually occurs, which is easily resolved with surgical excision of the fractured posterior talar shelf.

Following trauma, there may be accompanying decreased subtalar joint motion, with the posterior process of the talus articulating poorly with the adjacent portion of the calcaneus. This is called a posterior coalition of the subtalar joint; excision of this coalition usually results in improved function.

Stress Fracture of the Talus

Stress fractures of the talus are rare. I have not experienced any in my practice.

BONE LESIONS OF THE CALCANEUS

A bone lesion more commonly seen in the calcaneus in athletes is the unicameral bone cyst. This is seen in the body of the calcaneus; it is triangular in shape and lies immediately underneath the middle aspect of the subtalar joint. Seen radiographically, it is an embryonic void in the calcaneus. The danger of the unicameral bone cyst is that it may fracture with excessive activity. If a large cyst is present and the athlete is active, one might consider excising the cyst and packing the void with appropriate cancellous bone. I have had occasion to do this in two gifted teenage athletes with large cystic lesions extending to just under the subtalar joint. Both did very well, returning to full activity. These lesions are usually seen in teenagers.

Differentiation must be made between unicameral bone

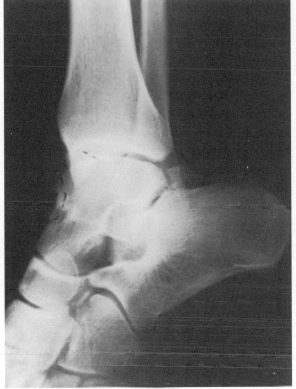

Figure 14-20 Lateral view of plantar-flexed foot showing posterior impingement at a fractured os trigonum. (From Marcus SA: Complications in Foot Surgery: Prevention and Management. 2nd Ed. Williams & Wilkins, Baltimore, 1984, with permission.)

cysts and aneurysmal bone cysts and other types of cystic bony lesions (i.e., giant cell tumor or fibrous dysplasia). More serious rare neoplasms or infective processes are also included in the differential diagnosis. A rare cystic lesion that may be found in the cuneiforms or the calcaneus is Ewing's sarcoma. I have treated one case of Ewing's sarcoma of the medial cuneiform in an athlete. This resulted in death 5 years after amputation. Bone lesions of the talus are rare, but one must realize that a bone lesion, whether benign or neoplastic, can occur in any bone in the foot.

SPURS AND EXOSTOSES OF THE CALCANEUS

Plantar Calcaneal Spurs

Plantar calcaneal spurs are termed *heel-spur syndrome*[75-77] (Fig. 14-21). The plantar condyles of the calcaneus are the origin of the plantar fascia and the deep intrinsic muscles of the foot. Chronic pulling of these muscles on the plantar

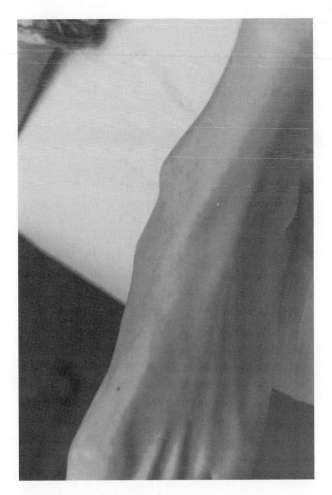

Figure 14-19 Fracture of the navicular tuberosity.

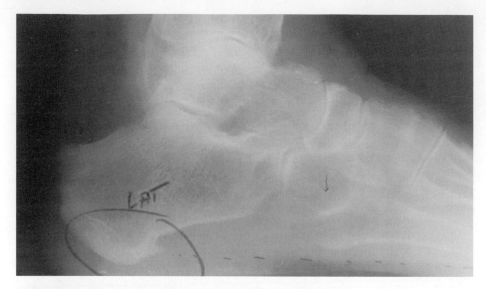

Figure 14-21 Plantar calcaneal spur.

condyles causes spur formation; usually the larger medial plantar condyle is affected as the forefoot abducts upon the rearfoot during pronation. The intrinsic muscles resist this motion through isometric or eccentric contraction. There is usually an enthesitis at the attachment of soft tissue to the bone. Heel-spur syndrome really is a combination of plantar fasciitis, intrinsic foot muscle myopathy and enthesitis, stress reaction of bone (a pre-stress fracture condition with inflammatory bone weakening and osteoporosis), and finally the heel spur itself. Pronation of a normal or hypermobile foot leads to excessive pulling of the medial plantar fascia and the intrinsic plantar musculature, resulting in a tension hyperostosis, the so-called heel spur. The high-arched cavus foot, which pronates as well, may also form a spur. Plantar heel pain may also be associated with a hypertrophic medial plantar condyle of the calcaneus.

Along with the bony spur or inflammatory bony process, there are soft tissue changes. There may be an abductor hallucis myositis at the medial plantar aspect of the heel. Likewise a medial calcaneal nerve entrapment or neuropathy may be present, although not as commonly as previously thought.[75–77] Adventitious bursitis is often present at the plantar aspect of the heel, as evidenced by a firm, palpable, painful plantar heel bursa that responds favorably to intrabursal injection. Plantar fat pad syndrome is usually more proximal than the heel spur and consists of plantar pain secondary to a soft tissue mass. This mass can be associated with a medial calcaneal neuroma or adventitious bursa. The true heel-spur syndrome is a bit more distal.

With stress reaction of bone, the entire calcaneus may be sore, especially on medial and lateral pressure, in contradistinction to the plantar spur or fasciitis, which is more painful to direct plantar pressure.

Bone scan or MRI will confirm the diagnosis. These patients need rest and, at times, non-weight-bearing cast immobilization, as well as calcium and magnesium supplementation along with associated trace minerals and remedies such as calcium fluoride or *Symphytum caucasicum* 12x, 4 tabs bid. If standard plantar fascia or heel-spur treatment has been tried and there is limited response and considerable pain with everyday activity, stress reaction of calcaneal bone, or stress fracture itself must be ruled out. Both tension and compression beyond physiologic tolerance, as is possible in sports, especially running or jumping on resistant surfaces, can cause bone failure directly or from increased osteoclastic activity triggered by the action and subsequent bone inflammation.

The heel-spur syndrome is classically associated with pain upon initial activity after periods of rest. During rest the forefoot hangs down upon the rearfoot, thus shortening the plantar intrinsic musculature and overlying plantar fascia. Like a rubber band, these structures contract. Upon initial weight bearing they create a stiff pain that can cause the patient to hobble about for 5 to 10 minutes until the tissue stretches out and warms up, hence the description, "worse initial motion, better continued motion." Then continued prolonged weight bearing again causes pain. Following even small periods of rest, such as driving a car or sitting at a desk, upon arising there is a "rusty gate" stiffness and pain upon initial weight bearing. This usually lessens upon warming up the foot by stretching the fascia and posterior leg muscles before full weight bearing. Night splints stretching out the plantar fascia and holding the leg and foot at 90 degrees are commercially available and most helpful. Another approach is taping the foot to rest the plantar fascia and prevent initial weight-bearing elongation.

As the foot warms up, collagen fibers, which become crisscrossed and entangled when there has been a tear and fibrosis, gradually become parallel. Thus a patient who has symptoms of heel-spur syndrome or plantar fasciitis may report that there can be pain for the first 15 to 30 minutes into a run that gradually goes away. They can then run comfortably for another hour, stop running, and then have pain and stiffness return 2 hours after the run. After any period of rest, there is pain and stiffness upon resumption of activity or weight bearing. Interestingly, this set of symptoms fits the characteristics of the arthritic homeopathic remedies *Rhus toxicodendron* and *Ruta graveolens*. *Rhus toxicodenron* produces more stiffness and restlessness than does *Ruta graveolens*, which is associated with more soreness and despair. These remedies, 6 or 12x, 3 tablets bid, are often surprisingly helpful, at times far more so than NSAIDs and certainly with fewer long-term side effects to the athlete.

The size or actual presence of a spur has no direct correlation with the amount of pain or symptoms present. Plantar heel spurs are often incidental radiographic findings, and may be asymptomatic. Many patients have bilateral heel spurs with only unilateral symptoms. Not uncommonly, I will treat one foot, at times with surgery being the end result; then the patient will resume running, only to return 2 years later with pain in the opposite heel. I then try an injection or two, as well as other conservative measures but if there is no encouraging response, I go immediately to surgery rather than prescribing a prolonged conservative course that, as evidenced by the opposite foot, will most likely end in surgery anyway.

Surgery for chronic plantar fasciitis with or without spur has evolved into a rather simple procedure with predictably good results. I prefer a small medial plantar incision allowing access to the medial plantar calcaneal condyle with first a #15 blade, then a meniscotome to release the intrinsics and fascia from the medial plantar condyle only. This preserves the lateral foot column stability and helps prevent subluxed cuboid. I remove the spurs with a Maltz rasp, percutaneously. Some of my colleagues use an endoscope

to guide them with this release. The surgery is done under local standby anesthesia, and patients are partially weight bearing within 5 to 7 days.

Certainly, large spurs are present from chronic pulling of the intrinsic plantar foot muscles and plantar fascia on the calcaneus during weight bearing. This may be more prevalent in an obese or heavy patient or when excessive pronation takes place. Static standing on hard surfaces appears to predispose to this problem. Like all hypertrophic osteoarthritic spurs, correcting the etiology is important.

Plantar Calcaneal Apophysitis   A traction apophysitis may appear on the plantar aspect of the calcaneus and present with pain similar to that of the heel-spur syndrome. This occurs in adolescent boys between the ages of 8 and 12. It may be aggravated by stress or trauma. It tends to be prevalent during soccer season and may be aggravated by utilizing thin-soled soccer shoes and running on hard surfaces. Pain with palpation on the plantar aspect of the calcaneus is usually present. Radiographs will show a plantar apophysis in the calcaneus, and there may be lines through the apophysis, suggestive of stress reaction of bone, stress fracture, or both. The treatment is conservative, using some form of soft orthosis to prevent excessive pronation if present and to provide for about one-quarter inch of heel lift. I prefer modifying an off-the-shelf Birkenstock orthotic shell, which has a good heel cup and can be easily posted with additional Korex material, similar to the Birkenstock rubberized semirigid material, and then covered with Spenco or Poron for shock attenuation. These are affordable and dispensed on the first visit. Return to sport may be as soon as the next day, if there is no pain—good news to players and coaches! I often use *Ruta graveolens* 12x, 3 tabs bid for 3 weeks, then calcaria phosphoricum 12x, 3 tabs bid (for healing of growing bones) for an additional 3 weeks.

In addition to orthotics, viscoelastic heel pads are often helpful. Taping of the heel to keep the fat under the plantar surface of the calcaneus and plantar-flex the forefoot on the rearfoot with low-dye strapping is quite helpful for acute cases when plantar fasciitis is present. The problems are self-limiting and almost always respond quite nicely with conservative therapy. The plantar calcaneal apophysitis is the counterpart of the posterior calcaneal apophysitis, termed *Sever's disease*, "pump bump," or "sock hop" heel pain, also seen in this age group. In the adult, the plantar lesion merely presents as a heel-spur syndrome.

Another form of the heel-spur syndrome is that of hypertrophy of the medial plantar condyle of the calcaneus.

A true traction enthesitis may be absent. However, there may be a hypertrophic medial plantar condyle of the calcaneus that impinges or digs into the underlying soft heel pad tissue during the impact of running. There is pain upon palpation of the tissue over the medial plantar condyle. An adventitious bursa may be present and abductor hallucis myositis or medial plantar fasciitis may coexist. The condition clinically appears to be more prevalent in the higher arched foot, which places more point pressure concentration on this condylar area. This type of foot is generally considered worse at absorbing shock than a normal arched, more flexible foot, with a broader plantar calcaneal contact area.

Contributing Factors, Diagnosis, and Treatment
Contributing factors leading to heel pain are direct trauma, such as acute pounding on the plantar aspect of the heel, or chronic repetitive stress, as seen in long-distance running on hard surfaces. One must rule out metabolic causes, such as seronegative arthritides and rheumatoid arthritis, or osteoporosis. Among the more notable of these conditions are Reiter's syndrome and ankylosing spondylitis.

Differential diagnosis includes medial calcaneal neuroma, systemic seropositive and seronegative arthritides, stress fracture, and soft tissue inflammatory diseases associated with the heel-spur syndrome, including plantar fasciitis and abductor hallucis myositis.

Diagnosis is made clinically and is substantiated with radiographs. A bone scan may be necessary to rule out stress fracture. Appropriate laboratory tests are indicated. A complete biomechanical test is necessary, and trial of soft temporary orthoses to control foot function and help disperse shock is helpful.

Acute heel-spur syndrome or plantar heel pain is treated with rest and acute physical therapy modalities, especially ice and compression. Shock-absorbent or dispersive devices, such as viscoelastic or silicon gel or Spenco heels, are helpful. These can be provided with a horseshoe heel-spur pad. Heel cups are helpful to keep the fat under the calcaneus and decrease the pressure on the bone. Low-dye foot strapping incorporating heel pads is very effective in acute cases, especially if preceded with an injection of a homeopathic cocktail or cortisone. Oral remedies, Traumeel or *Rhus toxicodendron*, or NSAIDs are most helpful, as are additional physical therapy modalities such as interferential stimulation or ice-cold whirlpool.

Chronic Problems Chronic problems are treated initially with a biomechanical approach to re-establish normal foot function and decrease abnormal shock or pressure distribution on the calcaneus. Temporary soft orthotics, taping, padding, and injections are all useful and generally necessary. Mobilization and manipulation help restore normal joint motion, which had been altered by the antalgic gait. Finally, the patient is fitted with neutral functional custom foot orthotics. In the case of plantar calcaneus apophysitis, an orthosis with a viscoelastic or Poron heel is especially helpful. A soft, flexible, cushiony temporary support is used in the initial phase of treatment. Taping of the foot is necessary to relax plantar soft tissue structures; a low-dye plantar fascial rest strap, using moleskin and tape, is advantageous to the patient. Another taping method that is well tolerated uses 2-inch Elastikon tape from above the ankle into the arch. This helps control both the subtalar and midtarsal joints while resting the plantar fascia. Of course, this can also be accomplished with a modified high-dye strapping with conventional Zonas tape. Either way, tape can be "waterproofed" by rubbing in paraffin wax, which makes showering easier than chancing it with plastic bags over the tape. Local treatment at home with ice massage and gentle stretching of the calf muscles is helpful. The patient must be told that the posterior musculature of the leg, when tight, can predispose to plantar foot pain. As previously mentioned, chronic cases of fasciitis with morning pain do well with posterior rest splints.

For established heel spurs that are inflamed and that have a mechanical etiology, injection therapy with a homeopathic cocktail with or without long- and slow-acting corticosteroids and anesthetics is essential. Three to five injections (ending with noncortisone homeopathic cocktail injections) about 1 week apart, followed by physical therapy and appropriate biomechanical devices, will give about a 90 percent success rate with chronic heel-spur syndrome.

Surgery has been necessary in only 10 percent of the many hundreds of cases that I have treated over the past 25 years. In addition, one can try oral *Rhus toxicodendron* 12x, 3 tabs bid for 3 weeks, followed by calcium fluoride 12x, 3 tabs bid for an additional 3 weeks, to complete healing of the bone. Zeel, 1 tab tid, may be used as a broad-spectrum homeopathic anti-inflammatory, and will often be effective even in those cases where single remedies, such as *Rhus toxicodendron*, are not. These natural remedies have no side effects and are surprisingly effective, as well as very affordable.

Posterior Hypertrophy and Spurs of the Calcaneus

Hypertrophy or pain at the posterior aspect of the calcaneus is often termed *Haglund's condition*. In adolescence, it is called Sever's aseptic necrosis or osteochondrosis of the

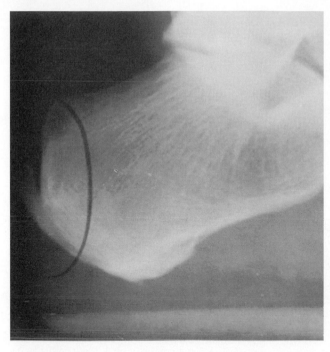

Figure 14-22 Retrocalcaneal hyperostosis with intratendinous calcification present.

Contributing Factors   Contributing factors include a rearfoot varus with compensatory pronation. As the foot spins in the shoe, the counter of the shoe applies pressure to the posterolateral aspect of the calcaneus, causing reactive hyperostosis, soft tissue pressure, and damage leading to adventitious bursitis. A red, inflamed area is seen clinically. Tight, ill-fitting shoes with a firm counter that rubs may likewise predispose to retrocalcaneal irritation or exostosis (Fig. 14-23).

There is a congenital predisposition to retrocalcaneal exostosis irritation, secondary to a high Fowler's angle.[53-55] This exists when the calcaneal inclination angle is such that the posterosuperior surface of the calcaneus is prominent posteriorly; thus the bone of the calcaneus is constantly irritated by foot gear and shoes.

Sever's Disease   Sever's disease is an osteochondritis of the posterior surface of the calcaneus, which may be predisposed for by tight Achilles tendons, rapid growth spurts, and repeated blows to the posterior surface of the calcaneus. It is usually self-limiting and resolves with the use

Figure 14-23 Inflamed retrocalcaneal exostosis caused by irritation from running shoes.

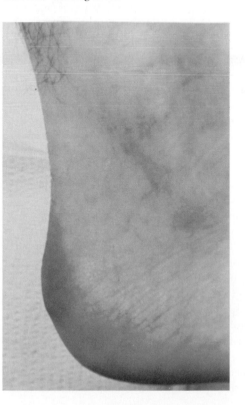

calcaneus. In lay terms, this may be called a "pump bump" or runner's bump. Skiers or skaters may call it skier's or skater's bump. The problem exists as hypertrophy of bone and pain around the posterosuperior surface of the calcaneus.

In its mild forms, retrocalcaneal hypertrophy or exostosis presents with pain at the posterolateral aspect of the calcaneus. In more severe forms, there is hypertrophy of bone and pain along the whole posterior one-third of the calcaneus. Variations in the shape, inclination, posterior protuberance, and varus tilt or "C" shape of the posterior portion of the calcaneus are all predisposing factors. In differentiated forms, there may be pain at the middle one-third of the posterior surface of the calcaneus, where there is intratendinous calcification or spurring, which is sometimes called a posterior calcaneal step. When this is present radiographically, there will be a step or spur of bone coming from the posterior surface of the calcaneus at the insertion of the Achilles tendon (Fig. 14-22). A true Haglund's condition or retrocalcaneal exostosis is a bit more superior to this area. Retrocalcaneal bursitis is commonly associated with retrocalcaneal exostosis. There may be supratendinous or infratendinous bursitis about the Achilles tendon over the posterior surface of the calcaneus.

of some form of orthosis to help balance a pronated foot and provide a one-quarter-inch heel lift. Of course, irritating shoe counters must either be softened by pounding with a hammer (to fracture the plastic in the counter) or remedied by removing the counter and replacing it with elastic and accommodative padding. At times a one-quarter-inch felt, viscoelastic, or rubber heel lift will suffice by elevating the irritated area above the offending portion of the shoe counter. Mild oral anti-inflammatory medications, homeopathics, herbal (white willow bark), or aspirin, are helpful. Local measures such as topical Traumeel, *Arnica* gel, Zeel, or ice massage help. Athletes and their parents must be told that they will most certainly outgrow this condition and that they can exercise to tolerance. It is surprising how many of these conditions coexist with the pronated foot, which causes abnormal pulling of the Achilles tendon on the calcaneus. These cases respond readily to an orthosis with appropriate heel lift.

Diagnosis and Treatment Differential diagnosis for acute posterior calcaneal pain includes stress fracture of the calcaneus, seronegative or seropositive arthritis, and gout. Chronic conditions must be differentiated from retrocalcaneal exostosis and bursitis, and Achilles tendinopathy. Retrocalcaneal bursitis or exostosis will become asymptomatic with an injection of local anesthetic, Wydase, and *Ruta graveolens* into the bursa or about the spur. Due to the adjacent tendon, I prefer to avoid cortisone in this area. With positive results, repeated homeopathic *Ruta*, Zeel, or Traumeel injections will often render the condition asymptomatic. If there is still pain, especially upon palpation of the Achilles tendon, one would suspect that most symptoms are coming from a tendinous lesion. MRI may help in regard to diagnosing a tendon problem, whereas a bone scan will help diagnose an acute bone problem.

Acute retrocalcaneal exostosis and bursitis are treated with anti-inflammatory medications and appropriate physical therapy. Ice, rest, and elevation are helpful, as are topical applications of Traumeel. Persistent pain responds to an injection of a homeopathic cocktail. Long-term treatment begins with appropriate biomechanical evaluation and a soft type of orthosis with a heel lift. A more permanent orthosis may be necessary in the later phases. Radiographs are taken, and a differential diagnosis is established. Injections (homeopathic or cortisone) into a bursa or about a spur are useful. Cortisone injection into the Achilles tendon is avoided inasmuch as this may predispose to central necrosis of the tendon, predisposing to rupture. Most posterior calcaneal problems will subside with conservative therapy, consisting of injections (homeopathic or corti-

sone) remedies, anti-inflammatory medicines, physical therapy, orthoses, and stretching and strengthening exercises. Attention should be placed upon stretching out the plantar fascia and posterior musculature. Good running form and avoidance of causative factors, such as overstriding and sprinting without an appropriate workout, should be emphasized.

Chronic resistant cases are usually those that present with a bony lesion, which may require surgical excision. When there is a true exostosis, simple excision through a small posterolateral incision will work well. When there is excessive posterior protuberance of the calcaneus, an osteotomy of the calcaneus with a dorsal wedge may be considered to bring the posterior two-thirds of the calcaneus forward and away from the Achilles tendon and counter of the shoe. There may be that rare case of posterior calcaneal apophysitis in a child, which will require a calcaneal dorsal wedge osteotomy to remove excessive pressure and functionally lengthen the Achilles tendon. I have had occasion to perform this in only two adolescents, both of whom had gratifying results. I have performed the calcaneal osteotomy upon adults several times. This functional lengthening of the Achilles tendon is also important in the older athlete who has intratendinous calcification or a true retrocalcaneal step.

EXOSTOSIS OF THE TALUS

Anterior impingement exostosis of the talus is a dorsal spur occurring on the talar neck. This is sometimes called footballer's or lineman's ankle. It may be present secondary to impingement of the talar neck on the anterior lip of the tibia, or to traction injury such as a plantar-flexion sprain. It can be associated with anterior tarsal tunnel syndrome or tenosynovitis of surrounding anterior structures. It presents with pain over the anterior aspect of the foot and ankle joint secondary to a dorsal bony protuberance. There may be limited ankle joint dorsiflexion. The spur may be palpable clinically but difficult to see to its full extent radiographically due to its position on the talus. There may be associated anterior tibial spurs (see Fig. 14–20).

Etiologic factors include impingement secondary to joint mechanics; traction spurs following injuries with capsular pulling on the talar neck; and prolonged cast immobilization, which results in joint narrowing and traction spurs because of the plantar-flexed position of the feet in the cast. Differential diagnosis includes coexistent ankle pathology, such as osteochondral fractures. Coexisting instabilities of the ankle joint are commonly seen with anterior impingement exostosis.

The acute symptoms present with a synovitis and pain at the anterior aspect of the ankle joint. This is treated with oral anti-inflammatory medications, homeopathic remedies, physical therapy, rest, and, in some cases, corticosteroid injection, or homeopathic cocktail injections. Appropriate plantar-flexory stretching exercises are prescribed. For limited ankle joint dorsiflexion due to impingement spurs that is interfering with athletic performance and causing overuse injuries in other parts of the body, surgical excision may be indicated. Likewise, for chronic pain that has not responded appropriately to conservative measures, including some form of foot balancing, surgery would be the treatment of choice, especially if there is overlying nerve impingement, which may be progressive.

Prior to surgery, one might consider arthrography or an arthroscopic examination if there is suspected intraarticular damage of the ankle joint. Osteochondral lesions should be ruled out, as well as instability of the ankle joint, which may need to be addressed at the time of surgery. When surgery is performed, the anterior talar neck exostosis is excised and delled down, and the talar neck is remodeled. When more proximal talar hyperostosis is associated with tibial hyperostosis or lipping, this is excised and remodeled through an anterior arthroplastic approach. The ankle joint itself should be inspected to rule out osteochondral lesions, which may need surgical ablation. When intraarticular lesions are present, or the anterior lip of the tibia is remodeled, the patient is kept non-weight bearing with early motion. Weight bearing may interfere with fibrocartilage formation on weight-bearing surfaces and should therefore be avoided for 4 to 6 weeks. Early motion is necessary to prevent narrowing of joints, atrophy, stiffness, and limited motion.

POSTERIOR TALAR SPURS

Spurs at the posterior aspect of the talus (posterior impingment) occur with the os trigonum syndrome or the talar posterior shelf syndrome. The os trigonum is a separate ossicle or united tubercle at the posterior lateral tubercle of the talus. It is usually a second center of ossification, which may not ossify completely with the main body of the talus, in which case it is attached by interosseus fibers. Since the posterior fibulotalar ligament attaches to it, it is vulnerable to avulsion with inversion sprains. Plantarflexion sprains can avulse or impact the os trigonum, causing fracture.

The posterior shelf of the talus occurs between the talus and the calcaneus at the posterior aspect of the posterior facet of the subtalar joint. Excessive posterior protuberance of bone may cause an incomplete posterior subtalar joint coalition with limited or painful inversion or eversion of the subtalar joint.[69-72] Both conditions are readily seen radiographically. The latter presents with a true shelf, whereas the former presents as a loose ossicle.

An os trigonum syndrome is present secondary to trauma, whereby the foot is plantar flexed and inverted. The posterior surface of the talus may abut against the posteroinferior surface of the tibia, thus causing a fracture (see Fig. 14-20). More commonly, however, the posterolateral tubercle of the talus, the os trigonum, is avulsed by the posterolateral collateral ligament. This occurs with a plantar-flexory inversion injury. There is pain upon palpation at the posterlateral aspect of the ankle and subtalar joint located in front of the tendo Achillis and behind the lateral malleolus. The pain is usually accentuated with motion of the flexor hallucis longus tendon, which runs along the inner aspect of the os trigonum; thus, when standing on the great toes in plantar flexion, the athlete experiences pain. With inversion, the pain is accentuated. With full plantar flexion, there is even more pain as the os trigonum or posterior shelf of the talus abuts against the tibia. These problems are more common in those sports that require more plantar flexion, such as gymnastics, basketball, and fast running.

Similarly, the posterior shelf condition presents with posterior subtalar joint pain. There may be more pain with inversion or eversion. There does not appear to be a position of comfort in these patients. Cast immobilization does render them asymptomatic since it stops all subtalar joint motion. With resumption of activity, the pain returns.

Differential diagnosis includes retrocalcaneal bursitis. This usually presents as a problem more posteriorly and is usually readily identifiable. The retrocalcaneal bursitis usually presents with more pain upon dorsiflexion, whereas the os trigonum or posterior talar shelf syndrome presents with pain upon plantar flexion. Stress fracture and metabolic causes must be ruled out.

The acute phase of an avulsion or fracture of an os trigonum or posterior shelf should be treated with immobilization and physical therapy. When practical, posterior fiberglass splint or cast boot, allowing physical therapy, should be used for 4 to 6 weeks while the fracture and injury hopefully heal. Daily periods of gentle range-of-motion exercises out of the splint, within the tolerance of discomfort, are helpful after 3 weeks of immobilization. Following this rest period of 4 to 6 weeks, gradual return to activity

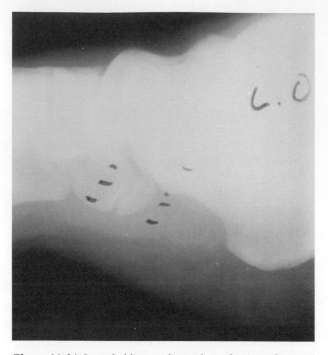

Figure 14-24 Lateral oblique radiograph confirming a fractured os naviculare. This avulsion fracture is similar in etiology and consequences to the avulsion fracture of the posterior process of the talus.

is allowed if the union is complete. If considerable pain persists, one might assume that the problem will be chronic, with either malunion of the avulsed portion or chronic fibrosis with posterior subtalar joint arthrosis.

Treatment of the chronic phase consists of physical therapy and injections if the fracture has united, or surgical excision if not. When a true posterior talar shelf or incomplete coalition exists, the injections will most likely give only temporary relief.

The definitive treatment is that of excision of the fractured or avulsed os trigonum or resection arthroplasty of the posterior shelf of the subtalar joint. This procedure is carried out through a longitudinal posteromedial approach. Most references in the literature show a posterolateral approach.[64,65] However, I find the posteromedial approach to be more satisfactory inasmuch as it allows for complete and direct visualization of the os trigonum and the adjacent flexor tendons, which can be easily retracted out of the way to provide for adequate resection, with the patient supine and the leg and foot in a "figure-of-four" position. The postoperative course includes early motion and physical therapy. Results of surgery are uniformly

good. Avulsion fractures similar to those of the os trigonum also occur with the os naviculare (Fig. 14-24) (see the discussion on p. 237).

SUBTALAR JOINT COALITIONS

Coalition of the subtalar joint will present in the athlete, often during adolescence. There may be a coalition of the posterior, middle, or anterior facet. There will be pain with range of motion of the subtalar joint. Usually the athlete complains of more pain and aggravation when performing on irregular surfaces; thus a youngster may present with pain at the beginning of football season after having a relatively uneventful summer. Limited or complete absence of subtalar joint motion will be present. CT scans can confirm the diagnosis.

Posterior facet coalitions present with posterior subtalar joint pain. They may be associated with pain in the midtarsal and ankle joints, which are providing abnormal, compensatory motion. With a subtalar joint coalition, especially of the posterior facet, there are usually hypertrophic bone changes at the dorsal aspect of the midtarsal joint. This presents as dorsal talar head lipping.

Treatment of the posterior subtalar joint coalition consists of the use of orthotics with a valgus rearfoot post to hold the foot somewhat pronated. This is usually the position of comfort. Cast immobilization may be necessary. Some of these children will be able to perform relatively well on even surfaces, despite the coalition. Others will need to have a subtalar arthrodesis when bone maturation is about 80 percent complete. This is usually the case past the age of 10. Posterior facet coalitions are seen on lateral radiographs and usually require arthrodesis.

Middle facet coalitions are more difficult to diagnose. They present with pain under the sustentaculum tali. The pain is present with activity on irregular surfaces. Although a lateral radiograph is helpful in making the diagnosis, a CT scan is more definitive.

Treatment of middle facet coalitions originally was a triple arthrodesis. Over the past several years I have operated upon a limited number of cases of middle or anterior facet coalition with resection arthroplasty, with acceptable results. I have limited experience with Silastic implants as spacers after resection. The implant is anchored dorsally, and serves as a spacer to deter intra-articular fibrosis.

The anterior facet coalition presents with pain at the anterolateral aspect of the midtarsal joint. Radiographs may show a coalition at the anterior facet, but often this is difficult to see. A tomogram or CT scan usually will be necessary. Treatment consists of excising the anterior facet of the subtalar joint by resecting a portion of the calcaneus. This surgery is similar to that performed for a midtarsal joint coalition. An extensor brevis arthroplasty is often performed as an adjunctive procedure. The procedure is done through an anterolateral approach. Early range of motion and activity are encouraged. The results have been quite satisfactory.

REFERENCES

1. Fredericson M: Common injuries in runners: diagnosis, rehabilitation and prevention. Injury clinic. Sports Med 21: 49, 1996
2. Shores M: Foot print analysis in gait documentation. Med Phys Ther 60:1163, 1980
3. Katoh Y, Chao EY, Laughman RK et al: Biomechanical analysis of foot function during gait and clinical applications. Clin Orthop 177:30, 1983
4. Schwab GH, Moynes DR, Jobe FW, Perry J: Lower extremity electro-myographic analysis of running gait. Clin Orthop 176:166, 1983
5. Subotnick SI: How I manage ingrown toenails. Physician Sportsmed 11, 1983
6. Drago JA, Jacobs AM, Oloff L: A comparative study of postoperative care with Phenol nail procedure. J Foot Surg 22: 332, 1983
7. Weinstock RE: Table plantar keratoses. J Am Podiatry Assoc 65:979, 1975
8. Hatcher RM, Goller WL, Weil LS: Intractable plantar keratoses. J Am Podiatry Assoc 68:377, 1978
9. Fielding MD: The Surgical Treatment of Intractable Plantar Keratoma. Futura, Mount Kisco, NY, 1974
10. Bart B: Plantar warts. Postgrad Med 72:251, 1982
11. Mullis DL, et al: A disabling sports injury of the great toe. Foot Ankle 1:22, 1980
12. Drago JJ, Oloff L, Jacobs AM: A comprehensive review of hallux limitus. J Foot Surg 23:213, 1984
13. O'Farrell TA, Costello BG: Osteochondritis dessicans of the talus, the late results of surgical treatment. J Bone Joint Surg [Am] 64:494, 1982
14. Rynn M, Fazekas EA, Hecker RL: Osteochondral lesions of the talus. J Foot Surg 22:155, 1983
15. Berndt AL, Harty M: Transchondral fractures of the talus. J Bone Joint Surg [Am] 41:988, 1959
16. Heppenstall RB: Constant direct current treatment for established non-union of the tibia. Clin Orthop 178:179, 1983
17. Basset CA, Mitchell SN, Gaston SR: Treatment of ununited tibial diaphyseal fractures with pulsing electromagnetic fields. J Bone Joint Surg [Am] 63A:511, 1981
18. Arangio GA: Proximal diaphyseal fracture of the 5th met base. Foot Ankle 3:293, 1983
19. Laurich LJ, Witt CS, Zielsdorf LM: Treatment of fractures of the fifth metatarsal bone. J Foot Surg 22:207, 1983
20. Stewart IM: Jones fractures: fracture of the base of the fifth metatarsal. Clin Orthop 16:190, 1960
21. Gilula LA, Oloff L, Caputi R, Destouet JM et al: Ankle tenography: a key to unexplained symptomatology. Radiology 151:575, 1981
21a. Subotnick SI: Update on common injuries of the lower extremity. Isr J Sports Med (Special Congress Issue) March: 36–37, Jerusalem, 1997
22. Subotnick SI: Sports and Exercise Injuries: Conventional, Homeopathic, and Alternative Treatments. North Atlantic Books, Berkeley, CA, 1991
23. Brantingham J: Plantar fasciitis. Chiropractic Tech 4:77, 1992
24. Brill PA, Macera CA: The influence of running patterns on running injuries. Sports Med 20:365, 1995
25. Zell J: Treatment of acute spasm of the ankle: controlled double-blind trial to test effectiveness of homeopathic ointment. Biol Ther VII(1):1–6, 1989
26. Macauley DI, Evans DM, Ansell BM: Assessment of tenosynovitis in rheumatoid arthritis. Rheumatol Rehabil 20:25, 1981
27. Myers BW, Masi AT: Pigmented villonodular synovitis and tenosynovitis. Medicine (Baltimore) 59:223, 1980
28. Eichelberger RP, Lichtenstein P, Brogden BG: Peroneal tenography. JAMA 247:2587, 1982
29. Cyriax J: Textbook of Orthopaedic Medicine. 10th Ed. Bailliere Tindall, London, 1980
30. Travell JG, Simons DO: Myofascial Pain and Dysfunction: The Trigger Point Manual: The Lower Extremities. 2nd Ed. Vol. 2. Williams & Wilkins, Baltimore, 1992
31. Johnson KA: Tibialis posterior tendon rupture. Clin Orthop 177:140, 1983
32. DeZwart DF, Davidson JS: Rupture of the posterior tibial tendon associated with fractures of the ankle. J Bone Joint Surg [Am] 65:260, 1983
33. Kelbel M, Jardon OM: Rupture of tibial posterior in a closed ankle fracture. J Trauma 22:1026, 1982
34. Bora FW Jr, Osterman AL: Compression neuropathy. Clin Orthop 163:20, 1982
35. Banerjee T, Coons DD: Superficial peroneal nerve entrapment. J Neurosurg 55:991, 1981
36. Stein JM, et al: Two entrapment neuropathies. Hosp Pract 18:100, 1983
37. Bralliar F: Electromyography: its use and misuse in peripheral nerve injuries. Orthop Clin North Am 12:229, 1981
38. Parkes JC, Hamilton WG, Patterson AH, Rawles JG: The anterior impingement syndrome of the ankle. J Trauma 20:895, 1980
39. Subotnick SI: Anterior impingement exostosis of the ankle. J Am Podiatry Assoc 66:958, 1976
40. Oloff LM, Jacobs AM, Jaffe S: Tarsal tunnel syndrome: a manifestation of systemic disease. J Foot Surg 22:302, 1983

41. Kaplan PE, Kernahan WT Jr: Tarsal tunnel syndrome: an electrodiagnostic and surgical correlation. J Bone Joint Surg 63A:96, 1981

42. Borges LF, Hallet M, Selkae DJ, Welch K: The anterior tarsal tunnel syndrome. J Neurosurg 54:89, 1981

43. Hoffman GS: Intra- and periarticular cortisone therapy. Am Fam Physician 23:106, 1981

44. Belkin SC: Stress fractures in athletes. Orthop Clin North Am 11:735, 1980

45. Meurman KO: Less common stress fractures in the foot. Br J Radiol 54:1, 1981

46. Goergen TG, Venn-Watson EA, Rossman DJ et al: Tarsal navicular stress fracture in runners. AJR 136:201, 1981

47. Batillas J, Vasilas A, Pizzi WF, Gokeebay T: Bone scanning in the detection of occult fractures. J Trauma 21:564, 1981

48. Torg JS, Pavlov H, Cooley LH et al: Stress fractures of the tarsal navicular: a retrospective review of twenty-one cases. J Bone Joint Surg [Am] 64:700, 1982

49. Moss A, Mowat AG: Ultrasonic assessment of stress fractures. Br Med J 286:1479, 1983

50. Voloshin A, Wosk J: Influence of artificial shock absorbers on human gait. Clin Orthop 160:52, 1981

51. Katoh Y, Chao EY, Laughman RK et al: Biomechanical analysis of foot function during gait and clinical applications. Clin Orthrop 177:23, 1983

52. Griffin ER: Heel pain in athletes. Am Fam Physician 28:23, 1983

53. Pavlov H, Heneghan MA, Hersh A et al: The Haglund syndrome: initial and differential diagnosis. Radiology 144:83, 1982

54. Rzonca EC, Shapiro P, D'Amico JC: Haglund's deformity. J Am Podiatry Assoc 74:482, 1984

55. Notari MA: An investigation of Fowler-Philips angle in diagnosing Haglund's deformity. J Am Podiatry Assoc 74:482, 1984

56. Kvist M: Achilles tendon injuries in athletes. Sports Med 18:173, 1994

57. Inglis AE, Sculco TP: Surgical repair of ruptures of the tendo Achilles. Clin Orthop 156:160, 1981

58. Nistor L: Surgical and nonsurgical treatment of Achilles tendon rupture. J Bone Joint Surg [Am] 63:394, 1981

59. Dugan RC, D'Ambrosia R: Fibular stress fractures in runners. J Fam Pract 17:415, 1983

60. Wing M: Phonophorsis with hydrocortisone in the treatment of TMJ. Phys Ther 62:32, 1982

61. Ketchum LD, Martin NL, Kappel DA: Experimental evaluation of factors affecting the strength of tendon repairs. Plastic Reconstr Surg 59:708, 1977

62. Bosworth DM: Repairs of defects in the tendoachilles. J Bone Joint Surg [Am] 38:111, 1956

63. Marcus SA: Complications in Foot Surgery: Prevention and Management. 2nd Ed. Williams & Wilkins, Baltimore, 1984

64. Kavros SJ, Shoenhäus HD, Jay RM: Fracture of the posterior process of the talus. J Am Podiatry Assoc 73:421, 1983

65. Giannestras NJ: Foot Disorders: Medical and Surgical Management. 2nd Ed. Lea & Febiger, Philadelphia, 1973

66. Earle AA, Moritz JE, Tapper EH: Dislocation of peroneal tendons at the ankle: an analysis of 25 ski injuries. N Engl J Med 71:108, 1972

67. Marti R: Dislocation of the peroneal tendons. Am J Sports Med 5:19, 1977

68. Jones E: Operative treatment of chronic dislocation of the peroneal tendons. J Bone Joint Surg [Am] 14:547, 1932

69. Wheeler R, Guevera A, Bleck EE: Tarsal coalitions: review of the literature. Clin Orthop 156:175, 1981

70. Chambers RB, Cook TM, Cowell HR: Surgical reconstruction for calcaneo-navicular coalition. J Bone Joint Surg 64:829, 1982

71. Deutsch AL, Resnick D, Campbell G: Computed tomography and bone scintigraphy in the evaluation of tarsal coalition. Radiology 144:137, 1982

72. Cowell HR, Elener V: Rigid, painful flatfoot secondary to tarsal coalition. Clin Orthop 177:54, 1983

73. Schmidt TL, Weiner DS: Calcaneal fractures in children. Clin Orthop 171:5, 1982

74. Omoto H, Sakurada K, Sugi M, Nakamura K: A new method of manual reduction for intra-articular fracture of the calcaneus. Clin Orthop 177:104, 1983

75. Michetti ML, Jacobs SA: Calcaneal heel spurs: etiology, treatment, and a new surgical approach. J Foot Surg 22:234, 1983

76. Rubin G: Plantar calcaneal spurs. Am J Orthop 5:38, 1963

77. McCarthy DJ, et al: The anatomical basis of inferior calcaneal lesions. J Am Podiatry Assoc 69:527, 1979

15

Ankle Injuries

STEVEN I. SUBOTNICK

The ankle joint is a hinge-type articulation between the inferior surface of the tibia, the tibial and fibular malleoli, and the trochlear surface of the talus and corresponding medial and lateral facets. The axis of the ankle joint is externally rotated and can be approximated by palpating the tips of the medial and lateral malleoli. Thus, because of the variability of the obliquity of the axis of the ankle joint, the hingelike motion of plantar flexion and dorsiflexion is accompanied by some degree of inversion with full plantar flexion and eversion with dorsiflexion.

The ankle joint works in conjunction with the subtalar joint, providing for smooth transmission of forces during gait. Thus the up-and-down as well as rotational forces taking place during gait are accommodated and adjusted for by the mutual alignment and arrangement of the ankle (superior ankle) joint and the subtalar (inferior ankle) joint. Whereas dorsiflexion and plantar flexion occur primarily in the ankle joint, pronation and supination with inversion and eversion occur in the subtalar joint. Furthermore, the rotation of fibers of the Achilles tendon inserting into the posterior one-third of the calcaneus accounts for inversion of the calcaneus with full plantar flexion and slight eversion of the calcaneus with dorsiflexion. The fibers of the Achilles tendon rotate approximately 90 to 100 degrees, with the medial fibers shifting posteriorly and the lateral fibers shifting anteriorly. In addition, the collateral ligaments of the ankle are arranged in such a way as to provide for dorsiflexion and plantar flexion at the ankle joint without restricting inversion or eversion of the subtalar joint. This is particularly true of the calcaneofibular ligament, which is biarticular, thereby influencing the motion of the subtalar and ankle joints. Because of the unique arrangement

of the lateral collateral ligaments, there is more inversion instability and increased talar tilt with full plantar flexion. More stress is also placed on the anterior talofibular ligament, which is under particular stress in the plantar-flexed attitude.

Whereas the axis of the subtalar joint averages 42 degrees of inclination on the sagittal plane and 24 degrees of medial deviation on the transverse plane, the axis of the ankle joint on the transverse plane is directed laterally and posteriorly; on the coronal plane, it is directed laterally and downward. The axis passes slightly distal to the tips of the malleoli. The amount of obliquity of the ankle joint can be appreciated by palpating the tips of the malleoli. With full dorsiflexion of the foot, a slight amount of posterior migration of the fibula is possible. Some movement is also available to the distal tibiofibular syndesmosis, but not much.

The anatomic confinements of the ankle joint are the strong posterior tibiofibular ligament at the back of the ankle, the medial deltoid ligaments with their deep and superficial portions, and the three distinct lateral collateral ligaments comprising the anterior talofibular ligament, the middle calcaneofibular ligament, and the posterior talofibular ligament. The anterior aspect of the ankle joint is bordered by the anterior tibiofibular ligament.

TERMINOLOGY

The inferior surface of the tibia that articulates with the trochlear surface of the talus dorsally is known as the plafond. The dorsal surface of the talus is called the trochlear surface or dome of the talus. The articular surface of the talus, medially, is the medial facet, which articulates with the corresponding medial facet of the medial malleolus; the lateral triangular articular surface of the talus is the lateral facet, which articulates with the corresponding lateral facet of the fibular malleolus. The lateral talar facet is a large triangle, whereas the medial talar facet is a small pear-shaped or tear-shaped articular surface. The dome of the talus is triangular, with the medial and lateral borders converging posteriorly. The lateral portion of the ankle joint is called the lateral gutter, whereas the medial portion is the medial gutter.

ANATOMY

There is an abundant capsule about the ankle joint. At the anterior aspect of the ankle joint, there is subcutaneous fat and an anterior neurovascular bundle containing the anterior tibial artery and nerve. The extensor tendons are at the anterior aspect of the ankle joint; the anterior tibial is medialmost, flanked by the flexor hallucis longus, the neurovascular bundle, and the extensor hallucis longus. The peroneus tertius is the lateralmost extensor tendon. Covering the extensor tendons is the extensor retinaculum, with the cruciate crurals inferiorly and the transverse crurals superiorly. At the medial aspect of the ankle joint is the medial neurovascular bundle, with the posterior tibial nerve and artery and two posterior tibial veins. This is covered by the laciniate ligament. Within the tarsal tunnel are the flexor tendons, beginning medially with the posterior tibial, then the neurovascular bundle, followed by the flexor digitorum longus and the flexor hallucis longus beneath the sustentaculum tali. At the posterior aspect of the ankle joint is the Achilles tendon, and at the lateral aspect of the ankle joint are the peroneal tendons, which pass beneath the fibular malleolus and are held in place by the superior and inferior peroneal retinaculum. Accompanying the peroneal tendons is the sural, or lateral peroneal, nerve. In the superficial soft tissue at the anterior aspect of the ankles, coursing from lateral to anterior, are the superficial peroneal nerves. They divide to provide sensation over the anterior aspect of the foot and dorsal aspects of the digits. The saphenous nerve is a sensory superficial nerve at the anterior aspect of the ankle, which follows the course of the saphenous vein.

Although the dorsalis pedis or anterior tibial artery is the main supplier of blood to the anterior aspect of the foot, there may be a lateral peroneal artery, which also supplies the dorsal aspect of the foot. The plantar aspect of the foot is supplied by the posterior tibial artery.

The collateral ligaments of the ankle include the medial deltoid ligament, with four bands that blend into a spring ligament anteriorly. The spring ligament inserts into the talus and navicular. The lateral collateral ligaments comprise three distinct ligaments, with the middle collateral ligament the longest, the anterior collateral ligament the weakest, and the posterior collateral ligament the strongest. The tibia and fibula are held together deeply by the interosseous ligament.

Because of the unique integrated mechanism and function between the subtalar joint and ankle joint, injury to one joint affects the function of the other, hence the causal relationship between a ball-and-socket ankle joint and subtalar joint trauma with resultant limited motion, or subtalar joint arthrodesis. There is also a causal relationship between ankle joint limited motion or fusion and pathology to the subtalar joint and midtarsal joints due to increased load in attempts to compensate for the decreased ankle joint motion. The degree of increased load on the subtalar or ankle joint is dependent on the axis of this joint. Thus, if the ankle joint axis were more oblique, more pronation and supination would be available for compensation of a pathologic subtalar joint, resulting in less abnormal strain at the ankle joint. In contradistinction, if the midtarsal joint oblique axis allowed for considerable dorsiflexion and plantar flexion, limited motion in the ankle joint would be less damaging to the foot.

SOFT TISSUE PATHOLOGY

The soft tissue about the ankle joint is composed of skin and subcutaneous tissue. Immediately beneath the subcutaneous tissue are the various fascial layers. Three fascial bands, which may be called ligaments, bind down the tendons about the ankle joint. Anterior to the ankle is the transverse crural; the cruciate crural is beneath the transverse crural. Both ligaments aid in stabilizing the antigravity extensor tendons. The laciniate ligament is a medial ligament over the tarsal tunnel that maintains the flexor tendons. There is a superior and an inferior peroneal retinaculum laterally for the peroneus longus and brevis tendons. The inferior peroneal retinaculum is the continuation of the lateral band of the cruciate crural.

Anteriorly in the subcutaneous fat are the superficial peroneal nerves, which supply sensation to the dorsal aspect of the foot. At the lateral aspect of the foot in the subcutaneous fat is the sural nerve and, medially, the saphenous nerve. All three of these nerves in the superficial tissue are sensory nerves, easily damaged with direct contusion or tension neurapraxia. Care must be taken to avoid them during surgical dissection. Tightness of the three thickened portions of fascia that form ligaments can cause considerable problems. Notable is the tarsal tunnel syndrome, secondary to tightness of the laciniate ligament or swelling from any cause (varicose veins, tendinitis, or edema from hypothyroidism) within the fibro-osseous tunnel. There may also be an anterior tarsal tunnel syndrome secondary to tightness of the cruciate ligament. Subluxation of the peroneal tendon may occur as a result of avulsion or rupture of the superior peroneal retinaculum.

Beneath the deep fascial layers about the ankle joint, between the anterior tibial tendon and the extensors, is the anterior neurovascular bundle, comprising the deep peroneal nerve and dorsalis pedis artery. Medially, beneath the laciniate ligament, are the contents of the tarsal tunnel: the flexor tendons and the posterior tibial artery, nerve, and veins. At the anteromedial aspect of the foot, in the subcutaneous tissue, is the saphenous vein, which accompanies the saphenous nerve; at the posterolateral aspect is the short saphenous vein, which accompanies the sural nerve.

The tendons about the ankle include the anterior tibial and extensors anteriorly; the flexor and posterior tibial tendons medially; the peroneal tendons, the longus and brevis, laterally; and the gastrocnemius–soleus complex, or the triceps surae with the gastrocnemius, soleus, and plantaris tendons posteriorly, inserting into the middle one-third of the calcaneus.

At the lateral aspect of the ankle joint, the collateral ligaments are three distinct entities known as the anterior talofibular, the calcaneofibular, and the posterior talofibular. At the medial aspect of the ankle joint is the thick, strong deltoid ligament, with its superficial and deep portions; at the posterior aspect of the ankle joint is the posterior tibiofibular ligament. At the anterior aspect of the ankle is the anterior tibiofibular ligament and an interosseous ligament between the tibia and fibula above the tibial plafond.

Consistently present bursae about the ankle joint include the supratendinous and infratendinous bursae about the Achilles tendon. The supratendinous Achilles bursa is between the Achilles tendon and the posterior skin of the foot and ankle at the level of the posterosuperior one-third of the calcaneus. It may become inflamed secondary to excessive shoe pressure. The infratendinous bursa is between the posterior one-third of the calcaneus superiorly and the Achilles tendon. It becomes symptomatic and inflamed secondary to excessive motion of the calcaneus or to excessive pressure from the counter of the shoe pressing on the Achilles tendon, impinging on the bursa between tendon and bone.

Blisters and Skin Irritation About the Calcaneus

Blisters and skin irritation about the calcaneus occur secondary to abnormal pressure from the counters or heel cups of shoes or boots. They are not uncommon in skiers and ice-skaters. The solution is to have the boots punched out or stretched over the malleoli and to pad the malleoli with various foam rubber cushions. Counters in athletic shoes can be modified, or removed. If there is excessive pronation of the foot within the boot, predisposing to medial malleolar rubbing, as well as excessive pressure on the lateral malleolus, realignment of the foot with an orthosis may help prevent abnormal strain on the malleoli. Additional help may be obtained by padding the malleoli with stirrups of felt cut out in a horseshoe shape. Abnormal boot pressure associated with tibial varum may be solved with cants. Fine tuning can be accomplished by shaving down the outsole of the boot.

Superficial Nerve Compression

Superficial compression of the nerves in the subcutaneous fat about the anterolateral and medial aspects of the ankle joint occurs most often secondary to tight-fitting boots. In skiing, the forward lean causes considerable pressure from the tongue, or anterior boot shell, on the anterior aspect of the ankle joint and foot. This may cause superficial nerve palsy. Athletes often complain of numbness in their toes that does not go away for several days or weeks after removal of the boots. Almost all of these pressure neurapraxias are reversible, although I have seen five cases, over the past 25 years, of irreversible scarring and damage to the superficial nerves of the foot secondary to ski boot pressure.

The solution is to find a boot with adequate flexibility at the ankle joint level to allow for forward lean without excessive anterior boot pressure. Initially, during the break-in period with new boots, foam rubber can be used at the anterior aspect of the ankle, placed beneath the tongue area of the boot. Care should be taken to avoid buckling the boots too tightly at the ankle joint level, to permit appropriate flexion.

Traction neuropathy may occur about the sural nerve secondary to plantar-flexion inversion sprains. Most of these palsies are reversible and will respond to rest and physical therapy. Local injection with lidocaine, vitamin B$_{12}$, and a *Hypericum perforatum* cocktail is beneficial to nerve recovery and allows for a fluid neurolysis of adhesions. In some cases, significant intractable superficial peroneal nerve damage may occur, requiring neurolysis. However, in the patient with very thin subcutaneous tissue, neurolysis may fail owing to inadequate fat to cover and protect the nerve, resulting in further postoperative scarring of the nerve, which then must be resected. This should be avoided if at all possible because it leads to superficial sensory nerve loss. The saphenous nerve is less often damaged by traction or compression at the anteromedial aspect of the foot.

Compression of the Anterior Deep Neurovascular Bundle

Anterior tarsal tunnel syndrome, or compression of the neurovascular bundle anteriorly, may occur secondary to impingement of the neurovascular bundle between underlying spurs on the talar neck and tight-fitting boots or shoe gear. The extensor retinaculum becomes a binding structure if involved with chronic repetitive stress, causing fibrosis of the tissue. Conservative treatment is that of physical therapy, appropriate shoe gear, lysis injection therapy, and "tincture of time." Surgical treatment consists of releasing the extensor retinaculum, decompressing the anterior tarsal tunnel, and removing underlying bone spurs. The surgery is usually successful and generally well tolerated by athletes.

Flexor Hallucis Longus Tendinitis

Tendinitis of the flexor hallucis longus may be secondary to excessive toe-off during sports. It may also be coexistent with trauma at the posterolateral tubercle of the talus—the os trigonum. At times, there may be an avulsed or fractured os trigonum secondary to excessive inversion or plantar flexion. During plantar flexion, the posterolateral shelf of the talus may abut against the posterior surface of the tibia, causing a fracture. Inversion may occur as a component of avulsion. When there is a damaged os trigonum, motion of the long flexors of the hallux causes pain at the damaged bone and a secondary tendinitis.

The differential diagnosis includes tarsal tunnel syndrome or tendinitis of the long flexor to the lesser toes. Radiographs are taken to rule out the presence of an os trigonum or an excessively large posterolateral tubercle of the talus (Fig. 15-1). During clinical examination, the long flexor is palpated as the great toe is taken through its range of motion.

Conservative treatment consists of the use of elastic straps around the hallux to decrease the amount of dorsiflexion. For excessive pronation, a temporary orthosis is used. Injection therapy using a homeopathic cocktail with Traumeel or a standard injection with long- and slow-acting local anesthetic and corticosteroids is beneficial. The injection may be placed around the os trigonum and around the tendon sheath, but not intratendinously. Physical therapy, ultrasound, or interferential electrotherapy is helpful.

If pain persists, exploratory surgery is indicated. I prefer a medial approach. An incision is made just posterior to the medial malleolus, with the patient supine. With careful Loupe magnification and dissection, the neurovascular bundle is identified and avoided. The long flexor tendon is easily seen; just lateral to this is the os trigonum or lateral posterior shelf of the talus. This is usually simply and easily excised with appropriate instrumentation, and the long flexor tendon can be checked. If there is fibrosis about the sheath, a tenolysis is carried out. The results for this surgery are uniformly excellent.

Posterior Tibial Tendinitis

Posterior tibial tendinitis can be coexistent with flexor tendinitis or it may be secondary to abnormal pronation. It is often found when there is an excessively large medial tubercle on the os naviculare. When this is the case, the posterior tibial tendon has an abnormal attachment to the medial aspect of the navicular and is excessively stretched as the foot pronates. The function of the posterior tibial tendon is to decelerate pronation at foot contact. Therefore, excessive or rapid pronation may cause excessive loading of the tendon and secondary degeneration or tenosynovitis. Partial or complete rupture may occur as well.

When crepitation is present, a more serious problem exists, and infection must be ruled out. If infection is not present, injection therapy to reduce the crepitation, followed by rest for 2 to 3 weeks, is indicated. During the rest period, physical therapy is helpful. If crepitation or stenosis persists, surgical decompression is indicated. At times, a subtalar or triple arthrodesis may be the end result

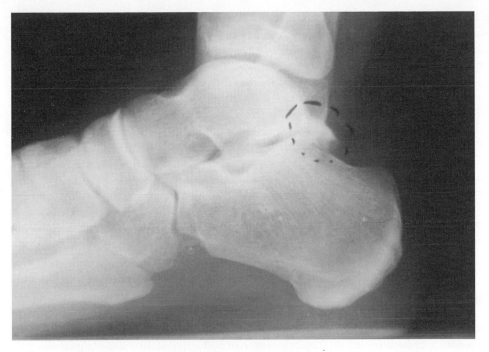

Figure 15-1 Lateral radiograph showing the os trigonum (circled).

of a ruptured posterior tibial tendon that is not quickly diagnosed and repaired.

Anterior Tibial Tendinitis

Anterior tibial tendinitis is associated with excessive pronation of the foot. The anterior tibial tendon inserts into the medial aspect of the foot at the medial plantar aspect of the first metatarsal–medial cuneiform articulation; thus excessive pronation stretches this tendon obliquely. The tendon may also become damaged secondary to overload or overstress with running on hard surfaces or overstriding. As the foot rapidly plantar-flexes, the anterior tibial muscle attempts to slow down the anterior plantar foot slap; this leads to excessive loading and degeneration.

Patients with anterior tibial tendinitis present with pain and swelling over the anterior aspect of the ankle. Upon dorsiflexion of the foot and palpation of the anterior tibial tendon, areas of tenderness and swelling are easily found. When anterior tibial tendinitis is present, foot imbalances must be ruled out or corrected with a full-length soft temporary orthosis. Anti-inflammatory measures, such as physical therapy, ice message, and oral anti-inflammatory medications, are used. For chronic problems (more than

3 weeks old) injection therapy with a homeopathic cocktail or a small amount of cortisone may be helpful. Injections into the tendon are to be avoided because they will cause intratendinous damage, necrosis, or both.

As with all tendon problems, tenosynovitis must be differentiated from partial rupture, and magnetic resonance imaging (MRI) may be required in questionable cases. Partial rupture requires rest for at least 4 to 6 weeks, and tenosynovitis requires reduced activity and aggressive physical therapy. Intratendinous damage of the anterior tibial tendon may eventually require surgery.

Extensor Tendinitis

Extensor tendinitis about the ankle is similar in onset to anterior tibial tendinitis and shows similar findings. The extensors and anterior tibial are eccentric decelerators of the foot and can be pulled or inflamed secondary to overuse or rapid foot loading, such as running downhill or unaccustomed race walking. The patient presents with pain at the anterior aspect of the ankle along the course of the extensor tendons. By selectively dorsiflexing all toes, the involved extensor tendon can be isolated and treated appropriately. Pressure (compressive or friction) extensor tendinitis is more prevalent in those who wear tight-fitting shoes or boots. The tendons become irritated secondary to abnormal shoe or boot pressure. Likewise, eyelets from foot gear can precipitate tendonitis. Treatment for the extensors is similar to that for the anterior tibial tendon. With foot gear problems, remedies include stretching the shoes, removing eyelets, or changing shoes or boots. Initially felt, foam, or viscoelastic pads are helpful. Treatment involves ruling out underlying dorsal exostosis, correcting biomechanical predisposing factors such as forefoot varus or anterior equinus, utilizing physical therapy, resting the foot with strappings, correcting training errors such as overstriding, and injecting with a homeopathic cocktail or dilute cortisone as needed. Remedies such as Traumeel or *Rhus toxicodendron* or nonsteroidal anti-inflammatory drugs (NSAIDs) are helpful.

Peroneal Tendinitis

In addition to cuboid subluxation with peroneal–cuboid syndrome, the peroneal tendons may be involved in tenosynovitis or tendinopathy from other causes. Tenosynovitis often occurs secondary to plantar-flexory inversion sprains. This maneuver can stretch the peroneal tendons, causing tenosynovitis. I have had occasion to treat numerous cases of peroneal tendinitis, with or without subluxed cuboid, that persist after treatment of lateral ankle sprains. Some of the patients have been disabled for months to years, only to respond completely and dramatically to proper treatment, including injections, manipulation, and an orthotic with a long lateral flange to keep the cuboid in place and prevent abduction of the forefoot on the rearfoot. Physical therapy, such as interferential electrotherapy, is also helpful adjunctive treatment.

Peroneal spasm may be present secondary to coalition or post-traumatic arthritis of the subtalar or midtarsal joints. The peroneal brevis is usually involved, and holds the foot abducted. Plantar flexion of the first ray usually indicates spasm of the peroneus longus. Tenograms may permit visualization of the tendon sheath (Fig. 15-2). MRI can be used when tenograms are difficult to interpret or inconclusive. Radiographs are helpful to rule out bony pathology. A computed tomography (CT) scan may be necessary when coalition or pathology of the anterior middle facet of the subtalar joint is suspected. Medial oblique radiographs usually suffice in ruling in or out midtarsal joint bony pa-

Figure 15-2 Arthrogram outlining the peroneal tendon sheath.

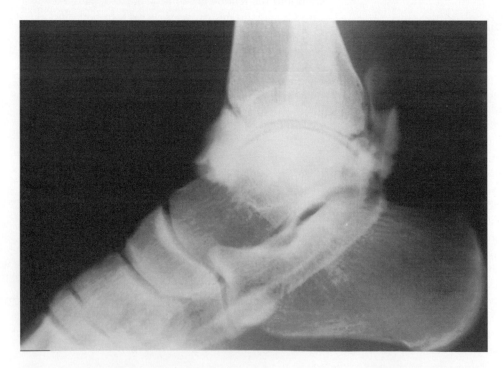

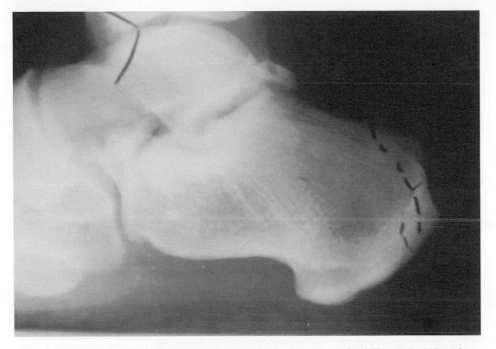

Figure 15-3 Lateral projection illustrating calcaneal step at insertion of Achilles tendon (dotted line).

thology, whereas MRI may be necessary to detect subtalar or midtarsal soft tissue fibrous pathology or coalition.

Bony pathology requires a surgical approach, whereas soft tissue pathology often responds to injections, usually cortisone with Wydase, followed by manipulation to restore joint function and range of motion. Physical therapy and anti-inflammatory medications or remedies may be useful.

Occasionally, tenolysis is necessary for chronic tenosynovitis of the peroneal tendons. I have seen patients with partial rupture of the peroneals secondary to trauma who responded well to using a portion of the peroneus brevis tendon to reinforce the partially ruptured peroneus longus tendon.

Achilles Tendinopathy

The Achilles tendon and calf muscles (triceps surae) function to stabilize the posterior aspect of the foot and ankle eccentrically, isometrically, and concentrically, throughout the various phases of walking, running, or jumping (Fig. 15-3). The Achilles tendon also mildly supinates the foot at contact due to its slightly medial insertion and the rotation of its fibers. Along with its supinating and stabilizing function during contact and midstance, it is also involved in propulsion at the toe-off phase. This muscle and tendon unit crosses three joints, the knee, the ankle, and the subtalar, thus mechanically predisposing to greater incidence of injury than muscle–tendon units that cross only one joint.

Achilles tendinopathy presents with pain at the posterior aspect of the ankle. Tenosynovitis is present secondary to overuse or may be present secondary to tight-fitting foot gear and excessive friction. When tenosynovitis is present, patients present with pain over the Achilles tendon, which has palpable point tenderness, edema, and sometimes crepitation. There is usually more pain upon forceful dorsiflexion of the foot. Likewise, there may be pain upon attempts to rise on the ball of the foot. When overuse is a contributing factor, there will be a characteristic history of gradual onset of pain. The pain may be accentuated by excessive pronation or supination. When pronation is present, the pain will be medial. When supination is present, the pain will be more lateral. The pain may also be associated with underlying hyperostosis of the posterior surface of the calcaneus. A congenital posterior tilt to the calcaneus may be observed with an increased Fowler's angle. In addition, there may be intratendinous calcification secondary to repeated pulling of the Achilles tendon. Retrocalcaneal spurs or exostoses may cause undue pressure on the overlying Achilles tendon during pronation, supination, or toe-off. Coexistent with tenosynovitis of the Achilles tendon may be an infratendinous or supratendinous bursa. Bursitis alone may be present and should be included in the differential diagnosis for posterior heel and ankle pain.

Also included in the differential diagnosis are os trigonum problems. If there is pain upon excessive plantar flexion, especially with palpation at the lateral posterior aspect of the ankle, an os trigonum should be suspected. If there is pain upon dorsiflexion, one is more apt to suspect pathology of the Achilles tendon or retrocalcaneal exostosis or bursitis. Radiographs are helpful. Likewise, intrabursal injections help differentiate the two problems.

Along with tenosynovitis of the Achilles tendon, more appropriately called paratenonitis, patients may present with pathlogy of the tendon itself (tendinosis). Tenosynovitis or paratenonitis is present with inflammation of the loose areolar sheath about the Achilles tendon (see Fig. 20-19). This sheath has an abundant blood supply; overuse causes inflammation and swelling of the sheath. The tendon itself has a rather poor blood supply, and central necrosis of the tendon, partial rupture, or tendinosis occurs secondary to trauma. The poor blood supply of the tendon also accounts for poor healing of intratendinous lesions. One must also realize that the fibroblasts of the adult Achilles tendon are inactive and incapable of healing. Healing of the Achilles tendon occurs secondary to metaplasia of the surrounding fat cells.[1]

Paratenonitis is symptomatic. There may be crepitation upon palpation, and pain is always elicited upon palpation. By contrast, tendinosis may be asymptomatic. Tendinosis without coexistent paratenonitis may go on to partial and then complete rupture without a prodromal syndrome. A presentation of considerable swelling and lumpiness of the Achilles tendon usually points to intratendinous damage. When there are superficial, isolated areas of pain and crepitation that are palpable, one may be more sure of the diagnosis of paratenonitis.

Paratenon lesions are treated with physical therapy, rest, and appropriate biomechanics. Transverse friction massage is also helpful. Cortisone injection therapy is usually not advised because inadvertent injection of the Achilles tendon itself leads to central necrosis and further tendon damage. Homeopathic cocktail injections, in contrast, are safe and often useful in reducing adhesion and encouraging healing. If the plan is to inject the paratenon tissue, the athlete should rest for 3 weeks following the injection. For extreme tenderness or swelling, one may administer oral NSAIDs, or use a decreasing-dose oral cortisone regimen, again with protective decreased activity for 3 to 6 weeks. When homeopathic injections or remedies, along with NSAIDs, fail to provide relief, I use an Aristo-pak Dose-Pack (Lederle Laboratories, Wayne, NJ) over a 6-day course. Chronic paratenon lesions that do not respond to appropriate physical therapy, rest, and other adjunctive measures will require a surgical tenolysis. This procedure is easily carried out with the patient under local anesthesia and in the prone position. The results are uniformly good.

Tendinosis or intratendinous lesions require surgical exploration. Necrotic tissue is curetted, and the tendon is repaired. If a considerable amount of tendon is involved, a tendon graft is used in the repair. The plantaris tendon may be used as a graft. We have also had success with woven Dacron (Meadox graft) for repairing partially to completely ruptured Achilles tendons.

BONY ASPECTS OF THE ANKLE JOINT

The ankle joint is involved with dorsiflexion and plantar flexion. Its oblique axis permits a small amount of inversion with plantar flexion and eversion with dorsiflexion about an arc depending on the precise axis of the ankle joint. The ankle joint works in conjunction with the subtalar joint as a torque converter, similar to the universal joint in an automobile, in allowing for forward gait progression as well as adaptation of the foot to varying irregular surfaces, such as slopes and the side hill lays of golf. Because of the unique biomechanics and functions of the ankle joint and its specialized interface between the foot and leg, it is quite vulnerable and often injured during sports. Foot gear and playing surfaces also play a role in injury of the ankle.[2]

Anterior Impingement Exostosis

Anterior impingement exostosis of the ankle joint occurs secondary to forceful dorsiflexion of the foot on the ankle. The dorsal aspect of the talus abuts against the anterior distal edge of the tibia. This "nutcracker syndrome" has been called "footballer's ankle"; a lineman on a football team is often positioned with a dorsiflexed everted foot, which impinges on the ankle, resulting in an impingement exostosis with hyperostosis of the talar neck and the adjacent tibial surface (Fig. 15-4). As the spurs become larger,

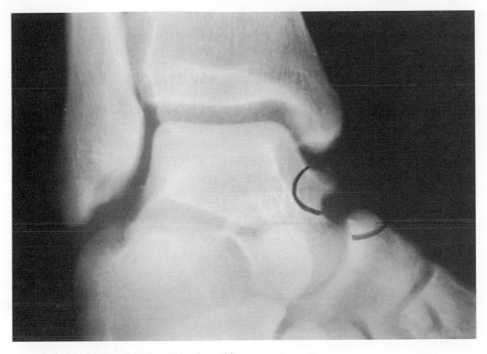

Figure 15-4 Talar neck exostosis in the ankle.

they impinge on overlying soft tissue and cause pain. The spurs can be seen radiographically. Special care in taking the radiographs is necessary because of the oblique nature of the spurs. Mildly symptomatic spurs are treated with physical therapy and appropriate balancing of the foot. Injection therapy may be helpful in reducing surrounding inflammation or adhesions. Persistent symptomatic spurs are excised. It is important to remove adequate amounts of bone from the talar neck and anterior leading edge of the tibia, to decrease the rate of recurrence.

Anterior spurring about the ankle joint may be secondary to traction rather than to compression; thus chronic plantar flexion of the ankle, such as might occur in ballet or gymnastics, will cause traction and microscopic bleeding and lead to spur formation. These spurs may form as sequelae to plantar-flexory inversion sprains. Spurring of the ankle joint also occurs secondary to cast immobilization for long periods of time. Casting the foot in a plantar-flexed position causes soft tissue traction and secondary spur formation. Inactivity also causes degeneration of the cartilage of the ankle joint and secondary narrowing of the joint, leading to arthritic changes. The diagnosis of anterior spurs is easily made on the basis of palpation, clinical findings, and radiographs. The treatment is that of surgical excision as described above. When chronic synovitis is present, a partial synovectomy is carried out.

Anterior Synovitis of the Ankle

Athletes may complain of painful chronic anterior synovitis of the ankle. This may be secondary to chronic repetitive strain at the ankle joint or pressure from ill-fitting foot gear. Physical therapy along with injection therapy and manipulation usually suffices, but occasionally arthroscopic exploratory surgery with a partial synovectomy is indicated. The synovium is usually inflamed and pathologic. Coexisting with the synovitis may be intra-articular lesions, such as osteochondritis or transchondral fractures. Meniscoid degeneration of the ankle joint may be noted at the anterolateral aspect. Arthrograms or MRI are useful for ruling out these lesions (Fig. 15-5). As with all inflammatory soft tissue lesions, metabolic causes must be ruled out.

Posterior Impingement of the Ankle Joint

Posterior impingement of the ankle joint is caused by impingement of the posterior talar process with the adjacent posterior aspect of the tibia. This occurs during rapid

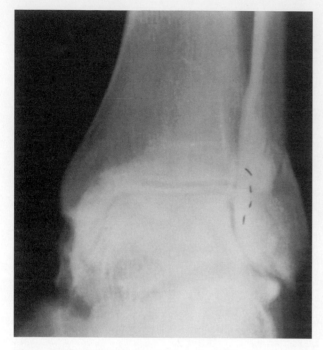

Figure 15-5 Ankle arthrogram is used to rule out meniscoid lesions. This one appears normal.

excessive plantar flexion. This type of activity is found during dance and gymnastics. The resultant posterior impingement causes a fracture of the posterior surface of the talus.

Clinically, the athlete complains of pain during push-off, as in running. Palpation medial and lateral to the posterior aspect of the subtalar joint causes pain. There may be pain with inversion or eversion; in fact, the foot is uncomfortable in any position. Forceful plantar flexion reproduces the pain. When there has been avulsion of a secondary center of ossification (the os trigonum), plantar flexion and inversion reproduces the pain. A sprained ankle may have been the inciting incident.

The diagnosis is made using appropriate radiographs. If the radiographs are not conclusive, an MRI bone scan or CT scan will help verify the diagnosis. Treatment consists of excision of fracture fragments. This is carried out through a posteromedial approach. Results of the surgery are most gratifying.

Anterolateral Impingement

Anterolateral impingement of the ankle joint may occur secondary to repeated sprains involving the anterolateral aspect of the ankle. These are usually plantar-flexory inversion sprains. A meniscoid lesion develops at the anterolateral aspect of the ankle joint in the anterolateral gutter, evidenced by shiny gray discolored tissue found at the time of arthroscopy or open arthrotomy. MRI also demonstrates these soft tissue lesions.

Patients complain of a catching sensation at the anterolateral aspect of the ankle joint. Pain with eversion or inversion and with plantar flexion or dorsiflexion is present; thus there is no real position of comfort during function. Since this is also the symptom complex of osteochondral talar lesions, which may coexist or present separately, they must be ruled out or in. If chronic repetitive sprains have been present, an anterior drawer or frontal plane stress test may be positive. In some cases, the ankle may be stable, yet the lesion persists. Injection therapy is often helpful initially, but the problems usually persist after the effect of the injection wears off.

Upon clinical examination, the athlete feels pain at the anterior aspect of the junction of the fibular malleolus to the dome of the talus. The facets of the lateral aspect of the talus and adjacent surface of the fibula may be involved. Radiographs can reveal bony impingement (see Figs. 15-5, 15-6 and 20–14) but will be negative with soft tissue impingement. Treatment consists of exploratory surgery. When a fibrotic meniscoid lesion is present, it is removed with soft tissue dissection and a pituitary rongeur, often transarthroscopically. Intra-articular pathology, such as transchondral fractures or osteochondral lesions, should also be looked for. Loose bodies may be found, which often are not seen radiographically (Fig. 15-6). Ruptured ligaments are surgically repaired, usually with a delayed primary repair being favored over a peroneal tendon-stabilizing procedure. The results of this surgery are uniformly good.

Osteochondral Defects

Osteochondral defects in the ankle joint may occur secondary to chronic inversion or eversion injuries.[3–5] Berndt and Harty suggest that these lesions are "transchondral fractures."[6] They found 44 percent of the lesions to be anterolateral and 56 percent posteromedial. These talar lesions are identified by stages of pathogenesis: stage I, compression; stage II, partially detached fragment; stage III, completely detached osteochondral fracture defect; and stage IV, displaced osteochondral fragment. Although symptomatic, stage I defects are usually written off as sequelae of sprains and not treated.

Lateral instability, therefore, leads to these lesions as the

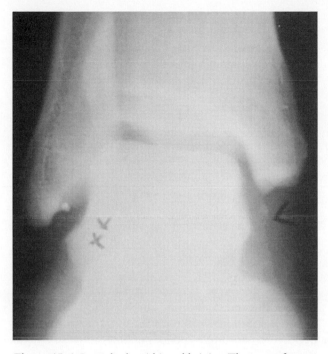

Figure 15-6 Loose body within ankle joint. These are often not seen on radiographs.

anterolateral border of the talus is compressed by the abutting fibula. The posteromedial lesions result from compressive or shear forces. The talus is medially tilted in its mortise when the ankle is plantar-flexed, explaining the predilection for osteochondritis dissecans at the posteromedial aspect of the trochlea of the talus. This injury appears to be secondary to combined shear and compression. Excessive jumping force may also cause a transchondral fracture. Portions of damaged cartilage may flip up and fail to unite.

The primary symptom is intra-articular pain at the ankle joint. The pain is deep in the ankle joint and may be present with or without instability of the joint, depending upon location. In most cases there is a history of ankle joint trauma. Standard radiographs may be helpful, but often do not delineate osteochondritis dissecans, osteochondral lesions, or transchondral fractures. A CT scan should be ordered if plain radiographs are inconclusive. I have seen several cases of painful transchondral fractures with normal radiographs and positive CT scans. At the time of arthroscopic surgery, large stage IV lesions were removed and the bed drilled. These patients have all done very well following initial non-weight bearing for 6 weeks followed by physical therapy and rehabilitation.

The treatment of choice for stage I and II lesions is conservative therapy with non-weight-bearing casts for 6 weeks, then physical therapy. Stage III lesions may respond to conservative treatment, but often require surgery. Stage IV lesions do best with surgical excision and drilling of the bed, usually transarthroscopically. With open or closed arthrotomy, the lesion is removed and the bed treated by abrasion arthroplasty, which includes removal of the first 2 mm of subchondral bone down to a bleeding surface. Then small holes are made in the abraded surface with a 0.045 Kirschner wire to promote bleeding and the formation of fibrocartilage. When abrasion arthroplasty is carried out, weight bearing should be deferred for 6 weeks. To encourage the formation of healthy fibrocartilage, which may be quite functional in its final form, early active motion is recommended. Whereas old transchondral fractures are usually excised, fresh stage II or III lesions may be treated by intra-articular pinning. The results of pinning are variable and, unless the lesions are quite large, I prefer excising them and doing abrasion arthroplasty. Newer fixation methods with absorbable pins and screws may prove useful in surgical fixation, eliminating the problems seen with metal intra-articular fixation devices.

Intra-articular lesions may be present with chronic instability of the ankle joint or anterolateral impingement. When this is the case, the ruptured ligaments should be repaired either by delayed primary repair or by lateral stabilization. Failure to correct the instability will lead to progressive articular damage of the trochlear surface of the talus.

Further intra-articular ankle joint damage may exist about the medial and lateral gutters and facets. Excessive pronation, or supinatory sprains, may cause lesions of the medial or lateral malleolar facets at the articulations with the trochlear surfaces and facets of the talus. Abrasion arthroplasties are generally helpful in treating these problems.

Lateral Ankle Joint Ruptures

The ankle joint is one of the most frequently injured joints of the body. It is estimated that each year 1 million people experience acute ankle injuries, most commonly plantar-flexion inversion sprains. These ankle sprains account for 15 percent of all sports injuries.[7]

Lateral ruptures of the ankle joint ligaments occur most often with plantar-flexory inversion injuries. Plantar flexion of the ankle joint leads to increased talar tilt with inversion stress. This instability laterally occurs secondary to the individual arrangement of the collateral ligaments. With full plantar flexion of the ankle joint, the anterior talofibular ligament is in a position in which it alone must withstand the inversion plantar-flexory force. Since it is the weakest lateral collateral ligament, it often stretches and ruptures completely or incompletely. When the foot is in dorsiflexion, however, the anterior talofibular ligament is more horizontal and less vulnerable. The middle collateral ligament is more vulnerable in this position.

When checking for laxity of the lateral collateral ligaments and comparing one ankle with the other, it is important to have the comparison foot in the same degree of plantar flexion or dorsiflexion as the injured foot. The degree of talar tilt is dependent on the extent of plantar flexion present and the tension on specific collateral ligaments. In plantar flexion, the anterior collateral ligament is stressed; in dorsiflexion, the middle collateral ligament is stressed. Thus one may differentiate between the pathology of these two ligaments. With plantar flexion and complete rupture of the anterior lateral collateral ligament, the next ligament to rupture would be the middle collateral ligament. With middle collateral ligament rupture, insta-

bility of the subtalar joint results, especially when the lateral calcaneotalar ligament is damaged.

Plantar-flexory inversion frequently damages the anterior lateral collateral ligament. Coexistent with this injury may be an injury to the bifurcate ligament between the lateral aspect of the calcaneus, talus, and cuboid. Excessive varus twisting of the foot results in rupture of the intraosseous talocalcaneal ligament, which lies in the sinus tarsi. This understandably results in subtalar joint postsprain instability and chronic synovitis. With rotation, injury to the anterior inferior tibiofibular ligament may also occur. With ligamentous damage, there is almost always capsular damage and subsequent bleeding.

The immediate treatment in ankle joint sprain at the lateral aspect of the ankle is that of PRICE (protection, rest, ice, elevation, and compression). Moist, cold Ace bandage wraps are helpful, as are ice packs secured with Ace wraps. Frozen peas conform well to the ankle and stay cold for 20 minutes or more while thawing. Care should be taken not to ice burn the skin; thus the ice is applied over a towel for limited periods of time (15 to 20 min/h) (Fig. 15-7). A grade I sprain exists when there is stretching

Figure 15-7 Ice burn on the fibular malleolus, sustained during ice treatment for an inversion strain.

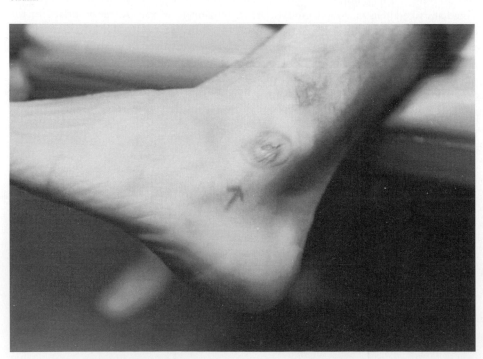

of the collateral ligaments but no tearing, a grade II sprain occurs with an incomplete tear, and a grade III sprain is present with a complete tear.

With a grade I sprain, at gameside, the athlete can usually safely return to competition after PRICE followed by protective taping of the ankle joint. A grade II sprain with a partial tear can be reduced to a grade I sprain by taping; competition is allowed if the athlete is able to jump up and down on the involved ankle and run without pain. With a grade III sprain with complete rupture, the athlete has difficulty walking and may need to be on crutches. Even with taping and icing, the athlete will be unable to return to competition. When ambulation is difficult following a sprain, radiographs should be taken to rule out fracture. Pain that persists beyond 2 months is suggestive of transchondral fracture, meniscoid lesion, or chronic synovitis.

DIAGNOSIS AND TREATMENT

The optimal time to examine an ankle joint is immediately after the injury. At this point, there has been very little reaction to the soft tissue damage, and all the ligaments can be palpated. Icing the ankle joint initially helps reduce the pain, after which one can selectively go through palpation of all the ligaments with the foot dorsiflexed, neutral, and plantar flexed. The anterior drawer test is very helpful in diagnosing instability. This will usually give a tentative diagnosis. The standard tests are as follows:

1. *Anterior drawer test.* With the anterior drawer test, the foot is plantar flexed, and the tibia is pushed posteriorly as the posterior aspect of the calcaneus is pulled forward. The amount of laxity at the ankle joint is determined by comparing one ankle with the other. When the anterior lateral collateral ligament has been ruptured, there will be a positive anterior drawer sign, because this is the only ligament maintaining the foot and ankle in anatomic position with the foot in a plantar-flexed attitude.

2. *Frontal plane or inversion stress test.* This test is carried out with the foot in a plantar-flexed position. The maneuver is performed first with the foot inverted, and then with the foot in a neutral position. The frontal plane tilt of the two ankles is compared; one can actually feel the rocking of the trochlear surface of the talus within the ankle mortise when there is significant lateral instability.

3. *Diastasis test.* This test is carried out with the superior aspect of the ankle held firmly as one pushes the calcaneus laterally to determine whether the fibula has separated from the ankle joint.

If persistent pain and swelling exist after an injury, radiographs are taken. If the radiographs are negative, a stress test is carried out (see Figs. 20–15, 20–16 and 20-22). Immediately after injury, local anesthesia is usually unnecessary for the stress test. After 1 to 2 hours, the pain cycle sets in; a local anesthetic block would then be necessary to give a valid result. A peroneal nerve block is carried out at the distal one-fourth of the fibula, where the superficial peroneal and sural nerves pierce the deep fascia and become superficial. This block is carried out rather easily with 5 ml of 2 percent lidocaine. Following the nerve block, an adequate push–pull (anterior drawer) test and frontal plane stress test are carried out, comparing the involved limb with the uninvolved limb. The peroneal nerve block followed by early active and passive protected motion decreases the chronic edema and painful stiffness associated with grade I and grade II sprains and is often very useful. Although the literature shows variable figures in regard to the significance of talar tilt, most reports state that, in an involved ankle with 5 degrees more talar tilt on the frontal plane than in the uninvolved ankle, at least the anterior lateral collateral ligament has been ruptured.[8][11] With more than 10 degrees of disparity, the anterior and middle collateral ligaments may be ruptured.[8-11]

When the athlete comes to the practitioner's office with a swollen, painful ankle following a sprain, it is often very difficult to evaluate the ankle adequately. On such occasions, the arthrogram is most helpful. An air-dye contrast arthrogram is carried out using 10 ml of a mixture containing 2 to 3 mg of Renografin 60, 1 to 2 ml of 1 percent Xylocaine plain, 1 to 2 ml of 0.5 percent Marcaine plain, 1 ml of Traumeel, and 1 to 2 ml of air. If bleeding is taking place, 1:200,000 epinephrine a vasoconstrictor may be given with the Marcaine. Traumeel aids healing and is used to decrease inflammation or reaction from the radiopaque dye. This solution is then injected into the anterior aspect of the ankle joint after a superficial nerve block is done. An adequate sterile preparation is carried out before the arthrogram injection. The arthrogram also allows the examining physician to inspect the cartilage of the ankle joint. If the dye leaks along the lateral aspect of the ankle joint and along the peroneal tendons, the capsule of the ankle joint and the middle collateral ligament have probably been torn. The middle collateral ligament is between the peroneal tendons and the lateral aspect of the capsule; therefore, when both the capsule and the middle collateral ligament are torn, the dye may flow easily along the course of the peroneal tendon sheaths. When the arthrogram is positive for dye leakage, there is usually a significant talar tilt of at least 15 to 20 degrees, indicating a double ligament rupture.

Conservative treatment of grade I sprains of the ankle is that of PRICE followed by peroneal nerve block and infiltration of the ankle joint with a Traumeel and Lymphomyosot homeopathic cocktail. Gentle mobilization and manipulation of the foot and ankle are carried out to restore normal joint function and reset the involved peripheral nerves. This greatly reduces pain and swelling while allowing rapid return of normal function. Physical therapy with electrogalvanic stimulation and microelectric nerve stimulation or interferential electrotherapy initiates healing and reduces edema and subsequent adhesions. For simple stable sprains an Ace bandage will suffice. With more painful or swollen ankles, the ankle is taped or an Unna boot applied and rehabilitative exercises, including proprioceptive balancing and range of motion, are begun. Topical Traumeel is helpful in reducing pain and promoting healing. Weight bearing is allowed as soon as it is comfortable, with the ankle protected with taping, an Unna boot, or an air splint, depending on the edema and stability. Return to activity is allowed when pain-free stability is exhibited. The ankle should remain protected for 4 to 6 weeks while the ligament is healing.

A stretched ligament may lead to chronic instability if the stretching is significant. This is especially true in the younger age group, in which stretching takes place before rupture does. If intra-articular pathology or chronic repetitive sprains secondary to an unstable ankle joint are noted, protective taping or bracing is indicated for participation in sports. One should look for foot imbalances as a reason for lateral instability. Rearfoot varus and forefoot valgus with a plantar-flexed first metatarsal are obvious causes. Orthoses with a lateral wedge or flange will help prevent reinjury. Other than this, a lateral stabilization would be the treatment of choice for persistent instability of the ankle joint with repeated sprain of the ankle, despite protective taping or bracing, resulting in chronic instability with continued stretching or progressive rupture of the ligaments. Without proper stabilization, serious intra-articular damage may result. For severe varus of the calcaneus, a valgus wedge (Dwyer) osteotomy of the calcaneus is preferred over lateral stabilization, because lateral stabilization restricts subtalar motion in the cavus foot with lateral instability (see Ch. 26).

With a grade II sprain of the ankle joint, there has been a partial rupture. These are treated essentially the same as grade I sprains, with the exception that more emphasis is placed on protective splinting, taping, or bracing. Initially a posterior splint may be necessary for 3 or 4 weeks. These sprains will usually heal with early and aggressive physical therapy three times a week, early protective range of motion exercises, weekly injection therapy, and strengthening of the peroneal tendons. Homeopathic–lidocaine injections about the ligaments create local inflammation and result in early fibrosis and healing of the ligaments. This has been termed *prolotherapy*. Some form of external support is necessary for about 2 months following healing of the injury, especially during rough competition or practice. Proprioceptive rehabilitation is of prime importance in preventing reinjury.

With a complete rupture or grade III sprain, one has the choice of conservative treatment with physical therapy, prolotherapy injection, protected function including posterior splints, or a below-knee (BK) cast for 4 weeks followed by physical therapy. The selected treatment depends upon the severity of the rupture, the amount of instability, history of prior sprains, and the compliance of the athlete. With cooperative, well-motivated patients, I prefer a posterior splint, weekly injections, mobilization and manipulation, oral remedies (Traumeel, Lymphomyosot, Zeel), and early return to activity with an air cast or protective taping. Later, lace-up braces can be used for 4 months after initial healing.

With athletes with a history of repeated serious sprains, I prefer surgical repair. If this is the first sprain, and very unstable, and if the athlete is gifted, I discuss the option of primary repair. The athlete will have a stable ankle and rapid recovery and return to sports, within 6 to 8 weeks following surgery. If opting to treat the sprain conservatively with physical therapy and rapid return to function when the ligament is protected initially using a posterior splint, the splint should be removed three to four times a day and sagittal plane motion gently carried out. This prevents atrophy of the surrounding dynamic stabilizers of the ankle joint and decreases the likelihood of narrowing of the ankle joint secondary to inactivity. Motion also allows for peripheral "pumping" to eliminate edema and reduce fibrous adhesions. Early weight bearing is allowed with the ankle joint protected either with an air cast, a posterior splint, or later a lace-up ankle brace. Physical therapy is carried out three times a week to daily for best results. Once ambulation is pain free, the ankle is protected with taping or a double upright brace; the athlete can gradually return to function, first doing straight-ahead running and then progressing from a large figure-eight to a narrower figure-eight course. Balance exercises are imperative to improve proprioception. Once the athlete is able to demonstrate a stork stand for at least 1 minute with the eyes closed, as well as agility, strength, and balance, return to practice is allowed. Return to competition is advised with the provision that the ankle is taped and protected for the remainder of the athletic career, during practice and competition. Should other plantar-flexory inversion sprains occur with disability and pain, a primary repair should be carried out immediately.

The more active the athlete and the more prolonged the athletic career is expected to be, the greater the indication for primary repair of ruptured ligaments. For sedentary people who happen to have sprained or ruptured an ankle joint, a conservative approach will suffice. For non-compliant patients, a BK cast for 4 weeks is advised. For the patient who has had chronic repetitive sprains with chronic lateral instability, a delayed primary repair is advised. When this procedure is done, the tissue around the ruptured ligament is used to form a new ligament. Both the anterior and middle collateral ligaments are checked and repaired as needed. If insufficient ligamentous structures remain for a delayed primary repair, a lateral stabilization is carried out. Various modifications of the Chrisman-Snook procedure are performed. Woven Dacron can be used to repair the ankle after the methods of Park. When this is done, a modified Watson-Jones procedure is used with the woven Dacron graft (see Ch. 26).

The results of delayed primary repair are quite satisfactory. The results of lateral stabilization using a peroneus brevis tenodesis procedure or the Dacron graft are also good. One must be careful when performing a lateral stabilization not to decrease subtalar joint motion excessively. A lateral stabilization should be performed with the subtalar joint 1 to 2 degrees everted to neutral. Maximum pronation should be avoided. Lateral stabilization should not be performed when there is excessive calcaneal varus, because this will limit the subtalar joint function significantly. A valgus calcaneal osteotomy is preferred.

MEDIAL SPRAINS OF THE ANKLE JOINT

The medial ligament of the ankle joint is the deltoid. The deltoid is made up of a strong, flat, triangular band of tissue attached at the anterior and posterior borders of the medial malleolus. It consists of two sets of fibers that are superficial and deep. Of the superficial fibers, the most anterior (tibionavicular) pass forward and insert into the tuberosity in the navicular bone and also blend into the calcaneonavicular ligament. The middle portion of the deltoid is the calcaneotibial, which inserts into the sustentaculum tali of the calcaneus. The posterior fibers (posterior talotibial) pass posterolaterally and are attached to the inner side of the talus as well as to the medial malleolus. The deep fibers (anterior talotibial) are attached from the anteromedial surface of the medial malleolus to the medial surface of the talus. The deltoid ligament is contiguous with the posterior tibial and flexor digitorum longus tendons.

Whereas the lateral collateral ligaments are three separate ligaments that are easily injured depending on the position of the foot, the deltoid ligaments constitute a strong, thick band that is difficult to injure. Injuries of the deltoid occur with plantar flexion and external rotation of the foot. These injuries often coexist with a push-off fracture of the lateral malleolus. Chronic instability may be the sequela of an ankle joint fracture. Acute instability is usually secondary to acute ankle joint pathology, and the treatment is dictated by clinical and radiographic findings.

ANKLE ARTHRITIS

Post-traumatic arthritis of the ankle joint may be the end result of chronic repetitive stress of the ankle joint with instability. When there is anterior impingement and arthritis of the ankle joint, the treatment of choice may be anterior arthroplasty. Radiographs will show significant spurring about the medial and lateral gutters of the ankle joint as well as its anterior aspect. Using an anterior surgical approach to the ankle, arthrotomy and debridement of the medial and lateral gutters, as well as the anterior aspect of the ankle joint, is usually quite helpful. Abrasion arthroplasties may be carried out where the cartilage is eroded, and hypertrophic synovium can be excised. These procedures may give an athlete, such as a lineman, an additional 5 years of competition. However, with chronic abuse of the ankle joint, spurs and anterior pathology may recur. Athletes must be made aware of this problem.

When anterior arthroplasties of the ankle joint fail or significant arthritis is present, one must entertain the possibility of an ankle joint fusion. Ankle fusions are carried out only when there is so much pain that complete elimination of joint motion is desirable to permit more normal function. Ankle implants have a poor record in the younger age group and should therefore be reserved for older patients who have less demand on the ankle joint.

REFERENCES

1. Inglis AE: Surgical repair of ruptures of the tendo Achillis. Clin Orthop 156:160, 1981
2. Barrett J, Bilisko T: The role of shoes in the prevention of ankle sprains. Sport Med 22:227, 1995
3. Naumetz VA, Schweigel JF: Osteocartilagenous lesions of the talar dome. J Trauma 20:924, 1980
4. Wray DG, Muddu BN: Lateral dome fracture of the talus. J Trauma 9:818, 1981
5. O'Farrell TA, Costello BG: Osteochondritis dissecans of the talus. J Bone Joint Surg 64:494, 1982
6. Berndt A, Harty M: Transchondral fractures (osteochondritis dissecans) of the talus. J Bone Joint Surg [Am] 41:988, 1995
7. Sitler M, Horodyski M: Effectiveness of prophylactic ankle stabilisers for prevention of ankle injuries. Sports Med 20: 53, 1995
8. Hughes J: The medial malleolus in ankle fractures. Orthop Clin North Am 11:649, 1980
9. Sheller AD, Kasser JR, Quigley TB: Tendon injuries about the ankle. Orthop Clin North Am 11:801, 1980
10. Reckling FW, McNamara GR, De Smet AA: Problems with diagnosis and treatment of ankle injuries. J Trauma 11:943, 1981
11. Sauser DD, Nelson RC, Lavine MH, Wu CW: Acute injuries of the lateral ligaments of the ankle. Radiology 148:653, 1983

16

Exercise–Induced Leg Pain

RICHARD T. BOUCHÉ

Sports-related leg pain can be classified as traumatic (overt trauma or macrotrauma) or nontraumatic in nature. Nontraumatic leg pain can further be broken down into exercise-induced and atypical (problems simulating sports-related leg pain). Exercise-induced leg pain encompasses a variety of problems, including overuse injuries, "claudication" syndromes, and miscellaneous entities secondary to sustained exercise:

Overuse Injuries
    Tibial fasciitis
    Stress fracture
    Muscle strain
    Tendinitis

Claudication syndromes
    Chronic compartment syndrome
    Popliteal artery entrapment syndrome
    Peroneal nerve entrapment

Miscellaneous disorders
    Muscle soreness
    Muscle cramps
    Muscle herniation

This chapter provides a brief but comprehensive overview of exercise-induced leg pain, emphasizing problems most likely to be encountered by the sports physician.

When faced with a patient with exercise-induced leg pain, a systematic evaluation should be performed to determine a definitive or tentative diagnosis. This is accomplished by obtaining a complete history, performing a thorough static and dynamic lower extremity physical examination (*not* just of the foot and ankle) and obtaining appropriate diagnostic studies to complement the history and physical examination. Common causes of exercise-induced leg pain should be considered first, followed by uncommon causes. Subtle traumatic or atypical causes should also be considered, especially if the leg problem defies diagnosis. Atypical causes can stimulate sports-related leg pain and include infections, systemic conditions, upper/lower motor neuron lesions, neoplasms, rheumatic conditions, pain dysfunction syndromes, dermatologic conditions, and superficial/deep vein thrombophlebitis. Once a diagnosis has been firmly established, a specific treatment plan can be determined. A multidisciplinary team approach to leg problems is most efficient and highly recommended. If the diagnosis is in doubt or initial treatment is unsuccessful, a consultation should be considered.

OVERUSE INJURIES

Exercise-induced leg pain secondary to overuse is commonly encountered by the sports physician. Stress fractures and tibial fasciitis (shin splints) predominate.[1] Muscle strains and leg tendinitis must also be considered.

Tibial Fasciitis (Shin Splints)

Tibial fasciitis (TF) is an inflammatory condition characterized by pain commonly localized to the posteromedial tibial crest and uncommonly to the anterior tibial crest. This condition is the most common cause of leg pain in athletes, especially those involved in running sports.[1] Many names have been used to refer to this entity, including anterior and posterior shin splints,[2] soleus syndrome,[3] medial tibial syndrome,[4] tibial stress syndrome,[5] and medial tibial stress syndrome.[6] Although often considered a minor problem, this condition can significantly affect athletic participation and performance.

ANATOMY

Anatomically, the crests of the tibia are attachment sites for the deep fascia of the leg which extends from the knee to the ankle (Fig. 16-1). Anterior compartment fascia extends from the anterior peroneal septa and encompasses the anterior compartment, inserting into the anterior crest of the tibia. Deep posterior compartment fascia inserts into the posteromedial crest of the tibia and generally intersects the deep transverse fascia, soleus fascia, and superficial posterior compartment fascia to form the intermuscular septum.

ETIOLOGY/PATHOGENESIS

Etiology of this condition is overuse (unaccustomed and excessive exertional exercise), typically associated with running sports. It is thought that excessive exercise results in fatigue failure at the deep fascial attachment sites of the tibia, especially involving the posteromedial crest. This fatigue failure commences as a fasciitis, progressing to periostitis and eventually developing endosteal activity if the leg continues to be stressed. This inflammatory response is probably due to excessive weight bearing on the tibia and to excessive tension force applied to the fascia by eccentrically contracting muscle-tendon units of the involved compartment. Pressure exerted by tendons on the fascia is directed to the fascial/periosteal attachment site on the tibial crest where this "stress reaction" occurs. Pronatory foot disorders and exercising on hard surfaces will also accentuate eccentric contractions of leg muscles and must be considered when discussing pathomechanics of this condition.[7]

Figure 16-1 Cross-section of right leg showing deep fascia and attachments. ACF, anterior compartment fascia; DPCF, deep posterior compartment fascia; SPCF, superficial compartment fascia.

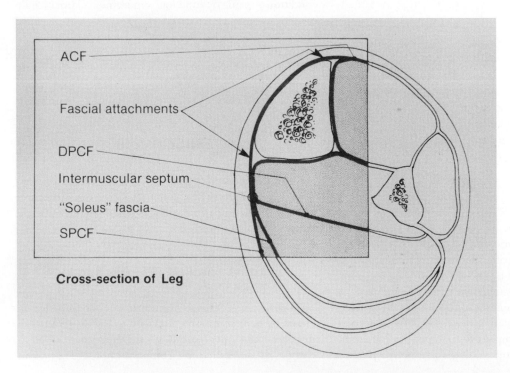

ACF

Fascial attachments

DPCF

Intermuscular septum

"Soleus" fascia

SPCF

Cross-section of Leg

CLASSIFICATION

TF is classified by duration, location, and severity of symptoms (using a functional pain rating). Duration of symptoms is divided into acute (<2 weeks), subacute (2 to 6 weeks) and chronic (>6 weeks) categories. Location of symptoms will be posteromedial, anterior, or combined. Severity of symptoms using a functional pain scale is classified grades 1 through 4. Grade 1 is characterized by pain in response to palpation of involved tibial crest with no symptoms during daily activity or running. Grade 2 indicates discomfort mainly after running but not during running. Some mild discomfort may be present initially but subsides with continued exercise. Grade 3 patients have pain during running and residual discomfort after running. Grade 4 patients are symptomatic with walking and unable to run comfortably.

CLINICAL EVALUATION

Clinically, patients will present with exercise-induced symptoms of a gradual, insidious onset that improve with rest. Pain is the chief complaint and may vary from dull to intense, being localized to the crests of the tibia. Tightness and cramping may also be related, especially if patients attempt to "run through" their discomfort. Training programs should be scrutinized because training errors (e.g., sudden increase in existing activity or participation in a new activity) are extremely common. Examination reveals pain in response to palpation of the anterior or, more commonly, the posteromedial tibia. Mild swelling can be present but is usually not obvious. No symptoms can be elicited on specific muscle testing, and neurovascular status is normal. Loading the involved extremity with a "one-legged hop test" can usually be performed without problems (in grade 4 patients symptoms become apparent with increased repetitions).

Radiographs are usually negative for bony changes, but localized cortical hypertrophy may be seen. Triphasic bone scanning has been helpful in differentiating TF from stress fracture. Radionuclide angiograms and blood-pool images are normal, with delayed images revealing variable longitudinal tracer uptake along the involved tibial crest (Fig. 16-2).[8] This bone scan finding probably indicates localized periostitis (stress reaction). Two other scintigraphic findings have been apparent in patients presenting with TF. Normal findings on bone scan would indicate fasciitis without bone involvement, and diffuse tracer uptake not just localized to the tibial crests would indicate diffuse periostitis. Endosteal activity can be documented with use of single-photon emission computed tomography (SPECT) imaging, which essentially has bone scan and CT scan capabilities. Magnetic resonance imaging (MRI) has also been used recently to more precisely define anatomic location and extent of injury.[9]

TF is commonly confused with stress fracture, tendinitis, muscle strain, and chronic compartment syndrome. Careful clinical examination should allow differentiation.

TREATMENT/PREVENTION

A four-phase treatment program is recommended. *Phase 1 (acute phase)* aims to decrease pain and inflammation. This is accomplished with use of relative (avoiding offending activity) or absolute (crutches) rest, immobilization, cryotherapy (icing), and anti-inflammatory medication. Phase I can last days to weeks and is critical in treatment of this injury.

Phase 2 (rehabilitative phase) focuses on further decreasing pain and swelling, decreasing/preventing scar tissue formation, strengthening the deep fascial–bone interface, and maintaining flexibility of surrounding soft tissue structures. Pain and swelling are addressed with continued cryotherapy, contrast baths, galvanic stimulation, neuroprobe, and other physical therapy modalities. Scar tissue can be treated with use of moist heat followed by deep transverse friction massage (manually or with instrumentation), local anesthetic/steroid injections, and phonophoresis. Strengthening the deep fascial–bone interface is accomplished by exercising deep compartment muscles, which direct a tension force to the deep fascial insertion. Strengthening should be performed after pain is adequately controlled. A graduated strengthening program is initiated with isometric exercises followed by isotonic and variable-resistance exercises, progressing to isokinetic exercises. Flexibility of the posterior group musculature of the leg is addressed with a comprehensive stretching program.

Phase 3 (functional phase) aims to functionally strengthen the fascial–bone interface and to protect the bone structure from excessive tension forces. Controlled plyometric-type strengthening exercises will prepare the patient for return to desired activity. Tension forces can be minimized by use of foot orthotics, taping, and Neoprene sleeves.

Phase 4 (return-to-activity phase) is designed to return the athlete to the desired sport and level of activity. This phase is based on many factors, including level of fitness, previous training program, and personal injury pattern. Return to desired sport should be gradual, systematic, and to tolerance. If pain is experienced and sustained, this phase of

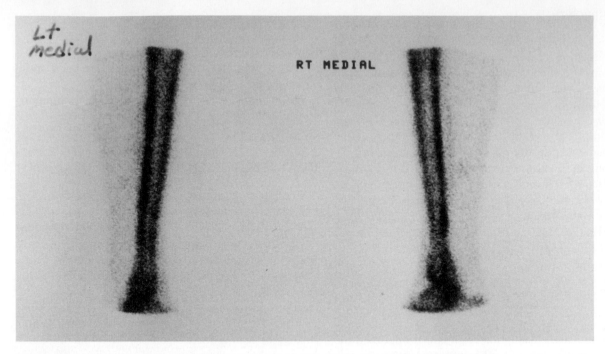

Figure 16-2 Delayed-image radionuclide scans showing longitudinal tracer uptake in patient with tibial fasciitis.

treatment should be discontinued and the patient re-evaluated. Protective and preventive measures should also be discussed and initiated when appropriate.

Conservative treatment is usually successful, but some cases become intractable, being resistant to all conservative measures. In these situations surgical release of the deep fascia should be considered.[4,10–12] My results in a limited series of patients have been excellent although conservative treatment is not a panacea.

TF can be prevented by (1) determining proper shoes for the biomechanical demands of each patient, (2) maintaining flexibility and range of motion through specific stretching exercises, (3) strengthening deficient muscle groups, (4) considering temporary and permanent orthotic therapy when indicated, and (5) following a sensible training program consistent with the athlete's abilities and goals.

Stress Fracture

Stress fracture of the leg is a potentially serious overuse injury prevalent in athletes and military personnel who participate in strenuous activity (especially running). The tibia and fibula are common sites of injury, with the tibia being one of the most frequent sites of stress fracture in the body.[13,14] Stress (or fatigue) fracture implies a disruption in the continuity of normal bone in response to repeated subthreshold forces. Stress fracture must be differentiated from insufficiency and pathologic fracture.[15] Insufficiency fracture occurs when normal stress is applied to abnormal bone (i.e., rheumatoid arthritis, osteoporosis, etc.). Pathologic fracture refers to any bone weakened by pre-existing neoplasm.

ETIOLOGY/PATHOGENESIS

Two theories have been set forth to explain the etiology of stress fracture.[16,17] The first theory hypothesizes that muscular fatigue secondary to stress overload causes a loss of shock absorption function, which allows excessive forces to be transmitted to the underlying bone.[16] The second theory contends that repeated muscular forces acting on a bone can produce a stress fracture.[17] The second theory is supported by the fact that stress fractures can occur in non-weight-bearing bones (i.e., humerus).[18] It is likely that both mechanisms play a role but the relative contribution of each is unknown and probably depends on types of activity (military vs. athletic population) and the specific bone being stressed.

Bone responds to stress (via Wolff's law) by a process of osteonal remodeling or osteonization.[19] In the normal sequence of remodeling, resorption of bone is followed by replacement. Replacement is a slow process, whereas resorption proceeds rapidly, producing a temporarily weakened cortex. Sufficient weakening leads to periosteal reinforcement until the refilling process has caught up and solidified the cortex. If continued stress is applied during the time when the cortex is temporarily weakened, accelerated remodeling occurs and ultimately a stress fracture may result. If stress is reduced or eliminated, there will be a shift favoring bone formation, thus achieving greater bone strength. Using this model of osteonal remodeling, it becomes evident that response of bone to stress is a dynamic process and not an isolated event. The term *stress reaction* is used to indicate bone remodeling responses of bone to stress that precede stress fracture.[20]

CLINICAL EVALUATION

Typically an athlete will present with localized pain and swelling exacerbated with weight bearing and improved with rest. Onset is gradual and insidious with no history of overt trauma. Historically, the athlete relates participating repeatedly in a strenuous activity that is either new or different. Recurrent stress fractures may represent insufficiency fractures and suggest osteoporosis. An in-depth history should be performed. Physical examination reveals a discrete area of pain on palpation, percussion pain, localized swelling and erythema, and an inability to perform the one-legged hop test because of pain. Significant muscle splinting and guarding may also be evident.

Initial screening radiographs (including oblique views) should be obtained, although they are frequently negative. Radiographs are insensitive early and late in the course of stress fracture healing. When positive, they are specific for stress fracture and exhibit characteristic findings including periosteal new bone formation, intracortical lucency, and endosteal new bone formation, although these findings may take weeks to months to be evident. Bone scan provides the most useful information. Technetium bone scan is highly sensitive but nonspecific for stress fracture, because other disease processes can cause similar findings. Bone scan findings for stress fracture reveal a sharply marginated, dense, fusiform uptake correlated to the area of involvement. A bone scan becomes positive within days of the stress fracture and can stay positive for over 1 year despite clinical healing. Asymptomatic areas of uptake may be found on bone scan, indicating subclinical sites of bone

remodeling.[21] False-negative findings have also been reported although only anterior and posterior views were obtained (oblique views should also be obtained).[22] Triphasic or triple-phase bone scans consist of angiographic, blood-pool, and delayed phases and can provide additional information (i.e., acute vs. chronic, soft tissue vs. bone involvement, stress fracture vs. stress reaction).[23]

Patients suspected of being osteoporotic with a history of recurrent stress fractures are candidates for bone mineral content studies. Three noninvasive and an invasive technique are available for assessing bone mineral density.[24] The noninvasive techniques include single/dual-photon absorptiometry,[25] quantitative CT, and a relatively new, inexpensive radiographic imaging technique called dual-energy x-ray absorptiometry. Iliac crest biopsy remains the primary invasive technique. Cortical and cancellous bone density can be measured with these techniques.

CLASSIFICATION

The classification scheme recommended for stress fracture takes into consideration the clinical symptom of pain and radiographic and bone scan findings. It is based on the concept of bone stress being part of a continuum that can vary from accelerated bone remodeling or stress reaction to bone fatigue and exhaustion.[26] Grade 0 indicates normal bone remodeling with no symptoms, negative radiograph, and bone scan findings. Grade I represents an asymptomatic stress reaction with the radiograph being negative and bone scan positive. Grade II represents a symptomatic stress reaction with pain present, radiograph negative, and bone scan positive. Grade III is characterized by marked pain and positive radiographic and bone scan findings indicating stress fracture. Most of the injuries are actually symptomatic stress reactions (grade II) but may represent occult stress fractures with the fracture not being evident radiographically. CT scanning or MRI may better elucidate grade II injury.[27]

TREATMENT/PREVENTION

Classically, treatment of stress fractures consist of relative or absolute rest depending on the clinical situation. The offending activity must be avoided for a period of time to prevent further injury. Cross-training emphasizing non-weight-bearing activity (i.e., swimming, biking, and water running with a wet vest) is recommended. If walking is painful, immobilization with a cast or functional leg brace may be indicated for a period of time. Certain "at-risk" fractures (bicortical) may require a period of non-weight bearing with use of crutches. Acute-phase treatment (ice, compression, elevation) and use of nonsteroidal anti-inflammatory agents may be helpful. When the "rest period" of the treatment program has been completed and the patient has been pain free for 2 weeks, a supervised rehabilitation program is initiated. The most common problem we encounter in patients with recurrent pain secondary to stress fracture involves an inadequate period of rest with a premature return to weight-bearing activity. A gradual, progressive return to full activity is recommended, allowing adequate rest periods between workouts. Care should be taken especially in the first 4 weeks following the reintroduction of activity because bone is most vulnerable to reinjury during this period, when bone resorption is greater than bone replacement.

Recently, a randomized, prospective study was performed stating that certain stress fractures of the leg (specific types of tibial stress fractures) can be managed functionally with a semirigid pneumatic leg brace, allowing athletes to return to their sport in a much shorter period of time compared to conventional treatment involving periods of relative and absolute rest.[28] This concept deserves further study and research.

Prevention involves identifying etiologic factors that may potentiate injury: for example, inappropriate shoewear, muscle imbalances, and structural abnormalities. Training programs should be thoroughly reviewed. Pronated feet and cavus feet have been associated with stress fractures of specific bones, but the role of orthotics has not been fully elucidated.[29–31] Further research is needed.

SPECIFIC STRESS FRACTURES OF THE LEG

Stress fractures of the leg can involve multiple sites, including the medial tibial plateau, tibial shaft (proximal, middle, and distal), medial malleolus, and fibula.

Injury to the *medial tibial plateau* has been infrequent in my experience but important because the fracture can extend into the knee joint. This injury must be differentiated from extra- and intra-articular knee involvement and pes anserinus tendinitis/bursitis. Radiographs (after at least 3 weeks) usually reveal endosteal callus or sclerosis just beneath the medial tibial plateau. Treatment for this problem is conservative and theoretically should take 6 to 8 weeks, but I have encountered four patients who clinically had delayed healing, with one patient requiring 4-plus months to return to athletic activity.

In my experience, *tibial shaft* stress fractures are most common and usually involve the posteromedial crest of the tibia at the junction of the middle and distal third of the leg. Proximal shaft fractures (involving the posteromedial tibial crest) occur less commonly. Healing can take up to 12 weeks with this injury, but usually 8 to 10 weeks is adequate. Radiographs for this injury should include the standard anteroposterior and lateral as well as oblique views. When obtaining a bone scan, it is also important to order oblique views to avoid a false-negative finding.

Anterior crest midshaft tibial stress fractures should be approached cautiously because this injury has been commonly associated with delayed union, nonunion, and complete fracture.[32–34] Pathogenesis of this injury suggests the tension role of the anterior tibial cortex, with its poor vascularity and inability to mount a healing response. Radiographs reveal a horizontal fissure extending into the cortex of the tibial crest that is surrounded by new bone formation or sclerotic bone; thus this injury has earned the name, "the dreaded black line" (Fig. 16-3).

Figure 16-3 Horizontal fissure involving anterior cortex of tibial crest indicating the presence of midshaft tibial stress fractures.

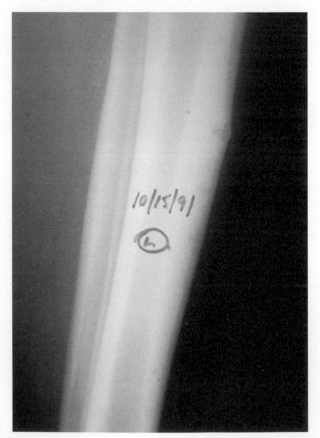

Bone scans obtained for this problem may be weakly positive or negative. This injury should be treated aggressively with a prolonged period of rest and electrical bone stimulation for a minimum of 4 to 6 months before considering surgical intervention, which can include either fracture excision with bone grafting, intramedullary rodding, or both.

Medial malleolar stress fractures should be considered in patients with medial ankle pain and localized swelling without history of injury or trauma.[35] Radiographs may be positive or negative, and bone scan reveals focal uptake to the medial malleolus. In one series of four patients (five stress fractures with one patient having bilateral involvement), all responded well to 4 to 6 weeks of relative rest with initial use of functional leg bracing until the patient could walk in regular shoewear without symptoms.

Fibular stress fractures commonly involve the lateral cortex of the distal third just proximal to the level of the distal tibiofibular articulation, and uncommonly the proximal third. In general, these injuries respond well to a period of relative rest, taking 6 to 8 weeks for complete healing.

Muscle Strain

Strains of muscle and muscle-tendon units are among the most common causes of injury and disability in sports.[36] A strain is defined as partial or total muscle fiber disruption caused by overstretching of muscle from an excessively applied tensile force. The entire muscle-tendon unit is susceptible to injury, with the musculotendinous junction being the most vulnerable site of injury.[37] Strain can also occur at the muscle origin, within the muscle substance, or at the tendon–bone junction. Strain injuries are most common in sports requiring rapid accelerations and sudden bursts of speed (i.e., court sports and sprinting).[38] Muscles at risk for strain are those that have a high percentage of fast twitch (type II) muscle fibers and cross two or more joints.[39]

ETIOLOGY/PATHOGENESIS

Muscle strain occurs in response to forcibly stretching a muscle either passively or, more commonly, when the muscle is undergoing an eccentric contraction. There is greater force production during an eccentric contraction; therefore, greater stress is exerted on the muscle-tendon unit with greater potential for injury.[38] Injury can result from a single tensile force that exceeds the critical limit of the muscle (traumatic) or from repetitive submaximal forces producing a cumulative fatigue failure of the muscle (nontraumatic or overuse). Factors that predispose a muscle-tendon unit to injury include lack of or insufficient warmup,[40] muscle fatigue,[41] muscle weakness,[42] muscle tightness,[43,44] and previous injury with scar formation.[37]

CLASSIFICATION

A useful classification scheme divides muscle strains into three grades.[45,46] Grade I (mild) strain is a stretch injury with few muscle fibers being disrupted. Grade I strains are considered muscle pulls in which the limits of the muscle have not been exceeded. Grade II (moderate) strain is a partial muscle tear. If the perimysium and fascia remain intact, a local hematoma will form (grade IIA). If the perimysium and fascia are disrupted, a diffuse ecchymosis will be evident (grade IIB). Grade III (severe) strain is a complete disruption of the muscle and fascia.

CLINICAL EVALUATION

An athlete with a muscle strain presents with localized pain and swelling of acute onset and an inability to use the involved muscle. A causal event is related usually involving eccentric contraction activity. Depending on the grade of injury, localized hematoma formation or diffuse ecchymosis can develop and is usually evident a day or more after the initial event.

Physical examination reveals localized pain on palpation and swelling (minimal or absent in type I). The involved muscle will be maintained in a position of least tension, and the athlete will exhibit significant muscle guarding and splinting on attempted joint range of motion. Pain is elicited on passive stretch and resistance to active contraction of the involved muscle. A palpable defect may be evident in a grade II or III strain. Depending on the length of time since the injury, bleeding may be evident.

Diagnosis can usually be established clinically with a thorough history and physical examination. Radiographs are obtained for suspected bony pathology. Ultrasonography,[47,48] soft tissue CT scanning,[49] or MRI[50] can be obtained when the diagnosis is in doubt or when additional information is desired.

TREATMENT/PREVENTION

The regeneration potential of injured muscle fibers is limited, with disrupted fibers being replaced by inelastic scar tissue.[37] The goal of treatment is a small, painless, supple scar not limiting muscle elasticity. Most muscle strains are grades I and II; grade III is seen only rarely. Grade III injuries may require open surgical repair to avoid a painful, extensive nonfunctional scar. Grade I and II injuries are treated similarly in a systematic fashion progressing through four phases of treatment.[51] Phase duration varies depending on injury type. Initial acute-phase treatment consists of relative rest, protection of the involved muscle, ice, compression, elevation, and the use of nonsteroidal anti-inflammatory agents. Interferential electrical stimulation can be used if swelling is present. Gentle muscle contraction to tolerance can also be started at this time. During the acute phase, massage is contraindicated to avoid further muscle injury. Patients with grade I strains can usually walk with protection (i.e., taping, Neoprene compression sleeve, etc.). Grade II injuries require non-weight bearing with crutch ambulation for a period of time.

During the rehabilitation (second) phase, degree of pain is used to determine treatment efficacy and rate of progression. If severe pain is present, treatment should be discontinued and the patient re-evaluated. Initially, passive range-of-motion exercises are performed, followed by active range-of-motion exercises. When range of motion is pain free, gentle passive stretching exercises are initiated. A strengthening program is then started, progressing from isometric to isotonic (first concentric then eccentric exercises) to isokinetic exercises. Physical therapy modalities and massage are also utilized during this phase.

The functional (third) phase consists of a variety of supervised therapeutic exercises (including plyometric training) stressing sports-specific activities and preparing the patient for return to activity. A final assessment of the patient is performed with consideration of strength, flexibility, general conditioning, biomechanics, and ability to perform sports-specific activities. In the return-to-activity (fourth and final) phase, the athlete is counseled on the beneficial effects of warmup, proper stretching, strengthening exercises, and equipment issues (e.g., proper shoewear). Strategies to continue to protect the involved area are also discussed, including the use of taping, Neoprene sleeves, and foot orthotics.

SPECIFIC MUSCLE STRAINS OF THE LEG

Strains commonly encountered involve the gastrocnemius, tibialis anterior, and peroneal muscles.

The most common strain involves a grade I injury to the *gastrocnemius* muscle at the musculotendinous junction. Activities involving repetitive eccentric loading are usually responsible. These injuries respond well to conservative treatment. Grade II and III injuries of the gastrocnemius muscle at the musculotendinous junction are known as "tennis leg".[52] Previously this injury was thought to represent a rupture of the plantaris muscle, but there is no evidence that a plantaris rupture has ever occurred and its existence is in doubt.[53] The onset of "tennis leg" is sudden, with sharp pain localized to the calf. Patients describe a sensation of being struck on the back of the leg and are unable to support themselves while standing on their toes. The mechanism usually involves knee extension with foot dorsiflexion associated with a stretching or lunging maneuver. Treatment is usually conservative, although grade III injuries may require surgical repair.

Injuries to the *anterior tibial* muscle are commonly seen in bicyclists (using toe clips), swimmers (training with fins), runners (excessive downhill running), and cross-country skiers (using the skating technique). All of these activities can load the anterior tibial tendon excessively, resulting in muscle strain, with grade I injuries predominating. This injury is most often confused with chronic anterior compartment syndrome.

Peroneal muscle strains (grade I) are prevalent in patients who (1) have an inverted resting calcaneal stance position due to various biomechanical abnormalities (partially compensated rearfoot varus, intrinsic heel varus, rigid plantarflexed first ray, rigid forefoot valgus, compensated genu valgum deformity, etc.); (2) compensate for a foot problem (i.e., sesamoid fracture or second metatarsophalangeal synovitis) by maintaining their foot in an unaccustomed inverted attitude to avoid bearing weight on the painful area; and (3) have excessively worn out the lateral sole of their shoe (especially the heel), resulting in an inverted attitude of the foot. Peroneal muscle strains usually respond well to conservative treatment addressing the aforementioned etiologic factors.

Tendinitis

Tendinitis literally means "inflammation of tendon," although historically it has been a general term describing all painful tendon structures, including bursae and synovial sheaths.[54] There is increased pathologic evidence that distinguishes between acute traumatic inflammatory response and the more insidious process of chronic tendon degeneration.[54–56] This differentiation has obvious treatment implications.

In my experience, tendon injury of the leg is uncommon compared to tendon injury of the ankle and foot (the

Achilles tendon is considered an ankle tendon and *not* a leg tendon in this discussion), which is common. Tendons of the leg course vertically with no change in direction, and they do not have to withstand high frictional forces (no retinacula). Tendinitis of the leg has been confused with other types of leg pathology and has been implicated, wrongly in my opinion, as a primary cause of "shin splints." I have encountered (uncommonly) acute and subacute forms of "true" leg tendinitis (and paratenonitis) most commonly involving the extensor digitorum longus, peroneal longus, and posterior tibial tendons. Chronic degenerative tendon disorders of the leg have not been encountered.

ANATOMY

Anatomically, two types of tendon arrangement can be identified. In locations where the tendon is subjected to high friction forces, a sheath lined with synovium surrounds the tendon. This situation is found in the ankle and foot, where there is a 90-degree change in direction as tendons course from the leg to the foot (passing under a retinaculum). In regions where frictional forces are minimal (e.g., tendons of the leg), only loose connective tissue surrounds the tendon.

ETIOLOGY

Tendons are injured when excessive tensile forces are applied, thereby causing breakdown of tendon substance. Tendon just as bone, is susceptible to fatigue where the resistance capacity is lowered when continual force is applied. The intensity of force may be below the threshold for a given load, but this threshold is lowered when repetitive load is applied (overuse). Factors affecting these loads may include age, tendon vascularity, body weight, intensity and duration of activity, muscle weakness, muscle flexibility, and biomechanics.

In my experience with leg tendinitis, the offending activity involves a repetitive, unaccustomed activity of high intensity and long duration. Based on speculation, the etiology may be a tethering force exerted against the deep fascia of the leg just proximal to the ankle retinacular structures (i.e., superior extensor retinaculum).

CLASSIFICATION

Based on previous observations,[55,56] four pathologic conditions of tendon are classically described, distinguishing between acute inflammatory processes and chronic de-generative changes. *Tendinitis* is a symptomatic degeneration of tendon with vascular disruption and inflammatory repair response. The old terminology was tendon "strain" or "tear." Acute (<2 weeks), subacute (2 to 6 weeks) and chronic (>6 weeks) subgroups are recognized. Histology can vary from acute hemorrhage and tear to calcification/pre-existing degeneration. In the chronic stage there may be interstitial microinjury, central necrosis, and partial or complete rupture. *Paratenonitis* is an inflammation of only the paratenon, whether lined by synovium or not. Older terms used to describe this condition included "tenosynovitis," "tenovaginitis," or "peritendinitis." *Paratenonitis with tendinosis* is paratenon inflammation with intratendinous degeneration. The old term was "tendinitis." *Tendinosis* refers to asymptomatic intratendinous degeneration due to atrophy caused by aging, microtrauma, and vascular compromise. The former term was also "tendinitis."

Although the aforementioned classification has generally been accepted, the terminology remains vague and confusing. Based on a recent histopathologic study of chronic Achilles tendinopathy[57] and personal experience with surgical treatment of Achilles insertional calcific tendinopathy, I propose that the term *tendinitis* not be used as it applies to chronic Achilles tendinopathy because an inflammatory process is unlikely to occur in the tendon structure itself. The term *tendinosis* refers to a process of tendon degeneration that can be asymptomatic or symptomatic. Therefore, I proposes two subtypes of tendinosis, type A being asymptomatic and type B being a symptomatic degenerative process involving tendon. Thus the classification of chronic tendinopathy would include paratenonitis, paratenonitis with tendinosis, tendinosis (two types), and calcific tendinosis. Further study is needed to confirm this proposed classification system, but I believe it is clinically useful, with the terminology being accurate and well defined.

CLINICAL EVALUATION

Clinically, patients present with localized symptoms of pain, redness, heat, and swelling and may have an impairment in performance. A helpful grading scheme is used based on a functional pain scale: grade 1—pain is present after but not during activity; grade 2—pain is present during and after intense exercise with mild impairment; grade 3—pain is present at the beginning, during, and after activity, with significant performance impairment; and grade 4—pain with daily activity, unable to compete.

Examination reveals tenderness/pain in response to palpation, and crepitation may be present. Ankle joint range of motion may be guarded due to pain. There will be pain on passive stretch and on resistance to active contraction of the muscle-tendon unit. MRI, by virtue of its unmatched soft tissue resolution capability, can probably provide the most information in trying to elucidate the different types of tendon pathology.[58]

TREATMENT

Treatment is based on grade of injury and individual expectations of the athlete. The goal of treatment is to achieve grade 0, which would indicate no pain during or after activity. Management parallels the treatment for muscle strain (see earlier) and includes four stages: acute, rehabilitative, functional, and preventive. The mainstay of treatment is the eccentric strengthening program.[59]

CLAUDICATION SYNDROMES

The term *claudication* is derived from the Latin word *claudicare,* meaning to limp.[60] Intermittent claudication (or limping) refers to a symptom complex characterized by pain in lower extremity muscles brought on with exercise and immediately relieved with rest. Classically, this symptom has been commonly associated with a vascular etiology (arteriosclerosis obliterans) presenting clinically as calf pain in the elderly. This symptom can also occur in the younger athletic population, although it is uncommon. When confronted with this presenting symptom, vascular and nonvascular etiologies must be considered:

Vascular
    Arterial
    Venous
    Chronic compartment syndrome
Nonvascular
    Systemic
    Neurogenic
    Muscle enzyme deficiency
    Vitamin B_1 deficiency

Chronic compartment syndrome, popliteal artery entrapment syndrome (arterial), and peroneal nerve entrapment (neurogenic) are important claudication syndromes that must be considered.

Chronic Compartment Syndrome

Although chronic compartment syndrome (CCS) has been recognized for 40 years,[61] only since 1975 has it received significant attention in the literature. CCS is now considered a well-defined clinical entity, but its uncommon occurrence and confusion with acute compartment syndrome (ACS) continue to make this diagnosis a mystery to many a clinician.

Simply defined, compartment syndrome is a condition in which increased pressure within a limited anatomic space compromises the circulation and function of the tissues within that space, resulting in temporary or permanent damage to muscles and nerves.[62] Acute and chronic forms of compartment syndrome exist in the leg.[63] ACS is secondary to trauma but can also be due to intense exercise (although rare). CCS is an exercise-induced condition that is recurrent, with symptoms subsiding when exercise is discontinued and returning when it is resumed.

ANATOMY

Anatomically, the leg is divided into four compartments: anterior, lateral, deep posterior, and superficial posterior. Each compartment has osseous and fascial boundaries except for the superficial posterior compartment, which has fascial boundaries only. By becoming familiar with the structures in each anatomic compartment (Table 16-1), clinical findings can be anticipated based on specific compartment involvement.

ETIOLOGY/PATHOGENESIS

Compartment syndrome appears to be caused by an increase in tissue pressure to a critical level resulting in a compromise in tissue perfusion.[62, 64-67] Increased tissue pressure may result from limited or decreased compartment volume (tight, thickened fascia); increased compartment content (muscle swelling and hypertrophy); or externally applied pressure (taping or casts).[68] Although many theories have been proposed to explain the compromise in tissue perfusion, the arteriovenous gradient theory correlates well with clinical findings.[62] According to this theory, an increase in tissue pressure increases local venous pressure, thus reducing the local arteriovenous gradient. This results in reduced local blood flow and oxygenation, compromising tissue function and viability. Because intracompartmental tissue pressure is usually less than arterial blood pressure, distal arterial blood flow and peripheral pulses remain intact. Thus peripheral pulses and digital cir-

Table 16-1 Structures in the Various Anatomic Compartments of the Leg

Compartment	Boundaries	Muscles	Nerves	Vessels
Anterior	Tibia	Tibialis anterior	Deep peroneal	Anterior tibial
	Interosseous membrane	Extensor hallucis longus		artery/vein
	Fibula	Extensor digitorium longus		
	Anterior intermuscular septum	Peroneus tertius		
	Deep fascia			
Lateral	Fibula	Peroneus longus	Superficial peroneal	
	Anterior and posterior intermuscular septum	Peroneus brevis		
	Deep fascia			
Deep posterior	Tibia	Tibialis posterior	Posterior tibial	Peroneal artery vein
	Interosseous membrane	Flexor digitorium longus		Posterior tibial
	Fibula	Flexor hallucis longus		artery vein
	Deep intermuscular septum			
Superficial posterior	Deep intermuscular septum	Gastrocnemius	Sural (before it exits the deep fascia)	
	Deep fascia	Soleus Plantaris		

(From Bouché RT: Chronic compartment syndrome of the leg. J Am Podiatr Med Assoc 80: 635, 1990, with permission.)

culation are poor indicators of blood flow within the compartment.

CLINICAL EVALUATION

Historically, patients relate chronic, recurrent tightness and pain that is disproportionate to the clinical situation. The clinical findings are localized to one or more of the four compartments of the leg. Symptoms are induced by exercise and relieved with rest. The type of exercise can range from walking to running, but symptoms can also be specific to one type of activity (e.g., dancing). Exercising through the pain is impossible. Other complaints may include leg weakness with an inability to control the foot, or footdrop; dorsal or plantar numbness and tingling of the foot; pain when stretching the involved muscles or tendons; and lump formation, or muscle herniation, of the leg. Swelling is usually not a complaint in isolated CCS.

Physical examination before exercise usually reveals few if any abnormalities, although muscle herniations (fascial defects) may be present. The patient is exercised specifically until symptoms are reproduced, and then placed in a supine position and re-examined. Muscle herniations are now more obvious if present. The vascular status is checked and, if pulses are absent, a vascular etiology is sought. The results of vascular examination are normal in CCS. Hypesthesia may be present in the distribution of the involved nerve. Palpation of the involved compartment reveals significant localized tenseness with pain. Passive stretch of compartment muscles is also quite painful. A strength deficit is noted on manual muscle testing. After exercise is completed, these clinical findings usually resolve in minutes to hours, depending on duration of exercise and severity of the problem.

Intracompartmental pressure measurement provides reproducible, quantitative documentation and is the most objective test available for confirming the presence of CCS. Some work is presently being done with MRI as a diagnostic tool for CCS.[68] Various systems are commercially available for measuring intracompartmental pressure (Fig. 16-4). These systems measure intracompartmental pressure statically at rest, before and after exercise, and dynamically during exercise depending on the system used. Criteria for confirming the diagnosis of CCS include (1) elevated resting pressure before exercise (greater than 15 mm Hg); (2) increased intracompartmental pressure during exercise (muscle relaxation pressure greater than 35 mm Hg); (3) increased postexercise pressure (5-minute postexercise pressure greater than 20 mm Hg); and (4) prolonged return to pre-exercise resting pressure values (normal patients will return to pre-exercise levels in 6 minutes or less after exercise).[69] Tissue pressure measurements should be evaluated in association with diastolic blood pressure, because tissue tolerances may vary in patients who are hypertensive or hypotensive. Regardless of the technique used to measure intracompartmental pressure, protocols should be standardized and instrumentation should be properly calibrated. Patients are instructed not to exercise before the test to avoid falsely elevated readings. Patient positioning is

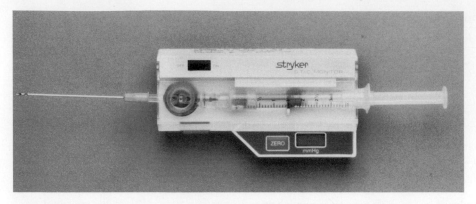

Figure 16-4 Instrument for measuring intracompartmental pressure. (Courtesy of Stryker, Inc.)

critical and must be standardized to obtain reproducible, accurate results. The recommended position is to have the patient in a supine position on a flat surface with heels supported and feet in a neutral position.

TREATMENT

Treatment options for patients with CCS include living with the problem or surgical intervention. Conservative treatment has been unsuccessful in patients who continue vigorous exercise. Patients who decide to live with the problem must either eliminate or limit the offending activity (usually running). Patients who are starting an exercise program may experience a transient compartment syndrome and will respond to rest, altering their training program, and appropriate conditioning of the lower extremity. In patients with confirmed CCS, surgical treatment involving decompressive fasciotomy of the involved compartment(s) is definitive and curative.[70–72] Although fasciotomy techniques vary, their purpose is to relieve pain and increase exercise tolerance.

Popliteal Artery Entrapment Syndrome

Popliteal artery entrapment syndrome (PAES) was first described in 1879,[73] but the presently used name was coined in 1965.[74] PAES is a condition resulting in compression/occlusion of the popliteal artery in the popliteal fossa. The popliteal vein and tibial nerve can also be involved.[75,76] PAES occurs in young patients, with the average age being less than 30 years old (range 12 to 60 years old) with a male-to-female ratio of 15 : 1.[77,78] Incidence varies from 0.17 to 3.5 percent, with 25 percent of cases being bilateral.[79,80]

ANATOMY

Anatomically, the femoral artery begins immediately distal to the inguinal ligament as an extension of the external iliac artery. Just inferior to the inguinal ligament, within the femoral (Scarpa's) triangle, the deep femoral artery branches off the femoral artery, which now continues distally as the superficial femoral artery (SFA). The SFA courses through the adductor (Hunter's) canal in the middle third of the thigh, exiting an opening in the adductor magnus muscle to become the popliteal artery. The SFA in the adductor canal is bounded by the vastus medialis anteriorly and laterally and the adductor longus and magnus medially and posteriorly. The popliteal artery continues through the popliteal fossa to the distal border of the popliteus muscle, where it divides into the anterior and posterior tibial arteries (popliteal trifurcation). The popliteal artery as it courses through the popliteal fossa is bounded lateral-proximally by the biceps femoris and lateral-distally by the plantaris and lateral head of the gastrocnemius. Medially, it is limited by the semitendinosis, semimembranosus, and medial head of the gastrocnemius.

ETIOLOGY/PATHOGENESIS

The etiology is intermittent compression of the popliteal artery as a result of an anatomic anomaly within the popliteal space. Anomalies involving the popliteal artery, medial head of the gastrocnemius (most common), popliteus muscle, and aberrant fibrous bands have been implicated.[81] Other causes must also be considered (e.g., space-occupying lesions and exostosis formation). Intermittent compression on the popliteal artery can ultimately cause an intimal tear of the vessel wall or a "stenosing arteriopathy," resulting in premature focal atherosclerosis and localized thrombosis.

CLASSIFICATION

Although many classification schemes have been proposed for PAES, I prefer the classification of Rich and Collins,[81] who describe five types of anatomic variants: type 1—medial deviation of the popliteal artery; type 2—lateral origin of medial gastrocnemius; type 3—accessory medial gastrocnemius; type 4—popliteal muscle, fibrous band, or tibial nerve involvement; type 5—popliteal vein entrapment.

CLINICAL EVALUATION

Clinically, patients present complaining of recurrent leg and foot pain with exercise. Onset of the problem can be sudden or gradual. The pain is severe (with patients being unable to continue their activity) and located most commonly in the calf (uncommonly the lateral or anterior leg, or both) and the arch of the foot. The offending exercise usually involves walking (or running). Rest provides immediate relief (in seconds to minutes), at which time exercise may be resumed until symptoms return once again. Patients may also relate coolness and blanching of the involved extremity, nonspecific tingling and numbness (especially of the foot), and muscle weakness with an "inability to control the foot." Physical examination at rest can reveal normal pulses, pulse alteration, or nonpalpable pulses. An unusually warm knee ("hot knee") may be present as a result of increase in local blood flow and development of collateral vessels.[82] After exercise, pulses are altered (usually being nonpalpable), foot pallor is evident, and the extremity is cool to touch. If pulses are palpable, provocative maneuvers may be necessary to occlude the pulse. These maneuvers include passive ankle dorsiflexion, active ankle plantar flexion, and knee hyperextension.[83] Superficial sensorium may be altered. Pain is elicited on palpation of the calf (and arch of the foot), on passive stretch (ankle dorsiflexion), and on resistance to active contraction of the calf muscles. PAES is often confused with chronic superficial or deep posterior compartment syndrome or both. It must also be differentiated from other arterial pathology, especially cystic adventitial degeneration (popliteal cyst), which is also prevalent in young athletes, although the condition is rare.

Diagnostic testing includes Doppler pulse recording, ankle/brachial pressures with exercise (extended treadmill testing), segmental leg pressures, segmental pulse volumes with pulse volume recorder and CT scanning. Arteriography and duplex scanning are definitive. Dynamic studies with provocative maneuvers may need to be performed to elucidate the pathology (Fig. 16-5).[84,85]

TREATMENT

Treatment for this problem is surgical, with the goals being to correct the anomaly and repair the damaged artery as necessary.[86]

RELATED CONDITION

Adductor outlet syndrome is a condition quite similar to PAES except that the SFA is involved instead of the popliteal artery. The SFA becomes occluded or compressed at the outlet of the adductor (Hunter's) canal because of an anatomic anomaly. It is caused by intermittent scissor-like compression on the SFA by the vastus medialis and adductor magnus muscle/tendons. Its incidence is rare. Clinical presentation and diagnostic work-up are identical to PAES. Treatment is surgical to correct the anomaly and repair the vessel as necessary.[87,88]

Peroneal Nerve Entrapment

Common peroneal nerve injury at the level of the fibular neck is a well-established clinical entity with various causes being elucidated. Common etiologies include traumatic (contusion, traction, etc.), external compression/irritation (sitting crosslegged, suitcase palsy, etc.), internal compression/irritation (space-occupying lesions, fabella syndrome, etc.) and miscellaneous conditions (systemic, neurologic, etc.). Exercise-induced peroneal nerve entrapment (PNE) caused by repetitive exercise (i.e., running and aerobics) is an unusual and uncommon entity that is one cause of neurogenic claudication in the athlete,[89–94] along with tibial nerve entrapment in the popliteal space[95] and nerve root compression in the cauda equina region.[96] Discussion here is limited to exercise-induced PNE.

When PNE occurs as a result of exercise or other causes, it is consistently localized to specific anatomic sites involving the leg and foot. The two common sites of entrapment involving the leg are the proximal fibular neck[89,90] and the deep fascial exit of the superficial peroneal nerve (SPN).[91–94] Fibular neck entrapment can involve the common peroneal nerve (CPN), SPN and deep peroneal nerve (DPN). The deep fascial exit site of the SPN classically is located in the lateral compartment, but it may be located

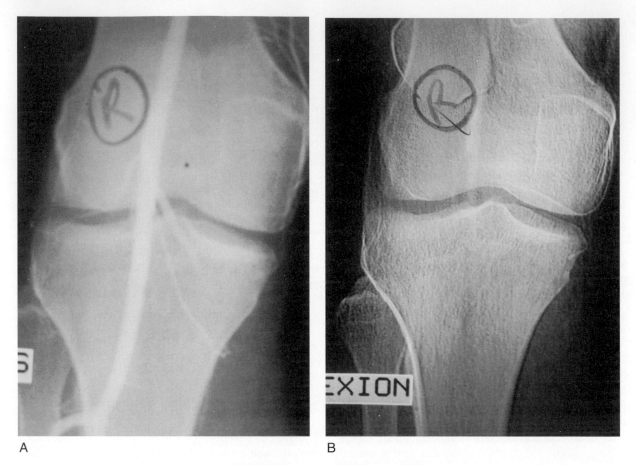

A   B

Figure 16-5 Popliteal artery entrapment syndrome. **(A)** Arteriogram in resting position. **(B)** Provocative maneuver involving active ankle plantar flexion reveals pathology on arteriogram.

in the anterior compartment in a certain percentage of patients.[97] Two potential entrapment sites of the foot are the dorsal aspect of the foot, affecting the terminal branches of the SPN, and the inferior extensor retinaculum, affecting the DPN (anterior tarsal tunnel). Entrapment sites on the foot can cause retrograde symptoms involving the leg.

ANATOMY

The sciatic nerve divides into the tibial nerve and CPN in the distal one third of the thigh. The CPN descends through the lateral aspect of the popliteal fossa, crosses over the lateral head of the gastrocnemius muscle, and courses around the lateral fibular neck. It then becomes superficial, piercing through the J-shaped origin of the peroneus longus muscle, where it divides into SPN and DPN. The SPN usually descends in the lateral compartment (sometimes the anterior) and exits the deep fascia in the distal one third

of the leg (10 to 12 cm proximal to the ankle). It then divides into two terminal branches (medial and intermediate dorsal cutaneous nerves) coursing to the dorsum of the foot. The DPN courses deep through the anterior compartment, dividing into two branches (medial and lateral terminal branches) just anterior to the ankle.

ETIOLOGY/PATHOGENESIS

With repetitive exercise (running, aerobics, etc.) PNE may occur. Proposed etiologies include (1) tethering at the fibular neck as a result of the normal fibrous J-shaped origin of the peroneus longus,[89] an anomalous origin of the peroneus longus, or an anomalous fascial band; and (2) tethering at the deep fascial exit of the SPN, especially with extreme ankle plantar flexion. Predisposing factors include hypermobility of the proximal tibiofibular joint, genu varum, genu recurvatum, and generalized ligamentous laxity.[90]

The pathophysiology, regardless of etiology, is conduction block (secondary to focal demyelination), axonal loss (the predominant injury), or both.[98] Neurapraxias are injuries involving conduction block in which the anatomic continuity of the nerve is preserved with only selective demyelination. Axonotmesis involves axonal loss with interruption of axons and myelin sheath, with preservation of contiguous connective tissue.

CLINICAL EVALUATION

Patients with PNE at the proximal fibular neck present with pain or fatigue of gradual, insidious onset localized to the anterior or lateral leg, or both. Pain is described as "weird sensations" with tingling, cramping, burning, and numbness. Footdrop may develop, with patients having difficulty controlling the foot. Ankle instability may be related. The exercise usually involves a repetitive weight-bearing activity. Symptoms occur after a definite period of time and may not preclude the patient from continuing exercise. Cessation of exercise resolves symptoms in minutes to hours. Physical examination at rest and especially after exercise may reveal a positive Tinel's sign on palpation of the fibular neck; decrease in sensorium over the anterior or lateral leg or both; weakness of the anterior or lateral muscle groups, or both, on manual muscle testing; and pain on provocative maneuvers (prolonged passive stretch with the foot in extreme plantar flexion/inversion and resistance to active foot dorsiflexion/eversion). During exercise, gait abnormalities may be appreciated (i.e., steppage gait).

Patients with PNE at the deep fascial exit site of the SPN will present complaining of tingling, burning, and radiating pain with numbness aggravated by certain positions of the foot (especially plantar flexion). Examination at rest and especially after exercise usually reveals localized pain with Tinel's sign elicited on palpation of the deep fascial exit site, reproduction of symptoms by maintaining the foot in a plantar-flexed/inverted position for a few minutes, and decrease in sensorium over the distal leg and dorsum of the foot.

Diagnostically, radiographs may be obtained to rule out bony abnormality, local anesthetic blocks to localize the problem, and electromyographyl nerve conduction studies (EMG/NCS) for further elucidation of the problem (dynamic studies may be revealing[1]). EMG/NCS delineates specific nerve pathology (conduction block vs. axonal loss vs. mixed), which can determine prognosis.[98]

TREATMENT

After confirming the diagnosis, treatment may include (1) cessation of the offending activity; (2) eliminating external factors that may aggravate the involved area (i.e., ski boots, shin guards, etc.), (3) "tincture of time," depending on the severity of nerve injury; (4) symptomatic treatment with transcutaneous electrical nerve stimulation and interferential therapy; and (5) surgery to relieve the entrapment and free up the nerve[89-94] (Fig. 16-6).

MISCELLANEOUS CONDITIONS

Various other leg problems exist that are exercised induced but do not fit the category of overuse injury or claudication syndromes. Muscle soreness, muscle cramps, and muscle herniation are common miscellaneous conditions that are briefly reviewed.

Muscle Soreness

Temporary pain (soreness) and stiffness of muscle that occurs following unaccustomed muscular exertion is called *delayed-onset muscle soreness* (DOMS).[99] Severity of symptoms is dependent on intensity and duration of activity.[100] Symptoms normally increase in intensity the first 24 hours after exercise, peak at 24 to 72 hours, then subside over the ensuing days. Overexertion of any skeletal muscle may result in DOMS. Most people have experienced episodes of DOMS after vigorous exercise, although few people seek medical care for this self-limiting problem.

In distinction to DOMS, there is an acute form of muscle soreness that occurs. In the acute form of muscle soreness, muscle pain occurs during exercise and is probably due to muscle ischemia with accumulation of metabolic waste products (i.e., lactic acid and potassium).[101]

ETIOLOGY/PATHOGENESIS

The pathophysiology of DOMS is still unclear; however, prolonged excessive exercise, especially eccentric muscle contractions, is definitely a causative factor.[102,103] Many believe excessive metabolite buildup (lactic acid) causes the pain, but this theory has been disproved in several studies.[99] There are presently three popular theories suggested to explain DOMS.[101] The "torn tissue hypothesis" of Hough concludes that, after high-intensity exercise, the diminution in the ability of muscles to produce tension and the soreness that develops is due to muscle damage

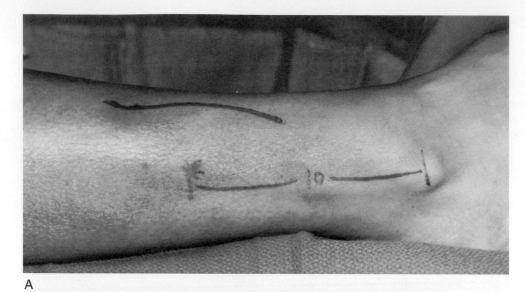

A

B

Figure 16-6 Treatment of PNE, **(A)** Marking the skin in preparation for surgery. **(B)** Release of entrapped superficial peroneal nerve.

either in the muscle itself or at the myotendinous junction.[104] The "spasm theory" of DeVries suggests that exercise promotes ischemia, which results in production of a particular pain substance ("P-substance"). This substance then stimulates pain receptors within the muscle, thus pro-

ducing more reflex spasms, which causes more ischemia.[105] The third theory is based on the work of Assmussen and Komi,[102,103] who noted diffuse soreness is more likely to develop with negative (eccentric) work than with positive (concentric) work. These investigators proposed that soreness arises because eccentric work places a greater strain on the muscle's elastic components (i.e., the connective tissue).

A model for DOMS has been proposed based on available information and with the assumption that high local tensions in muscles cause structural damage.[99] The model is as follows: (1) mechanical forces during exercise (especially eccentric) work cause disruption of muscle fibers and connective tissue; (2) disruption of muscle causes increase in intracellular calcium ions, which leads to proteolytic enzyme release and degradation of muscle; and (3) monocytes are attracted and mast cells are activated, leading to accumulation of inflammatory products and nociceptor activation. This sequence of events is hypothetical, and further research is needed to elucidate the mechanisms involved in DOMS.

CLINICAL EVALUATION

A patient presenting with suspected DOMS will give a history of performing an unaccustomed level of exercise days before presentation without history of injury or trauma. Decreased performance with additional exercise is related. Symptoms can vary from slight stiffness to debilitating pain that interferes with movement. Physical examination will reveal pain or tenderness on palpation of the involved muscle without obvious inflammation. Patients may have pain with active joint range of motion, passive stretch, and resistance to active muscle contraction. There is *no* weakness on manual muscle testing. DOMS should be differentiated from grade 1 muscle strain and other causes of muscle pain without contraction (myalgia).

TREATMENT/PREVENTION

The best initial treatment to date for patients with DOMS is low intensity/duration exercise—specifically, the same exercise that caused the symptoms.[99,104] Upon completion of the exercise, symptoms may return but are usually less severe. Massage with application of liniments, ointments, and creams (containing methyl salicylate, menthol, thymol, and/or camphor) can also be effective and is widely used. It is thought that tactile stimulation and the sensation of warmth imparted by the medication may inhibit pain transmission through the "gating" mechanism of Melzack and Wall.[106] Anti-inflammatory medication,[107] ultrasound, and stretching[108,109] are other commonly used empiric techniques that may also prove helpful.

Preventative measures include a gradual systematic conditioning program starting with light loads/minimal repetitions and progressing slowly by increasing repetition while keeping loads relatively constant. Large incremental increases in load and duration should be avoided. Training should specifically involve eccentric contractions.[110] Warmup, cooldown, and stretching probably will not prevent DOMS but may aid in injury prevention.[99]

Muscle Cramps

Muscle cramps are common occurrences that affect athletes and nonathletes alike. The term *cramp* is often used to describe many different muscle conditions involving contraction, pain, or both. A true muscle cramp is characterized by an involuntary, painful, visible contraction having a sudden onset with resolution in seconds to minutes.[111] Muscle cramp is a symptom, not a diagnosis, and may require further investigation to establish a diagnosis.

ETIOLOGY/PATHOGENESIS

Exercise-induced muscle cramps may be caused by transient hypoglycemia, inadequate conditioning, fatigue, electrolyte imbalances (rare), overexertion, and dehydration (aggravated by high temperatures).[112] Although all athletes can be affected, the poorly conditioned individual who sporadically exercises is probably at greatest risk.

The pathophysiology of cramps involves sustained hyperactivity of the motor unit causing sustained involuntary contraction, which usually occurs when the muscle is in a maximally shortened position.[111,113] Although many researchers believe cramps are neurogenic in origin, the true cause is unknown.

CLINICAL EVALUATION

Clinically, it is important to differentiate between exercise-induced cramps that are benign and those that may require further investigation. Patients with benign muscle cramps usually relate a clear history of occasional episodic cramping (without muscle weakness) that usually occur at rest, especially after athletic activity. A history reviewing the athlete's training program, fluid intake patterns, diet, and medical history, including medications, may be revealing.

Intensely painful involuntary contraction of muscle should suggest cramp, spasm, or contracture. *Spasm* is identical to a cramp except that it occurs secondary to an injured or inflamed structure. *Contracture* is a rare condition caused by metabolic myopathy occurring during exercise (not at rest) and accompanied by weakness. In distinction to a muscle cramp, a muscle contracture is electrically silent as determined by electromyography.[111] *Myalgia* (muscle pain without contraction) and *tetany* or *occupational cramp* (contraction without muscle pain) should also be differentiated.[111,113]

Recurrent muscle cramps may involve underlying disease and require further investigation, including an in-depth history, complete physical examination (by an internist), and appropriate diagnostic testing. Diagnostic testing may include blood tests, EMGINCS, and tissue analysis (muscle and nerve biopsy).[111,114]

TREATMENT/PREVENTION

The best treatment for an acute muscle cramp is sustained stretching (and active contraction of the antagonist) and pressure application/massage to the affected muscle.[111] Immediate fluid replacement (preferably water or a dilute electrolyte sport drink) is paramount. Salt tablets are contraindicated and can actually enhance fluid loss.[112]

The superficial application of ice or heat is controversial and may depend on environmental conditions.[112] The popular technique of firmly pinching the athlete's upper lip may, empirically, be helpful.[112] Potassium supplements (oranges, bananas) have been shown to be ineffective in the treatment of muscle cramps. Continued exercise with severe muscle cramps should be discouraged because further injury (i.e., falling) can result.

Prevention of muscle cramps includes proper conditioning, nutritious diet, warmup, stretching, adequate hydration, appropriate clothing for conditions, and avoidance of overexertion.

Muscle Herniation

Muscle can bulge or herniate through normal fascial openings of the leg or through congenitial or traumatic fascial defects. These herniations occur in the deep fascia (fascia cruris) of the leg. Normal fascial openings of the leg include the distal exit on the lateral (or anterior) compartment for the SPN and the fascial openings in the deep posterior compartment for communication between the superficial and deep veins. Congenital and traumatic herniations are common in the anterior and lateral leg and uncommon over the medial and posterior leg.

Fascial defects may be unilateral or bilateral, solitary or multiple, and can be seen in patients who are symptomatic and asymptomatic.[115] They have been commonly associated with CCS, with 30 to 60 percent of patients with compartment syndrome having muscle herniations.[115,116] There have been multiple case reports on symptomatic muscle herniation through the normal fascial exit of the

SPN,[91–94] with one case associated with a chronic anterolateral compartment syndrome as well.[117]

ETIOLOGY

Pain, induration, and prominence occur with exercise as the herniated portion of muscle prolapses through the fascial opening and is constricted by the edge of the unyielding fascia, resulting in a localized ischemia.

CLINICAL EVALUATION

Patients usually relate no pain at rest. After exercise, severe pain and swelling is related and can worsen with continued exercise. Rest improves the condition in minutes. On examination before exercise, the fascial defect can be palpated and its borders easily appreciated. In stance, the herniation is usually apparent, although it may be subtle. After exercise, the muscle herniation becomes obvious and well deliniated (Fig. 16-7). Severe pain is elicited on

Figure 16-7 Appearance of muscle herniation after exercise.

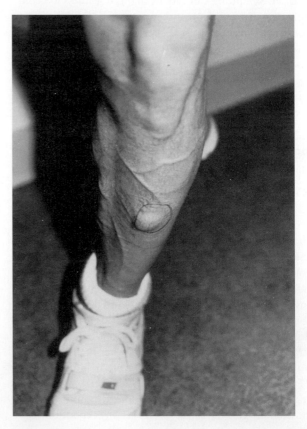

palpation, with the involved muscle being indurated. Palpation can also elicit distal paresthesias if there is nerve involvement (i.e., SPN at the distal fascial exit). Muscle herniation must be differentiated from a soft tissue tumor, and CCS should be ruled out.

TREATMENT

Definitive treatment for patients with symptomatic muscle herniation is complete fascial release, with particular attention directed to the relationship of the fascial defect and superficial sensory nerves. Fascial release should be extensive and complete to relieve the herniation and nerve entrapment if present. If a small, limited release is performed, a larger symptomatic herniation may result. Primary fascial closure of the defect should be avoided because an ACS or CCS can be precipitated. The deep fascia functions to maintain muscle force of the leg; therefore, a theoretical concern following fascial release would be loss of strength. Although I have not encountered this complication, it should be considered.

REFERENCES

1. Orava S, Puranen J: Athlete's leg pains. Br J Sports Med 13:92, 1979
2. Siocum DB: The shin splint syndrome—medical aspects and differential diagnosis. Am J Surg 114:875, 1967
3. Michael RH, Holder LE: The soleus syndrome—a cause of medial tibial stress (shin splints). Am J Sports Med 13:87, 1985
4. Puranen J: The medial tibial syndrome—exercise ischemia in the medial fascial compartment of the leg. J Bone Joint Surg [Br] 56:712, 1974
5. Clement DB: Tibial stress syndrome in athletes. J Sports Med 2:81, 1974
6. Mubarak SJ, Gould RN, Lee YF et al: The medial tibial stress syndrome—a cause of shin splints. Am J Sports Med 10:201, 1982
7. Richie DH, De Vries HV, Endo CK: Shin muscle activity and floor surfaces in dance exercise: an electromyographic study. J Am Podiatr Med Assoc 83:181, 1993
8. Holder LE, Michael RH: The specific scintigraphic pattern of "shin splints in the lower leg": concise communication. J Nucl Med 25:865, 1984
9. Fredericson M, Bergman AG, Hoffman KL et al: Tibial stress reaction in runners—correlation of clinical symptoms and scintigraphy with a new magnetic resonance imaging grading system. Am J Sports Med 23:472, 1995
10. Jarvinnen M, Aho H, Niittymaki S: Results of the surgical treatment of the medial tibial syndrome in athletes. Int J Sports Med 10:55, 1989
11. Akermark C, Ljungdahl M, Johansson C: Long-term result of fasciotomy caused by medial tibial syndrome in athletes. Scand J Med Sci Sports 1:59, 1991
12. Wallensten R: Results of fasciotomy in patients with medial tibial syndrome or chronic anterior-compartment syndrome. J Bone Joint Surg [Am] 65:1252, 1983
13. Bennell KL, Malcolm SA, Thomas SA et al: The incidence and distribution of stress fractures in competitive track and field athletes—a twelve-month prospective study. Am J Sports Med 24:211, 1996
14. Matheson GO, Clement DB, Mckenzie DC et al: Stress fractures in athletes: a study of 320 cases. Am J Sports Med 15:46, 1987
15. Daffner RH: Stress fracture: current concepts. Skeletal Radiol 2:221, 1978
16. Stanitski CL, McMaster JH, Scranton PE: On the nature of stress fractures. Am J Sports Med 6:391, 1978
17. Taunton JE, Clement DB, Webber D: Lower extremity stress fractures in athletes. Physician Sports Med 9:77, 1981
18. Allen ME: Stress fracture of the humerus: a case study. Am J Sports Med 12:244, 1974
19. Sweet DE, Auman RM: RPC of the month from AFIP. Radiology 99:687, 1971
20. Jones BH, Harris JM, Vinh TN et al: Exercise-induced stress fractures and stress reactions of bone: epidemiology, etiology and classification. Exerc Sports Sci Rev 17:379, 1989
21. Matheson GO, Clement DB, McKenzie DC et al: Scintigraphic uptake of 99m Tc at non-painful sites in athletes with stress fractures: the concept of bone strain. Sports Med 4:65, 1987
22. Milgrom C, Chisin R, Giladi M et al: Negative bone scans in impending tibial stress fractures. Am J Sports Med 12:488, 1984
23. Rupani HD, Holder LE, Espinola DA et al: Three-phase radionuclide bone imaging in sports medicine. Radiology 156:187, 1985
24. Snow-Harter C, Marcus R: Exercise, bone mineral density and osteoporosis. Exerc Sport Sci Rev 19:351, 1991
25. Benson JW, Hanelin LG: Place of bone density measurement in the management of osteoporosis. Bull Mason Clin 39:61, 1985
26. Roub LW, Gumerman LW, Henley EN et al: Bone stress: a radionuclide imaging perspective. Radiology 132:431, 1979
27. Yousem D, Fishman EK, et al: Computed tomography of stress fracture. J Comput Assist Tomogr 10:92, 1986
28. Swenson EJ, DeHaven KE, Sebastianelli WJ et al: The effect of a pneumatic leg brace on return to play in athletes with tibial stress fractures. Am J Sports Med 25:322, 1997
29. Milgrom C, Giladi M, Kashtan H et al: A prospective study

of the effect of a shock-absorbing orthotic device on the incidence of stress fractures in military recruits. Foot Ankle 6:101, 1985

30. Simkin A, Leichter I, Giladi M et al: Combined effect of foot arch structure and an orthotic device on stress fractures. Foot Ankle 10:25, 1989

31. Milgrom C, Burr DB, Boyd RD et al: The effect of a viscoelastic orthotic on the incidence of tibial stress fractures in an animal model. Foot Ankle 10:276, 1990

32. Orava S, Hulkko A: Stress fracture of the mid-tibial shaft. Acta Orthop Scand 55:35, 1984

33. Green NE, Rogers RA, Lipscomb AB: Nonunions of stress fractures of the tibia. Am J Sports Med 13:171, 1985

34. Rettig AC, Shelbourne KD, McCarroll JR et al: The natural history and treatment of delayed union stress fractures of the anterior cortex of the tibia. Am J Sports Med 16:250, 1988

35. Shelbourne KD, Fisher DA, Rettig AC et al: Stress fractures of the medial malleolus. Am J Sports Med 16:60, 1988

36. Kibler WB: Clinical aspects of muscle injury. Med Sci Sports Exerc 22:450, 1990

37. Nikolaou PK, Macdonald BL, Glisson RR et al: Biomechanical and histological evaluation of muscle after controlled muscle strain injury. Am J Sports Med 15:9, 1987

38. Garrett WE: Muscle strain injuries: clinical and basic aspects. Med Sci Sports Exerc 22:436, 1990

39. Garrett WE, Califf JC, Bassett FH: Histochemical correlates of hamstring injury. Am J Sports Med 12:98, 1984

40. Safran MR, Garrett WE, Seaber AV et al: The role of warmup in muscular injury prevention. Am J Sports Med 16:123, 1988

41. Mair SD, Seaber AV, Glisson RR et al: The role of fatigue in susceptibility to acute muscle strain injury. Am J Sports Med 24:137, 1996

42. Garrett WE, Safran MR, Seaber AV et al: Biomechanical comparison of stimulated and nonstimulated skeletal muscle pulled to failure. Am J Sports Med 15:448, 1987

43. Taylor DC, Dalton JD, Seaber AV et al: Viscoelastic properties of muscle-tendon units—the biomechanical effects of stretching. Am J Sports Med 18:300, 1990

44. Wiktorssib-Moller M, Oberg B, Ekstrand J et al: Effects of warming up, massage, and stretching on range of motion and muscle strength in the lower extremity. Am J Sports Med 11:249, 1983

45. Zarins B, Ciullo JV: Acute muscle and tendon injuries in athletes. Clin Sports Med 2:167, 1983

46. Glick JM: Muscle strains: prevention and treatment. Physician Sports Med 8:73, 1980

47. Fornage BD, Touche DH, Segal P et al: Ultrasonography in the evaluation of muscular trauma. J Ultrasound Med 2:549, 1983

48. Slasky BS, Lenkey JL, Skolnick ML et al: Sonography of soft tissues of extremities and trunk. Semin Ultrasound 3:288, 1982

49. Garrett WE, Rich FR, Nikolaou PK et al: Computed tomography of hamstring muscle strains. Med Sci Sports Exerc 21:506, 1989

50. Fleckenstein JL, Shellock FG: Exertional muscle injuries: magnetic resonance imaging evaluation. Techniques Orthop 7:50, 1991

51. Herring SA: Rehabilitation of muscle injuries. Med Sci Sport Exerc 22:453, 1990

52. Garrick JG: Tennis leg—how I manage gastrocnemius strains. Physician Sports Med 20:203, 1992

53. Severance HW, Bassett FH: Rupture of the plantaris—does it exists? J Bone J Surg [Am] 64:1387, 1982

54. Leadbetter WB: Cell-matrix response in tendon injury. Clin Sports Med 11:533, 1992

55. Clancy WG: Tendon trauma and overuse injuries. p. 609. In Leadbetter WB, Buckwalter JA, Gordon SL (eds): Sports-Induced Inflammation: Clinical and Basic Science Concepts. American Academy of Orthopedic Surgeons, Park Ridge, IL, 1990

56. Puddu G, Ippolito E, Postacchini F: A classification of Achilles tendon disease. Am J Sports Med 4:145, 1976

57. Astrom M, Rausing A: Chronic Achilles tendinopathy—a survey of surgical and histopathological findings. Clin Orthop Rel Res 316:151, 1995

58. Mink JH, Deutsch AL, Kerr R: Tendon injuries of the lower extremity: magnetic resonance assessment. Techniques Orthop 7:23, 1992

59. Curwin S, Stanish W: Tendinitis: its Etiology and Treatment. The Collamore Press, Lexington, MA, 1984

60. Webster's New World Dictionary. 2nd College ed. The World Publishing Company, New York, 1970

61. Mavor GE: The anterior tibial syndrome. J Bone J Surg [Br] 38:513, 1956

62. Matsen FA: Compartment syndrome—a unified concept. Clin Orthop 113:8, 1975

63. Mubarak SJ, Hargens AR: Compartment Syndromes and Volkmann's Contracture. WB Saunders, Philadelphia, 1981

64. Eaton RG, Green WT: Epimysiotomy and fasciotomy in the treatment of Volkmann's ischemic contracture. Orthop Clin North Am 3:175, 1972

65. Ashton H: The effect of increased tissue pressure on blood flow. Clin Orthop 113:15, 1975

66. Burton AC: On the physical equilibrium of small blood vessels. Am J Physiol 164:319, 1951

67. Hargens AR, Akeson WH, Mubarak SJ et al: Fluid balance within the canine anterolateral compartment and its relationship to compartment syndromes. J Bone Joint Surg [Am] 60a:499, 1978

68. Amendola A, Rorabeck CH, Vellet D et al: The use of magnetic resonance imaging in exertional compartment syndrome. Am J Sports Med 18:29, 1990

69. Pedowitz RA, Hargens AR, Mubarak SJ et al: Modified

criteria for the objective diagnosis of chronic compartment syndrome of the leg. Am J Sports Med 18:35, 1990

70. Martens MA, Baeckaert M, Vermaut G et al: Chronic leg pain in athletes due to a recurrent compartment syndrome. Am J Sports Med 12:148, 1984

71. Rorabeck CH, Fowler PJ, Nott L: The results of fasciotomy in the management of chronic exertional compartment syndrome. Am J Sports Med 16:224, 1988

72. Styf JR, Korner LM: Chronic anterior-compartment syndrome of the leg. J Bone J Surg [Br] 68b:1388, 1986

73. Stuart TPA: A note on variation in the course of the popliteal artery. J Anat Physiol 13:162, 1879

74. Love JW, Whelan TJ: Popliteal artery entrapment syndrome. Am J Surg 109:620, 1965

75. Rich NM, Hughes CW: Popliteal artery and vein entrapment. Am J Surg 113:696, 1967

76. Podore PC: Popliteal entrapment syndrome: a report of tibial nerve entrapment. J Vasc Surg 2:335, 1985

77. Hamming JJ, Vink M: Obstruction of the popliteal artery at an early age. J Cardiovasc Surg 6:516, 1965

78. Berg-Johnsen J, Holter O: Popliteal entrapment syndrome. Acta Chir Scand 150:493, 1984

79. Bouhoutsos J, Daskalakis E: Muscular abnormalities affecting the popliteal vessels. Br J Surg 68:501, 1981

80. Gibson MHL, Mills JG, Johnson GE et al: Popliteal artery entrapment syndrome. Ann Surg 185:341, 1977

81. Rich NM, Collins GJ, McDonald PT et al: Popliteal vascular entrapment. Arch Surg 114:1377, 1979

82. Chavatzas D, Barabas A, Martin P: Popliteal artery entrapment. Lancet 2:181, 1973

83. Darling C, Buckley CJ, Abbott WM et al: Intermittent claudication in young athletes: popliteal artery entrapment syndrome. J Trauma 14:543, 1974

84. McDonald PT, Easterbrook JA, Rich NM et al: Popliteal artery entrapment syndrome—clinical, noninvasive and radiographic diagnosis. Am J Surg 139:318, 1980

85. Williams LR, Flinn WR, McCarthy WJ et al: Popliteal artery entrapment: diagnosis by computed tomography. J Vasc Surg 3:360, 1986

86. Whelan TJ Jr: Popliteal artery entrapment syndrome. p. 493. In Haimovici H (ed): Vascular Surgery. McGraw-Hill, New York, 1976

87. Balaji MR, DeWeese JA: Adductor canal outlet syndrome. JAMA 245:167, 1981

88. Lee BY, LaPointe DG, Madden JL: The adductor outlet syndrome. Am J Surg 123:617, 1972

89. Leach RE, Purnell MB, Saito A: Peroneal nerve entrapment in runners. Am J Sports Med 17:287, 1989

90. Moller MN, Kadin S: Entrapment of the common peroneal nerve. Am J Sports Med 15:90, 1987

91. Styf J: Entrapment of the superficial peroneal nerve—diagnosis and the results of decompression. J Bone J Surg [Br] 71b:131, 1989

92. Lowdon IMR: Superficial peroneal nerve entrapment—a case report. J Bone J Surg [Br] 67b:58, 1985

93. Kernohan J, Levack B, Wilson JN: Entrapment of the superficial peroneal nerve—three case reports. J Bone J Surg [Br] 67b:60, 1985

94. McAuliffe TB, Fiddian NJ, Browett JP: Entrapment neuropathy of the superficial peroneal nerve—a bilateral case. J Bone J Surg [Br] 67b:62, 1985

95. Ekelund AL: Bilateral nerve entrapment in the popliteal space. Am J Sports Med 18:108, 1990

96. Abramson DI: Symptomatology of organic and vasospastic arterial disorders. p. 1. In: Circulatory Problems in Podiatry. Karger, Switzerland, 1985

97. Adkinson DP, Bosse MJ, Gaccione DR et al: Anatomical variations in the course of the superficial peroneal nerve. J Bone J Surg [Am] 73a:112, 1991

98. Katirji MB, Wilbourn AJ: Common peroneal mononeuropathy: a clinical and electrophysiologic study of 116 lesions. Neurology 38:1723, 1988

99. Armstrong RB: Mechanisms of exercise-induced delayed onset muscular soreness: a brief review. Med Sci Sports Exerc 16:529, 1984

100. Tiidus PM, Ianuzzo CD: Effects of intensity and duration of muscular exercise on delayed soreness and serum enzyme activities. Med Sci Sport Exerc 15:461, 1983

101. Abraham WM: Exercise-induced muscle soreness. Physician Sports Med 7:57, 1979

102. Assmussen E: Observations on experimental muscle soreness. Acta Rheumatol Scand 1:109, 1956

103. Komi PV, Buskirk ER: The effect of eccentric and concentric muscle activity on tension and electrical activity of human muscle. Ergonomics 15:417, 1972

104. Hough T: Ergographic studies in muscular soreness. Am J Physiol 7:76, 1902

105. DeVries HA: Quantitative electromyographic investigation of the spasm theory of muscle pain. Am J Phys Med 45:119, 1966

106. Melzack R, Wall PD: Pain mechanisms: a new theory. Science 150:971, 1965

107. Hasson SM, Daniels JC, Divine JG et al: Effect of ibuprofen use on muscle soreness, damage, and performance: a preliminary investigation. Med Sci Sport Exerc 25:9, 1993

108. DeVries HA: Prevention of muscular distress after exercise. Res Q 32:177, 1960

109. DeVries HA: Quantitative electromyographic investigation of the spasm theory of muscle pain. Am J Phys Med 45:119, 1966

110. Newham DJ, Mills KR, Quigley BM et al: Muscle pain and tenderness after exercise. Austr J Sports Med Exerc Sci 14:129, 1983

111. Simchak AC, Pascuzzi RM: Muscle cramps. Semin Neurol 11:281, 1991

112. Benda C: Outwitting muscle cramps—is it possible? Physician Sports Med 17:173, 1989

113. McGee SR: Muscle cramps. Arch Intern Med 150:511, 1990

114. Felmus MT: A neuromuscular approach to muscle aches, cramps and pains. Arizona Med 41:169, 1984

115. Renemans RS: The anterior and the lateral compartmental syndrome of the leg due to intensive use of muscles. Clin Orthop 113:141, 1975

116. Mubarak SJ, Owen CA: Double incision fasciotomy of the leg for decompression in compartment syndrome. J Bone J Surg [Am] 59a:184, 1977

117. Garfin S, Mubarak SJ, Owen CA: Exertional anterolateral compartment syndrome: case report with fascial defect, muscle herniation and superficial nerve entrapment. J Bone J Surg [Am] 59a:404, 1977

17

Knee and Thigh Injuries

JAMES D. KEY
DONALD JOHNSON
GARY JARVIS
DAVID PONSONBY

KNEE INJURIES

Cartilaginous Injuries

Cartilaginous injuries to the knee, which is one of the largest joints in the body, produce lesions that are painful, debilitating, and difficult to diagnose and treat. The challenge of injury to the articular cartilage is that cartilage lacks the ability and blood supply to heal itself. Yet a great deal of research into the fluids of the joint and the healing capacity of the articular surface of the knee has yielded many breakthroughs. New treatment options include synthetic synovial fluid, cultured cell transplants, autografts, meniscal stapling, and laser arthroscopic and multi-electrode surgery.

TRENDS IN CARTILAGE REPAIR

Cultured Cells and Synthetic Synovial Fluid

Research into the makeup of cartilage and advances in cell culturing techniques has added a new dimension to knee cartilage resurfacing. Chondrocytes and hyaline cartilage can now be taken from the injured individual and sent to specialty laboratories for growing a culture of the cells. This technique allows reimplantation of the patient's own cells back into the knee joint. Currently, in relatively small defects (i.e., no more than 1 to 1.5 cm), the cultured cells can be inserted through an arthrotomy incision under a membrane sewn to the surface cartilage of the knee. With protection from weight bearing for a period of weeks, good results of regrowth of cells has been obtained. The advantage of this technique is that the patient's own cells are reproduced and reintroduced to the articular surface, rather than relying on scar tissue to cover this surface. Scar tissue has been proven to last only 3 to 4 years before breaking down again. Cultured hyaline cartilage should last many times longer than this, perhaps as long as the joint itself. The disadvantages of this procedure are that it requires an open arthrotomy of the knee with moderately prolonged disability in a non-weight-bearing position for the cartilage cell regeneration. The technique, and the theory itself, offer promise for future cartilage resurfacing treatment of small to moderate defects in the knee joint.

The study of proteoglycans and other substances in the joint have led to the development of a substance called Synv-Hyaluron, a synthetic synovial fluid that has proven successful in trials and has received Food and Drug Administration approval. This fluid is injected into a deteriorating knee joint once a week for a period of 3 weeks; in a high percentage of patients it has produced pain relief for in excess of 9 months. The increase in the normal amount of proteoglycans produced in the patient's knee may in the future prove to be a tool to help salvage a failed total knee joint replacement.

Meniscal Repair Techniques and Autografting

Repair of the meniscus, especially in more peripheral tears or separations in relatively young athletes and patients who are still active, has become relatively commonplace. Transplantation and repair of menisci was pioneered by German physicians in the late 1970s and early 1980s and has become a standard method of treatment; artificial menisci are currently being researched. Techniques for meniscal repair have improved over the last decade and a half. Dissolvable pins are now available for pinning the meniscus back into place, ending the need for suture removal and long periods of disability associated with the old method of meniscal repair. The meniscal stapler is now available for repair of the torn meniscus rather than removal of the entire torn portion. By obviating the need to pass sutures from the inside to the outside of the joint, or vice versa, it has speeded up the average surgeon's ability to repair the torn meniscus. The use of the meniscal stapler should also greatly shorten the length of required immobilization of the knee for the meniscus to heal.

The transplantation of cadaver cartilage into the knee joint, although holding much early promise, has fallen into some disfavor with the rise of various viral communicable diseases. Although the likelihood of any such transmission is slight, the ever-present fear of such an occurrence has caused most surgeons to shy away form using cadaver cartilage because of the possible long-term catastrophic results. An alternative procedure known as the osteochondral autograft transfer system (OATS) has been introduced into the surgical armamentarium. It provides an arthroscopic method for treating full-thickness cartilage lesions by transplanting 13- to 15-mm-long osteochondral autograft cores into matched recipient sockets created in the defect. Tube harvesters are used to harvest hyaline cartilage from a well-defined rim and socket wall away from the weight-bearing surface of the knee joint. Precise drilling into the defect then allows the transplantation of these harvested cores into the weight-bearing surface of the knee in a mosaic pattern. The transplanted hyaline cartilage then is able to resurface a good portion of the articular defect, both relieving pain and producing a longer wearing joint than was possible with the previous methods of chondroplasty or abrasion arthroplasty used in an attempt to cause the joint to form scar tissue.

Laser Arthroscopic and Multi-electrode Surgery

Since the homium laser has been introduced into the arthroscopic treatment of both the shoulder and knee joints, it has proven especially effective in treating fibril-lated cartilage under the patella and over the femoral condylar surface. The technique has proved reliable for reducing the debris and smoothing the surface cartilage of the patella, and femoral condyle without removing as much of the normal cartilage as is removed using cutting instruments.

A simpler, less expensive technique of "melting" the fibrillated hyaline cartilage by means of an electrical current passed through a multi-electrode system using bipolar multi-electrode technology allows surgeons both to work with precision and safety in the knee and to control arthroscopic treatment of the fibrillated cartilage. One of the manufacturers of such systems, Arthro-Care, has wide experience with the technique, with 30,000 procedures having been done to date. The multi-electrode instrument is easily used to ablate meniscal tissue and cauterize simultaneously. It has good tactile feedback for fine sculpting of the meniscus and soft tissue, even in hard-to-reach places. It has proven satisfactory for sculpting fibrillated hyaline cartilage as well.

Summary

The 1990s have seen rapid advances in methods of treating the surface cartilage of the knee joint. However, it remains obvious that we have not completely met the challenge of resurfacing the damaged articular cartilage of the knee joint, in that most of the major sports medicine orthopedics meetings still include full discussions, panels, and papers on treating articular injuries to joint surfaces. As we enter the new millennium with the next decade, continuing advances in research on the surface articular cartilage and synovial fluid should prove very exciting to present and future surgeons. We should be able to better protect surface articular cartilage and be able to treat with many more tools than we have had in the past the unavoidable damage that is attendant on vigorous athletic activity, as well as the trauma of everyday living. The cloning of body parts appears to be technically feasible sometime in the not-too-distant future, but this treatment option will not be available until the science is reconciled with political, moral, and religious opinion. Currently, surgeons will continue using the tried and true methods discussed in the remainder of this chapter, but this brief overview of some of the different types of treatment now available should whet the reader's appetite for further research and development in this field.

OSTEOCHONDRAL FRACTURES

Frequently, when athletes fall against hard surfaces or receive a severe impact to the joint, a piece of bone with its underlying cartilage is sheared off (Fig. 17-1). This con-

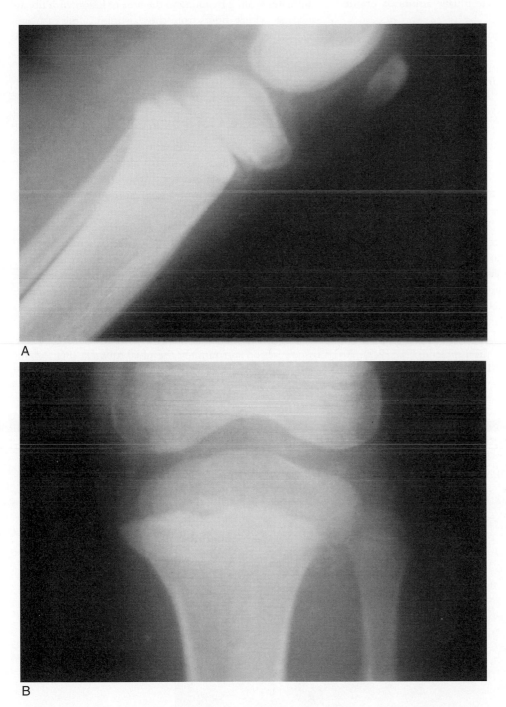

A

B

Figure 17-1 Anteroposterior (B) and lateral (A) radiographs of fractured tibial epiphysis.

dition immediately develops into a hemarthrosis, or blood in the knee joint. The athlete usually assumes a position of flexion.

Treatment consists of immobilizing the affected part, using the PRICE acronym (pressure, rest, ice, compression, elevation). Arthroscopy permits first-hand assessment of the damage, particularly in the knee joint. At that point, the examining surgeon can decide on management of the condition. The area is likely to be probed for determination of the extent of damage and is then abraded to remove the damaged surface and promote the development of a new surface.

OSTEOCHONDRITIS DISSECANS

Osteochondritis dissecans is a separation of the osteocartilaginous portion of the joint surface from subchondral bone. Osteochondritis dissecans is often seen in adolescent athletes presenting with lesions of the medical femoral condyle near the insertion of the posterior cruciate ligament. The defect is believed to be associated with growth variance resulting from obstruction of blood flow to that region. Athletes often complain of pain, catching, and recurrent swelling. Arthroscopy may provide the opportunity for immediate diagnosis of the problem (Fig. 17-2). Arthroscopic treatment would remove the fragment, then

drill the osteochondral lesion down to bleeding bone. This stimulates healing by filling in the area of lesion with fibrocartilage, which differs from the existing hyaline cartilage but is preferable to the defect. The patient is immobilized in a tight cylinder cast or splint for up to 8 weeks, during which the cast may be periodically removed for range-of-motion exercises. Straight leg raises and electrical stimulation are used to prevent quadriceps atrophy.

OSGOOD-SCHLATTER DISEASE

In children, the tibial tubercle is formed by a cartilaginous, tongue-shaped, downward elongation of the tibial epiphysis. During adolescence, toward the end of growth, centers of ossification begin to appear in this tubercle, rendering it most vulnerable to the effects of repeated forceful traction via the patellar tendon. A partially avulsed portion of the growing tibial tubercle will suffer avascular necrosis.

Osgood-Schlatier disease is usually found in very active boys between the ages of 10 and 15, occuring unilaterally or bilaterally[1-3] (Fig. 17-3). The child usually complains of local pain, which is aggravated by kneeling, direct blows, running, or bicycle riding. Clinically, a prominent subcutaneous swelling is evident, some of which is due to a soft tissue reaction surrounding the tibial tubercle (Fig. 17-4). Pain may be reproduced by having the patient extend the

Figure 17-2 Arthroscope in use.

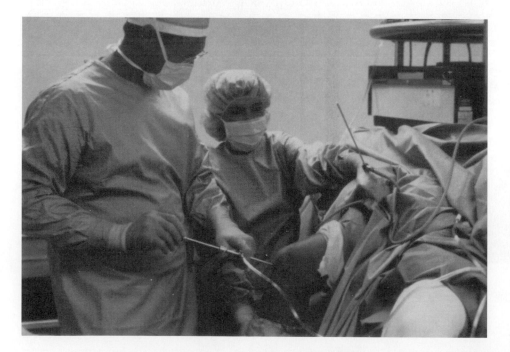

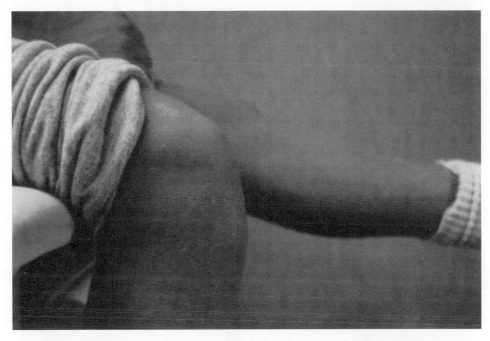

Figure 17-3 Patient with bilateral Osgood–Schlatter disease.

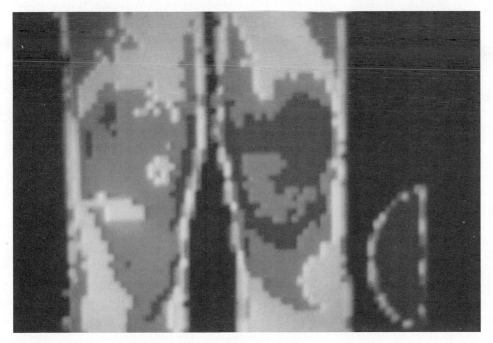

Figure 17-4 Thermogram of patient with bilateral Osgood–Schlatter disease showing subcutaneous dwelling.

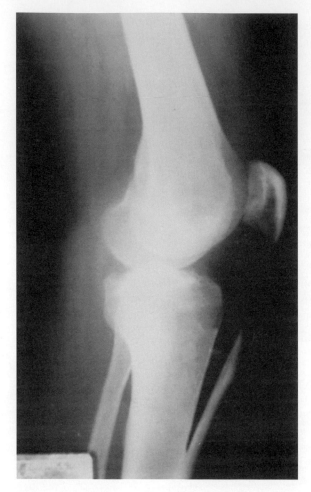

Figure 17-5 Maquette radiograph showing elevated tibial tubercle.

knee against resistance. Again, it is the pull of the quadriceps muscle, in addition to the elongation of the patellar tendon in the flexed position, that causes a traction lesion at its insertion. Radiography shows the proximal part of the tibial tubercle to exhibit irregular changes of bony deposition and bone reabsorption (Fig. 17-5).

This disease is usually self-limiting; once recognized, the treatment is uncomplicated. We have recommended cryotherapy (ice massage) for the tender area, stretching of the hamstring muscles, excluding the child from participating in sports that require a vigorous knee extensor mechanism (e.g., kicking a soccer ball), and strengthening the quadriceps using straight leg raises. Some athletic participation may be tolerated but, if pain recurs, activity must be reduced or stopped completely until the symptoms resolve.

In extreme cases, we generally find it necessary to immobilize the knee in full extension. Residual nonunion of the proximal fragment with the tibial tubercle will not heal, and symptoms will continue (Fig. 17-6, 17-7). Under these circumstances, excision of the nonunited fragment is indicated after the epiphysis is closed and growth is complete. Skin healing is facilitated if a vertical rather than a horizontal incision is made.

MENISCAL INJURIES

The menisci of the knee are C-shaped cartilaginous wedges covering 30 percent of the medial and 50 percent of the lateral tibial plateau. These mobile buffers absorb shock and also help guide and synchronize knee motion by providing stability. Meniscal tears are one of the most frequently sustained sports injuries.[4,5]

Meniscal injuries usually follow acute trauma. The athlete may have felt something give way in the knee, followed within 12 hours (and frequently immediately) by swelling. Initial physical signs besides effusion include joint-line tenderness, localized pain with full extension, and possible locking. The knee may appear to recover from the first episode; if locking, giving way, and repeated swelling persist, a torn mensicus is the possible diagnosis.

Diagnostic methods range from McMurry's test, which manually produces an audible "pop" when there is a tear in the posterior horn of the medial meniscus; to an arthrogram, a radiologic examination of the knee following injection of a radiopaque dye; to arthroscopy, which permits direct visualization of every portion of the knee joint, providing 100 percent accuracy in diagnosing knee pathologies. Most knee surgeries are now performed using arthroscopic techniques, which, because they involve only small puncture wounds and minimal surgical trauma, have earned the name of "Band-Aid surgery" and tend to be done on an outpatient basis (Fig. 17-8). Arthrotomy is only resorted to for major derangements.

Knee Plicae

A plica is an embryonic fold or septum, normally separating the suprapatellar pouch from the major part of the knee. This usually disappears but may become a fiberous band due to trauma. Intra-articular plicae are now known to be a major source of knee pain in runners.[6] Diagnosis is usually made arthroscopically. The plica, especially if it is the medial fibrous one, may also mimic a meniscal tear. The medial plica originates from the undersurface of the quadriceps tendon just above the patella and extends transversely across the

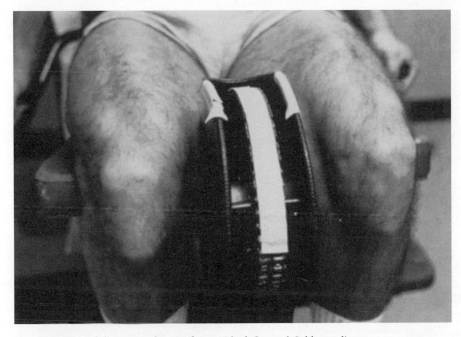

Figure 17-6 Adult man with pain-free residual Osgood-Schlatter disease.

joint to insert into the medial aspect of the infrapatellar fat pad. During knee flexion and extension, the fibrous plica rubs across the medial femoral condyle, causing pain that mimics a medial meniscus tear as well as degenerative changes in the medial femoral condyle.

The shelf may be felt by the examiner with the knee flexed about 40 degrees and the thumb rolled over the medial side of the patella; just above the joint line, the round, cylindrical body of the plica is felt. This is called the "thumb roll" test. Arthroscopic examination of the knee may reveal a normal meniscal pattern; however, thickening of the synovial fold constitutes a fibrotic plica. This may be excised arthroscopically, which has proved highly successful in resolving pain in athletes (Fig. 17-9).

Ligamentous Injuries

COLLATERAL LIGAMENTS

The knee is encased in a fibrous capsular sleeve within which the major collateral stabilizing ligaments are found.

Medial Compartment

On the medial side of the knee, the medial capsular ligament has three parts: an anterior capsule, medial capsular ligament, and posterior oblique ligament. The medial collateral ligament extends to the medial mensicus via the coronary ligament, a meniscofemoral and meniscotibial junction. This medial, or tibial, collateral ligament originates high in the medial femoral condyle, crosses the joint line connecting the medial meniscus, and inserts into the medial tibial condyle beneath the pes anserinus. It is the key medial stabilizer of the knee, withstanding excessive external rotatory as well as vagus forces. Injuries to the medial collateral ligament are classically graded: grade I means a stretch of the capsular fibers; grade II, stretching and tearing of the capsular fibers; and grade III, a complete tear.

Medial collateral ligament sprains may be initially protected naturally by a spasm of the adductor muscles. Further protection is afforded by using a knee immobilizer and possibly by non-weight bearing for 3 weeks, with crutches prescribed. Straight leg raises and other progressive resistance exercises help maintain muscular size and condition; therapeutic modalities such as ice, compression wraps, and cool whirlpools, as required, control inflammatory responses. Range of motion is always an important consideration. This protocol has proved successful with first-, second-, and third-degree medial collateral ligament sprains and tears.

Lateral Compartment

The lateral complex of the knee consists of the iliotibial band, the lateral collateral ligament, the popliteus tendon, and the biceps femoris. The iliotibial band is a dynamic

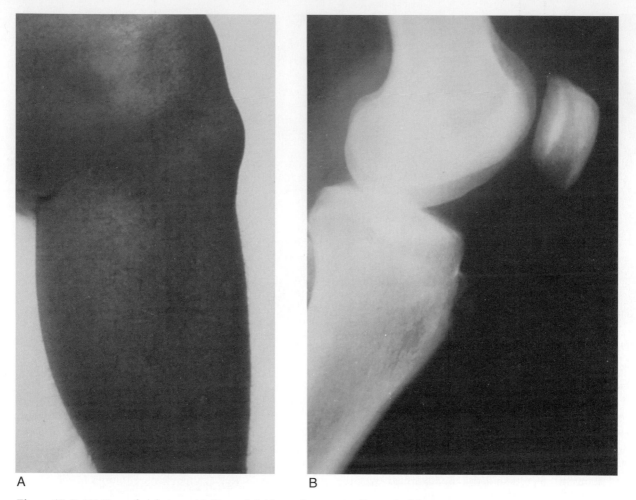

A

B

Figure 17-7 (A) Knee of adult man with Osgood-Schlatter disease caused by avulsed fragments.
(B) Radiograph showing avulsed fragments.

structure originating proximally at the fascial extension of the tensor fasciae latae muscle and attaching to the intermuscular septum at the level of the lateral tibial tubercle of Gerdy. This band also provides static lateral stabilization; with the lateral collateral ligament, it constitutes the main stabilizer of the lateral knee. The lateral collateral ligament is a cord-shaped structure arising from the lateral femoral condyle and inserting on the fibular head. This ligament is tight in extension but relaxes as the knee flexes.

CRUCIATE LIGAMENTS

Anterior Cruciate Ligament

The anterior cruciate ligament (ACL) is both an intracapsular and an extrasynovial ligament. It has a crescent-shaped origin at the lateral femoral condyle behind the intercondy-lar shelf and extends forward and medially into the medial plateau of the tibia in front of the intercondylar eminence. The ACL is known to have at least three bundles: anteromedial, intermediate, and posterolateral. In extension, the anterior bundle is tight against the intercondylar shelf of the femur. In flexion, the anterior bundle relaxes while the posterolateral becomes tight. The bundles of the ACL fibers spiral from one insertion to the other. For this reason, the geometry of the ligament is difficult to reproduce synthetically. The ACL is tightest at extremes of motion: full extension and full flexion. In midrange, it is tight when the tibia is internally rotated but otherwise remains lax. The ACL prevents forward subluxation of the tibia on the femur and abnormal internal rotation of the tibia, which would tighten and twist the posterior cruciate ligament.

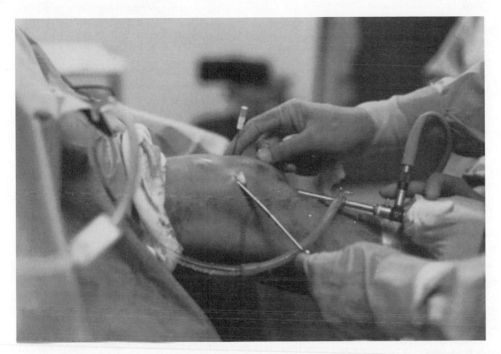

Figure 17-8 Arthroscopic removal of loose body.

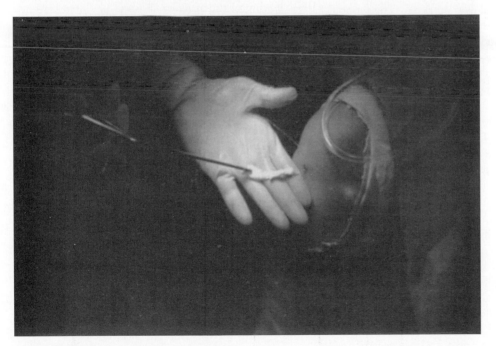

Figure 17-9 Meniscus removed by arthroscopy.

Posterior Cruciate Ligament

The posterior cruciate ligament differs from the ACL in being solely an extrasynovial ligament with a crescent insertion on the medial femoral condyle. It works reciprocally with the ACL; at all points in the range of motion, one of these ligaments is tight.

Popliteal or Baker's Cyst

The popliteal or Baker's cyst usually occurs in response to a problem in the knee joint, such as a torn meniscus.[7] Damage causes synovitis, which produces secondary effusion that fills the joint capsule, which then herniates between the heads of the gastrocnemius muscle. Its presence can be confirmed by arthrogram or ultrasound studies. The treatment of choice is arthroscopy, to identify the underlying pathology. Removal of the source of the problem usually allows the cyst to resolve itself; otherwise, surgical removal is necessary.

Subluxing Patella

Subluxing patella may result from biomechanical misalignment of the knee as well as trauma.[8–10] The pushoff phase of a sidestep cut, or extension with valgus force on the knee, may cause the patella to slide laterally, especially in female athletes who have a weak vastus medialis obliquus muscle. Female athletes characteristically have a wide pelvis, anteverted hips, a shallow femoral groove with a flat lateral femoral condyle, and high-riding patellae, along with ligamentous laxity and recurvatum of the knee with an externally rotated tibia. These conditions, particularly in combination, favor subluxation of the patella. The male athlete may also sublux the patella when higher forces are applied, from trauma, or with cutting, for example. The athlete with a subluxing patella reports catching, giving way, and some medial knee pain, mimicking a medial meniscus tear. In the past, this misdiagnosis led to unnecessary meniscectomies.

Treatment of the acutely subluxed or dislocated patella (when the patella is prominently off the lateral aspect) usually begins with reduction. Gentle extension of the lower leg results in spontaneous reduction of the dislocation. The leg needs to be immobilized in a straight position in order for radiographs to be taken to rule out a fracture. Application of ice and a compression wrap to control swelling is also mandatory. The PRICE principle should be employed. Quad-setting exercises, straight leg raises, and continued cool whirlpool baths should be used along with gentle range-of-motion exercises to prevent quadriceps atrophy. Exercises progress to short-arc leg extensions and, finally, to full-range progressive resistance exercises to build up the vastus medialis obliquus muscle.

In the malalignment syndrome, the patella does not properly track in the patellofemoral groove, and there is a flattening of the lateral femoral condyle. Surgical intervention may be necessary; releasing the lateral retinaculum is the most basic method. Continued strengthening of the vastus medialis obliquus muscle is essential for proper tracking. Patients with patella problems often suffer chondromalacia as well.[11–13] This condition has been increasingly recognized as the major knee condition affecting athletes of both sexes.

Chondromalacia Patellae

Chondromalacia represents a form of degenerative arthritis; progress between onset and advanced stages is rapid:

I—Softening or degeneration of the articular cartilage

II—Cleaving of the articular cartilage

III—Cleaving and fronds of the articular cartilage

IV—Wearing away of the articular cartilage to subchondral bone

During knee flexion and extension, the patella normally tracks up and down the femoral groove smoothly and silently, like ice sliding on ice. When the knee is fully extended, the patella is above the level of the femoral condyles and in contact with the fat pad of the suprapatellar pouch. As the knee flexes, there is greater contact between the articular surfaces of the patella and the groove of the femoral condyles. Forces increase within the patellar tendon and the patellofemoral joint as the knee flexes. The patella is maintained within the femoral groove by

Height of the medial and lateral condyles (the lateral being higher)

Muscular balance between the transverse and oblique fibers of the vastus medialis and lateralis muscles

Ligamentous support of the medial and lateral retinaculum

Iliotibial band

Certain biomechanical factors affect normal tracking of the patella. An imbalance tends to result in lateral movement of the patella as the knee flexes, producing pain when the patella overrides the lateral femoral condyle.

The literature reports that a Q angle greater than 15 to 20 degrees constitutes a malalignment syndrome. The Q angle is measured between the intersection of two lines, one drawn vertically through the patella and the patellar tendon, and the other forming a tangent along the shaft of the femur along the anterior iliac spine. An increased Q angle produces a bowstring effect of the quadriceps, pulling the patella laterally as the quadriceps forcefully contract and the tibia rotates internally on the pronated foot during the stance phase.

Aided by the running boom, surgical treatment of chrondromalacia is now the most commonly performed operation on the North American continent. However, chondromalacia patellae can be treated conservatively with straight leg raises, preferably from a sitting position; with shorts arcs, from 30 degrees to full extension; and with quadriceps/hamstring-setting exercises. This approach achieved good results in 85 percent of DeHaven's patients (K. DeHaven, personal communication). We like to add stretching of the antagonist hamstring muscles to permit full extension.

Physical therapy modalities of ice and electrical stimulation support these exercise periods. Securing the patella with a brace is also helpful. These braces can range from a "horseshoe belt pad," held on with an Ace wrap, to a custom-made Neoprene knee sleeve that contains a buttress to help tracking (Fig. 17-10). Most now have a cutout to reduce patellofemoral compression.

In some runners who overpronate, excessive external rotation of the tibia may be controlled with medial longitudinal arch supports or a custom orthosis. In the exercise program, the patient should be given ample time to try to reach 30 repetitions of sitting straight leg raises, with a resistance of 15 to 20 pounds, in a month. This produces a powerful vastus medialis muscle, which contributes significantly to medial tracking.

When conservative treatment does not satisfy the surgeon or the athlete, arthroscopic examination of the knee affords a "look-and-see" rather than a "wait-and-see" approach. It positively documents the grade of chondromalacia appearing on the retropatellar surface and facilitates a prognosis for a lateral retinacular release. Where a lateral release may prove ineffective, we now recommend a modified Maquet procedure, instead of a patellectomy. This procedure uses a bone graft to elevate the insertion of the

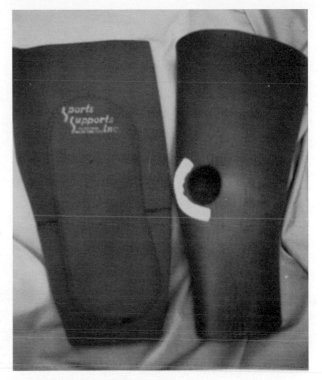

Figure 17-10 Neoprene knee supports. Inside view shows patellar buttress.

patellar tendon, allowing the patella to ride farther away from the femoral condyles, with a resultant reduction of patellofemoral compressive forces.

Chondromalacia patellae is a difficult pathology to manage, particularly if the patient is very active. Just as the wear and tear of the teeth show the age of a horse, the patella indicates the age of the runner or athlete.

Tendon Injuries

QUADRICEPS AND PATELLAR TENDINITIS

Patellar tendinitis, or jumper's knee, is found in a considerable number of athletes, especially volleyball and basketball players. Jumping stresses the extensor mechanism and is localized to the bone–tendon junction. It can affect either the quadriceps or the patellar tendon.

During the early stages, conservative treatment is usually sufficient to alleviate the symptoms. This involves ice massage for 20 minutes per session, phonophoresis (driving in cortisone ointment with ultrasounds), quadriceps strengthening, rest, and a Neoprene knee sleeve. The sleeve is buttressed with an upright felt U-shaped felt piece for patellar tendinitis and an inverted U-shaped felt piece for quadriceps tendinitis.

Severe and chronic cases may require a local steroid injection. However, repeated local injections of corticosteroids to any tendon area brings the possibility of mucoid degeneration, fibrinoid necrosis, mineralization, and areas of fibroblastic degeneration and capillary proliferation within the patellar tendon. This picture is similar in most respects to patellar tendinitis, except that it is localized at the insertion of the quadriceps tendon into the patella.

POPLITEUS TENDINITIS

The popliteus muscle originates from the lateral femoral condyle. Its tendon passes under the fibular collateral ligament in a recess of the lateral meniscus before inserting as a conjoined tendon on the fibula and tibia just anterior to the fibular collateral ligament. This muscle stabilizes the femur against forward displacement on a relatively fixed tibia during the stance phase and especially when running downhill.

A runner may experience pain in the lateral aspect of knee, especially when the training can be related to some recent downhill work. Banked surfaces produce oblique internal lateral rotatory stress that places more traction on the popliteus muscle. Pain is localized, with point tenderness over the insertion of the popliteus tendon.

The examiner should have the athlete sit in a figure-four position, with the lateral side of the ankle of the affected leg resting on the opposite knee. This position makes the lateral part of the ligament more prominent for the examiner to palpate just above the joint line. Popliteal tendinitis will not produce the "giving way" or locking characteristic of a torn lateral meniscus. Nonsteroidal anti-inflammatory medication, as well as phonophoresis (10 percent cortisone with ultrasound), is the treatment of choice. A Marcaine (bupivacaine) and Celestone (betamethasone) solution may also be instilled into the bursa about the tendon, and the athlete's training should preclude running downhill. Changing sides of the road in training also is helpful, because the typical 14-degree cant places excess stress in relationship to hyperextension.

Overuse Synovitis

Some athletes develop chronic knee synovitis without any apparent intra-articular pathology or history of injury, other than increased activity.[14] Typical histories would be increased mileage or a faster pace. Oral anti-inflammatory medication over several weeks, combined with decreased mileage or an easier pace, utilizing cryotherapy (cool whirlpools) afterward, usually controls the synovitis. In some cases, injection of an intra-articular steroid is indicated; unfortunately, steroids can damage the articular cartilage, so we dislike using them. The injection upsets the acid balance within the joint capsule, although a new type of drug, Feldene piroxican helps neutralize this process.

SOFT TISSUE THIGH INJURIES

Thigh Strains

Strains to the groin, the quadriceps, and especially the hamstring muscles are commonplace in sports. Some athletes never seem completely free from them. Such chronic problems are usually traceable to insufficient healing of an original injury followed by repeated re–injury and the accumulation of scar tissue at the same spot, which usually heals in a contracted state, causing pain and microbleeding when suddenly stretched and traumatized.

Upon clinical examination, the muscle group will be extremely tender and swollen and will have limited range of motion. Recovery as well as a more meaningful diagnosis are facilitated if a cold compression pad is used to stabilize the injured muscle and control microbleeding posttrauma. Strains can be mild, moderate, or severe, taking days or weeks to heal. Ecchymosis becomes increasingly apparent in grade III strains and can be large and colorful, indicating the contused area. The muscle defect may be palpable, although this is not likely to be instructive, only painful.

Treatment is straightforward: rest, immobilization, nonweight bearing with crutches, ice massage followed by contrast baths, gentle stretching, and mild strengthening. Ultrasound can be added if soreness continues once activities are resumed (Table 17-1). Administration of an anti-inflammatory agent such as Indocin (indomethacin) has been shown to decrease the occurrence of myositis ossificans in the injured muscle.

Thigh Contusions

Contusions of the thigh are very common injuries in contact sports. They can be classified as mild, moderate, or severe according to the rating for pain, swelling, and range of motion. *Mild* contusion is characterized by mini-

Table 17-1 Treatment Suggestions for Thigh Strain

Modality	Days						Weeks				Comments
	1	2	3	4	5	6	1	2	3	4	
Rest	X	X	X								
Ice				X		X	X				
Hydrotherapy				X		X	X	3X	3X	3X	Or moist heat after day 3, as indicated
Ultrasound											Possibly
Exercise		X	X	X	X	X	X	X	X	X	Daily, including stretching
Strapping		X	X	X	X	X	X	X	X		

mal pain, tenderness, and swelling and no limitation of motion. *Severe* contusion causes intense pain, especially on attempting range of motion. Tenderness is present over a wide area, and swelling is pronounced. Range of motion is severely limited. *Moderate* symptoms fall somewhere between these two extremes.

Immediate treatment is crucial. As soon as the contusion is recognized, the player should be pulled out of the game or practice, preventing further aggravation of the injury. Continuing would increase bleeding into the muscle, causing a large hematoma. Ice packs are used initially with the knee flexed, so as to keep the thigh muscles stretched. This treatment is repeated as required. The scar tissue then heals in an elongated, rather than a contracted, state, maintaining range of motion during the healing process. An elastic bandage containing a compression pad also helps control bleeding during the rehabilitation stages. The patient may require crutches to decrease strain from weight bearing. Neither heat (either superficial and deep) nor massage is be employed, because they increase circulation, which may exacerbate hemorrhage and edema, adversely affecting the resolution of the contusion. Exercise stimulates circulation without these side effects, if not carried to extremes. Radical techniques such as aspiration of the hematoma or injection of enzymes carry risk of infection or of producing a draining sinus tract. Oral enzymes have been used with apparent success but remain controversial. Indocin may be given to safeguard against formation of myositis ossificans.

Myositis Ossificans

Myositis ossificans is a formation of bone within a muscle.[15] It originates with a blow to the soft tissues, typically in the frontal thigh, causing bleeding into the muscle and producing a hematoma. Repeated trauma, without proper treatment or protective padding, prevents the hematoma

from resolving, and the calcification process begins. A calcified hematoma has the capacity for growth after attaching itself to the diaphysis of the bone. Surgical excision may be necessary if pain, restricted range of motion, or loss of muscular strength is present. If pain persists for 3 or 4 weeks after any contusion, radiographic investigation should be routinely instituted. The growth will not be apparent on the radiograph until this time. Football players in particular should wear secure padding in vulnerable regions such as the frontal thigh and the lateral aspect of the humerus (when calcified tissue occurs here, it is known as "blocker's knots"). Surgical removal of the mature calcified growth can be done successfully.

Iliotibial Band Friction Syndrome

The iliotibial band is a fascia strip that passes down the lateral aspect of the thigh from the crest of the ilium, inserting in Gerdy's tubercle of the lateral tibial condyle. As the knee flexes and extends during running, this band repeatedly rubs over the lateral femoral condyle, which may cause an inflammatory response. The resultant knee pain is just above the joint line. Runners who extend their training program suddenly or who incorporate some hill work tend to develop this syndrome. Runners with a biomechanical abnormality such as tibia varus who tend to overpronate are susceptible to this condition as well.

Treatment for a mild condition includes adequate stretching and warming, with a topical ointment, for example, before the run and more stretching but ice massage afterward. More sophisticated modalities are available at therapy clinics. We have found phonophoresis of a cortisone preparation very effective. The ointment is used topically but is driven in with ultrasound. Steroid may also be injected into the area for severe cases. Biomechanical problems may require simply a longitudinal arch support

Table 17-2 Treatment Suggestions for Iliotibial Band Friction Syndrome

Modality	Days						Weeks				Comments
	1	2	3	4	5	6	1	2	3	4	
Cold	X	X	X	X	X	X	X				As necessary in weeks 2–4
Ultrasound	X	X	X								Use phonophoresis
Braces	X	⟶									Shoe orthotic
Exercise	X	X	X	X	X	X	X				Include stretching
Orthotics	X	X	X	⟶							Medial longitudinal arch support with lateral buildup

and building up the medial aspect, thereby reducing the stresses on the lateral side of the knee (Table 17-2).

ACKNOWLEDGMENT

We would like to thank Dr. David Ponsonby for the use of the illustrations.

REFERENCES

1. Mital MA, Matza RA, Cohen J: The so-called unresolved Osgood-Schlatter lesion. J Bone Joint Surg [Am] 62:732, 1980
2. Jakob RP, Von Gumppenberg S, Englehart P: Does Osgood-Schlatter disease influence the position of the patella? J Bone Joint Surg [Br] 63:579, 1981
3. Levine J, Kashyap S: A new conservative treatment of Osgood-Schlatter disease. Clin Orthop 158:126, 1981
4. The knee: athletic injuries. Phys Ther (Special Issue) 60: 1553, 1980
5. Wirth CR: Meniscus repair. Clin Orthop 151:153, 1981
6. Munzinger U, Rickstahl J, Scherrer H, Gshwerd W: Internal derangement of the knee joint due to pathologic synovial folds. Clin Orthop 155:59, 1981
7. Patrone NA et al: Baker's cyst and venous thrombosis. South Med J 74:768, 1982
8. Paulos L, Rusche K, Johnson C, Noyes FR: Patellar malalignment. Phys Ther 60:1624, 1980
9. Slocum B, Slocum DB, Devine T, Boone E: Wedge recession for treatment of recurrent luxation of the patella. Clin Orthop 164:48, 1982
10. Larsen E, Lauridsen F: Conservative treatment of patellar dislocations. Clin Orthop 171:131, 1982
11. Livingstone BN: Clinical tests for chondromalacia patella. Lancet 2:210, 1982
12. Osborne AH, Fulford PC: Lateral release for chondromalacia patella. J Bone Joint Surg 64:202, 1982
13. Brown DE, Alexander AH, Lichtman DM: Elmsue-Trillat procedure: evaluation in patellar dislocation and subluxation. Am J Sport Med 12:104, 1984
14. Subotnick SI: Orthotic foot control and the overuse syndrome. Physician Sports Med 3:75, 1975
15. Rothwell AG: Quadriceps hematoma. Clin Orthop 171:97, 1982

18

Hip, Pelvis, and Low Back Injuries

JAMES D. KEY
DONALD JOHNSON
GARY JARVIS
DAVID PONSONBY

The hip, pelvis, and low back areas play a vital role in athletic injuries. These areas form the strength and support for the rest of the lower extremity. Many of the major muscles have their origin in these areas, particularly the quadriceps and hamstrings. Stresses often begin with impact and are transmitted to these areas, resulting in injury. The hip joint is the largest joint in the body, and has a wide range of motion derived from major muscle groups. One group is often overdeveloped, causing an imbalance, which can lead to injury.

Weakness of the quadriceps musculature and hip extensors remains one of the most common afflictions of injured athletes and is widely affecting an aging American population (the Baby Boomers). Weakness of the quadriceps frequently results in a prolonged disability in the injured athlete, or ultimately even the inability to rise from a seated position in a chair. The complicated motion around the hip joint itself is a combination initiated by the quadriceps muscle first around the knee (from its origin on the pelvis) and then aided by the strong extensors of the hip (originating on the pelvis and inserting into the proximal femur) and the large extensors of the spine. Weakness of these muscles has been determined to be responsible for injured athletes not being able to rehabilitate themselves, as well as for the prolonged disability of the senior or adult population, resulting in approximately 50 percent that population having difficulty rising from a chair.

A recent study of the aging population shows that that 50 percent can be helped dramatically by simple exercises for the quadriceps mechanism, hip extensors, and low back. Well-documented research has been done by Dr. Michael Pollock, Ph.D., at the University of Florida in Gainesville for the MedX Corporation in isolation and strengthening of low back musculature with the MedX equipment. Miriam Nelson Ph.D., and Sarah Wernick, Ph.D., have published a great deal of documented research on this same mechanism of getting athletes and patients active and out of the seated, debilitated position. Nelson's publication *Strong Women Stay Young* has been a well-received addition to the literature for anti-aging physicians, podiatrists, and orthopedic surgeons. If our patients are not ambulatory, they are not as capable of participating in all of the activities that they should to enjoy a full and active life. Nelson was able to get a high percentage of wheelchair-bound patients up out of the chairs, active and walking, restoring not only their strength but their balance (which prevented falling), restoring bone density, reducing osteoporosis, and increase muscular strength. She continued the research that Arthur Jones, the researcher who invented both Nautilus and the MedX equipment, had

313

begun some two and a half decades earlier. Both proved that strength influenced balance and bone metabolism and that, to increase strength in the proximal and distal quadriceps muscle groups, strengthening the hamstrings, the flexors and extensors of the hip group, and the spine was one of the most important things that could be done to help facilitate continued athletic activity and rehabilitation. This research has contributed significantly not only to rehabilitation of injured athletes, but to the strengthening and prevention of debilitation of the aging Baby Boomer population.

Treatment of spine injuries has taken giant steps forward in the surgical arena with the recognition of segmental instability of the spine, spinal stenosis, and stabilization of the spine with fixation with various innovative types of hardware. The treatment of spondylolisthesis in the athlete (or even simple segmental instability in the average population after rupture and collapse of the disc) has taken a giant step forward in stabilization with the development of pedicular screws, rods, plates, and hooks, which have been used effectively for this type of fixation and rehabilitation. The introduction of the anterior and posterior lumbar interbody fixation with titanium cages filled with the patient's own bone (from either the posterior approach or the anterior approach) has greatly reduced the tendency of interbody fusions to collapse and has aided in the prevention of neuroforaminal stenosis. The technical expertise now exists to implant these cages anteriorly through the endoscope (and possibly intrathoracically via the thoracoscope), and work is being done on the cervical spine as well. These types of innovations hold initial excellent promise for stabilization of the entire spine through the anterior or posterior approach (especially from the anterior approach) without the danger of injury to the nerve root or spinal cord elements. Fixation of the injured facet joint and pedicles posteriorly enters a second decade of use for widespread treatment of spinal instability in the United States. The fixation of the lumbar and thoracic spine is now widely performed using pedicular screws and rods or plates for fixation. It is believed to be one of the best methods of producing fusion and fixation of the spine, as evidenced by the official policy statement of the North American Spine Society.

With continued progress in treatment of the lumbar spine, more and more refinements in decompression and fixation will continue to unfold with each passing decade. The use of arthroscopic decompression of the disc from the posterior aspect has produced a significant reduction of disability related to lumbar spine and disc surgery. The introduction of the nomium laser and other lasers for use in removing intradiscal lesions has helped decrease morbidity to the lumbar spine. The proteoglycans of the joints and spine itself are actively being studied by biochemists to determine exactly what role they may play in production of spinal disc, facet, and nerve root pain. The frankly ruptured lumbar disc is easily recognizable and treatable. The additional burden of spondylosis in an aging population, along with nerve root decompression and medial facet removal, has added an importance tool to the armamentarium of the orthopedic surgeon for relieving spinal stenosis and biomechanical low back pain.

Increased exercise tolerance has been demonstrated by treadmill tests and other quantifiable exercise programs to demonstrate the efficacy of decompression laminectomy and decompression of spinal stenosis in this aging population. An explosion in the treatment of nerve root pain and disc pain by pain specialists in the fields of general practice, anesthesiology, surgery, and orthopedics has seen widespread use of injection of epidural steroids into the lumbar and cervical facets, with improvement in some patients with minor anatomic deformity, and has become a recognized first line of defense in acute disc and low back pain before resorting to surgical intervention. The widespread application of magnetic resonance imaging and computed tomography (CT) (both with and without contrast material) and the use of the C-arm in the office have made possible many of the advances in spinal intervention.

Although these modern technologies have greatly added to the armamentarium of the podiatrist, the internist, the surgeon, and the pain control specialist, all of these techniques are still enhanced by the oldest known standby for treatment of the lumbar spine—progressive resistive exercise. Progressive resistive exercise is believed by many purists to be the only type of rehabilitation that produces ultimate permanent changes in the structure of the lumbar spine. It is also the only consistently prescribed regimen that appears to have little or no undesirable side effects. Certainly the side effects from lumbar spinal exercise remain much less than those from the above-mentioned treatments (surgical intervention, oral medication, or injections). As recently noted at the annual meeting of the Anti-Aging Society, approximately 50 percent of the medications being advocated at this time (if statistics hold true) will have fallen into disfavor or have been recognized to have serious side effects within a decade. As much as a 50 percent improvement in rehabilitation of the injured lumbar, thoracic, or cervical spine can be produced with progressive resistive exercise. Studies continue to be carried out at many academic institutions, and a graphic analysis of the areas of pathology and documentation of improvement in spinal muscular strength has greatly aided its widespread acceptance in the medical community. Pioneers in exercise for the last three decades have continued to call our attention to what we have basically known all of this time—that progressive resistive exercises alone is a potent tool against injuries of the lumbar spine, hip, and thigh.

This chapter deals with basic injuries and symptomatology about the hip, pelvis, and low back. Problems often develop in this area early in an athletic career, as much of our growth occurs at this area. It is important to be aware of pediatric problems in this area. The chapter is a brief overview that touches on a wide variety of ailments. If problems do develop in these areas, expert advice should be sought.

HIP INJURIES

Trochanteric Bursitis

The greater trochanter has a bursa immediately underneath the iliotibial band that contains the powerful quadriceps muscles. Bursitis is usually initiated in this area from a direct blow or uneven gait. Traumatic incidents are commonplace on football fields and racketball courts, while runners are vulnerable if they have a leg length discrepancy, a scissor style, or a muscular imbalance (especially with fatigue) or choose to run on uneven terrain, including the camber of a road or track.

Cycling motions can be used to reproduce the symptoms for clinical review. One distinguishing characteristic of some bicyclists has been referred to as "frog's legs." This refers to their appearance, owing to the greatly developed vastus lateralis musculature.

Trochanter bursitis responds well to accurate bursal aspi-

ration and injection with (Xylicaine lidocaine) and hydrocortisone, as well as rest, ice, and, later, heat. Rest, ice, and contrast baths are the first modalities to try, but the condition is generally chronic, requiring oral anti-inflammatory agents or local steroid injection for resolution. Strengthening for muscular balance and endurance offers a long-term solution, while an orthosis would also overcome any structural inequities.

Legg-Perthes Disease

In young, active children, especially boys, pain and limitation of hip movement may be linked to aseptic avascular necrosis of the femoral head. Many parents first bring their child to the physician with a complaint of knee pain. There is usually marked disuse atrophy of the upper thigh, and abduction and internal rotation are limited. The child tends to walk with an antalgic, or protective, limp, splinting his legs against the pain. This diagnosis is confirmed radiographically. The goal of treatment is to prevent deformity of the femoral head, which if it occurs speeds degenerative changes during adult life. Destruction can be considerable and the joint will be arthritic. A total hip replacement is a possibility, although other surgical options include resurfacing the femoral head and replacing it with a prosthesis.

The most common treatment consists of a brace, worn for up to a year, to permit the femoral head to revascularize and the bone to heal (Table 18-1). In the brace used at Scottich Rite Children's Hospital, the legs are abducted 45 degrees to prevent subluxation of the hip, but the child continues to have knee motion and can walk effectively.

Acute Fractures of the Hip

Acute hip fractures are usually the result of trauma. The three types of hip fracture are intertrochanteric, subtrochanteric, and subcapital.[1,2] These fractures are usually dis-

Table 18-1 Treatment Suggestions for Legg-Perthes Disease

Modality	Days						Weeks				Comments
	1	2	3	4	5	6	1	2	3	4	
Rest	———————————————————————————→										Patient must not put weight on joint for up to 1 year
Brace	———————————————————————————→										Traction
Exercise	X	X	X	X		——————————————→					Continue until other modalities are ended

placed and comminuted. Open reduction and internal fixation techniques are used to stabilize the fracture for healing. In some cases, undisplaced hairline intertrochanteric fractures can be treated conservatively with traction and non–weight-bearing status. Severe fractures of the subcapital type demand the replacement of the head of the femur using a prosthetic implant. In all these types of fracture, one must always worry about avascular necrosis of the head and malunion at the fracture site.

Slipped Femoral Capital Epiphysis

Endomorphic teenage athletes can suffer from a slipped femoral capital epiphysis.[3,4] The usual age for this type of fracture is from 9 years to the end of growth; it is more common in boys than girls. The femoral epiphysis usually slips slowly and progressively, leading to a progressive coxa vara deformity. The head of the femur on radiography looks like an ice cream cone that is melting and tilting off to the side. When the epiphysis becomes separated from the femoral neck, its precarious blood supply may be severely damaged, and avascular necrosis may result.

Usually the child first complains to parents of mild discomfort from the hip and deep in the groin. This may also be referred to the knee in later stages of the slippage. As the slip progresses, the child develops a Trendelenburg gait (the child's trunk leans toward the affected side as weight is borne on the affected limb). The lower limb becomes externally rotated. Further examination reveals limitation of internal rotation and abduction of the hip, when the hip is passively flexed and the thigh rotates externally. The diagnosis may be suspected but can only be confirmed by radiographic examination of the hip joint.

Treatment for slipped femoral capital epiphysis in the early stages is to prevent further slippage. If there has been a minimal slip, it should be stabilized surgically with threaded pins followed by non–weight-bearing status until the epiphysis has healed to the neck, which will require several months. Resumption of sports activities is the long-term treatment goal. Complete reunion of the fracture site, evidenced by radiography, is mandatory. For the athlete, rehabilitation is most important to regain full range of motion, muscular strength, and flexibility before resuming full activities.

Stress Fractures of the Hip

Stress fractures are frequently attributed to overuse or to inadequate conditioning. Today, instead of a handful of elite athletes training for the Olympics, thousands of people train to complete marathons, ultramarathons and triathlons. Their training may be suddenly increased to match their new goal, or slightly raised from an already massive total, usually around the magic figure of 100 miles. Stress fractures are explainable as an incomplete attempt by the bone to remodel itself, whereby bone is deposited in sites subjected to stress and reabsorbed from sites where there is no excessive stress. This phenomenon is known as Wolff's law. There is rarely any history of acute trauma.

The athlete usually presents symptoms of pain deep in the groin at clinical examination. Patrick's test will be positive.[5] The pain may interrupt sleep (as well as running), and consumption of aspirin will be at the maximum recommended level. Without athletic participation, the athlete is no longer invincible and eagerly seeks a medical solution.

The delay aids the physician in providing an immediate tangible diagnosis, because the stress fracture requires time to become visible on radiography (Fig. 18-1). The first radiograph may reveal some elevation of the periosteum, which evokes a high index of suspicion for a stress fracture site, but the physician is likely to instruct the patient to stop running, just in case, and to come back for serial radiographs to monitor the condition.[6-8] Early confirmation may also be sought from a bone scan[9] or ultrasound.[10] Athletes are impatient, and "wait and see" is not a satisfactory state of affairs. Treatment is rest and non–weight bearing with crutches. We encourage our athletes to keep up their cardiovascular endurance by using a stationary bike, swimming, and maintaining their strength in the upper extremity and the noninvolved limb where the stress fracture is unilateral (Table 18-2).

During rehabilitation, the yearn to resume running is almost overpowering, especially as they athlete begins to feel good again. A prescribed training program may be necessary to protect the athlete from overdoing things again. It is also important at this time to rule out other contributory factors that might otherwise lead to recurrence of the injury, such as unsuitable shoes, a harsh running surface, or a biomechanical predisposition in need of orthotic correction.

Actually, pain can disappear during a run because the body produces its own β-endorphins (chemically related to morphine). Bearing all these factors in mind, we encourage and counsel our runners to resume training very slowly and easily. At times the progression may seem too easy, but this generally means it is working. Bone is a living tissue that can adapt to tremendous stresses, given time.

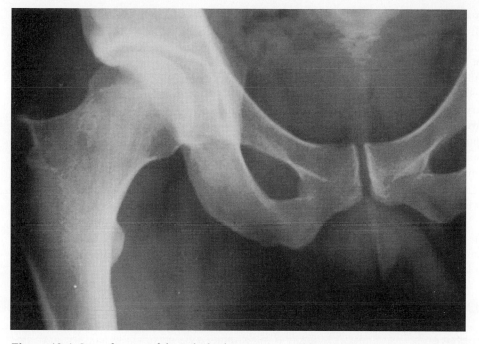

Figure 18-1 Stress fracture of the ischial tuberosity in a middle-aged distance runner.

Running for health should not be painful before, during, or afterward.

Hip Pointer

The injury known as hip pointer is a contusion on the rim of the iliac crest caused by a blow, probably from a helmet, knee, or elbow. A particularly severe blow, as when colliding with an artificial turf surface, can result in some separation, or possibly complete detachment, of the muscle fibers from the iliac crest. The abdominal and oblique muscles attach to the inner margin of the iliac crest and the muscles of the thigh attach to the cover margin. When these muscles are injured, everyday as well as athletic movements become painful. The injured area becomes discolored because as the hematoma lies in the sparse layer of adipose tissue covering the iliac crest.

When hip pointer injury occurs, after examination the athlete's hip should be radiographed to rule out fracture of the iliac crest, avulsion fracture, or apophysitis. This is especially important in the growing athlete, because a significant avulsion of the apophysis needs to be reattached by open reduction and internal fixation.

These injuries should be treated initially by immediate application of ice and compression. The swelling and tenderness usually resolve with the application of ice. Aspiration is not recommended, but it may be necessary to inject the area with lidocaine during the healing phase. Analgesics and anti-inflammatory agents greatly reduce discomfort. An elastic wrap is worn between treatments of ice massage for compression. This continues until the ecchymosis, swelling, and soreness subside. At this time, contrast baths could begin. Treatment can cease once activities are pain free. Rehabilitation consists of strengthening the muscula-

Table 18-2 Treatment Suggestions for Stress Fractures

Modality	Day 1–7	Week 1–4	Comments
Brace	⟶		Splint/cast as indicated
Exercise	⟶		Range of motion; gentle exercise as tolerated

ture surrounding the iliac crest and reestablishing mobility of the hip and waist.

Prevention is a problem in many sports that do not use protective padding as part of the standard uniform or equipment, wrestling, basketball, soccer, and baseball being prime examples. A protective pad is desirable when possible to prevent early reinjury. A football knee pad may be used, or Orthoplast, lined with felt, can be form fitted.

A more severe problem, apophysitis of the iliac crest, exists but is not recognized as such by the American Medical Association's (AMA's) Committee on Standard Nomenclature. The AMA defines apophysitis as a contusion of the iliac crest. We believe it becomes apophysitis when radiographs demonstrate displacement of the iliac apophysis requiring surgery. The hip pointer usually clears up within 4 to 6 weeks, with recommended treatment. Apophysitis may take 8 months to heal.

PELVIC INJURIES

Pelvic Fracture

Pelvic fractures require extreme trauma, such as an automobile accident, falling from a horse, or falling down a mountain. The fracture tends to be over-shadowed by associated complications: extensive internal hemorrhage, rupture of the bladder or of the urethra, and similar internal injuries. Physical examination reveals local swelling, abdominal tenderness and rigidity, and possibly instability and deformity of the hips as well. The patient is likely to be in shock and must be watched closely for life-threatening blood loss.

Treatment of the fracture is aimed at correcting significant deformities in order to prevent malunion and resultant disturbances of function. If the fracture does not pass through the pelvic ring, the pelvis can retain some stability, allowing it to heal so long as the patient refrains from weight bearing on the affected side. Disruption of the pelvic ring requires closed or open reduction with fixation (with Hoffmann external fixation system or ASIF system.)

Osteltis Pubis

Inflammation is not always restricted to soft tissues, as with bursitis. Running and bicycling can impose excessive shear forces when the pelvis rotates and shifts in see saw fashion, to accommodate the up-and-down pumping action of the legs. Symptoms may be reproduced clinically with both abduction and adduction movements of the hip. Radiographs of the ischium may, in time, demonstrate sclerosis (seen as hardening of the bone with white appearance on radiography) on both sides at the attachment of the adductor muscles. This finding would confirm an inflammation of the pubis.

A typical treatment program would begin with rest, ice, and massage, progressing to hydrotherapy (contrast baths and whirlpool), and followed by mild stretching and low-intensity muscular exercises to preserve muscular strength and tonus. Anti-inflammatory agents may be necessary, especially to facilitate swimming or stationary bicycling. Because cycling could also aggravate the condition, care must be taken with regard to saddle position and smooth riding style, using resistance within the capabilities of the patient, who must not overexert during the pedal motion.

Avulsion Fractures

Avulsion fractures are most commonly seen around the pelvis at the origins of the adductor magnus, hamstrings, and sartorius muscles. Clinical evaluation usually indicates restricted mobility and point tenderness; radiographs are positive. The avulsed fragment may be large enough to require open reduction and internal fixation. Otherwise, the use of rest, ice, and oral anti-inflammatory agents is sufficient.

Ischial Bursitis

A bursa is a soft sac-like structure that provides lubrication and some cushioning between tendon and bone. It can become inflamed with point tenderness when irritated, hence the term *bursitis*. One such area is the ischial tuberosity. Ischial bursitis usually develops in adolescent runners doing speed work, especially given the additional impetus of coming down a slope. This injury is even aggravated by excessive sitting, so other forms of rest are required to promote healing.

Treatment typically comprises ice, massage, and stretching and strengthening exercises, as tolerated. Emphasis should be given to the adductor and hamstring groups. Oral nonsteroidal anti-inflammatory agents may prevent the condition from becoming chronic, which happens occasionally, in which case the bursa must be injected locally with steroids. Standard and specialized radiographs of the femur, pelvis, and acetabulum should be a part of the work-up, along with aspiration and analysis (fluid smear).

Blood work for uric acid or rheumatoid antibody or later antibody factors is important. Technetium scan or cineradiography might help reveal any occult idiopathic avascular necrosis. Athletic activity must be suspended until diagnosis is completed.

Groin Strain

Groin pain may be brought on suddenly by a single injury or gradually by multiple traumas caused by overuse. Athletes in many sports may develop groin pain, but it is especially common in soccer and football and in track and field events. A variety of structures may be affected in groin injuries, including the pubis symphysis and ramus; the bellies, origins, and insertions of the adductor muscle group; and the gracilis.

The groin injury may be caused by sudden powerful overstretching of the leg in abduction and external rotation, especially if there is an opposing force. These forces may overstretch the fibers of the muscles or tendons, the bony tissue of the pelvic ring and pubis symphysis.

Groin pain may develop suddenly or gradually, and it may be sharp or dull. It may be strong enough to stop players from playing and force them to limp off the field. The pain may be localized or may be diffuse. Pain often radiates in different directions, usually down along the adductors, and laterally to the hip and often the back.

Rest usually relieves and may eliminate the pain. Motion, especially abduction with external rotation of the hip, aggravates it. To test the source of pain, passive and active assisted motion of the patient's hip with the leg extending is used in all directions, especially abduction and external rotation. Careful palpation of the groin structures will help localize the pain.

After clinical examination, radiographs should be taken (anteroposterior, lateral, and oblique views of the pubis and symphysis). Four stages of radiographic changes have been seen in the source of serious groin strain. Stage 1 is osteolytic changes in the os pubis and ischium and may be evident around the insertion of the gracilis and adductor longus and brevis muscles. At stage 2, the symphysis is more affected. At stage 3, the symphysis is more deformed and erosion is well developed. By stage 4, myositis ossificans, may be evident in the adductor longus and brevis and gracilis muscles at their insertions.[11]

Rest is the best treatment for groin pain. When the player stops playing, the condition will resolve. Rest, routine physical therapy, medication, and rehabilitation are a must for the athlete to be able to return to competition.

Initial treatment on the field or in the training room would consist of immediate rest of the area and ice application. Analgesics and anti-inflammatory agents are used to eliminate pain. The painful area may be infiltrated with 5 to 10 ml of 0.5 to 1 percent lidocaine. Cortisone is not recommended as an injectible agent for the site.

The patient is put on crutches, and a groin wrap or spica with compression pad is used. Rehabilitation begins with range-of-motion exercises of the affected extremity. Exercises should increase gradually to progressive resistive exercises as the athlete can tolerate them. The athlete is encouraged to swim or ride a stationary bike and to use endurance training to preserve cardiovascular endurance.

By the time the athlete regains full range of motion, and is doing progressive resistive exercises with full weight bearing, he or she may begin a jogging and running program. As rehabilitation proceeds, sports-specific exercises will be incorporated. To prevent groin injuries, the pelvis and lower extremities must be carefully conditioned to withstand the forces encountered in sports. To develop strength in all the groin muscles, exercises should be performed against resistance to the maximum range of motion and with repetitions to build strength as well as endurance. To maintain range of motion, special stretching exercises of the groin implementing proprioceptive neuromuscular facilitation techniques should be used.[12] The thigh muscles, especially the adductors and lower back and abdominal muscles, need special attention. The athlete must endeavor to develop flexibility and agility of the entire body, with special emphasis on areas that have been previously injured.

LOW BACK INJURIES

Lumbosacral Strain

Lumbosacral strain is a catchall term, covering any back condition in a patient who has no readily identifiable source of low back pain. Most athletes are young and their resilient ligaments can compensate for many of the stresses imposed during activities. These ligaments become more fibrous after age 35 and less able to rescue the typically declining musculature and deteriorating posture. In women, hyperlordosis is often related to the wearing of high heels and the stresses of pregnancy. Overcoming flabby musculature is the best course of action.

Football involves collisions, the confrontation of linemen being especially likely to generate a chronic back condition, while receivers are likely to be hit from behind, causing acute injury. The linemen, because they are down in their stance, come up to a standing position against resistance. This causes extreme stress on the lumbosacral area. When these players have a lumbosacral strain episode, they may become completely incapacitated and experience excruciating discomfort. This pain is usually due to the extreme muscle spasm and tightness caused by the spasms. Physical therapy modalities, strengthening, stretching, and lumbosacral supports are helpful in the treatment of lumbosacral strain. Antispasmodic medications such as Flexeril (cyclobenzaprene) are also useful in controlling the muscle spasm and in making the patient more comfortable. Anti-inflammatory agents, such as Feldene (piroxicoin) or Motrin (ibuprofen) are also available and useful for these conditions.

Herniated Disc

Intervertebral discs are subject to constant stress and are susceptible to degenerative tears and dehydration. The most vulnerable disc lies between L4 and L5. The mechanism of injury is usually a sudden blow or twist that places abnormal strain upon the lumbar region. Biomechanical calculations put the multiplier effect for this disc level at 10 to 15 times the weight being lifted. The disc must therefore withstand forces of 1,000 to 1,500 pounds when 100 pounds are lifted.

The disc may become herniated and impinge upon the spinal cord or spinal nerves. This nerve root compression syndrome manifests itself in identifiable patterns, according to the location of impingement. Routine neurologic examination, along with testing the patient's flexibility and muscle strength, are used to assess the clinical picture and history for athletes. CT scan shows the precise extent of the problem. A more conventional myelogram may also be used as a diagnostic tool.

Treatment for herniated disc often starts conservatively with bed rest in the hospital and pelvic traction. As time progresses, if the patient does not receive relief from this type of treatment and diagnostic tests have revealed a bulging disc at the appropriate nerve level that corresponds with clinical findings, surgical intervention must be considered. As the literature has stated, 70 percent recovery is a good estimate for most persons undergoing a discectomy. We have found this percentage to be reliable in our own hands. Postsurgical treatment includes physical therapy modalities and encouragement for the patient to

do a lot of walking and to refrain from prolonged sitting. It may take 6 to 9 months, or up to 1 year, before satisfactory results are shown.

Spondylolysis/Spondylolisthesis

Spondylolysis refers to a defect in the lamina, or neural arch, of the vertebra.[13] There is an 85 percent probability that the lumbar vertebrae will be involved. The condition is never present at birth but has been noted as early as 4 months. Heredity plays a significant role but, while severe stresses are inevitable in an upright animal, the inadequacy may not prove critical until exceptional forces are added from football, wrestling, or gymnastics. These sports involve hyperextension of the back against resistance, significantly stressing the vertebrae and causing a stress fracture of the lamina.

The diagnosis is usually suspected clinically from symptoms and history provided by the athlete. Complete back films, including oblique views, are essential in making this diagnosis. In the oblique view, the Scotty dog formation will appear to have a collar, indicating the area of stress fracture. Tomograms or bone scans are also helpful in making the diagnosis if regular radiographs are negative for pathology, but clinically the symptomatology is indicative of a spondylolysis. Clinical tests to reproduce the symptoms include leg extension, with the patient standing and hyperextending the leg on the involved side. Clinically, the history reported is that of low back pain, spasm of the erector spinae muscles, and loss of range of motion, usually of forward flexion and lateral flexion. The usual physical therapy modalities include rest, a possible warm-and-form corset to support the back, exercises, and stretching.

When the defect occurs bilaterally, slippage of the vertebra is almost inevitable. Forward displacement of the deficient vertebra is referred to as spondylolisthesis. It is even possible for the vertebra to move without any bony disruption, which is known as a pseudospondylolisthesis. Treatment is similar for both spondylolysis and spondylolisthesis; radiographs can distinguish between the two diagnoses by forward subluxation of L5 vertebra onto S1. Symptoms usually subside with rest, although some sort of lumbosacral support is helpful in the treatment of both entities, as is the Boston brace. This is used, along with conservative care, in more resistant cases in which the pain progressively worsens but for which surgery is not indicated. Spondylolysis and spondylolisthesis occasionally require surgery.

This would involve the removal of the pseudoarthrosis and fusion in spondylolysis. For spondylolisthesis, the procedure of choice is usually posterior fusion, to stabilize the spine.[14]

REFERENCES

1. Berger EY: More on diagnosing fractures of the hip or pelvis. N Engl J Med 306:366, 1982
2. Sotos JG: Diagnosis of fractures of the hip or pelvis. N Engl J Med 308:971, 1983
3. Boyer DW, Mickelson MR, Poldseti IV: Slipped capital femoral epiphysis: long-term follow up study of one hundred and twenty one patients. J Bone Joint Surg [AM] 63:85, 1981
4. Kulick RG, Denton JR: A retrospective study of 125 cases of slipped capital femoral epiphysis. Clin Orthop 62:87, 1982
5. Belkin SC: Stress fractures in athletes. Orthop Clin North Am 11:735, 1980
6. Meurman KO: Less common stress fractures in the foot. Br J Radiol 54:1, 1981
7. Goergen TG, Venn-Watson EA, Rossman DJ et al: Tarsal navicular stress fracture in runners. AJR 136:201, 1981
8. Torg JS, Pavlos H, Cooley D et al: Stress fractures of the tarsal navicular: A retrospective review of twenty one cases. J Bone Joint Surg 64:700, 1982
9. Batillas J, Vasilas A, Pizzi WF, Gokcebay T: Bone scanning in the detection of occult fractures. J Trauma 21:564, 1981
10. Moss A, Mowat AG: Ultrasonic assessment of stress fractures. Br Med J 286:1479, 1983
11. Zeanah WR, Hudson TM: Myositis ossificans. Clin Orthop 168:187, 1982
12. Pink M: Contralateral effects of upper extremity proprioceptive neuromuscular facilitation patterns. Phys Ther 61:1158, 1981
13. Klinghoffer L, Murdoch MG: Spondylolysis following trauma: a case report and review of the literature. Clin Orthop 166:72, 1982
14. Cloward RB: Spondylolisthesis: treatment by laminectomy and posterior interbody fusion. Clin Orthop 154:74, 1981

IV

Treatment of the
Lower
Extremity

19

History and Physical Examination

STEVEN I. SUBOTNICK

The lower extremity history and physical is an orderly, progressive means of evaluating the athlete's lower extremity as it relates to the whole body on many levels. It enables the practitioner to appreciate any localized pathology that may be present, and its relationship to as well as impact upon the total body system. There is usually a correlation between the area of chief complaint, with its localized malfunction, and areas of secondary compensatory imbalance with their own regional symptoms. This alters the function of the whole body. Often, for example, an area of hypomobility secondary to acute pain splinting will cause proximal or distal areas of hypermobility with discomfort or pain. More subtle are joint movement restrictions necessitating hypermobility in adjacent joints. These secondary areas are often symptomatic while the, "triggers" those areas of reduced or altered joint motion, are asymptomatic. It therefore behooves the practitioner to seek out the cause of imbalance or pain, and to eliminate these triggers. When combined with a biomechanical examination, the lower extremity examination helps the practitioner correlate pathology with function and deformity, injury, or both. An injury or biomechanical imbalance in one part must affect the whole in gross as well as subtle ways. The body is truly an integrated system wherein every part is in communication with every other part for the synergistic good of the collective whole.

INSTRUMENTATION

The instruments needed for the lower extremity history and physical are the same as for the biomechanical examination. A tractograph, as well as a goniometer and tape measure, is used. For gait analysis, either a gait platform, along hallway, or a treadmill, along with videotaping equipment, is used. Nerve trauma requires pinwheels, a neurologic hammer, and a vibratory fork. For advanced problems, nerve conduction studies as well as electromyography may be helpful. Vascular examination is aided with Doppler ultrasound equipment. Pressure studies for compartment syndrome use the Striker system.

PROCEDURES

The same procedures for a localized history and physical examination are used as for the general examination. More emphasis is placed on local pathology in regard to examination, palpation, and evaluation. Since there is a high correlation between foot injury or malfunction and low back pain, motion palpation of the low back, including the sacroiliac joints, should be part of a screening examination. Examiners must remember to ask their patients, and themselves, about concomitant areas that are affected by the primary focus: "How does your sore heel affect other parts of your body? What else has bothered you since the foot, leg, or knee problem?"   An orderly progressive way to proceed is as follows:

I. Chief complaint
   A. Primary problem
   B. Secondary concomitant problems
   C. Overall effect of injury on athlete as a whole

II. History of present illness
  A. Onset
    1. Activity
    2. Mechanism of injury
      a. Acute
      b. Overuse
      c. Reinjury
  B. Environment
    1. Surfaces
    2. Foot gear
  C. Duration
  D. Course
  E. Previous treatment
    1. Self
    2. Professional
  F. Related factors—areas of compensation, functional limitations
  G. Other injuries
    1. Contralateral injuries
    2. Ipsilateral injuries
III. Sports history
  A. Evaluation of activity, level and intensity of training, years in various sports, and other injuries with various sports
  B. For distance runner, determination of mileage, speed, and type of terrain
  C. Evaluation of foot gear (history of abnormal foot gear important)

STANDARD PHYSICAL EXAMINATION OF THE LOWER EXTREMITY

An orderly, progressive evaluation of the lower extremity enables the practitioner to evaluate each patient systematically and to compile and compare data. In this way, a differential diagnosis can be reached and a comfortable routine maintained to minimize oversights.

While the patient is in each of the evaluating positions, it is important to observe, palpate, and measure range of motion and quality of motion in major joints. Function is measured statically and dynamically.

Static Evaluation

SITTING POSITION (POSITION 1)

With the patient seated after the history has been taken (position 1), the localized physical begins with observation. The area of chief complaint or maximum tenderness is observed. Color is evaluated, and the presence or absence of erythema is noted, as well as yellow discoloration, ecchymosis, and color or consistency—for example, vasospasm or avascular appearances (such as a white, shiny appearance, which would be present with a compartment syndrome). Presence or absence of asymmetry or obvious atrophy is noted. Next, the examiner touches the injured portion, and temperature is recorded. The extremity or area of chief complaint may be hot, cold, sweaty, or dry. This will give some clues as to the status of the injury, that is, whether it is inflammatory, overuse, or chronic in nature. The vascular status of the extremity should be evaluated, as well as the neurologic status. The soft tissue around the area of the chief complaint should be palpated gently to find the area of maximum tenderness. If a fracture is suspected, radiographs should be taken. If a fracture is not suspected, the joints may be taken through a range of motion proximal and distal to the area of chief complaint. If the area itself is bony or a joint, gentle range of motion and evaluation should be undertaken.

If there is not an acute problem, the various joints of the lower extremity can be taken through a range of motion. The hips, knees, legs, ankles, and feet are evaluated in a systematic manner (this is covered in the section on biomechanical evaluation, below). The feet can be evaluated by observation and palpation for deformity, such as bunions, hammertoes, callosities, or ingrown toenails. The patient then sits with no support for the back, with the feet hanging over the table. The back is inspected for gross asymmetry, scoliosis, or kyphosis. The patient then assumes position 2.

SUPINE POSITION (POSITION 2)

Position 2 is the supine position, with the patient on the back. The back of the chair is lowered, and the patient lies down in a flat position. Further localized palpation and examination may be carried out in this position. The hips, thighs, knees, legs, ankles, and feet are then evaluated. Tightness as well as weakness of the hamstrings are evaluated in this position. Straight leg raises may be carried out to rule out sciatica. Stress tests of the knee are accomplished easily in this position. The ankle joint is evaluated, and anterior push–pull and frontal plane stress tests may be carried out. Dorsiflexion of the ankle joint is easily evaluated. Malleolar torsion should be noted to see if there is gross asymmetry between internal or external rotation of one ankle versus the other. Attention is then focused on position 3.

PRONE POSITION (POSITION 3)

Position 3 is the prone position, with the patient lying stomach-down. With the patient in the prone position, the back is again inspected for gross asymmetry, abnormality, or spasm. Systematically, the hips, thighs, knees, and ankles may be evaluated. A biomechanical examination is carried out on the ankle, subtalar, and midtarsal joints. This is correlated with any asymmetry or restricted motion at the various proximal joints (see the section on biomechanical evaluation for details).

When the ankles and feet are evaluated, palpation of areas of chief complaint or soreness oftentimes reveal the diagnosis. The plantar fascia may be palpated for plantar fascial partial rupture or nodular fasciitis. Likewise, the feet may be palpated for intermetatarsal neuromas; the severity of submetatarsal lesions, such as keratomas, is noted. Once the static non-weight-bearing examination is accomplished, provided there is no acute injury, a dynamic evaluation is carried out.

Dynamic Evaluation

With the patient standing in a relaxed stance wearing a pair of shorts and a T-shirt, the body is scanned quickly. During relaxed stance, the attitude of the shoulders, back, hips, and pelvis are noted. From behind, the examiner evaluates whether there is recurvatum at the knees or gross calcaneal valgus at the ankle level. Excessive pronation of the feet or lowering of the subtalar and midtarsal joints with pronation are noted. From the front, valgus at the knees, malposition of the patella (coxa varus, genu valgum), excessive internal rotation of the lower extremities, and/or miserable malalignment syndrome are noted. Miserable malalignment syndrome is pronation and external rotation of the feet, internal rotation of the legs, valgus of the knees, internal rotation of the hips, and lordosis. There is a functional valgus at the knees with secondary lateral subluxation of the patellas. These patients are particularly susceptible to injury.

The patient is then evaluated in neutral stance; the calcanei and feet are place in a neutral position, with the feet pointing straight ahead and the bisection of the calcaneus parallel to the lower one-third of the leg. In neutral stance, the back is examined from posterior to make sure there is no anatomic limb length discrepancy. Scoliosis and lordosis are noted. The knees and legs are evaluated for varus or valgus, and the relative amount of forefoot varus or valgus is recorded. The body is then evaluated from the front and

the attitude of the lower extremity is re-evaluated. As a quick reference, the patellas should be straight ahead, and the midline of the patellas should line up with the second toes when the feet are neutral. Atrophy or asymmetry is noted and recorded with a tape measure, so that a physical therapy and rehabilitation program can be monitored.

The examination proceeds to the functional evaluation. The patient is examined walking. Balance is then evaluated with the patient standing first on one foot and then on the other foot, with the eyes first open and then closed. If there has been an injury, kinesthetic sensations are easily lost and there is difficulty in balancing. These sensations must be rehabilitated with various balance and flexibility exercises. The walking evaluation then proceeds to a treadmill evaluation with videotaping. The athlete first walks, then runs slowly, and then runs faster if applicable. Video playback is used to compare the athlete's performance barefooted, then in normal running gear, and then in running shoes with the feet held neutral with a soft temporary orthosis. A correlation is made between abnormal function and biomechanical abnormalities.

On the basis of findings from the static and dynamic evaluations, various tests may be ordered, including laboratory tests to rule out inflammatory or infectious disease, tests to rule out metabolic disease, and radiographs to rule out fractures, arthritis, or other problems. Stress tests may be indicated. This is correlated with the biomechanical examination, described later in this chapter.

THE SPORTS MEDICINE HISTORY AND PHYSICAL EXAMINATION

The sports medicine history and physical examination can be the key to establishing a working differential diagnosis for an atheletic injury. This is true for the acute or the overuse incident. When taking a history, forms may be used, allowing the athlete to make an outline of the complaints while seated in the waiting room (Fig. 19-1).

The history and physical examination not only provide information about the athlete's body limits and capacities, but also alert the physician to problems that may occur during the competitive season. If muscular or ligamentous weakness in the body is noted, preventive exercises may be instituted, decreasing the likelihood of injury. If excessive stiffness is noted, flexibility exercises can be prescribed.

Examination should include a complete evaluation of the physical status, with special emphasis on the body areas directly related to the specific sport. However, examina-

Date: _____   Occupation: _____

Vital Statistics: Sex: M F   Age: _____ Ht: _____ Wt: _____ BP: _____ / _____ P: _____ T: _____

Chief Complaint: 1) Primary:

                          2) Secondary:

History of Present Illness: Onset:

                          Duration:

                          Type of Discomfort:

                          Previous Treatment:

Past Medical History: Childhood:
                          Adult:
                                  Arthritis   Foot Problems
                                  Cancer   Gout
                                  CV disease   Hypertension
                                  Diabetes
                          Adverse Reactions to Medications:
                          Allergies:
                          Surgeries (date, procedure, surgeon, result):

                          Present Physician:

                          Present Medications (name, dosage, physician):

Review of Systems: HEENT:
                          CVR:
                          GI:
                          GYN/GU:
                          Back & Extremities:
                          Neurologic:
                          Skin & Nails:

Familial History: Mother:
                          Father:
                          Siblings:
                          Arthritis: Foot Problems:
                          Cancer: Gout:
                          CV disease: Hypertension:
                          Diabetes: Other:

Figure 19-1 The form used in our office to record a patient's general history and the results of examination. (*Figure continues.*)

```
┌─────────────────────────────────────────────────────────────────────────────────┐
│ Social                                                                            │
│ History:      Marital:                        Alcohol:                            │
│               Employment:                      Drugs:                             │
│               Sports:                          Tobacco: Never  Yes _____ Packs/day│
│                                                         Previous  When quit? _____│
│                                                                                   │
│ Physical                                                                          │
│ Findings:     Neurologic:                                                         │
│                   Reflexes          Sensations           Vibratory                │
│                                                                                   │
│               Vascular:                                                           │
│                   A.T.              P.T.                 Veins                     │
│                                                                                   │
│               Deformity:                                                          │
│                   Right             Left                                          │
│                                                                                   │
│ Comments:                                                                         │
└─────────────────────────────────────────────────────────────────────────────────┘
```

Figure 19-1 (*Continued*)

tion should never be restricted to only the area involved in the sport. A limb length discrepancy with scoliosis of the back may be the key to an injury in the foot. A foot imbalance may be associated with radiculopathy and imbalance of the back.

The most important laboratory test for a female athlete would be the hemoglobin and hematocrit. This test will determine whether the athlete is receiving enough iron to meet her daily demands. Chronically fatigued athletes may be suffering from overuse or some form of mononucleosis, and appropriate laboratory tests may be indicated. Inflammatory disease may suggest seropositive or seronegative arthritis as well as gout.

The Sports Medicine History

A detailed history aids the physician in knowing the patient and establishes criteria for further diagnosis and examination. It indicates associated problems that may have considerable importance in the presenting chief complaint. In my experience, the use of forms is helpful. Drawings of various portions of the body are included on the form used in our office, and the athlete, while in the waiting room, indicates the primary as well as associated injuries on these diagrams (Fig. 19-2). The type of pain is described as sharp, dull, intermittent, or continuous.

A pain scale of 1 to 10, the Visual Analogue Scale (VAS), is very useful in documenting symptomatic improvement. A VAS score of 5 is moderate continous pain that affects the athlete's ability to walk comfortably. This would be seen in a moderate-intensity plantar fasciitis. A VAS score of 9 or 10 would follow an acute grade III ankle sprain or a fractured fibular maleollus. A VAS score of 3 or 4 might accompany an interdigital neuroma. Associated factors are indicated by the athlete. The athlete should record a VAS score in the morning, in the afternoon, after work, and before retiring for bed. Standard VAS rulers with color intensity codings are readily available.

The history should also include an athletic history. The form in Figure 19-3 explores the body type, running activity, terrain, surface, time of day that the injury occurs, shoe style, shoe brand, socks, mileage, duration of running, maximum mileage, competition, past forms of treatment, and the athlete's own statement of the primary injury and associated injuries. The parts of the body involved are indicated, as well as the severity of pain. The patient's basic approach to training is explored. Past treatment is indicated, and additional comment space is allowed for the athlete. The combination of the injury diagram and the athletic history form allows the examiner to readily focus on what may be the primary, as well as secondary problems.

The importance of associated problems cannot be overemphasized. Has the athlete had an injury on the contralateral side? If so, this injury may have caused more stress to be applied to the now-injured area. For example, a runner may have sprained the hamstrings on the right side, placing more force on the left leg, leading to an eventual stress fracture.

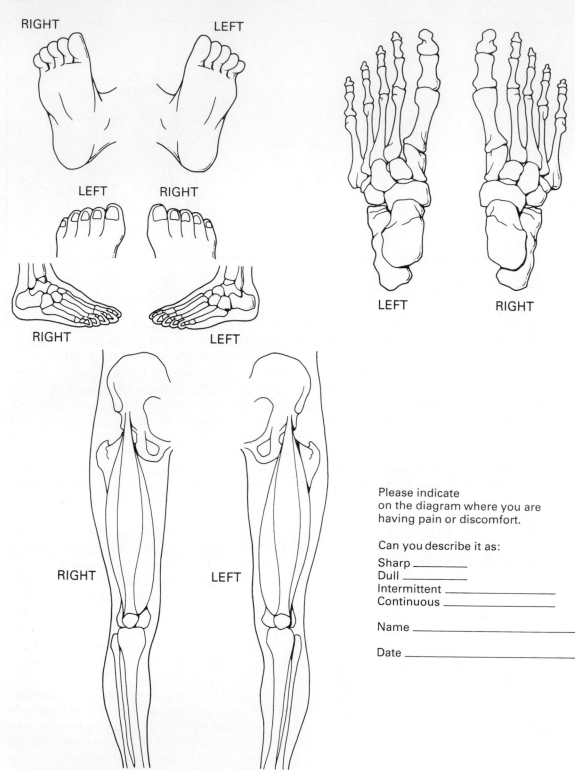

Figure 19-2 The patient uses a chart like this to indicate where symptoms occur.

ATHLETIC HISTORY FORM

(Please complete by circling or filling in blanks)

Name: _____ **Age:** _____ **Height** (inches): _____

Weight (pounds): _____

Sex: M   F   **Shoe Length:** _____ **Shoe Width:** _____

Dominant Hand: R   L   **Dominant Foot:** R   L

Body Type: Thin   Muscular   Overweight   **Body Frame:** S   M   L

Athletic Activity:

Sport or Sports _____

Intensity:

Terrain: Level   Hill   Track   Other (specify)

Surface: Paved road   Sidewalk   Dirt   Grass   Soft sand   Packed sand   Artificial track
Combinations

Time of Day: Morning   Afternoon   Evening

Shoe Style: Walking   Aerobic   Cleated   Distance running   Sprinting   Court shoes
Other (specify)

Shoe Brand: Adidas   Brooks   Converse   Nike   New Balance   Turntec   Tiger   Rockport
Others (specify)

Socks: Yes   No   If yes, pairs   1   2

Runners: **Mileage per week**   0–20   20–40   40–60   60–80   80 +

How Long Have You Been Running? Less than 3 months   Less than 6 months   Less than 1 year
Less than 5 years   More than 5 years

What is the Most Mileage Ever Run at One Time?   0–2   3–4   5–6   7–10   10–20   Greater than 20

Have You Ever Run a Marathon? Yes   No   If yes, how many?

Do You Use Orthotics? Yes   No   If yes, rigid or flexible?

How Would You Classify Your Foot Structures? Flatfoot   High arch   Normal

Athletic Injury Statement

_____
_____
_____
_____
_____

Figure 19-3 The athletic history form. (*Figure continues.*)

Body Part Involved: Forefoot Midfoot Rearfoot Ankle Fibula Tibia Femur Knee Hip Back

Severity: Pain only after running
Pain before, during, and after running, but able to perform workout
Workout compromised by pain
Unable to work out—self-imposed rest

Please write in own words the type of pain and where it hurts. _____
_____

Symptomatic Side: Right   Left   Both

Reinjury? Yes   No

What is Your Basic Approach to Training? _____
_____

Do You Regularly Change Directions of Your Runs? Yes   No

Do You Stretch (Warm Up) Before Workouts? Yes   No

If Yes, How Long? 5 minutes   10 minutes   15 minutes

If you follow a different warm-up/warm-down routine before or after running competitively, please explain.
_____
_____

Past treatment, this injury: Yes   No

Describe: _____
_____

Previous injuries: Yes   No

Describe: _____
_____

Name of Doctor or Facility: _____
_____

Type of treatment: Rest   Pills   Injections   Tape   Cast   Physical therapy   Other (specify)

Did treatment help? Yes   No

Additional Comments: _____
_____
_____

Figure 19–3 (*Continued*)

It is important to explore the goals and level of fitness of the athlete. Are the goals realistic? Has a rapid acceleration in training pace and duration caused an overuse injury? Is fatigue present? Is malnutrition present? Has there been a rapid gain or loss of weight? The past level of fitness is also important.

The pain experienced by the athlete, as well as the pain-related disability, must be assessed. Does the pain occur during runs or after runs? Is there swelling, locking, or popping associated with the pain? Is the pain made worse by running uphill or downhill? Does a short stride or a long stride alter the pain or injury? The level of the disability may range from pain with walking to pain with activity only. The ranges in between include pain after 30 minutes of exercise to pain beginning 2 hours after exercise and lasting 3 to 4 hours. The pain may be present with partial weight bearing, or weight bearing may be impossible. There may be pain with or without function.

The onset of the injury is crucial to the history. Was it sudden or gradual? A sudden onset may indicate a rupture or partial rupture. A stress fracture could be sudden. Gradual onset usually indicates chronic repetitive stress and overuse. If microtrauma, increased shock absorbance, or biomechanical imbalances is the cause of the injury, the onset may be sudden, semichronic, or chronic. Related factors include training, speed, surfaces, racing, foot gear, and terrain. The mechanism of injury may be impact, collision, violent twist or torque with a sprain or strain, or accumulated microtrauma (overuse).

The history of injury is also important. When was the athlete first injured in sports? Have there been previous or similar injuries, or previous adjacent or associated injuries? What has been the past treatment (self-treatment or prescribed by another professional)? What were the results? Has physical therapy been used in the past? Have orthoses or shoe adjustments been used? Have there been changes in the training program that have helped or hindered the problem? Is there any indication of full complete recovery of strength and flexibility? Has balance been reestablished? What has the athlete done in response to the injury: reduced mileage, increased mileage, used tape, bought new shoes, changed running style, taken medications, or sought professional help? What has worked? Past medical history is taken as in any examination and includes medical problems, surgical injuries, allergies, and medications. Familial history may be important, especially if it indicates a tendency to develop arthritis or gout. A familial history of cardiovascular disease or diabetes indicates the need for education of the patient.

Finally, the social history can be important. The patient may be going through a separation or divorce and be under unusual stress. He or she may be running to escape emotional or school-related problems. Occupation may indicate excessive stress. Type A behavior or activity may be transferred to an exercise program, predisposing to injury. Information on the patient's goals in life and sports may be helpful in fully evaluating the patient and the patient's problems. Athletes are not immune from alcohol abuse, and some may be taking drugs.

The Physical Examination

The physical examination must encompass the entire lower extremity and back. Evaluation of posture is important. Head carriage and arm swing in running may influence lower extremity biomechanics. Examination should be carried out with the patient standing, sitting, lying prone, and in a supine position. If possible, the athlete should be examined walking and running. The utilization of a videotaped treadmill exam with slow-motion playback is most helpful. For difficult cases, an electrodynogram-computed evaluation of forces, motions, and time sequences in gait can be helpful.

General physical findings should include height, weight, blood pressure (sitting), and pulse. If an inflammatory process is present, temperature should be taken. A complete physical examination is usually deferred unless indicated by the history.

STANCE

With the patient standing on a gait platform, posture is observed. The symmetry of the shoulders and scapulas is noted. Arm length is noted. The spine is inspected, and scoliosis is noted. The level of the pelvis is inspected, and limb length discrepancies are ruled in or out. The back is checked for an increase in lumbar lordosis, which may be associated with weakened abdominal muscles. Scoliosis may be associated with functional or anatomic limb length discrepancy or malalignment of the spine. The patient is asked to bend over and touch the floor; the flexibility of the hamstrings is noted. The patient leans forward with the knees extended toward the wall, and the flexibility of the calf muscles is noted. The overall alignment of the knees is noted, and variations such as coxa varus/genu valgum are observed. Gross abnormalities of the patella may be noted, such as lateral subluxation or patella alta. Excessive internal rotation of the knees with internally deviated patellas are noted. Atrophy of the vastus medialis may be noted. Recurvatum of the knee should be ruled out. The legs are then inspected for excessive varus or valgum. The ankles are inspected for excessive lateral or medial instability. With the patient in relaxed stance, one can assess the foot for excessive calcaneal pronation and laxity of the foot with increased pronation. The patient is asked to stand on the outsides of both feet to assess lateral instability. The legs are then maximally internally rotated to assess maximum pronation. The athlete stands on the balls of the feet, walks, and then walks on the heels. Weaknesses are noted. The athlete is then examined in neutral stance. The perpendicular bisection of the calcaneus should be parallel to the lower one-third of the legs. The middle of the kneecap should approximately line up with the second and third toes. The disappearance of functional valgus at the knee with neutral foot position may suggest faulty biomechanics as the cause of a chief complaint centered about the knee. Functional limb length discrepancies may be ruled out if the pelvis is level with the feet balanced, and not level with the feet in relaxed stance. Asymmetry is noted with more pronation or supination in one foot versus the other foot and concomitant increased rotation in the lower extremity.

Inversion and eversion of the feet are helpful in evaluating subtalar joint and midtarsal joint range of motion. Dorsiflexion and plantar flexion of the foot helps in evaluating the ankle joint and subtalar and midtarsal joints. Raising up and down on the ball of the foot may indicate limited range of motion of the metatarsophalangeal joints.

Next, the general appearance of the foot and ankle is recorded. Are there obvious lumps and bumps or exostoses? Are ganglia present? Are there contractures of the toes, or is hallux valgus with bunion deformity present? Are tailor's bunions present? Are the toenails discolored secondary to subungual hematomas or perhaps to tight shoes?

Balance is then assessed. The patient is asked to stand on one foot and then the other foot with the eyes closed and the arms outstretched. Lack of proper kinesthetic balance indicates lack of full rehabilitation from a strain or sprain. Neurologic pathology could be present.

WALKING EXAMINATION

The athlete is then asked to walk and, depending on the circumstances, a walkway or treadmill with a videotape system may be used. The trained observer should watch for premature heel-off or a guarding-type gait. A quick liftoff of an injured foot indicates alteration of normal bio-mechanics for guarding. Excessive internal or external rotation of the foot or leg is important to note. Deviations from the normal line of progression are recorded. Inequality of stride length is noted. An antalgic gait must be recorded. Excessive contact and midstance pronation with lack of normal resupination is an important finding. Apropulsive gait indicates lack of proper biomechanical sequential function. Depending on the circumstances, the patient is then asked to jump up and down on each foot, to assess the severity of imbalance or injury.

The patient is then examined running. While running, the back is observed for imbalance or asymmetry. The thighs as well as the hips are examined for excessive internal or external rotation. Excessive anteversion with valgus at the knees is associated with increased risk of knee or medial leg problems. Function of the knees is observed as well as the angle of gait. Excessive pronation is observed, as well as lack of delayed sequential resupination.

SITTING EXAMINATION

In the sitting position, leg length is again observed by having the patient place the back flat against the wall or chair and then extend the knees. This is correlated with the limb length observed when the patient is standing in neutral stance position on a gait platform. It is also helpful to have the athlete in a sitting position place the heels against the buttocks to see whether there is asymmetry in the height of the knees. This may indicate a limb length discrepancy. Measurements from the anterior superior iliac crest to the tip of the medial malleolus can be helpful. If scoliosis is absent when the patient sits but present when the patient stands, a functional imbalance of the back may be present. Pelvic obliquities are likewise evaluated in the sitting position. This is correlated with what is seen in the standing relaxed stance and neutral stance positions.

When noting leg length, with the back straight and the knees extended, tightness of the posterior musculature of the legs and the hamstrings may again be observed. Flexion contracture is easily seen. Excessive sciatic nerve tightness may also be evaluated in this way.

The patient's knee alignment is then checked in the sitting position. Patella alta or lateral subluxation of the patella is noted. The tone of the vastus medialis is noted with the quadriceps contracted and then relaxed. The medial and lateral undersurface of the patellas may be palpated when chondralgia patella is present. The general laxity of the patella is evaluated. The knee is tested for recurvatum and medial and lateral instability. In special cases, a drawer test may be carried out, and tests for anterior, medial, and lateral rotatory instability performed. A positive apprehension test (pain with pressure over the superior pole of the patella with the patient doing a full contracture) indicates chondralgia patella or malalignment syndrome of the patella. Any areas of tenderness about the knee are carefully examined. Appropriate tests are carried out for intra-articular damage of the knee, such as McMurray's test for meniscal damage.

Internal and external rotation of the hips is evaluated. With the knees and the hips neutral, the relationship between the malleoli and the knee is assessed. Excessive internal or external malleolar torsion is noted. The bilateral symmetry of the foot, ankle, leg, and knee is noted.

The ankle joint is examined for dorsiflexion and plantar flexion, with the knee both extended and flexed. The subtalar joint and midtarsal joint are then evaluated for symmetry and range of motion. (See the discussion of position 2 in the section on lower extremity examination for further details.)

SUPINE EXAMINATION

The athlete is then examined in the supine position. Range of motion of the hips and knees is checked. If there is radiating or low back pain, straight leg raises are carried out to assess the sciatic nerve. The ankle joint is examined for inversion, eversion, and dorsiflexion. Dorsiflexion is checked with the knee both flexed and extended. Subtalar joint and midtarsal joint range of motion and position can be evaluated, as well as the relationship between the forefoot and the rearfoot.

Any specific area that is tender is examined in detail. An example is a painful knee with an effusion. A further example would be a painful foot with redness or swelling over a metatarsal, indicating a possible stress fracture.

PRONE EXAMINATION

With the patient in the prone position, once again, range of motion of the hips is assessed for internal and external rotation. Tightness of soft tissue structures is noted, so that appropriate rehabilitative exercises may be prescribed. The knees are checked for excessive recurvatum. Asymmetry in the thighs is noted. The calves are checked for tenderness or asymmetry. The Achilles tendon may be carefully examined for peritendinitis or intratendinous damage. The ankle joint may again be examined for dorsiflexion and plantar flexion. This is done with the knee extended and flexed.

The subtalar joint is examined for range of motion. Both calcanei are inverted and everted, and symmetry and quality of motion are evaluated. The neutral position of the subtalar joint is assessed, and the amount of motion in eversion and inversion from this position is measured (see the section on examination of the lower extremity). The relationship between the forefoot and rearfoot is assessed. Range of motion of the metatarsal–cuneiform joints, especially of the first ray, is assessed. The balance between the metatarsals and the plantar surface of the calcaneus is assessed to rule out anterior, lateral, or medial equinus. The general foot configuration is noted in the non-weight-bearing position (e.g., normal, cavus, or valgus). Any change in configuration that may occur with weight bearing is recorded. Depending on findings, radiographs may be necessary.

EXAMINATION WITH A TEMPORARY ORTHOSIS

If a soft temporary foot orthosis is indicated, the athlete is reassessed using the device in the shoe. Various types of shoes with various degrees of stiffness and control are helpful. One may see that the athlete is stable with a soft temporary support in one type of shoe while still unstable in the present shoe. This would indicate the need for obtaining new shoes. One might also note a perfectly normal running style in one brand of shoe without an orthosis, but poor or faulty biomechanics in the athlete's current shoe. This again would indicate the need for a different type of shoe.

Additional Procedures

On the basis of the history and physical findings, one might recommend the use of a soft temporary support, different shoes, or both. Although soft temporary supports are helpful, they often lose their efficiency or effectiveness and pain returns; a more permanent orthosis is indicated when this occurs. Radiographs would be indicated if an arthritic joint or loose intra-articular bodies are suspected. Radiographs might be helpful to indicate malformation or lateral subluxation of the patella when knee pain is present. Radiographs would be indicated to rule out longstanding stress reaction of bone, stress fractures, or chronic periostitis. Radiographs might also show foot abnormalities, such as coalitions, that are responsible for limited ranges of motion. Fractures and arthritis will be seen on radiographs. Occasionally, a bone lesion indicative of arthritis or neoplasm is seen.

Soft tissue radiographic technique may be indicated in the face of partial rupture. Occasionally, a bone scan may be indicated when stress reaction of bone or stress fracture is not seen on regular or coned-down radiographs but is suspected. Stress views and arthrograms may be necessary for knee or ankle problems. Specific patellar skyline views are helpful for subpatellar pain. Radiographs of the pelvis or hip are mandatory when an avulsion or stress fracture is suspected in this region. X-ray films of the back are indicated when discogenic disease is suspected.

The usual course of treatment for overuse injuries is that of soft temporary supports with foot gear change and training modifications to decrease the intensity of training while allowing continuation of sports. Physical therapy is usually necessary. When the patient does not respond to a logical course of rehabilitation and therapy, more specific tests are ordered to rule out autoimmune disease, collagen disease, or other systemic causes of extremity pain.

Summary

The goal of the athletic history and physical is to assess the athlete as an individual, to aid athletes in achieving their realistic potential, to reestablish a rational training program that includes appropriate flexibility and strengthening exercises, to advise as to appropriate gear, and to protect against further injury. The history should concentrate not only on the chief complaint, but on associated problems that could alter the normal athletic pattern, predisposing the contralateral limb to injury. Full rehabilitation of all injuries is necessary to allow for complete rehabilitation of the athlete. The goal of the athletic history and physical is to educate the patient, as well as treat the immediate problem.

BIOMECHANICAL EVALUATION OF THE LOWER EXTREMITY

Biomechanics is the evaluation of the efficiency of human locomotion. Relationships between various components of the lower extremity as a whole are evaluated, and the pathomechanics of injury may be appreciated. The biochemical evaluation is an orderly method of evaluating the weight-bearing and locomotive structures of the body to allow one to appreciate the functional efficiency, balance, and character of the body as a whole and in relationship to its component parts.

This examination enables the practitioner to correlate biomechanical abnormalities with injury or inefficient function. It is helpful in organizing a treatment plan that allows for functional therapeutic correction of imbalances. Injured parts may be rehabilitated by balance, strength, and flexibility. This examination helps the practitioner teach proper motion and instruct the athlete on choosing proper foot gear and improving performance while decreasing risk for injury. If the injury is chronic and due to overuse secondary to biomechanical imbalance, correcting these imbalances greatly aids the rehabilitation from injury and helps decrease the likelihood of recurrence.

Instrumentation

The following instruments are clinically necessary in an outpatient setting:

Tractograph: a measuring device that permits measurement of the angular ranges of motion or degrees of deformity in a joint

Goniometer: similar to a tractograph; measures ranges of motion about an axis

Tape measure: permits evaluation of limb length discrepancies and of muscle mass for the presence or absence of atrophy

Gait platform: helpful in observing the patient on a long runway

Treadmill: helpful in evaluating runners

Videotape equipment: used with slow-motion analysis to permit recording data and analysis of data otherwise unseen with the naked eye

Electrodynogram: an instrument available from the Langer Group that permits quantification and qualification of pressures and forces going through the foot, helps in evaluating the effectiveness of orthotics in establishing normal locomotive patterns, and measures interface between foot and shoe

Procedures

STATIC NON-WEIGHT-BEARING EXAMINATION

Sitting Examination

After the lower extremity history and physical are completed, the patient is seated in a chair and the function of the various joints of the lower extremity are evaluated.

The patient moves forward on the chair so that the knees are flexed, and the legs are internally and externally rotated to evaluate range of motion at the hips. When the legs are externally rotated, internal rotation of the hips is measured; the opposite is done with internal rotation of the legs, which allows measurement of external rotation of the hips. Thus the flexed range of motion at the hips is evaluated with the knees likewise flexed and the hamstrings relaxed (Fig. 19-4).

With the patient in the same position, the relationship between the ankle joint and knee is evaluated. One can palpate the medial and lateral malleoli and approximate the amount of malleolar torsion in relationship to the frontal plane bisection of the knee. Excessive internal or external rotation of the foot can then be evaluated as a function of tibial internal or external torsion (Fig. 19-5).

With the knee flexed and the ankle relaxed, the degree of dorsiflexion at the ankle can be measured using a tractograph. The tightness of the gastrocnemius–soleus complex can be evaluated by having the patient extend the knee with the foot in dorsiflexion. If the foot plantar-flexes markedly during the last 15 degrees of knee extension, there is probably tightness of the posterior musculature of the leg. Runners often have functional equinus, and it may be necessary to dorsiflex and plantar-flex the foot repeatedly before a true evaluation of the relaxed-knee dorsiflexion at the ankle can be obtained (Fig. 19-6).

In this same flexed-knee position, the anterior and posterior drawer signs of the knee joint may be evaluated, and the test for lateral instability performed (see Ch. 17). The ankle joint itself can be evaluated for frontal plane and sagittal plane stability with the anterior push–pull test and frontal plane inversion–eversion test (Fig. 19-5).

The patient then sits upright in the chair with the knees extended, and the examiner can again determine the range of motion at the hips with the legs extended and the back flexed. The knees may then be evaluated for soft tissue or bony problems. The patella can be palpated at the medial and lateral undersurfaces for plica, facet syndrome, or both. The patella apprehension test can be used. Flexion and extension of the knee may elicit crepitation, which is characteristic of chondralgia patella. The medial aspect of the knees can be palpated to rule out inflammation of the pes bursa; likewise, the lateral aspect of the knee can be evaluated for laxity of the lateral collateral ligament or for iliotibial band syndrome. The legs may be evaluated for gross abnormality or point tenderness.

The ankles are then evaluated for range of motion, laxity, or lack of stability. The feet are palpated and evaluated for gross abnormality. The metatarsals can be dorsiflexed and plantar flexed, and one can get an appreciation of the lateral and medial columns of the foot. The toes are evaluated, and the first metatarsophalangeal joint is taken through a range of motion. The quality of motion, degree of motion, and any deformity are recorded. Symmetry or lack of symmetry between pathologic and nonpathologic structures is noted. Toenails are evaluated.

Supine Examination

The second part of the examination is in the supine position, with the back of the chair lowered. The patient lies flat on the back, and the hips are again evaluated. The thighs are then evaluated. The knees are evaluated further for medial or lateral instability; if internal derangement is suspected, a McMurray's test is carried out. The legs are then evaluated. Areas of point tenderness may be palpated to rule out periosteal or soft tissue problems or bony problems. The ankle is again evaluated, if necessary, as are the feet.

Prone Examination

The third portion of the static examination is done in the prone position, with the patient lying down. The back is again examined and evaluated as in the sitting position. Presence or absence of lordosis, scoliosis, or kyphosis is noted. The paraspinal muscles are evaluated, and spasm is noted. The posterior aspects of the thighs and knees are then evaluated; the legs are evaluated, and the gastrocnemius–soleus complex is evaluated for tightness, weakness, or pathology.

Dorsiflexion at the ankle joint is again checked with the knee flexed and then extended. This is recorded on the biomechanical form (Fig. 19-4). Attention is then focused on evaluation of the subtalar joint. The calcaneus is inverted and everted, and the range and quality of motion of both calcanei and subtalar joints are recorded. The calcaneus is taken into full eversion and then brought back between one-fourth and one-third of the total range of motion of the subtalar joint in the direction of inversion. This is the neutral position of the subtalar joint (Fig. 19-7). The foot is dorsiflexed and plantar flexed; as long as the bisector of the calcaneus does not invert or evert, all motion takes place at the ankle joint, and one can assume that the subtalar joint is in a neutral position. When the subtalar joint is in neutral position, the calcaneus everts through one-third to one-fourth of the total range of mo-

MORPHOLOGICAL DATA CHART

LEFT   RIGHT

SUBTALAR JOINT:

- SUPINATION — INVERSION
- PRONATION — EVERSION
- TOTAL R.O.M.
- NEUTRAL POSITION — VARUS / VALGUS

MIDTARSAL JOINT:

- VARUS / VALGUS

ANKLE JOINT:

- RANGE OF DORSIFLEXION — DORSIFLEXION
- RANGE OF PLANTARFLEXION — DORSIFLEXION   } WITH KNEE EXTENDED
- RANGE OF DORSIFLEXION — DORSIFLEXION
- RANGE OF PLANTAR FLEXION — DORSIFLEXION   } WITH KNEE FLEXED

ANKLE TO KNEE:

MALLEOLAR TORSION

ABNORMAL TRANSVERSE KNEE ROTATION

INTERNAL	
EXTERNAL	
INTERNAL	
EXTERNAL	

HIP JOINT:

RANGE OF INTERNAL ROTATION

RANGE OF EXTERNAL ROTATION

TOTAL R.O.M.

NEUTRAL POSITION

GENU DEVIATION:

WITH HIP FLEXED	WITH HIP EXTENDED

VARUM	VALGUM	RECURVATUM

I.M. DISTANCE _____ cm.

STANCE CORRELATION:

FRONTAL PLANE TIBIA

ANGLE OF GAIT

CALCANEAL STANCE POSITION IN STATIC ANGLE OF GAIT

CALCANEAL POSITION TO FLOOR SUBTALAR JOINT NEUTRAL

RESULTANT ABNORMAL SUBTALAR JOINT POSITION

VARUM	
VALGUM	
ADDUCTION	
ABDUCTION	
INVERTED	
EVERTED	
INVERTED	
EVERTED	
PRONATION	
SUPINATION	

Figure 19-4 Range of motion is measured and recorded on a data chart like this one.

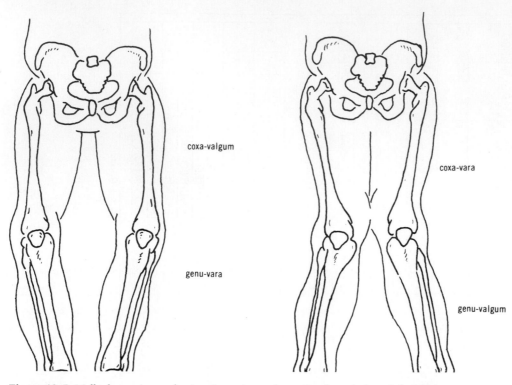

coxa-valgum

genu-vara

coxa-vara

genu-valgum

Figure 19-5 Malleolar torsion evaluation. Inversion and eversion frontal plane deformities are diagnosed at this stage. (From Subotnick SI: Podiatric Sports Medicine. Futura Publishing, Mt. Kisco, NY, 1975, with permission.)

tion and inverts through three-fourths to two-thirds of the total range of motion from this position (Fig. 19-8).

When first beginning biomechanical evaluations, it is helpful to bisect the lower one-third of the posterior aspect of the leg with a marking pen and to bisect the posterior surface of the calcaneus. Three marks are made on the calcaneus: one at the inferior aspect, one at the midaspect, and one at the superior aspect. That portion of the bisector of the calcaneus between the middle and superior mark changes when the calcaneus is maximally inverted or everted relative to the amount of inversion or eversion present (Figs. 19-9 and 19-10). Degrees of range of motion are recorded on the biomechanical form.

Attention is then focused on evaluation of the midtarsal joint. With the subtalar joint in a neutral position, the midtarsal joint is maximally pronated. This is accomplished by pushing up the fourth or fourth and fifth metatarsals. The calcaneus, cuboid, and fourth and fifth metatarsals constitute the lateral column of the foot. The medial column of the foot is the medial aspect of the calcaneus, beginning with the middle facet of the subtalar joint and including the talus, the navicular, the cuneiforms, and the first, second, and third metatarsals. The relationship between the medial and lateral columns is noted, as is the relationship between the metatarsal heads and the plantar aspect of the calcaneus. It can be seen whether there is depression of the metatarsal heads with a localized equinus present. A foot with forefoot varus may be plantar flexed at the fourth and fifth metatarsals or lateral column. This is noted when the fourth and fifth metatarsals are below the level of the plantar surface of the calcaneus. A forefoot valgus may be present with a localized plantar-flexed first ray. It is important to observe the position of the forefoot and various metatarsals in relationship to the plantar surface of the calcaneus, as well as the position of the metatarsals in relationship to each other.

In general, with the midtarsal joint maximally pronated and the subtalar joint in a neutral position, one would expect to see the metatarsals plantarly level to the plantar surface of the calcaneus and parallel to the frontal plane of the examiner when the patient is in the prone position. This would mean that, in static stance, the metatarsals

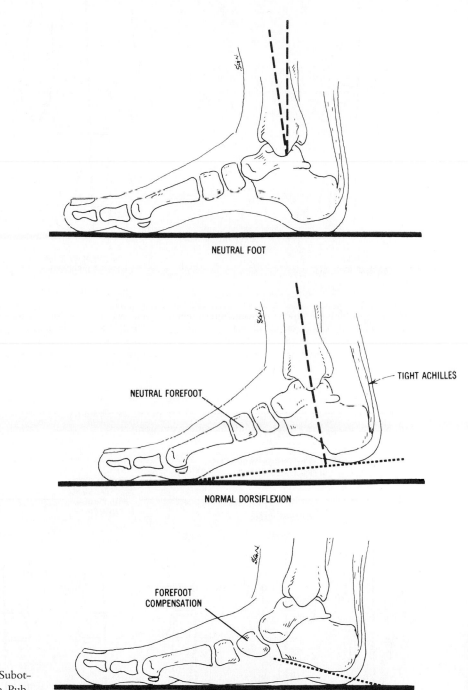

NEUTRAL FOOT

TIGHT ACHILLES

NEUTRAL FOREFOOT

NORMAL DORSIFLEXION

FOREFOOT
COMPENSATION

ABNORMAL DORSIFLEXION

Figure 19-6 Equinus deformity. (From Subot-nick SI: Podiatric Sports Medicine. Futura Publishing, Mt. Kisco, NY, 1975, with permission.)

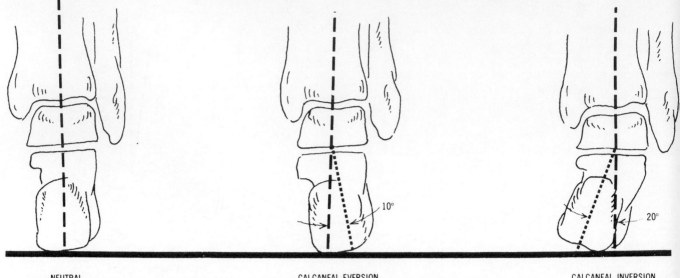

NEUTRAL
SUBTALAR JOINT (STJ)

CALCANEAL EVERSION
WITH S.T.J. PRONATION

⅓ TOTAL R.O.M.

CALCANEAL INVERSION
WITH S.T.J. SUPINATION

⅔ TOTAL R.O.M.

Figure 19-7 Skin lines used for evaluation of subtalar joints in a prone position. (From Subotnick SI: Podiatric Sports Medicine. Futura Publishing, Mt. Kisco, NY, 1975, with permission.)

Figure 19-8 Subtalar joint range of motion. (From Subotnick SI: Podiatric Sports Medicine. Futura Publishing, Mt. Kisco, NY, 1975, with permission.)

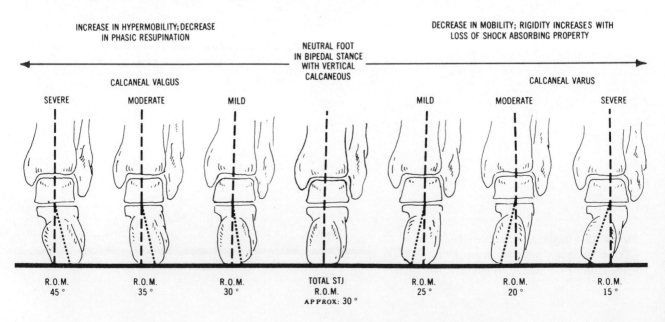

INCREASE IN HYPERMOBILITY; DECREASE
IN PHASIC RESUPINATION

DECREASE IN MOBILITY; RIGIDITY INCREASES WITH
LOSS OF SHOCK ABSORBING PROPERTY

NEUTRAL FOOT
IN BIPEDAL STANCE
WITH VERTICAL
CALCANEOUS

CALCANEAL VALGUS

CALCANEAL VARUS

SEVERE | MODERATE | MILD | | MILD | MODERATE | SEVERE

R.O.M.
45°

R.O.M.
35°

R.O.M.
30°

TOTAL STJ
R.O.M.
APPROX: 30°

R.O.M.
25°

R.O.M.
20°

R.O.M.
15°

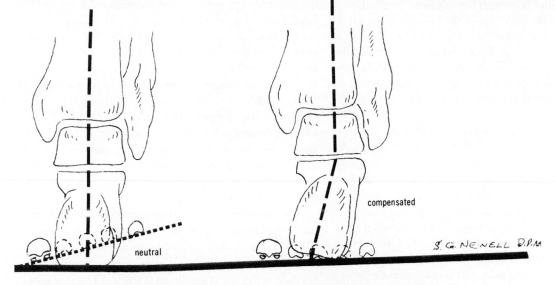

Figure 19-9 Forefoot valgus. (From Subotnick SI: Podiatric Sports Medicine. Futura Publishing, Mt. Kisco, NY, 1975, with permission.)

Figure 19-10 Forefoot varus. (From Subotnick SI: Podiatric Sports Medicine. Futura Publishing, Mt. Kisco, NY, 1975, with permission.)

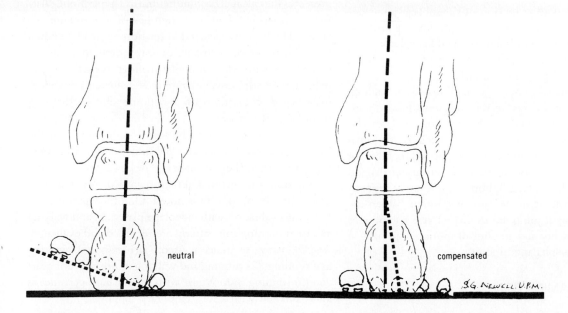

would all be on the floor with the calcaneus perpendicular to the floor, and the posterior of the bisector of the calcaneus parallel to the lower one-third of the leg. This is roughly approximated in stance when the talonavicular joint is congruous and the midaspect of the patella lines up with the second or third toe. Ideally, in neutral static stance, little muscular control is necessary to maintain the integrity of the arches of the feet.

The midtarsal joint is then evaluated for quality of motion. It is dorsiflexed, plantar flexed, adducted, and abducted with the heel held neutral. The midtarsal joint function evaluates the relationship between the forefoot and the rearfoot. Forefoot varus is evaluated as a relative dorsiflexion of the medial column and plantar flexion of the lateral column. Forefoot valgus is present when there is a plantar flexion of the medial column and dorsiflexion of the lateral column. When forefoot valgus is present, the range of motion of the midtarsal joint is narrow. When forefoot varus is present, there is an increased range of motion of the midtarsal joint. When the subtalar joint is neutral, there is greater motion in the midtarsal joint than when it is inverted or supinated. A supinated subtalar joint causes convergence of the axis of the midtarsal joint and disallows motion. A pronated subtalar joint allows a parallel relationship of the various components of the midtarsal joint and causes increased motion and decreased stability. This hypermobility with subtalar and midtarsal joint laxity allows for prolonged pronation and gait abnormalities in sports. Limited range of motion of the subtalar joints decreases the shock-absorbing ability of the lower extremity, which is present with normal pronation. Lateral instability of the foot or ankle may be a direct result of subtalar joint varus with limited pronation available.

Once the midtarsal joint has been evaluated and findings are recorded, one focuses on the metatarsal heads themselves. They are evaluated for abnormalities, and correlation is made between plantar lesions, such as keratomas under metatarsal heads, and metatarsal length, mobility, or both. Range of motion of the toes and metatarsophalangeal joints can again be reevaluated but is more easily appreciated with the patient in the supine position. When the metatarsophalangeal joints are evaluated, it is a good idea to record the quality and amount of motion, especially at the first metatarsophalangeal joint.

DYNAMIC EXAMINATION

In static stance, with the patient wearing a pair of gym shorts and T-shirt, the general posture is evaluated. With the patient in relaxed stance, the position of the shoulders, back, pelvis, hip, thighs, knees, legs, ankles, calcanei, and medial malleoli is noted. The foot itself is evaluated in static stance for abnormality or balance and medial and lateral longitudinal arches. The medial aspect of the foot is observed for bulging or abnormality of the talonavicular joint, which occurs with excessive pronation of the subtalar and midtarsal joints. The lateral aspect of the foot is likewise evaluated for excessive abduction or adduction of the forefoot upon the rearfoot. The amount of calcaneal inversion or eversion is recorded. The balance between the calcaneus at the posterior aspect and the lower one-third of the leg is evaluated.

Neutral stance is then evaluated; with the patient standing on a gait platform, the calcanei are put in a neutral position. This is determined by congruency of the talonavicular joint and by the bisection of the calcaneal posterior surface in relationship to the lower one-third of the leg. The foot may be pronated and supinated and the talonavicular joint palpated. When the head of the talus rests firmly in the navicular articulation, the subtalar and midtarsal joints are in neutral. The difference between these relationships in both the relaxed stance and neutral stance is recorded. One might note a functional valgus of the knees with internal rotation of the femurs and tibias during relaxed stance in the pronated foot, which reduces by a rather significant amount with the calcanei in neutral position. Recurvatum at the knees may be present as the calcanei become neutral in a hypermobile flatfoot. This may be secondary to tightness of posterior musculature. The back is evaluated in relationship to the neutral foot. The presence or absence of limb length discrepancies or scoliosis is noted. In a similar manner, with the feet in neutral, the entire lower extremity is evaluated and abnormalities or correction of functional abnormalities is recorded in the chart.

Balance and agility may be tested as described for the lower extremity history and physical examination. One then proceeds to the gait analysis. The character of walking locomotion is observed and then recorded. Antalgic limp or asymmetry of motion is noted. One then proceeds to treadmill evaluation with videotape playback, and walking and then running gait patterns are recorded and evaluated. The following sequence is used: (1) barefooted, walking and running; (2) running and walking in normal foot gear; and (3) running in foot gear with proper biomechanics as approximated with a soft temporary support.

If there is only minor abnormality or variances from good athletic form in regard to walking and running, appropriate patient instruction may be used and an orthosis may be avoided. If foot gear is inappropriate, changing to other foot gear would be advisable. Tightness or weakness of muscles is noted, and appropriate stretching and strengthening exercises are prescribed. For advanced cases, an electrodynogram or a similar computerized force plate motion analyzing system may be used to identify precise pressure points and provide for more graphic representation of the gait pattern and interface between the foot and the shoe.

Summary

Biomechanical evaluation of the lower extremity permits correlation of the presence or absence of imbalance in the lower extremity; this may preclude abnormal soft tissue, bone, or joint function that might be responsible for the injury. Once joint restriction or abnormal motion occurs, there will be concomitant proximal and distal areas of compensation that will need rehabilitation and restoration of normal motion, in the same way as the primary area of injury. Proper diagnosis and evaluation allows for a rehabilitation plan that treats the entire person, returning the athlete back to participation or competition in better overall condition than before the injury. Correlating the function of the lower extremity with a pattern for injury permits reversal of this pattern and full rehabilitation of the patient. No part stands alone from the whole.

SUGGESTED READINGS

Costill DL: Scientific approach to distance running. Track Field News 1979

Cyriax J: Textbook of Orthopaedic Medicine. Vol 5.1 and 2. Bailliere Tindall, New York, 1980

Harita I Jr: The Doctor and the Athlete. 2nd Ed. JB Lippincott, Philadelphia, 1974

Haycock CE: Sports Medicine for the Athletic Female. Medical Economics, Oradell, NJ, 1980

Hoppenfeld S: Physical Examination of the Spine and Extremities. Appleton & Lange, Norwalk, CT, 1976

Nicholas JA, Hershman EB: The Lower Extremity and Spine in Sports Medicine, 2nd Ed. CV Mosby, St. Louis, 1995

O'Donohue D: Treatment of Injuries to the Athlete. WB Saunders, Philadelphia, 1970

Subotnick SI: Podiatric Sports Medicine. Futura Publishing, Mt. Kisco, NY, 1975

Subotnick SI: Sports and Exercise Injuries. North Atlantic Press, Berkeley, CA, 1991

Subotnick SI: The podiatric history and physical. J Am Podiatry Assoc 63:538, 1973

Subotnick SI: The subtalar joint extraarricular arrhroereisis. J Am Podiatry Assoc 67:157, 1977

Travell JG, Simons DG: Myofascial Pain and Dysfunction. Vols. 1 and 2. Williams & Wilkins, Baltimore, 1992

Travell JG, Simons DG: The Trigger Point Manual Vol. 1, 2nd Ed. Williams & Wilkins, Baltimore, 1994

Travell JG, Simons DG: The Trigger Point Manual. Vol. 2. Williams & Wilkins, Baltimore, 1992

Williams JGP, Sperryn PN: Sports Medicine. Edward Arnold Publishers, London, 1976

Zier BG: Essentials of Internal Medicine in Clinical Podiatry. WB Saunders, Philadelphia, 1990

20

Diagnostic Imaging

STEVEN I. SUBOTNICK
YVONNE SUN

Since the first edition of this text, there have been great advances in diagnostic imaging techniques. Initial assessment of possible bone injury or deformity remains is still best accomplished with conventional radiography. Bone scans are helpful to detect stress fractures, but may lack spatial resolution. Conventional tomography, with computer-aided three-dimensional reconstruction, is a great advance in evaluating complex fractures. It helps sports surgeons to plan for complex reconstructive surgery.

Magnetic resonance imaging (MRI) has allowed us to visualize tissues and see body parts in ways that were never before possible. It provides for excellent soft tissue contrast in the evaluation of muscles, ligaments, tendons, blood vessels, and bone marrow. (The reader is referred to Schweitzer and Resnick[1] for a review of the normal MRI anatomy of the foot and ankle.) MRI is sensitive in detecting stress fractures, early avascular necrosis, transchondral fractures, and bone contusions, but may not detect small cortical avulsions.

In experienced hands, ultrasonography is useful in the assessment of tendon injuries, particularly to the Achilles tendon,[2,3] and in differentiating between tendon damage that requires surgery and damage that can be treated conservatively.[4] European orthopedic surgeons use ultrasonography in the operating room to help facilitate surgery and accurately locate lesions of tendons with less surgical exposure. Although popular in Europe, ultrasound has not yet gained widespread acceptance as a means of diagnosing tendon injuries in the United States. Certainly with the advantage of real-time, on-the-spot information, portabil-ity, and low cost, it will come into its own. Experience is required to interpret ultrasound scans, and MRI, for most practitioners, is easier to interpret. Yet with the current constraints in health care spending, it is only a matter of time before ultrasonography becomes routine for first-line evaluation of tendon injuries, especially to the Achilles and posterior tibialis.[5–7]

With these new advances, practitioners have had to learn not only how to interpret this new information, but also how not to rely solely upon it in making clinical and surgical decisions. The fact that an abnormality appears on an imaging study does not mean it is clinically significant or needs aggressive treatment. There are many asymptomatic athletes with abnormal MRIs, and there are many symptomatic athletes with minimal MRI pathologic findings. As with all forms of diagnostic testing, interpretation and correlation with clinical findings must prevail. The most important part of any sports medicine work-up remains the history, followed closely by the physical examination.[8–10]

This chapter covers the basic radiographic views used in evaluating the lower extremity. Information on special procedures, such as stress tests, arthrograms, bone scans, and computed tomography (CT) is also presented. Of added interest is the new section on MRI physics with cases, by radiologist Yvonne T. Sun. Dr. Sun presents cases of bone trauma, bone infection, bone tumors and cysts, tendon lesions, ligament lesions, cartilage lesions, and soft tissue masses. She also provides helpful suggestions for radiologic and imaging studies within the context of these categories that will be useful as a reference to the sports physician.

RADIOLOGIC EVALUATION

Standard Radiographic Projections of the Foot

Standard radiographic examination of the foot should be done with the foot bearing weight in the angle and base of gait, and in the normal position the feet assume during bipedal stance.

ANTEROPOSTERIOR PROJECTION

The anteroposterior (AP) projection of the foot is carried out with the central beam angled 15 degrees from the vertical. The central ray is directed at the navicular, pointing toward the calcaneus.

When functional views are preferred, one foot at a time is imaged. When functional evaluation is not important, both feet may be imaged at the same time with the central beam angled midway between the two feet. In cases of trauma, non-weight-bearing radiographs are advisable.

The AP view permits accurate visualization of the phalanges, metatarsals, navicular, cuboid, and medial, middle, and lateral cuneiforms. The distal talus and calcaneus, as well as the midtarsal joint, Lisfranc's joint, metatarsophalangeal joints, and interphalangeal joints, may all easily be observed (Fig. 20-1).

LATERAL PROJECTION

Whereas with the AP view the patient is standing on the radiographic plate, with the lateral view the cassette is placed vertically in the lead-lined orthoposer. The patient places one foot on each side of the film, with the medial aspect of the foot being radiographed in contact with the film. It is important to rotate the foot that is not being radiographed in the appropriate positions so that the angle and base of gait are maintained for functional evaluation of the foot. The central ray is angled 90 degrees from the vertical, pointed toward the lateral cuneiform. The lateral view depicts the talus, calcaneus, cuboid, navicular, and medial cuneiform. The metatarsals and phalanges overlap to varying degrees (Fig. 20-2). The hallux may be elevated above the other digits when evaluating for subungual exostosis or osteochondroma (Fig. 20-3).

MEDIAL OBLIQUE PROJECTION

The medial oblique projection is taken with the central ray entering the foot from a lateral oblique position. In

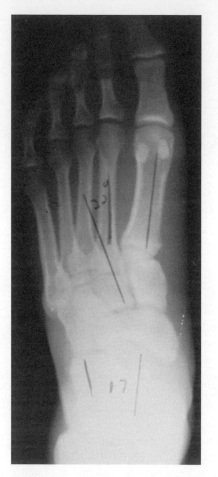

Figure 20-1 Anteroposterior projection of the normal foot.

practice, the patient stands on the radiographic cassette with the lateral aspect of the foot against the edge of the cassette. The central ray is angled 45 degrees from the vertical in the frontal plane and is aimed at the cuboid, perpendicular to the long axis of the foot from lateral to medial.

A non-weight-bearing medial oblique projection is similar to an AP projection. The foot rests on the radiographic plate, and the patient adducts the knee until the lateral portion of the foot is 45 degrees off the radiographic plate, with the medial portion being in contact with the plate. The central ray is aimed perpendicular to the film and directed toward the lateral cuneiform.

The medial oblique view is helpful in visualizing the digits, metatarsophalangeal joints, first metatarsal head, sesamoids, cuneiform–metatarsal joints, cuboid–metatarsal articulations, calcaneocuboid joint, midtarsal joint, ante-

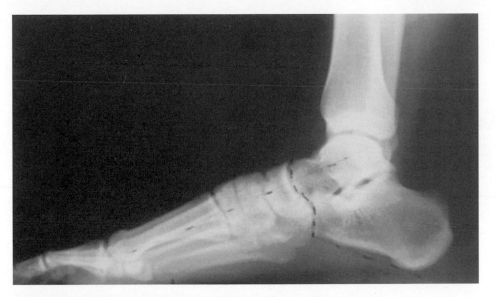

Figure 20-2 Lateral projection of the normal foot. Note congruous cyma line.

rior subtalar joint, posterior subtalar joint, and posterior aspect of the calcaneus (Fig. 20-4).

LATERAL OBLIQUE PROJECTION

The lateral oblique view is the opposite of the medial oblique projection. The weight-bearing lateral oblique projection is taken with the central ray at 45 degrees from the vertical, pointed at the navicular, angled from medial to lateral. The non-weight-bearing lateral oblique projection is taken with the patient sitting and the lateral border of the foot in contact with the film with the medial aspect of the foot raised 45 degrees. The central ray is perpendicular and aimed at the first cuneiform. This view is beneficial for evaluating most of the medial structures of the foot, including the first and second metatarsals, first and second cuneiforms, navicular, medial condyle of the calcaneus, and both sesamoids (Fig. 20-5).

Figure 20-3 Raised hallux, lateral projection.

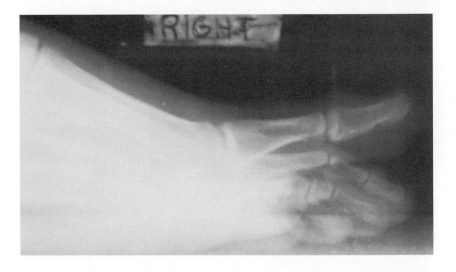

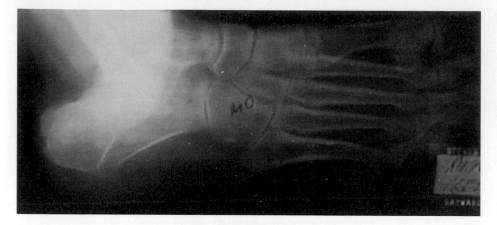

Figure 20-4 Medial oblique projection.

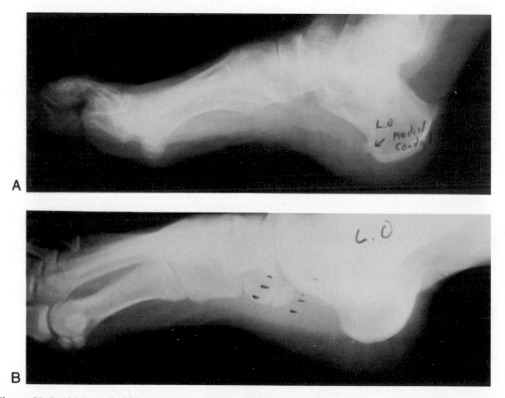

Figure 20-5 **(A)** Lateral oblique projection. Note medial condyle calcaneal spur. **(B)** Lateral oblique projection. Note fracture of navicular tuberosity.

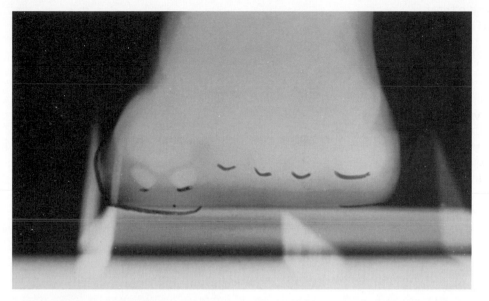

Figure 20-6 Axial sesamoid projection. Note plantar-flexed first ray.

AXIAL SESAMOID PROJECTION

The axial sesamoid view is taken with the film placed in the vertical position and the patient facing the film while standing on a special device that elevates the heel and extends the toes at the metatarsophalangeal joints. This same view may be taken without the device, with the patient facing the film standing on the ball of the foot with the toes dorsiflexed against the film. The central ray is perpendicular to the film and parallel with the long axis of the foot, directed from posterior.

This view is helpful when evaluating the sesamoids and their relationship to the first metatarsal head, when evaluating the lesser metatarsal heads and their relationship to one another, and when looking for hypertrophy of the metatarsal condyles or irregularities associated with various plantar lesions. The axial view alone, however, cannot determine to what extent any one metatarsal is involved with a plantar lesion because the mobility of the ray, as well as its length and function during gait, all contribute to plantar lesions (Fig. 20-6).

CALCANEAL AXIAL PROJECTION

The calcaneal axial projection is taken with the central ray directed 45 degrees to the posterior aspect of the calcaneus. The patient stands on the film with the knees slightly flexed. This view is helpful in evaluating the calcaneus for irregularities or excessive varus or valgus deformity (Fig. 20-7).

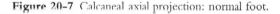

Figure 20-7 Calcaneal axial projection: normal foot.

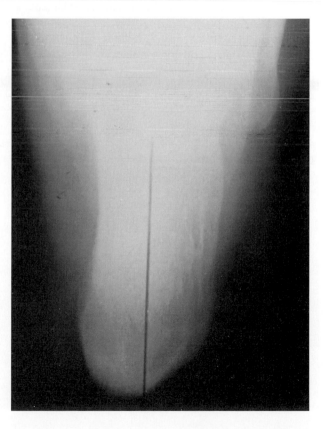

HARRIS AND BEATH PROJECTION: SUBTALAR JOINT COALITION VIEW

The Harris and Beath projection is taken similarly to the weight-bearing calcaneal axial projection. A scout lateral radiograph should be taken first to approximate the declination of the posterior facet of the subtalar joint in reference to the weight-bearing plane. Three projections are then recommended: one at 10 degrees above, one at 10 degrees below, and one at the measured angle of the posterior facet declination. The patient should flex the knees and ankles slightly before the film is taken. This projection gives an axial view of the calcaneus and the inferior aspect of the talus, as well as the middle and posterior facets of the subtalar joint (Fig. 20-8).

Standard Radiographic Projections of the Ankle

ANTEROPOSTERIOR PROJECTION

An AP projection of the ankle is carried out with the ankle bearing weight whenever practical. The radiographic cassette is vertical in the orthoposer. The patient stands with the posterior aspect of the heel against the film and the foot pointed straight ahead. The central ray is directed perpendicular to the film, entering midway between the malleoli. In the non-weight-bearing projection, the patient is sitting with the leg extended over the cassette and the foot placed flat on the table. The central ray is directed perpendicular to the film. This projection gives adequate representation of the ankle joint, including the distal aspects of the tibia and fibula as well as the trochlear surface of the talus. (Fig. 20-9).

MORTISE PROJECTION

The mortise projection is similar to the AP, except that the leg is internally rotated 15 degrees, placing the malleoli on a plane parallel to the film. This projection shows a better representation of the lower tibiofibular articulation and ankle joint mortise (Fig. 20-10).

MEDIAL OBLIQUE PROJECTION

The medial oblique is similar to the mortise view, with the leg internally rotated 45 degrees (Fig. 20-11).

LATERAL OBLIQUE PROJECTION

The lateral oblique projection is taken with the leg externally rotated 45 degrees.

Figure 20-8 Harris and Beath projection (coalition view). Note visualization of subtalar joint.

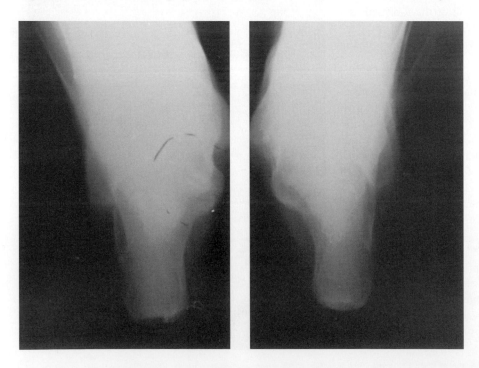

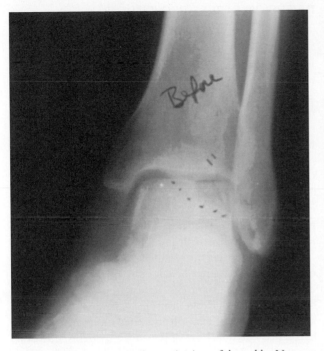

Figure 20-9 Anteroposterior projection of the ankle. Note osteochondral defect of talar dome.

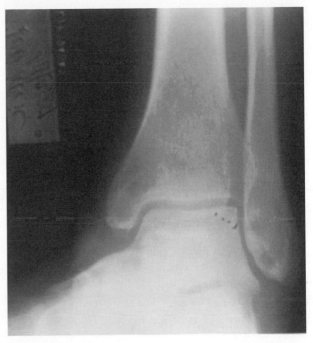

Figure 20-10 Mortise view of the ankle. Note talar dome defect.

Figure 20-11 Medial oblique projection of the ankle.

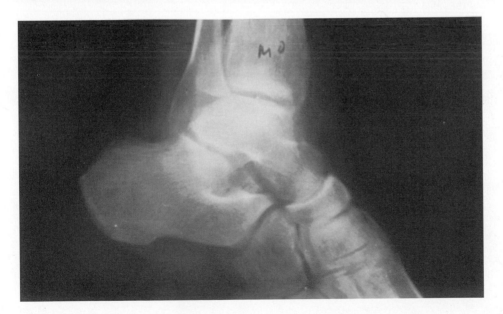

LATERAL PROJECTION

When a lateral ankle projection is taken, the medial aspect of the foot is placed in contact with the radiographic cassette. The central ray is directed perpendicular to the film. The film is positioned vertically so that more of the ankle and leg are shown. The lateral view shows the trochlear surface of the talus the talar neck, and the retrocalcaneal area (Fig. 20-12).

PLANTAR-FLEXOR LATERAL PROJECTION

A plantar-flexor lateral view is taken with the ankle bearing weight or non-weight bearing and shows the relationship between the posterior aspect of the talus and the tibia. This is a helpful view when one is evaluating for os trigonum or posterior impingement at the ankle joint (Fig. 20-13).

STRESS LATERAL PROJECTION

A stress lateral projection of the ankle joint is carried out similarly to a standard lateral with the exception that the patient maximally flexes at the ankle joint. This view is helpful when evaluating for anterior impingement exostosis of the ankle. (Fig. 20-14)

INVERSION STRESS PROJECTION

An inversion stress view is carried out when evaluating lateral stability of the ankle following ankle plantar-flexory inversion sprains. A standard radiograph is taken first to rule out bony pathology, which would be disrupted with a stress view. This view is taken with the posterior aspect of the heel and leg resting on the radiographic plate. The foot is mildly plantar flexed with the central ray aimed from vertical through the middle of the ankle joint. The examiner uses lead-lined radiography gloves. The calcaneus is inverted while the leg is externally rotated.

In acute injury, local anesthesia must be used. Either a local infiltration around the area of pain or a common peroneal block is carried out. The uninjured side is examined for comparison with the injured side (Fig. 20-15).

In general, a talar tilt of about 15 degrees is indicative of rupture of the anterior talofibular ligament; 15 to 30 degrees of talar tilt indicates rupture of the anterior talofibular as well as the calcaneal fibular ligament; and more than 30 degrees of talar tilt indicates rupture of all three ligaments. This does not hold true for all patients, however, inasmuch as the uninvolved ankle may have as much as 10 to 15 degrees of talar tilt without laxity or symptomatology. When the injured side has 5 to 10 degrees more talar tilt than the uninjured side, this is significant. A negative stress test does not rule out pathology inasmuch as the

Figure 20-12 Lateral projection of the ankle.

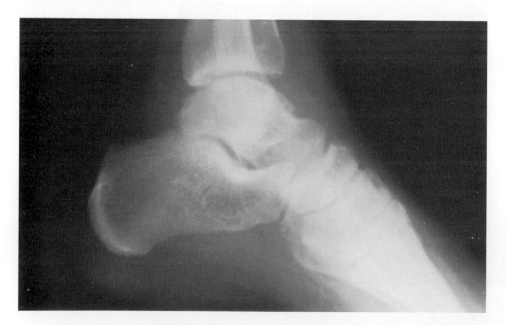

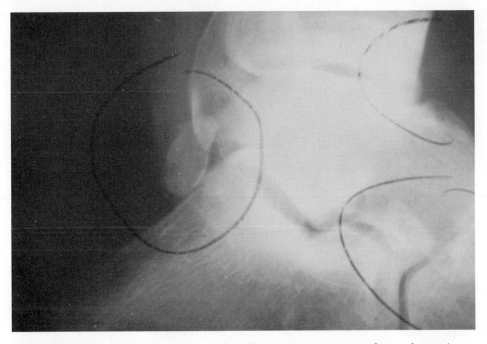

Figure 20-13 Plantar-flexory lateral projection illustrating os trigonum or fractured posterior process.

patient could be guarding even when local anesthetic blocks are used. A stress test is conclusively diagnostic only under general or spinal anesthesia. Nonetheless, when there is marked asymmetry in the stress test between the injured and uninjured ankle, one can assume that there is ligamentous laxity and/or rupture. An eversion stress test is helpful when evaluating the deltoid ligament. When there is over 10 degrees of tilt, pathology is usually present.

ANTERIOR DRAWER TEST OF THE ANKLE: PUSH–PULL STRESS PROJECTION

The anterior drawer test is used to evaluate the ankle after a plantar-flexion inversion sprain. With the patient seated in a chair level with the top of the orthoposer, the heel is placed on a block of rubber about an inch off the top of the orthoposer. The film is in a vertical position with the leg parallel to the top of the orthoposer. The tibia is then stressed in a posterior direction, toward the orthoposer, while the foot is held neutral to the ankle or slightly plantar flexed (Fig. 20-16).

An alternative method is to have the medial aspect of the foot and ankle parallel to the film with the examiner pushing the anterior aspect of the tibia posteriorly while

pulling the calcaneus forward. The central ray is directed toward the medial malleolus. The amount of anterior displacement is measured from the midpoint of the trochlear surface of the talus as compared with the midpoint of the articular surface of the tibia. More than 2 mm of displacement of the abnormal side versus the normal side is considered pathologic. There is great variance with the anterior drawer test; in general, however, when there is considerable difference between the uninjured and the injured side, rupture of at least the anterior lateral collateral ligament is present. Whereas there may be splinting with the frontal plane inversion stress test, the anterior push–pull test appears to be more reliable, with fewer false-negative results.

SPECIAL PROCEDURES

Bone Scanning

Technetium-99m (^{99m}Tc) bone scanning is useful in sports medicine in making an early diagnosis of stress reaction of bone or stress fracture. Technetium-Labeled methylene diphosphate is injected intravenously, and the patient is imaged 2 to 4 hours following injection. There is usually

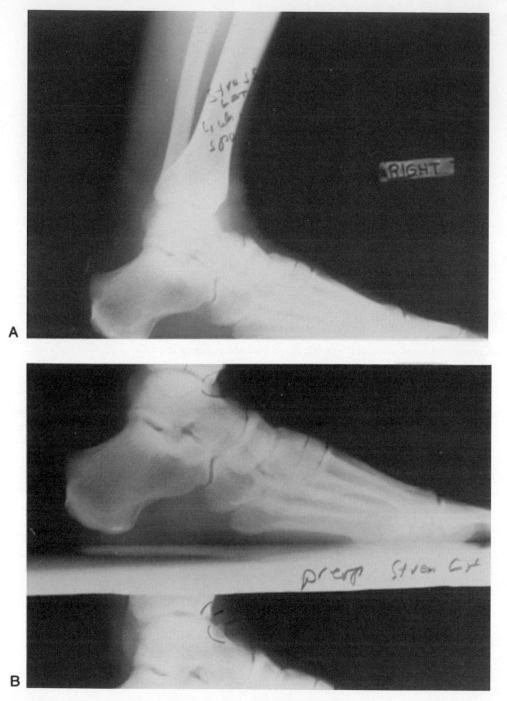

Figure 20-14 (A) Stress lateral projection of the ankle. **(B)** Comparison of stress lateral and relaxed lateral projections illustrating anterior ankle impingement.

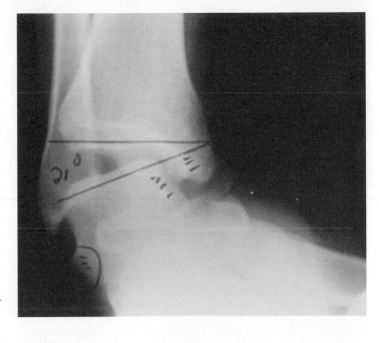

Figure 20-15 Inversion stress projection showing 21-degree talar tilt.

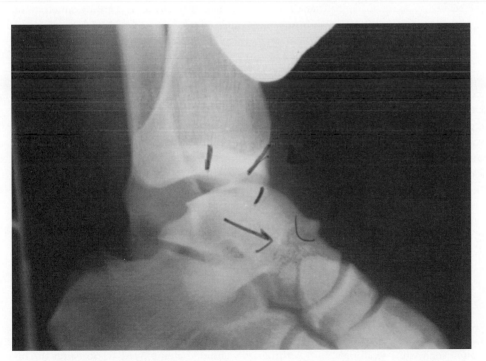

Figure 20-16 Anterior drawer projection (push–pull stress). Note talar neck exostosis.

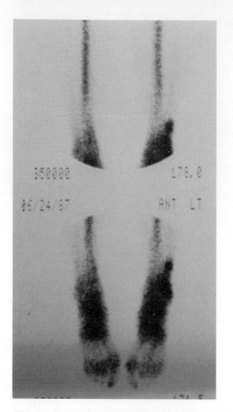

Figure 20-17 Bone scan illustrating fibular stress fracture of the left leg.

increased uptake at areas of stress or overuse. Thus consistent hot spots will be seen at the attachments of tendons to bone. Whereas with plane radiographs, a fracture may not be seen for 3 to 6 weeks, with the ^{99m}Tc scan, fractures can be revealed within 7 hours following injury. Focal uptake takes place at the area of inflammation or trauma, such as the fracture site. When a bone scan is ordered, sometimes a primary stress facture is seen along with otherwise secondary areas of stress fracture or stress reaction of bone[11-13] (Figs. 20-17 and 20-18).

Xerography

Soft tissue imaging via xerography is most helpful when evaluating tendon integrity or when looking for irregularity or stress fracture of small bones, such as the sesamoids. The xerogram gets unusually fine-quality resolution of soft tissue, such as the tendo Achillis[14-16] (Figs. 20-19 and 20-20).

Computed Tomography

CT is helpful in isolating tumors or coalitions of the foot and ankle. Arthritic conditions of joints may also be evaluated using a CT scan[17,18] (Fig. 20-21).

Arthrography

Arthrography is useful in evaluating the integrity of the joint capsule, as well as joint cartilage. Plain films are taken first to rule out fracture or obvious pathology. Renographin 60 is used as a contrast medium. This water-soluble iodinated medium should not be used in patients with an allergy to iodine or shellfish (which may contain iodine). Arthrography can be carried out in virtually any joint but is most useful in the ankle joint.

TECHNIQUE

The ankle joint is prepped with Betadine (povidone-iodine) solution. The skin and soft tissue down to the joint is anesthetized with a small amount of 1 percent Xylocaine (lidocaine). A 10-ml syringe is then filled with 2 ml Renografin 60, 2 ml 2 percent xylocaine, 1 ml dexamethasone phosphate (4 mg), 2 ml 0.5 percent Marcaine (bupivacaine), and 3 ml of air. An air-contrast arthrogram is carried out. The solution is injected using a 22-gauge needle through the anterolateral aspect of the ankle. During the injection, the foot is slightly distracted plantarly on the ankle to open up the ankle joint. A 1½-inch-long needle is used. As the fluid is injected, the ankle joint capsule is palpated for the development of distension. In most joints, the entire 10 ml can be injected. In some, only part of this amount can be injected because of the resistance of the capsular tissue, which is usually intact. After the injection of this solution, the needle is removed, and the ankle is taken through a range-of-motion exercise to spread the injected material throughout the joint. Any tears in the capsule will be readily visualized by dye leakage. Anterior posterior, oblique, and lateral projections of the ankle are taken. Stress films may also be taken with the radiopaque dye within the joint.

INTERPRETATION OF RESULTS

Arthrography should be employed as soon after the injury as possible because delays may produce false-negative results once clots or adhesions have sealed tears in the capsule or formed links between the calcaneofibular ligament

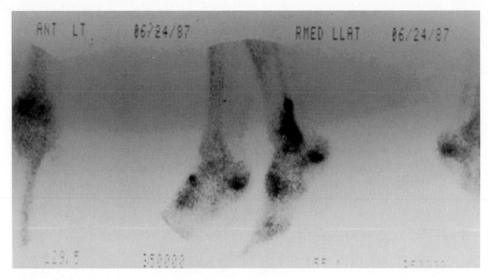

Figure 20-18 Bone scan illustrating ankle stress fracture.

Figure 20-19 Xerogram of Achilles peritendinitis.

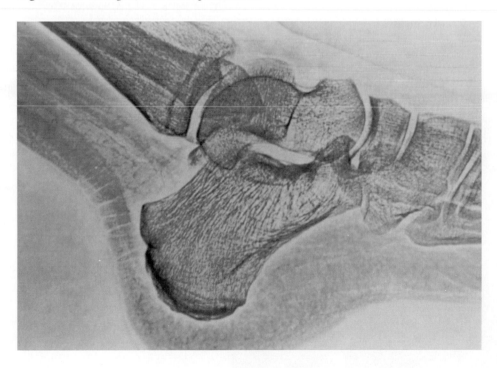

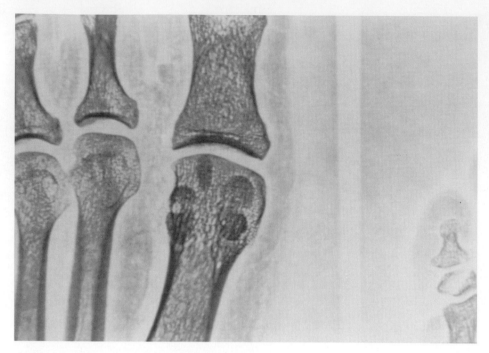

Figure 20-20 Xerogram of fractured sesamoids.

Figure 20-21 CT scan showing subtalar middle facet coalition.

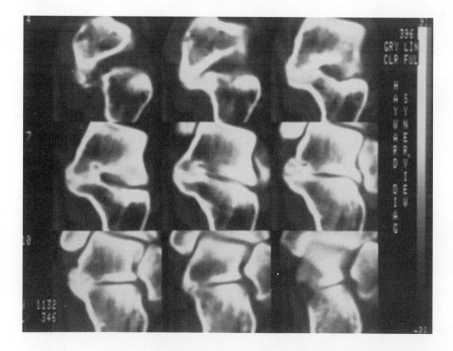

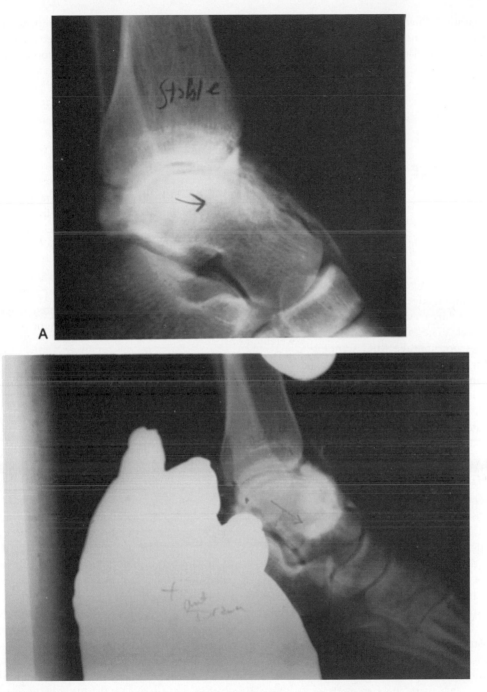

Figure 20–22 Arthrograms of ankle joint with stress test. **(A)** Stable joint. **(B)** Positive anterior drawer test.

and the peroneal tendon sheaths. When there is dye leakage along the peroneal tendon sheaths, this may indicate either a tear of the middle lateral collateral ligament with dye leakage from the joint into the peroneal sheath or an anatomic connection. Instability on the stress test, along with leakage along the peroneal sheath, is usually indicative of rupture of the anterior middle lateral collateral ligaments[19–23] (Fig. 20-22).

MAGNETIC RESONANCE IMAGING

Magnetic resonance imaging is a valuable cross-sectional multiplanar modality that utilizes magnetic fields and radiofrequency waves that are resonant with the hydrogen protons in the body. It provides excellent soft tissue contrast in the evaluation of muscles, ligaments, tendons, blood vessels, and bone marrow. There is no exposure to ionizing radiation and no known adverse biologic effect; thus MRI poses less risk to children and pregnant women when certain criteria are met. (The Food and Drug Administration currently does not approve MRI scanning during pregnancy.) MRI is generally noninvasive or minimally invasive with intravenous contrast injection or sedation. MRI is contraindicated in patients with aneurysm clips, pacemakers, metallic orbital foreign bodies, or implanted battery-operated devices.

The Physics of MRI

In conventional radiography, the relative contrast of a tissue is determined by density, thickness, and atomic number, which, in turn, is related to the amount of x-ray blocked or recorded by the image receptor. In MRI, subject contrast is related to the tissues' intrinsic parameters, such as proton density, T_1 and T_2 constants, flow of protons, and effects from paramagnetic contrast agents.

When subjected to a strong magnetic field, the body's hydrogen protons behave like tiny bar magnets and spinning tops. The primary component of magnetic resonance system is a strong external magnetic field, which aligns the protons along its longitudinal axis and thus generates a longitudinal magnetization. (Magnetic field strength in MRI is measured in teslas [1 tesla equals 10,000 gauss]. By comparison, the magnetic field of the earth is between 0.3 and 0.7 gauss.) Another component of the system, a radiofrequency (RF) transmitter coil, then generates a resonant RF pulse, which causes the protons to precess, or wobble, in phase, and thus generates a new magnetic vector, or transverse magnetization. A moving magnetic field induces an electric current, which can be detected and amplified by a receiver coil or antenna. As soon as the RF pulse is turned off, the newly established energy is dissipated, that is, the protons wobble out of phase and the transverse magnetization starts to disappear or relax. The longitudinal magnetization returns to its original value in a process called "longitudinal relaxation."

T_1 is the longitudinal relaxation time when 63 percent of the original longitudinal magnetization is reached. T_2 is the time when transverse magnetization is decreased to 37 percent of its original value. T_1 constants range from 300 to 2,000 msec while T_2 constants range from 30 to 150 msec. T_1 is dependent on the magnetic field strength and the tissue's molecular lattice, or microenvironment. T_2 is caused by inhomogeneities of the external and local magnetic fields. Water or similar liquids have a long T_1 and a long T_2. Fat has a short T_1 and a short T_2. Tissues that have a short T_1 appear bright on T_1-weighted images, and tissues that have a long T_2 also appear bright on T_2-weighted images.

By manipulation of extrinsic sequence parameters, T_1 and T_2 differences between tissue type can be minimized or maximized. A T_1-weighted spin-echo sequence is obtained with a short repetition time (TR) of 0.5 second or less between successive 90-degree RF pulses and a short echo time (TE) of 30 msec or less. A T_2-weighted spin-echo sequence is obtained with a long TR of 2 seconds or more and long TE of 60 msec or more. T_1-weighted sequences render "anatomic" definition of the musculoskeletal system by outlining fat or bone marrow, which is bright; water, which appears dark; and tendons and ligaments, which also appear dark. T_2-weighted sequences render "physiologic" information by outlining tumors, abscesses, edema, inflammation, and fluid collections, which appear bright because of increased water content, or hyperemia associated with these processes. Suppression of signal from fat can also improve conspicuity and sensitivity of bright lesions obscured by adjacent bright fat in a normal spin-echo sequence. Some fat-suppression techniques include the subtraction method, the chemical shift method, short tau inversion recovery (stir), and fat presaturation.

In addition to manipulation of TR, TE, and TI, tissue contrast and image appearance can be affected by RF pulse flip angle, as in gradient echo imaging with less than 90 degrees' flip angle. Spatial resolution is in part determined by slice thickness, field of view, and voxel size.

Magnetic field gradient coils produce additional linear variations to make slice selection possible in the x, y, and z

planes. (The banging of these coils against their anchoring devices causes the "knocking" noise heard during the scan.) Conventional two-dimensional MRI requires slice selection in the slice direction, as well as spatial position in a phase-encoding direction and in a readout direction. The volume averaging, lack of contiguous slices, and thicker slice scan obscure pathology. Three-dimensional MRI can produce 1-mm or submillimeter contiguous slices with near-isotropic voxels, which can provide high-spatial-resolution detail viewed from any plane from a single three-dimensional data set.

Fast scanning techniques differ by means of data collection for reconstruction. These techniques use a small RF tip angle and gradient refocusing to acquire a gradient echo. These images are similar to T_1 or T_2 weighting depending on the choice of TR, TE, and type of magnetization spoiling, type of echo acquired, and type of RF pulse. These images also have a low signal-to-noise ratio.

"Turbo" fast scans employ short TR acquisitions in a continuous mode where image contrast is a complex function. Fast spin echo is typically used to obtain two-dimensional proton density and T_2-weighted images by reducing the scan time; however, fat generally appears brigher than on standard spin-echo T_2 sequences unless some form of fat suppression is used. The use of MRI, in angiography and spectroscopy, as well as more detailed discussions of the fundamentals of MRI, are beyond the scope of this introduction, and can be found in other sources.[8,24]

Practical Applications

MRI of the lower extremity should be tailored to the exact body part scanned. There are trade-offs between the chosen field of view, matrix, section thickness and desired degree of spatial resolution, signal-to-noise ratio, and scan time. Plane selection is also important. For example, coronal and sagittal slices are useful in evaluating the talus and subtalar joint, while axial and sagittal slices are useful in imaging the Achilles tendon. Immobilization of the body part during scanning is also essential.

Case Studies

BONE TRAUMA

Initial assessment of possible fractures is accomplished with conventional radiography, followed by conventional tomography for complex fractures. Radioisotope bone scanning is helpful to detect stress fractures, but may lack spatial resolution. MRI is sensitive in detecting stress fractures, early avascular necrosis transchondral fractures, and bone contusions, but may not detect small cortical avulsions.

Case 1:   Avascular Necrosis of the Hip

A T$_2$-weighted coronal image reveals avascular necrosis of the right femoral head in a 34-year-old woman with right hip pain and normal radiographs of the right hip.

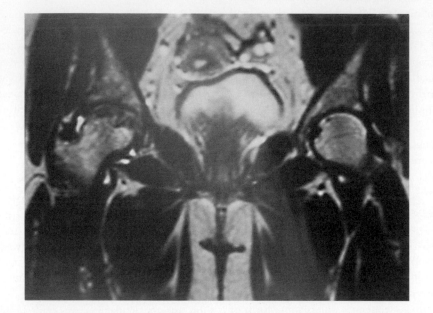

Case 2:   Fracture of the Ankle

In a 62-year-old woman with right ankle pain and swelling, a field–echo oblique sagittal image shows a medial talar dome transchondral fracture that is also seen on a T_1-weighted coronal image (B) and a T_2-weighted axial image (C).

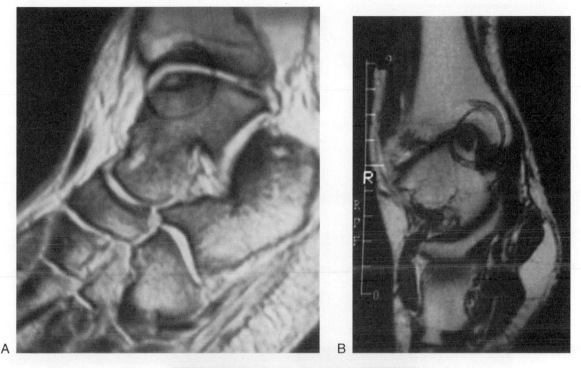

A   B

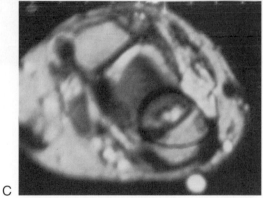

C

Case 3:   Contusion and Stress Fracture of Metatarsal

A T$_1$-weighted axial image (A) and a T$_1$-weighted coronal image (B) reveal bone edema compatible with bone contusion of the second metatarsal with stress fracture at the base in a 53-year-old man with persistent pain exacerbated by walking.

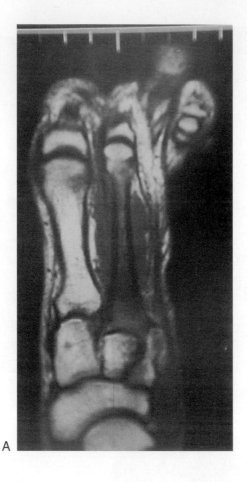
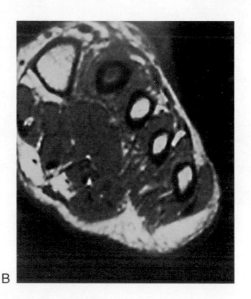

Case 4: Fracture of the Calcaneus

A T$_1$-weighted image shows a comminuted fracture of the calcaneus in a 23-year-old man with heel injury.

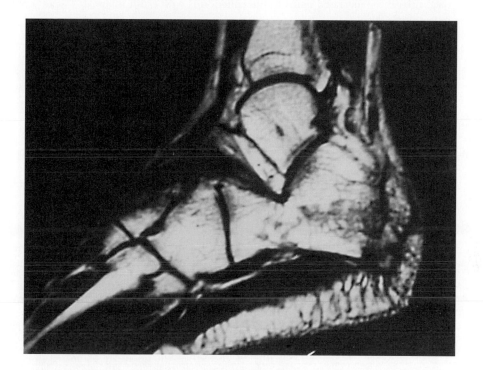

Case 5:   Crush Injury of the Midfoot

In a 26-year-old man with a crush injury to the right midfoot 5 weeks ago, T_1-weighted axial images (A) show a slightly mottled appearance of the cuneiforms. Inversion recovery axial images (B) show increased signal in the cuneiforms with crush injury. CT scan would show better bone detail.

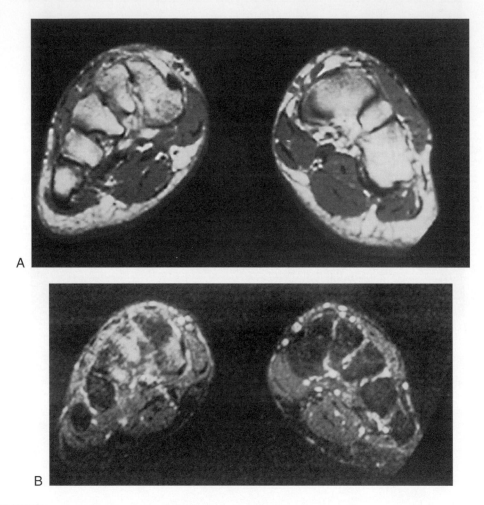

A

B

BONE INFECTIONS

Clinical history and laboratory studies (white blood cell count, sedimentation rate) usually determine the diagnosis of septic arthritis or osteomyelitis. Conventional radiography may reveal bone resorption, periosteal new bone formation, or joint space widening. Technetium or indium radionuclide bone scan is helpful for confirmation. MRI may help to delineate extent of infection for debridement with fat suppression scan technique.

Case 6: Diabetic Osteomyelitis of the Foot

In a 62-year-old diabetic man with osteomyelitis of the distal second phalanx, a T_1-weighted axial image (A) shows decreased signal in the bone marrow of the distal second phalanx with cortical erosion. An inversion recovery coronal image (B) shows increased signal in the marrow of the distal phalanx.

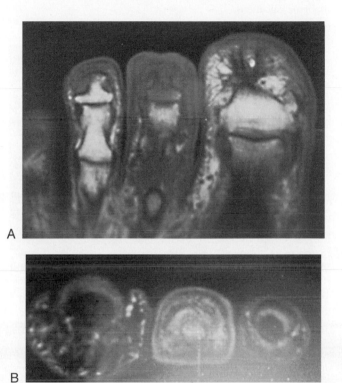

BONE TUMORS/CYSTS

Case 7: Aneurysmal Bone Cyst

In a 30-year-old man with left ankle and foot pain, a field-echo sagittal image (A) reveals a lesion with multiseptated fluid, also seen on a T_2-weighted coronal image (B) and a T_2-weighted axial image (C). The fluid levels are consistent with an aneurysmal bone cyst involving the superior calcaneus.

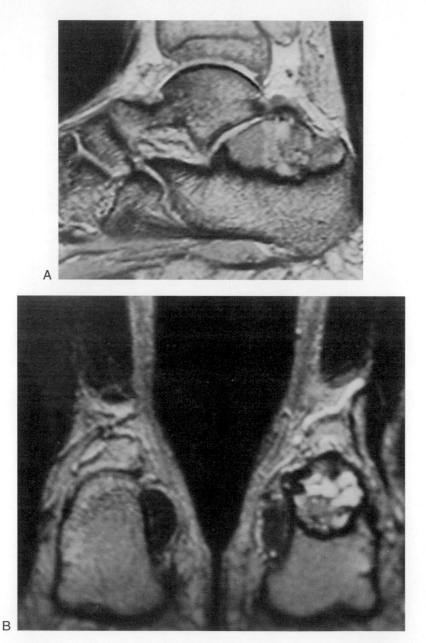

A

B

(Case continues.)

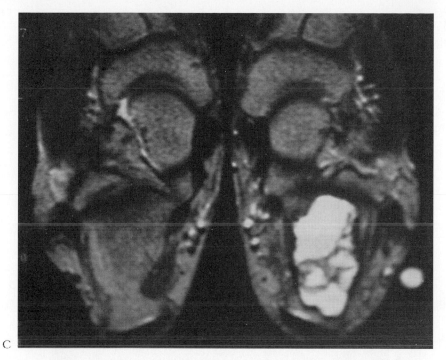

C

Case 7 (*Continued*)

TENDONS

Tendinous ruptures, tears, tendinitis, and tenosynovitis are well demonstrated by MRI.

Case 8:   Rupture of the Achilles Tendon

A T_2-weighted sagittal image shows a rupture of the Achilles tendon in a 33-year-old man with pain and swelling of the ankle for 10 months.

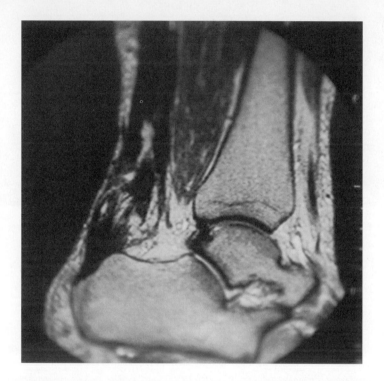

Case 9:   Mucinoid Degeneration of the Achilles Tendon

In a 32-year-old man with pain and swelling after running 7 miles, MRI shows chronic tendinitis with mucinoid degeneration of the left Achilles tendon on (A) a T_1-weighted sagittal image showing faint increased signal and thickening of the tendon and (B) a T_1-weighted axial image.

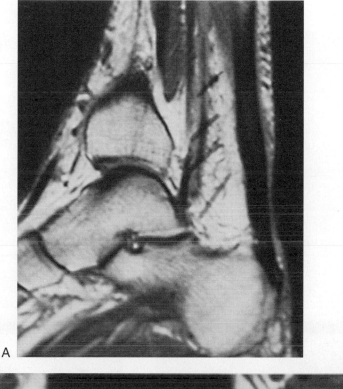

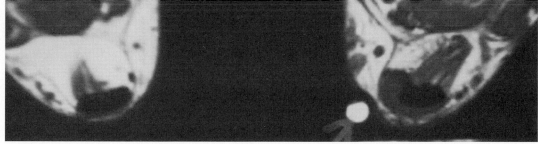

LIGAMENTS

Tears are well demonstrated by MRI.

Case 10: Calcaneofibular Ligament Tear

MRI demonstration of a calcaneofibular ligament tear on (A) a T_1-weighted axial image and (B) a T_2-weighted coronal image.

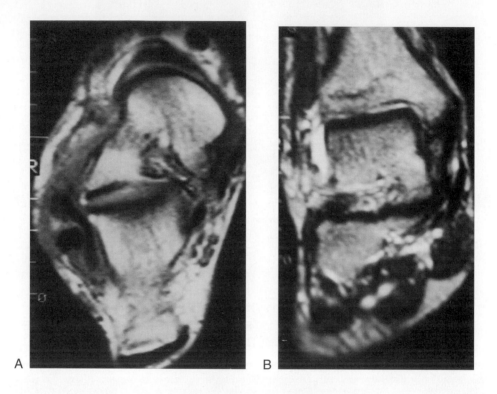

CARTILAGE

Mensical tears, chondromalacia, and osteochondral defects are well demonstrated by MRI.

Case 11:   Meniscal Tear

In a 31-year-old man with right knee "catching" when walking, MRI shows a complex tear of the posterior horn of the medial meniscus on (A) a T$_1$-weighted sagittal image and (B) a field-echo sagittal image.

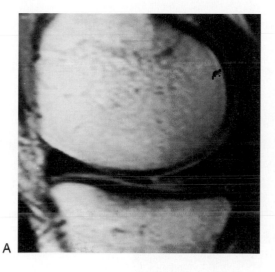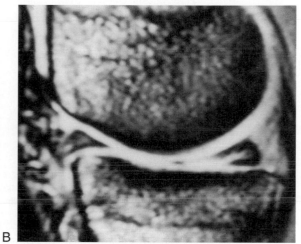

A   B

Case 12:   Osteochondral Defect

In a 44-year-old man with medial knee pain, popping, and clicking, a T_2-weighted sagittal image (A) shows a suprapatellar crescent-shaped loose body that originated from an anterior osteochondral defect in the medial femoral condyle, which is also seen on a field-echo axial image (B) and a T_1-weighted coronal image (C).

SOFT TISSUE MASSES

MRI or ultrasound can be used to determine the solid or cystic nature of masses as well as aid in the localization of such masses and adjacent tissue planes.

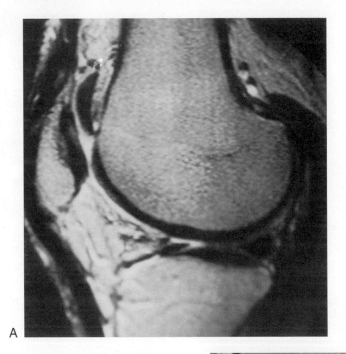

A

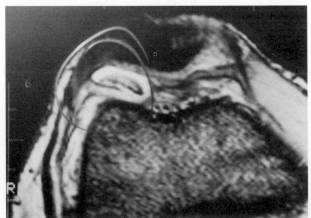

B

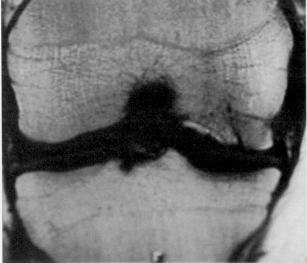

C

Case 13: Ganglion Cyst

In a 54-year-old man with recurrent ganglion cyst, a T_2-weighted axial image (A) shows a multilobulated cystic mass adjacent to the lateral malleolus without involvement of the peroneus brevis tendon or extension into the ankle joint, as is also seen on a T_1-weighted coronal image (B) and a T_2-weighted axial image (C) of the talus taken more caudal to that in A.

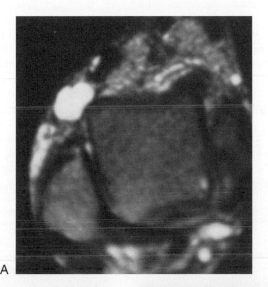

A

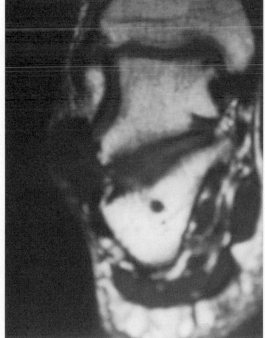

B

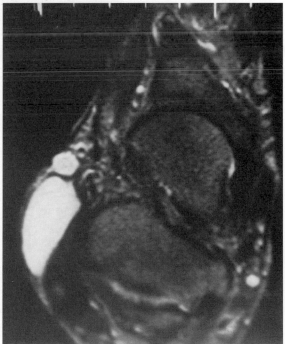

C

REFERENCES

1. Schweitzer ME, Resneck D: Normal anatomy of the foot and ankle. p. 33. In Deutch AL et al (eds): MRI of the Foot and Ankle. Raven Press, New York, 1992
2. Blei CL et al: Achilles tendon: US diagnosis of pathological conditions. Radiology 159:765, 1986
3. Fornage BD, Rifkin MD: Ultrasound examinations of tendons. Radiol Clin North Am 26:87, 1988
4. Mathison JR et al: Sonography of the Achilles tendon and adjacent bursae. Am J Roentgenol 151:127, 1988
5. Fornage BD, Rifkin MD: Ultrasound examination of tendons. Radiol Clin North Am 26:87, 1988
6. Kaplan PA, Anderson JC, Norris MA et al: Ultrasonography of post traumatic soft tissue lesion. Radiol Clin North Am 27:973, 1989
7. Therman H et al: The use of ultrasonography in the foot and ankle. Foot Ankle 13:386, 1992
8. Stark DD, Bradely WG (eds): Magnetic Resonance Imaging. CV Mosby, St. Louis, 1988
9. Stiller DW et al (eds): MRI in Orthopaedics and Sports Medicine. Lippincott-Raven, Philadelphia, 1988
10. Barrington NA: Radiology. p. 57. In Helal B, Rowley DI, Cracchioliol. A III, Myerson MS et al (eds): Surgery of Disorders of the Foot and Ankle. Martin Dunitz Limited, London, 1996
11. Geslien GE, Thrall JH, Espiosa JL, Older RA: Early detection of stress fractures using 99m-Tc polyphosphate. Radiology 121:683, 1976
12. Norfray JF, Schlachter L: Early confirmation of stress fractures in joggers. JAMA 243:1647, 1980
13. Schlefman BF, Arneson DJ: Recurrent tibial stress fracture in the jogger. J Am Podiatry Assoc 71:577, 1981
14. Winiecki DG, Biggs EW: Xeroradiography and its application in podiatry. J Am Podiatry Assoc 67:393, 1977
15. Wolfe JN: Xeroradiography in bones, joints, and soft tissues. Radiology 93:583, 1969
16. Pagliano JD, Wexler CE: Xeroradiography: detection of neuromas in podiatry. J Am Podiatry Assoc 68:38, 1978
17. Melincoff RH: Computerized tomography—the CT scanner. J Am Podiatry Assoc 70:161, 1980
18. Heatherington VJ: Special studies: bone scans and computerized axial tomography. p. 442. In Weisman SD (ed): Radiology of the Foot. Williams & Wilkins, Baltimore, 1983
19. Callaghan JE, Percy EC, Hill RO: The ankle arthrogram. J Can Assoc Radiol 21:74, 1970
20. Olson RW: Arthrography of the ankle: its uses in the evaluation of ankle sprains. Radiology 92:1439, 1969
21. Bonstrom L: Sprained ankles. III. Clinical observations in recent ligament ruptures. Acta Chir Scand 130:560, 1965
22. Lindholmer E, Blolged N, Jensen JT: Arthrography of the ankle. Acta Radiol 19:595, 1978
23. Reinherz RP: Contrast media in the foot. J Am Podiatry Assoc 72:569, 1982
24. Stiller DW, (ed): MRI in Orthopedics and Sport Medicine. Lippincott-Raven, Philadelphia, 1997

SUGGESTED READINGS

Felson (ed): Seminars in Roentgenology, Vol. 4: The Foot. Stratton, New York, 1970
Subotnick SI: Radiographic studies. In Subotnick SI (ed): Podiatric Sports Medicine. Futura, Mt. Kisco, NY, 1975

21
Physical Therapy

GEORGE J. DAVIES
DONALD A. CHU

This chapter describes the role of physical therapy and rehabilitation as an integral part of the health-care team approach in treating sports-related injuries. The focus of this chapter includes an introduction to rehabilitation, to physical therapy examination concepts and techniques, and to physical therapy treatment techniques (e.g., exercise, assistive devices, flexibility, manual therapy, and physical therapy modalities).

Rehabilitation often makes the difference between successful participation following an injury or compromised performance and reinjury. Furthermore, rehabilitation prevents the recurrence of injury, leading to continued safe and successful performance.

All rehabilitation techniques must be based on an accurate diagnosis by the physician/podiatrist or physical therapist. The physical therapist also performs a comprehensive examination, similar to that described by Davies and co-workers,[1,2] to establish a database. From this database, the patient's problems are identified and listed.

An example might be the athlete who has the following problems:

1. Pain (L) medial knee; (L) semitendinosus hamstring
2. Excessive compensatory pronation on (L)
3. Short leg syndrome
4. Decreased flexibility of (L) gastrocnemius–soleus
5. Decreased flexibility of (L) and (R) hamstrings
6. Decreased muscular strength (L)

7. Decreased muscular power (L) and (R)
8. Decreased muscular endurance (L) and (R)

After the problem list is developed for the athlete, goals are established. Short-term, long-term, and terminal goals are developed (see Box).

SHORT-TERM, LONG-TERM, AND TERMINAL GOALS FOR REHABILITATION

Short-Term Goals

1. Protect the involved area
2. Rest or decrease activity level
3. Decrease pain
4. Decrease inflammation
5. Decrease swelling
   a. Intracapsular effusion/synovitis
   b. Extracapsular edema
6. Increase joint range of motion

Long-Term Goals

7. Increase musculotendinous flexibility
8. Increase muscular strength
9. Increase muscular power
10. Increase muscular endurance

(Continues)

Long-Term Goals

11. Maintain cardiovascular endurance
12. Restore normal biomechanical functioning
13. Increase balance, proprioception, kinesthesia
14. Progressively return athlete back to functional activities

Terminal Goals

15. Increase musculotendinous flexibility to within normal limits for sport-specific requirements
16. Increase muscular strength to WNL for sport-specific requirements
17. Increase muscular power to WNL for sport-specific requirements
18. Increase muscular endurance to WNL for sport-specific requirements
19. Increase functional activities to WNL for sport-specific requirements
20. Prevent reinjury

In a problem-oriented approach to rehabilitation, each problem is listed and specific treatment techniques are identified to treat each problem. Examples from the above problem list include the following:

1. Cryotherapy, ultrasound
2. Orthotic appliances
3. Heel lift
4. Static stretching, wedge board
5. Static stretching, proprioceptive neuromuscular facilitation contract–relax, spray and stretch
6. Progressive resistive exercises (weight training), slow-speed isokinetic exercises
7. High-speed isokinetic exercises, plyometries, functional exercises
8. High-speed isokinetic exercises, bicycling, swimming, functional exercises, plyometries

The treatment techniques identified must be based on an examination and rational treatment programs predicated on biomechanics, physiology, kinesiology, and pathology. The rehabilitation program is based on a comprehensive examination and database that will be continually reas-

sessed to evaluate the effectiveness of the treatment/rehabilitation program.

A problem-oriented medical record (POMR) is used, following the SOAP (*subjective, objective, assessment, plan*) format. On each clinical visit, the SOAP format is followed. The patient describes the *subjective response* subsequent to the previous treatment up to the present time. Specific subjective questions can be asked to expedite the process. We use a subjective pain rating scale from 0 (no pain) to 10 (worse pain). On each clinical visit, the patient reports the pain rating. This can be compared with previous pain scores to monitor subjective improvement as well as the pain response relative to objective signs and changes. Next, certain objective parameters are measured to determine the effectiveness of the prior treatment. Various *objective measurements* should be used, such as goniometric range-of-motion (ROM) measurements, Isokinetic tests, functional tests, and objective balance tests for time. On the basis of the patient's subjective and objective responses, an *assessment* of the patient's present status is formulated. Is the patient better, worse, or the same after the previous treatment? Is the treatment used, such as the mobilization technique, the proper one, in the proper direction, at the proper force? Is the amount of exercise appropriate? Does the patient understand the home exercise program, and is it being performed properly? The physiologic, neurophysiologic, mechanical, and psychological effects of the treatment are assessed.

Depending on the subjective and objective assessment, predicated on the aforementioned considerations, the *treatment plan* is developed. The treatment plan consists of the particular treatment techniques, including the important details. Throughout the remainder of this chapter, specific treatment techniques that have proved clinically effective are presented.

EXERCISE

The emphasis should be on exercise in all rehabilitation programs. Exercise consists of four types: passive, active-assistive, active, and resistive. Most exercise programs consist of active exercise, with particular emphasis on active-resistive exercises. Preparatory to active and active-resistive exercise, either passive exercises, active-assistive exercises, or both may be used. The specifics of this approach are discussed later in this chapter.

ETIOLOGY (MECHANISM OF INJURY)

When dealing with athletes, particularly those with overuse syndromes, it is important to treat the etiologic factors and not just the signs and symptoms. For example, if a runner develops medial knee pain, the focus should be not only on the knee and its treatment but on the entire patient as well. This holistic approach enables the clinician to focus *in* on and treat the symptoms to relieve the immediate discomfort, but to also focus *out* and treat the etiologic factors.

HOLISTIC REHABILITATION

When an injury occurs, clearly the emphasis is placed on rehabilitating the injured area. The holistic approach takes into consideration the rehabilitation of the entire kinetic chain and total body conditioning. Prevention of deconditioning of the cardiovascular–respiratory system, the upper body, and the uninvolved lower extremity must be considered as an integral part of all rehabilitation programs.

A problem oriented approach to rehabilitation is far more accurate and appropriate than a time-oriented program. Having a time frame for rehabilitation is necessary as a guideline (particularly with soft tissue healing constraint times); however, the ultimate decisions should rest on a problem-oriented approach.

OBJECTIVE EXAMINATION

A comprehensive objective examination can be performed by the sports physical therapist to establish a database and perform serial testing and final tests for discharge (see Box).

COMPONENTS OF THE OBJECTIVE EXAMINATION

Vital signs

Posture and observation (shoes)

Gait evaluation

Anthropometric measurements

Leg length measurements

Referral-related joints

(Continues)

Palpation

Circulation/skin

Neurologic
　　Sensation
　　Reflexes
　　Balance

ROM testing Active

ROM testing Passive

Flexibility testing

Neurologic-resisted testing [manual muscle testing (MMT)]

Special tests

Isokinetic Tests

Functional tests [activities of daily living (ADL); sports specific]

Correlation with medical tests

PHYSICAL THERAPY TREATMENT TECHNIQUES

A number of physical therapy treatment techniques and modalities are discussed in this section; these are listed in Table 21-1.

Our philosophy is to develop a specific treatment program, apply treatment techniques separately, and evaluate the effectiveness of each treatment procedure before multiple modalities or multiple treatments are applied. The simultaneous application of hot packs, ultrasound, massage, manual therapy, and exercise has no place in sports rehabilitation. The shotgun approach (treat the patient with everything and hope that something will work) is totally inappropriate and has no place in a problem-oriented rehabilitation program. The reasons are the costs, clinical time, treatment time for equipment, and unnecessary treatments. Modalities have a role in decreasing the patient's symptoms but have limited effectiveness otherwise. The emphasis certainly must be oriented toward exercise as the treatment program progresses.

When a treatment is applied, the effectiveness of that treatment should be evaluated. If the treatment is effective and has not produced any negative effects from its application, the treatment is the correct one for that patient at that time but should be continually reassessed. Additional treatment techniques can be individually added, but each

Table 21-1 Physical Therapy Treatment Techniques and Modalities

TECHNIQUES	Combined ultrasound and electrical stimulation
Assistive devices	Phonophoresis
Crutches	Superficial thermotherapy
Canes	Whirlpools
Taping and wrapping	Hydrocollator packs
Sleeves and braces	Moist air
Orthotics	Paraffin
Flexibility exercises	Infrared
Static stretching	Ultraviolet
Proprioceptive neuromuscular facilitation	Topical counterirritants
Cryotherapy and stretch	Electrotherapy
Myofascial techniques	Low-voltage therapy
Ballistic stretching	Iontophoresis
Functional flexibility	High-voltage therapy
Balance/proprioception/kinesthesia	Electromyography
Manual therapy	Nerve conduction velocity studies
Joint mobilization	Transcutaneous electrical nerve stimulation
MODALITIES	Microelectrical nerve stimulation
Massage	Exercise
Cryotherapy and cryokinetics	Isometrics
Cryotherapy	Isotonics
Cryokinetics	Concentric
Contrast baths	Eccentric
Intermittent compression units	Variable resistance
Penetrating (deep) thermotherapy	Isokinetics
Ultrasound	Submaximal exercises
Pulsed ultrasound	

technique should be continually evaluated or the combination of treatments assessed.

Factors that can be monitored continually in patient treatments include (1) subjective comments, involving pain (pain-rating scale) and functional ability; (2) anthropometric measurements (i.e., swelling); (3) ROM-goniometric measurements; (4) MMT[3] and isokinetic testing; (5) gait evaluation; (6) functional performance in ADL; and (7) functional performance in sports activities.

Use of Assistive Devices

CRUTCHES

An athlete should use crutches under the following conditions:

1. If protection of the involved area is necessary
2. If an area should be rested
3. If pain is present

4. If swelling is present creating a reflex inhibition of the surrounding muscles
5. If ROM is significantly restricted
6. If muscular strength, power, and endurance are significantly decreased
7. If an area is non-weight bearing or partially weight bearing to permit tissue healing
8. If the athlete limps

Protection of a joint and prevention of intracapsular effusion or extracapsular edema can only be accomplished by using crutches, not by the use of a cane, which affords limited protection. Aten[4] provides a brief overview of the uses, indications, and contraindications for crutches. Basmajian[5] describes the types of crutches, crutch-fitting procedures, and crutch gaits.

CANES

Canes should not be used in place of crutches because canes do not offer adequate protection or support.

TAPING AND WRAPPING

Several books and chapters in books[6-9] are devoted to taping and wrapping procedures (see Ch. 25). There are a variety of considerations with taping and wrapping, including purpose, tape selection, supplies, skin preparation, positioning, tape application, and tape removal. Taping is useful for many reasons:

1. Prevents injury
2. Prevents reinjury
3. Limits extremes of ROM
4. Limits ROM and enables patient to exercise in the healthy part of ROM
5. Applies compression to decrease pain, swelling, and spasms
6. Immobilizes or rests the involved area so that healing can occur, especially during the fibroblastic stage of healing
7. Provides proprioception and biofeedback
8. Provides stabilization to area
9. Serves as an external reminder
10. Gives psychological support and a sense of security
11. Applies resistance
12. Supplies assistance
13. Holds dressings in place
14. Holds pads in place
15. Holds equipment in place

It is beyond the scope of this chapter to discuss the variety of taping procedures currently in use as adjunctive measures in treatment and rehabilitation of lower extremity injuries (see Ch. 25). Because there are specific indications for taping injuries or anatomic areas, the procedure should be done selectively. The most important point to be stressed concerning taping and wrapping is to use these techniques to complement and facilitate the rehabilitation program, and not in place of rehabilitation.

Sleeves and Braces

A variety of commercially available sleeves and braces can be selected as part of the rehabilitation program. It must be emphasized again that these devices are used to complement, and not replace, rehabilitation. Devices available include the Levine strap (Jack Levine, M.D., Brooklyn, NY), Cho-Pat Strap (Fig. 21-1) (Cho-Pat, Inc., Hainesport, NJ), Pro Knee Sleeve, and Pro Knee Sleeve with retainer (Pro Orthopaedic Devies, Inc., King of Prussia, PA), Lenox Hill Derotation Brace (Lenox Hill Brace Shop, Inc., New York, NY), Jose Bands (Jose Bands, Inc., Eugene, OR), and Palumbo Patellar Stabilization Brace (P.M. Palumbo, M.D., McLean, VA).

Figure 21-1 Cho-Pat chondromalacia strap.

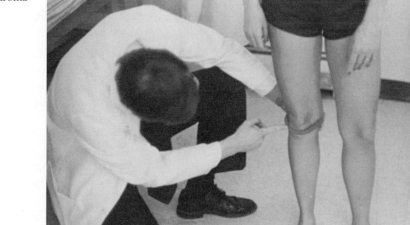

Flexibility Exercises

After the flexibility tests during the examination are performed and specific deficits identified, the athlete should be placed on a flexibility/stretching program. There is limited information in the literature documenting the most effective methods of increasing flexibility of the musculotendinous unit. More research is needed to document the anatomic, physiologic, and neurophysiologic responses to various stretching techniques. Anatomic and physiologic considerations for various muscle groups should be considered when designing a flexibility program. For example, the length of time required for increasing flexibility of the hamstrings is usually shorter than that for the gastrocnemius–soleus complex. There may be several reasons, one of which is probably attributable to the anatomic structures involved. For example, there is more dense fascia in the posterior lower leg than in the hamstring area, so the former will require prolonged stretching. Clearly, the anatomic type and quantity of tissue present in an area may provide clues for future research. These considerations may dictate the time spent with the stretching procedures. Neurophysiologic considerations such as the myotatic (stretch) reflex should also be considered.[10]

There are at least three reasons for incorporating flexibility exercises into a rehabilitation or conditioning program: (1) prevention of injury or reinjury, (2) increased efficiency of performance, and (3) decreased residual muscular soreness following exercise.

Nicholas[11] and Glick[12] reported the role of flexibility in the prevention of injury. If the flexibility of the musculotendinous unit is increased, this should decrease the passive resistance of soft tissue that occurs with functional movements. Increased flexibility should permit freer movement through a greater ROM, which should increase performance. DeVries[13] demonstrated that stretching following exercise decreases the subjective complaints of muscular soreness and decreased electromyographic (EMG) activity in the muscles. Several principles can be applied for increasing flexibility as described by Uram.[14]

STATIC STRETCHING

Static stretching techniques are the most effective and safest procedures to increase musculotendinous flexibility. Static stretching or yoga-type stretching, in which the athlete stretches to the end of the ROM and then a little beyond (but short of creating pain or reflex responses), is

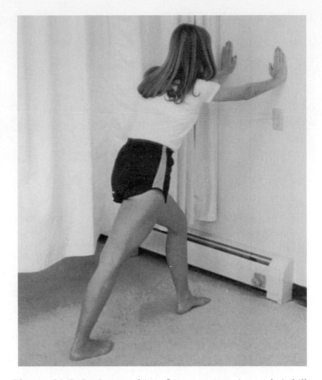

Figure 21-2 Static stretching for gastrocnemius and Achilles tendon.

preferred (Fig. 21-2). Admittedly, little evidence is available in the literature to demonstrate the most effective duration of hold positions but, on the basis of empirical clinical observation and experience, prolonged holds of 30 seconds appear to be more effective.

PROPRIOCEPTIVE NEUROMUSCULAR FACILITATION

Proprioceptive neuromuscular facilitation (PNF) techniques, described by Voss et al.,[15] are effective in increasing the flexibility of the musculotendinous unit (Fig. 21-3). Contract–relax and hold–relax are particularly effective and are the most commonly used procedures in clinical practice.

Contract–relax: Isotonic contraction of antagonistic pattern, with no ROM allowed, followed by passive motion of agonistic pattern

Hold–relax: Isometric contraction of antagonist pattern followed by free active motion of agonist pattern

Additional beneficial components of PNF procedures

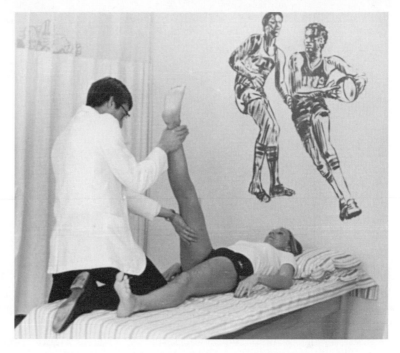

Figure 21-3 Proprioceptive neuromuscular facilitation for hamstring flexibility.

are muscle contractions, which increase muscular strength through increasing ROM. Rehabilitation involves not only increasing ROM but using PNF to strengthen the muscle through the ROM. Two-person PNF techniques at practice sessions are particularly useful. However, any assistive PNF techniques should also be complemented with prolonged passive stretching.

CRYOTHERAPY AND STRETCH

Spray and stretch, described by Travell and Rinzler[16] and Mennel,[17] or ice and stretch are additional procedures found clinically effective in increasing musculotendinous flexibility (Fig. 21-4). Knight[18] has written the most comprehensive overview regarding the techniques and effectiveness of cryotherapy.

MYOFASCIAL RELEASE

One of the techniques being taught in many continuing education courses in physical therapy, as well as being used regularly in the clinic by many therapists, is myofascial release. This is a soft tissue technique designed to mobilize the fascial connective tissue. However, no scientific reports have yet been published that definitely demonstrate the efficacy of this technique.

BALLISTIC STRETCHING

Ballistic or dynamic stretching should be avoided because of the tendency to elicit the myotactic stretch reflex and produce microtrauma muscle strains. If ballistic stretching is performed, the opposite of the intended effect for the musculotendinous unit may result. The myotactic reflex occurs to act as a protective mechanism to prevent an injury to the musculotendinous unit and consequently splints and shortens the unit. Furthermore, repeated dynamic stretching producing microtrauma muscle strains, which may cause scar development and lead to musculotendinous shortening, since cicatrix collagen fibers are not as elastic as the initial musculotendinous fibers.

FUNCTIONAL FLEXIBILITY

Although ballistic flexibility is contraindicated, we would like to emphasize the importance of functional flexibility or controlled dynamic flexibility (Fig. 21-5). Clinically it does not make sense for the athlete to perform passive stretching and to then directly participate in a dynamic sports-related activity. A functional flexibility, controlled dynamic flexibility, or a "transition flexibility" activity leading from static stretching to dynamic sports performance appears to be a reasonable approach in the flexibility regimen. These controlled dynamic flexibility

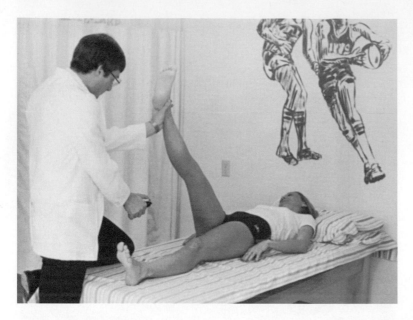

Figure 21-4 Spray and stretch technique for hamstring flexibility.

Figure 21-5 Functional (controlled dynamic) flexibility.

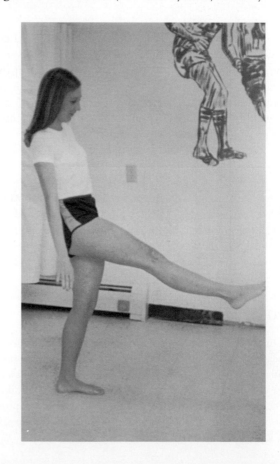

activities have been more commonly referred to in the past as direct active warmups.

The first author (G.J.D.) is involved in the martial arts and shall describe a typical workout session. For a 1-hour workout, the initial 10 minutes are spent on static stretching, followed by approximately 5 minutes of controlled dynamic flexibility exercise specifically replicating the skills (kicks and punches) to be used during the skill performance or sparring sessions. This transition phase acts to prepare the musculotendinous unit for additional demands to be placed on it by increasing blood flow, increasing internal temperature, and decreasing passive internal resistance of soft tissues.

Balance/Proprioception/Kinesthesia

Not only are the terms *balance, proprioception,* and *kinesthesia* frequently used to describe skills necessary for successful sports performance, but they have become a significant part of lower extremity and spine rehabilitation programs. Wyke[19] demonstrated that injuries to a joint (ligament, capsule, or both) result in injury to, and loss of, the mechanoreceptors of that joint. The chronic injury may be due to various factors, such as muscular weakness (dynamic stabilizers) and joint instability (static stabilizers), but also to joint proprioceptive (neural stabilizers) loss. Wyke[19] also demonstrated that the patient's balance improves with participation in activities designed to stimulate these mechanoreceptors (Fig. 21-6).

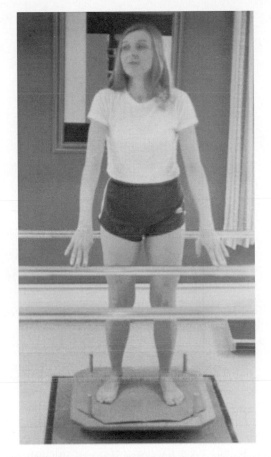

Figure 21-6 Proprioceptive board activity.

Therefore, every patient with a lower extremity or spine injury should be tested for balance (static and dynamic) in order to identify deficits. If deficits are observed, this becomes a clinical problem and treatment techniques designed to increase balance should be implemented. Many types of activities can be used, including rocker boards, tilt boards, balance beams, standing on one foot, hopping on one foot, throwing and catching a ball against the wall while standing on one foot, and agility drills.

Manual Therapy

JOINT MOBILIZATION

If the athlete is found to have restrictions in the noncontractile structures, manual therapy techniques are designed to promote motion in these structures. Inevitably, if an area is immobilized through the use of casting, bracing,

or protective devices, adaptive shortening of surrounding tissues as well as fibrous adhesions develop. Several books[20,21] deal specifically with mobilization techniques of the lower extremity. It is beyond the scope of this chapter to discuss manual therapy in detail, but an overview of the application of manual therapy techniques is presented.

The use of manual therapy procedures is predicated on a careful and meticulous physical examination, particularly passive ROM testing. Various concepts can be applied when using manual therapy:

1. End feel
2. Paris's joint mobility scale (from 0, for ankylosed, to 6, for hypermobility)
3. Pain-resistance sequence
4. Concept of convex/concave treatment technique
5. Maitland's grades of movement

Paris's classification of joint mobility dictates the appropriate treatment of the joint. Grade 0 requires a surgical procedure. Grades 1 and 2 are indications for joint mobilization or manipulation, provided the limitations (end feels) are capsular or ligamentous. Grade 3 is normal. Grades 4 and 5 require taping or bracing. Grade 6 usually requires surgery. Grades 4 through 6 are similar to the joint instability classification used by the American Academy of Orthopaedic Surgeons (AAOS). As an example, the AAOS ranks the accessory movement from 1 + to 3 +. The correlations would be as follows:

AAOS	Paris's scale
1 +	4
2 +	5
3 +	6

The AAOS does not have a classification ranking for joint hypomobility. Therefore, if a grade 1 or 2 mobility exists in the joint, passive joint mobilization techniques are indicated to facilitate restoration of joint ROM. The end feel, joint mobility, and pain-resistance sequence will dictate the grades (Maitland's) of movement to be used in treating the patient.

Concept of Convex/Concave Treatment

Every joint in the body has both a convex and concave surface. This forms the basis for the application of passive movements. The concept of convex/concave treatment is based on joint arthrokinematics for treating the noncontractile structures surrounding a joint. The clinical application of these concepts is illustrated by the following two examples:

Concave/convex treatment: tibia/femur surfaces

Convex/concave treatment: talus/tibia–fibula surfaces; femur/tibia

If one mobilizes a concave articular surface (tibia) on a stationary convex articular surface (femur), the treatment force at the joint is in the same direction as the desired arthrokinematic and osteokinematic movement (Fig. 21-7). Therefore, if one were to mobilize the tibia on the stationary femur, the application of the treatment force arthrokinematically would be in the same direction as the desired osteokinematic movement. For example, to increase knee flexion, the tibia would be passively mobilized toward flexion, with a resultant increase in flexion.

By contrast, if one were to mobilize a convex articular

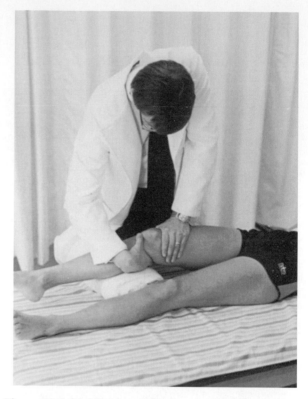

Figure 21-8 Mobilization of femur to increase knee flexion.

surface (femur) on a stationary concave articular surface (tibia), the direction of force arthrokinematically would be in the opposite direction of the desired osteokinematic movements. For example, to increase knee flexion, the femur would have to be passively mobilized toward extension, with the resultant osteokinematic motion of increasing knee flexion (Fig. 21-8).

In addition to applying the force in the proper direction on the basis of joint arthrokinematics, there are additional treatment guidelines for the application of grades of movements, as described by Maitland.

Summary

To reiterate, the purpose of joint mobilization techniques is to restore joint ROM. This includes restoration of the physiologic joint movements as well as the component joint motions. Loss of these component motions is often the limiting factor in regaining full pain-free ROM. Being cognizant of the component joint movements rather than just the obvious physiologic joint motions can enhance joint functioning.

Figure 21-7 Mobilization of tibia to increase knee flexion.

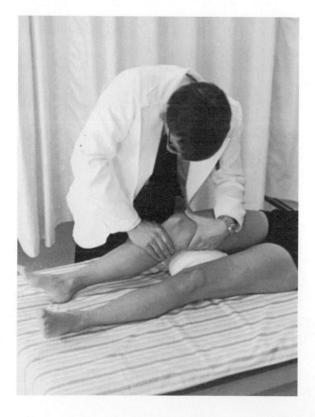

PHYSICAL THERAPY MODALITIES

Physical therapy modalities are certainly an important adjunct to a rehabilitation program, but the actual indications and effects should be carefully evaluated. Physical therapy modalities are particularly effective, especially early in a rehabilitation program. One must not become dependent on modalities, however, but instead should use modalities as adjunctive techniques as part of the rehabilitation program.

Several books[22-27] are available for detailed descriptions of various modalities. Such considerations as the types of modalities; appropriate positioning; treatment dosage; patient preparation; the physiologic, neurophysiologic, and mechanical effects; treatment precautions; anticipated treatment results; indications; contraindications; and review of literature may be found in these sources.

The specific diagnosis, type of anatomic structures involved, severity, location of lesion, contraindications, special instructions, and the prescription for the treatment should be outlined before therapy begins. The area to be treated should be carefully inspected both before and after the treatment. Particular attention to inspecting the area after the application of the modality is necessary to determine the immediate results. Often, the effects of the modalities are latent, or the results continue for a long period of time.

Modalities are particularly effective during the early rehabilitation stages of a program. During the acute phase, modalities can decrease pain, retard the inflammatory process, decrease swelling, and facilitate the healing process.

These modalities include massage, heat, water, ice, sprays, and electricity for the primary purposes of controlling (retarding) the inflammatory response, facilitating the healing responses, and assisting the rehabilitation program. Exercise is also a therapeutic modality, in fact the most important one.

Modalities should be used as adjunctive techniques during the rehabilitation program to complement the exercise program. As the rehabilitation program progresses to the intermediate and advanced phases, there should be less reliance on modalities and greater emphasis on exercise.

Massage

Massage is the systematic application of the hands to manipulate soft tissues. The five categories of massage include effleurage (stroking), petrissage (kneading), topotement (percussion), vibration, and friction. We use the cross-transverse friction massage much more frequently than any other massage technique. Cross-transverse friction massage is a deep massage applied perpendicularly to the anatomic fibers in the area (Fig. 21-9). Cross-transverse friction massage is clinically effective when applied over muscle bellies or tendons affected by muscle strain or tendinitis. This massage is also quite effective in chronic strains (particularly of the hamstrings) when scar tissue develops and either limits ROM, causes pain, or both. The purpose of this massage is to try to produce a more mobile functional scar or prevent the development of more scar tissue. If an area, such as a knee, has been immobilized for several

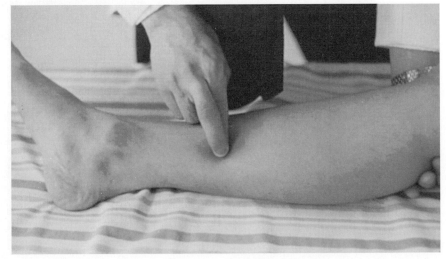

Figure 21-9 Cross-transverse friction massage to posterior tibialis tendon.

weeks, cross-transverse friction massage on the medial collateral ligaments will assist in breaking up fibrous adhesions and mobilizing the tissue.

When treating a musculotendinous unit, we generally use a sequence of ultrasound or phonophoresis first to make the scar tissue more malleable, followed by cross-transverse friction massage, followed by high-speed submaximal or maximal isokinetic exercises to produce a functional (mobile) flexible scar. This is a primary goal when treating musculotendinous injuries.[28]

Cryotherapy and Cryokinetics

CRYOTHERAPY

We use cryotherapy procedures extensively during rehabilitation. The effectiveness of the old theory of ice for the first 24 to 72 hours followed by heat is not well documented. If one intends to use heat, we recommend that it not be applied for a minimum of 72 hours. If heat is applied too soon and the inflammatory process is still active, increased swelling results. Specific clinical parameters to determine when the actual inflammatory process has ceased are generally not reliable. Therefore, continuing with cryotherapy procedures until there is no longer a positive clinical response from the patient seems like a rational approach to treatment. Often one can use cryotherapy throughout a rehabilitation program without resorting to heating techniques. Exercise promotes the local physiologic effects to increase healing as effectively as the application of passive heating.

Cryotherapy can be applied by several procedures: cold immersion baths, cold slush (water and ice) baths, cold whirlpools, cold hydrocollator packs, ice massage, ice chips in a bag, cold compression units, spray and stretch with fluoromethane spray, and ethyl chloride spray (Fig. 21-10). Each of these cryotherapy applications has specific indications based on locations of dysfunction, purpose of cryotherapy, and desired results. Clinical experience will dictate appropriate selection.

CRYOKINETICS

The application of cryotherapy followed by active movements is an effective procedure to assist in increasing ROM and in increasing the patient's exercise tolerance during a clinical treatment session. Following treatment, particularly exercise bouts, the area is inspected; we then have almost all patients apply cryotherapy to decrease any treatment soreness that may develop.

Contrast Baths

Once the acute phase has passed, if residual swelling remains in a joint, contrast baths are indicated. The purpose of contrast baths is to use alternating heat (vasodila-

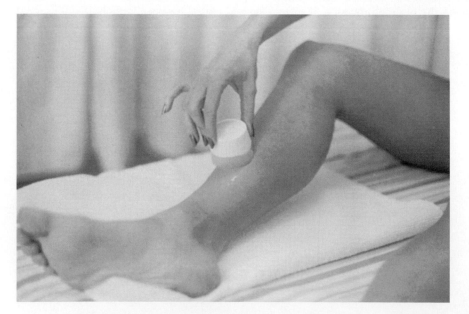

Figure 21-10 Ice massage.

tion) and cold (vasoconstriction) to create an alternating mechanical force that will decrease the swelling (i.e., externally induced pumping mechanism by the alternate use of heat and cold). Contrast baths are applied by alternating from heat (95 to 105°F) to cold (55 to 65°F).

The procedure begins with hot baths for 3 minutes, switching immediately to cold for 1 minute; when the extremity is in the cold, cryokinetics can also be employed. In addition to the mechanical effects of going from heat to cold, the active cryokinetics serves as an assistive muscular pumping device that decreases the swelling; a potentiation effect of the cold and of the active movements decreases the swelling. This sequence is repeated approximately seven to eight times for about 28 to 32 minutes. If the injury is still in the subacute phase with minimal swelling but the athlete still requires assistive devices because of the limp, we recommend ending in a cold bath to bring about vasoconstriction and decrease the likelihood of increased swelling. For a chronic condition, we recommended ending in heat to increase blood flow, which brings nutrients to promote the healing process.

Intermittent Compression Units

Intermittent compression units are effective in decreasing swelling. Often, with residual swelling or chronic swelling resistant to other physical therapy modalities, intermittent compression units are effective. Newer commercial units have combined intermittent compression with cryotherapy for the simultaneous application of compression and cryotherapy.

Penetrating (Deep) Thermotherapy

There are two types of deep thermotherapy: ultrasound and ultrasound phonophoresis. The recurrent theme with both modalities is a high-frequency current that produces deep heating effects.

ULTRASOUND

Ultrasound is an acoustic vibration that creates a conversion of ultrasonic wave energy to heat in the body tissues. It is the deepest heating modality and is selectively absorbed by various tissues, with the most absorption occurring in high-protein tissue (muscle). The physiologic effects include elevation of tissue temperature, decreased pain through decreased nerve conduction velocity, increased blood flow, increased membrane permeability, and

increased local metabolism. Ultrasound also produces mechanical effects in various tissues. Ultrasound is indicated in joint contractures in order to decrease symptoms in various musculoskeletal injuries, provide pain relief, and increase scar malleability; it is also used to treat calcific tendinitis conditions. The application and specific details of the ultrasound prescription vary from patient to patient, depending on the purpose of the ultrasound application.

PULSED ULTRASOUND

The flow of ultrasound current is interrupted when there is an increase in energy without the accumulation of heat. When less heating effect is desired and more of the mechanical effects are desired, pulsed ultrasound is indicated.

COMBINED ULTRASOUND AND ELECTRICAL STIMULATION

The combination of the muscular massage and relaxation effects of electrical stimulation with the deep heating effects of ultrasound are frequently used clinically. However, no studies have unequivocally demonstrated the efficiency of this technique.

PHONOPHORESIS

The technique of phonophoresis[29] is used when a topical medication is introduced by dispersion. Topical medications are applied to the skin and used as a coupling agent for ultrasound. This causes the medication to penetrate more deeply (Fig. 21-11).

Superficial Thermotherapy

There are various superficial heating modalities. These include whirlpools, hydrocollator packs, moist air, paraffin, infrared (IR), ultraviolet (UV), and topical counterirritants.

WHIRLPOOLS, HYDROCOLLATOR PACKS, MOIST AIR, AND PARAFFIN

These are all superficial modalities and cause increased temperature, increased local rate of metabolism, increased local circulation, analgesic effect, increased phagocytosis, sedation, and a reflex vasodilation. Indications include various musculoskeletal conditions, although the clinical efficacy is not well documented.

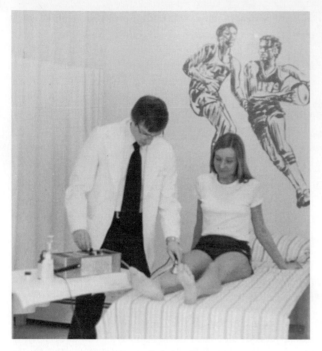

Figure 21-11 Application of phonophoresis.

INFRARED

Infrared is superficial heating by radiant energy. Therapeutic effects of IR include relief of pain (through counterirritation), muscle relaxation, and increased blood supply; it is also a preliminary adjunct to other forms of physical agents.

ULTRAVIOLET

Ultraviolet is also a radiant energy superficial heat. Physiologic effects of UV are erythema, pigmentation, bactericidal effects, and wound healing. Its primary application in sports medicine is for various dermatologic conditions.

TOPICAL COUNTERIRRITANTS

Topical counterirritants produce superficial heating and counterirritation. These agents stimulate pain receptors in the skin; a reflex is thereby stimulated that counteracts the athlete's perception of pain. Several neurophysiologic reactions occur that are not well understood. Topical counterirritants include such products as Cramergesic and Atomic Balm (Cramer Products, Inc., Gardner, KS).

Electrotherapy

Several electrotherapy modalities are currently in use, including electrical stimulation [low-volt therapy using alternating (AC) or direct (DC) current], iontophoresis, high-(galvanic) voltage stimulation, transcutaneous electrical nerve stimulation (TENS), microelectrical nerve stimulation (MENS), EMG, nerve conduction velocities, and biofeedback. Electrotherapy is the application of current into the body, flowing from an area of increased electrons to one of fewer electrons. Low-voltage DC stimulation is commonly used. The effects of DC on tissue are primarily chemical, while AC has contractile effects on muscles.

Various types of electrical currents are used in physical therapy: low-voltage DC, high-voltage DC, AC interferential current, and faradic current.

LOW-VOLTAGE THERAPY

Clinical application of electrical currents (electrical stimulation) is used to produce contraction in an individual muscle or muscle group.[30-33] With careful selection of current form, strength, and duration, one stimulus will be as physiologic as possible. Electrical stimulation can be a useful adjunct in a patient's rehabilitative program,[34] but its limitations should be kept in mind: (1) it may be used with, but should not replace, voluntary exercise; and (2) in past experiences, it has not been more effective in maintaining or developing strength than resistive exercises.

Several studies[35,36] have indicated that strength increases with electrical stimulation.

The uses of electrical stimulation are to aid in re-education and as a form of massage for reduction of edema and relaxation of muscle spasm. The details regarding the exercise prescription (method of application waveforms, dosage, time duration) will vary with the objective of the treatment.

Some of the clinical effects of AC stimulation have been described as follows:

1. Tone is restored to muscles in cases of injury or weakness.

2. Atrophy is halted in cases of prolonged immobilization.

3. Blood supply to injured tissues is increased, and rate of repair may be stimulated.

4. Relaxation is obtained in skeletal muscle spasms through inhibition.

IONTOPHORESIS

Iontophoresis is the injection of ions into the body by the use of continuous DC stimulation for therapeutic purposes. The advantages of iontophoresis include the following:

1. Consistent drug delivery and controllable dosage localized to precise tissue area
2. No risk of infection
3. Does not traumatize underlying tissue
4. Low systemic dose delivered with fewer side effects than with injections
5. Has greater penetration than systemic therapy and topical application
6. Decreased anxiety or fear of patients during the performance of a painful medical treatment
7. Decreased expense

Various ions are used for iontophoresis, depending on the desired clinical results of the treatment.

HIGH-VOLTAGE THERAPY

High-voltage therapy is designed to create an impulse with enough potential to enter the body with (1) a minimum of sensory disturbance, and (2) as little distortion of the impulse as possible. There are several uses, including acute trauma (since there is no heat buildup in the tissues); decreasing swelling; exercising muscles weakened due to postsurgical conditions, disuse atrophy, or injuries; increasing circulation; and increasing wound healing.

ELECTROMYOGRAPHY

Electromyography[33] is an audio and visual representation of the electrical activity of muscle. EMG is clinically used (1) as a diagnostic aid, (2) in kinesiologic studies, and (3) as biofeedback to facilitate muscle re-education. During kinesiology studies, the electrical activity of one or more muscles may be observed during activity in the normal or pathologic subject. EMG is not a measure of muscle strength but can be related to magnitude and pattern of participation in the activity being investigated.

NERVE CONDUCTION VELOCITY STUDIES

Nerve conduction velocity is used as part of the electrodiagnostic examination.[33] It involves the study of the distance an impulse travels along a nerve per unit of time, expressed in meters per second. Nerve conduction velocity measurements involve stimulating a nerve at one point and recording the response of either the muscle (motor nerve conduction) or the nerve (sensory nerve conduction) at a distant point.

TRANSCUTANEOUS ELECTRICAL NERVE STIMULATION

TENS[37] involves the use of low-voltage or low-amperage current to produce electroanalgesia by a process of differential sensory nerve excitation. TENS is a process of sensory modulation; the primary objective of this approach is the modulation of pain—that is, treatment by counterirritation.

It has been proposed that TENS current most specifically elicits increased activity in the afferent (A) fibers. Afferent fibers are primarily divided into two major classifications based on size and function. Large myelinated A fibers tend to be epicritic mechanoreceptors that conduct nonpainful stimuli. The thick A fibers require phasic input for stimulation; thus sustained activity in the A fibers has a net effect of abating the sensation of pain. There are many considerations when applying TENS, similar to those associated with any other modality. These considerations include type, size, current, size of electrodes, application of electrodes, placement of electrodes, the specific condition, and diagnosis.

MICROELECTRICAL NERVE STIMULATION

MENS is one of the newer physical therapy modalities used in the treatment of a variety of musculoskeletal dysfunctions. Although it is a relatively "hot" item, it is controversial at this time whether MENS is a valid means of treatment for pain control, because minimal research has been performed with MENS therapy.

The difference between the standard TENS units and the MENS units is the current used. TENS units utilize milliamperage currents, whereas MENS units use microcurrent (microamps). A microamp is only one millionth of an amp and is 1/1,000th of a milliamp. Since the currents used in MENS are so small, they are usually subsensory and are described as being similar to the body's own "natural electricity."

MENS has several proposed uses, including:

1. Reduction of chemical pain
2. Reduction of mechanical pain

3. Reduction of creatine phosphokinase (CPK, a muscle enzyme) levels when applied following exercise

4. Direct effect on nociceptive fibers to reduce pain

5. Diagnostic tool to identify trigger points

6. Relax muscles

7. Stimulate muscles

8. Enhance muscle re-education

9. Regenerate healing of damaged tissues

10. Reduce edema, effusion, and inflammation

Of course, more controlled experimental clinical trials must be performed to demonstrate the effectiveness of MENS in treating various conditions of the lower extremities.

Exercise

Exercise is the key factor in any rehabilitation program. Exercise is usually directed toward (1) cardiovascular–respiratory exercise and conditioning, (2) general total-body musculoskeletal exercise and conditioning, and (3) local musculoskeletal exercise and conditioning directed toward the area of pathology.

Various types of exercises can be performed:

Passive Exercise: performed by the therapist and not by the athlete. Passive exercise can be performed as joint mobilization to increase joint ROM of the noncontractile structures. Furthermore, passive stretching is an effective procedure for increasing musculotendinous flexibility. Passive movements can also be used to help align collagen tissue formation and maturation according to Davis's law of soft tissue modeling, producing a more functional flexible scar. Passive movements are indicated early in a rehabilitation program to prevent degenerative changes in the soft tissues and promote healing.

Active-Assistive Exercise: most commonly used in early postsurgical or post-traumatic conditions. An example of a variation of active-assistive exercises is eccentric exercise. In immediately postoperative knee rehabilitation, the therapist can passively lift the hip, and the athlete lowers the leg eccentrically (with active assistance), performing an eccentric straight leg raise.

Active Exercise: incorporated into an exercise program while ROM is gained. Active exercises are also used to maintain ROM once it has been achieved. Active exercise combined with ice is known as cryokinetics.

Resistive Exercise: designed to increase muscular strength, power, and endurance. Manual resistance by the therapist, using such techniques as PNF, can also be incorporated as a resistive exercise.

Muscle strength, endurance, and power are the parameters that should be developed through an exercise program. Muscle strength is developed by using isometric contractions, isotonics with high weight (resistance) and low repetitions (one to eight repetitions) at slow speeds (approximately 60/second), or isokinetic slow-contractile-velocity exercises (60/second or slower). Muscle endurance is enhanced through isotonics with low weight (resistance) and high repetitions (eight, ad infinitum) and isokinetics using fast-contractile-velocity exercises (60/second or faster). Muscle power is developed isotonically through faster movements with weights and isokinetically with fast-contractile-velocity exercises (180/second or faster), plyometrics, or functional exercises.

MODES OF EXERCISE

Isometric Exercises

These exercises are performed at 0 degrees speed (no observable joint movement or functional movements); they are designed to strengthen the muscles at the specific point of application of force in ROM. In most instances, we have considered isometrics specific to the joint angle. Knapik and colleagues[38] demonstrated a 20-degree physiologic overflow from the specific joint angle. Therefore, one can use multiple-angle isometric contractions every 20 degrees through ROM and still strengthen the muscles throughout ROM.

Isotonic Exercises

These exercises are performed with fixed resistance at variable speed. Isotonic exercises are also referred to as progressive resistive exercises or weight training (Fig. 21-12).

Concentric Isotonic Exercises　　These exercises cause a shortening of the muscle fibers, and the muscle's origin and insertions approximate.

Eccentric Isotonic Exercises　　These exercises cause a lengthening of the muscle fibers, and the muscle's origin and insertion separate.

When the three types of contractions are evaluated for the tension they generate, the contractions produce the greatest to the least tension in the following order: eccen-

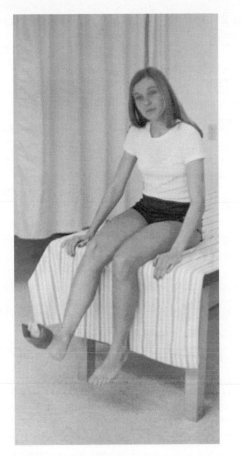

Figure 21-12 Progressive resistive exercises for ankle dorsiflexors.

tric isotonic contractions, isometric contractions, concentric isotonic contractions. There are three popular weight-training/isotonic training programs: De Lorme,[39] Oxford,[40] and DAPRE.[41]

Variable Resistance   Another variation of exercise is variable isotonic resistance such as the Nautilus (Nautilus Sports/Medical Industries, Deland, FL) with the cam shaft and the Universal Gladiator (Universal, Cedar Rapids, IA).

Isokinetic Exercises

Another form of exercise used extensively in sports medicine rehabilitation is isokinetic exercise. Commercially available isokinetic equipment includes the Cybex isokinetic Dynamometer, Orthotron, Fitron, and Kinetron (all from Cybex, Ronkonkoma, NY), Kin Com (Chattecx Corp., Chattanooga, TN), and Biodex (Biodex,

Shirley, NY). Isokinetic exercises have fixed speed with accommodating resistance. There are many advantages of isokinetic exercises:

1. Efficiency—the only way to load a dynamically contracting muscle to its maximum capacity through full ROM.
2. Safety—athletes never meet more resistance than they can lift, since it is accommodating resistance
3. Accommodating resistance that varies according to the length–tension ratio (Blix curve) of a muscle and also due to skeletal leverage changes (biomechanics), permitting accommodation to pain and fatigue so the athlete can exercise through the full ROM
4. Ability to exercise at fast functional velocities of limb speeds
5. Decreased joint compressive forces at faster speeds
6. Physiologic overflow of tension increases from faster speeds to slower speeds (i.e., specific adaptation to imposed demands)

SUBMAXIMAL EXERCISES

Little literature is available concerning the indications and effectiveness of submaximal exercises. We often integrate this concept into resistance programs in the following sequence: submaximal multiple-angle isometric exercises, maximal multiple-angle isometric exercises, submaximal short-arc (partial ROM) exercises, maximal short-arc exercises, submaximal full ROM exercises, and maximal full ROM exercises (see Box).

SUBMAXIMAL AND MAXIMAL EXERCISES AS REHABILITATION

Early rehabilitation
    Submaximal multiple-angle isometrics
    Maximal multiple-angle isometrics
Intermediate rehabilitation
    Maximal multiple-angle isometrics
    Submaximal short-arc exercises
    Maximal short-arc exercises
Late rehabilitation
    Maximal short-arc exercises
    Submaximal full ROM exercises
    Maximal full ROM exercises

PARAMETERS TO MONITOR EXERCISE RESPONSE

Once a patient is placed on an exercise program, the effects of the exercise must be continually monitored and assessed. Several parameters can be efficiently monitored on a regular basis in the clinic:

1. Subjective complaints of pain (pain rating scale: 0 to 10) or stiffness
2. Palpable increase in cutaneous temperature
3. Anthropometric measurements
4. ROM
5. ADL
6. Functional performance during exercise program

These parameters must be continually monitored to assess the effectiveness of the rehabilitation program and to determine whether there are any negative training effects, such as a resultant joint synovitis. Exercise programs should be initiated as soon as possible, taking into consideration any contraindications, such as joint effusion, limited ROM, or pain.

Most exercise programs can begin with submaximal to maximal isometric exercises. The isometric exercises can decrease joint effusion through mechanical compression by the muscle contractions. Through muscle contractions, they also provide a stimulus to the mechanoreceptors of the joints.

As pain and effusion decrease, submaximal and maximal exercises can be performed through partial ROM. A general rule of thumb is to improve muscular strength through the existing ROM, never mobilizing anything that cannot be stabilized.

As normal ROM is established, submaximal and maximal full ROM exercises are initiated. The emphasis with full ROM exercises should progress from muscular strength to muscular power and endurance. In other words, high-speed isokinetic training is functional training because of the angular velocities of lower extremities during sports performance. Biomechanical studies indicate that the angular velocity of the knee during gait is 233 degrees/s. In reviewing National Football League films, Rockwell and Garrick,[42] indicated that most medial collateral ligament injuries occur within 62.5 ms or 320 degrees/s angular velocity of the knee.

Davies et al.[43] presented specificity Cybex testing data on U.S. Olympic cross-country ski team members. The Cybex testing speeds were predicated on biomechanical

Table 21-2 Average Angular Velocities of Lower Extremity in Cross-Country Skiers

Motion	Flat Surfaces (deg/s)	Hills (deg/s)
Hip flexion/extension	469	202
Knee flexion/extension	242	241
Ankle flexion/extension	371	268

studies of films taken during actual cross-country ski competition. The angular velocities of the lower extremities are listed in Table 21-2.

Besides using fast contractile velocity exercises, we emphasize power–endurance as the hallmark of the exercise program. We emphasize a velocity-spectrum rehabilitation program at high speeds (i.e., 180 to 300 degrees/s). Furthermore, because jogging or running for 1 mile requires approximately 1,500 steps, we emphasize high numbers of repetitions or endurance training.

FUNCTIONAL REHABILITATION

Kinetic chain exercise does more than stabilize the knee joint . . . . The concurrent shifts that occur during such exercise cause unique muscular contraction and intricate muscular interactions that cannot be reproduced with joint isolation exercises.[44]

There has been a controversy of sorts in various approaches to the rehabilitation of the lower extremity following injury or surgery. This controversy has grown largely from a questioning of the benefits of machine devices creating isolated joint movements, versus those benefits of functional exercises that simulate the movements of athletes in their sport. Since one of the ultimate goals in rehabilitation is to return the injured athlete to the field in the shortest amount of time, with the lowest probability of a re-injury, this controversy has merit and deserves consideration.

Rehabilitation of the lower extremity that utilizes exercises or movements specific to those that occur in the sport activity may be termed *functional* in nature. These functional exercises or movements have been more elaborately called "closed kinetic chain" exercises.[44–51] The specificity of these exercises allows for the constant testing of the joint in a manner that has direct application to the court or playing field. Since most racquet sports, for example, rely heavily upon footwork, and speed of movement for positioning oneself for effective swings and groundstrokes, it is imperative that rehabilitation of the lower extremities consider functional and specific exercises in the rehabilitation process.

The kinetic chain, as it relates to the human body, has been defined as a combination of successively arranged joints that, when working in synchrony, constitute a motor complex.[44] The "kinetic chain" is a reference to the biomechanical link within a series of joints in which action at one joint has an effect on the joints proximal and distal to it. In the lower extremity this would include the hip, knee, and ankle. In opposition to the "closed" kinetic chain is the "open" kinetic chain. The primary difference between open and closed kinetic chain exercises is the position of the end segment. Since the end segment of the lower extremity is the foot, in closed kinetic chain activities, the foot is fixed against the ground or a groundlike platform, thereby restraining its freedom of movement. In open kinetic chain activities, the foot is free[48]; thus an isolated joint movement occurs at the knee.

The use of open kinetic chain exercises in rehabilitation of the lower extremity is often based on the rationale that an injured individual should avoid weight bearing. Similarly, available ROM may be judged insufficient, or the joint activity classification may be that it is not antigravity in function. In other words, when the lower extremity is not capable of resisting gravity through full weight bearing, open kinetic chain exercises are indicated.

Yack et al.[51] found that open kinetic chain exercises (knee extension) caused greater anterior tibial displacement than closed kinetic chain exercises (parallel squat). This finding has been supported by other investigators as well.[50,52] It was concluded that the open kinetic chain exercises placed repetitive stress on already injured tissue and on tissue not primarily involved in control of anterior tibial displacement.

Shelbourne and Nitz[52] pointed out the importance of facilitation via the return of kinesthetic awareness in their knee patients. Limited activities such as shooting basketballs or hitting tennis balls were permitted as soon as tolerated by their anterior cruciate ligament injury patients even though return to competition did not occur for 4 to 6 months postsurgery. These authors point out that closed kinetic chain exercises were emphasized in their accelerated rehabilitation protocol and open kinetic chain exercises were avoided. An important point cited by these researchers was that postoperative anterior knee pain was decreased and subjective stability of the involved knee, as well as patient confidence, were improved following the accelerated rehabilitation program. Total rehabilitation time was reduced for this group.

Lutz et al.,[47] citing rehabilitation programs used at the Mayo Clinic for anterior cruciate ligament-deficient athletes, describe a "sport-specific agility training" stage. Much of this activity is based on the development of the anterior cruciate ligament "mechanoreceptor reflex arc" involving the hamstring muscle group. This neuromuscular arc is believed to be responsible for the recruitment of the hamstring by a method of co-contraction, thus reducing pivot shift. This recruitment is stimulated through the use of balance board activities. These activities are begun in a seated position in an attempt to regain proprioception, stabilization, and muscle recruitment in a functional manner.

Gooch et al.[46] cited information on the patellofemoral compression forces during knee extension exercises. Since the surface area of contact between the patella and the femur decreases, patellofemoral compression forces are increased as the knee extends against a load. This situation can result in damage to the articular cartilage surfaces. In closed kinetic chain activities (e.g., squats, leg press), increased force occurs with knee flexion but the contact area between patella and femur is greater and offsets the increased force. Thus, weight-bearing exercises may be more beneficial than non-weight-bearing exercises for athletes with patellofemoral pain.

For the purpose of this chapter, the terms *closed kinetic chain exercises* and *functional exercises* are synonymous. Functional exercises are often specific to, or related to, both everyday life and sports-oriented activities. Those principles that apply to this type of rehabilitation include:

1. The elimination of muscle or joint isolation exercises (e.g., prone hamstring curls).
2. The initiation of all exercises with the legs, including upper body strengthening (e.g., push–press).
3. The majority of emphasis on leg work utilizing multijoint movements (e.g., squats versus seated knee extension).

The equipment utilized for functional rehabilitation of the lower extremity is primarily that known as "free weights." These free weights have the ability to allow the patient to mimic sport-specific movements under resistance-trained conditions. They allow for a large variety of exercises to be performed, thus increasing the exercises of choice available for the therapist to use. Finally, they create a need for the patient to develop "stabilizing" musculature versus agonists or prime movers only. This co-contraction of other muscles around a joint will lead to increased stabilization and serve a protective role for the joint as well as enhancing performance

In sport activities, stabilization of the body by the athlete may be a crucial factor in developing skills such as leaping, bounding, cutting, starting, and stopping. Resistive exercise utilizing machines is often classified as open kinetic chain activity. Machines may or may not be multi-joint usage in their orientation, but they certainly do not create the proprioceptive stimulation or need for balance and stabilization that free weights do.

Practical Applications

The onset of functional rehabilitation is not always a clear-cut event. Closed kinetic chain activities can be used from the very beginning of the rehabilitation process. The transition from "basic rehabilitation" to "functional rehabilitation" can often be a function of the volume and intensity variables of exercise, rather than just the choice of exercises.

Ankle, knee, or hip areas will be affected simultaneously when performing functional rehabilitation. It is possible, however, to emphasize one joint over the others through the selection of the appropriate exercises.

Minimum criteria for beginning functional exercises should include 90 to 95 percent of complete ROM in all directions available to the joint in question. At this point, it is obvious that functional rehabilitation can take many forms. Some of the following are examples of exercises used to build strength through the use of a closed kinetic chain.

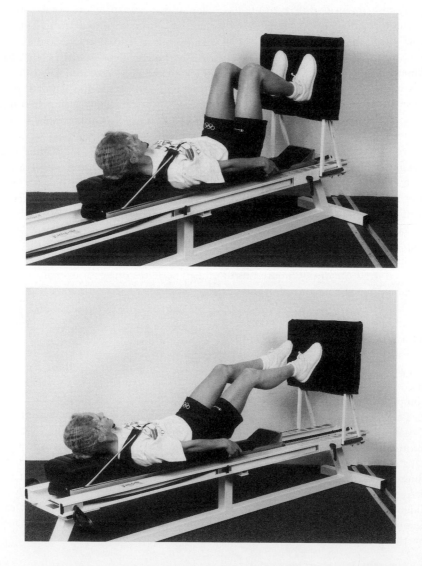

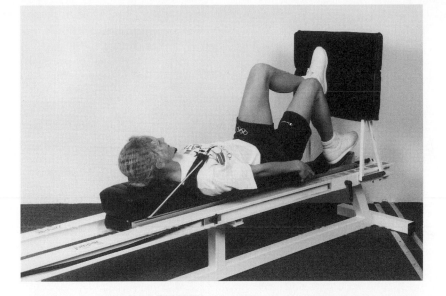

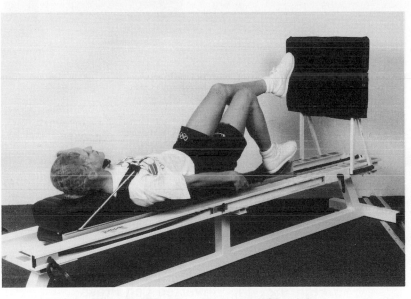

Figure 21-13: Jumper/Shuttle

The jumper/shuttle is a sledlike device in which resistance is provided through rubber tubing. Exercises can be performed with the foot/feet fixed against the base platform or, in advanced situations, where the feet break contact with the platform in a jumping motion. Table 21-3 outlines a protocol for rehabilitation using this device (see below). (© 1996 by Nancy Hines.)

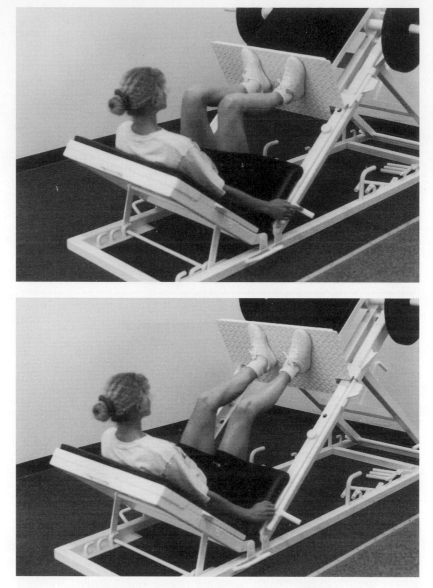

Figure 21-14:   Inverted Leg Press

This exercise is performed with the back stabilized against a floor surface. The feet are fixed against the platform of a specialized stack machine with the body in an inverted position. As the legs extend, the hamstrings and gluteal muscles are worked both concentrically and eccentrically. Stabilization of the back against the floor reduces the technical requirements of a free-weight lift. (© 1996 by Nancy Hines.)

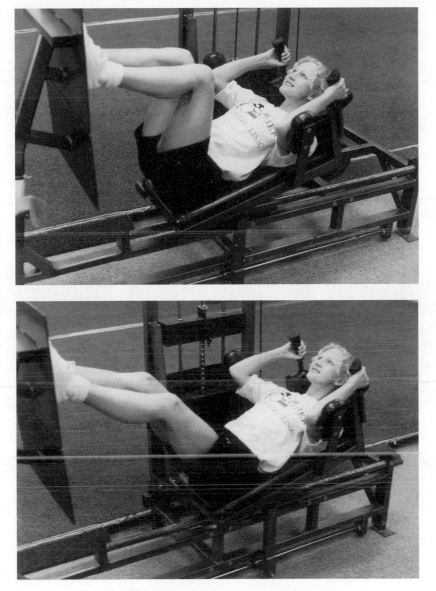

Figure 21-15:   Leg Press

This device is a machine or selectivized stack device that allows for resistance provided to a sled with the feet fixed against a platform. The resistance applied can be considerable. (© 1996 by Nancy Hines.)

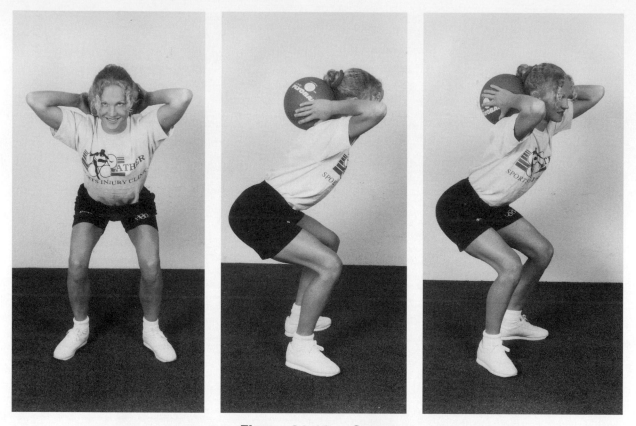

Figure 21-16:   Squat

The squat is a free-weight exercise that is a staple in most performance-oriented strength training programs. This exercise is performed with the low back in slight extension, thus "locking" the lumbar vertebral facets in a secure position. The hips move backward while the shoulders and upper body counter this movement to balance the body. Shear stress at the knee is minimized by keeping the knee at or over the toes, and not in front of the toes, from a sagittal view. (© 1996 by Nancy Hines.)

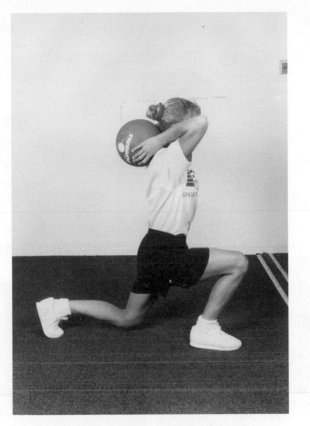

Figure 21-17:   Split Squat

Split squats are free-weight exercises performed with a front-to-back distance between the feet of 4 to 5 feet depending upon the height of the individual. The upper body is positioned in a near vertical position over the base of support. The athlete raises and lowers the center of gravity vertically. The feet are reversed to complete the exercise. (© 1996 by Nancy Hines.)

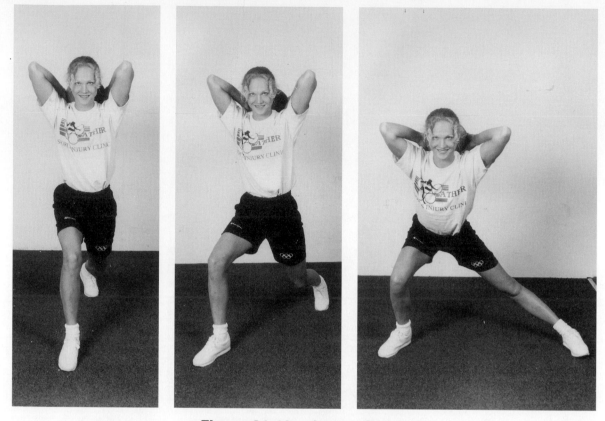

Figure 21-18:   Lunge Series

The lunge series is a free-weight exercise performed form a two-foot starting position. The athlete steps directly forward, then recovers, then steps forward on a 45-degree angle and recovers, then steps laterally and recovers. This series presents the athlete with specific activities similar to those performed in sport-specific situations. The resistance used can be relatively light but, when held behind the head, elevates the body's center of gravity, creating an even greater involvement of stabilizing musculature. (© 1996 by Nancy Hines.)

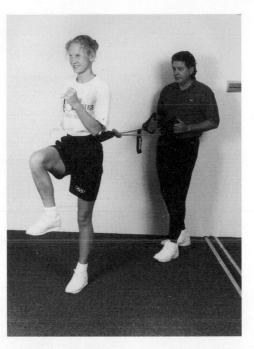

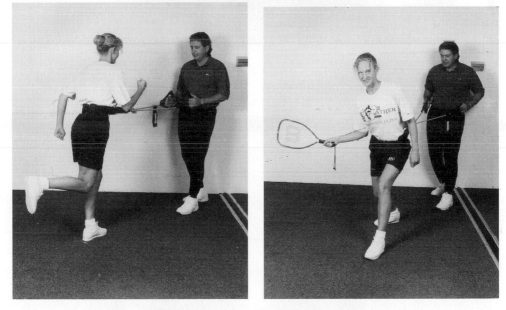

Figure 21-19: Rubber Tubing

This form of resistance allows for not only greater general closed kinetic chain activities, such as concentric and eccentric gait patterns, but resisted specific sport movements as well. Movements such as step patterns for volleys and ground strokes are also feasible. (© 1996 by Nancy Hines.)

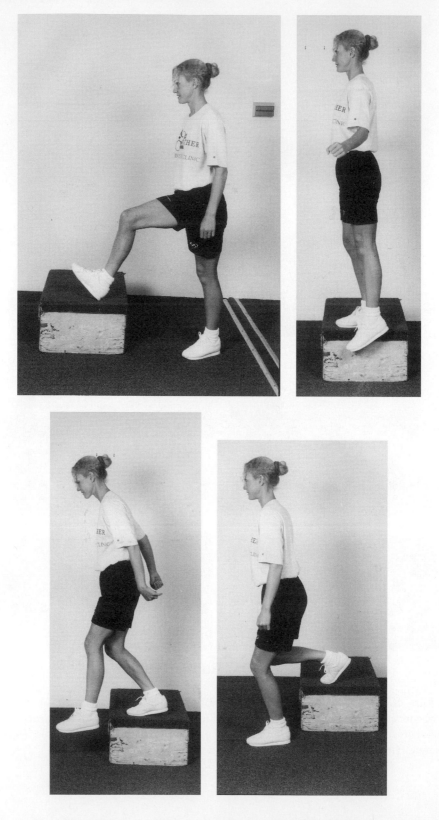

Figure 21-20: Step-Up/Downs

Boxes can be utilized for closed kinetic chain activities such as step-ups. The box shown is a 12-inch high box that is 20 inches wide. The athlete begins this exercise with the involved leg up on the box resting on the heel and the ankle dorsiflexed. The movement is initiated by digging the heel in and forcing the body forward through vigorous contraction of the hamstring muscles. The foot goes flat at midstance and the athlete moves forward and eccentrically contracts the quadriceps muscles to decelerate the body as it comes to a landing. This path of movement requires an initiation of the body movement with the hamstrings followed by deceleration of the body with the quadriceps. (© 1996 by Nancy Hines.)

Program Development

Exercises for strength development are generally begun utilizing a moderate-volume, low-intensity format, for example, two sets of 10 to 12 repetitions for a 2 to 3 week preparation cycle (Fig. 21-21). Intensity in this phase may be nothing more than body weight during this cycle. Three to six exercises may be selected from those listed in Figure 21-21 to form the core of the rehabilitation program. In addition to these core exercises, a low-intensity plyometric training program is begun utilizing the shuttle device (Table 21-3). In plyometric activity, the mechanical output of muscle increases with the speed of the prestretching of muscle and decreases with the amount of time elapsed after the stretch stimulus. This stimulates the type of contractile activities occurring in sport activities and must begin as early in the rehabilitation process as possible for re-education and training effects leading to maximum success.

Continuing along the periodization continuum, it can be noted that volume of exercise drops per each cycle, even though the number of exercises remain the same or may even increase. Intensity or load now becomes a more crucial variable, and the theories of adaptation and overload must be considered. Each cycle is marked by the use of core exercises for the lower extremities, accompanied by exercises designed to stress the "stretch-shortening cycle"[53] in the form of plyometric exercises (Tables 21-4 and 21-5). It is thought that these types of exercises can be used to simulate many of the exact forces that the athlete will encounter in competition following return to play.

An important phase in the rehabilitation process is the reassessments conducted to ensure individual progress. These may be considered an ongoing process and are employed at intervals along the periodization scheme.

Return to Play

One of the major difficulties in carrying out closed kinetic chain exercises is the quantification of the results of the program, since isokinetic testing has been used as a mainstay of quantifying strength and power development. The lack of correlation between this form of testing and closed kinetic chain results has caused some concern with clinicians. However, when one considers that testing specificity is just as important as the specificity of the rehabilitation program, it is clear the situation calls for testing that is specific to closed kinetic chain rehabilitation.

"Return to play" evaluations comprise mainly functional or field tests. Since return to activity is considered to be the endpoint of rehabilitation, it appears crucial that this system be progressive and sports specific in nature. Tegner et al.[49] described a test protocol that requires a 10-minute warmup on an ergometer, running figure-eight patterns for time, a single-leg hop three times for distance comparing the involved to the noninvolved extremity, running up and down a staircase, and sloped runs for time. Meeting standards for time and distance serve as indicators for return to play.

The single most important activity that the athlete must accomplish successfully prior to return to play is change of direction (i.e., the cutting mechanism). Andrews et al.[54] first described the cutting mechanism as early as 1977. They defined two separate cutting techniques as follows:

1. *Sidestep cut*—planting the foot opposite to the direction of intended movement.

2. *Crossover cut*—planting the foot on the same side as the new direction and then crossing the opposite leg in front to provide acceleration in the new direction.

Since both of these techniques have common applications in sport activities, it appears that these types of maneuvers are both specific and unique enough to command attention during both the rehabilitation and evaluation processes.

The value of simulating cutting maneuvers has been demonstrated by Tibone et al.[50] in evaluating the anterior cruciate ligament-deficient knee. Of interest in this study

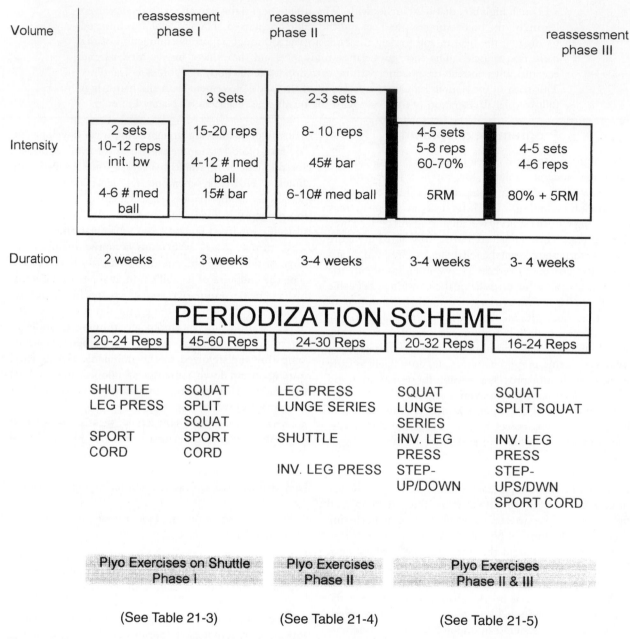

Volume

| reassessment phase I | reassessment phase II | | | reassessment phase III |

Intensity

| 2 sets 10-12 reps init. bw 4-6 # med ball | 3 Sets 15-20 reps 4-12 # med ball 15# bar | 2-3 sets 8- 10 reps 45# bar 6-10# med ball | 4-5 sets 5-8 reps 60-70% 5RM | 4-5 sets 4-6 reps 80% + 5RM |

Duration

| 2 weeks | 3 weeks | 3-4 weeks | 3-4 weeks | 3- 4 weeks |

PERIODIZATION SCHEME

| 20-24 Reps | 45-60 Reps | 24-30 Reps | 20-32 Reps | 16-24 Reps |

| SHUTTLE LEG PRESS SPORT CORD | SQUAT SPLIT SQUAT SPORT CORD | LEG PRESS LUNGE SERIES SHUTTLE INV. LEG PRESS | SQUAT LUNGE SERIES INV. LEG PRESS STEP-UP/DOWN | SQUAT SPLIT SQUAT INV. LEG PRESS STEP-UPS/DWN SPORT CORD |

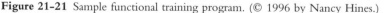

Plyo Exercises on Shuttle Phase I	Plyo Exercises Phase II	Plyo Exercises Phase II & III
(See Table 21-3)	(See Table 21-4)	(See Table 21-5)

Figure 21–21 Sample functional training program. (© 1996 by Nancy Hines.)

Table 21-3 Ather Sport Injury Clinic Low-Intensity Plyometric Protocol—Phase 1: Jumper/Shuttle

ANTERIOR CRUCIATE LIGAMENT

Purpose:	Increase range of motion to 90+ degrees (bilateral/single leg)
Volume:	30–50 repetitions; repetition to fatigue; time interval 30–90 s
Intensity:	5–8 cords
Frequency:	Daily preferred

MEDIAL COLLATERAL LIGAMENT

Purpose:	Increase range of motion to 120+ degrees (bilateral/single leg)
Volume:	50–100 repetitions; repetitions to fatigue (three times); time interval 60–120 s
Intensity:	6–8 cords
Frequency:	Daily preferred

MENISECTOMIES

Purpose:	Develop eccentric strength in lower extremities
Volume:	24–50 repetitions
Intensity:	2–8 cords
Technique:	Push off with straight/locked knees to simulate an "ankle hop"; "catch" yourself when landing on the footplace so as to lower body weight slowly to desired angle of knee flexion
Frequency:	Three times each week

PATELLAR–FEMORAL SYNDROMES

Purpose:	Develop ballistic strength in the lower extremities
Volume:	30–100 repetitions; time interval 30–90 s; sets to fatigue
Intensity:	6–8 cords
Technique:	Push off bilaterally or on single leg so as to attain maximum distance between the foot pad and the feet of the user; anticipation of the landing is a must; "touch and go" attitude is a priority; note the movement of the shuttle sled—it must not be allowed to travel to the resting position
Frequency:	Three times each week

is the fact that 17 of 20 subjects had only a 4 percent or less value for hamstring strength differences when tested on Cybex equipment. Despite most of the subjects having virtually normal hamstring strength scores as tested isokinetically, the authors concluded that the hamstrings could not compensate for the deficient anterior cruciate ligament. They further concluded that "cutting" maneuvers of a crossover nature may be used to objectively document functional pivot shift problems in the anterior cruciate ligament-deficient knee. With these concepts in mind, the functional "return to play" testing procedure must include those activities that stress and test the athlete's ability to change direction. These measures may be accomplished using hand stopwatches, tape measures, and boxes or cones for various tasks. A typical evaluation might resemble the one used at the Ather Sport Injury Clinic (Fig. 21-22).

Table 21-4 Ather Sport Injury Clinic Plyometric Protocols—Phase II: Box and Cones

BOX PLYOMETRICS (with 6- to 12-inch-high box)
Routine (20- to 30-s time intervals):
1. Right foot on box; push up to get clearance; "touch and go" at landing
2. Repeat with left foot
3. Repeat alternating feet
4. Side-to-Side: start with two feet on one side of box and exchange feet while moving laterally; change direction and repeat
5. Box Drill: Start with two feet on one side of box and move laterally across, touching the box top with both feet; upon landing on the other side, reverse direction and repeat
6. Hands behind the head to eliminate the use of the arms: jump repeatedly from the ground to box top

Any part of this routine can be used as an individual exercise or combination to form a plyometric circuit.

CONE DRILLS
Volume: 3–6 times over six cones; increase to 10 times over 10 cones
Intensity: 8- to 12-inch cone
Frequency: 2–3 times per week

Forward Movement—Space cones approximately 3–4 feet apart. Hop forward, spending a minimal amount of time on the ground between cones.

Lateral Movement—Repeat as above in both right and left directions.

Forward-Backward Combinations—Hop forward over one cone, then backward over the cone; hop forward over two cones and backward over one; forward over three cones and backward over one.

Lateral Combinations—Hop laterally over cones with both feet; change direction at each end so that the cones are transversed three times. Variation: land on the outside of the cones on one foot and change direction.

180-Degree Turns—Hop over the cone and turn a 180-degree turn in the air. Immediately upon landing, reverse direction; repeat over each cone.

Table 21-5 Ather Sport Injury Clinic Plyometric Protocols—Phase III: Cone Drills and Shuttle Runs

Recommended Time Volumes: 30–120 S

Single Leg Hops—Done with a distance of 3–6 feet for the advanced candidate. Individual takes off and lands on one foot over each cone.

Cone Hops with Medicine Ball Throw—Three cones are set in a single row. Individual jumps back and forth laterally. Therapist throws medicine ball to the same side as individual lands. Individual catches and returns ball, then resumes hopping in opposite direction and repeats for prescribed number of repetitions.

Cone Hops with Sprints Left–Right—As above; individual is directed to a mark set approximately 10–25 feet away. Sprints back and resumes hopping. Repeat for prescribed time volume.

Cone Exchange Drill—Two cones are placed approximately 25–30 feet away from a single cone. Individual grasps one cone and sprints to other side, exchanging cones; this action is continued for prescribed time volume.

Timing devices with switch mats may serve as excellent indicators of consistent movement abilities. Cybex has developed a sophisticated timing device (Fig. 21-23) that allows the tester to evaluate differences in ground reaction times, transit speeds, and stabilization times. Furthermore, it allows one to evaluate each limb individually. It is of interest that preliminary data suggest consistent differences between involved and noninvolved extremities on stabilization, transit speeds, and ground reaction times for nonsurgical anterior cruciate ligament-deficient knees. Involved extremities have been consistently deficient in each of these categories when tested on the reactor at the Ather Sport Injury Clinic. The involved extremity has demonstrated difficulty with eccentric forces and stabilization during landing and with developing concentric forces during push-off.

This form of testing, along with maneuvers such as those described by Tibone et al.,[50] will help to define the status of the athlete who desires to return to play. As each activity is accomplished and the athlete demonstrates normal movement patterns, they will also show increased confidence and a willingness to return to activity.

Summary

Rehabilitation of the lower extremities has fallen into two basic categories known as "open" and "closed" kinetic chain activities. Closed kinetic chain exercises are functional exercises that are specific to sport movement patterns. Exercises performed with a variety of equipment may be classified as closed kinetic chain. Program development should include a variety of functional exercises utilizing variable volumes and intensities of resistance for maximum results. "Return to play" evaluations should utilize "field tests" that are specific to sport movement patterns and consistent with closed kinetic chain rehabilitation.

COMMON RUNNING PROBLEMS AND REHABILITATION: REGIONAL APPROACH

The following brief comments about specific running problems are not meant as a cookbook approach to each injury. They simply provide clinical guidelines we have found effective. The etiologic factor must be treated, and not just the signs and symptoms present at the moment. Again, a problem-oriented approach to rehabilitation is advocated.

To prevent redundancy, with a holistic problem-oriented rehabilitation program, the following components should be integrated into the rehabilitation program at the appropriate times:

1. To prevent deconditioning, total body musculoskeletal conditioning should be away from the injured area. With a lower extremity injury, the upper body, trunk musculature, and uninvolved lower extremity are continually exercised. Although controversial, there is some evidence of cross-transference of positive musculoskeletal gains. Therefore, working on the uninvolved lower extremity may actually help improve the involved side.

2. On the injured lower extremity, since we are dealing with a kinetic chain, the proximal and distal musculature must be exercised.

3. Exercises to promote cardiovascular–respiratory endurance, such as circuit weight training (CWT),[55] cycling, and swimming, are encouraged as part of the rehabilitation program (Fig. 21-24). Costill[56] demonstrated additional benefits of cycling to the musculoskeletal system.

4. Cryotherapy in the form of ice massage or ice packs is generally included post-treatment to decrease potential treatment soreness or inflammation.

5. The athlete is taught how to avoid training errors.

6. A progressive gradual return to functional activities is part of the rehabilitation program. The discharge pa-

Name:_____ Dx:_____ Dr._____

Phase I Test:

Heel raises X 15_____ Heel walk X 15ft._____ Toe walk X 15ft._____

Stork stand: Eyes open (sec.)_____ Eyes closed (sec.)_____

Step-ups: forward (3 X 10)_____ lateral (3 X 10)_____

Hops: BL10X _____ Side-Side 30X_____ Circle 5X_____

Hops: SL 5X _____ Side-Side 10X_____ Ladder 5X_____

Phase II Test:

(Timed in seconds)

Walk/Jog 10yds - 1/2 speed_____ 3/4 speed_____ full speed_____

30yds - 1/2 speed_____ 3/4 speed_____ full speed_____

60yds - 1/2 speed_____ 3/4 speed_____ full speed_____

Sprinting:

Technique_____

Forward (distance)_____

Backward (distance)_____

Carioca (distance)_____

Phase III Test:

Hexagon test: T1_____ T2_____ T3_____

Quick Foot Drill_____ _____ _____ _____ _____ _____ Tt_____

Amortization phase: Depth Jumps _____ T1

_____ T2

_____ T3

Cutting:

135 degree cut 1/2 speed_____ 3/4 speed_____ full speed_____

90 degree cut 1/2 speed_____ 3/4 speed_____ full speed_____

Phase IV Test:

Other Activities Cleared:

Swimming:_____

_____

Biking:_____

_____

NEEDS ANALYSIS:(Sports Specific)

_____

_____

LIMITATIONS/COMMENTS:

Drills only:_____ Non-contact_____ Full

Practice:_____ Competition:_____

_____

_____

_____

_____

Figure 21–22 The "return to play" evaluation used at the Ather Sport Injury Clinic in Castro Valley, California. (© 1996 by Nancy Hines.)

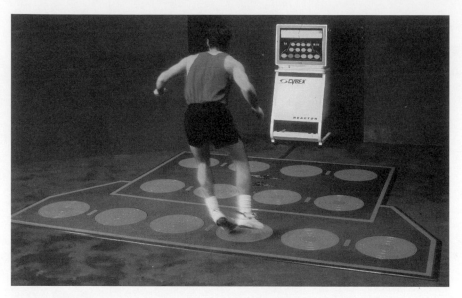

Figure 21-23 The Reactor (Cybex, Ronkonkoma, NY, with permission).

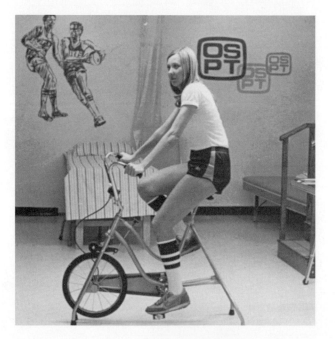

Figure 21-24 Cycling for cardiovascular endurance.

	R	L			
Anthropometric measurements	___	___	Functional rehabilitation		
	___	___	1. Toe/heel raises	___	
	___	___	2. Jog slowly, start	___	
	___	___	3. Jog faster	___	
	___	___	4. Jog faster; stop and start	___	
Pain	___	___	5. Run on track	___	
AROM	___	___	6. Sprinting	___	
PROM	___	___	7. Jog figure-eights	___	
Biomechanical corrections	___	___	8. Run figure-eights	___	
Assistive devices (taping, braces)	___	___	9. Cariocas	___	
Flexibility			10. Cutting: half-speed	___	
Achilles/gastrocsoleus	___	___	11. Cutting: full-speed	___	
Hamstrings	___	___	12. Increase distance; cross-country running	___	
Low back	___	___	13. Continue weight training	___	
Abductors	___	___	14. Return: drills	___	
Adductors	___	___	15. Return: noncontact	___	
Iliotibial band	___	___	16. Return: practice	___	
Hip flexors	___	___	17. Return: competition	___	
Rectus femoris	___	___	18. Cybex tests: S,P,E	___	
Quadriceps	___	___	Follow-up	___	
Balance/proprioception	___	___	1 month	___	
Cybex			6 months	___	
Strength			12 months	___	
Quadriceps	___	___			
Hamstrings	___	___			
Power					
Quadriceps	___	___			
Hamstrings	___	___			
Power					
Quadriceps	___	___			
Endurance	___	___			

Figure 21-25 Checklist for discharge from sports physical injury: lower extremity injuries.

rameters for athletes who have sustained a lower extremity injury are listed in Figure 21-25. Furthermore, in most instances, the PRICE formula is the basis of immediate or acute care treatment:

*P*rotection of the area from further injury with use of crutches and bracing or casting (protected exercises can be continued whereby the involved area is protected, but other areas can be maintained through CWT, swimming, cycling, and upper extremity exercises)

*R*est from exertion of the area to prevent further damage but not from protected (limited) functional movement

*I*ce or cryotherapy

*C*ompression

*E*levation and *E*ducation

This convenient formula is used to educate athletes about the injury and inform them of the mechanism, immediate treatment, prognosis, and expected requirements and performance during the rehabilitation program. Athletes are warned that they will pay the PRICE with prolonged morbidity and possibility of reinjury if they do not cooperate, demonstrate compliance, and follow rehabilitation recommendations. The athlete will thereby increase the chances of returning to the former level of competition without negative sequelae.

The following list indicates common sports injuries of the lower extremity and specific rehabilitation programs that we have found clinically effective.

REHABILITATION OF COMMON SPORTS INJURIES OF THE LOWER EXTREMITY

Lumbar Spine

Muscle strains
  PRICE
  Ultrasound/phonophoresis
  Cross-transverse friction massage
  Stretching exercises
  Active exercises
  Resisted exercises (from flexion to extension); abdominal exercises

Facet sprains
  PRICE
  Mobilization (Fig. 21-26)
  Active exercise
  Resistive exercises (flexion to extension)

Ligamentous sprains
  Treatment same as for facet sprains

Sciatica from disc injury
  PRICE
  Passive hyperextension[57] (Fig. 21-27)
  No passive flexion exercises
  Active exercise
  Resisted exercises

Mechanical dysfunctions
  PRICE
  Mobilization
  Active exercise
  Resisted exercises

Sacroiliac Joint

Torsion dysfunction
  PRICE
  Mobilization for correction (Fig. 21-28)
  If hypermobile, sacroiliac belt support
  Active exercises
  Resisted exercises

Short leg
  Mobilization for correction
  If hypermobile, sacroiliac belt for support
  Heel lift, if indicated

Pes cavus foot
  Shoes with good rearfoot and forefoot cushioning
  Soft orthotics for cushioning
  Training recommendations
    Continually switch sides of road
    Train on soft level surfaces

Road crown training error
    Continually switch sides of road

Hip

Hip flexor strain
  PRICE
  Ultrasound/phonophoresis
  Cryotherapy and flexibility exercises
  Active exercises
  Resisted exercises
  Wraps (Fig. 21-29)
  Prevent training errors

Rectus femoris strain
  Treatment same as for hip flexor strain

Iliotibial band syndrome (hip) (greater trochanteric bursitis)
  PRICE
  Phonophoresis to hip
  Cryotherapy and flexibility exercises
  PNF to iliotibial band
  Active exercises: hip abductor
  Resisted exercises: lateral step-ups; adductors (Fig. 21-30)
  ADL: lean-in standing position to involved side
  Prevent training errors: change sides of road
  Orthotics, if indicated
  Heel lift, if indicated

High hamstring strain
  PRICE
  Phonophoresis
  Cross-transverse friction massage
  Cryotherapy and flexibility exercises
  Active exercises
  Resisted exercises
  Prevent training errors

Adductor strain
  Treatment same as for hamstrings

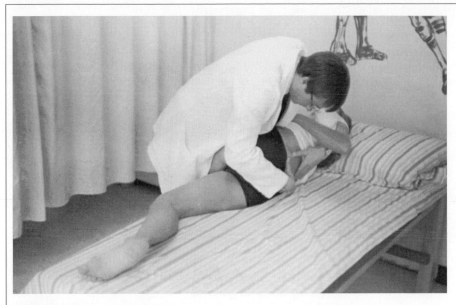

Figure 21-26 Mobilization technique for lumbar spine facet joints.

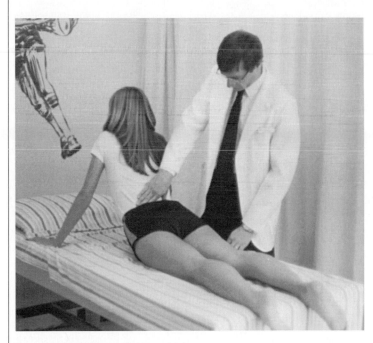

Figure 21-27 Passive hyperextension.

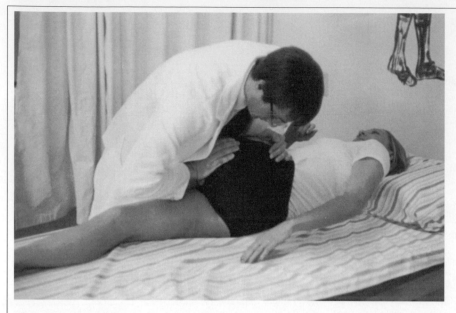

Figure 21-28 Mobilization technique for anterior torsion of iliac bone at sacroiliac joint.

Thigh

Quadriceps strain
    Treatment same as for hamstrings

Hamstring strain
    Treatment same as for high hamstrings

Knee

Patellofemoral problems
    PRICE
    Cryotherapy
    Flexibility exercises
    Orthotics, if indicated
    Knee appliances, taping
    Quad sets
    Straight leg raises (Fig. 21-31)
    Short arc (terminal extension exercises)
    Full-ROM submaximal to maximal high-speed
      isokinetics

Iliotibial band syndrome
    Treatment same as for hip, except phonophoresis,
      flexibility, and exercises are directed toward knee;
      orthotics, if indicated (Fig. 21-32)

Popliteus tendinitis
    PRICE
    Phonophoresis
    Orthotics, if indicated
    Prevent training errors; prevent downhill running

Medial plica syndrome (Fig. 21-33)
    PRICE
    Phonophoresis
    Cross-transverse friction massage
    Flexibility exercises
    Active exercises
    Resisted exercises
    Knee appliance
    Orthotics, if indicated

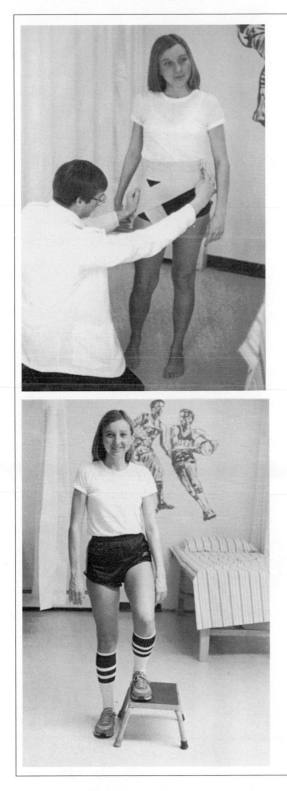

Figure 21-29 Ace bandage for hip strain

Figure 21-30 Lateral step-up exercises.

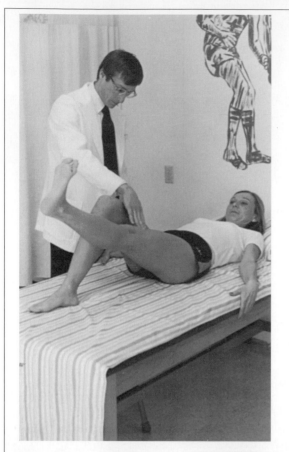

Figure 21–31 Straight leg raise.

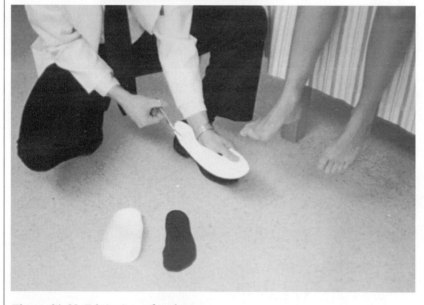

Figure 21–32 Fabricating soft orthotics.

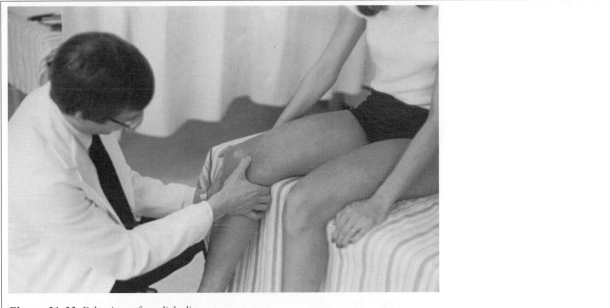

Figure 21-33 Palpation of medial plica.

LIGAMENTOUS/CAPSULAR INJURIES

Because of the tremendous complexity and controversy regarding the classification of knee ligamentous/capsular injuries, the specific details of various rehabilitation programs are also a matter of controversy. One very important concept when dealing with ligamentous/capsular injuries and rehabilitation is the biomechanics of ligamentous healing. Noyes et al.[58-68] produced some fascinating work to provide a scientific basis for rehabilitation of ligamentous injuries based on soft tissue healing.

Many variables are involved in knee rehabilitation, including mechanism of injury, structures involved, severity of involvement, type of immobilization, time frame, surgical procedure, and philosophical approach. An overview of the knee in sports as well as information on rehabilitation programs is given by Malone and Blackburn.[69] Rehabilitation for each specific injury or surgical repair as well as the patient's needs require modifications and individualization of the rehabilitation program. An understanding of normal joint structures and their reaction to injury[70-72] is useful in designing a rehabilitation program. An important consideration and goal following a ligamentous injury, particularly after prolonged immobilization, is to protect the articular cartilage of the patellofemoral joint and prevent the creation of an iatrogenically induced patellofemoral joint problem. Prolonged immobilization leads to a number of adverse effects from disuse,[73-80] making several structures more vulnerable to injury. Consequently, the rehabilitation program must initiate controlled motion[80-83] as soon as possible and yet protect the articular cartilage and the collagen tissue maturation during the biomechanics of soft tissue healing.

Some very general guidelines for ligamentous/capsular exercise rehabilitation are described below. Quadriceps sets and straight leg raises are included in most programs.

Collateral ligament sprains: exercise through mid-ROM with short-arc exercise, 70 to 30 degrees.

Anterior cruciate ligament insufficiency: exercise program emphasizes hamstrings and rotary muscles at the knee. The quadriceps is de-emphasized because of the anterior subluxation of the tibia with quadriceps contractions, which increases the instability, unless performed in CKC position.

Anteromedial rotary instability: emphasis is placed on medial hamstrings for flexion work to about 20 degrees of flexion to prevent the tibia from going to external rotation and further stretching the mid third of the medial capsule and posteromedial oblique ligament. The medial rotators (pes anserine muscles) are also emphasized.

Anterolateral rotary instability (ALRI): emphasis is placed on lateral hamstrings for flexion work from 20 degrees to flexion. Quadriceps extension exercises are encouraged from 30 to 0 degrees to emphasize external tibial rotation to tighten and reinforce the mid third of the lateral capsule and arcuate complex. the cause of the ALRI must be determined, because this may be modified if the primary instability is due to the primary restraint (anterior cruciate ligament) and its functional status or the secondary restraint (midthird of the lateral capsule). *Posterolateral rotary instability:* emphasis is placed on quadriceps exercises from 90 to 20 degrees to prevent tibial external rotation and placing excessive pressure on the arcuate complex.

KNEE REHABILITATION

PRICE

Flexibility exercises

Electrical stimulation

Quadriceps sets, if indicated

Straight leg raise, if indicated

Active exercises

Mobilization of the patella (Fig. 21-34)

Balance, proprioceptive exercises (Fig. 21-35)

Resisted exercises (submaximal to maximal)
    Multiple-angle isometrics
       to
    Short arc exercises
       to
    Full ROM exercises isokinetically

Plyometrics

Functional exercises

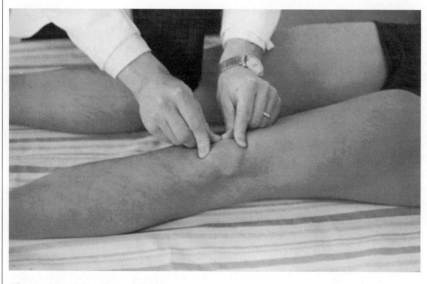

Figure 21-34 Patella mobilization.

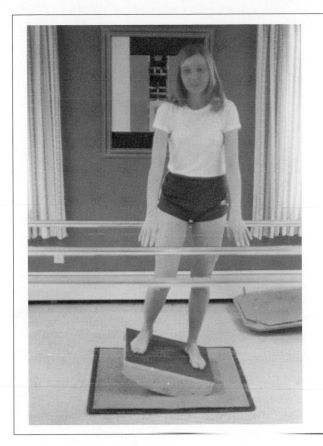

Figure 21-35 Balance/proprioceptive exercises.

LOWER LEG

When dealing with lower leg problems, it is necessary to rule out particular conditions that may mimic signs and symptoms of "shin splints." Conditions to be ruled out include stress fractures, intermittent claudication, medial tibial stress syndrome, and chronic compartment syndromes.

Anterolateral "Shin Splints"

Shin splints is a "garbage-can" term and has no place in defining an injury. As emphasized throughout this chapter, the specific structures involved as well as the etiology must be identified before an injury can be treated and rehabilitated. Therefore, with anterolateral "shin splints," we are primarily referring to inflammatory reaction to microtrauma to the anterior tibialis muscle. There are several causes, including forefoot varus, poorly conditioned muscles, tight posterior muscle groups, running on hard sur-

faces, and running with shoes that have poor forefoot cushioning. Cavanaugh[84] identified this as the area of highest impact between interfaces (see Box).

TREATMENT OF ANTEROLATERAL "SHIN SPLINTS"

PRICE

Orthotics, if indicated

Active exercises

Resisted exercises

Flexibility exercises—posterior muscle groups

Encourage softer running surfaces

Shoes with good forefoot cushioning[84]

Posteromedial "Shin Splints"

Posteromedial "shin splints" primarily represent a posterior tibialis tendonitis/periostitis/myositis (see Boxes).

TREATMENT OF POSTEROMEDIAL "SHIN SPLINTS"

PRICE

Taping (low-dye strap, Herzog)

Orthotics, if indicated

Phonophoresis/ultrasound

Cross-transverse friction massage

Proper flexibility for posterior muscles with supinated foot position

Active exercises

Resisted exercises—non-weight bearing to prevent further stretching of posterior tibialis; usually high-speed isokinetic exercises

TREATMENT OF OTHER LOWER LEG CONDITIONS

Tendinitis Conditions

PRICE

Ultrasound/phonophoresis

Cross-transverse friction massage

Flexibility

Active exercises

Resisted exercise

Orthotics, if indicated

Gradual return to functional activities (Fig. 21-36)

Tenosynovitis Conditions

Treatment same as for tendinitis conditions

Achilles Tendinitis

Treatment same as for tendinitis

Add bilateral heel lifts to decrease stress and stretch on Achilles tendons (Fig. 21-37)

Bursitis

Ultrasound/phonophoresis

Eliminate etiologic factor

Ankle Sprains

PRICE

Contrast baths

Active exercises

Resistive exercise

Flexibility

Balance exercises

Taping and wrapping (Fig. 21-38)

Plantar Fasciitis (Heel Spur Syndrome; Bursitis)

PRICE

Ultrasound/phonophoresis

Orthotics (with modifications if heel spur is present)

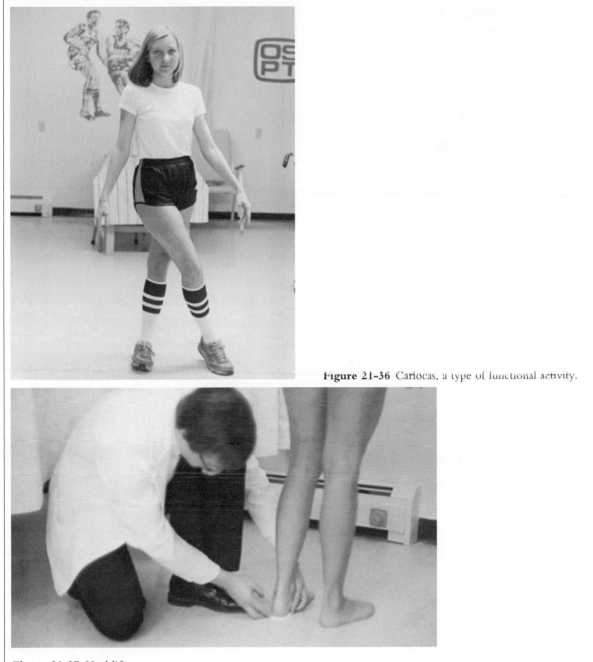

Figure 21–36 Cariocas, a type of functional activity.

Figure 21-37 Heel lifts.

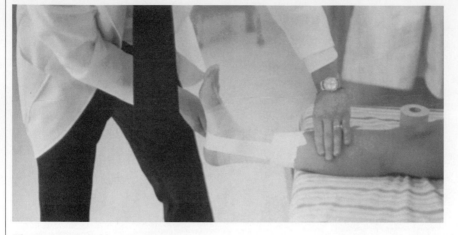

Figure 21-38 Ankle taping.

PREVENTION

Although this chapter has been primarily oriented to treatment and rehabilitation, the most important area of the health care delivery system is prevention. Many of the aforementioned techniques used as rehabilitation, if applied before the injury, can also serve as preventive measures. Many deficiencies can be identified in preseason screening programs and preventive prehabilitation to prevent or reduce injuries. The Sports Physical Therapy Section of the American Physical Therapy Association[85] has published a book to provide guidelines for screening programs. Sports physical therapy does not have to be only an ex post facto profession whereby we intervene after an injury occurs; we also have many skills and the knowledge base to help prevent injuries.

Various preventive techniques include

1. Breaking the inflammatory/injury cycle

2. Appropriate and properly performed warmups

3. Cooldown

4. Appropriate and properly performed flexibility exercises

5. Maintenance of total body muscular strength, power, and endurance

6. Maintenance of cardiovascular–respiratory endurance

7. Modification of biomechanical dysfunctions

8. Maintenance of joint proprioception and balance

9. Use of judicious training programs

    a. Avoidance of mileage mania

    b. Training intensity

10. Athletic footwear

11. Appropriate training surfaces

12. "Reading" the body, educating the athlete

SUMMARY

This chapter provides an introduction to rehabilitation, sports physical therapy examination concepts and techniques, and rehabilitation concepts and techniques. Physical therapy rehabilitation involves the use of general assistive devices, assistive devices (appliances) for the knee, flexibility exercises, balance/proprioception exercises, manual therapy (mobilization) techniques, various physical therapy modalities, and exercises. Rehabilitation techniques that have proved effective in treating various lower-extremity injuries are briefly identified. Finally, since the most important area of health-care delivery is prevention, several preventive techniques are outlined.

ACKNOWLEDGMENTS

We would like to thank Carol Davies for serving as the model, Mrs. Lillian Smith for typing the manuscript, and Doug Ross for the photography.

REFERENCES

1. Davies GJ, Larson RL: Examining the knee. Physician Sportsmed 6:49, 1978
2. Davies GJ, Malone T, Bassett FH: Knee exam. Phys Ther 60:1565, 1980
3. Daniels L, Worthingham C: Muscle Testing. 5th ed. WB Saunders, Philadelphia, 1986
4. Aten D: Crutches: essential in caring for lower extremity injuries. Physician Sportsmed 8:121, 1980
5. Basmajian JV: Crutch and cane exercises and use. p. 228. In Hoberman M (ed): Therapeutic Exercise. Williams & Wilkins, Baltimore, 1978
6. Cody J (ed): Techniques of Taping. Texas Kurik Kare Products, 1974
7. Athletic Uses of Adhesive Tape. Johnson & Johnson, New Brunswick, NJ, 1973
8. Dixon D: The Dictionary of Athletic Taping. Bloomcraft Central Printing, IN, 1965
9. Arnheim DD, Prentice WE: Principles of Athletic Training. 8th ed. CV Mosby, St. Louis, 1993
10. Guyton AC: Textbook of Medical Physiology. WB Saunders, Philadelphia, 1976
11. Nicholas JA: Injuries to knee ligaments: relationships to looseness and tightness in football players. JAMA 2:2236, 1970
12. Glick JM: A study of ligamentous looseness in football players and its relationship to injury. p. 34. In Abbott Proceedings 1, 1971
13. DeVries HA: Prevention of muscular distress after exercise. Res Q 32:177, 1961
14. Uram P: The Complete Stretching Book. Anderson World, Bolinas, CA, 1980
15. Voss DE, Ionta MK, Myers BJ: Proprioceptive Neuromuscular Facilitation. 3rd Ed. Harper & Row, Philadelphia, 1985
16. Travell J, Rinzler SH: The myofascial genesis of pain. Postgrad Med 11:425, 1952
17. Mennel JM: Spray and stretch treatment for myofascial pain. Hosp Physician, p. 1, 1973
18. Knight K: Cryotherapy: Theory, Technique and Physiology. Chattanoga Corporation, Chattanooga, TN, 1985
19. Wyke B: Neurology of Joints. APTA Instructional Course, presented at the 55th Conference of the APTA, Atlanta, June 1979
20. Maitland GD: Peripheral Manipulation. Butterworth, London, 1979
21. Kaltenborn FM: Manual Therapy for the Extremity Joints. Olaf Horbis Bokhandel, Oslo, 1976
22. Griffin JE, Karselis TC: Physical Agents for Physical Therapists. Charles C Thomas, Springfield, IL, 1979
23. Shriber WJ: A Manual of Electrotherapy. Lea & Febiger. Philadelphia, 1975
24. Prentice WE: Therapeutic Modalities in Sports Medicine. Times Mirror/Mosby. St. Louis, 1990
25. Krusen FH, et al: Handbook of Physical Medicine and Rehabilitation. WB Saunders, Philadelphia, 1971
26. Rogoff JB (ed): Manipulation, Traction, and Massage. Williams & Wilkins, Baltimore, 1980
27. Michlovitz SL: Thermal Agents in Rehabilitation. FA Davis, Philadelphia, 1990
28. Krejci V, Koch P: Muscle and Tendon Injuries in Athletes. Year Book Medical Publishers, Chicago, 1979
29. Quillen WS: Phonophoresis: a review of the literature and technique. Athletic Training 15:109, 1980
30. Kahn J: Low Volt Technique. J. Kahn, Syosset, NY, 1978
31. Notes on Low Volt Therapy, Teca Corp, NY
32. Burdick, Inc.: Low Voltage Currents. Burdick Corp, Milton, WI, 1969
33. Brown I: Fundamentals of Electrotherapy. American Printing and Publishing, Madison, WI, 1974
34. Eriksson E, Hazzmark T: Comparison of isometric muscle training and electrical stimulation supplementary isometric muscle training in the recovery after major knee ligament surgery. Am J Sports Med 7:169, 1979
35. Johnson DH, Thurston P, Ushcroft, PJ: The Russian technique of faradism in the treatment of chrondromalacia patella. Physiotherapy 29, 1977
36. Garrett TR, Laughman RK, Youdas JW: Strengthening brought about by a new Canadian muscle stimulator: a preliminary study, abstracted. Phys Ther 60:617, 1980
37. Lampe G: A Clinical Approach to TENS in the Treatment of Chronic and Acute Pain. Med General, Minneapolis, MN, 1978
38. Knapik JJ, Ramos MU, Wright JE: Non-specific effects of isometric and isokinetic strength training at a particular joint angle, abstracted. Med Sci Sports Exerc, 12:120, 1980
39. De Lorme TL: Restoration of muscle power by heavy resistance exercises. J Bone Joint Surg 27:645, 1945
40. Zinovieff AN: Heavy resistance exercise. the Oxford techniques. Br J Phys Med 14:29, 1951
41. Knight KL: Knee rehabilitation by the daily adjustable progressive resistance exercise technique. Am J Sports Med 7: 336, 1980
42. Rockwell J, Garrick J: High speed training is the secret to successful isokinetic training. Physician Sportsmed 7(12):13, 1979
43. Davies GJ, Halback J, Wilson P et al: A descriptive muscular power analysis of U.S. cross-country ski team, abstracted. Med Sci Sports Exerc 12:141, 1980
44. Palmitier R, An K, Scott S, et al: Kinetic chain exercise in knee rehabilitation. Sports Med 11:6, 1991
45. Curl W, Markey K, Mitchell W: Agility training following anterior cruciate ligament reconstruction. Clin Orthop Rel Res 172:133, 1983
46. Gooch J, Geiringer S, Akau C: Sports medicine: three lower extremities injuries. Arch Phys Med Rehab 74:S438, 1993
47. Lutz G, Stuart M, Sim F: Rehabilitative techniques for ath-

letes after reconstruction of the anterior cruciate ligament. Mayo Clin Proc 65:1322, 1990

48. Panariello R: The closed kinetic chain in strength training. Nat Strength Conditioning J 13:29, 1991

49. Tegner Y, Lysholm J, Lysholm M, et al: A performance test to monitor rehabilitation and evaluate anterior cruciate ligament injuries. Am J Sports Med 14:156, 1986

50. Tibone J, Antich T, Fanton G, et al: Functional analysis of anterior cruciate ligament instability. Am J Sports Med 14:276, 1986

51. Yack H, Collins C, Whieldon T: Comparison of closed and open kinetic chain exercise in the anterior cruciate ligament-deficient knee. Am J Sports Med 21:49, 1993

52. Shelbourne K, Nitz P: Accelerated rehabilitation after anterior cruciate ligament reconstruction. Am J Sports Med 18:292, 1990

53. Bobbert M, Huijing P, Gerrit J: Drop jumping II: the influence of dropping height on the biomechanics of drop jumping. Med Sci Sports Exerc 19:339, 1987

54. Andrews J, McLeod W, Ward T, et al: The cutting mechanism. Am J Sports Med 5:111, 1977

55. Gettman LR, Pollock ML: Circuit weight training: a critical review of its physiological benefits. Physician Sportsmed 9:44, 1981

56. Costill D: Knee rehabilitation. Physician Sportsmed, 1972

57. McKenzie R: Treat Your Own Back. Spinal Publications, Waikanae, New Zealand, 1980

58. Noyes FR, DeLucas JL, Torvik PJ: Biomechanics of anterior cruciate ligament failure: an analysis of strainrate sensitivity and mechanisms of failure in primates. J Bone Joint Surg [Am] 56:226, 1974

59. Noyes FR, Torvik PJ, Hyde WB, DeLucas JL: Biomechanics of ligament failure. II. An analysis of immobilization, exercise and reconditioning effects in primates. J Bone Joint Surg [Am] 56:1406, 1974

60. Noyes FR, Grood ES: Strength of the anterior cruciate ligament in humans and rhesus: age and species-related changes. J Bone Joint Surg [Am] 58:1074, 1976

61. Grood ES, Noyes FR: Cruciate ligament prosthesis: strength, creep and fatigue properties. J Bone Joint Surg [Am] 58:1083, 1976

62. Noyes FR, Grood ES, Nussbaum NS, Cooper SM: Effect of intra-articular corticosteroids on ligament properties: a biomechanical and histological study in rhesus knees. Clin Orthop 123:197, 1977

63. Noyes FR: Functional properties of knee ligaments and alterations induced by immobilization: a correlative biomechanical and histological study in primates. Clin Orthop 123:210, 1977

64. Butler DL, Zernicke RL, Noyes FR, Grood ES: Biomechanics of ligaments and tendons. p. 125. In Hutton R (ed): Exercise and Sports Science Review. Vol. 6. The Franklin Institute Press, Philadelphia, 1978

65. Butler DL, Noyes FR, Grood WS: Ligamentous restraints to anterior-posterior drawer in the human knee. J Bone Joint Surg [Am] 62:259, 1980

66. Noyes FR, Grood ES, Butler DL, Paulos LE: Clinical biomechanics of the knee—ligament restraints and functional stability. In Funk J (ed): American Association of Orthopedic Surgeons, Symposium on the Athlete's Knee. CV Mosby, St. Louis, 1980

67. Noyes FR, Bassett RW, Grood ES, Butler DL: Arthroscopy in acute traumatic hemarthrosis of the knee—incidence of anterior cruciate tears and other injuries. J Bone Joint Surg [Am] 62:687, 1980

68. Grood ES, Noyes FR, Butler DL, Suntay WJ: Ligamentous restraints in the intact human knee: straight medial and lateral laxity. J Bone Joint Surg [Am] 63:1257, 1981

69. Malone T, Blackburn TA (eds): The knee—athletic injuries. Phys Ther 60, 1980

70. Hettinga DL: Normal joint structures and their reaction to injury. I. JOSPT 1:16, 1979

71. Hettinga DL: Normal joint structures and their relation to injury. II. JOSPT 1:83, 1979

72. Hettinga DL: Normal joint structures and their relation to injury. III. JOSPT 1:178, 1980

73. Akeson WH: An experimental study in joint stiffness. J Bone Joint Surg 43A:1022, 1961

74. Akeson WH, Amiel D, LaVilette D: Connective tissue response to immobility. Clin Orthop 51:183, 1967

75. Finsterbush A, Friedman B: Early changes in an immobilized rabbit knee joint. Clin Orthop 92:305, 1973

76. Mooney V, Ferguson AB: The influence of immobilization and motion on the formation of fibrocartilage in the repair granuloma after joint resection in the rabbit. J Bone Joint Surg [Am] 48:1145, 1966

77. Viidik A: Effect of training on the tensile strength of isolated rabbit tendons. Scand J Plast Reconstr Surg 1:141, 1967

78. Laros GS, Tipton CM, Cooper RR: Influence of physical activity on ligament insertions in knees of dogs. J Bone Joint Surg [Am] 53:275, 1971

79. Cooper RR, Misol S: Tendon and ligament insertions. J Bone Joint Surg [Am] 52:1, 1970

80. Jack EA: Experimental rupture of the medial collateral ligament of the knee. J Bone Joint Surg [Br] 32:396, 1950

81. Dehne E, Torp RP: Treatment of joint injuries by immediate mobilization. Clin Orthop 77:218, 1971

82. O'Donoghue DH: Reconstruction for medial instability of the knee. J Bone Joint Surg [Am] 55:941, 1973

83. Salter RB, et al: The biological effect of continuous passive motion on the healing of full thickness defects in articular cartilage. J Bone Joint Surg [Am] 62:1231, 1980

84. Cavanagh PR: The Running Shoe Book. Anderson World, CA, 1980

85. Blackburn TA (ed): Guidelines for Pre-Season Athletic Participation Evaluation, Sports Medicine Section, American Physical Therapy Association, LaCrosse, WI, 1984.

22

Manipulation of the Lower Extremity

Chiropractic
DANA J. LAWRENCE

A SHORT HISTORY

By now, the basic history of the chiropractic profession is well known. Daniel David Palmer, who lived from 1845 to 1913, came to the United States from Port Perry, in Ontario, Canada, in the year 1865. His next 20 years were spent in various occupations such as farming, beekeeping, and store sales. In 1885, he opened a practice as a magnetic healer in the city of Davenport, Iowa, although he had no formal training in any healing art.

The story of the first chiropractic adjustment, rendered to Harvey Lillard in September 1895 (coincidentally and significantly, the same year that Roentgen discovered the x-ray), has moved beyond that of a simple tale to that of legend. A manual adjustment was given to a fourth thoracic vertebrae and as a result, the hearing of Mr. Lillard was restored. From this reasoning, "Palmer then applied similar techniques to other individuals with a variety of problems, each time using a spinous process of a vertebra as a lever to produce the adjustment. This constituted the initiation of chiropractic as an art, a science, and a profession."[1]

From this nearly chance opportunity came the outlines of the profession almost as it exists today. Palmer was re-sponsible for formulating the concept of a "subluxation" as a causal factor in disease, through the pressure by which such "displacements" would affect nerve roots. "Within 2 years of the initial discovery, Palmer had started the Chiropractic School and Cure, and soon had his first student enrolled. By 1902, Palmer's son, Bartlett Joshua (usually simply referred to as B. J.), had enrolled in his father's school; 2 years later, B.J. had gained operational control of the institution and was, by 1907, the President." This post he maintained until his death in 1961.[1]

This also created animosity between the father and the son. The elder Palmer left the school of his name and traveled around the country, forming at least four other chiropractic colleges (in the states of California, Oregon, and Oklahoma). He was also placed in jail for a short time for the crime of practicing without a license from the Board of Medical Examiners. While he might have been able to avoid jail by paying a small fine, he believed there was a more important principle to uphold. Palmer was not the last to be jailed for this "crime."[1]

D. D. Palmer died in 1913 after enjoying only a short reconciliation with his son. B. J. had, by that time, led the original Palmer College for nearly 7 years. In 1906, the elder Palmer had already forsaken education at the original Palmer College. That year was also significant because it marked the first time that there were philosophical differences within the fledgling chiropractic profession. John Howard, one of the first graduates of the Palmer School,

---

* Some material in this chapter is reprinted by permission from Bergmann T, Peterson D, Lawrence DJ: Chiropractic Technique. Churchill Livingstone, New York, 1993.

was unable to accept many of the philosophical beliefs relative to health care that B. J. Palmer was now openly espousing. B. J. had, by then, begun to preach that subluxation was the cause of all disease, in opposition to his father's initial beliefs. Howard therefore left the Palmer School and founded the National School of Chiropractic not far from the Palmer School in Davenport. These two schools (now colleges) still exist today and, in the minds of many, still typify the differences within the chiropractic profession.[2]

As Beideman[3] noted, Howard wanted to teach chiropractic "as it should be taught" and, therefore, moved the school to Chicago, feeling that Davenport was inimically against the development of a rational form of chiropractic care. This form of chiropractic necessitated access to laboratory, dissection, clinics, and the like.

By this time, chiropractic colleges were being founded all over the country, and there was more and more internecine warfare among practitioners. B. J. Palmer had set himself up as the protector of a fundamental form of chiropractic (usually referred to today as "straight" chiropractic). During the years 1910 to 1926, Palmer lost many important administrators, most of whom went on to form their own colleges. Regardless of the philosophical issues that arose then, and that still divide the profession today, it is undoubtedly sure that, without Palmer's missionary zeal and entrepreneurial brilliance, the chiropractic profession would likely not exist today. B. J.'s role as the "developer" of chiropractic was honestly earned.

While organized medicine rejected chiropractic from its outset, events within medicine had a major impact upon the development of the chiropractic profession. The Flexner Report, released in the year 1910, had a profound effect upon chiropractic education.[4] This report was highly critical of the status of medical education in the United States. It recommended that medical colleges affiliate with universities to gain educational support. As Beideman noted, it took the chiropractic profession nearly 15 years from the time of that report to begin the same types of changes that medicine underwent to improve its education.[5]

However, the changes were not long in coming once their need was recognized, and these improvements ultimately led to the creation of the Council on Chiropractic Education, which later became recognized by the U.S. Department of Education (actually, the Department of Health, Education, and Welfare) as the accrediting agency for the chiropractic profession.

Dr. John Nugent was largely responsible for ensuring that educational improvements would occur within the chiropractic profession. In 1935, Dr. Nugent was made the first Director of Education for the National Chiropractic Association (NCA). In the study performed by Dr. Nugent and brought to the delegates of the NCA, Nugent reported that there were 37 active chiropractic colleges, all of which were proprietary and all of which apparently followed different educational standards. It took Nugent the better part of the next two decades to begin to standardize the chiropractic educational process. Part of this standardization process included the initiation of the Council on Chiropractic Education (CCE). This occurred in 1947. In 1963, the NCA reformed itself as the American Chiropractic Association (ACA). By the late 1960s, the CCE had required its accredited colleges to use a 2-year preprofessional educational experience as a requirement for matriculation. In 1968 the Doctor of Chiropractic (D.C.) became a recognized first professional degree, and in 1971 the CCE became an autonomous body.

The educational process noted above allowed the chiropractic colleges to upgrade their professional standards to an unprecedented degree. The requirements of the CCE govern the entire educational spectrum of chiropractic education, mandating that certain information must be imparted to the student body, and providing for a way in which to monitor compliance and to provide guidance to an individual college. The effect has been quite salubrious. Today, all CCE-accredited colleges teach a comprehensive program, incorporating elements of basic science (such as physiology, anatomy, and biochemistry), clinical science (such as laboratory diagnosis, radiographic diagnosis, orthopedics, and nutrition), and clinical experience (where experience in patient management, involving therapeutic intervention, is gained).

What is interesting in this approach is that, indeed, the curriculum is standardized so that a member of the public can be assured that most graduates of CCE colleges have been provided competent educations. Yet each college must teach its students chiropractic manipulative therapy of some sort; that is, they must teach their students to adjust. The procedures taught at one college may be different from those taught at other colleges. The National College of Chiropractic may focus its curriculum upon teaching diversified technic, while the Palmer College may offer the Palmer Package, and Logan College may focus upon the Logan Basic Procedure. While all these forms of chiropractic adjustive techniques have many elements in common, there can be substantial differences and disparities in their approaches. A graduate of one college may find it difficult to share information with the graduate of a different college that teaches some alternate form of adjustive procedures.

The majority of chiropractic technique systems were started by interested and probing doctors who noticed a regularity in their results, and began to ask why those results occurred. This was largely a bootstrapping effort, where the impetus to gain new knowledge and then disseminate it was largely self-driven. However there has been some divisiveness as a result.

A COMMENT ON CHIROPRACTIC PHILOSOPHY

Books and journal articles have been written that discuss chiropractic philosophy in all its ramifications (indeed, Lawrence[6] argues that there is no specific chiropractic philosophy; rather, there is a philosophy of chiropractic), so it is well beyond the scope of this chapter to provide such lengthy discussion. However, it is apparent that "chiropractic philosophy" is based upon four major considerations: that the body has an innate ability to heal itself and desires to maintain balance; that the nervous system has influence over the rest of the body and must therefore play a role in maintaining health; that joint dysfunction, no matter how defined (as subluxation or fixation) interferes with the nervous system's ability to maintain that health; and that chiropractic care is based upon appropriate diagnosis and therapy designed to detect those dysfunctions.[7] It is for this reason that manual procedures are primary in chiropractic, for both diagnosis and treatment. The chiropractic adjustment is therefore critically significant in clinical practice.

THE SUBLUXATION

The concept of the subluxation is at the core of the chiropractic profession. While the term itself has been present for hundreds of years, being defined in 1746 by the physician Hieronymus as "lessened motion of the joints, by slight change in position of the articulating bones and pain,"[8] its existence within the chiropractic profession has been one of contention, controversy, and debate. Often, the term is defined operationally, since there is no clear consensus for one exact meaning of the term.

Early medical definitions almost universally centered upon the static nature of the subluxation: an incomplete dislocation, a semiluxation, or a partial or incomplete separation. Within chiropractic, the term first gained common

Table 22-1 Four Criteria Used by B. J. Palmer To Define Subluxation

1. Misalignment of a vertebra relative to the one above or below (positional alteration) occurs
2. This misalignment then occludes the intervertebral foramen
3. This occlusion then creates pressure upon the spinal nerve roots
4. This pressure leads finally to interference with the transmission of the nerve impulse

usage through the work of D. D. and B. J. Palmer. It was their insight to tie the nervous system in with the positional alteration, stating that the structural disrelationship of the bones compromised nerves, leading to abnormal neural function.[9,10] Indeed, B. J. Palmer used four criteria help define subluxation (Table 22-1). These criteria represent the first time that subluxation by definition involved interference with the nervous system.

This initial definition evolved over time, and today there are a number of definitions in general use. Perhaps the one most well accepted grew out of the National Institute of Neurological and Communicative Disorders and Stroke Conference of 1975. "Subluxation is the alteration of the normal dynamics, anatomical or physiological relationships of contiguous articular structures."[11] This particular definition could make everyone happy, inasmuch as it is at least relatively general and nonspecific. This fact led to consensus panels being developed to attempt a better profession-wide definition. After a series of Delphi and nominal group meetings, a definition was developed that read: "Subluxation: a motion segment in which alignment, movement integrity, and/or physiologic function are altered though contact between the joint surfaces remains intact." Even this definition lacks reference to the nervous system, making it unpalatable to some within the profession. Thus the concepts of the subluxation complex and the subluxation syndrome were also devised. The subluxation complex comprises a model of segmental dysfunction incorporating the complex interaction of pathologic changes in nerve, muscle, and ligamentous, vascular, and connective tissues,[12] while the syndrome is that constellation of signs and symptoms that indicates the presence of dysfunction in spinal or extraspinal motions segments.[13]

However, notwithstanding the continual, and healthy, debate, there is one concept that lies at the core of all definitions: subluxation alters the normal neurophysiologic balance in the body. Leach[14] notes that four secondary hypotheses develop naturally from this key concept (Table

Table 22-2 Major Subluxation Concepts

Primary Hypothesis: subluxation alters the normal neurophysiologic balance in the body

Secondary Hypotheses:
1. Subluxation may cause spinal cord compression
2. Subluxation may cause nerve root compression
3. Subluxation may lead to vertebrobasilar arterial insufficiency
4. Subluxation may cause somatic afferent bombardment of dorsal horn cells in the spinal cord

22-2). These help preserve and expand upon the involvement of the nervous system in subluxation.

Of course, defining subluxation leads to the challenge of how to locate it. A large number of procedures exist for this purpose, but chief among them is palpation and motion palpation, discussed elsewhere in this text. This implies that yet again evolution of the term has occurred, since motion palpation is designed to locate fixation alone.

THE LOWER EXTREMITY AND CHIROPRACTIC

There are differences in how a podiatrist and a chiropractor approach involvement of the lower extremity. The podiatrist is likely to consider the root cause of a lower extremity condition to be located in the lower extremity and will therefore direct therapy solely to it (of course, taking into account the license of the podiatrist). The chiropractor may look outside the lower extremity, in recognition of the role that the lower extremity plays in spinal health. Postural analysis has always been an important part of the chiropractic assessment procedure; postural misalignments in the lower extremity can manifest themselves in the spine. Indeed, abnormal pedal biomechanics will likely have effects all the way up the lower kinetic chain; problems in the foot may cause problems not only in the knee and hip, but in the lumbar and cervical spine as well. As an example, consider the pronated foot. It may lead to the development of genu valgus and coxa vara, placing stress on the lumbar spine, which then creates abnormal stress patterns in the spine, causing cervical subluxations. Correction in such a case would require attention to the flatfoot as well as adjustment of the cervical and lumbar spine, so that neurologic integrity is enhanced. In particular, upper cervical integrity is critical to overall health.

This raises an interesting "chicken or egg" question: does abnormal pedal biomechanics lead to abnormal cervical integrity, or does abnormal cervical integrity (cervical subluxation) lead to later pedal dysfunction? This question cannot be easily answered without substantial research, but both optimal biomechanics and cervical integrity are key to better health and function. Schafer has said that spinal subluxations will be reflected in the upright posture and that spinal distortions result in the development of subluxation syndromes.[15]

One possible explanation for the involvement of the cervical spine in pedal abnormalities may be ascribed to the dentate ligament cord distortion theory, which was most recently advanced by the late John Grostic.[16] He describes two mechanisms for how the dentate ligaments may adversely affect the conduction of neural impulses in the spinal cord, and these two mechanisms may be a result of problems arising from lower in the spine (from problems arising even lower in the lower extremity). The two mechanisms include direct irritation due to dentate ligament traction, and venous occlusion and vascular stasis (and even ischemia) in the upper cervical spinal cord. Small cervical misalignments may lead to substantial compression on the cord.[17]

More than just posture must be examined; gait is also important in assessing the relationship between pedal function and cervical biomechanics. A number of phases of gait should be assessed: stance and swing phases, heel strike to foot flat, foot flat to midstance, midstance to heel-off, heel-off to toe-off, toe-off to midswing, and midswing to heel-off. This may be done by visual observation, or if possible through force plate analysis on a gait platform.

Finally, this implies that chiropractic therapy must be directed at the whole athlete or patient; it cannot simply be regionally directed. The approach is more global in nature, looking not just at the injured or involved body part (foot, knee, etc.) but at how those problems are manifest throughout the patient's body. This is a holistic method of health care.

POTENTIAL COMPLICATIONS OF MANIPULATIVE PROCEDURES

Like any therapeutic procedure, the use of a high-velocity thrust carries with it certain risks, especially in the cervical spine. While the incidence of adverse reactions following manipulation are exceedingly rare, estimated by at least one individual at less than one death per tens of millions of manipulations,[18] the amount of notoriety these accidents have received has been extensive. With proper caution and careful investigation and diagnosis, the chances of such accidents can be substantially minimized.

The accident that is generally considered to be most potentially serious is that of vascular compromise, especially involving the vertebral artery. Patency of the vertebral artery can be tested by various orthopedic tests, such as extension–rotation or George's test. The vertebral artery itself ascends through the transverse foramina of C6 to C1, then passes over the posterior arch of the atlas in the vertebral artery sulcus. Once in the skull, the artery runs forward alongside the medulla into the lower pons, where it meets its other branch to form the midline artery. The artery is poorly protected in the area where it leaves the atlas and before it enters the skull. As the head is rotated, the artery on one side is kinked while the artery on the other side is stretched against the transverse process of the atlas. In that artery, blood flow may be decreased by a variety of processes, such as tortuosity, congenitally small arteries, and atherosclerosis.

Certain chiropractic techniques for adjusting the upper cervical region initially used a combination of rotation and extension; this position is one that can cause decrease in blood flow in an already compromised vertebral artery and, for that reason, testing of the vertebral arteries prior to adjusting the cervical spine is absolutely necessary. Jaskoviak[19] was able to identify 45 cases of vertebral artery syndrome following cervical manipulation, and certainly not all were chiropractic cases. The truly unfortunate cases, in which 11 patients died, might have been avoided had more extensive procedures been used or proper care rendered. However, the incidence remains extremely low, and can be avoided entirely by proper diagnostic work-up.

PROFESSIONAL CLINICAL OVERVIEW

What types of patients seek chiropractic care, and who do chiropractors treat? Without doubt, the major reason people seek chiropractic care is for the treatment of musculoskeletal conditions. Typically, such conditions represent about 80 percent of chiropractic cases, with lumbosacral strain ranking as most common; other common conditions include thoracic and cervical strains, headache, and various sprain conditions. Intervertebral disc prolapses are infrequent.[20] Visceral conditions account for perhaps 5 percent of chiropractic cases.

Chiropractors are uniquely qualified to treat such conditions, since the educational system is built around appropriate training. Educational requirements for chiropractic

training are mandated by the appropriate accrediting agency, both regional and professional. The accreditation process has helped to standardize, as well as set standards relating to, treatment and diagnosis. In initiating a referral network with local chiropractors, one important factor to consider would be whether that chiropractor is a graduate of an accredited chiropractic institution, which at least ensures a particular level of training. Other factors include what types of patients the chiropractor sees, whether he or she uses standard techniques (typically those taught within the colleges), and whether he or she has advanced training (such as in radiology or orthopedics). Chiropractors cannot use drugs or surgery, and will refer when their patients require such care. In addition to the manipulative procedures used by all chiropractors, other treatment procedures may include the use of physiotherapeutic modalities, exercise, nutritional supplementation, and orthotics.

THE FUTURE

The chiropractic profession has labored long and hard to get to where it is. What does the future portend for the profession? There are both the chance for opportunity and advancement, and the chance to lose many of our hard-gained privileges. The outcome of the Wilk case, which began several years ago, will have a large impact upon our future.

On February 7, 1990, the Seventh Circuit U.S. Court of Appeals found the American Medical Association (AMA) guilty of an illegal conspiracy to destroy the competitive profession of chiropractic. The impetus for this decision arose from a suit brought by five chiropractors, alleging that the AMA, along with several other organizations involved in health care, conspired to restrain the practice of chiropractic through a sustained and unlawful boycott of the chiropractic profession. This was in spite of the fact that chiropractic care had been found to be, in many cases, more effective in treating certain kinds of health problems.

The effects of the boycott were to severely limit the potential effectiveness of chiropractic in offering itself as a viable alternative to allopathic medical care. The trial took over 12 years to complete, and was upheld by the U.S. Supreme Court in their refusal to hear arguments in the case, thus upholding the decision by Judge Susan Getzendanner in the Seventh Circuit Court.

This decision opens many avenues of health care long thought closed to chiropractors. While there had already been inroads made into gaining hospital privileges for individual chiropractors, the decision makes it easier for this to occur. It should be noted that while the Joint Commission on the Accreditation of Hospitals was named in the original suit, they were soon separated from the suit. Thus it is entirely possible that pressure could still be brought to bear upon any hospital that accepts a chiropractor on staff. Indeed, it seems likely that this will occur, at least during the short term.

The effects of medical propaganda upon chiropractors will take many years to overcome; evidence suggests that in many ways this process is already starting. There are still suits brought by chiropractors against medical practitioners who refuse to have anything to do with the chiropractic profession. In one notable case, the use of the RICO laws was proposed in an attempt to punish several medical doctors who successfully caused the removal of a neurosurgeon from the hospital that granted him privileges, because of his association with a local chiropractor. The ball, however, rests mainly with the chiropractic profession, and it is likely that, over the long term, more and more chiropractors will gain hospital privileges.

This must come, in part, by our successfully defending chiropractic techniques, and by testing and refining them. Presently, this is a process in its infancy. The profession is now involved in developing standards of care; these standards have a mechanism for testing chiropractic methods and then classifying them as experimental, mainstream, and so forth. In early 1990, the profession held its first Consensus Conference on the Validation of Chiropractic Methods. The conference brought together researchers, academicians, technique developers, politicians, and others from all walks of chiropractic life for the purpose of developing systems to test the validity of chiropractic procedures through a consensus process. In this particular program, the first day was given over to invited speakers talking on a variety of topics relating to technique, while the second day had several roundtable and panel discussions relating to the ways such validation might occur. It is exciting to see how many technique developers were involved. The history of chiropractic technique is largely one of individual drive and bootstrapping rather than hard scientific research prior to the release of information.

The science of chiropractic is now beginning to investigate the art of chiropractic. In such a manner, the profession will better be able to define itself for the continual debate regarding national health insurance. There can be no doubt that the potential to lose all that was won in the Wilk case exists in this emerging national health care debate. The nation has become increasingly cost conscious, and many decisions regarding health care no longer rest with those involved in delivering that care. Instead, these decisions rest with insurance company executives, politicians, and governmental agencies. These groups are not likely to support methods of health care in a national health insurance plan that lack any scientific credibility. The need to continue scientific research is paramount to maintaining chiropractic practice rights, and the process initiated by the Consensus Conference must be ongoing.

If national health insurance becomes a reality, practitioners of manual therapy must ensure that they are in the accepted procedures covered by the plan. The chiropractic profession is rapidly gaining increasing acceptance. It now has a body of credible research to document much of what it claims; it supports several fine scientific journals (at least one of which is indexed worldwide in Index Medicus, with several others indexed in the Cumulative Index to Nursing and Allied Health Literature); it has an increasing number of high-quality textbooks; it has developed teaching techniques in its educational curriculum (many of which are moving toward problem-based learning); and it has increasing legislative clout.

A challenge for the future is to place all chiropractic techniques into a framework that allows us to determine whether any of them has a basis in fact. The profession can then begin to weed out unacceptable procedures that are promoted largely on the strength of the cult of personality that arises around the founder of the system. We can all appreciate the effort and drive that led so many chiropractic pioneers to devise their systems, but to allow those systems to flourish solely because of those efforts is to do a grave disservice to those who come after. Serious investigation into many of these systems is now underway.

Manipulation
DON G. DAVIS

The intent of this section is to acquaint the reader with a rationale of manipulative treatment in dysarthrosis (joint misalignment), and the rudiments of actual lower extremity manipulation. The purpose is not to report on the etiology, biomechanics, clinical anatomy, or complete treatments of the syndromes listed. Clearly, other forms of treatment are necessary and, in fact, required to ensure quick, uneventful, and full recovery. It is important to recognize that several treatment approaches must coexist. I use many other treatment modalities in my practice, and hope that the reader also will use the full armamentarium that is described extensively in the other chapters of this book.

With this in mind, we are concerned first with elucidating the diagnosis of proper joint configuration, joint play, and specific joint range of motion; and second, with the proper utilization of manipulative therapeutics. Normal range of motion may incorporate several specific improper or decreased articular motions within the joint in question. These problems must be considered when locating the site of pain and malfunction. Manipulation is intended to correct abnormal motion (dysarthrias), allowing the lower extremity to function normally within its environmental and morphologic limits.

MANIPULATION

According to Sandoz,[21] "a joint adjustment can be defined as a passive manual maneuver during which an articular element is suddenly carried beyond the usual physiological limit of movement without, however, exceeding the boundaries of anatomical integrity." Often a "clicking" sound accompanies the adjustment thrust.

In order to portray the physiology of manipulation more accurately, it is helpful to explain graphically the mechani-

Figure 22-1 Joint mobilization and adjustment in one plane (see text). (From Sandoz R: Some physical mechanisms and effects of spinal adjustments. Ann Swiss Chirop Assoc 6:91, 1976, with permission.)

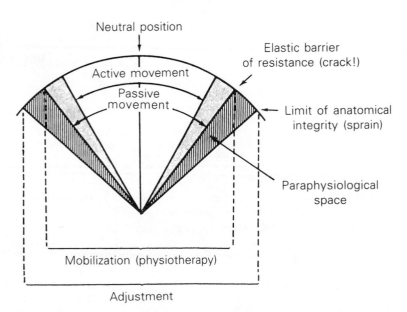

cal events that occur within the joint space. Figure 22-1 depicts the range of movement of mobilization and manipulation in a diarthrodial joint in one plane.

The central area shows a range of active motion that, when mobilized passively, increases until it meets an elastic barrier of resistance. This range is commonly used in physical therapy for stretching soft tissue structures. If this barrier is surpassed by assistance from the physician, a slight give is perceived with an audible click, and the movement is slightly increased beyond the normal passive range into the paraphysiologic space. If manipulation is forced beyond this anatomic limit, disruption of joint integrity occurs, resulting in sprain.

The physician must take the utmost care not to force the joint outside the anatomic limit while still overcoming the elastic barrier of resistance. This is done by slowly taking the slack out of the joint motion and, when the elastic barrier is encountered, adding a slight thrust, increasing the motion just beyond the passive range.

Two groups of researchers have described the mechanical aspects of manipulation.[22] In these studies, the metacarpophalangeal joint was subjected to axial traction and, at various intervals, the joint spaces were observed by radiography. A graph correlating the results was developed by Sandoz, depicted in Figure 22-2.

Preliminary tension results in only a slight separation of the articular cartilage (what one might expect, considering the strength of the joint capsule), until about 8 kg of force. This is followed by a dramatic increase in joint space relative to tension, and a click is heard. This click is explained by the release of gases from the synovial fluid under negative pressure, and may be seen as a radiolucent area within the joint space on radiographs. This process is called *cavitation*. When the tension is gradually decreased, we see a sloping decrease in articular separation. When another manipulation is attempted shortly thereafter, there is no second cavitational phenomenon. This evidently will only occur once the gases have completed a reverse-phase

Figure 22-2 Adjustment of carpometacarpal joint under axial stretch (see text). (From Sandoz R: Some physical mechanisms and effects of spinal adjustments. Ann Swiss Chirop Assoc 6:91, 1976, with permission.)

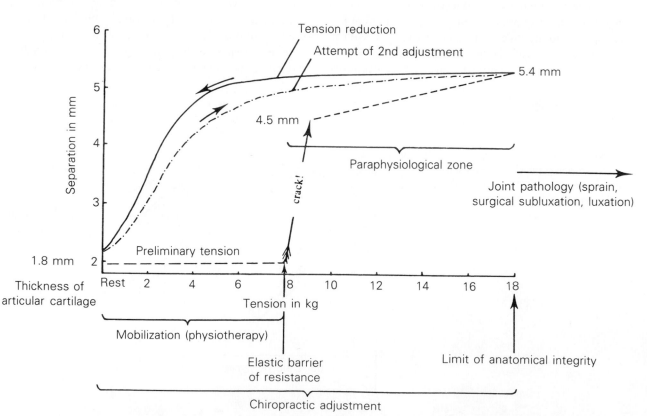

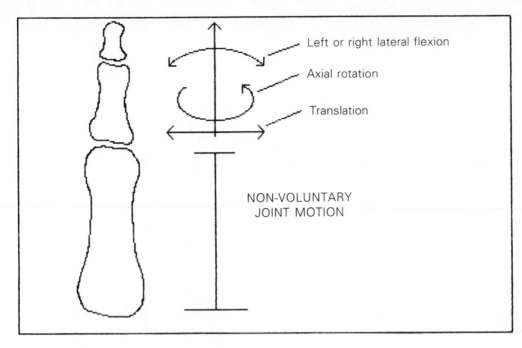

Figure 22-3 Nonvoluntary joint motion.

change and have been resorbed, in about 15 to 20 minutes. Attempts at further manipulation run the risk of joint injury, because the motion of the paraphysiologic space is temporarily added to the active and passive movement. It should also be kept in mind that, during this refractory period, the joint is relatively unstable, and, therefore, should not be stressed or exercised for about 1 hour after manipulation.

Manipulation is an art and, as such, requires talent and considerable practice. It is highly effective in relieving patient discomfort, but, as in other therapies, correct application is crucial.

MOTION PALPATION

Indications for manipulation are best derived through the technique of joint play assessment, championed by Mennell.[23,24] The concept of joint play is similar to that of manipulation. In manipulation, the goal is to barely transcend the elastic barrier, whereas in joint play, the goal is to access the qualitative texture of the elastic barrier. Here, the joint is examined by moving it in a plane that is not under voluntary control. As in machinery, a defined tolerance exists in each moving part. When this is perceived

as decreased in comparison with the opposite limb, or with what would be considered "normal," joint play is compromised, along with the normal range of motion, and manipulation is indicated. For example, of the nonvoluntary motions of a joint, consider the metatarsophalangeal joint of the great toe. This articulation has palpable joint play motion along the long axis in traction, anteroposterior translation, medial and lateral side tilt, and rotation (Fig. 22-3).

Palpatory dysfunction in a joint can be in the form of decreased motion (hypomobility) or of increased motion (hypermobility).[25] One can imagine that hypomobility would result from chronic injuries, such as degenerative arthritis or surrounding soft tissue contracture, from surgery, or from nonuse. Muscle shortening may also occur across the joint line; muscle stretching (mobilization) with other therapeutic modalities such as ultrasound would therefore be the most prudent therapeutic approach. However, in hypermobility, by definition, the joint already has its full complement of motion, and then some. Unfortunately, a joint in this condition has inadequate baseline proprioceptive feedback, along with an inordinately long neutral-to-barrier phase. The elastic barrier resides deep in the paraphysiologic space close to the limit of motion. Here, manipulation is not indicated and could, if forced, result in even further hypermobility, joint instability, and damage.

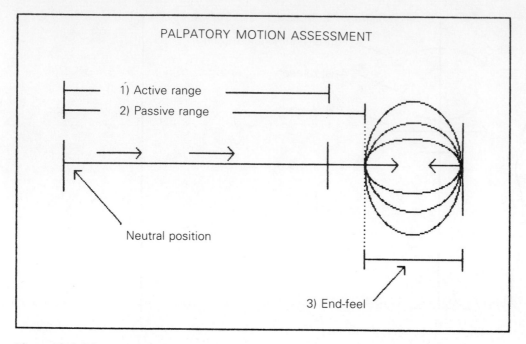

Figure 22-4 Palpatory motion assessment.

The quantitative assessment of movement is divided into two stages: first, that of motion from neutral position to the elastic barrier, and second, "end feel," which is the texture felt by the examiner just beyond the passive arc of motion (Fig. 22-4).

The first stage of passive range should be smooth and free of pain. Only enough force is applied as is necessary to ease the joint to full motion. Deviations from normal can be detected easily through this stage, and very often when the limb is simply held by the examiner.

The second stage, known as "end feel," is better understood if thought of in terms of three characteristics:

Soft end feel—resistance met by musculature

Firm end feel—resistance met by capsular and ligamentous structures

Hard end feel—resistance provided by actual bone limitations.

Motion palpation is the ability to feel all three aspects of end feel within the elastic barrier in order that the subtle and sometimes cryptic characteristics of the joint are realized.

Mennell provides an extensive discussion of the specific joint-play motions of the foot and knee.[24] The most clinically significant articulations are outlined. These important studies should be reviewed before any attempt is made to manipulate suspected joint dysfunction.

Appropriate manipulation is often simply the continuation of joint play motion into the paraphysiologic space. Because manipulation is kept within physiologic limits, there is no trauma to the joint, and hence minimal pain. In order to examine and manipulate the lower extremity fully, one can see that a thorough knowledge of normal range of motion of the examined articulation is required.

The physician will eventually become proficient in palpating aberrant motion in the lower extremity joints. Proficiency in this subtle technique takes a great deal of practice. Listed below are some common ailments in sports medicine that have proved amenable to manipulation. These are outlined only as possible approaches to treatment and are intended as an organized guide to prevent possible oversight. The sequelae surrounding these syndromes (e.g., erythema and edema) may actually be secondary to primary causal pathomechanics. This possibility must be taken into account by the physician and corrected. To ignore them is to permit a definite increase in the length of healing time, if, indeed, healing occurs at all.

Equally important in delineating which approach one should take in the manipulative procedure is to ascertain the vector of heel stress. Some runners tend to hit the heel and then slide, creating a certain amount of anteroposterior shear. In this case, the adjustment of choice drives the calcaneus forward (the posterior calcaneous). Others, such as race walkers, tend to dig in, placing anterior-directed stress on the calcaneus and possibly overloading the shock-neutralizing factors in the rearfoot. In this case, anteriorly directed manipulation or a general mobilization maneuver is more appropriate. This can be done by stabilizing the forefoot and then rocking the calcaneus in eversion and inversion.

In the manipulations described in the following sections, reference is made to a stabilization hand and a contact hand. The stabilization hand is the hand that is utilized to hold the part in base position, while the contact hand usually delivers a particular force to the part in question.

RIGID CAVUS FOOT

FOOT AND ANKLE

Plantar Fasciitis

Plantar fasciitis is usually caused by irritation ensuing from dramatically increased fascial stress. This can be attained by a rigid cavus foot with its limited range of subtalar excursion and distributed shock—stress to the adjacent soft tissues. The pronated foot, with its hypermobile first metatarsal ray, can result in elevated tensile stress and microtears at the plantar fascial origin. The following discussion first outlines the manipulations germane to the rigid cavus foot (Figs. 22-5 through 22-7), followed by a description of the hypermobile pronated foot (Figs. 22-7 through 22-10).

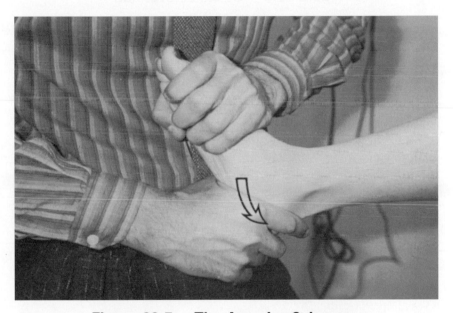

Figure 22-5:   The Anterior Calcaneus

The patient lies supine with the involved leg flexed 30 degrees. The forefoot is held firmly with the stabilization hand, while the webbed portion of the contact hand is placed around the anterior aspect of the calcaneus. The contact hand delivers a short, quick thrust to the anterior aspect of the calcaneus.

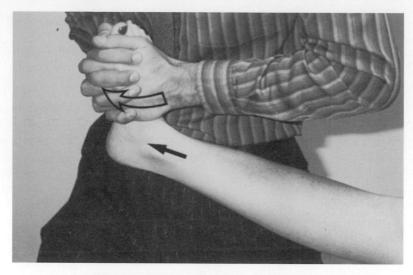

Figure 22-6:   Subtalar Eversion

The patient lies supine, with the involved leg extended. The midfoot is grasped with fingers interlaced at its medial region. A sharp tug is applied in both traction and eversion.

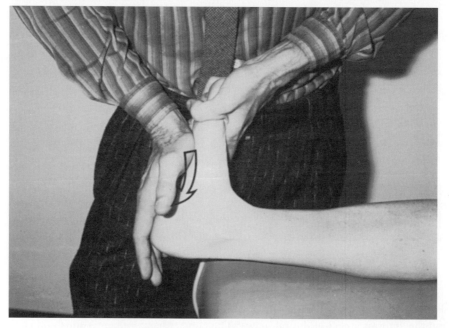

Figure 22-7:   Plantar Palming

The patient lies supine with the involved leg extended. The foot is dorsiflexed with the stabilization hand. With the thenar eminence or base of the hand, frictional pressure is applied to the plantar fascia close to its insertion at the metatarsal heads. This contact is slid slowly to the fascial origin.

HYPERMOBILE PRONATED FOOT

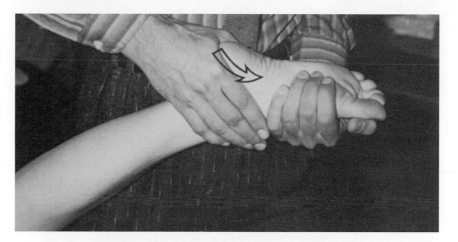

Figure 22-8:   The Posterior Calcaneus

The patient lies prone with the involved leg flexed at 30 degrees. The dorsal aspect of the foot is stabilized with the stabilization hand, while the contact hand cups the calcaneus and applies a posterior-to-anterior thrust.

Ankle Sprain

The ankle sprain may involve many different structures, depending on the degree of injury or the direction of disrupting force. This sprain can involve more than the lateral or medial ligaments of the ankle. The mechanics of the injury may result in disrelationships of surrounding joints, such as those illustrated in the following pages, along with adjacent soft tissue elements of the ankle mortise. Since the involved ankle joints and bones may not always return to their neutral position after injury, manipulation may be required in order to ensure correct mechanical function of the ankle.

The Inferior Navicular

Treatment is identical to that for the pronated foot, described and pictured above (Fig. 22-8).

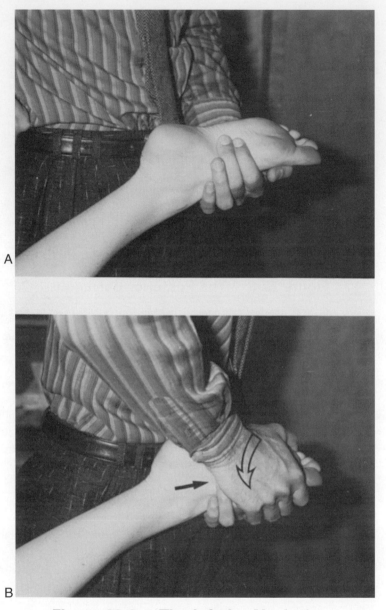

Figure 22-9: The Inferior Navicular

The patient lies prone with the involved leg flexed at 30 degrees. The second and third fingers of the stabilization hand are placed over the medial and inferior aspect of the navicular (**A**). With the base of the contact hand, inferior pressure is placed over the finger contact. A downward thrust is delivered with the contact hand (**B**).

Plantar Palming

This is performed in the same manner as plantar palming for the cavus foot, described and pictured in Figure 22-7.

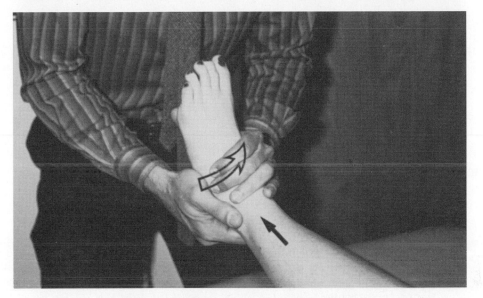

Figure 22-10:   The Lateral Talus

The patient lies supine with the involved leg extended. The stabilization hand cups the calcaneus, while the third and fourth fingers of the contact hand apply pressure at the anterolateral aspect of the talus. A slight tractional eversion thrust is then applied.

INVERSION SPRAIN

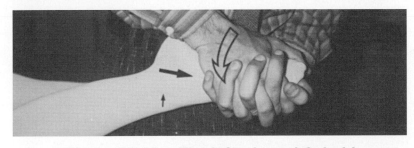

Figure 22-11:   The Inferolateral Cuboid

The patient lies prone with the involved leg flexed at 30 degrees. The heel of the contact hand is placed over the inferolateral aspect of the cuboid, and the fingers are interlocked. A tractional plantar-flexion thrust is then provided. It is helpful to support the dorsal aspect of the ankle on the physician's upper thigh to give added support and to prevent excess plantar flexion of the ankle.

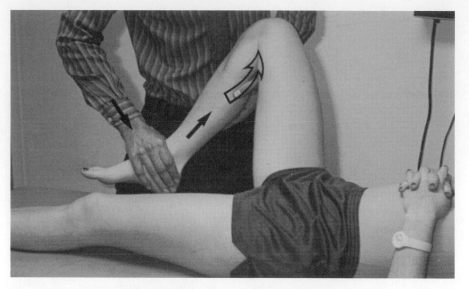

Figure 22-12:   Inferior Fibula

The patient lies supine with the involved leg flexed 140 degrees. The stabilization hand grasps the anterior aspect of the ankle, while the contact hand is placed in the popliteal fossa, with the base of the thumb just medial to the fibula. The thrust is made with the contact hand, pulling and lifting the fibula superiorly.

EVERSION SPRAIN

The Inferomedial Talus

This manipulation is performed exactly as for the lateral talus (Fig. 22-10), except that the hands are switched to apply pressure to the medial aspect of the talus, and an inversion thrust is applied.

Metatarsalgia

The prime cause of metatarsalgia is loss of transverse arch, along with the attendant disproportionate increase in metatarsal stress. Over time, the metatarsal bones can sublux inferiorly, increasing the chances of plantar interdigital nerve neuroma, and mechanical irritation of the metatarsal heads. Even if surgery is required, manipulation is suggested in order to reduce the secondary fibrositis from spasm and joint dysfunction.

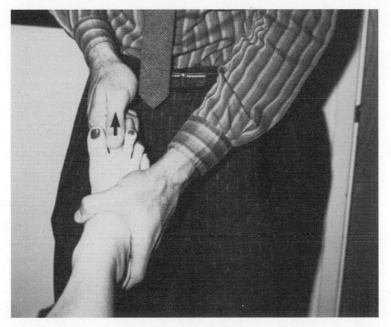

Figure 22-13:   Metatarsophalangeal Decompression

The patient lies supine with the involved leg extended. The stabilization hand grasps the lateral aspect of the midfoot, while the contact hand holds the phalanx with the thumb and forefinger. A tractional and plantar-flexing tug is applied at the metatarsophalangeal joint.

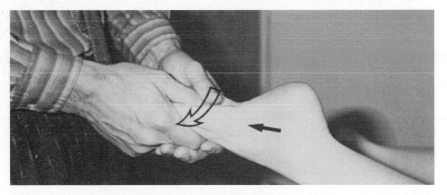

Figure 22-14:   Metatarsal Whip

The patient lies prone with the involved leg flexed 30 degrees. Crossed thumbs are placed over the involved metatarsophalangeal head, with the dorsum of the foot resting on the overlapping fingers. The thrust is given with a traction and plantar-flexion whip to the entire foot.

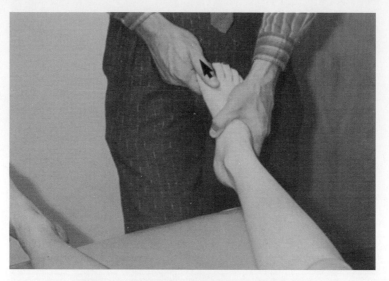

Figure 22-15:   Abducted Hallux

The patient lies supine with the involved leg extended. The stabilization hand holds the midfoot securely, while the thumb and forefinger of the contact hand grasp the first phalanx at the metatarsophalangeal joint. A tractional and adduction motion is then initiated.

Hallux Valgus

Hallux valgus, or bunion, is usually caused by improper fitting foot gear or has a genetic origin. Because of this, the treatment of choice is mechanical, such as bracing, orthotics, or surgery. However, along with this, mobilization and manipulation should be used in order to help increase the adduction of the first MP joint.

Postsurgical Syndrome

After surgery, and the appropriate healing period, mobilization can be used effectively to speed rehabilitation and prevent adhesions. This is accomplished by using the postsurgical mobilization techniques. The maneuvers shown assume that the motion abnormality is within the ankle mortice.

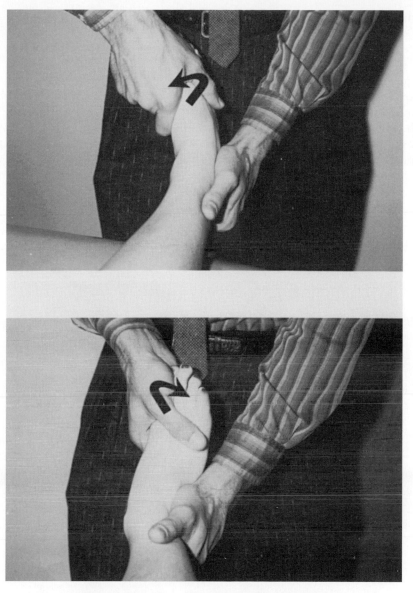

Figure 22-16:   General Mobilization

The patient lies supine with the involved leg extended. The stabilization hand grasps the calcaneus, while the contact hand holds the forefoot. The mobilization is delivered by a figure-eight motion. Careful attention should be given to any uneven motion or crepitation.

PRIME DIRECTIVE VECTOR

Postsurgical mobilization requires a certain amount of creativity. Because many surgical procedures are tailored to the individual needs of the damaged joint, mobilization should be oriented toward that particular joint. The prime directive vector is simply a reminder that the instability inherent in surgery should always be considered and proper care taken to realize the direction of that instability. It also means that, when surgical intervention is directed toward increasing joint range of motion, mobilization should be used early in the treatment plan to reinforce this new motion.

Postorthotic Syndrome

An orthotic device can be helpful in normalizing total foot motion. However, if the foot is not accustomed to the altered position provided by the orthotic, an inexperienced physician may misinterpret the increased pain after orthotic prescription. Motion errors and degenerative changes take a considerable length of time to develop and heal. Therefore, some assistance should be given in coping with their newfound, neutral position. Manipulations such as those described in Figure 22-16 can be used to help speed this process. Time should be taken to consider how mobilization might reinforce this neutral position.

KNEE

Knee pain has a plethora of causes. The origins of knee pain generally are ligament sprains or muscular strains. These are usually treated effectively with physical therapy modalities. Within the context of manipulative success, the most amenable are small cartilage tears and loose bodies (joint mice) or synovial plica. Motion palpation, in tandem with the required orthopedic tests, is effective in diagnosing the offending cause. When isolated decreased motion is noted, these manipulations can be effective in restoring full range.

Medial Knee Syndromes

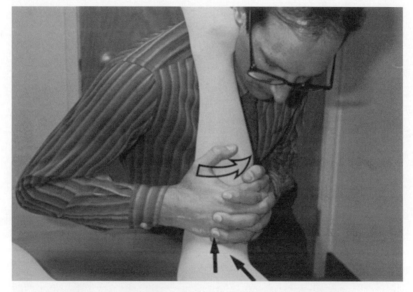

Figure 22-17:   External Rotated Tibia

The patient lies prone with the involved leg flexed at 90 degrees. The fingers are locked behind the uppermost portion of the calf. The contact hand grasps the gastrocnemius and rotates the posterior tibia internally; a tractional thrust is then applied.

Lateral Knee Syndromes

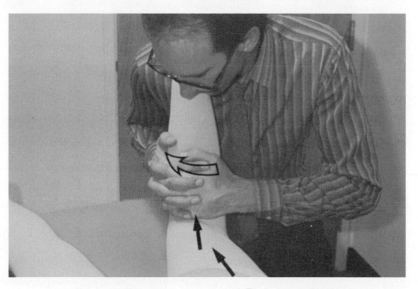

Figure 22-18: Internal Rotated Tibia

The patient lies prone with the involved leg flexed at 90 degrees. The fingers are locked behind the uppermost portion of the calf. The contact hand grasps the gastrocnemius and rotates the posterior tibia externally; a tractional thrust is then applied.

Patellofemoral Syndrome

Patellofemoral disorders may have lateral tracking errors linked to their etiology. As we know, this can be caused by genu valgum or faulty foot mechanics, but a tight lateral retinaculum is a common cause of lateral deviation and subsequent pain. The manipulation below attempts to stretch these lateral structures.

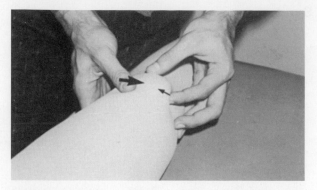

Figure 22-19:   Lateral Translated Patella

The patient lies supine with the involved knee extended. The stabilization hand is placed on the medial aspect of the patella, guarding against upward or downward motion. The contact hand is placed at the lateral patella. The patella is then pressed medially with the thumb.

HIP AND PELVIS

The hip and pelvis are extremely complicated structures, deserving more attention than can be afforded in this chapter. The field of chiropractic has researched these areas, and much of what is known clinically is based on the considerable work in that discipline. Research has unequivocally shown that motion does occur in the sacroiliac joint, and that there is a certain directional predictability to that movement.[26,27] The syndromes below are listed together because they tend to occur with other pelvic or hip dysarthrias. In other words, it is common to see more than one of these problems occurring at the same time. This happens because there is an anatomic, mechanical, and functional link between these two structures and their adjacent soft tissues.

Piriformis Syndrome

Piriformis syndrome can be a troublesome ailment, especially in long-distance runners and athletes in sports requiring repetitive external rotation of the hip. The patient often describes discomfort as imprecise hip, buttock, groin, or coccygeal pain that can be accompanied by sciatic neuralgia. This condition can lead to greater trochanteric bursitis because of the key role of the piriformis in external rotation, and its attachment on the medial aspect of the greater trochanter.

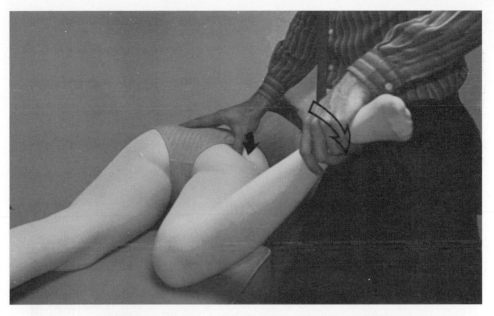

Figure 22-20:   Piriformis Mobilization

The patient lies prone with the involved leg flexed 90 degrees. The stabilization hand grasps the ankle and internally rotates the hip. The physician then applies pressure to the belly of the piriformis with the thumb of the contact hand. Both hands work in a pumping motion to massage the piriformis muscle.

Piriformis Mobilization

This manipulation is identical to that performed for piriformis syndrome (Fig. 22-20).

Gluteus Medius Syndrome

Gluteus medius syndrome arises in part because of other trochanteric ailments and in part because of referred pain and muscle spasm from facet and nerve root irritation. It should be evident that, since most causes of gluteus medius pain and spasm are from other structures, correct and specific diagnosis is paramount is ensuring a lasting cure. The manipulation shown below is provided to facilitate the treatment of this syndrome by directly neutralizing muscle hypertonicity.

Greater Trochanteric Bursitis

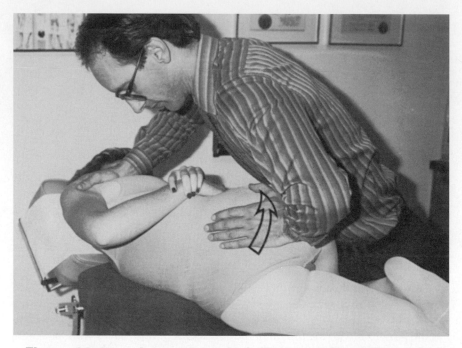

Figure 22-21: Anterosuperiorly Rotated Sacroiliac Joint

The patient lies on the side opposite the involved sacroiliac joint. The stabilization hand is placed on the ipsilateral shoulder to secure the patient and to provide tension to the involved sacroiliac joint. The base of the contact hand applies an anterior thrust to the ischial tuberosity.

Hip Syndromes

Hip dysarthria and sprain can manifest with pain in a variety of locations. The patient commonly presents with a sharp catching pain in the hip or groin, with radiating pain down the front or back of the thigh. A dull general pain may be experienced at the low back as well. Because of the extremely strong acetabular capsule, even minor swelling can result in disabling pain from increased intra-capsular pressure. Traction and mobilization of the hip joint in this case will help relieve this added irritation.

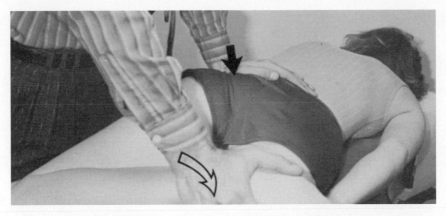

Figure 22-22:   Gluteus Medius Mobilization

The patient lies prone with the involved leg flexed 90 degrees. The stabilization hand grasps the ankle and externally rotates the hip. The physician then applies pressure to the belly of the gluteus medius with the base of the contact hand. Both hands work in a pumping motion to massage the muscle.

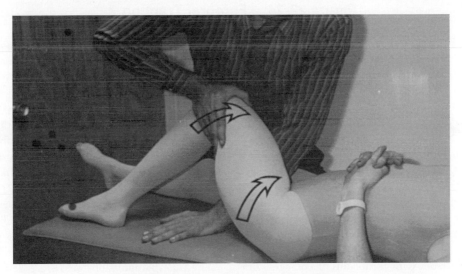

Figure 22-23:   Femoral Traction 1

The patient lies supine with the involved leg flexed 30 degrees. The stabilization hand is placed on the table with the doctor's forearm medial to the patient's proximal femur. The contact hand grasps the lateral knee and internally rotates the hip over the fulcrum of the forearm.

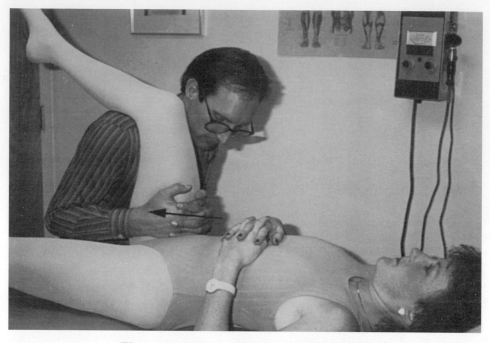

Figure 22-24:   Femoral Traction 2

The patient lies supine with the involved hip flexed 90 degrees. The knee is draped over the doctor's shoulder. The fingers are interlocked at the anterior proximal thigh and an inferior, pulling thrust is applied.

Sacroiliac Joint Syndrome

Sacroiliac joint syndrome is a complex subject, and its differential diagnosis is not within the scope of this chapter. However, its strong role in low back pain, as well as in other lower extremity complaints, cannot be ignored. Decreased sacroiliac movement requires additional motion from the hip joints, along with changing the entire gait motion. Runners seem to be the most sensitive to this gait alteration. They present with complaints of a dragging hip or with increased internal or external foot rotation. They also state that there is less hip extension and therefore a tendency for a shorter stride. Because of these gait aberrations, it is prudent to employ treadmill analysis with videotape slow-motion replay, if possible, to analyze the subtleties. The sacroiliac joint is mechanically linked to the entire lower extremity; therefore, it can affect compensatory changes in those structures, as well as being affected by lower extremity. This means that a sacroiliac joint refractory to treatment may have its symptoms perpetuated by other lower extremity problems and vice versa.

The two manipulations below are designed to correct the most common sacroiliac motion errors: anterosuperior fixation and posteroinferior fixation.

Anterosuperiorly Rotated Sacroiliac Joint

This manipulation is identical to that described and pictured for greater trochanteric bursitis (Fig. 22-21).

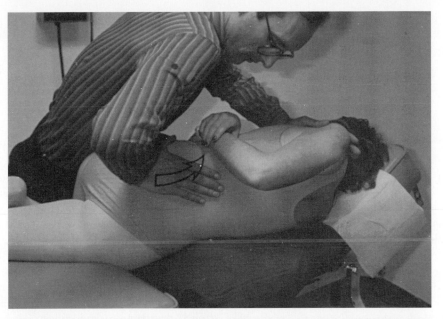

Figure 22-25:   Posteroinferiorly Rotated Sacroiliac Joint

The patient lies on the side opposite the involved sacroiliac joint. The stabilization hand is placed on the ipsilateral shoulder to secure the patient and to provide tension to the involved sacroiliac joint. The base of the contact hand applies an anterior thrust to the posterior superior iliac spine.

CONCLUSION

These manipulations should be attempted only when the physician has mastered the application of motion palpation for accurate diagnosis. Many more manipulations are cited throughout the literature. Those readers desiring a more thorough discourse of the various lower extremity manipulations are invited to consult the suggested readings provided at the end of this chapter.

Sports Chiropractic
JAN M. CORWIN

Chiropractors have been present at Olympic Games as part of the United States Medical Staff for the United States since the 1980s. There have also been chiropractors present treating athletes for numerous other countries from around the world. From the Virgin Islands to Australia, chiropractors have been providing care for the athletes of the world. Primarily used as specialists, sports chiropractors have served athletes as an adjunct to their training and for performance enhancement. Many world-class athletes use chiropractors routinely during their training and at competitions, as I can attest to personally.

During my 20 years as a practicing chiropractor, I have had the opportunity to treat and care for many Olympic athletes and aspiring Olympic athletes. This opportunity was galvanized during the late 1980s when I was selected to be part of the United States Olympic Medical Staff. In 1988 I traveled with the Olympic Team to Seoul, South Korea as the chiropractor for the U.S. team. The importance of my presence on the staff was best described when one of the senior members of the U.S. Track Team informed me that "I was NOT to offer my services to members of any other country." I was part of their armamentarium and was there to provide them with the added benefit of chiropractic care.

During the 1988 Olympics, it was my opinion that, of all the participants for the U.S. teams, the track athletes demanded and utilized chiropractic care the most. My records reveal that 80 percent of the track athletes requested and utilized chiropractic care. Many had already been under the care of a chiropractor prior to their Olympic experience.

It should be strongly emphasized that these athletes were not seeking care because of an injury, because any significant injury would have prevented them from being there in the first place. They were constantly seeking chiropractic services for "tune-ups" as well as care that they considered an integral part of their training. To further elucidate, I will describe the most common scenarios that required treatment.

Almost all track athletes (not field) requested manipulation of their lower extremities. Manipulations of the tarsal bones, the subtalar joint, and the cuboid were constantly requested. These athletes, who obviously demanded much of their feet (52 tarsal bones and the extensive network of supporting tendons and ligaments), constantly would require attention to these structures. In addition to overcoming normal effects of gravity, these structures are subjected to the forces that incorporate acceleration, controlled deceleration, and concentrated contractions that provide ballistic movements that allow these athletes to run and jump faster and higher than most other bipeds.

Subluxations, fixations, malalignments, and scenarios of dysfunctional biomechanics of these structures that could detract from an optimal performance were cared for daily. Most individuals never realized or appreciated the effects that such functional abnormalities could have on performance or ability to compete at the highest level.

Athletes have always demanded that their anatomy perform at levels that could easily cause breakdowns or scenarios of dysfunctional biomechanics. These breakdowns or functional alterations of normal biomechanics are what the chiropractor addresses or corrects when providing manipulative skills to the athletes' anatomy. In the case of track athletes, these subtle dysfunctions in the lower extremities and spinal column must be reduced or eliminated to allow for optimal performance.

Spinal manipulation to the spine and its supporting structures is required by all athletes for optimum performance. Athletes require optimum structural integrity of their entire anatomy for optimum performance. Any breakdown along the kinetic chain can detract from the optimization of the entire kinetic chain. There have been many world-class athletes, as well as "weekend warriors," who have had careers shortened or performances that have never achieved desired results because of nagging injuries or altered biomechanics and anatomy. Besides the obvious detriment to performance, an injury can cause an interruption of valuable training time, which is the lifeblood to any athlete.

Like no other segment of the population, the athlete is also most likely to be the patient who is the most demanding when care is to be administered. The practitioner who is able to provide biomechanical improvement to an athlete becomes invaluable to that athlete's career, especially when the improvement does not involve drugs or surgery. This is what prompted the athletes of the world to incorporate chiropractic care into their training regimen.

REFERENCES

Chiropractic

1. Gibbons RW: The evolution of chiropractic: medical and social protests in America. In Haldeman S (ed): Modern Developments in the Principles and Practice of Chiropractic. Appleton-Century-Crofts, New York, 1980

2. Caplan R: Chiropractic. In Salmon J (ed): Alternative Medicines. Tavistock Publications, New York, 1984

3. Beideman RP: Seeking the rational alternative: the National College of Chiropractic from 1906 to 1982. Chirop History 3:17, 1983

4. Flexner A: Medical Education in the United States and Canada. Bulletin of the Carnegie Foundation for the Advancement of Teaching, No. 4, 1910

5. Beideman RP: A short history of the chiropractic profession. In Lawrence DJ (ed): Fundamentals of Chiropractic Diagnosis and Management. Williams & Wilkins, Baltimore, 1990

6. Lawrence DJ: Can chiropractic be a philosophical discipline? Philos Constr Chirop Profession 1:25, 1991

7. Lawrence DJ: Chiropractic. In Rubik B, Pavek R, Ward R et al (eds): Manual Healing Methods. In Alternative medicine: Expanding Medical Horizons. A Report to the National Institutes of Health on Alternative Medical Systems and Practices in the United States (NIH publication no. 94-0666). National Institutes of Health, Washington, DC, 1994

8. Hieronymus JH: De luxationibus et subluxationibus. Thesis, Jena, 1746

9. Palmer DD: The Science, Art and Philosophy of Chiropractic. Portland Printing House, Portland, OR, 1910

10. Palmer BJ: Fight to Climb. Palmer School of Chiropractic, Davenport, IA, 1950

11. Goldstein M (ed): The Research Status of Spinal Manipulative Therapy (NINCDS Monograph no. 15). National Institute of Neurological and Communicative Disorders and Stroke, Washington, DC, 1975

12. Lantz C: The vertebral subluxation complex. ICA Int Rev Chirop Sept/Oct: 37, 1989

13. Gatterman M: Foundations of Chiropractic: Subluxation. Mosby–Year Book, St. Louis, 1996

14. Leach R: The Chiropractic Theories. 2nd ed. Williams & Wilkins, Baltimore, 1986

15. Schafer RC: Clinical Biomechanics: Musculoskeletal Actions and Reactions. Williams & Wilkins, Baltimore, 1987

16. Grostic JD: Dentate ligament-cord distortion hypothesis. Chirop Res J 1:47, 1988

17. Jarzem PF, Quance DR, Doyle DJ et al: Spinal cord tissue pressure during spinal cord distraction in dogs. Spine 17(suppl 8):S227, 1992

18. Maigne R: Orthopedic Medicine: A New Approach to Vertebral Manipulation. p. 169. Charles C Thomas, Springfield, IL, 1972

19. Jaskoviak PJ: Complications arising from manipulation of the cervical spine. J Manipulative Physiol Ther 3:213, 1980

20. Nyiendo J, Haldeman S: A critical study of the student interns' practice activities in a chiropractic college teaching clinic. J Manipulative Physiol Ther 9:197, 1986

Manipulation

21. Sandoz R: Some physical mechanisms and effects of spinal adjustments. Ann Swiss Chirop Assoc 6:91, 1976

22. Unsworth A, Dowson D, Wright V: Cracking joints, a bioengineering study of cavitation in the metacarpophalangeal joint. Ann Rheum Dis 30:348, 1971

23. Mennell J: History of the development of medical manipulative concepts. p. 19. In The Research Status of Spinal Manipulative Therapy, (NINCDS Publication no. 15). US Department of Health and Human Services, Washington, DC, 1975

24. Mennell JM: Foot Pain. Little, Brown, Boston, 1969

25. Kaltenborn FM: Mobilization of the Extremity Joints. Olaf Norlis Bokhandel, Oslo, 1980

26. Frigerio NA, Stowe RR, Howe JW: Movement of the sacroiliac joint. Clin Orthop Rel Res 100, 1974

27. Gillet H: Clinical measurements of sacro-iliac mobility. Ann Swiss Chirop Assoc 6:59, 1976

SUGGESTED READINGS

Berman DL: Etiology and management of hallux valgus in athletes. Physician Sports Med 10(8), 1982

Cailliet R: Foot and Ankle Pain. FA Davis, Philadelphia, 1968

Christensen KD: Extremity Adjusting. Copybreak Printing, Portland, OR, 1978

Gertler L: Illustrated Manual of Extravertebral Technic. Gertler, Oakland, CA, 1978

Hollinshead WH: Textbook of Anatomy. Harper & Row, New York, 1974

Keskinen K, Eriksson E, Komi P: Breaststroke swimmer's knee. Am Orthop Soc Sports Med 8(4), 1980

Kirkaldy-Willis WH, Burton CV: Managing Low Back Pain. 3rd ed. Churchill Livingstone, New York, 1992

Noble BH, Hajek MR, Porter M: Diagnosis and treatment of iliotibial band tightness in runners. Physician Sportsmed 10(4), 1982

Potter GE: Diagnosis and manipulative management of postpartum back pain: a case study. J Manipulative Physiol Ther 2:99, 1979

Roston JB, Haines RW: Cracking in the metacarpo-phalangeal joint. J Anat 81:165, 1947

Sandoz R: Newer trends in the pathogenesis of spinal disorders. Ann Swiss Chirop Assoc 5:93, 1971

Schafer RC: Chiropractic Management of Sports and Recreational Injuries. Williams & Wilkins, Baltimore, 1982

Schultz AL: Athletic and Industrial Injuries of the Foot and Ankle. Argus, Stickney, SD, 1979

Schultz AL: The Knee, Femur, and Pelvis. Argus, Stickney, SD, 1976

Scranton PE: Metatarsalgia: diagnosis and treatment. J Bone Joint Surg [Am] 62, 1980

Seimon LP: Low Back Pain. Appleton & Lange, Norwalk, CT, 1983

Southmayd W, Hoffman M: Sports Health. Quick Fox, New York, 1981

Stierwalt DD: Extremity Adjusting. Stierwalt, Davenport, IA, 1976

Tepoorten BA: The piriformis muscle. J Am Orthop Assoc 69(150/78), 1969

23

Anti-inflammatory Medications, Analgesics, and Anesthetics

C. MICHAEL NEUWELT

In recent decades, exercise has been proven to be a prescription for good health,[1,2] and interest in sporting activities has grown proportionally. Ten percent of all traumatic injuries treated in emergency rooms of hospitals in industrialized countries are sustained in sports.[3] Principles of sports medicine treatment are no longer applicable only to young athletes but also apply to middle-age recreational athletes, as well as to the elderly. High-intensity resistance exercise training is a feasible and effective means of counteracting muscle weakness and physical frailty in the very elderly.[1] Regular exercise increases oxygen delivery to the heart by several physiologic adaptations, and regular exercise over time has proven protective against coronary artery disease and triggering of myocardial infarction.[2]

Injury is inevitable in exercise. Sports injury prevention is paramount and should be emphasized prior to injury. Primary prevention at the individual level includes medical screenings; protective equipment, including adequate running shoes; flexibility and strength training; and nutrition.[3] Once injury occurs, expectations of the athlete, regardless of age, are high for fast wound healing and prompt return to full capacity.[4] These expectations make the sports medicine setting difficult. Patients with exercise-induced injuries must be educated on further prevention and, as progressive treatment modalities are employed, the risk/benefits ratio must be carefully explained. As older and older patients do more vigorous exercise and consequently sustain injury, the pressure for fast wound healing and prompt return to full capacity must be resisted, and more conservative and even slower but safer modalities employed.

Prior to the use of anti-inflammatory medications, anesthetics, analgesics, and other nonpharmacologic therapies, rest, ice, compression, and elevation (RICE) remain the traditional recommendation for initial treatment.[5,6] These modalities are widely accepted in the sports medicine arena, lack major side effects, and effectively reduce swelling and decrease pain.[6] Anti-inflammatory medications, both nonsteroidal and steroidal, are widely used in sports today,[7] but their roles are much more controversial, and safety issues with each individual injury must be weighed. Anesthetics, analgesics, and other nonpharmacologic therapies are taking on new roles, and their use is greatly increased as athletes age and are more susceptible to chronic injury and secondary osteoarthritis. This chapter explores the use and application of all these medications, emphasizing patient education, safety issues, and tailoring the treatment to the individual injury and the age of the patient/athlete.

ANTI-INFLAMMATORY MEDICATIONS

Nonsteroidal Anti-inflammatory Drugs

In an attempt to provide for fast wound healing and prompt return to full capacity, sports medicine physicians often use nonsteroidal anti-inflammatory drugs (NSAIDs) to minimize inflammation and to speed the healing process. Although short-term studies suggest NSAIDs do not delay the healing process after an acute injury, only modest benefits are seen in most studies compared to placebo controls.[4] Consequently, since NSAIDs are almost universally used by sports and team physicians for injury, they must be used cautiously in individual injuries since in many cases the risk/benefit ratio may be slight.

Many recreational runners and athletes try to prevent delayed-onset muscle soreness (DOMS) by use of NSAIDs. Although DOMS can be prophylactically prevented by proper training, NSAIDs are not effective in avoiding DOMS[5,8] and there are no objective scientific data to support using NSAIDs to prevent injury in general.[6] Since gastrointestinal side effects of NSAIDs are frequent and runners especially tend to perform on an empty stomach, runners put themselves at risk for major gastrointestinal complications with no proven benefit if they take NSAIDs prior to performing to prevent soreness or injury. There is also an increased risk of decreased kidney function if an athlete becomes dehydrated, and in rare cases end-stage renal failure can be caused by regular use of anti-inflammatory analgesic medication.[9] Prophylaxis should not be confused with pre-existing chronic injury, where certainly reasonable doses of NSAIDs are indicated. Depending on the age of the athlete and pre-existing medical conditions, if NSAIDs are used chronically for injury, laboratory checks of blood counts and chemistries should be performed every 3 to 6 months.

For stretch-induced muscle injuries, after RICE for initial treatment, NSAIDs should be started as soon as possible after injury. They should be used for a relatively short period of time since they may interfere with subsequent repair and remodeling.[5] Early mobilization is important, and this goal is augmented by treatment with anti-inflammatory agents. In rare circumstances, steroid injections and proteolytic enzymes are used for acute muscular injuries (Table 23-1).[5] Treatment modalities should be combined for maximum early benefit. For example, physiotherapy (ultrasound and cross-transverse friction massage) together with combined analgesic/anti-inflammatory medication is superior to any modality alone for early management of iliotibial band friction syndrome.[10]

In choosing an NSAID, differences and similarities exist, and an understanding of these widely used medications is important to maximize their benefit and minimize side effects in the patient/athlete. NSAIDs tend to divide into two groups on the basis of their plasma elimination half-life: those with a short half-life (less than 6 hours) and those

with a long half-life (more than 10 hours) (Table 23-2).[11] Both groups have been extensively studied and compared in clinical trials. Etodolac (Lodine), a safe short half-life NSAID in a dose of 300 mg tid, was compared to naproxen (Naprosyn), a time-honored long half-life NSAID in a dose of 500 mg bid, in a double-blind, parallel-group evaluation. Both medications, when used for several days beginning within 48 hours of injury, were comparable, and significant relief of symptoms was observed with both drugs.[12] However, when these drugs are used for longer than several days, steady-state plasma concentrations are achieved only after a period of dosing extending for three to five half-lives, and NSAIDs with a long half-life do not achieve plateau concentrations in plasma and maximal clinical effects as fast as NSAIDs with short half-lives unless a loading dose regimen is used.[11]

Based on half-life and other factors, further differences exist between NSAIDs, and these differences are compounded as athletes age and develop concomitant medical problems. Phenylbutazone and indomethacin are more frequently associated with agranulocytosis and aplastic anemia than are other NSAIDs.[13] Piroxicam (Feldene and

Table 23-1 Summary of Modes of Treatment for Acute Muscular Injuries

Mode of Treatment	Period	Effect
Rest	24–48 hr in grades I–II 3–5 weeks in grade III unless repaired	Decrease swelling Decrease hemorrhage Allow bridging of the defect
Ice	24–48 hr	Decrease swelling Slow metabolism Analgesic
Compression and elevation	24–48 hr	Decrease swelling
NSAIDs	3–5 days	Pain control Decrease inflammation
Steroid injection	Within 24 hr	Decrease inflammation
Proteolytic enzymes	Within 24 hr	Decrease hematoma
Mobilization	After 24–48 hr in grades I–II	Stimulate repair Prevent contracture Prevent weakness

(From Almekinders LC: Anti-inflammatory treatment of muscular injuries in sports. Sports Med 15:139, 1993, with persmission.)

Table 23-2 Mean (± SD) Plasma Half-Lives of Different NSAIDs

Drug	Half-Live (hr)
Short Half-Life	
Aspirin	0.25 ± 0.03
Diclofenac	1.1 ± 0.2
Etodolac	3.0; 6.5 ± 0.3[a]
Fenoprofen	1.4; 9.0[a]
Flufenamic acid	
Flurbiprofen	3.8 ± 1.2
Ibuprofen	2.1 ± 0.3
Indomethacin	4.6 ± 0.7
Ketoprofen	1.8 ± 0.4
Pirprofen	3.8; 6.8[a]
Tiaprofenic acid	3.0 ± 0.2
Tolmetin	1.0 ± 0.3; 6.8 ± 1.5[a]
Long Half-Life	
Apazone	15 ± 4
Diflunisal	13 ± 2
Fenbufen	11.0
Nabumetone	26 ± 5
Naproxen	14 ± 2
Oxaprozin	58 ± 10
Phenylbutazone	68 ± 25
Piroxicam	57 ± 22
Salicylate	2–15[b]
Sulindac (sulfide)	14 ± 8
Tenoxicam	60 ± 11

[a] Elimination of this drug occurs in two phases (indicated by semicolon), of which the first is generally the most important.

[b] Elimination of this drug is dose dependent.

(From Brooks PM, Day RO: Drug therapy—nonsteroidal anti-inflammatory drugs—differences and similarities. N Engl J Med 324:1716, 1991. Copyright 1991, Massachusetts Medical Society, with permission.)

others), which has a longer half-life and may cause a higher incidence of gastrointestinal bleeding than other NSAIDs, should be avoided in elderly patients.[14]

Unfortunately, since NSAIDs inhibit prostaglandin biosynthesis, they also cause common and occasionally severe side effects such as hypertension, congestive heart failure, hyperkalemia, renal insufficiency, and most commonly gastrointestinal side effects.[15] However, more recently, we now know that there are two distinct cyclo-oxygenase (COX) molecules, COX-1 and COX-2 (Fig. 23-1). COX-1 is expressed in most tissues, is constitutive, and is synthesized at a constant rate. It is involved in cellular homeostasis, synthesizing prostaglandins in response to physiologic stimuli at a rate in proportion to the availability of the substrate, arachidonic acid. Prostaglandins in the gastrointestinal tract have an important protective role in the maintenance of microvascular integrity, the regulation of cell division, and the production of mucus.

COX-2, by contrast, is undetectable in most tissues under normal physiologic conditions. It is inducible at sites of inflammation through the action of cytokines and endotoxins. Macrophages and other inflammatory cells have abundant COX-2 activity. Therefore, the products of COX-2 may drive inflammation and the prostaglandins so formed may be important mediators for pain. Selective COX-2 inhibition has become a target for treatment, based on the promise of gastrointestinal tolerability. Although the assays for COX-1 and COX-2 at this time vary, and there is not a pure COX-2 NSAID available, Sir John Vane, who discovered this system, stated to the American College of Rheumatology that etodolac nabumetone and ibuprofen products had favorable profiles (i.e., marked COX-2 selectivity over COX-1). Meloxicam, not yet available in the United States, is under further investigation and is the closest NSAID studied that approaches pure COX-2 selectivity.[17] Celecoxib (SC-58635) and MK-0966 are even newer agents that are undergoing Phase III trials.[18,19]

Tenidap sodium is a new anti-inflammatory, an oxindole with other novel properties, that is not yet approved by the Food and Drug Administration (FDA) (side effect issues may further delay approval). Like other NSAIDs, tenidap inhibits cyclo-oxygenase, and therefore provides direct analgesic activity and acute anti-inflammatory activity associated with inhibition of prostaglandin synthesis. However, other anti-inflammatory activities of tenidap are similar to those of corticosteroids and have been associated with cytokine-modulating activity.[20] This dual mechanism of action (inhibition of cyclo-oxygenase plus modulation of cytokines) may give tenidap an important role in more serious active and chronic injuries in sports medicine. Tenidap has analgesic properties advantageous in sports injury as tested in experimental animals, but its COX-1/COX-2 selectivity has not been adequately studied in human clinical trials.[20]

Nonacetylated salicylates (generic sodium salicylate) do not inhibit platelets[13] yet have mild anti-inflammatory properties not based on prostaglandin inhibition, and should probably have an expanded role in sports medicine. In injuries where there is concern about hemorrhage in the first 48 hours, such as a severe ankle sprain, nonacetylated salicylates are good drugs if anti-platelet effects are to be avoided; in the elderly exercise participant, in whom long-term antiplatelet effects are desired for cardiac and neurologic risk factors, aspirin should be used. In a patient with

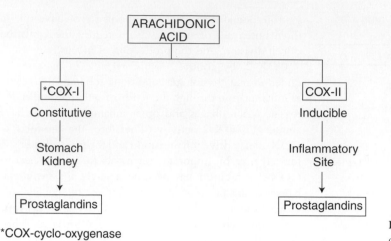

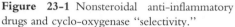

*COX-cyclo-oxygenase

Figure 23-1 Nonsteroidal anti-inflammatory drugs and cyclo-oxygenase "selectivity."

a history of gastrointestinal ulcer, NSAIDs with a short serum half-life may be used to minimize the duration of antiplatelet effects.[13] Besides concerns about gastrointestinal, kidney, hematologic, and platelet effects, NSAIDs may have an effect on bone resorption relevant to osteoporosis. Bone density in long-term runners is a major concern, and studies have shown a decrease in bone density over a 2-year period for runners who decrease their running habits.[21] As postmenopausal women who run age, and suffer from chronic injuries, perhaps NSAIDs will play a further role. Diclofenac sodium (Voltaren) was found to inhibit bone resorption in postmenopausal women, but whether this nonsteroidal agent will effectively prevent long-term loss of bone mass in postmenopausal women remains to be determined.[22]

Compliance is a major issue with NSAIDs and must be balanced with the side effects in choosing a medication for the patient/athlete, especially in the older patient. Once-a-day dosing is convenient for younger patients, but NSAIDs with longer half-lives raise concerns in older patients.[14] Sustained-release preparations of NSAIDs that maintain the advantages of those with short half-lives, such as ketoprofen (Oruvail), indomethacin (Indocin),[11] diclofenac extended release (Voltaren-XR), and the newest such drug etodolac extended-release (Lodine XL), have been developed. A new formulation of naproxen sodium (Naprelan) is now available that takes a time-honored NSAID and converts it to once-a-day dosing, consequently increasing compliance. However, indomethacin in particular can interfere with the pharmacologic control of hypertension.[11]

NSAIDs are so commonly used in sports medicine that, because of the desire to minimize side effects, they have been administered by routes other than oral. A popular current approach has been the use of gel forms of NSAIDs, which can be applied topically onto the affected area of injury. Many studies suggest that topical NSAIDs may indeed be significantly better than placebo in treating acute injury without subjecting the athlete to the myriad of adverse events associated with oral administration of NSAIDs. Further studies conducted in the United States should be performed in well-controlled settings to determine if topical nonsteroidal agents are efficacious after acute athletic injury.[4] The American College of Rheumatology advisory committee to the FDA has suggested further studies to determine if topical NSAIDs have significant anti-inflammatory properties,[23] but with topical agents there is a high placebo response rate, and it is difficult to find appropriate placebo treatments.[14] If efficacy is clearly demonstrated in rigorous clinical trials, the mechanisms responsible for pain relief should be considered, including diffusion of NSAIDs directly into target tissues, as well as possible effects on sensory nerve function or products (e.g., substance P).[24]

Corticosteroids and Anesthetics

Cortisone is one of the most effective anti-inflammatory agents used in sports medicine, but it has serious side effects that demand judicious use and judgment.[25] Oral cortisone should rarely be used because of a marginal long-term risk/benefit ratio in athletes, but it is occasionally used for conditions such as tenosynovitis of the Achilles tendon. Injections of cortisone around the Achilles tendon are generally accepted as dangerous, and there have been reports that injections into the tendon may lead to central necrosis and partial or complete rupture.[7] Most patients with Achilles tendonitis do well with time and conservative treatment. However, there are two indications for corticosteroid injections: symptoms secondary to a retrocalcaneal bursitis and diffuse tendonitis when the tendon sheath is involved. Retrocalcaneal bursitis is the most common Achilles tendon insertional problem. Treatment with ice, stretching, NSAIDs, and 2 to 3 weeks of complete rest may be necessary to reduce the inflammation and the pseudo-synovial thickening. Injectable steroid should be used once if there is no involvement of the Achilles tendon as demonstrated by magnetic resonance imaging.

Plantar fasciitis is another common lower extremity injury in runners. When conservative treatments have been exhausted with no measurable relief obtained, some recommend a steroid injection administered at the site of the attachment of the plantar fascia to the medial calcaneal tubercle.[26] In resistant plantar fasciitis, a single injection that includes 1.5 ml of lidocaine and an appropriate small amount of steroid into the plantar fascia origin is a second step.[27] If not successful within 6 weeks, a possible single reinjection of the injectable steroid and casting should be considered,[24] but no more than three injections should be given in any one series.[28] After an injection, a runner must allow time for tissue healing. The injections increase the possibility of plantar fascia rupture because of the tissue reaction to the steroid preparations (e.g., decreased tissue tensile strength). The most recalcitrant cases of plantar fasciitis may require surgical release of the fascia from its attachment at the medial tubercle of the calcaneus.[28] As mentioned, local anesthetics are commonly used with injectable steroidal preparations; these include 0.75 to 4 ml of 1 percent lidocaine plain, as well as 0.75 to 1 ml of 0.5 percent bupivacaine plain.[7] The local anesthetic not only has immediate therapeutic value but diagnostically reassures the sports medicine physician that the pain is coming from that anatomic site—especially when secondary psychological factors are involved.

Local corticosteroid injections also play a role in ligamentous injury with ankle sprains but should not be substituted for a well-managed rehabilitation program. The local corticosteroid injection can facilitate the rehabilitation process when there is slow resolution of the symptoms.[27]

Besides the rare use of oral cortisone and the frequent but cautious use of injectable corticosteroid preparations, fluorinated cortisone creams also play a role in sports medicine. The creams, when used with ultrasound, may decrease superficial inflammation around tendons or bursas or within the skin itself through the process of phonophoresis.[7]

ANALGESICS AND NONMEDICINAL THERAPIES

The principal mechanism of action of NSAIDs is cyclo-oxygenase inhibition and interference with the synthesis of prostaglandins. Cyclo-oxygenase inhibition through actions on other mediators may in turn have secondary effects, including inhibition of neutrophil activation, T- and B-cell proliferation, and leukotriene production.[13] Brooks and Day[11] have summarized the processes influenced by NSAIDs (see Box). These processes also control and reduce pain, which many times may be the primary goal in sports medicine, since not all sports injuries are accompanied by inflammation. The ideal NSAID controls pain at a low dose with minimal side effects. Diclofenac and indomethacin are potent inhibitors of leukotrienes, perhaps more important in pain modulation.[11]

Pure analgesics that do not inhibit prostaglandins can spare side effects yet control pain. Although acetaminophen (e.g., Tylenol) can cause serious hepatotoxicity, in the absence of other hepatotoxic agents this occurs only with a daily dose exceeding 10 g (2.5 times the maximum recommended dose). Although most physicians initiate

---

PROCESSES INFLUENCED BY NSAIDs

Prostaglandin production

Leukotriene synthesis

Superoxide generation

Lysosomal enzyme release

Neutrophil aggregation and adhesion

Cell-membrane functions
 Enzyme activity (NADPH oxidase, phospholipase C)
 Transmembrane anion transport
 Oxidative phosphorylation
 Uptake of arachidonate

Lymphocyte function

Rheumatoid factor production

Cartilage metabolism

(From Brooks PM, Day RO: Drug therapy—nonsteroidal anti-inflammatory drugs—differences and similarities. N Engl J Med 324:1716, 1991. Copyright 1991, Massachusetts Medical Society, with permission.)

treatment with an NSAID, a current trend in osteoarthritis suggests acetaminophen should be prescribed initially in a dose as high as 4 g/day, in parallel with implementation of nonpharmacologic measures.[15] In sports medicine injuries, especially in the elderly, the same principles apply. Except for severe, acute injuries, narcotic analgesics should be avoided. Tramadol (Ultram) is a recently released "atypical" opioid analgesic that has a low abuse potential and low dependency when used chronically, is unscheduled, yet is indicated in chronic pain. Its mechanism of action is mediated by opioid and nonopioid mechanisms[29] and, because of its low potential for abuse and addiction, it can be used for severe, chronic sports medicine injuries to control pain.

In patients/athletes with underlying osteoarthritis aggravated by sports injuries, cold applications are preferable because an increase in intra-articular temperature is undesirable. If heat is preferred by the patient, application should last no more than 5 to 10 minutes.[30]

Capsaicin cream (Zostrix-HP) is effective in managing numerous conditions, including painful diabetic neuropathy, postherpetic neuralgia, postmastectomy pain syndrome, reflex sympathetic dystrophy, and musculoskeletal pain syndromes, including osteoarthritis.[24] Sports medicine conditions such as tendonitis, bursitis, and epicondylitis have also responded favorably to therapy with topical capsaicin. Purified capsaicin depletes substance P, a neurotransmitter of pain, from type C neurons.[31] Data on other nonpharmacologic therapies, including transcutaneous electrical nerve stimulation, pulsed electromagnetic fields, and acupuncture, are sparse.[24]

SUMMARY

Anti-inflammatory medications, anesthetics, analgesics, and nonpharmacologic therapies are frequently used in sports medicine. Conservative measures should always be employed first, with early consideration of analgesics to supplement NSAIDs and consideration of nonacetylated salicylates, especially as the sports medicine population broadens and ages. Corticosteroids, whether oral or injectable, should always be used cautiously, but timely institution can facilitate the rehabilitation process. The pressure for fast wound healing and prompt return to full capacity should be resisted in sports medicine, especially as the patient/athlete ages. In addition, education and injury prevention should be emphasized and the risk/benefit ratio carefully explained for all treatment modalities.

REFERENCES

1. Fiatarone MA, O'Neill EF, Ryan ND et al: Exercise training and nutritional supplementation for physical frailty in very elderly people. N Engl J Med 330:1169, 1994
2. Curfman GD: Editorial—is exercise beneficial or hazardous to your heart? N Engl J Med 329:1730, 1993
3. Renstrom P, Kannus P: Prevention of sports injuries. p. 307. In Strauss RH (ed): Sports Medicine. 2nd ed. W.B. Saunders, Philadelphia, 1991
4. Weiler JM: Medical modifiers of sports injury: the use of nonsteroidal anti-inflammatory drugs (NSAIDS) in sports soft-tissue injury. Clin Sports Med 11:625, 1992
5. Almekinders LC: Anti-inflammatory treatment of muscular injuries in sports. Sports Med 15:139, 1993
6. Sellers RG: Sports injuries: practical diagnostic and management concerns for primary care physicians. Postgrad Med 14:31, 1992
7. Subotnick SI: Anti-inflammatory medications, analgesics, and anesthetics. p. 420. In Subotnick SI (ed): Sports Medicine of the Lower Extremity. Churchill Livingstone, New York, 1989
8. Donnelly AE, Maughan RJ, Whiting PH: Effects of ibuprofen on exercise-induced muscle soreness and indices of muscle damage. Br J Sports Med 24:191, 1990
9. Griffiths ML: End-stage renal failure caused by regular use of anti-inflammatory analgesic medication for minor sports injuries—a case report. S Afr Med J 81:377, 1992.
10. Schwellnus MP, Theunissen L, Noakes TD, Reinach SG: Anti-inflammatory and combined anti-inflammatory/analgesic medication in the early management of iliotibial band friction syndrome. S Afr Med J 79:602, 1991
11. Brooks PM, Day RO: Drug therapy—nonsteroidal anti-inflammatory drugs—differences and similarities. N Engl J Med 324:1716, 1991
12. D'Hooghe M: Double-blind, parallel-group evaluation of etodolac and naproxen in patients with acute sports injuries. Clin Ther 14:507, 1992
13. Furst DE: Are there differences among nonsteroidal anti-inflammatory drugs? Comparing acetylated salicylates, nonacetylated salicylates, and nonacetylated nonsteroidal anti-inflammatory drugs. Arthritis Rheum 37:1, 1994
14. Abramowicz M (ed): Drugs for rheumatoid arthritis. Med Lett Drugs Ther 36:101, 1994
15. Brandt KD: NSAIDS in the treatment of osteoarthritis: friends or foes? Bull Rheum Dis 42:1, 1993
16. Hayllar J, Bjarnson I: NSAIDS, Cox-2 inhibitors, and the gut. Lancet 346:521, 1995
17. Auvinet B, Rainer Z, Appleboom T et al: Comparison of the onset and intensity of action of intramuscular meloxicam and oral meloxicam in patients with acute sciatica. Clin Ther 17:1078, 1995
18. Hubbard RC, Mehlisch DR, Jasper DR et al: SC 58635, a

highly selective inhibitor of Cox-2, is an effective analgesic in an acute post-surgical pain model. J Invest Med 44, 1996

19. Ehrich E, Schmitzer T, McIlwain H et al: MK-966, a highly selective COX-2 inhibitor is effective in the treatment of osteoarthritis in a 6-week pilot study. Osteoarthritis Cartilage 5 (suppl A), 1997

20. Moore PF, Larson DL, Otterness IG et al: Tenidap, a structurally novel drug for the treatment of arthritis: anti-inflammatory and analgesic properties. Inflamm Res 45:54, 1996

21. Lane NE, Bloch DA, Hubert HB et al: Running, osteoarthritis, and bone density: initial 2-year longitudinal study. Am J Med 88:453, 1990

22. Bell NH, Hollis BW, Shary JR et al: Diclofenac sodium inhibits bone resorption in postmenopausal women. Am J Med 96:349, 1994

23. Weisman MH, Furst DE, Paulus HE: FDA Arthritis Advisory Committee meeting: Analgesics guidelines; topical NSAIDS; extracorporeal photochemotherapy in scleroderma. Arthritis Rheum 34:931, 1991

24. Puett DW, Griffin MR: Published trials of nonmedicinal and noninvasive therapies for hip and knee osteoarthritis. Ann Intern Med 121:133, 1994

25. Kerlan RK, Glousman RE: Injection and techniques in athletic medicine. Clin Sports Med 8:541, 1989

26. Leach RE, Schepsis AA, Takai T: Achilles tendinitis—don't let it be an athlete's downfall. Physician Sports Med 19:87, 1991

27. McBryde AM: Disorders of the ankle and foot. p. 474. In Grana WA, Kalenak A (eds): Clinical Sports Medicine. W.B. Saunders, Philadelphia, 1991

28. Warren BL: Plantar fasciitis in runners—treatment and prevention. Sports Med 10:338, 1990

29. Raffa RB, Friderichs E, Reimann W et al: Opioid and nonopioid components independently contribute to the mechanism of action of tramadol, an "atypical" opioid analgesic. J Pharmacol Exp Ther 260:275, 1992

30. Oosterveld FJ, Rasker JJ: Treating arthritis with locally applied heat or cold. Semin Arthritis Rheum 24:82, 1994

31. Deal CL: The use of topical capsaicin in managing arthritis pain: a clinician's perspective. Semin Arthritis Rheum 23: 48, 1994

24

Orthoses

RONALD VALMASSY
STEVEN I. SUBOTNICK

Most athletes, especially those who run, will, at some point in their running career, develop a lower extremity problem that prevents them from continuing with their athletic endeavors. Although most of us can easily appreciate a marathoner developing a foot or leg problem that prevents running, we must also appreciate that golfers, bowlers, walkers, and skiers, to name but a few, also get crippling lower extremity injuries. In many instances, the injury is short lived and is nothing more than a minor nuisance that can be readily linked to overzealous training, improper warmup exercises, or inappropriate shoe gear. In other instances, minor discomfort may steadily increase to chronic pain that fails to respond to conservative measures or changes in running habits. These more chronic problems are often associated with the abnormal mechanics and function of the athlete's lower extremity in general, and of the foot in particular. It is in these cases, in which lower extremity injury stems from abnormal foot mechanics, that a sports podiatrist will often attempt to alter foot function through the use of a functional orthosis.[1,2]

Just what is an orthotic device? What does it do and why? To the orthopedist, an orthosis is a foot brace that supports the foot and limits unwanted motion. Examples are the UCBL molded device and the old Roberts plate foot braces. To the family practitioner, a foot orthotic is a fancy name for an arch support. To the chiropractor, an orthotic is a semiflexible device, made of leather, cork, and rubber using a weight-bearing foot impression foam box, that is designed to help balance the pelvis. These devices are not biodynamic according to podiatric param-

eters, yet may suit the needs of the chiropractor, although not the podiatrist. To the ski boot fitter, an orthosis is a molded foot bed made of cork and rubber, designed to improve boot fit while increasing comfort and edge control. To the pedorthotist, an orthosis can be arch "cookies" in the shoe, an ankle–foot polypropylene drop foot spring loaded device, an HA pad in the shoe, or flexible plastic UCBL molded foot devices. To the podiatric diabetic specialist, an orthotic is an accommodative device that shifts pressure away from areas of potential neuropathic ulceration. To the podiatric arthritic foot specialist, an orthotic cushions, pads, accommodates, and supports to prevent further subluxation and breakdown of tissue. Orthotic foot devices might pad a bunion, protect a toe, or accommodate a plantar-flexed metatarsal.[3] To the sports podiatrist, a foot orthosis is a biodynamic device that guides the foot through the various weight-bearing portions of the gait cycle to promote a generally biomechanically efficient movement pattern.

A foot orthotic is not a brace—far from it. It provides stable fulcrums that allow the intrinsic stabilizers and extrinsic prime movers to effectively do their job, thereby creating a stronger, more efficient foot even when the orthosis is not being used. With a well-designed foot orthosis, function is centered around a neutral midstance foot position. This theoretical neutral point exists at the middle of midstance. From this point in time and space, supination and propulsion proceed phasically and with the least necessary expenditure of energy. The orthotic decreases the speed and, to a lesser extent, the amount of impact pronation, and appears to function by a combination of mechanical control and biofeedback.[4–6] Certainly it teaches the athlete good foot mechanics, because it is uncomfortable if not painful to run improperly with the foot orthotic in the shoe. Biofeedback is as important as mechanical control in guiding the foot through the various phases of gait. Balanced forefoot and rearfoot shims, cants, or posts and custom-molded medial and lateral arches help to decrease excessive or abnormal motion. The heel cup must be deep, 16 to 17 mm, to keep the calcaneal fat pad under the heel for impact shock attenuation and rearfoot control. The importance of the lateral arch, the calcaneocuboid joint, is often not fully appreciated.[7,8]

Given the multitude of variables (body type, shoes, surfaces, and speed), how effective are most foot orthotics? When well designed, foot orthoses are impressively effective in reducing biomechanically induced overuse pain, and restoring normal gait and foot function.[4,9] Many orthotic devices, however, are far from effective. Why is this? Often it is because many foot orthotic prescribers are unclear as to what a true sport-specific foot orthotic is. Most do not test the effectiveness of their devices with treadmill and video, and, furthermore, with computer-assisted devices such as the f-scan dynamic three-dimensional computer-imaging gait analysis, (*Note*: This has replaced and far upgraded the once-popular Langer EDG) or the AMTI force platforms and Accusway balance and postural sway evaluation system. The orthosis designs are often faulty, and all too often walking orthotics are dispensed for runners or, worse, running orthotics are dispensed for golf or tennis players. When designed properly, over a neutral cast of a foot that has been adjusted and stretched out of soft tissue adaptive changes, these orthotics can do a marvelous job of realigning the foot, leg, and knee while providing a stable platform for the pelvis and spine. Any change in foot position affects the posture of the entire body above it. The somatovisceral changes, and vice versa, can wreak havoc on the entire body. Dananberg has clearly demonstrated gait style to be an etiology of chronic postural pain.[9,10]

An orthotic device is generally recommended following a thorough evaluation of the runner's lower extremity, as well as the back and spine, in both weight-bearing and non-weight-bearing positions.[11] Computerized gait analysis (f-scan data) is often helpful in assessing orthosis function. Of prime importance is evaluating the athlete barefooted, then with shoes. Surprisingly, most athletes walk and run more efficiently without shoes.[12] The shoes often promote excessive motion in their attempt to attenuate shock. While good walking shoes with a firm counter are far superior to higher heeled shoes, the barefooted gait is still a bit more stable for walking. Lateral counter instability causes lateral foot instability with excessive supination. Medial counter weakness, fracture, or breakdown at the midsole–counter interface leads to excessive contact and midsupport pronation.

The weight-bearing examination will include not only static evaluations but a dynamic functional walking and running examination as well, the latter often performed on a treadmill and analyzed through slow-motion videotape playback.[13,14] If, following these extensive measures (which generally include radiographic evaluation and thorough evaluation and inspection of the running shoes), the practitioner believes there is a problem regarding foot function, the recommendation will be made to alter the foot's function. Depending on the extent and severity of the biomechanical malfunction, the practitioner will recommend one of several different types of in-shoe orthotic devices. Other factors that will be evaluated are the type of activity the athlete participates in, the level of participation anticipated, and whatever personal performance goals the athlete has established. All these factors are carefully weighed in determining whether an orthosis is to be used, as well as what materials should be incorporated and the degree of correction required. The differentiation between unidirectional and multidirectional sports is essential. Edge-control sports are differentiated from rebound or jumping sports. The base of gait and center of gravity must be taken into account.[15]

In the short term, soft temporary orthoses are often used in order to improve foot function immediately, evaluate shoe function, and act as an indicator of necessity for permanent foot orthoses. These softer temporary devices are not made from a neutral cast; rather, they are made from a tracing of the foot and fabricated in the office biomechanics lab of softer heat-molded, compression-set materials. They may be posted, and various arch cookies, metatarsal pads, and accommodations may be built in. They are generally inexpensive and provide immediate first-visit foot treatment. Their effectiveness is checked by videotaped treadmill analysis. Although not a biodynamic, sport-specific, sophisticated biomechanical device, they are surprisingly effective.

In most cases, the permanent orthotic device will be fabricated over a plaster impression of the foot. With this more common neutral casting method, once the appropriate impression is taken, an orthosis laboratory will fabricate the device according to the practitioner's prescription. Computer scanning and imaging of the foot is available now and will do away with plaster casting in the near future. This allows the podiatrist to design custom orthoses with flanges, accommodation, and posts, cants, and counter balances on the computer screen, and then e-mail the design to the central computer of a milling Laboratory, which will fabricate the orthosis and store the foot image and prescription for further modification or replacement.

The type of device fabricated will most likely be a functional orthosis, that is, one that alters the mechanics of an individual's foot function. This type of biomechanical device is in no manner analogous to an arch support, in that it does not merely elevate the arch of the foot; it actually attempts to restore an element of normal foot function. In eliminating the need for the abnormally functioning foot to continue to compensate, the device functions in a fashion similar to a contact lens. When the device is worn during a particular activity, foot function is altered so that the lower extremity functions in a more normal fashion. Once the orthotic is removed from the shoe, foot function often remains more efficient as the foot remembers what to do from the biofeedback effect, and the general strengthening of intrinsic and extrinsic muscles. Unfortunately this does not last, and, after the device is removed, foot function slowly returns to its pre-existing state. Therefore, the orthosis generally has no long-term corrective qualities; it works efficiently primarily during the time it is being worn. In the younger athletic patient with a growing foot, changes may be more permanent and lasting.

Although the various types of orthoses are often modified for specific sports, it is not uncommon for some athletes to require different devices for various activities.[16] If an athlete's problem is only precipitated during the athletic activity, and there is no problem associated with normal day-to-day activities, one pair of devices may be all that is necessary. However, if the extent of foot malfunction is such that daily standing and walking exacerbates the problem, a second pair of devices, better suited to that purpose, may become appropriate. A running orthosis usually has too much varus control for everyday use. In any event, the overall goal of using "functional orthoses" is primarily what the name implies—that is, to alter the mechanics of the foot significantly to the point where normal foot and leg function can occur.[14,17–22] When used properly, the orthotic device is an efficient method whereby normal function can be restored, permitting the athlete

to resume appropriate levels of performance[13] (C. Smith, personal communication, 1979).

The remainder of this chapter deals with the various types of casting techniques currently available for obtaining appropriate negative casts. Some of the more common types of orthoses and modifications are examined.

CASTING TECHNIQUES

The practitioner has four widely used casting techniques to choose from in obtaining negative impressions of the patient's feet. Each is an acceptable method of obtaining a neutral-position cast, and may be used after evaluating several variables. These variables include the patient's foot type, foot structure, and extent of deformity, as well as foot gear.[23,24]

Suspension Casting

Suspension casting is the classic technique and the principal method of casting as described by Root et al.[23] (Fig. 24-1). This method places the patient in the treatment chair in the supine attitude. Two strips of plaster are applied to the foot. The foot is moved through its full excursion of inversion and eversion and is maintained in the neutral position. The subtalar joint neutral position may then be determined via three methods.[11] First, the head of the talus may be palpated as the foot is moved through its range of motion. The point at which the head of the talus is slightly palpable as it begins to emerge from behind the navicular reflects the neutral position. This can be confirmed by two methods. The skin lines superior and inferior to the lateral malleoli should be neither taut nor folded. Taut skin is indicative of a supinated foot, whereas excessive folding of the skin lines in these two areas reflects a pronated foot position. We should therefore strive for a relaxed position of the skin lines. Also, the concavities formed superior and inferior to the lateral malleolus should be equal in appearance. A discrepancy in concavity size is, again, indicative of a supinated or pronated position of the foot's subtalar joint. The subtalar joint is placed in its neutral position after the plaster is in place. Several factors must be considered to maintain the foot in this position with the midtarsal joint locked. Care must be taken to grasp the foot only by the fourth and fifth digits; the practitioner should not allow the thumb to encroach onto the second and third digits, because it is possible to introduce a supinatory force into the drying plaster cast (Fig. 24-2). A properly locked

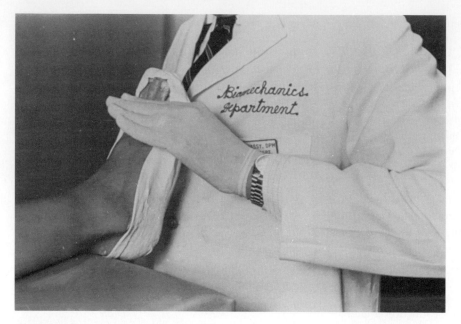

Figure 24-1 Suspension casting.

midtarsal joint is established by moving the forefoot in a dorsiflexory direction only to resistance. Furthermore, to ensure that the midtarsal joint is locked (fully pronated and stable against the rearfoot), the forefoot is slightly abducted while maintaining the neutral position of the subtalar joint. Obtaining a cast according to these guidelines will enable the practitioner to reproduce consistently good, accurate negative casts. When properly taken, this type of cast will duplicate the abnormal amount of forefoot varus or valgus present and should closely correspond to the pathology noted during the musculoskeletal examination.

Overall, the advantages of this casting technique are that it (1) effectively locks the midtarsal joint, (2) maintains an appropriate forefoot–rearfoot relationship, (3) facilitates visualization and palpation of the neutral position of the subtalar joint, and (4) produces proper elongation of soft tissue.

Prone Casting

The prone casting method places the patient in the prone position with the examiner positioned above the foot, sighting down the rearfoot to the forefoot (Fig. 24-3). Plaster is applied in the customary manner. The foot is then placed in its neutral position with the midtarsal joint locked. This is accomplished via two methods. First,

a dorsiflexory force may be applied against the fourth and fifth metatarsal heads with the examiner's thumb; this maintains the midtarsal joint locked by applying a dorsiflexory force to the forefoot. S.I.S. prefers this technique because it allows casting in the position of evaluation. The neutral rearfoot position is visualized and maintained as the forefoot is corrected relative to the rearfoot. He pushes up under the fourth metatarsal head to lock the midtarsal joint. Supinatus around the midtarsal joint longitudinal axis can be corrected for by downward pressure on the first metatarsal. Functional hallux limitus correction can be provided for by slightly dorsiflexing the hallux, thereby depressing the first metatarsal. Because distortion of this segment may be an artifact of the thumb's indentation, the area must be considered and corrected with accuracy either on the negative or positive cast. Generally this is easily done on the wet slipper cast.

A second method that may be used to maintain the foot in a neutral and locked position is to grasp the foot as in the supine technique, that is, by the fourth and fifth digits. In this way, the forefoot will not only be dorsiflexed and abducted relative to the rearfoot, but the examiner will also be able to direct a downward force on the foot. Such elongation is provided in the supine technique by the force of gravity as the foot is lifted slightly from the chair.

Advantages of this casting technique are (1) desired cast-

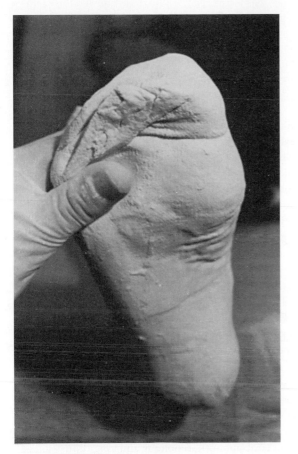

Figure 24-2 Appropriate thumb position for neutral suspension cast technique.

ing alignment of the forefoot to the rearfoot by locking the midtarsal joint, (2) the ability to judge subtalar joint neutral position through visualization and palpation, and (3) ease of cast corrections.

Semi-Weight-Bearing Technique

The semi-weight-bearing technique is best suited to creating a more pronated type of orthosis for those patients who have an equinus, coalition, or primary or secondary arthritic limitations of motion (Fig. 24-4). It may also be used for patients who possess a high degree of flexible forefoot valgus or in those who possess both types of deformity. Even if done with the foot maintained in a neutral position, this type of casting technique is not as satisfactory as either of the two preceding methods of obtaining a cast. It is, however, an excellent method for the broken-down

splay foot, which needs a very wide, semirigid device. It is also a good method for the compromised foot needing the exceptional control afforded by a UCBL or type C adult heel stabilizer (Fig. 24-5).

The plaster is placed on the foot in the customary fashion, with the foot then placed into the foam casting block with the subtalar joint in its neutral position. As the weight of the forefoot comes into contact with the casting block, a dorsiflexory reactive force of gravity is placed against the foot, which in turn supinates the longitudinal axis of the midtarsal joint. The net effect is inversion of the forefoot relative to the rearfoot, decreasing the amount of the flexible forefoot valgus or possibly increasing the amount of forefoot varus captured in the cast.

It should be noted that, when a neutral suspension cast of a patient with a flexible forefoot valgus is compared with a semi-weight-bearing cast of the same foot, a significant difference exists. The differences occur primarily with a

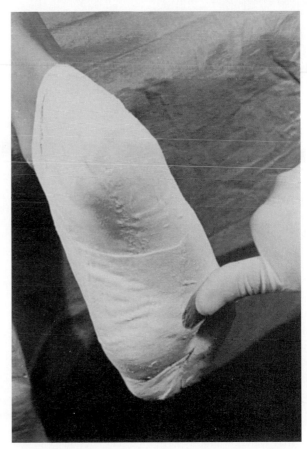

Figure 24-3 Prone casting technique.

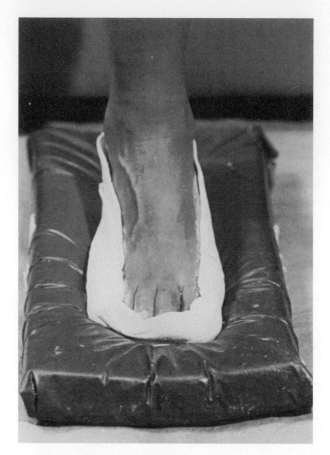

Figure 24-4 Semi-weight-bearing technique.

flexible type of forefoot valgus, one in which most of the compensation occurs within the longitudinal axis of the midtarsal joint. This is distinguished from the rigid type of forefoot valgus, which compensates primarily by subtalar joint supination and oblique axis midtarsal joint adduction and plantar flexion throughout gait.

Advantages of this casting technique are (1) ease of casting and positioning the patient, (2) ability to judge subtalar joint neutral position through visualization and palpation, and (3) locking of the oblique axis of the midtarsal joint by placing a reactive force of gravity against body weight. Some disadvantages of this particular technique also warrant mention: (1) the longitudinal axis of the midtarsal joint becomes supinated; (2) secondary to the supinated position of the midtarsal joint, there is a decrease in forefoot valgus and often an increase in forefoot varus; and (3) the first ray may function in a hypermobile state secondary to the supinated position of the midtarsal joint.

In-Shoe Vacuum Cast

The in-shoe vacuum cast technique is a relatively new system. The plaster is applied in the same manner as with the previous techniques. Following this, a plastic bag is applied over the foot, and a vacuum tube is inserted (Fig. 24-6). The system is sealed and the vacuum engaged to pull the plaster to the foot. A good, loose-fitting shoe, preferably a running shoe, is then applied over the plastic bag. The subtalar joint is placed in its neutral position, and a dorsiflexory force is placed on the lateral aspect of the foot in the area of the fifth metatarsal head[25] (Fig. 24-7). This system is relatively easy to operate, even for those not fully educated in the biomechanics of the foot. Therefore, office personnel can be trained to take accurate casts.

Advantages of this casting system are (1) the ease with which the techniques employed by this system are performed, and (2) the ease of judging subtalar joint position through visualization and palpation.

SELECTION OF THE CASTING TECHNIQUE

The key element in selecting the casting technique is that the more precise and accurate one's casting ability, the better the orthosis will function. For that reason, the supine, prone, and vacuum methods will most often faithfully reproduce the foot's pathology with the midtarsal joint locked about both its oblique and longitudinal axes.[24] The practitioner should use whichever of these methods is personally preferred when it has been decided that the patient's problem should be controlled with a truly functional orthosis. If a rigid device is chosen, the technical casting skills must be as precise as one's surgical skills. An orthotic device will only be as effective as the negative cast permits.

PRESCRIPTION WRITING

Once the appropriate cast has been obtained from the patient, the practitioner must determine the amount of correction to be requested, as well as the type of materials to be used, in construction of the orthotic device. Both variables will be affected by the type of sports activity engaged in, along with the nature of the patient's problem and the intrinsic foot pathology.

In most cases, the practitioner will not fabricate the device unless complete laboratory facilities are readily available. When using a professional laboratory, adequate information should be provided in order to obtain the best

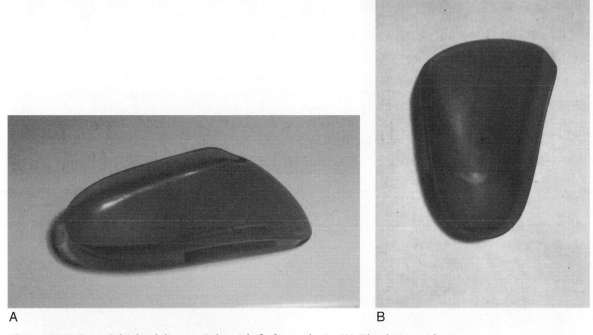

A   B

Figure 24-5 Type C heel stabilizer or Subotnick flatfoot orthosis. (**A**) The device with an accommodation for the second metatarsal head. Note the deep heel cup and extended medial and lateral flanges, which lock the subtalar joint in a neutral position. (**B**) Lateral photo of the type C heel stabilizer showing the high lateral extended wall to support the calcaneocuboid joint and midtarsal. Note also the high medial wall supporting the medial column and talonavicular joint.

possible orthosis. Each of the following variables must be considered when using orthoses for the athlete: (1) type of material, (2) material thickness, (3) amount of forefoot correction, (4) rearfoot posting, (5) posting elevator, (6) top cover, (7) temporary measures, (8) heel cup depth, (9) lateral flange for cuboid support, (10) medial flange for talar–navicular control, (11) width, and (12) accommodations and extensions.

Type of Material

Probably the most commonly asked question regarding orthoses for the athlete is: "What type of material should I use?" Although there is no black-and-white answer to this question, there are numerous guidelines that may be followed in assisting the practitioner to make a final choice.

Our first statement is one that some would probably disagree with. The only truly functional orthosis—that is, one capable of fully correcting foot pathology via a locking of the midtarsal joint—is one fabricated of fiberglass, graphite, polypropylene, or another minimally yielding material. This is not to say that every patient with some type of lower extremity pathology requires an inflexible device; it merely means that this type of device will generally provide the highest degree of control of abnormal foot and leg motion.

The peak stress in an orthotic device is in the heel. This is where the sharp impact spike of running, and to a lesser extent walking, occurs. Certainly a durable deep heel should be considered when treating the athlete with a high-demand foot.[26]

Many practitioners rely heavily on more flexible devices because of their more yielding nature and generally higher level of initial patient acceptance. However, in many instances these softer, more yielding devices control the patient's pathology inadequately when sufficient abnormal motion is present. Essentially, there is nothing wrong with using an orthosis fabricated of Polydor (thermal molded polymere; Allied OSI Lab, Indianapolis, IN), graphite, or fort and shock attenuation. Ethyl vinyl acetate (EVA) of 40 to 60 durometers, the same as used in the heels of running shoes, is excellent for rearfoot posting and forefoot wedging. It will, of course, "bottom out" and must be replaced often, at about 750 running miles. Crepe is far less durable and effective than EVA.

In some specific cases related to the abnormal pathomechanics of the subtalar and midtarsal joints, only a more rigid material will be appropriate. Symptoms associated with a progressing hallux abductovalgus, tailor's bunion, hallux limitus, heel-spur syndrome, retrocalcaneal exostosis, and posterior tibial tendinitis will often respond fully only to rigid orthotic therapy, because more flexible devices will not control the foot adequately. Again, this type of device will function only within certain parameters. For example, a sub-5-mph runner with one of the above pathologies would not benefit from a flexible device, due

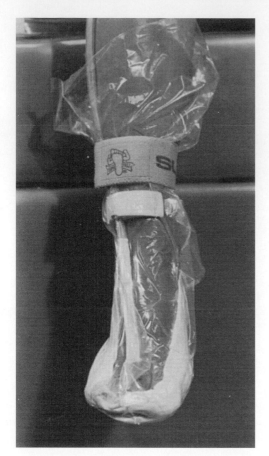

Figure 24-6 In-shoe vacuum cast technique.

polypropylene for a long-distance runner, a basketball player, a tennis player, or a skier, if the device is fabricated over an appropriate negative cast.

The old rohadur devices were generally well tolerated, yet they are seldom available or used now that more modern and forgiving materials are available. Subotholene, although easy to work with and well tolerated, is usually not stiff enough for the high-demand athletic foot. It is more suited for the low-demand foot. All materials must be chosen with consideration given to longevity and material creep. Polypropylenes and ethyly vinyl chlorides tend to creep over time and loose their initial integrity. Graphite does not appear to creep as much, but it too can suffer material failure, especially at the edges of the heel cup. Polydur appears to have the workabilty of the old rohadur and the comfort of polypropylene, but lacks the durability of graphite. New shock-absorbing materials, such as PPT (Poron) can be used for arch and heel fill for greater com-

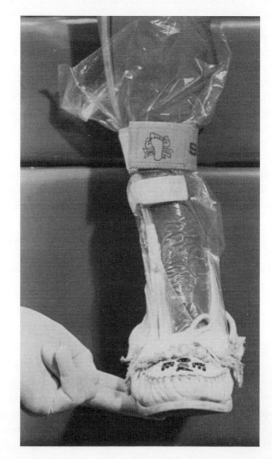

Figure 24-7 Proper positioning of foot using vacuum casting technique.

to the mechanics inherent in the activity. If the patient's sporting event does not provide heel contact, midstance, and toe-off phases of activity, a more functional device will not be used to its fullest capability. In those cases, alternative methods of foot control via flexible devices with correction distal to the metatarsal heads, such as a runner's forefoot wedge of EVA, may be appropriate.

There are some instances, however, in which the patient's activity, size, or degree of activity may make the more rigid materials inappropriate. In these cases, a suitable type of more flexible material should be employed. Even if a more yielding material is used, however, the practitioner should still use an appropriate neutral cast and employ proper forefoot and rearfoot corrections.

The following are some specific considerations that will be beneficial when using rohadur, Polydur, graphite, polypropylene, fiberglass, or other rigid devices. For the excessively pronated foot that demonstrates marked calcaneal eversion, a higher heel cup is recommended. If room in the athletic shoe permits, an 18-mm heel cup is appropriate. If there is minimal room, 18 mm medially and 14 to 15 mm laterally is sufficient. It should be remembered that the height of the heel cup includes the thickness of the particular material ordered. That is, heel cup height for any orthosis is measured from the outside of the device to the top of the heel cup (Fig. 24-8).

If the patient has a foot that functions in a markedly inverted or supinated attitude, a higher lateral heel cup is most useful. In this instance, 18 to 20 mm laterally and 14 to 15 mm medially would be appropriate. This is essential for the subluxed cuboid or peroneal cuboid syndrome, and is most commonly used in patients being treated for chronic ankle instability or a retrocalcaneal exostosis. The pathology would most likely be due to an uncompensated or partially compensated rearfoot varus, rigid forefoot valgus, or rigid plantar-flexed first ray. These types of symptoms and function most commonly require the above-stated modifications in basketball, racquetball, tennis, and any other mixed-motion or lateral-motion sport in order to increase the level of lateral stability. With the tendency to lateral ankle sprains in jumping or rebound sports, a long forefoot EVA lateral wedge extending from behind to beyond the metatarsal heads is most helpful. A lateral "dutchman" can also be added to the shoe, with a lateral heel extension in the case of rearfoot instability. Too often we fail to consider shoe modifications when dealing with foot orthotics, trying to do too much from within the shoe. Nothing takes the place of a reinforced heel counter, or counter modifications for Haglund's disease "pump bumps." An anterior metatarsal roller bar works well for metatarsalgia or hallux limitus.

Depending on the sporting activity, one pair of orthoses is often not enough. For example, if the patient enjoys doing running speedwork during the week and plays tennis on the weekend, two pairs may be needed.

Golf requires an orthosis that allow pronation and supination while providing for subtalar and midtarsal stability. Skiing requires an orthosis with the medial arch bent away from the foot to allow for forward bend at the ankle with medial edge control, without irritating the foot. Long-distance runners need 5 to 7 degrees of varus forefoot and rearfoot canting or wedging to accommodate the functional varus. Football, with its wide base of gait, requires minimal rearfoot control.

Material Thickness

As a general rule, the heavier the patient, the more significant the pathology, and the more strenuous the activity, the greater the likelihood that the orthotic device will creep or bottom out and need replacement, so the positive casts must be saved. Therefore, all these factors must be gauged in determining the appropriate thickness and flexi-

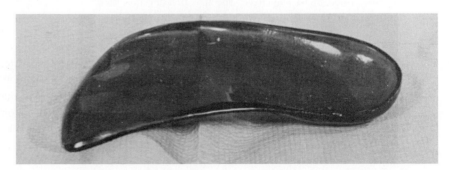

Figure 24–8 Rohadur appliance demonstrating deeper heel cup.

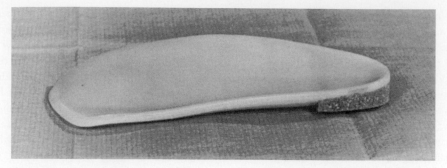

Figure 24-9 Flexible orthosis.

bility of the material. Rohadur or polypropylene thicknesses of 4.0 and 5.0 mm may be necessary for some athletes with extensive pathology and difficult-to-control abnormal forces. By contrast, a fairly flexible device of any material may be all that is necessary for the patient suffering from plantar fasciitis or metatarsalgia during a jazzercise or aerobics class (Fig. 24-9).

Forefoot Correction

In most cases, the general rule in forefoot correction is to post or cast-correct the entire amount of forefoot pathology in the patient. Failing this, the orthotic device will not be capable of "locking" the midtarsal joint properly, thereby providing the patient with nothing more than a costly arch support.

When patients are being properly evaluated and casted, there will not be many instances in which the patient will demonstrate an inverted attitude of the forefoot relative to the rearfoot, when the midtarsal joint is locked about both its axes and the subtalar joint is in neutral position. Most athletes have a flexible forefoot valgus with a plantar-flexed first ray when the foot is in neutral and the calcaneo-cuboid joint is locked, providing the peroneus longus with a stable fulcrum to *plantar-flex* the first metatarsal. Often chiropractic-type foot adjustments and precasting soft tissue streching help to eliminate the unwanted functional supinatus so often misinterpreted as forefoot varus. However, if a forefoot varus or supinatus is observed and captured in the cast, the laboratory should be instructed to correct it fully.

If most patients demonstrate a forefoot varus, the examination and casting technique is more than suspect. The most common error in casting is supinating either the longitudinal or oblique axis of the midtarsal joint, introducing

an error of excessive varus into the patient's foot. By contrast, if patients are being properly evaluated and casted, most will demonstrate an everted position of the forefoot relative to the rearfoot when the midtarsal joint is locked about both its axes and the subtalar joint is in its neutral position. In this case, however, it may be inappropriate to correct the entire amount of forefoot valgus captured. If the patient demonstrates a marked rearfoot varus along with a forefoot valgus, the calcaneus should be checked to see whether it is capable of attaining a vertical attitude. If not, the laboratory should not be requested to correct the forefoot valgus fully, because this will precipitate subtalar joint or calcaneocuboid pain in the athlete. For example, if a patient is found to have 25 degrees of inversion with supination, 3 degrees of eversion with pronation, and 7 degrees of tibial varum for the subtalar joint and 6 degrees of forefoot valgus for the midtarsal joint, this patient's maximally pronated position is still 4 degrees inverted. Therefore, a device with a 6-degree forefoot valgus correction would not be tolerated; this would attempt to force the subtalar joint to function in a position that it could not attain. This patient's device should only have a 2-degree forefoot valgus correction introduced into it.

In cases in which the patient is complaining of pain plantar to the first metatarsal, it should be determined whether the valgus attitude is associated with a structurally plantar-flexed position of the first ray. If so, a functional orthosis will most likely be inefficient in dealing with the pain. In this case, an accommodative device or surgical correction will be most appropriate.

If a rigid material such as polypropylene or graphite is used, the laboratory may be instructed either to cast-correct (i.e., plaster-balance) the forefoot deformity or to add on a forefoot post. The latter option is less desirable, however, because the overall device becomes excessively in-

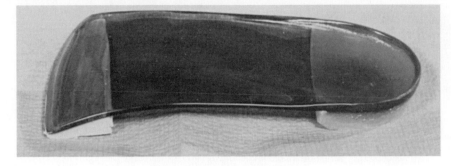

Figure 24-10 Functional orthosis with both forefoot and rearfoot positioning.

flexible, making it more susceptible to fracturing (Fig. 24-10). However, if one of the more flexible materials is chosen, it is advisable to request external posting, which will allow for better foot control. Orthoses for runners are typically cast-corrected for forefoot deformity, then given additional compressible medial forefoot wedging to correct midstance and propulsive pronation. They must be full length to control propulsion. If the patient is participating in interval training or primarily performs speedwork, a standard rigid posted orthosis is obviously inappropriate. The orthosis must be full length and flexible under the ball of the foot. In these cases, an extremely flexible material, with the forefoot correction extending beyond the metatarsal heads of either a varus or valgus deformity, will be more beneficial, because it will attempt to control the foot primarily during the propulsive phase of gait.

Rearfoot Posting

Most devices work with greatest efficiency when ordered with a rearfoot post. This ensures proper positioning of the subtalar joint at heel contact and decreases excessive abnormal frontal plane movement of the device in the shoe. The rearfoot post, however, has little chance to be effective if the calcaneus is not controlled with a deep heel cup. In addition, the orthosis is at a disadvantage with a shoe that has a loose-fitting, weak, or sloppy heel counter. In most cases, a 4- to 7-degree compressible EVA varus rearfoot post is most commonly used, depending on the anatomic and functional extent of the rearfoot varus component (Fig. 24-11). In running, the pendulum effect of the lower limb exaggerates the amount of functional rearfoot varus commonly found in walking, thereby creating a functional varus that requires greater pronation.

With foot orthotics, some lateral knee pain may be precipitated, specifically an iliotibial band syndrome, if the device does not allow for enough rearfoot movement. Therefore, if the patient returns to the office with a new complaint of lateral knee pain initiated through the use of the orthosis, the post should be checked for excessive medial rearfoot control.[27]

In most cases, if a rigid post is preferred, it should either be 4 degrees with 4 degrees of motion or 6 degrees with 6 degrees of motion. While the rigid posting may be more effective, it has the disadvantage of not damping impact shock, and may be more jarring to the athlete. The motion introduced by the laboratory into the rearfoot post via grinding of the distal medial aspect of the post is essential to permit normal pronation with the rigid rearfoot post, although not necessary or desirable with the semirigid EVA post. Most sports podiatrists prefer varus compressible rearfoot posts. These do not normally need medial grinding inasmuch as medial compression of the EVA posting material provides ample motion. When this normal amount of pronation is allowed and supported through the initial 25 percent of stance with the post, normal shock absorption occurs, and the entire orthotic plate contours to the shoe properly. An additional correction that may be requested from the laboratory is for a medial or lateral flare on the rearfoot post. If the patient exhibits marked subtalar joint eversion past perpendicular, a medial flare to the post will assist in controlling that motion. If the patient functions in a markedly inverted position, a lateral flare added to the rearfoot post will improve lateral ankle stability.

Patients should be informed that the posting will most likely be altered and worn down through excessive use; annual evaluation of the post is essential to ensure continued control. This is especially true for compliant, compressible posts and wedges.[28] Some specifics regarding posting for sports that require the use of rigid boots are

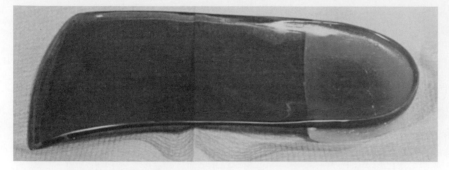

Figure 24-11 Functional orthosis with rearfoot post.

worth reviewing. If the athlete is participating in skiing, ice skating, or roller skating, a more rigid device is generally more effective. These athletes do not require the same degree of subtalar joint motion required by most other athletes in their activities. Therefore, 4 or 6 degrees of subtalar joint motion is not necessary in designing their devices. Depending on the degree of rearfoot varus present, these orthoses could be either flat posted, or posted 4 or 6 degrees but without any motion introduced into the post. Therefore, an additional forefoot post would be added to assist in inverting the entire orthotic plate inside of the boot, in order to provide a rigid 4- or 6-degree inverted surface in the boot. Orthoses for edge-control sports may need to be bent away from the medial dorsal arch to prevent impingement during forceful pronation.

Posting Elevator

The posting elevator is used by the laboratory to fabricate the device properly for a shoe's inherent heel-to-ball angulation. The elevator is placed under the rearfoot post as the post is added; it ensures that the device clears the shank of the shoe properly. For most athletic shoes, a 4- or 8-mm elevator should be requested. Obviously, if no rearfoot post is requested, a posting elevator height should not be ordered.

Top Cover

Several commercially available top-cover materials can be used to enable the athlete to wear an orthosis comfortably. If possible, the top-cover material should be added following the initial break-in sequence, in the event that some modification of the orthosis becomes necessary. If this cannot be easily accomplished, the cover may be added at the time that the device is dispensed. In most cases, the material will not interfere with the function of the orthotic device and will generally aid in the control of blisters or hyperkeratoses. Top covers include those made of Poron, Viscolas (Chattanooga Corporation, Chattanooga, TN), and Spenco (Spenco Medical Corporation, Waco, TX).

Temporary Measures

In many instances, it is necessary to fabricate some type of temporary device for the patient either to decrease symptoms initially or to be used in a diagnostic fashion.[14] This type of on-the-spot orthosis may be fabricated from any number or combination of materials and is intended to alter the patient's gait only minimally. Effective combinations have been made from Spenco and Korex (Mayflower Podiatry Supplies, Los Alamedes, CA) (Fig. 24-12), PPT, and Nickelplast (Alimed, Dedham, NJ) (Fig. 24-13) and Plastizote with a synthetic leather covering (Steinmold) with Vylyte (Stein Foot Specialties, Hackensack, NJ), as well as by adding accommodative materials to an athletic shoe's removable innersole (Fig. 24-14). In some instances, commercially available devices can be recommended for a patient's use, but only on an interim basis to determine whether even a minimal response may be elicited by altering foot function (Fig. 24-15). Viscolas Underdogs are inserts that can be modified with modular wedges and additions to fabricate shock-attenuating on-the-spot orthoses. The Spenco cross-trainer is a generally well-accepted, accommodating store-bought device.

Although these temporary devices may be beneficial in some cases, they are in no way intended to replace the use of an appropriately fashioned permanent orthosis. Even if the temporary device is beneficial, the practitioner should proceed with more definitive therapy.

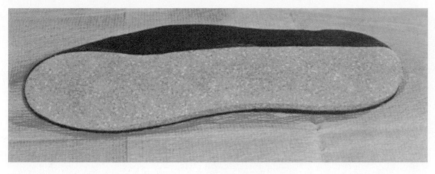

Figure 24-12 Spenco and Korex temporary orthosis.

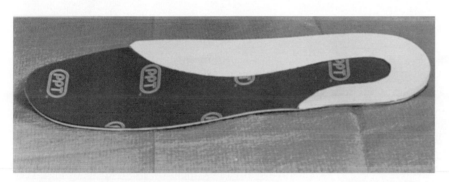

Figure 24-13 PPT and Nickelplast temporary orthosis.

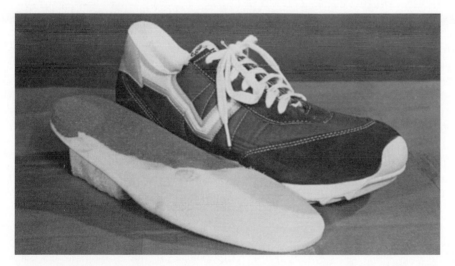

Figure 24-14 Korex added to removable innersole of running shoe in order to create varus wedge effect.

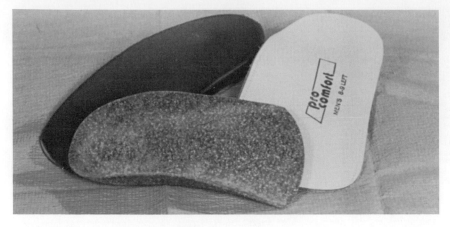

Figure 24-15 Commercially available arch supports.

CONCLUSION

The thoughts, recommendations, and observations presented here should prepare the practitioner to deliver orthotic therapy for each patient's athletic endeavors. Successful orthotic therapy can only be instituted by following careful evaluation and examination principles used in conjunction with the appropriate casting technique.

If an orthosis is uncomfortable or not providing the desired effects, the practitioner should re-evaluate, represcribe, or recast. We should never give up, always attempt to do better, and not be afraid to experiment. The patient can be told that, if the orthotic does not work, it will be replaced at no charge. Sports medicine and foot orthotic work is an art that takes trial and error as well as humility and a dedication to providing the very best of care, never settling for less. Many sessions of "fine tuning" may be required for optimal results.

Generally, a full-length foot orthotic with a deep heel cup, a stable lateral column with a lateral extension, and forefoot and rearfoot compressible posts and runners wedges works wonders. At times a type C heel stabilizer or UCBL device is required, when greater control is needed. Practitioners must remember that they are the athletes' advocates.

REFERENCES

1. Subotnick SI: The biomechanics of running: implications for the prevention of foot injuries. Sports Med 2:144, 1985
2. Fredericson M: Common injuries in runners: diagnosis, rehabitation and prevention. Sports Med 21:49, 1996
3. Conrad KJ, Budiman-Mak E, Roach KE et al: Impact of foot orthoses on pains and disability in rheumatoid arthritis. J Clin Epidemiol 49:1, 1996
4. Nawoczenski DA, Cook TM, Saltzman CL: The effect of foot orthotics on three-dimensional kinematics of the leg and rearfoot during running. J Orthop Sports Phys Ther 21: 317, 1995
5. Cornwell MW, McPoil TG: Footwear and foot orthotic effectiveness: a new approach. J Orthop Sports Phys Ther 26:337, 1995
6. Guskiewicz KM, Perrin DH: Effect of orthotics on postural sway following inversion ankle sprain. J Orthop Sports Phys Ther 23:326, 1996
7. Bosjen-Moller F: Calcaneocuboid joint and stability of the longitudinal arch of the foot at high and low gear push off. J Anat 129:44, 1979
8. Kitaoka HB, Lundberg A, Luo ZP: Kinematics of the normal arch of the foot and ankle under physiologic loading. Foot Ankle Int 16:492, 1995
9. Saggini R, Giamberardino MA, Gatteschi L et al: Myofascial pain syndrome of the peroneous longus: biomechanical approach. Clin J Pain 2:30, 1996
10. Dananberg HJ: Gait style as an etiology to chronic postural pain, parts I and II. J Am Podiatr Med Assoc 83:433, 615, 1993
11. Root ML, Orien WP, Weed JH: Biomechanical Examination of the Foot. Clinical Biomechanics, Los Angeles, 1971
12. Kadawa A et al: Effect of walking shoes and higher heel shoes compared to barefoot walking for maximum balance in older women. J Am Geriatr Soc 44:429, 1996
13. Sgarlato T: A Compendium of Podiatric Biomechanics. California College of Podiatric Medicine, San Francisco, 1971
14. Subotnick SI: Orthotic foot control and the overuse syndrome. Physician Sports Med 3:75, 1975
15. Subotnick SI: Variation of the angle of gait in runners. Physician Sports Med 7:75, 1975

16. Subotnick SI: Variations in angles of gait in running. Physician Sports Med 7:110, 1979

17. Close RJ, Inman VT: The Action of the Subtalar Joint (Prosthetic Devices Research Project, Series II, Issue 24). Institute of Engineering Research, University of California, Berkeley, 1953

18. Close RJ, Inman VT: The Action of the Ankle Joint (Prosthetic Devices Research Project, Series II, Issue 22). Institue of Engineering Research, University of California, Berkeley, 1952

19. Elftman H: Transverse tarsal joint and its controls. Clin Orthop 16:41, 1960

20. Hicks JLH: Mechanics of the foot. 1. The joints. J Anat 87: 345, 1953

21. Maner JT: Movements of the subtalar and transverse tarsal joints. Anat Rec 80:397, 1941

22. Root ML, Orion WP, Weed JH: Normal and Abnormal Function of the Foot. Clinical Biomechanics, Los Angeles, 1977

23. Root ML, Orien PO, Weed JH: Neutral Position Casting Techniques. Clinical Biomechanics, Los Angeles, 1971

24. Valmassy RL: Advantages and disadvantages of various casting techniques. J Am Podiatry Assoc 69:707, 1979

25. Brown D, Smith C: Vacuum casting for foot orthosis. J Am Podiatry Assoc 66:422, 1976

26. Chu TM, Reddy NP, Padovan J: Three-dimensional finite element stress analysis of the polyprophylene ankle-foot orthosis: static analysis. Med Eng Phys 17:372, 1995

27. Subotnick SI: The abuses of orthotic devices. J Am Podiatry Assoc 65:1025, 1975

28. Subotnick SI: Foot orthosis in ski boots. Physician Sports Med 10:61, 1982

25

Accommodation, Strapping, and Bracing

WILLIAM L. VAN PELT

Knowing what and when to tape or pad is a science; a well-done "tape job" is the art form of an athletic trainer. Like any other treatment regimen, its success depends on accurate diagnosis and precise application. A professor once cautioned, as he demonstrated classic low dye strapping, "tape is the medicine, tension is the dose." Sixty percent of all athletic injuries are foot and ankle related. Well over 75 percent of these injuries are primarily to the soft tissues: the skin, tendons, and ligaments. Many of these injuries can be treated with, or prevented by, the use of noninvasive mechanical modalities.

Shielding, supportive padding, strapping, and bracing are mechanical methods of applying materials under, around, or on the foot and ankle. All these methods attempt to eliminate or minimize extrinsic friction and pressure, redistribute weight-bearing forces, or replace or reinforce the stabilizing structures of the foot and leg. *Shields* are appliances fashioned from natural or synthetic fabrics. They are applied for the purpose of relieving pressure or friction or to protect a tender part of the foot. Examples are felt pads for a painful bunion (Fig. 25-1) or a sponge rubber "donut" pad for a painfully blistered "pump bump" on the back of the heel.

Supportive paddings (accommodative paddings) are used to re-establish weight-bearing forces or to realign structural abnormalities. They may be applied to the foot using an innersole in the shoe or applied directly to the skin. Examples are a Vylyte (Stein Foot Specialties, Hackensack, NJ) first-ray padding, to compensate for a forefoot varus defor-

mity (Fig. 25-2), or a felt varus heel wedge glued to the bottom of the shoe, to realign the calcaneus in a neutral (varus) attitude.

Strappings are made of various adhesive tapes or fabrics that are supportive and compressive. They are applied either alone or in conjunction with supportive pads in an effort to realign the structural abnormalities of the foot. Examples are Campbell's reststrap for strained arch or the time-proven low-dye strapping for plantar fascial strain with or without heel spur padding (Fig. 25-3).

Braces are used to replace or reinforce an injured or lost ligament or tendon. The purpose is to provide external support and to stabilize unstable parts. An example of brace strapping is the classic ankle tape with or without heel lock for an acutely sprained ankle. Another is a double upright lace-up brace for a chronic unstable ankle. A contemporary version of the classic ankle brace is the Airsplint (Air Cast, Summit, NJ) (Fig. 25-4).

MATERIALS AND SUPPLIES

A wide variety of materials and supplies are available for the fabrication and application of shields, pads, straps, and braces used in the treatment of athletic injuries. The materials most often used for shielding and accommodative padding are adhesive-backed moleskin and felt.

Adhesive moleskin is particularly useful because of its adaptability for shaping and its quick application. A shield of adhesive moleskin consists of one, two, three, or more

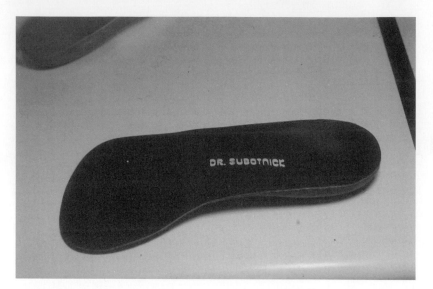

Figure 25–1 Dr. Scholl's advanced cushioning polymer gel shields. (Courtesy of Schering-Plough Healthcare Products, Inc., Memphis, TN.)

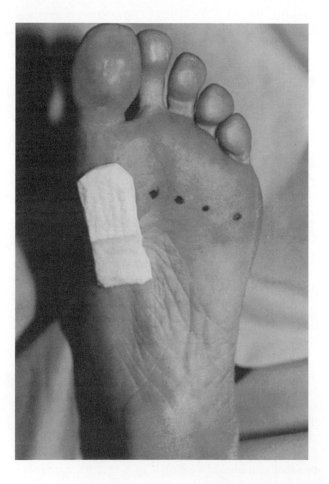

Figure 25–2 Forefoot varus accommodative padding of 1/4-inch adhesive felt.

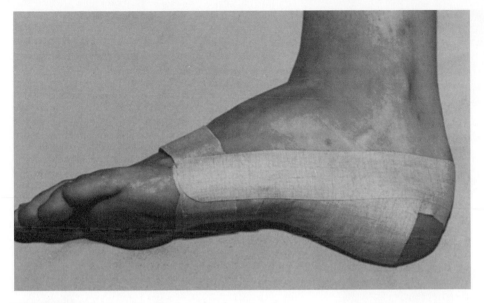

Figure 25-3 Classic application: low-dye foot strapping.

layers, depending on the thickness desired. Felt comes with or without adhesive backing. It ranges in thickness from 1/16 to 1 inch. Various grades of felt are available. However, standard podiatric felt is the best quality and is used most often. Foam rubber and sponge rubber are also used for shielding and accommodative padding. Foam rubber is lighter and more breathable; sponge rubber is denser, heavier, and sturdier. Both products come in 1/16- to 1-inch thickness. They can also have adhesive or nonadhesive backing.

White or flesh-colored adhesive tape is used most for bracing and strapping. It is also used in conjunction with paddings or to hold them in place. Adhesive tape is available in widths of 1/8 to 3 inches. Some other types of tapes are nonallergenic, 3M or "paper tape," and Johnson & Johnson tape. The most versatile and time proven is the Johnson & Johnson flesh-colored Zonus tape.

Other products used for accommodative padding are lamb's wool, moldable podiatry compound, tube gauze with silicone gel, and Spenco Second Skin (Spenco Medical Corporation, Waco, TX). Aliplast and Plastizote (Alimed, Dedham, MA) have also been used to fabricate various types of paddings.

Elastoplast, Elasticon, self-adhering gauze, tube gauze, and Coban (elastized nonadhesive compression wrap by 3M), are products used to strap or retain paddings or to apply compression to the involved part.

Some materials are used for accommodative balance padding. They are applied to an innersole or to a shoe. There is great variety: felts (both adhesive and nonadhesive), cork, Korex, foam, sponge rubber, polyurethane, polypropylene, Vylyte, Plastizote, Aliplast, Spenco Second Skin, PPT, and viscoelastic polymers or Viscolas (Chattanooga Corporation, Chattanooga, TN). Materials used for bracing include elastic (with or without Velcro), Neoprene, stainless steel, aluminum, plasticized rubber, polyurethane, and polypropylene. These are only a few of the materials used today to prefabricate or custom mold ankle–leg–knee or hip orthotic devices.

The list of materials available for strapping, padding, and bracing is almost endless. Whether we choose to use a generic sponge or Vylyte, the freshness and quality is important. It is worth the few extra pennies to purchase high-quality materials from reputable and knowledgeable supply houses. Good supply houses understand the use of these materials and are willing to ensure that the materials purchased are fresh and of the finest quality. Once these materials are received, it is important to rotate the stock, using the oldest first. Materials should be stored in a cool, dry environment. Adhesive tape stays freshest in the refrigerator. It deteriorates fastest in the trunk of a car.

Rubber compounds are widely used for accommodative padding, strapping, and bracing. Spenco, a nitrogen-impregnated rubber similar to the wetsuit material used by underwater divers, provides for cushioning and decreasing sheer forces. It is excellent for blister prevention and is

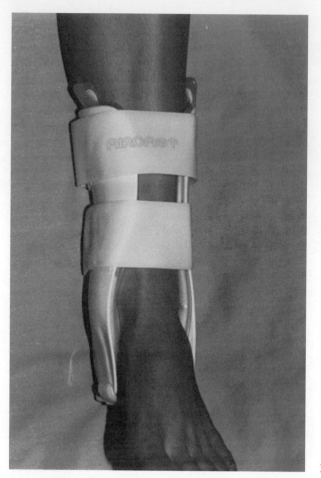

Figure 25-4 Darco splint.

used in full-length innersoles, off-the-shelf arch supports, or heel lifts. The material is also used in bicycle cushions and in handlebar grips.

PPT is another material that absorbs shock and decreases pressure. It is available through the Langer Group Corp. It too is often used as insert material or in prefabricated arch supports. Various forms of polyurethane and polyethylene are used for the fabrication of temporary or permanent orthotic devices. They are flexible, yet moldable and durable. For the most part they are lightweight. These are all important characteristics for today's athletic equipment.

Plastizote is a softer material than those in the polyethylene or polypropylene group. This takes a compression set and is used for accommodating or shielding lesions as well as for support and balance. It is often used in the fabrication of soft accommodative orthotic devices.

Korex (Mayflower Podiatry Supplies, Los Alamedes, CA) is a rubber–cork mixture that is relatively firm. It is stable and somewhat flexible and can be readily shaped with a grinder. Korex maintains a basic shape for a longer period of time than does Plastizote, but does not take a compression set and is not moldable.

Vylyte is a rubber material. It is used for various forms of padding, shielding, and bracing. Mostly it is used as an innersole material for posting or balancing temporary orthotic devices. It is extremely useful in devices designed to decrease motion or absorb shock. It takes a grind easily and is extremely durable and lightweight.

Viscoelastic polymers such as Viscolas are used as soft tissue supplements. They have excellent shock-absorbing qualities and provide an excellent supplement for an atrophic or painful fat pad in the forefoot and heel. Disadvantages are that they are heavy and hot and are difficult to bond to other materials.

Neoprene braces provide compression and support. Like wetsuits, they increase body heat, which aids in the

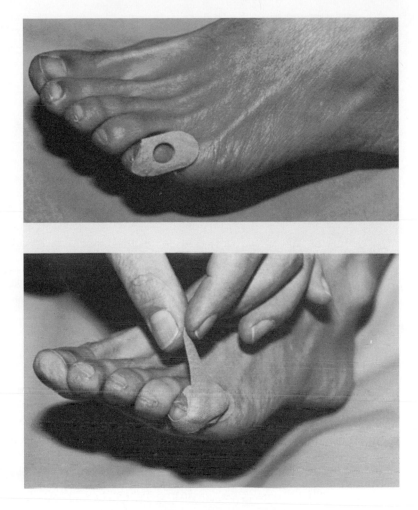

Figure 25-5 (Top) Application of an aperture pad to the fifth toe, using 1/8-inch felt. The pad should be slightly larger than the lesion and modeled so that there is no pressure on the nail groove or nail bed. The edges are skived for better contour. **(Bottom)** Aperture pad should then be held in place with properly applied adhesive tape or Elastoplast.

healing and comfort of damaged tissue and joints. Neoprene braces are available for ankle, leg, knee, and back.

Other useful braces are the Cho-pat strap (Cho-pat Inc., Hainesport, NJ) for peripatellar tendonitis and the Airsplint system. The Airsplint (Fig. 25-4) uses a polypropylene stirrup with an air-filled rubber bladder. Airsplint manufactures a variety of ankle and knee braces that have proved very successful. Improved versions of the ankle support system have been developed by the Darco Company. Their rubber bladders contain gel that can be heated or frozen for appropriate additional physical therapy.

APPLICATION METHODS

Knowing how to use the materials is as important as the diagnosis. Before applying any type of padding or strapping, it is extremely important to cleanse the skin with soap and water, followed by alcohol swabbing. This is an excellent routine that provides antisepsis and removes the skin oils.

The type of skin adhesive can make a big difference in the ease of application and durability. Tincture of benzoin is cheap and readily available and is the longtime standard for pretape adhesion. However, some people are allergic to it, and it can be a bit messy. For these reasons, some companies have developed aerosol pretape sprays that are easy to use and that tend to be less allergenic. They also seem to provide more adhesion.

There are a few rules to follow that will make padding and taping jobs more comfortable and professional looking. When applying padding to relieve or transfer pressure, it is important to make sure that the aperture hole is slightly larger than the lesion or bony prominence to be accommodated (flat aperture pads can be stretched before application).

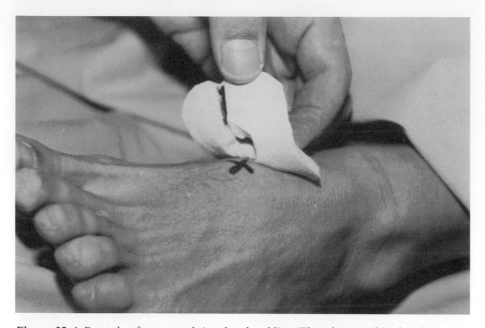

Figure 25-6 Example of accommodative dorsal padding. The edges are skived and cut-out grooves are fashioned to accommodate the extensor hallucis longus tendon.

It is best to fashion the primary aperture slightly smaller than the lesion, then to stretch the felt to a point at which the aperture is slightly larger than the area to be shielded. Foam rubber or sponge rubber paddings are not stretchable, so the aperture holes should be cut to exactly the correct size.

The surrounding structure must be considered. When a corn on the fifth toe is being padded, the pad should not rest on the nail or nail groove (Fig. 25-5). When padding around a joint, it is important to make sure the bulk of the padding does not transfer weight to an underlying nerve. When applying a dorsal (bump) pad (Fig. 25-6), cutout grooves should accommodate the extensor hallucis longus tendon. The goal is to try to distribute weight away from the injured part without transferring it to an underlying vital or painful area.

This principle also applies to taping done in a cerclage manner. Whether it is taping around a fractured toe or around the ball of the foot, any circumferential taping must be applied with some slack to compensate for weight-bearing swelling (see Fig. 25-3).

All shields and pads should be skived to a feathered edge for contour so that they will adhere to the underlying skin and bony prominences (see Fig. 25-13A). The ends of the tapes should be rounded to prevent rolling (Fig. 25-7).

When applying tapes, adhesive or compressive, or ankle straps, Unna boots, or hard casts (for that matter, whenever a flexor surface is to be encircled), the foot must be placed in a functional position. In the case of an ankle at right angles (Fig. 25-8), that position should be maintained while the tape is being applied. The placement of pretape wrapping or gauze pads over the tendons and skin crease will prevent cutting or compression injury of the underlying skin, tendons, and nerves. Cast padding, felt pads, or sponge rubber pads may also be used over bony prominences. For example, padding should be used over the lateral malleoli before taping or cast application.

Materials handling is also important. Sharp scissors or a skiving knife are a must for proper skiving or feathering of felt, sponge rubber, or cutting tape and moleskin with rounded edges. A good grinder with a belt sander and exhaust system is also necessary for the proper handling of such materials as Korex, Vylyte, rohadur, or polypropylpylene. Good-quality rubber or barge cement must be readily available and fresh.

To avoid delays in waiting for glue to dry, a highpowered hairdryer is very useful. It can also be used to spot-mold certain acrylics, polyethylene, or polypropylene materials, as well as Plastizote. Velcro can be purchased in variable widths. It is used for a variety of closures, to modify a surgical shoe, or to hold an insert in place in an open-backed shoe.

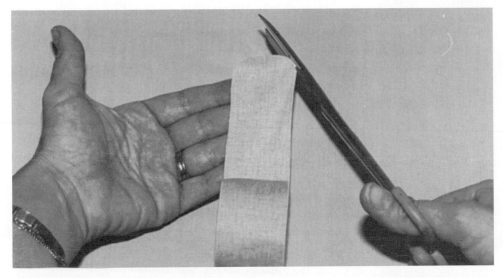

Figure 25-7 To prepare tape for application, the corners are rounded by cutting with scissors.

Figure 25-8 Tape should be applied with the ankle held at 90 degrees to the leg.

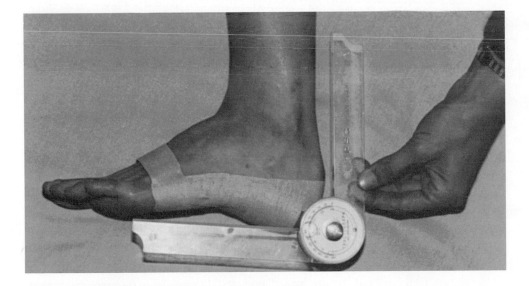

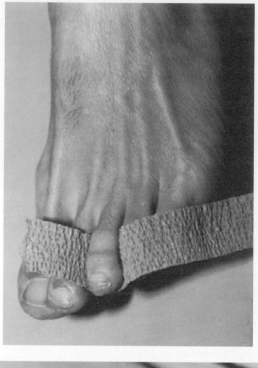

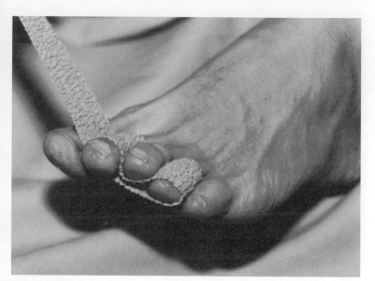

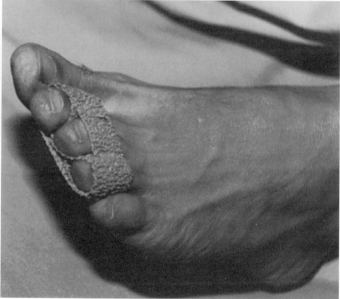

Figure 25-9 Digital injuries, such as contusions, sprains, dislocations, and fractures, may be managed by "buddy" taping the affected digit to the next toe.

USES IN ATHLETIC INJURIES

The applications of these materials to athletic injuries are numerous. Good imagination, manual dexterity, and concern for returning the athlete to action as soon as possible are the motivating factors in practicing good mechanical podiatry. Figures 25-9 through 25-19 illustrate the conditions that can be treated with the various materials.

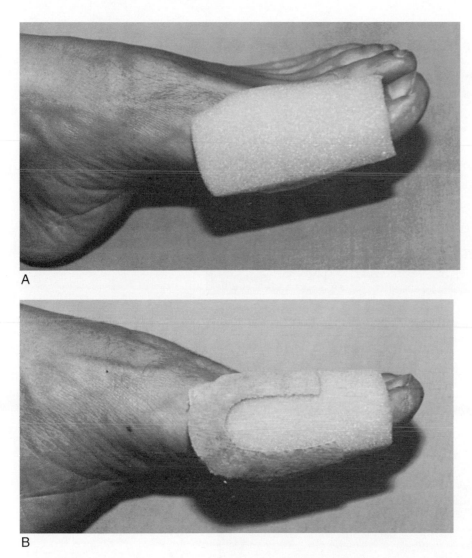

A

B

Figure 25–10 Painful first metatarsal. (**A**) Removable tubefoam shield is used to relieve a painful first metatarsal. (**B**) Removable tubefoam shield with an accommodative horseshoe pad made of adhesive-backed felt may be covered with Elastoplast. (*Figure continues.*)

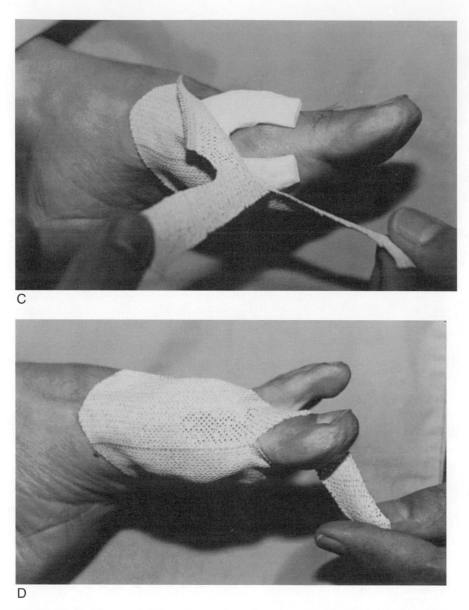

Figure 25–10 (*Continued*). (**C**) Accommodative horsehoe pad of adhesive-backed 1/8-inch felt has an Elastoplast cover. (**D**) Applying Elastoplast cover over an accommodative felt horseshoe-shaped pad.

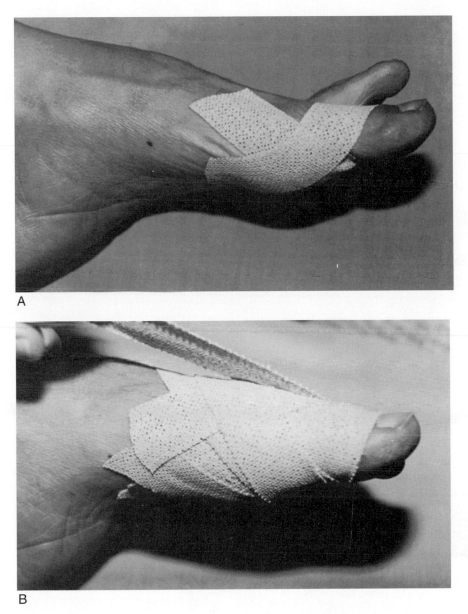

A

B

Figure 25-11 Ligament injuries. (**A**) A hallux lock is a strapping applied to the great toe joint. This criss-cross method is used for any injury to the ligaments around the joint, including turf toe and sesamoid pain. (*Figure continues.*)

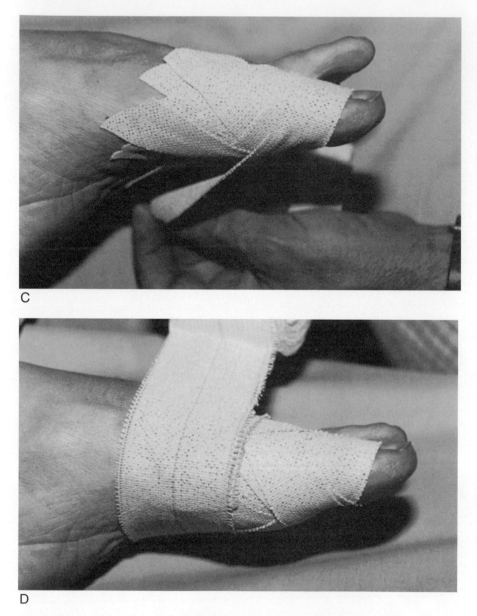

C

D

Figure 25-11 (*Continued*). (**B & C**) The hallux should be held in a plantar-flexed position when the strapping is applied. (**D**) Moleskin, Zonus tape, or Elastoplast can be used to secure the strap proximal to the great toe joint.

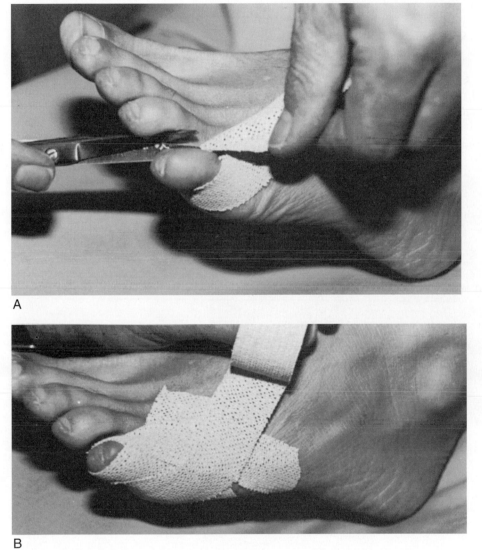

A

B

Figure 25-12 (**A & B**) When using the locking strap, it is important to narrow the Elastoplast to fill the interdigital space and avoid wrinkling or strangulation of the digit. (*Figure continues.*)

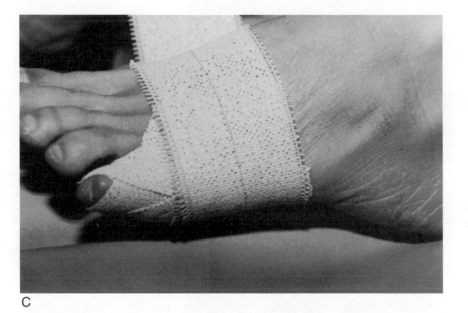

C

Figure 25–12 (*Continued*). (**C**) After wrapping the digit, wrapping is applied to the entire fore-foot–metatarsal area.

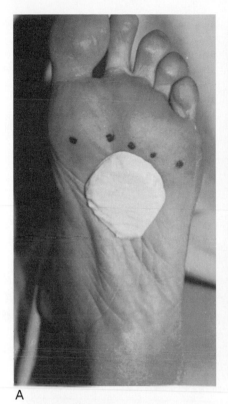

A

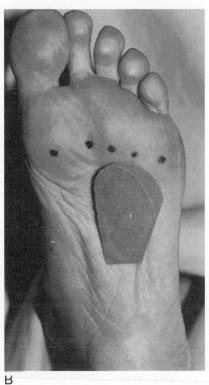

B

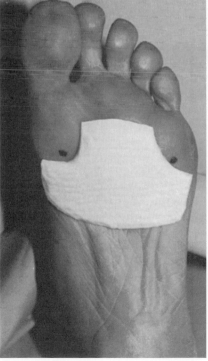

C

Figure 25-13 A variety of painful metatarsal conditions can be treated with forefoot padding. (**A**) This classic metatarsal pad of 1/4-inch adhesive felt is placed just proximal to the second, third, and fourth metatarsal heads. (**B**) This dense rubber metatarsal pad is similar to the classic one. It is used to accommodate a neuroma and is placed just proximal to the fourth metatarsal head. (**C**) An accommodative first and fifth metatarsal adhesive felt 1/4-inch cut-out pad may be used for painful calluses beneath the metatarsal heads or for a painful sesamoid and fifth metatarsal capsulitis. (*Figure continues.*)

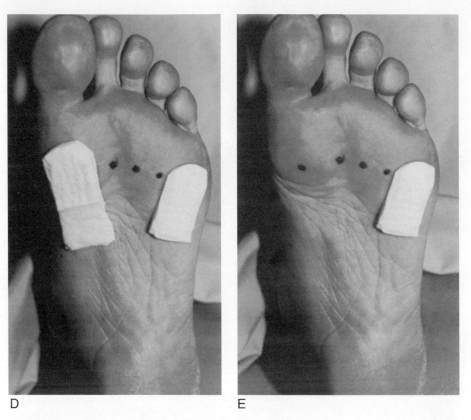

D   E

Figure 25-13 (*Continued*). (**D**) Classic biplanar padding is often used to transfer weight to the first and fifth metatarsal heads to relieve painful calluses or capsulitis of the second, third, and fourth metatarsals. (**E**) A lateral balance pad accommodates forefoot valgus deformity. This pad will increase weight bearing under the fifth metatarsal head.

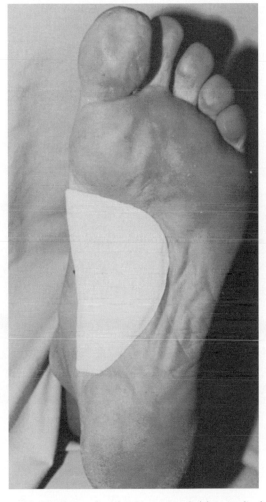

Figure 25-14 Plantar fascial strain. A medial longitudinal arch pad can be fabricated from 1/4-inch adhesive felt. This classic arch pad is used for plantar fascial strain or symptoms associated with flexible flatfoot. The pad can be applied directly to the bottom of the foot or incorporated into an arch support.

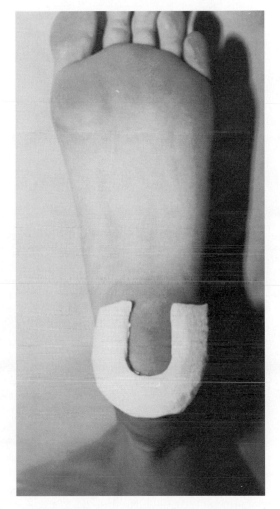

Figure 25-15 Heel spurs or plantar fasciitis. A plantar, horse-shoe-shaped 1/4-inch adhesive felt heel spur pad decreases pressure under the tuberosity of the calcaneus by increasing peripheral pressure. It is often used in heel-spur syndrome or plantar fasciitis. It can be applied directly to the skin, incorporated into a functional foot orthotic device, or fashioned and glued directly into the shoe.

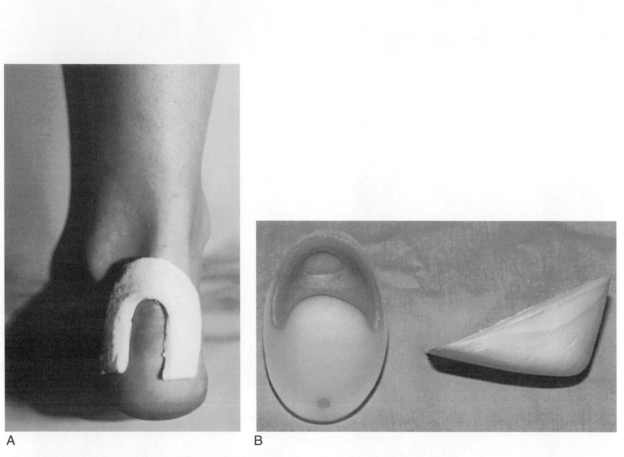

A   B

Figure 25-16 "Pump bump." (**A**) A 1/4-inch adhesive felt horseshoe-shaped pad is designed for painful retrocalcaneal exostosis or bursitis (pump bump). (**B**) It can be constructed of a variety of materials and applied directly to the foot orthotic device, or glued directly into the shoe.

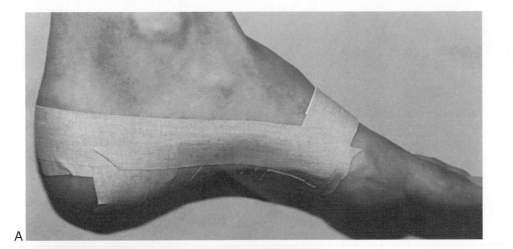

A

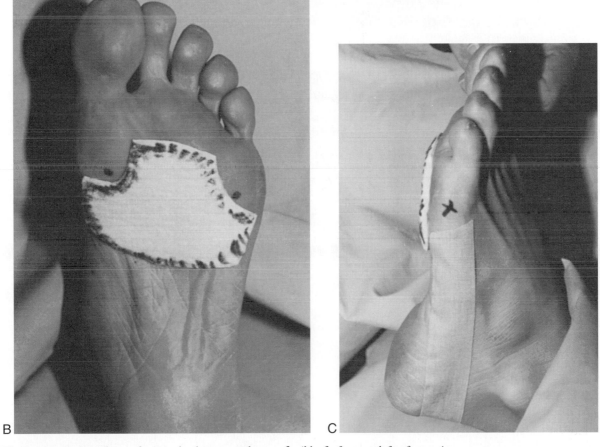

B   C

Figure 25-17 (**A**) Plantar fasciitis, heel–spur syndrome, flexible flatfoot, and forefoot pain secondary to excessive rearfoot motion. The classic low-dye strapping is used in a wide variety of acute and chronic foot conditions. (**B**) An accommodative first and fifth metatarsal adhesive felt pad is one variety of forefoot padding that can be incorporated into a low-dye strapping. (**C**) The first strap should begin just proximal to the fifth metatarsal head, extending from distal-lateral to proximal-lateral around the posterior aspect of the heel. The foot should be held in a neutral position and the tape applied without wrinkles. Tape is placed just superior to the posterior calcaneal fat pad. (*Figure continues.*)

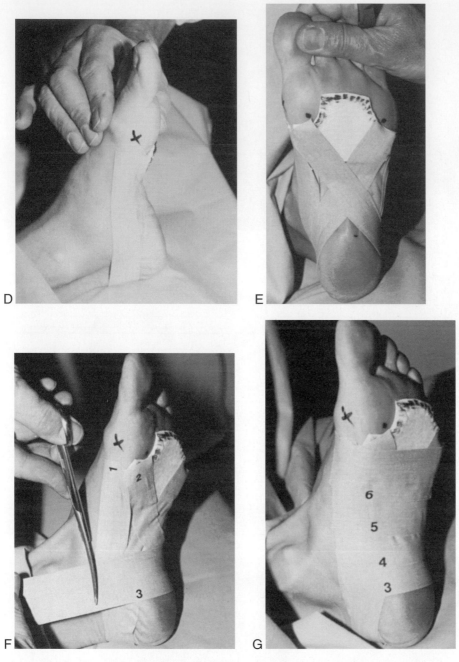

Figure 25-17 (*Continued*). (**D**) With the foot held in neutral position, the first metatarsal should be slightly plantar-flexed with the index finger. The tape is brought distal to just proximal to the first metatarsal head. This step is repeated two to three times, depending on the weight and degree of activity of the patient. (**E**) An additional two or three tapes may be criss-crossed on the plantar surface from the first and fifth metatarsals. (**F**) For stirrup strapping, tape #3 extends from just inferior to the lateral malleolus across the plantar aspect of the foot, then extends superior to just beneath the medial malleolus to the level of the superior aspect of tape #1. (**G**) Tapes #4 to #6 demonstrate application of plantar stirrup straps. Each succeeding tape is overlapped approximately 1/2-inch and extends distal to just behind the first and fifth metatarsal heads. (*Figure continues.*)

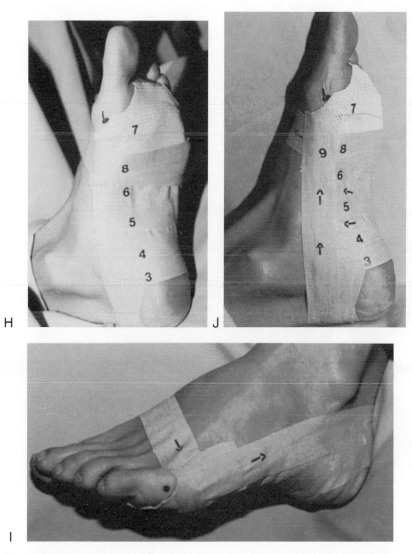

H

J

I

Figure 25-17 (*Continued*). (**H**) On the plantar surface, a 3-inch Elastoplast strip secures the distal portion of the accommodative pad. (The Elastoplast was trimmed just proximal to the first metatarsal head.) Also, tape #8 is applied in a cerclage manner as a retaining tape for tapes #1 and #2. This tape was applied plantar-medially in a superior direction across the dorsum of the foot and around the lateral aspect of the foot. It ends on the plantar aspect. It is important to leave some slack in the dorsal application of this strap. (**I**) The securing tape is drawn across the dorsum of the foot. (**J**) This shows the taping in its entirety and the direction of the application for tape #9. It follows the same course as tape #1.

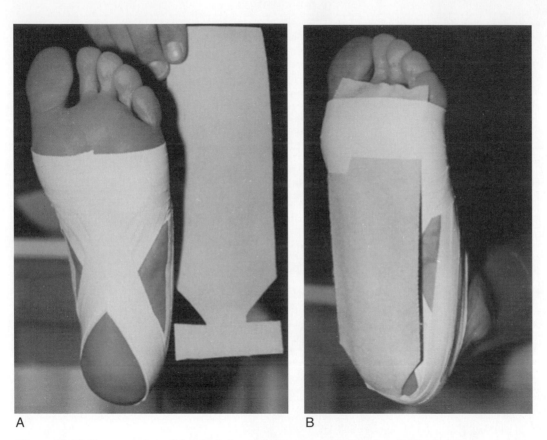

A

B

Figure 25–18 For a variation of the classic low-dye strapping, a T-shaped moleskin plantar fascial support strap is used.

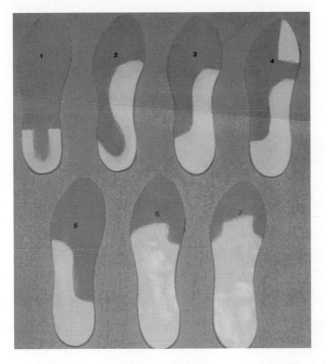

Figure 25-19 Uses of balance and accommodative paddings incorporated into temporary orthotics. (1) Plantar heelspur accommodation used for plantar calcaneal spurs, plantar fasciitis, or painful lesions that occur plantar to the heel, such as bruises or apophysitis. (2) Cobra pad for rearfoot control and supporting a forefoot varus deformity. (3) Medial heel–medial sole. The lateral aspect of this pad is skived to create a varus attitude to the rearfoot. This is designed to compensate for a rearfoot varus–forefoot varus deformity and to support the medial arch. (4) Medial heel Morton's extension, created similar to the medial heel–medial sole insole, with the same indications. Also, this enhances a great toe position and is mostly used in hallux limitus/rigidus and Morton's foot. (5) Medial heel–lateral sole, designed to stimulate out-toe gait. (6) Medial heel–first ray cut-out pad used to accommodate a plantar-flexed first metatarsal that is generally found with a high-arched cavus-type foot. The pad should be skived to create a 4- to 6-degree varus wedge on the rearfoot and to accommodate and allow the first metatarsal to sit in its neutral position. (7) Medial heel–first and fifth ray cut-out pad, commonly used in a high-arched cavus foot, with painful lesions below the first and fifth metatarsal heads.

CONCLUSION

Behind the sleight-of-hand show of the athletic trainer is a science that is an intricate and important part of athletic medicine. Shielding, supportive padding, strapping, and bracing are mechanical skills requiring study and practice. Material selection and handling, their application, plus anatomic study and a knowledge of clinical sports medicine all must be mastered. This body of information is used daily to prevent and treat acute and chronic athletic injuries at all levels of sport.

ACKNOWLEDGMENTS

I would like to thank Kenrick J. Dennis for taking the photographs used in this chapter, and Ed Stein for his assistance.

26

Surgical Intervention in the Foot and Ankle

HAROLD W. VOGLER
STEVEN I. SUBOTNICK

Musculoskeletal surgery performed on athletes requires special considerations and a different philosophy compared to such surgery on nonathletes. This is due mainly to their competitive personality profile as well as the significant physiologic demand on their locomotor system. They are always interested in a "quick fix" solution to their problem along with increased performance. Interestingly, athletes often self-treat rather effectively prior to presentation to a surgeon for evaluation of their condition. By the time they present to the surgeon, the condition is often well focused and defined. It is the surgeon who must decide whether the patient is best served with an operative approach for an acute or chronic problem, without being influenced by undue pressure from the athlete. Conservative care plays a critical role in sports medicine and should be applied when possible. Obviously, certain acute conditions preclude conservative treatment, and decision making becomes easier.

As a general rule, elective surgery in the athletic patient should be deferred or avoided while assessing the results of conservative treatment. In some situations, however, immediate surgical care may be the treatment of choice. Although a particular surgical procedure may give a very acceptable result in the general nonathletic population, the increased demands placed on the foot, ankle, and leg in the athletic patient can compromise even the most meticulous surgical procedure. The result can be an untoward postoperative outcome that can interfere with the optimum per-

formance of the athlete. This is particularly true if the proposed surgical plan alters a joint complex, musculotendinous unit, or individual bony link in the locomotor apparatus of the foot and ankle. Operative procedures on these musculoskeletal structures necessitate functional and positional changes in the "podiatric apparatus" that are ultimately reflected in postural biomechanical changes throughout the multiple lower extremity links.

Acute ruptures of major motor tendon units, such as the Achilles tendon, anterior and posterior tibial tendons, extensor hallucis longus, flexor hallucis longus, and peroneus longus, require primary repair in the athlete. Unstable grade III double ligament ruptures of the lateral ankle complex and recurrent ankle sprains with lateral instability require a surgical solution to optimize return to performance. There are several common "athletic fractures" that require surgery as a first-line approach, including the Jones fifth metatarsal base stress fracture, unstable ankle fracture, navicular tuberosity fracture, and posterior talar process fracture. Lisfranc joint fracture–dislocations can occur in athletes participating in sports that involve atypical landings, particularly basketball and soccer. These injuries are often occult and can be very disabling even if recognized early and treated aggressively initially. The tibial sesamoid fracture in the ballet dancer is often the professional "kiss of death" because it frequently goes unrecognized. These fractures represent a class of injuries that require immediate repair to reduce the morbidity of down time and allow the most anatomic restoration of the tissues and resumption of athletic performance.

There are myriad other chronic and post-traumatic musculoskeletal problems that lend themselves to surgical repair in the athlete when conservative treatment has failed; they can run the entire spectrum from simple to complex. Symptomatic subungual exostosis and ingrown toenails are basic problems but can be disabling to an athlete. More complex biomechanical conditions occur frequently, such as anterior and posterior ankle impingement syndrome, post-traumatic ankle compartment arthrofibrosis with chronic synovitis, midfoot boss formation (metatarsal–cuneiform exostosis), chronic posterior tibial tendon dysfunction, tarsal tunnel syndrome, achillodynia and tendinosis with or without paratenonitis and calcific tendinitis, chronic anterior compartment syndrome, plantar fasciitis with or without heel-spur syndrome, and Morton's neuroma. These conditions can all cause serious impairment for competitive athletes and, at times, end their careers. Surgery can often resolve or improve these conditions in athletes when practiced judiciously and in perspective.

Structural biomechanical forefoot problems, such as hallux valgus, hallux limitus and rigidus, hammertoes, and metatarsal angular deviations with painful plantar keratomas and bursitis, represent a class of common conditions that can disable an athlete for extended periods of time postoperatively. Midfoot, hindfoot, and ankle problems are commonly represented by conditions such as midfoot boss formation (metatarsal–cuneiform exostosis), Haglund's deformity with or without retrocalcaneal bursitis, and varus and valgus deformities of the hindfoot with pes cavus and flatfoot, ankle impingements, or acute traumatic ligament or fracture events. These deformities and problems produce complex compensation mechanisms that require careful consideration prior to surgical intervention in as much as the surgical solutions are often likewise complex and major.

Before surgery is undertaken in the athlete, careful assessment should be given to a number of factors. These include the nature and extent of injury or deformity, specific biomechanical considerations, the competitive level of performance, the long-term and short-term goals of the athlete, the functional demands of the patient's activity, and the anticipated level of compliance. It is frustrating when the results of a surgical procedure have been compromised by failure to follow postoperative instructions, such as not bearing weight on an extremity during the healing process or not adhering to specific prescribed activity modifications. Most athletes are highly motivated and share a common desire to recover as quickly as possible, and they recognize the importance of physical therapy and rehabilitation during the recuperative phase.

When considering surgery in the athlete, it is crucial that both the surgeon and patient have realistic expectations as to what can be accomplished by operation and what functional limitations may occur or be anticipated. Obviously, the patient should be well aware of the possible risks of surgery and the normal postoperative course, as well as alternatives to surgery. Once the decision to perform surgery has been made, a fundamental blueprint should be created. The general rule is to keep it practical and objective oriented. This means undertaking the minimal amount of surgery necessary to achieve the desired postoperative functional objective. At times, the condition will mandate significant and major surgery depending on the severity of the condition and the amount of interference with function and athletic performance. The surgeon should not attempt to correct every abnormal radiographic angle or biomechanical finding that is not interfering with performance. If osteosynthesis is necessary, proper planning for simple removal of fixation devices should be exercised at the time of delivery. Hardware is not psychologically and functionally acceptable to some athletes and can be the source of future problems, such as metal and bone fatigue pain, subcutaneous irritation, and interference with tendon gliding mechanisms. Kirschner wires K-wires are simple to remove, leaving no metal behind, but carry the risk of pin tract infection. When the operative plan calls for metallic instrumentation, the athlete should be advised of the possible need for future removal.

This chapter is not intended to be comprehensive or representative of the only acceptable approach to surgery in the athlete. It is intended to present a practical view of operative treatments in the athlete based on established current scientific information and recognized principles. Several surgical options often exist in each situation, and a selection can be made based on individual surgeon experience and training. The intent of this chapter is to provide clear, forthright surgical information presented in a usable format to serve as a convenient guide for the foot and ankle sports surgeon. The focus is surgical care when the mandate for surgery at a given point is manifest, and thus nonsurgical treatments are often not emphasized or discussed in detail; however, nonsurgical treatments must be recognized and practiced prior to undertaking many of the discussed index surgical treatments.

TOENAIL PROBLEMS

Onychocryptosis

Onychocryptosis is most frequently encountered in the hallux. Incurvation of the medial and lateral borders of the hallux nail with paronychia is seen in approximately equal proportions. In most instances, simple removal of the offending nail border and performance of a partial matrixectomy using the CO_2 surgical laser is all that is required. This may be performed even in the presence of mild infection with distal cellulitis. When there is abscess formation or frank pus, the offending nail border is removed and the infection is resolved with appropriate soaks, antibiotics, or both; the matrixectomy is performed at a later date. If access to a CO_2 surgical laser is unavailable, a phenol or NaOH chemical ablative matrixectomy may be performed, even with low-grade infection. Sharp blade procedures such as the Winograd, Suppan, and Ritchlin onychoplastics heal quickly with no drainage and are indicated only in the absence of infection.[1] The use of a sharp nail technique in these instances can provide a very satisfying result, avoiding the necessary and sometimes prolonged soaking regimen involved with the phenol or NaOH chemical matrixectomy, but carries a greater risk of postoperative infection and is associated with a greater degree of postoperative discomfort than a laser procedure or chemical ablation. When the Suppan plastic procedure is used, sutures are unnecessary.[1-3]

Subungual Exostoses and Osteochondroma of the Phalanges

Excessive pressure exerted against the dorsal aspect of the nail plate may lead to the development of a subungual bony exostosis or hematoma. This may be the result of direct trauma, as in football or soccer kicking injuries, or of chronic repetitive pressure, as in ill-fitting athletic foot gear or downhill running with increased extensor muscle activity, and is most common in the hallux.[4,5] A subungual hematoma is relieved by preparing a hole in the nail plate with either a small drill, a red-hot paper clip, or the CO_2 laser. Pain relief can be instantaneous. Radiographs are taken to rule out fracture.

The bony problems fall into the category of either a subungual exostosis or osteochondroma and are best treated by simple surgical excision under local anesthesia. The subungual exostosis is typically due to repetitive distal tuft trauma in shoe gear jamming, whereas the osteochondroma is a true neoplasm, comprising about 35 to 50 percent of all benign bone neoplasms. The osteochondroma is usually larger, with a differing appearance on the radiograph. A small distal skin incision (below the distal leading nail edge) can be used for exposure if the nail is not deformed. Temporary total avulsion of the nail plate more easily facilitates ostectomy if the bone lesion is central distal. Partial onychoplasty can be used also depending on whether the lesion is peripheral or central under the nail plate. Overlying soft tissues are gently freed from the exostosis spur or osteochondroma with the use of an elevator. Care must be taken to avoid damage to the nail bed, keeping dissection at a minimum. The bone lesion is then easily removed with the use of a rongeur or small oscillating saw blade. The wound is then flushed and closed primarily with one or two sutures. Alternatively, a closed osteotripsy technique can be used through a small dorsal distal stab incision with a low-speed, high-torque drill. Nonpermanent nail plate avulsion is often helpful even with this procedure to facilitate complete bone removal; the plate will regenerate subsequently.

In rare cases, osteochondroma can undergo malignant change to chondrosarcoma.[6] It might be prudent to send the specimen to pathology if it has any atypical appearance at excision.

NERVE LESIONS

Morton's and Interdigital Neuroma

Most reports indicate that the vast majority of neuromas occur in the third interspace, followed by the second, first, and fourth interspaces.[7-10] First-interspace neuromas are sometimes associated with fibular sesamoid fracture or dystrophy. This can be determined both radiographically and clinically. Occasionally, neuromas may occur in multiple interspaces at the same time. This has been determined to have a very low incidence—about 3 percent[11]—with the most common being in the third and second interspaces.

Various etiologies have been suggested,[7-9,12,13] including neuritis secondary to overpronation with traction placed on the nerve, intermetatarsal bursitis secondarily involving the nerve,[4] entrapment or irritation of the nerve as it passes beneath the deep transverse intermetatarsal ligament, injury to the nerve secondary to plantar impact or torque forces, and rheumatoid diseases.[11] Predilection for the third intermetatarsal space may be attributable to decreased mobility of the third plantar common digital nerve as a result of its lateral communication with the fourth common plantar digital nerve. The location of the third plantar common digital nerve in the vestigial cleft, which is the natural longitudinal separation of the lateral and medial columns of the foot, may also play a role. Second intermetatarsal space neuromas may be found in association with a hypermobile first ray and/or a long second metatarsal, both of which may result in increased weight-bearing loads to the second metatarsal–phalangeal joint and may lead to excessive shearing forces at the interspace. In athletes, interdigital neuromas are often attributable to a combination of faulty biomechanics with excessive pronation, excessive plantar twisting and shearing forces, and compression of the interspace secondary to foot gear and impact forces. Examples include pointed-toe bicycle shoes and thin-soled track spikes.

The diagnosis is established when palpation of the affected interspace reproduces the patient's symptomatology (Mulder's sign).[12] Palpation sensitivity is enhanced by the use of a topical lubricating cream. The patient may feel pain with palpation and compression of the affected interspace and may complain of a radiation of pain, numbness, or paresthesias into the adjacent toes. Mulder's sign or click can often be produced.[12] At times, a soft tissue mass may be palpable at the plantar aspect of the interspace, especially in a very flexible foot when the metatarsals are compressed medially and laterally. This displaces the neuroma plantarly, making it palpable and easy to reproduce the patient's symptomatology.

Interdigital neuromas usually respond favorably to conservative treatment consisting of custom-molded orthoses created from a balanced cast, with a metatarsal or neuroma pad, and injection therapy. This consists of a series of three injections, using a combination of long-acting local anesthetic with long-acting corticosteroid and vitamin B_{12} (neurolytic cocktail), to the affected interspace. These injections are given at at intervals of about 3 weeks. Physical therapy following the injection may be be helpful, combining electrogalvanic stimulation (EGS) and ultrasound plantarly. Oral nonsteroidal anti-inflammatory drugs (NSAIDs) are occasionally used. The success rate using this treatment regimen has been about 70 to 85 percent. Surgery is only recomended after this trial of conservative treatment has been unsuccessful.

When a single interspace neuroma is present, a dorsal longitudinal incision is the preferred surgical approach. The web space is avoided because of delayed healing as a consequence of natural inversion of the skin edges, in-

creased tissue moisture, and maceration. The transverse intermetatarsal ligament can be transected to decompress the intermetatarsal tunnel or left intact depending on surgeon discretion (Fig. 26-1). Dissection should be meticulous to avoid unnecessary damage to the vasculature and intrinsic digital musculature and associated tendons.

Adjacent interspace neuromas require a decision regarding incisional approach for appropriate exposure and resection. The third digit is subject to increased risk of vascular compromise because of its position. If both interspaces are to be operated simultaneously, a plantar transverse incision is preferred.[11,14] Staging can be considered in these situations. Recurrent neuroma is a difficult problem, and more recently the plantar approach has gained popularity for revisions. Plantar approaches must be placed distal to the weight-bearing area and proximal to the sulcus of the toes. Incisions in the weight-bearing area may produce painful

Figure 26-1 Classic Morton's neuroma excision, third interspace.

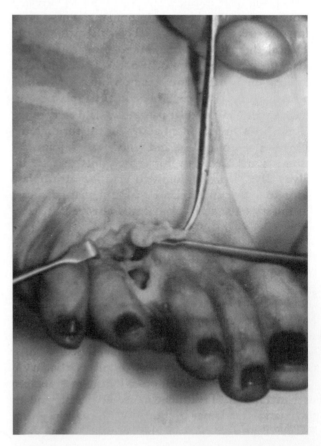

plantar scarring, causing more symptomatology than the original problem.

Solitary and adjacent interspace neuromas may be associated with plantar flexion of the adjoining metatarsal and a plantar keratoma. A concurrent distal metaphyseal elevation osteotomy might be considered to avoid secondary surgery. Osteosynthesis may be necessary depending on the adjacent metatarsal relationships, and can be achieved with a small screw or K-wire. If the situation requires an elevation osteotomy as well as dual interspace neuroma excision, osteosynthesis becomes more important, coupled with very judicious microdissection techniques under loupe magnification control. The surgeon must bear in mind that the more complex the surgery in a focused area, the longer the recovery and the greater the possibility of complications. Simple transverse intermetarsal ligament desmoplasty, either percutaneously or endoscopically, has recently as a surgical option. There are no long-term studies on this latter approach, although it is gaining popularity.

About 7 to 16 percent of patients may not achieve any significant relief whatsoever from neuroma exision.[10,11] Additionally, some residual symptoms can be anticipated to persist in about 40 percent of patients for up to 6 months or longer, although these patients are improved considerably over their preoperative status.[15] Recurrent neuromas can occur in as many as 24 percent of cases and present difficult challenges as well. A plantar revisional approach has become popular for secondary resection of these lesions.[16,17]

Superficial Nerve Compression

Any of the superficial nerves of the foot and ankle can be involved in nerve entrapment syndromes and can produce localized neuropathic radiating pain, numbness, or tingling in the distribution of the affected nerve. Superficial nerve entrapment syndromes may be the result of the nerve crossing over adjacent bony spurs or prominences. This is particularly common with the deep peroneal or anterior tibial nerves at the level of the first metatarsal–cuneiform joint when a first metatarsal–cuneiform exostosis is present. These syndromes may also be a secondary consequence of traction neuritis, especially following inversion-type ankle sprains with involvement of the sural nerve, branches of the superficial peroneal nerves, or both. The intermediate dorsal cutaneous nerve (Lemont's nerve) is commonly subject to shoe gear irritation or blunt truama and has the unique distinction of being the only nerve in the body that demonstrates traction visibility clinically. Superficial nerve entrapment may also be produced by scarring secondary to improper placement of skin incisions.

In the absence of a history of trauma or of obvious entrapment secondary to scar formation or improper placement of an incision, the athlete's foot gear should be considered. Simple manuevers such as changing the lacing pattern of shoes so that the laces do not cross a compressed anterior tibial nerve at the metatarsal–cuneiform joint may relieve symptomatology. A Joplin's neuroma may result from excessive pressure at the plantar medial aspect of the hallux or the first metatarsal–phalangeal joint area, especially in combination with bunion formation and axial rotation of the great toe.[13] This condition is more commonly seen in hyperpronatory athletes with hallux valgus and "pinch callous" deformity of the great toe.

When conservative treatment attempts fail to relieve the patient's symptomatology, a neuroplasty under loupe magnification may be considered to mobilize and decompress superficial nerves. This approach must involve resection of any underlying impingement exostosis, such as a metatarsal–cuneiform boss, or revision of any associated scar tissue formation. The procedure is less likely to be successful in thin patients, who have less subcutaneous tissue to provide protection of the superficial nerve, which minimizes the risk of postoperative adhesions and recurrent entrapment or compression neuropathy.[18]

An important differential diagnosis is occult diabetic neuropathy and reflex sympathetic dystrophy (RSD), which can masquerade as any of the above scenarios. RSD is an extensive subject beyond the scope of this chapter; however, the sports surgeon must be aware of the emergence of this phenomenon and institute early and aggressive intervention.

Tarsal Tunnel Syndrome

Tarsal tunnel syndrome (TTS) can be a frequently occurring neurologic entity in a busy foot and ankle surgical practice. Diagnosis depends on a high index of suspicion and careful history and physical examination. Anatomically, the tarsal tunnel extends from the proximal border of the laciniate ligament or flexor retinaculum distally to the porta pedis, which is bounded superiorly by the medial tarsal bones and inferiorly by the abductor hallucis muscle belly. Entrapment or compression of the posterior tibial nerve or any of its three branches may occur anywhere within this confined space, but most often occurs in the region of the laciniate ligament. Entrapment of the first branch of the lateral plantar nerve (Baxter's nerve) has been recognized as a frequent source of idiopathic inferior heel pain and should also be considered as part of a TTS differential.

There are many possible etiologies of compression of the neurovascular bundle within the tarsal tunnel.[19] These conditions generally fall into two categories: (1) decreased total volume of the tarsal tunnel or (2) space-occupying lesions within the tarsal tunnel. Examples of the former would be functional types of TTS resulting from excessive pronation with secondary heel valgus and excessive tension in the laciniate ligament. This produces compression of the tarsal tunnel and hypertrophy or spasm of the abductor hallucis muscle belly, placing pressure on the posterior tibial nerve branches and causing engorgement of the venous system in this confined region, occluding the potential space of this fibro-osseous canal.

Functional TTS often responds to orthotics and physical therapy. Injection of steroid and local anesthetic combinations is a necessary and useful treatment. Functional TTS with positive pathologic findings and nerve conduction and electromyographic (EMG) changes can occur.[20,21] The use of orthotics can reverse symptomatology, and repeat neurologic consultation and tests have shown normal electrodiagnostic findings.

Entrapment of Baxter's nerve is a form of distal tarsal tunnel syndrome (DTTS) that can be encountered following heel-spur surgery when the plantar fascia is released but not the deep fascia undersurface of the abductor hallucis muscle belly. Subtle lengthening of the foot and slight instability of the medial column can be produced by plantar fascia release and can produce a tension strain on the posterior tibial nerve and its branches. Often the first branch of the lateral plantar nerve becomes entrapped beneath the tight abductor hallucis muscle belly and its fascia, which has not been completely decompressed on its undersurface where it impinges against the quadratus plantae and medial slip of the plantar fascia.

A variety of conditions can produce TTS secondary to space-occupying lesions. These include vascular congestion secondary to local or metabolic vascular disease, such as (1) deep venous insufficiency with dilated and thrombosed veins or arteriovenous fistula; (2) ganglionic cyst originating from any of the tendon sheaths of associated tendons within the tarsal canal or the ankle or subtalar joints; (3) fusiform swelling of tendons or their associated sheaths secondary to chronic tenosynovitis (posterior tibial tendon dysfunction) or partial or complete tendon rupture

and associated scar tissue formation; (4) direct trauma to the tarsal tunnel region resulting in fusiform swelling or neuroma formation of the posterior tibial nerve or branches; and (5) a variety of metabolic or hormonal disturbances that can produce vascular engorgement within the tarsal canal, such as myxedema.

DIAGNOSIS

Clinically, tenderness to palpation of the tarsal canal in the area of entrapment or compression with percussion over the point of entrapment will usually result in a positive Tinel's sign with distal radiation represented by pain, numbness, or paresthesias. Turan's sign can also elicit distal radiation with inversion and dorsiflexion of the foot and hallux. Subjective areas of distal radiation are important in determining which nerves are being compressed. This may be either the entire proximal posterior tibial nerve, the medial or lateral plantar nerves, the medial calcaneal nerve, the first branch of the lateral plantar nerve or any combination of these. In the case of a unilateral TTS, it is important to check for palpation tenderness on the contralateral side as well as for Tinel's sign on the unaffected side. The absence of Tinel's sign on the contralateral extremity helps support the diagnosis of TTS. Clinical bilateral Tinel's sign can be elicited in the absence of a tarsal tunnel compression, especially in thin persons who lack abundant subcutaneous tissue. This can be a normal finding in the absence of other painful symptoms. The surgeon can often detect tenderness to palpation of the nerve trunk, both proximal and distal to the point of entrapment. This is known as a Villeaux phenomenon and does not refer to proximal radiation of symptomatology during the percussion test.[22]

TTS is essentially a clinical diagnosis. Neurologic consultation can be helpful to support the diagnosis in the face of multiple condition overlay, such as concurrent occult diabetic neuropathy, spinal stenosis, or radiculopathy. Neurologic consultation is often obtained to rule out systemic causes of increased or decreased nerve sensation, muscle strength, or both. "Normal" electrodiagnostic tests do not necessarily rule out a pathologic TTS. Unfortunately, normal electrodiagnostic test results are often the end result of outside consultation and must be interpreted in perspective. Magnetic resonance imaging (MRI) can identify space-occupying lesions or other fibrous or tendinous abnormalities in the canal and represent another option for preoperative evaluation.

When nerve conduction studies and EMG are undertaken in order to lend support to the diagnosis of TTS, particular attention is paid to denervation of the intrinsic musculature of the foot, as well as increased distal latency of the posterior tibial nerve. Distal latencies can exceed 6.1 msec for the medial plantar nerve and 6.7 msec for the lateral plantar nerve in pathologic situations. The abductor hallucis is innervated by the medial plantar nerve and the abductor digiti quinti by the lateral plantar nerve. The height and duration of the motor potentials are polyphasic and spread out over 15 to 20 msec or more with entrapment.[23,24] Nerve conduction velocity proximal to the point of entrapment or compression is normal in TTS. Sensory disturbance normally precedes motor weakness. Therefore, the presence of wasting or weakness of the intrinsic musculature suggests a more progressive disease. Intrinsic motor disturbance is sometimes implicated by the presence of digital contractures on the involved side. Whenever the patient is being evaluated for neuropathic distal pain in the extremities, pathology more proximal in the superstructure should be ruled out, such as nerve root compression secondary to traumatic or degenerative changes of the lower spine or even proximal nerve lesions in the leg. This is the major indication for nerve conduction or EMG studies.

When a patient's subjective complaints and objective findings are consistent with those of TTS, the appropriate diagnosis can be made in the absence of more proximal disease as described earlier. Neurologic studies are used adjunctively but not exclusively for diagnosis. It must be stressed that they are not used to rule out TTS, because functional TTS may coexist in the absence of notable findings.

TREATMENT

TTS may respond to conservative treatment, consisting of biomechanical control with orthoses or injection therapy to the area of entrapment using a combination of a long-acting local anesthetic with a long-acting corticosteroid, or both. Vitamin B_{12} can be added to the injection therapy empirically, especially if the TTS is of a functional nature. If this form of treatment fails to resolve or improve the patient's symptomatology and the symptoms are severe, or if there is evidence of motor disturbance (denervation, atrophy, or weakness of intrinsic musculature), decompression of the tarsal tunnel should be carried out, making certain the classic sites of compression are adequately released, often under magnification. RSD should always be considered and ruled out as well.

Tarsal Tunnel Decompression

The operation is preferably done under general anesthesia, using a thigh tourniquet. A posteromedial curvilinear incision is made, beginning just proximal to the superior border of the flexor retinaculum, coursing posteriorly and inferiorly to the medial malleolus and extending distally and inferiorly to the talonavicular joint at the superior margin of the abductor hallucis muscle belly. The incision is carefully deepened through the subcutaneous tissue, taking care to identify and preserve the greater saphenous vein distally. The deep fascia is identified and found to be taut and continuous with the laciniate ligament more distally. The full-thickness skin and subcutaneous flap is then retracted anteriorly, easily demonstrating the laciniate ligament, which can be appreciated as a well-defined thickening of the deep fascia with tight, obliquely oriented fibers. Decompression of the tarsal tunnel involves sectioning of the deep fascia in the distal aspect of the leg, extending to the porta pedis of the foot. In addition, a 1-cm-wide portion of the laciniate ligament can be excised. The divisions of the posterior tibial nerve are identified and followed distally. Any obvious fibrous adhesions are meticulously released. Loupe magnification is helpful, and any associated pathology is addressed at this time (e.g., a ganglionic cyst, fibro-osseous canal abnormalities or impingements, tortuous or constricting venous branches, or thrombosed veins are excised or ligated). A fluid epineurolysis can be carried out at the same time, using several milliliters of saline. A small amount of soluble steroid can be injected carefully into the epineurium at the completion of the neurolysis, which is also facilitated under magnification. The wound may then be flushed with the remainder of the irrigant solution. Meticulous attention must be paid to hemostasis. Prior to wound closure, the thigh tourniquet is released and bleeders are carefully ligated. Closure is accomplished in one thick layer. The laciniate ligament and deep fascia are not reapproximated.

Postoperatively, a Jones compression cast is applied to the leg with the foot in neutral position for 5 to 7 days to help control postoperative edema. The patient is then allowed to bear weight in a removable below-knee cast brace for 3 weeks. The use of a posterior splint or removable cast brace allows for adequate wound inspection when necessary and early rehabilitation at the 10th postoperative day. Physical therapy includes the use of gentle dorsiflexion, plantar flexion, inversion, and eversion of the foot within the limits of passive tension. It should be stressed that this is a very gentle range of motion in order to permit some flexibility of the foot and ankle and thereby lessen postoperative periarticular fibrosis. This may be combined with physical therapy modalities, such as EGS and ultrasound, if desired. Aggressive early range-of-motion and therapeutic exercises can cause disruption of capillary bed regrowth and may result in excessive fibrosis and scar tissue formation, which could lead to failure of the tarsal tunnel decompression. The overall success rate of the procedure is on the order of 60 to 75 percent.[19] TTS can recur following early apparently successful outcome. Trauma to the site is typically responsible, contributing to recurrent fibrosis in the tarsal canal.[25]

When the posterior molded splint or cast brace is discontinued at the end of 3 weeks, more aggressive range-of-motion and therapeutic exercises are begun with active range of motion against progressive resistance, allowing gradual return to activity over the next 2 to 3 months. Orthotic biomechanical control is a helpful adjunct in the rehabilitation process, particularly when the condition was a functional type of TTS.

Following surgery, patients are often initially better but, with continued healing and maturation of the healing scar tissue, the patient's condition may deteriorate. Continued rehabilitation may be indicated in these situations, and it should be recognized that maximal medical improvement (MMI) could take up to 1 year to achieve. Physical therapy is most helpful in the postoperative course to maintain reduction of edema in the limb and inhibit overgrowth of scar tissue. Occasionally, injection of a local anesthetic and long- and short-acting corticosteroid into the scar tissue formed by the surgery is necessary if the scar tissue is determined to be contributing to a delayed successful outcome.

Anterior Tarsal Tunnel Syndrome

Anterior tarsal tunnel syndrome (ATTS) may occur in two locations. The first anatomic site is the area dorsally over the first metatarsal–cuneiform articulation (type I). The second site is the anterior ankle region, where ATTS is associated with anterior impingement exostosis of the ankle joint frontier, with hyperostosis impingement of the overlying neurovascular bundle or superficial nerves, or both (Type II).

Type I ATTS

In type I ATTS, the anterior tibial (deep peroneal) nerve may become involved in entrapment or compression syndromes similar to those seen in medial TTS. The patient's presenting complaint is usually pain at the dorsal aspect of

the forefoot, usually in the midfoot region. This may be accompanied by distally radiating pain, numbness, or paresthesia, which may be subjectively located at the distal aspect of the first intermetatarsal space dorsally over the adjacent side of the first and second toes. A positive Tinel's sign may be elicited with percussion at the point of entrapment or compression. This condition is frequently associated with functional instability of the medial column, resulting in pronatory dorsal jamming at the first metatarsal–cuneiform articulation. Radiographically, this may be seen as osteophytic lipping or spur formation at the metatarsal–cuneiform articulation and often is associated with a navicular–cuneiform breach. Spurring or beaking of the talonavicular joint, as seen in tarsal coalition, may contribute to type I ATTS. ATTS can also be related to post-traumatic compression of the anterior tibial nerve as a result of direct trauma to the area or ill-fitting shoe gear. This is more common in high-instep cavus feet with rigid plantar flexion of the first metatarsal. The patient's clinical symptomatology is produced by compression of the anterior tibial nerve as it courses beneath the inferior extensor retinaculum over underlying bony prominences or spur formations. The neurovascular bundle actually travels in a fibro-osseous canal as it passes the ankle and enters the foot.

ATTS may respond to conservative measures consisting of functional orthotic control to minimize hypermobility of the first ray and associated dorsal jamming. The use of injection therapy with steroid and local anesthesia in the region of the entrapped nerve beneath the extensor retinaculum is often efficacious. Appropriate physical therapy modalities, such as EGS and ultrasound, may be used following injection therapy. The patient's shoes are evaluated for fitting problems and are modified accordingly. Often, shoelaces or ringlets of shoes cause compression of deep superficial nerves in the foot. They may enhance the symptoms of hyperostosis at the first metatarsal–cuneiform joint with overlying compression of the superficial or deep peroneal nerves. Removing the ringlet or alternate lacing of the shoes to avoid pressure on the hyperostosis is often all that is necessary to resolve the problem.

Type I Decompression: First Metatarsal–Cuneiform Hyperostosis with Superficial and Deep Nerve Compression   Failure of the patient's symptomatology to subside following orthotic control and a series of up to three injections with physical therapy may indicate surgical decompression of the anterior tarsal tunnel. Adjunctive nerve conduction or EMG is usually unnecessary because localized pathology is readily identified clinically. If a generalized neuropathy is suspected, neurologic consultation can be considered.

A dorsolinear incision overlying the first metatarsal–cuneiform articulation 5 cm in length is the usual approach. Preoperative planning is necessary in order to map the course of the neurovascular bundle accurately. This stage is crucial to avoid placement of the incision directly over the anterior tibial nerve; otherwise, postoperative scar tissue formation could result in failure of the decompression. The procedure may be performed under local anesthesia or local anesthesia with intravenous standby and ankle tourniquet for hemostasis. The oblique inferior medial band of the extensor retinaculum is identified as a well-defined thickening of the deep fascia of the foot, and obliquely oriented transverse fibers running proximal laterally to distal medially are found just proximal to the medial cuneiform. More distally, another band of the extensor retinaculum may be encountered dorsal to the metatarsal–cuneiform joint region, with obliquely oriented transverse fibers coursing toward the second metatarsal base. The fascia is incised, and the band of the inferior extensor retinaculum is sectioned between the tendons of the extensor hallucis longus and the extensor digitorum longus. The neurovascular bundle is located beneath this layer. Following meticulous dissection under magnification, the nerve is identified and gently freed from surrounding adhesions with microvascular dissection technique. The anterior tibial or dorsalis pedis artery is not always visualized. Great care must be taken to avoid arterial or venous injury; this is ensured with microvascular dissection technique under magnification. After adequate mobilization of the anterior tibial nerve, a fluid epineurolysis is performed in a fashion similar to that used in medial TTS. Adequate fluid is gently instilled in the epineurium to make certain all adhesion sites have been decompressed. A small amount of soluable corticosteroid is used to bathe the neurolysis site when the procedure has been completed.

If nerve compression is associated with a dorsal metatarsal–cuneiform exostosis, bone resection will enhance decompression. The tendon of the extensor hallucis longus is now retracted laterally or medially to expose the dorsal surface of the first metatarsal–cuneiform articulation. The associated bony hypertrophy is resected with the use of an osteotome and mallet. It is important to remove adequate bone, creating a concavity by directing bone removal concentrically toward the joint from the adjacent sides of the hypertrophy. Cavitation in this region helps compensate for new bone formation and dense fibrous tissue that often

regenerates in this region following resection of the impingement exostosis. The medial tarsal tunnel retaining system of the inferior extensor retinaculum is not reapproximated as in other closed tunnel decompressions. Following the procedure, the patient is placed in a below-knee Jones compression dressing or posterior splint for 5 to 7 days to maintain tissue stability. This is subsequently followed by a removable below-knee cast brace for 2 to 3 weeks. Physical therapy and early range of motion are thus facilitated. Orthotic stabilization of the tarsus will be helpful postoperatively to control any existing hyperpronation.

Type II ATTS

Type II ATTS results when the anterior tibial nerve becomes compressed over a dorsal talar neck bone impingement or anterior tibial frontier impingement exostosis of the ankle. Anterior frontier impingement of the ankle often presents as a syndrome, including proliferative bony changes at the anterior aspect of the ankle joint, chronic synovitis, and capsulitis of the ankle with entrapment or compression of the anterior tibial nerve. Anterior frontier impingement of the ankle can be tibial dominant, talar dominant, or combined.[26] Anterior frontier ankle arthroplasty is required as a necessary step in decompression of this entrapment and is best and most conveniently accomplished with an anterolateral ankle arthrotomy and arthroplasty. Spontaneous decompression results following arthroplasty in as much as the pathology is essentially an impingement syndrome and not a true nerve entrapment. A detailed discussion of anterior ankle arthroplasty and anterior frontier impingement is presented subsequently in this chapter.

CONDITIONS AFFECTING THE HEEL

Acute and Chronic Rupture of the Plantar Fascia

Plantar fascial rupture is an uncommon entity.[27-29] It can occur in athlete and nonathlete populations and can result in chronic disabling pain that interrupts athletic training. It can be an obscure form of dysfunctional pain resulting from spontaneous or minimal recreational activity. Acute rupture presents as sudden-onset pain in the arch region, usually distal to the tuberosity insertion, with ecchymosis and a palpable lump. MRI or sonography can easily further define the acute event if desired. This is an underdiagnosed occult form of plantar heel and arch pain. It should be suspected in sudden-onset arch pain scenarios with or without heavy activity.[30] This leads to the concept of both acute and chronic degenerative ruptures. Prior injury to the area is common, and steroid injections near the site have also been implicated.

It is interesting that this phenomenon is not more common with the high incidence of cortisone-like injections used to treat chronic heel pain conditions. There is no clear relationship between the use of occasional cortisone-like injections for heel pain and acute or chronic rupture, although some cases have been reported. Caution in treating chronic heel pain and a high index of suspicion are required in the diagnosis of this condition.

Treatment is usually conservative, with casting in the acute phase if considerable pain and ecchymosis are present. As the injury subsides, orthotic supports for up to 1 year are required to prevent propagation or re-rupture. If pain is chronic and persistent in spite of physiotherapy, orthotics, oral NSAIDs, and fascial stretching following subsidence of the acute event, surgery could be required. Macroscopically abnormal tissue must be removed at the site of the "lump" and pain. Interestingly, the literature also suggests fasciotomy for relief in these chronic cases following excision of scar tissue.[31–33]

Plantar Fasciitis and Heel-Spur Syndrome

Plantar heel pain is an extremely common clinical complaint in both the athletic and nonathletic populations. It is not always due to a heel spur, however. The presence of an inferior calcaneal spur is a radiographic finding and uncommonly the solitary cause of the associated pain. Heel spurs form as part of a biomechanical scenario in response to traction of the plantar fascia and intrinsic musculature of the hindfoot. The syndrome may be a self-limiting process over the course of 18 to 36 months. As the inferior spur enlarges, the origin-to-insertion distance of the plantar fascia is effectively reduced, possibly reducing tension on the plantar fascia as well as the patient's symptomatology. Progressive formation of an inferior calcaneal spur can also be associated with progression of patient's pain and disability.[34]

Plantar heel pain is part of a symptom complex and not necessarily associated with any radiographic evidence of heel spur formation. An accurate history and physical examination are paramount in determining the source of the heel pathology. Common culprits manifesting as heel pain syndrome are (1) inferior calcaneal bursitis, (2) plantar fasciitis and abductor hallucis myositis, (3) incomplete TTS with Baxter's nerve entrapment, (4) a partial tear of the plantar fascia, and (5) stress fracture of the os calcis (Fig. 26-2). The latter can be assessed by the appropriate imaging studies. These conditions may present separately or in combination. For example, it is not uncommon for a patient with plantar fasciitis to also have abductor myositis or Baxter's nerve entrapment in the same heel.[35] Inferior tuberosity heel spurring can be present with all three of these same findings as well.

Classic plantar inferior fasciitis clinically presents with pain upon palpation of the plantar medial calcaneal tuberosity, as well as the plantar medial aspect of the calcaneus at the origin of the abductor hallucis. It is commonly described as postdykinesia pain. Heel spur pain, if real, also presents at the same location. Distal pain associated with the plantar fasciitis may be evident at the medial or central band of the plantar fascia midarch in addition to its origin at the plantar medial calcaneal tuberosity. This combination is frequently seen in athletes who spend a lot of time on the ball of the foot while the calcaneus is being suspended between the Achilles tendon and the plantar fascia. This may occur in aerobics, ballet, sprinting, basketball, cycling, or similar activities and can manifest as the solitary reason for intractable heel pain in as many as 15 percent of patients.[35] Fortunately, conservative therapy consisting of biomechanical control of excessive pronation with the use of orthoses, taping, below-knee casting, NSAIDs, steroid injection therapy, and plantar fascial stretching night splints has a high rate of success (Fig. 26-3A & B). Below-knee casting with the ankle slightly dorsiflexed is probably the most effective treatment in recalcitrant cases.[36] Physical therapy is an important adjunctive modality and should be used if possible.

Patients who fail this regimen after at least 6 months or more of conservative care can fall into the category of surgical candidates. This group is larger than previously believed, based on a study by Gill and Kiebzak.[36] The exceptions are the focused medial hindfoot nerve entrapments, which can be operated sooner because their pathology is less likely to resolve with nonsurgical care. Partial plantar fasciotomy is the most common procedure used for true plantar fasciitis. It involves detachment of the medial band of the plantar aponeurosis from its insertion at the plantar medial calcaneal tuberosity, along with partial detachment of the abductor hallucis from its origin on the plantar medial aspect of the calcaneus. Subtotal endoscopic

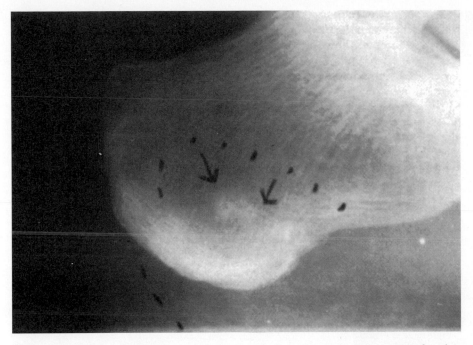

Figure 26-2 Increased bone density is indicative of calcaneal stress fracture, a cause of recalcitrant heel pain.

plantar fasciotomy is popular and perceived to be less traumatic and more accurate in the amount of plantar fascia actually severed. The outcome studies comparing standard techniques with endoscopic release are comparable in general, however. Plantar fasciotomy can cause destabilization of the foot[37] and must be undertaken carefully and in perspective, often with the use of a postoperative below-knee cast for 3 to 4 weeks.

PLANTAR FASCIOTOMY, BAXTER'S NERVE DECOMPRESSION AND HEEL SPUR EXCISION

The procedure is conveniently done under local or general anesthesia with or without an ankle tourniquet, according to surgeon preference. A low medial plantar longitudinal skin approach is used for exposure. An alternative 3-cm vertical incision medially is an excellent approach, developed about one fingerbreadth posterior and inferior to the medial malleolus. This exposure allows good access for Baxter's nerve decompression simultaneous with the spur excision and partial plantar fasciotomy if desired (Fig. 26-4). Both approaches cross the insertion of the abductor hallucis as well as the attachment point of the plantar aponeurosis in the region of the inferior calcaneal tuberosity.

A smooth periosteal elevator or endoscopic channeling elevator is used to create two pathways—one inferior to the origin of the plantar aponeurosis and one just superior. Curved Mayo scissors or a #11 blade may then be used to release the desired amount of plantar fascia at its attachments to bone, with care being taken to avoid the first branch of the lateral plantar nerve to the abductor digiti quinti. The tips of the scissors are directed posteriorly, and the contour of the plantar calcaneal tuberosity is followed medially to laterally. If an inferior calcaneal exostosis is present, it is resected with a rongeur or Maltz rasp. High-speed air drills and osteotomes must be used cautiously in this area, avoiding the incline of the undersurface of the os calcis, resection of which would produce a stress riser predisposing to pathologic fracture. Additional release of the inferior fibers of the plantar fascia can be conveniently and safely accomplished with a scissors or surgical blade, staying close to the medial tuberosity. The fascia on the deep side of the abductor hallucis should be delicately released at the same time to prevent nerve tethering against its rigid, deep, taut surface. This is recommended to avoid isolated cases of DTTS secondary to compression of the medial or lateral plantar nerves, or both, distal to the abductor hallucis.

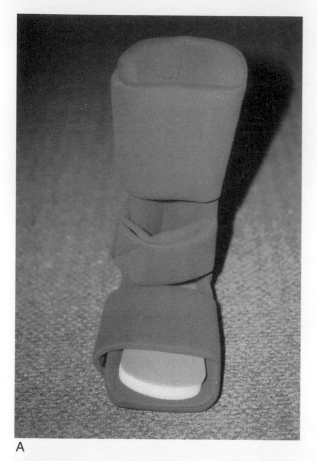

A

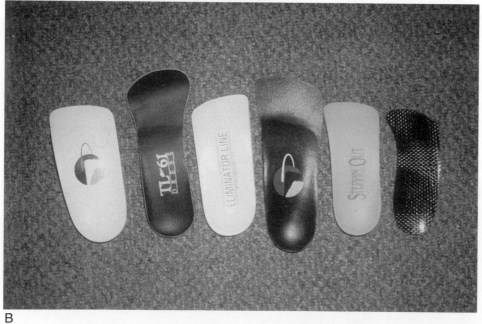

B

Figure 26–3 (**A**) Plantar fascial–stretching night splint. (**B**) Biomechanical orthotics for chronic plantar fasciitis and heel–spur syndrome.

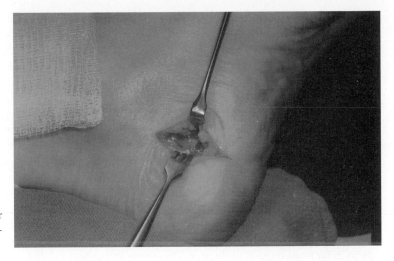

Figure 26-4 Vertical medial heel approach for decompression of Baxter's nerve and heel spur surgery if desired.

Release of the plantar fascia will allow for some positional changes in the foot (lowering and lengthening of the medial longitudinal arch). This may result in entrapment or compression of the medial or lateral plantar nerves, or both, between a taut abductor hallucis muscle belly and the adjacent tarsal bones and the medial slip of the plantar fascia and the actual heel spur. There is no real agreement on how much plantar fascia requires release in these procedures, and most surgeons perform subtotal fasciotomy unless they are dealing with a pes cavus foot architecture.

Neurectomy of the medial calcaneal nerve is often accomplished accidentally, particularly with the longitudinal medial approach, which almost always crosses this nerve. Occasionally, intentional transection of this nerve has been performed when neurolysis or other conservative measures have failed.[13] This will produce a certain degree of permanent numbness on the plantar aspect of the heel. If an inferior calcaneal bursitis is encountered at this time, it may be excised. Care must be taken not to disturb the plantar calcaneal fat pad. One thick layered closure is performed. Patients are allowed to walk in a fiberglass foot cast, below-knee cast brace, or short-leg cam walker for about 3 to 4 weeks depending on their weight and activity level. Orthotic control subsequently can be utilized for additional bracing; this decision may also be related to the same considerations of weight and anticipated activity level.

Heel spur resection with fasciotomy can sometimes have a protracted recovery process. Spur recurrence can occur; however, it does not seem to influence the outcome of the operation. An interesting study also failed to find any change in arch architecture following fasciotomy.[38] Patients tend to fall into one of three groups:

1. Those who return to normal activity level at about 6 weeks, which is uncommon, account for perhaps less than 25 percent of these patients. This group consists of those athletes who are in excellent physical condition prior to surgery.

2. Approximately half of the patients operated on will require about 3 to 6 months to regain full return to activity without associated pain or limitations. This group tends to comprise heavier patients, such as walkers, golfers, and bowlers.

3. Twenty percent of these patients may take up to 12 months to plateau or become symptom free, returning to their previous level of activity. These patients tend to have had longstanding chronic heel-spur syndrome or plantar fascial pain. This group tends to comprise heavier patients with thick, broad feet. Because of their prolonged course of heel pain, they tend to be out of shape.

Patients in this third group also tend to develop secondary acquired problems, such as neuromas in the second or third interspaces or "calcaneal cuboid instability syndrome." It is believed these problems are secondary to gait alteration with abnormal weight transfer to the lateral or distal aspect of the foot as a guarding mechanism. Lateral column instability or calcaneal cuboid fault syndrome can also occur with total or near-total plantar fasciotomy. This iatrogenic complaint can be chronic and require 12 months to improve or resolve. Loading studies have demonstrated considerable weight transfer to the lateral column following plantar fasciotomy, and this is believed to be the source of this problem. Orthotics with perpendicular-to-valgus rearfoot control and cuboid pads are necessary for peroneal cuboid syndrome. Cuboid manipulations, injections underneath the cuboid in the peroneal groove, or both may provide some relief.

Unfortunately, there is a small subgroup comprising perhaps 5 to 8 percent of patients who never attain significant relief of their preoperative symptoms and can even be worse.[39] We believe this to be due to inadequate release of the medial fascia at the tuberosity or the undersurface of the abductor hallucis, contributing to continued Baxter's nerve entrapment. Inferior calcaneal tuberosity heel pain surgery is far from refined, and optimal outcome probably depends most on diagnosis-specific surgery in this anatomic region.

Inferior Calcaneal Bursitis and Generic Inferior Heel Pain

Like plantar fasciitis and abductor myositis with or without heel spur formation, inferior calcaneal bursitis often responds well to conservative measures. This pathology is the result of impact forces produced by heel contact and is commonly seen in such activities as medium- and long-distance running on hard surfaces, downhill running, or acute trauma to the plantar tuberosity as in falling from a height. It may be seen in association with atrophy of the plantar calcaneal fat pad, especially in older athletes. Clinical examination will demonstrate pain on palpation directly inferior to the central weight-bearing aspect of the heel. A mass may also be palpable in this region and may even produce crepitation.

If we are to treat this problem successfully, it is important to be able to attenuate impact shock forces at heel contact. Viscoelastic polymer materials in the form of heel cups and lifts can decrease vibratory pathology and subsequent collagen tissue breakdown and be quite helpful. An inflamed inferior calcaneal bursa can be injected with a combination of long-acting local anesthetic and corticosteroids. Injections are followed by physical therapy to enhance the effect of the injections. Oral anti-inflammatory medications can be helpful concurrently. In nonarthritic patients, ice massage can reduce the symptomatology, especially when palpable swelling is present. Arthritic patients respond better to heat application. Abductor myositis and

inferior calcaneal bursitis respond initially to decreased activity and avoidance of hard surface and downhill running.

The differential diagnosis is similar in all chronic heel pain patients and must include radiculopathy and nerve root compression secondary to degenerative disk disease in the lower back. Myofascial pain syndrome may produce distally radiating pain symptoms as a result of compression or entrapment of the sciatic nerve in the region of the sciatic notch, piriformis muscle belly, gluteal muscles, or proximal aspects of the hamstrings. TTS with distal branch entrapment can simulate these same symptoms as well. Systemic diseases to consider include any of the collagen or vascular disorders, autoimmune disease, rheumatic or seropositive arthropathies, or inflammatory seronegative disease. Examples include Reiter's syndrome, psoriatic arthritis, ankylosing spondylitis, arthropathy associated with bowel disease, or sacroiliitis and low back disease. Laboratory tests, including sedimentation rate, uric acid, rheumatoid factor, and human leukocyte antigen B-27, are helpful in making a definitive diagnosis. Presence of one of these systemic diseases does not preclude surgical intervention. Such disease can influence the outcome, however, and knowledge of its presence aids the surgeon and rheumatologist in planning appropriate postoperative care.

Most cases of plantar fasciitis, abductor hallucis myositis, and inferior calcaneal bursitis will respond to conservative treatment. In some cases, however, a surgical approach is required.

EXCISION OF INFERIOR CALCANEAL BURSITIS OR HYPERTROPHIC MEDIAL CALCANEAL TUBERCLE

The skin incision and deeper dissection are identical to those used in heel spur surgery—either the posteromedial vertical incision or low medial longitudinal incision. When excising an inferior calcaneal bursa, it is crucial to leave the inferior calcaneal fat pad in place. Likewise, if a hypertrophic medial tuberosity of the calcaneus is being remodeled, the soft tissue should be carefully removed from the bone prior to remodeling. In some cases, a "hatchet-shaped" calcaneus may need remodeling to shift the concentrated weight-bearing area from the medial plantar aspect to encompass more of the total surface of the plantar aspect of the calcaneus (Fig. 26-5). This is done using an osteotome and mallet or an oscillating saw blade. Care must be taken to avoid disturbing or reducing the thickness of the fat pad; otherwise the fat pad will fail to attenuate heel strike forces. The surgeon should assess the area for pathology of the medial calcaneal nerve and its branches

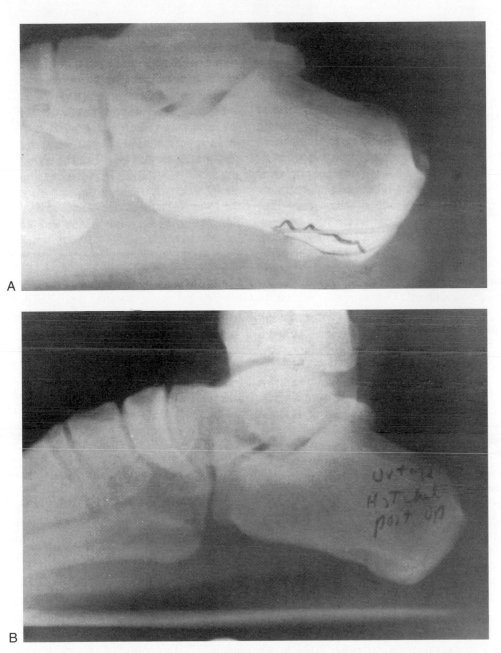

Figure 26-5 (**A**) Preoperative and (**B**) postoperative views of hatchet calcaneus with heel spur.

when excising a medial plantar symptomatic calcaneal bursa. At times the nerve will go directly into the bursa, and a neurobursitis may be present.

TENDINOPATHIES ABOUT THE FOOT AND ANKLE

Anatomy and Pathologic Changes in Tendons and Supporting Structures

Tendon is the anatomic component that transmits motor torque between bony links in the musculoskeletal system. As a result, tendons produce movement or stability, depending on their required function at the moment of muscle contraction. They can function isotonically, producing significant stability, and they can also function concentrically and eccentrically, producing both approximation of their linkage systems with movement (concentric function) and deceleration if distended while in an active state of contraction (eccentric contaction).[40] The morphologic composition of the various tendons indicates their ultimate function and load capabilities. Thicker, heavier, dense tendons imply a greater workload capacity compared to slender, more elastic tendons, which imply considerable elastic kinetic energy capacities. The histologic composition of tendon is defined mainly by densely packed connective tissue with a matrix of type I collagen fiber bundles with relatively parallel axial orientation. This design characteristic confers their ideal ability to sustain tensile loading and transmit elastic and kinetic energy when and as needed. Interspersed between the collagen fiber bundles are fibroblasts that create and maintain the matrix composition of the actual collagen connective tissue.

Paratenon is a peritendinous connective tissue membrane that surrounds nonsheathed tendons such as the Achilles. The Achilles tendon is unique among the major extrinsic foot–leg tendons in that it does not possess a true sheath but rather a paratenon (Fig. 26-6). It is composed of two layers: an inner visceral and an outer parietal layer. Mesotenon connects these layers periodically along their course; it typically lies on the nonfriction surface of a tendon unit and carries a considerable vascular arcade for nourishment. In the case of the Achilles tendon, this structure is on the anterior surface. This fact forms an important basis for various surgical procedures on this powerful tendon. When synovial fluid forms between the layers of paratenon, it is characterized as tenosynovium; when absent it is known as tenovagium. Synovial sheaths develop

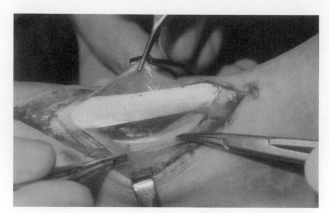

Figure 26-6   Paratenon of Achilles tendon.

around tendons that are exposed to angular changes and pulley systems. They are designed to dissipate friction and reduce strain during excursions around these rigid pulley mechanisms. The podiatric orthopedic apparatus manifests several sheathing and pulley mechanisms (Fig. 26-7A & B). All major extrinsic tendons crossing the ankle, either retrotibial or pretibial, possess complex tenosynovial sheathing mechanisms.[41] The digital flexors actually possess two—a proximal sheath at the ankle level and a distal sheath at the metatarsophalangeal joints as well.

Tendinitis is a generic term used loosely by clinicians to describe nonspecific tendon pain. Histologic intrinsic changes are in reality what produces the pain and tendinopathy, however.[42,43] Inflammatory changes usually fail to reveal significant histopathologic findings because of the paucity of macrophages in tendon tissue. The changes are more commonly mucoid degenerative, related to either age, gender (male more common), or activity type and intensity. The term most proper for defining this degenerative process is *tendinosis*. It refers to disorganized matrix with fibers that lack axial morphology, tightly woven collagen bundles, and a fatty, mucoid degeneration or hyaline composition. Originally, there was significant basis to believe the underlying pathology in Achilles tendinopathy was avascularity, induced by multiple factors including intrinsic paucity of vascular perfusion at the midportion of the Achilles tendon.[44–49] This concept now appears incorrect, as demonstrated clearly by Astrom and Rausing.[42] To the contrary, the vascular perfusion is now recognized as being hypervascular.[43,50] The so-called watershed area of the Achilles tendon is indeed the most common site of acute and chronic ruptures and degenerations, but hypovascularity cannot explain this lesion based on the most

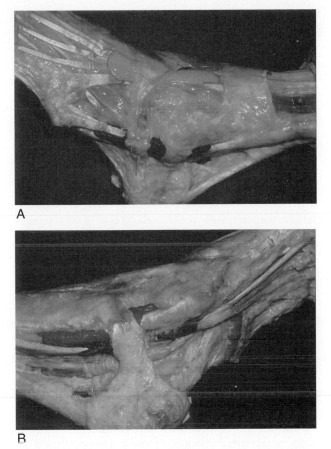

Figure 26-7 (**A**) Lateral view of the podiatric apparatus sheathing and pulley mechanisms of the extensor digitorum longus and peroneals about the foot and ankle. (**B**) Medial ankle view of the flexor tendon sheaths and laciniate ligament.

recent available research. Vascular proliferation in tendon lesions is a well-known phenomenon, and Astrom and Rausing believe this helps explain their findings of increased perfusion. These same studies also demonstrated a remarkable lack of paratenonitis or other pathology of this structure in symptomatic case of Achilles tendinopathy. As a result of these studies, male gender predominance is recognized as a factor in the development of Achilles tendinopathy, along with normal aging, which does factually decrease perfusion in the Achilles tendon. Tendinosis of other commonly dysfunctional tendons, such as the posterior tibial and peroneals, may not pursue the same course of degeneration because of inherent differences in the anatomic composition and sheathing mechanisms of these other tendons. However, it is not unreasonable to extend these same concepts to other major loaded tendons.

Achilles Tendinopathy and Related Retrocalcaneal Problems

Probably the most disabling chronic condition a performance athlete can develop is the "syndrome" of Achilles tendinitis or paratenonitis.[51] It has an athletic prevalence estimated at 11 to 20 percent in runners.[52,53] This syndrome represents a group of conditions that are poorly understood and can be disabling, interfering with performance even in noncompetitive athletes, often referred to as "weekend warriors." It has been reported that Achilles tendinitis is the most common athletic injury, occurring especially in middle- and long-distance runners. The areas most commonly involved are (1) the myotendinous junction of either the medial or lateral gastrocnemius muscle; (2) the portion of the Achilles tendon proximal to the distal insertional region and ankle joint, sometimes referred to as the "watershed area"; and (3) the insertion of the Achilles tendon into the posterior aspect of the os calcis. Conditions considered in this category are medial or lateral gastrocnemius strain at the myotendinous junction, Achilles paratenonitis, central rupture or degeneration (also known as tendinosis) of the Achilles tendon, and insertional Achilles tendinitis with or without calcinosis. Many of these problems can be related to training errors or overuse syndromes. The athlete will usually relate a history of sudden increase in either intensity or duration of athletic activity, a sudden change in the type of terrain, or an attempt to return to a high level of participation following a period of relative inactivity. Injury to the specific site has also been implicated.

Biomechanical influences may be implicated in the development of Achilles tendinopathy, such as pes cavus or hyperpronation flatfoot deformity with compensated gastrocnemius equinus or short heel cord. A fixed equinus of the forefoot on the rearfoot will result in compensation at the ankle joint. The tibiotalar articulation will function in a relatively dorsiflexed position to permit contact of both the forefoot and the rearfoot on the ground during midstance. This can result in overuse of the triceps surae and Achilles tendon and possibly predispose to tendon injury. Heel lifts are used in these cases to permit neutral midstance ankle position and eliminate excessive pull on the Achilles tendon. Heel lifts are also used when a short heel cord is present for similar reasons.

Other compensating biomechanical abnormalities, such as forefoot varus, rearfoot varus, and forefoot valgus with varus in metatarsals two through five and a rigid, plantarflexed first ray, may predispose to Achilles tendinopathy.

It has been suggested that any forefoot-to-rearfoot biomechanical imbalance that results in subtalar joint compensation producing either an inverted or everted calcaneus can result in force concentrations at either the medial or lateral side of the Achilles tendon. For example, a compensated forefoot varus deformity would result in eversion of the calcaneus, which could produce excessive tension located at the medial side of the tendon as compared to the lateral side.[54] Orthotic control of the forefoot varus with a medial forefoot post would then eliminate this abnormal compensatory mechanism, thereby reducing strain to the Achilles tendon. In the case of rigid plantar flexion of the first metatarsal, which results in inversion of the calcaneus and excessive strain to the lateral fibers of the Achilles tendon, orthotic control with forefoot valgus posting would be indicated.

The center of the insertion of the Achilles tendon into the os calcis has been shown to be invariably medial to the axis of the subtalar joint.[55] The triceps surae is therefore the most powerful supinator of the subtalar joint. Biomechanical deformities that result in excessive subtalar pronation may result in overuse with longitudinal shearing strain within the tendon fibers or at the tendon–peritenon interface. The tranverse plane rotation of the fibers might play a role in the syndromes that comprise the entity of Achilles tendinitis.

Active shock attenuation (running on the ball of the foot) with secondary dissipation of vibratory frequencies causes collagen tissue fatigue and disruption and, finally, breakdown. When forces or time periods are excessive, degeneration and scar tissue are the end result. Thus training errors may lead to Achilles tendinopathy. Preventive eccentric strengthening and stretching exercises should be used. Because most injuries occur during eccentric contracture, it makes little sense to rehabilitate these injuries with concentric exercise. Viscolas heel lifts help attenuate heel strike vibratory and shock forces and decrease the amount of these shock waves that must be absorbed by the musculoskeletal system, permitting the collagen tissue and structures to heal. Partial tears of this nature invariably heal with scar tissue formation. Eccentric stretching is therefore imperative to maintain proper length while strengthening and stretching the posterior musculature following injury.

ACHILLES PARATENONITIS

The most common presenting complaint referable to the Achilles tendon is pain and tenderness about the narrow portion of the tendon proximal to the insertion just behind the ankle joint.[54] Cases of pure paratenonitis without tendinosis degeneration usually do not manifest obvious clinical or imaging findings of fusiform swelling or degeneration of the tendon.[43]

The Achilles tendon, which pursues a relatively straight course from origin to insertion, lacks a true tendon sheath.[40,42,45,47,53] It is covered by a thin membrane known as paratenon, which forms the mesotenon anterior to the Achilles tendon. These thin structures carry the tenuous blood supply of the Achilles tendon, the so-called watershed area.[44,45] The underlying pathology in Achilles paratenonitis is an inflammation of the paratenon believed to be induced by overuse. A fusiform swelling of the actual Achilles tendon usually is not present, but tendon crepitus may exist. Insufficient treatment may allow swelling to progress to chronic edema with fibroadhesions that ultimately transform into chronic Achilles paratenonitis.[51] This is now known to be rather uncommon based on histologic studies by Astrom and colleagues in symptomatic patients with Achilles tendinopathy.[42,51] This impression has subsequently been confirmed by Movin and associates.[43] At this stage, there is little that can be done if pain persistently interferes with performance, other than perform surgery; however, one must carefully examine the tendon at surgery to determine small areas of degeneration–small macroscopic assessment might be inadequate.

Bilateral Viscolas heel lifts are used except in cases of unilateral Achilles paratenonitis and tendinosis secondary to short leg syndrome. In this instance, a Viscolas lift would be appropriate selectively for the short side only. Treatment for Achilles paratenonitis, as with all sports medicine injuries of the lower extremity, requires that the pelvis be level during the treatment phase. This is accomplished with an appropriate heel lift, orthosis, or both depending on the cause of limb length discrepancy. In addition to their roles as dynamic stabilizers and effectors of skeletal segment motion, the muscles of the lower extremity are also important in attenuation and transmission of ground reaction forces. Heel strike on a short leg, especially during strenuous athletic activity, results in increased ground reaction vibratory shock waves, as well as aftershock waves, that are transferred not only through the skeletal segments but through the musculotendinous units as well. In addition, overstriding on the involved shorter leg may place increased functional demands on the Achilles tendon of the short side. The short leg overstrides to keep up with the long leg. Contact is often farther back on the heel. This may place the contact foot on the short side in front of the center of gravity, increasing retrograde forces of the

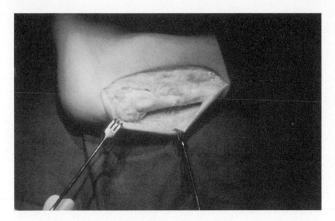

Figure 26-8 Chronic Achilles paratenonitis. (Courtesy of Dr. Mats Astrom, Malmö University Hospital, Malmö, Sweden).

contact surface. Appropriate heel lifts and physical therapy usually balance out this stride discrepancy.

The presence of palpable and audible crepitation surrounding the Achilles tendon with active or passive range of motion denotes the presence of a more advanced degree of inflammation. High levels of fibronectin and fibrinogen has been found in the connective tissue and vascular walls of the paratenon in chronic paratenonitis, indicating an immature form of scar tissue.[56] Such an inflammatory infiltrate of the paratenon has a significant potential to undergo fibrotic changes from fibrin organization, resulting in chronic Achilles paratenonitis (if not treated appropriately) characterized by chronic edema and hyperplasia of portions of the paratenon, fibrous adhesions, and chronic pain and disability [57,58] (Fig. 26-8). Athletic performance is restricted for about 3 weeks during this phase of disability. Swimming, cycling, and low-impact aerobics may be substituted to maintain cardiovascular fitness, followed by a gradual progressive return to activity. Subtle weaknesses may be detected and rehabilitated with the use of the Cybex dynamometer. Resistant cases of Achilles paratenonitis in the athlete are treated with weight bearing in a posterior molded splint or cast brace locked at the ankle at 90 degrees. Physical medicine and rehabilitation modalities, including range of motion and gentle stretching, are instituted under supervised programs initially.

The criterion for surgery has generally been accepted as failure of 6 to 12 months of aggressive conservative treatment with physical medicine and oral anti-inflammatory agents. It is now believed earlier surgical intervention might be beneficial because the condition appears to be chronic, with no significant histologic improvement oc-

curring spontaneously. Selective Achilles paratenon stripping, avoiding the anterior surface and the mesotenon, is the procedure of choice, with histologic examination if the problem can be demonstrated to lack tendinosis pathology with imaging studies. All chronic inflammatory or hypertrophic tissue surrounding the Achilles tendon is carefully dissected away, releasing any fibrous adhesions interfering with tendon gliding.[59] Palpation of the tendon by the surgeon is necessary to rule out the presence of pathologic tendinosis or nodules within the tendon.[54] It may be advisible to incise the tendon longitudinally to further examine the deeper substance, because it is now known that actual paratenonitis is not a common finding in symptomatic heel cords.[42]

ACHILLES TENDINOSIS

Achillodynia with central necrosis with partial internal rupture is characterized by a degeneration of the deep substance of the Achilles tendon (Fig. 26-9). Parallel fiber structure is lost with pathologic hyalinization, with increased vascularity and perivascular hemosiderin deposition. This process is gradual and results in decreased tensile strength along with a paradoxical thickening of the tendon and occasionally palpable nodules along the course of the tendon. This condition usually exists independently of Achilles paratenonitis. The development of central necrosis of the Achilles tendon seems to parallel the overall condition of the patient's connective tissues. There is an increased incidence of central necrosis with advanced age, collagen vascular and connective tissue disease, and generalized arthritis and overuse syndromes.[59] The precise etiol-

Figure 26-9 Central necrosis with partial degenerative rupture. (Courtesy of Dr. Mats Astrom, Malmö University Hospital, Malmö Sweden).

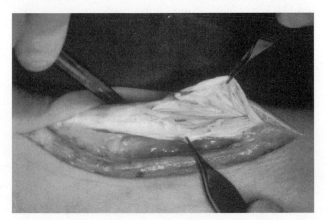

ogy is uncertain but seems related to functional demand, male gender predominance, and advancing age.[42]

The Achilles tendon is essentially a conjoined tendon, receiving contributions from both the soleus and the gastrocnemius muscle bellies (and to a lesser extent the plantaris). These muscle groups have somewhat different phasic activities. The situation is further complicated by the well-documented rotation of the fibers of the Achilles tendon.[60,61] As the proximal posterior fibers derived from the gastrocnemius muscle belly travel distally, they also course laterally and anteriorly. Similarly, the proximal anterior fibers derived from the soleus course medially and posteriorly as they descend toward the os calcis. There can be up to a 90-degree internal torsion of the tendon fibers, although individual variability does exist. It has been postulated that central necrosis of the Achilles tendon is the result of a concentration of shear stresses between the tendon fibers of the gastrocnemius and soleus in the so-called avascular watershed zone just proximal to the insertion. This zone was demonstrated only in the external vascular arcades of the tendon, however, and not internally. However, it has been shown that the rotation of the Achilles tendon fibers acts to eliminate such shearing stresses by equalizing the asymmetric tension forces that would otherwise be produced in the Achilles tendon as a consequence of calcaneal inversion or eversion. Thus the functional and internal structural demands of the Achilles tendon are complex and may predispose the patient to tendon injury.[54,59]

Clinically, it can be difficult to differentiate central necrosis partial rupture from peripheral paratenonitis. Central necrosis is not directly detectable radiographically, although thickening of the Achilles tendon shadow may be seen using soft tissue radiographs or xerograms. Thorough clinical examination supplemented with appropriate imaging studies (MRI, sonography) is often required to make a definitive diagnosis. Imaging techniques using ultrasound and MRI have evolved to a high state of accuracy, as verified at surgery, and are now the diagnostic state of the art.[40,50,62,63]

Isolated central necrosis or degeneration without associated paratenonitis may be suspected when there is asymptomatic palpable or visible thickening of the Achilles tendon without crepitus along the surface at examination. The presence of central necrosis predisposes to an increased risk of Achilles tendon rupture.

Surgical Treatment of Tendinosis With Central Necrosis

Central necrosis with partial rupture in combination with, or without, peripheral paratenonitis defines the entity of tendinosis.[50] The athlete is often subjected to considerable nonsurgical treatment, which probably is a waste of time in this scenario. If the athlete is disabled because of this painful chronic condition (often persisting for up to 3 years), surgery should be considered early during the treatment regimen in an effort to restore competitive performance. Surgery offers the patient the possibility of return to activity, whereas persistence of the painful condition without operation simply leads to continued disability, pain, and possible ultimate rupture if competition continues. The surgeon must engage in thorough discussion with the athlete prior to operation so that the athlete develops an understanding of the realistic outcome of any operative procedure. The athlete should also recognize that the outcome may be dependent on the magnitude of tendinosis determined intraoperatively, in as much as imaging studies are not 100 percent accurate or predictive of outcome. The recovery can be long and demoralizing to the competitive athlete, taking up to 1 year or more of rehabilitation. Recurrence of the tendinosis can develop several years subsequently, and it is prudent to warn of this outcome as well.

The operation can be performed under general or local anesthesia with sedation. Tourniquet hemostasis is recommended, but dilute epinephrine may be employed along with the local anesthesia if a tourniquet is not used. A linear longitudinal incision 5 to 7 cm in length is made over the medial posterior or lateral posterior aspect of the lower leg toward the insertion of the Achilles tendon. The approach is deepened through the subcutaneous tissue to the level of the paratenon. All chronic inflammatory tissue surrounding the Achilles tendon is carefully assessed and then sharply resected as indicated. Fibrous adhesions are delicately released when identified. The subcutaneous tissue surrounding the Achilles tendon must be preserved by using suture string retraction. Normal-appearing paratenon tissue is preserved, especially on the anterior surface of the tendon where the mesotenon is located.

Following debridement of visibly abnormal paratenon and adhesions, the tendon proper can be examined for nodules or mushy degeneration, which can often be palpated between the surgeon's fingers. If tendinosis pathology has been previously imaged or is palpated intraoperatively, an incision is made into the central portion of the Achilles until the degenerative pathologic substance or nodule is encountered. Chronic mucoid degeneration and abnormal-appearing material within the substance of the tendon are carefully and sharply excised and the tendon remodeled[54] (Fig. 26-10). Multiple longitudinal internal tenotomy[64] incisions may be required on all major surfaces

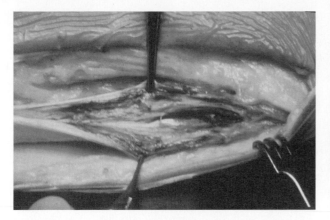

Figure 26-10 Extensive infratendinous Achilles degeneration and debridement in chronic tendinosis case. (Courtesy of Dr. Mats Astrom, Malmö University Hospital, Malmö Sweden).

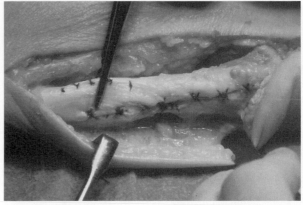

Figure 26-12 "Tubing" repair of Achilles following debridement of degenerative tissue. (Courtesy of Dr. Mats Astrom, Malmö University Hospital, Malmö, Sweden).

except the anterior, depending on the extent of the degenerative process or the number of nodules within the substance (Fig. 26-11). Longitudinal incisions into the Achilles tendon are not closed in order to facilitate migration of metaplasia cells to become fibroblasts within the tendon, thereby creating a new collagen matrix. The tendon is then repaired with a "tubed buried suture technique" if considerable central substance has been excised as a result of collagen disorganization and degeneration (Fig. 26-12). A novel percutaneous technique was described by Testa and associates[65] consisting of local anesthesia and delivery of a Q11 blade into several locations peritendinously at and near the site of clinical symptoms. The patient is then asked

to move the leg to induce tendon excursion and longitudinal tenotomy is accomplished by the natural range of tendon excursion during firing.

If the tendinosis has been extensive, with considerable degeneration that requires excision, a gastrocnemius recession advancement or a proximal aponeurotic "turndown" flap may be required to reinforce the reconstruction site and allow adequate length restoration (Fig. 26-13). This can also be accomplished using the local plantaris tendon for reinforcement, or even peroneus brevis transfer for augmentation (Fig. 26-14A & B). Alloplastic materials such as Dacron and allogeneic tendon implants are available for consideration in full-thickness degenerations that require

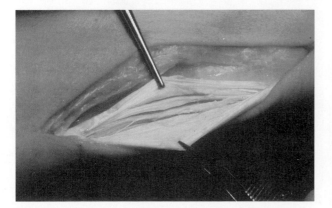

Figure 26-11 Testa technique of longitudinal tenotomy of the Achilles. (Courtesy of Dr. Mats Astrom, Malmö University Hospital, Malmö, Sweden).

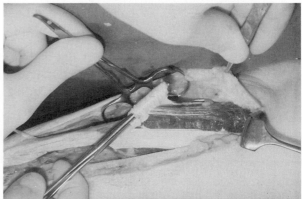

Figure 26-13 "Sardine can" turndown augmentation technique with gastrocnemius aponeurotic proximal flap.

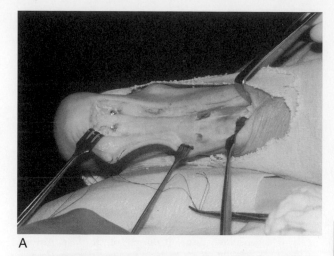

A

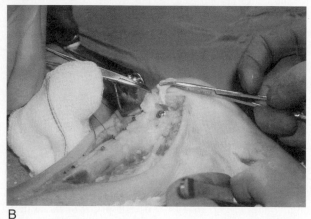

B

Figure 26-14 (**A**) Tongue-in-groove gastrocnemius recession for distal advancement when the terminal tendon is degenerative and requires excision. (**B**) Augmentation reinforcement with peroneus brevis tendon transfer.

an entire cross-sectional excision. Closure is accomplished with 5-0 absorbable suture in subcutaneous tissue and 5-0 skin suture of the surgeon's choice. In distal lesions demonstrating insertional calcific tendinosis, the abnormal tendon is remodeled and the calcific deposition is removed concurrently.[66] This may necessitate partial avulsion of the tendo Achillis, or at times avulsion of the entire insertion depending on the extent of the calcific tendinitis. Reimplantation with bone anchors or spiked washers and screws may be required (Fig. 26-15A & B).

Postoperative care consists of a cast brace or below-knee cast for 4 to 6 weeks, depending on the extent of the reconstruction or surgery required. The cast brace may

initially be hinged in mild plantar flexion. After 2 to 3 weeks, the brace is placed in a near-neutral position. Four weeks of brace protection or casting is sufficient for mild to moderate repair. When extensive degeneration and reconstruction has occurred, 6 weeks of cast brace immobilization is preferable, starting rehabilitation after the third week.

Figure 26-15 (**A**) Resection of a large global Haglund's deformity and calcific tendonitis that required total avulsion of the heel cord with "cleansing" of the insertion. (**B**) Reimplantation with 4.0-mm A-O screws and polyacetyl spiked A-O washers.

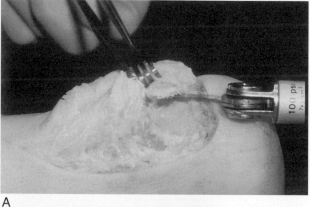

A

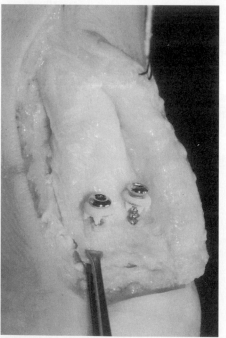

B

INSERTIONAL ACHILLES TENDINITIS AND CALCIFIC TENDINOSIS

Pain at the insertion of the Achilles tendon into the os calcis is often associated with alteration of the bony contour of the calcaneus. It may be seen with a prominent posterosuperior angle of the calcaneus, increased Phillips-Fowler angle, or retrocalcaneal exostosis.[54,67-69] A calcaneal "step" or insertional traction hyperostosis may be present, essentially transforming the condition into calcific tendinosis. A retrocalcaneal exostosis or a long posterior aspect of the calcaneus results in an increased lever arm of the Achilles tendon as measured from its insertion to the joint axis of the ankle. This is equivalent to a functional shortening of the Achilles tendon, yet presents an increased mechanical advantage. It may also place increased strain on the Achilles tendon as well as extra shoe pressure against the tendon, with chronic irritation. Excessive pressure applied by a firm shoe counter may result in an inflamed retrocalcaneal bursa. Superiorly orientated spur formation in the tendon may be evident radiographically. Such traction spurs are often associated with a calcaneal step. They may also be the result of excessive traction forces with microavulsions at the level of the insertion[18-20] (Fig. 26-16).

Conservative treatment of insertional tendinitis is essentially the same as that for the other forms of retrocalcaneal problems. This includes the use of physical therapy modalities, ice, oral anti-inflammatory medications, stretching and strengthening exercises, and viscoelastic heel lifts, cast bracing, or even total below-knee cast immobilization. An inflamed retroachilleal bursa may be carefully injected with

a short-acting corticosteroid one time. If there is a posterior prominence of the calcaneus, accommodative padding may be necessary to afford comfort within the shoe. When conservative treatment has failed to alleviate the athlete's symptoms and performance is affected, surgical intervention becomes necessary.

The incisional approach for surgical repair depends on the nature of the condition. If retrocalcaneal spurring is present at the insertion, a midline Achilles tendon–splitting approach is good and can provide adequate access to resect the spur.[70,71] Any enlargement at the posterior surface of heel can also be remodeled through this approach at the same time with minimal disruption of the insertional fibers. An axial radiograph or transverse plane computed tomography (CT) scan can demonstrate the extent of posterior spurring and assist in surgical planning. If the pathology is central and lateral, such as a Haglund's deformity with calcific tendonitis, then a lateral approach would better serve the surgeon. Occasionally, global calcific tendonitis requires an L approach, most often medially hinged with total avulsion of the insertion, thorough remodeling of the back of the heel, and replantation of the heel cord with anchors or spike washer and screws (see Fig. 26-15).

The tendo Achillis insertion is most profound on the posterior medial side of the heel. When retrocalcaneal spurring is present, the insertion of the heel cord fibers occurs anterior to the spur between the posterior wall of the calcaneus and the deep surface of the spur.[72] If there is a morphologic bone deformity in the region, such as Haglund's deformity, retrocalcaneal exostosis, or global hypertrophy at back of the heel, this is repaired at the same time. This finding can be exploited when resecting these painful spurs, which allows the surgeon to maintain most of the major posterior and medial insertional fibers of the heel cord. Haglund's deformity is usually most prominent along the posterolateral corner of the os calcis, and thus repair and resection at this site requires only partial avulsion of the tendon fibers to gain good access to the bone deformity for resection. If a chronically inflamed or calcific bursitis at the retrocalcaneal bursa is present, this may be surgically excised. There may be concomitant tendinosis or paratenonitis, which should be addressed simultaneously. Calcific tendonitis may require near-complete avulsion of the heel cord with "cleansing" of the calcified insertional region and re-implantation. The back of the heel is remodeled at the same time. Bone anchors or spiked washers with screws may be necessary if the required replantation is total (Fig. 26-17). This can occasionally require a small

Figure 26-16 Insertional Achilles calcific tendinosis with fragmentation.

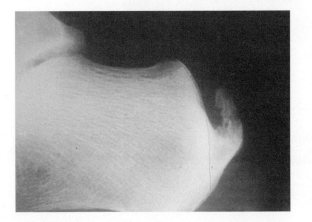

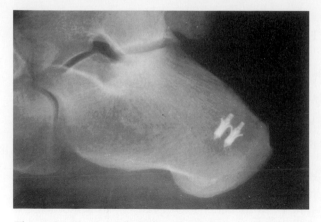

Figure 26-17   Reimplantation of Achilles with double bone anchors.

gastrocnemius advancement manuever to gain adequate length for replantation.

Disability time can be considerable with these operations, and down time for a competitive athlete can be up to 1 year. Total replantation operations require the longest periods of recuperation time, and sometimes athletes cannot resume their original preoperative competitive level; they need to understand this preoperatively.

RETROCALCANEAL EXOSTOSIS (HAGLUND'S DEFORMITY)

An enlarged or prominent posterosuperior angle of the calcaneus can result in posterior heel pain secondary to chronic irritation from the heel counter of shoes. It is usually associated with a painful retrocalcaneal bursitis and may secondarily affect the Achilles tendon as it courses over the bony prominence, resulting in chronic pain and inflammation in the area near the insertion[50,68] (Fig. 26-18). In some cases, vertically oriented osseous spurs may be evident within the substance of the Achilles tendon as it inserts into the os calcis (calcific tendonitis). This may predispose to avulsions of the Achilles tendon should a large spur be exposed to a traction overload and fractures. The precise etiology of retrocalcaneal spurring or calcific tendonitis is not known; however the condition is believed to be related to age, overuse, trauma, and enthesiopathies and has a high occurrence rate.[71]

Certain biomechanical deformities that compensate at the subtalar or ankle joint, or both, may predispose to retrocalcaneal exostosis. Examples such as compensated rearfoot varus, rigid forefoot valgus, and cavovarus deformities result in repeated irritation of the posterosuperior lateral aspect of the os calcis against the heel counter. An unpublished anatomic study by Vogler and Bojsen Møller (Panum Institute, University of Copenhagen, Denmark) has demonstrated the lateral side of the os calcis to be longer than the medial side in structural or positional tuber varus. Thus the posterolateral corner of the os calcis becomes prominent, resulting in a clinical Haglund's deformity (Fig. 26-19). This may be an incidental finding. It is uncertain whether this form of chronic repetitive irritation would result in bony hyperplasia, but it is a common clinical finding. This repetitive compensatory motion could result in chronic inflammation of the posterolateral corner of the os calcis, retrocalcaneal bursa, or retroachilleal bursa, which is superficial to the Achilles tendon, and therefore transform an otherwise normally contoured os calcis into a source of posterior heel pain.

The development of a retrocalcaneal exostosis (or Haglund's deformity) may be the result of a separate center of ossification at the posterosuperior angle of the os calcis.[73] This could represent a small portion or fragment of the calcaneal apophysis or may actually develop independently of the calcaneal apophysis.

The rounded posterior surface of the calcaneus acts as

Figure 26-18   Typical Haglund's deformity with posterolateral corner prominence, bursitis, and pain with a compensated rearfoot varus deformity.

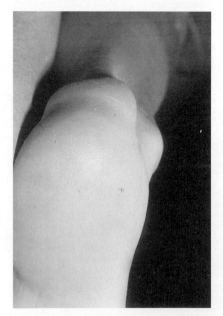

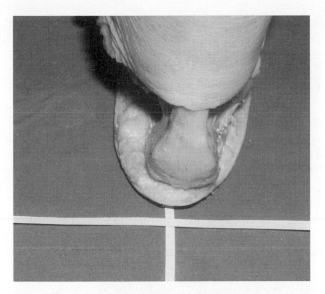

Figure 26-19 An anatomic model demonstrating the longer lateral wall of the os calcis compared to the medial wall in tuber or positional heel varus, making the posterolateral corner prominent.

a pulley system on the Achilles tendon. As the foot is dorsiflexed at the ankle joint, the anterior surface of the Achilles tendon comes into contact with more superior portions of the calcaneus, maintaining a relatively constant distance between the axis of the ankle joint and the effective insertion of the Achilles tendon. Thus the posterior surface of the os calcis acts to maintain the lever arm of the Achilles tendon at the ankle joint. If the posterosuperior angle of the calcaneus proximal to the Achilles tendon insertion were not present, as the foot dorsiflexed at the ankle joint there would be a progressive shortening of the distance between the ankle joint axis and the effective insertion of the Achilles tendon. As the lever arm shortens, the biomechanical advantage of the tendon function at the ankle joint would also be affected significantly. Conversely, an abnormally prominent posterosuperior angle of the os calcis would actually increase the lever arm of the Achilles tendon as the foot was dorsiflexed at the ankle joint, resulting in a relative functional shortening of the Achilles tendon. When the deformity is severe, chronic insertional Achilles tendinitis may result.

Clinically, the patient will present with pain localized to the posterior aspect of the heel and possibly the terminal portion of the Achilles tendon; typically a reddened and tender soft tissue swelling secondary to a retrochilleal or retrocalcaneal bursitis will be detected. The bony prominence of the posterosuperior angle of the os calcis is usually tender to palpation, especially on the lateral aspect but possibly also on the medial aspect.

The extent of bony involvement is evaluated radiographically. The Phillips-Fowler angle may be measured on the lateral view.[67,74] Also, the presence of any traction exostosis within the Achilles tendon may be detected on the lateral view. The relative obliquity of the bony prominence may be assessed with a special dorsal plantar projection of the posterior surface of the os calcis. This is done with the patient bearing weight, with the radiographic central beam posterior to the leg, which is dorsiflexed on the foot. The film cassette is placed beneath the plantar aspect of the foot, which is perpendicular to the central beam of the x-ray machine. The central beam is then directed vertically at the posterosuperior aspect of the os calcis.

Retrocalcaneal exostosis may be managed conservatively in a fashion similar to that used for Achilles paratenonitis. Ice massage is used on the painful inflamed area in nonarthritic patients. When a retroachilleal or retrocalcaneal bursitis is present, it may be carefully injected with a combination of short-acting corticosteroid and long-acting local anesthetic. This maneuver should be performed very cautiously and perhaps only one time, exercising caution to avoid injecting the actual tendon. At no time is the injection introduced into the substance of the Achilles tendon or its insertion, because this is well known to predispose to rupture. Following an injection effort, physical therapy modalities such as combined EGS and ultrasound are used over the area of inflamed bursa, retrocalcaneal exostosis, and posterior distal aspect of the Achilles tendon. Multiple physical therapy treatments two to three times a week, for 2 to 3 weeks, can be quite effective. The athlete is instructed on gentle stretching and strengthening exercises of the posterior musculature. Viscoelastic-type heel lifts are used to attenuate heel contact and vibratory shock waves and to compensate for the functional heel cord shortening that is produced by having a prominent posterosuperior angle of the calcaneus. Bony prominences at the posterior aspect of the heel are accommodated with moleskin in an attempt to relieve shoe pressure. The athlete must avoid running or jumping maneuvers for a period of approximately 3 weeks following the last injection. Activity modification is employed for this time, with cycling, swimming without fins, and/or the use of a wet vest to maintain tone and cardiovascular fitness. In resistant cases, a well-padded weight-bearing posterior molded splint or removable cast is used. It is removed on a daily basis for the application of physical therapy modalities, icing, and gentle stretching exercises.

Surgery is recommended when conservative measures have failed and when symptomatology is interfering with or defeating the athlete's ability to perform or compete. Patient positioning is determined by the incisional approach, with the two most common options being prone or lateral supine. The procedure may be performed under general or local anesthesia with intravenous sedation. The thigh tourniquet is used in the case of a general anesthetic, and a midcalf tourniquet is used when local anesthesia under intravenous sedation is used.

Operative Technique

A lateral longitudinal incision, approximately 6 cm in length, is placed just anterior and lateral to the lateral border of the Achilles tendon, centered at the superior surface of the calcaneus. An additional longitudinal medial incision may be made when there is excessive medial bone that cannot be adequately resected from the lateral incision.[75,76] This is preferable to a transverse incision or a lazy-S incision, which offers adequate exposure but can interrupt the superficial nerves, creating distal numbness at the posterior aspect of the heel. Care is taken to avoid the lesser saphenous vein and sural nerve, should they be encountered. The surgical site is then deepened directly down to the enlarged bone site. The periosteum is incised longitudinally overlying the prominence and elevated from the lateral posterior surface deep to the Achilles tendon. Soft tissue must also be mobilized from the medial aspect of the calcaneus. This is accomplished by plantar-flexing the foot, creating some redundancy and thus gaining access more easily. If there is difficulty in completely freeing the medial portion of the calcaneus and excessive hypertrophy of bone is noted, an ancillary medial longitudinal incision is indicated to facilitate appropriate dissection and avoid "blind" dissection. Care is taken to avoid interrupting the insertion of the Achilles tendon.

The posterolateral portion of the calcaneus is first removed generously and the clinical prominence of the area evaluated. Often this is sufficient. The posteromedial aspect of the calcaneus is removed with the second resection only if clinically prominent and a source of preoperative symptoms. The resection can be accomplished with an osteotome or power instrumentation (Fig. 26-20). Any remaining rough surfaces are remodeled as necessary. Posterior decompression dorsal closing wedge osteotomy can be performed with an inferior apex just below the Achilles

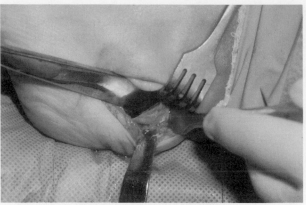

A

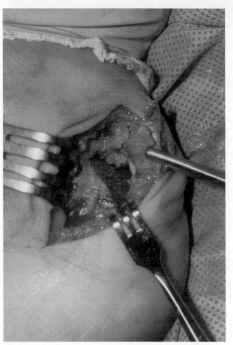

B

Figure 26-20 (**A**) Lateral exposure of entire posterior "wall" of heel in preparation for global resection. (**B**) Lateral resection of entire posterior wall for global Haglund's deformity. Heel cord fibers are left intact.

insertion, carried forward and upward and fixated with one 4.0-mm lag screw and washer. The posterolateral corner resection is still performed concurrently. This particular osteotomy is considered when the posterior prominence is very large (Fig. 26-21A, B, C). Postoperative failures occur when inadequate resection of the posterolateral prominence has been performed or insuffucient bone

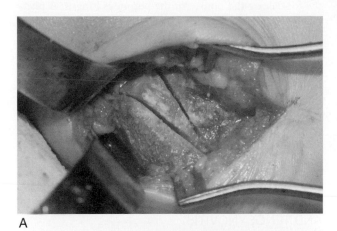

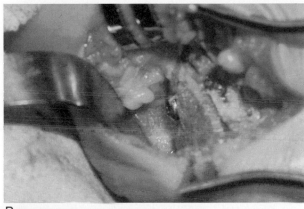

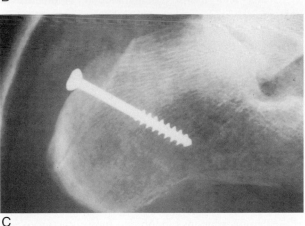

Figure 26-21 (**A**) Posterior tuber decompression wedge osteotomy from lateral approach. (**B**) Osteotomy completed, along with prominent posterior resection and site fixation with 4.0-mm lag screw. (**C**) The radiographic appearance.

wedge osteotomized. These two problems represent the most common surgical undersights. This is especially true with posterior or posteromedial hypertrophy of the calcaneus.

The wound is then flushed with copious amounts of a normal saline antibiotic solution. Attention is focused on the retrocalcaneal bursa, which may be excised if it appears clinically pathologic. Portions of the insertion of the Achilles tendon disrupted during resection are repaired at this time, occasionally with osteosuture and drill holes or anchors. The wound is then closed in two layers. A drain is optional and depends on good hemostasis achieved upon release of the tourniquet. On completion of the procedure, a fluffy compressive dressing is applied to the posterior aspect of the heel, and the leg is placed in a Jones compression cast. This is left in place for 5 to 7 days in order to control postoperative edema. The patient is non–weight bearing at this time.

Following removal of the Jones compression cast, the patient is placed into a well-padded weight-bearing posterior molded splint or cast brace, which is worn for approximately 3 weeks. If a significant portion of the insertion of the Achilles tendon was interrupted and repaired, casting is continued longer (up to 4 weeks). The splint or cast brace is removed on a regular basis to permit wound inspection and the application of physical therapy, such as gentle range of motion of the ankle, beginning on the 7th to 10th postoperative day. Following discontinuation of bracing, a sensible progressive return-to-activity program is instituted over the next 3 months. The athlete should be forewarned, however, that it may take anywhere from 3 to 12 months for a full recovery and resumption of previous athletic level.

MYOTENDINOUS JUNCTION AND PLANTARIS RUPTURE

Athletes who have strains or partial tears at the myotendinous junction of the medial or lateral head of the gastrocnemius, or both, usually present with pinpoint tenderness over the injured area high on the calf. The plantaris tendon can undergo an elastic overload and fail with an audible snapping sound that mimics a myotendinous gastrocnemius partial tear. The pain will always be along the medial edge of the gastrocnemius myotendinous junction or posterior calf region. Higher levels of pain intensity associated with a palpable rift or defect with diffuse swelling overlying the myotendinous junction usually imply a clinical diagnosis of partial tear. Myofascial pain and Achilles tendon pain syndromes are not common with generalized calf myalgia.

Differential diagnosis may require MRI in chronic troublesome cases.[77] Surgery is not indicated in these syndromes.

These injuries usually respond favorably to conservative treatment consisting of (1) local applications of ice, or both; heat, (2) compression; (3) bilateral ¼-inch heel lifts made of a viscoelastic polymer (e.g., Viscolas); (4) oral anti-inflammatory medications; and (5) local myofascial massage and gentle exercise.

Peroneal Tendon Compartment and Associated Pathology

The peroneal tendons and synovial components can manifest a variety of conditions that result in pain, swelling, inflammation, or instability at the lateral ankle and lower leg.[77,78] These problems in the athlete form a constellation of conditions that can interfere with performance. They are often the result of overuse, improper training, and injury in activities such as skiing, running, tennis, football, basketball, or any torsional sport activity that generates considerable tension in the peroneal tendon compartment and lateral ankle ligamentous complex.

The peroneal tendons are enclosed in a common synovial sheath under the superior peroneal retinaculum but develop separate sheaths more distally. The peroneus longus actually has a second synovial sheath between the cuboid sulcus and the base of the first metatarsal on the undersurface of the skeletal structure of the foot. A thin mesomembrane separates the two sheaths at the area of the peroneal sulcus. Anatomic communication between the two sheaths occurs about 33 percent of the time. The floor of the common sheath shares an intimate relationship with the lateral talocalcaneal and calcaneofibular ligaments. Traumatic disruption of these ligaments can cause extravasation into the common peroneal tendon sheaths or other synovial injury that can be demonstrated with contrast arthrography. Disruption of the peroneal retinacular structures can result in anterior dislocation or periodic subluxation of the peroneal tendons during certain phsyiologic exercises. Peroneal tendon attrition or longitudinal degenerative rents can occur, causing "idiopathic" pain. MRI and sonography can image many of these problems and assist in more accurate diagnosis and treatment.

Biomechanical imbalance, such as a plantar-flexed lateral column, may lead to chronic subluxing cuboid or peroneal cuboid syndrome or both. This condition is characterized by pain and tenderness at the lateral and plantar aspect of

the foot along the course of the peroneus longus. A plantar-flexed lateral column can adversely affect the ability of the peroneus longus to control stability of the first ray. Forced dorsiflexion–eversion injury to the foot can result in traumatic subluxing peroneal tendons. This condition is manifested as chronic peroneal tendinitis, pain, and clinical instability of the ankle. Subluxing peroneal tendinitis is more prevalent in accidents that occur in sports, such as skiing, basketball, or volleyball. An os peroneum accessory ossicle may lead to peroneal tendon pain secondary to enlargement, avulsion of a fibrocartilaginous union with the cuboid, or direct trauma.

PERONEAL TENDINITIS AND TENOSYNOVITIS

Postinversion peroneal tendinitis generally responds favorably to conservative treatment, which is essentially the same as conservative treatment of an ankle sprain. Patients will often relate a history of having had an inversion-type ankle sprain that was not severe enough to cause them to seek medical care at the time of injury. Clinically, there is pain and tenderness along the lateral aspect of the foot and ankle over the peroneal tendons. There may be diffuse mild synovial swelling in this area. This area contains the common sheath of the peroneal tendons, and thus testing of either the peroneus longus or peroneus brevis muscle function may produce discomfort. Either or both tendons may be involved in inversion peroneal tendinitis. NSAIDs, ice massage, and physical therapy, such as combined EGS and ultrasound, are employed over the tender, painful tendons. Physical therapy may be employed two to three times per week for about 3 to 4 weeks. Ice massage and gentle peroneal stretching as well as eccentric strengthening exercises are performed on a daily basis. If the patient is particularly symptomatic, immobilization may be accomplished with a weight-bearing cast brace or molded splint, maintaining the foot in a slightly everted position for a period of 3 to 4 weeks. The cast brace is removed on a routine basis for the application of physiotherapy and stretching and strengthening exercises.

If a subluxed cuboid or peroneal cuboid syndrome is present, cuboid manipulation is carried out.[79] The portion of the peroneus longus tendon that runs in the groove of the cuboid and travels toward the insertion at the base of the first metatarsal is surrounded by a separate tendon sheath and can manifest tenosynovitis independently of the more proximal sheath. If there is pain with palpation along the plantar aspect of the foot from the cuboid to the base of the first metatarsal, a peroneal cuboid syndrome is present. A temporary soft accommodative orthosis is fabricated that incorporates a $\frac{1}{4}$-inch heel lift, a felt cuboid pad, and a cutout under the first metatarsal head. This allows for a relative shortening of the distance between the origin and insertion of the peroneus longus, creating relative lengthening of the tendon. Multiple cuboid manipulations may be necessary. In resistant cases, a below-knee walking cast brace can be applied in a manner similar to that for tenosynovitis conditions for a period of 4 weeks following manipulation of the cuboid. Instability of the ankle joint should be ruled out by performing provocation inversion and anterior drawer tests of the ankle. Arthrography or peroneal tenography can be considered in these situations and are readily available modalities.

Imaging the lateral ankle region with sonography or MRI will provide intimate anatomic definition, allowing a high degree of accuracy for the diagnosis of chronic peroneal tenosynovitis, stenosis of the common compartment, or tendon attrition pain. Standard radiographs with axial calcaneal views can demonstrate an enlarged peroneal tubercle that can cause impingement pain and synovitis. Provocation testing with forced eversion–dorsiflexion will demonstrate peroneal tendon subluxation easily, which can be viewed and heard as, an audible click. CT imaging will allow clear definition of fibular groove anatomy to help design an appropriate surgical procedure for chronic subluxation. Acute peroneal tenosynovitis may progress to a chronic form with stenosing tenosynovitis refractory to conservative care and require operative decompression.

Surgery

When symptoms are not reversible by means of conservative measures as outlined, a simple tenolysis and sheath decompression is performed. This may be done under local anesthesia with the patient in a supine or lateral recumbent position. Hemostasis is not normally necessary because the tendon sheath is readily accessible subcutaneously, especially in thin patients. A small linear longitudinal incision approximately 2.5 cm in length is made overlying the common peroneal tendon sheath posterior to the fibular malleolus. Delicate dissection is used to identify the common peroneal sheath and to avoid damage to the lesser saphenous vein or sural nerve. Subcutaneous release of the common peroneal sheath can easily be accomplished with the use of blunt Metzenbaum scissors, removing any hypertrophic and discolored synovial tissue. The sheath is not reapproximated, and the peroneal retinacula are not violated. The wound is lavaged and then closed in two layers. A

compressive dressing is applied, and the patient is allowed to bear weight. Range-of-motion exercises are encouraged early to promote unrestricted gliding of the peroneal tendons. Physical therapy, such as combined EGS and ultrasound, may be instituted postoperatively. A gradual return-to-activity program begins approximately 3 weeks after surgery.

In the case of a chronically unstable cuboid or peroneal cuboid syndrome, or both, secondary to a plantar-flexed lateral column that has not responded to conservative treatment, various procedures have been recommended in the literature, ranging from calcaneocuboid arthrodesis to calcaneal osteotomy or regrooving of the peroneal cuboid groove. Peroneal cuboid syndrome is difficult to treat. Dorsal wedge arthroplasty of the cuboid and fourth–fifth metatarsal base articulation can produce good results in patients who have disabling chronic painful peroneal cuboid syndrome. This surgical concept allows adaptation to the lateral column of principles routinely applied to the medial column. Arthrofibrosis develops in this interval similar to that seen in a painless pseudoarthrosis. Alternatively, a dorsal cuboid wedge osteotomy can be considered, especially in the absence of fourth–fifth metatarsal base cuboid joint symptomatology. These procedures are not well documented.

Postoperative weight bearing allows the lateral column to dorsiflex to a level more consistent with that of the medial column, thereby eliminating a plantar-flexed lateral column or lateral cavus deformity. This dorsiflexion occurs at the lateral tarsal-metatarsal articulation and allows for a decrease in the calcaneal pitch angle and more even weight distribution across the medial and lateral column's of the forefoot.

SUBLUXING PERONEAL TENDONS

Aggressive tension developed in the peroneal tendons during maximal dorsiflexion–eversion force on the foot may result in an acute subluxation of the peroneal tendons with rupture of the superior retinaculum. This may be quite painful and swollen upon initial presentation. Active dorsiflexion and eversion of the foot against manual resistance of the examiner will usually reproduce a subluxation of the peroneal tendons as they are seen to snap anteriorly across the lateral surface of the fibular malleolus.[80] As the contraction is relaxed, the peroneal tendons are seen to return to their normal position. Chronic luxation is often accompanied by an audible popping as the tendons dislocate and relocate themselves in performance. A feeling of ankle instability is often reported with this condition. Diagnosis usually does not require sophisticated imaging techniques and is an easy clinical determination.

The retrofibular positioning of the peroneal tendons is crucial to their function. The peroneus brevis restrains external tibial-fibular rotation with subtalar joint supination during late midstance and after heel-off. Once the peroneus brevis moves or dislocates anterior to the fibular malleolus, this important function is lost. Similarly, the ability of the peroneus longus to stabilize the first ray is compromised when anterior subluxation exists.

The superior peroneal retinaculum is responsible for maintaining the retrofibular position of the peroneal tendons. This thickening of the deep fascia of the ankle extends from the fibular malleolus to the lateral surface of the os calcis, forming a fibro-osseous tunnel retaining the common peroneal tendon sheath. The biomechanics of acute lateral ankle injury causing rapid peroneal muscular contraction against a rapidly and forcefully dorsiflexing foot can rupture the superior retinaculum, contributing to dislocation. Insufficient treatment at the time of the acute injury and traumatic subluxation can result in chronic subluxation. Generalized ligamentous laxity can also predispose to acute or chronic peroneal tendon subluxation. Acute peroneal tendon subluxation may present with a small periosteal lift or "fleck fracture" of the lateral fibular malleolar attachment of the peroneal retinaculum.

Conservative treatment may be attempted in acute injuries. A right-angle cast brace is used incorporating a felt buttress over the injured peroneal tendons inferior and posterior to the lateral malleolus. This provides further restraint against recurrent subluxation in the cast brace. Bracing is discontinued in 4 weeks. If painful or disabling subluxation persists following cast removal, surgical peroneal retinaculoplasty is recommended. Chronic subluxation usually requires surgical repair. Repair of the superior peroneal retinaculum may be combined with other procedures, such as primary repair of acute lateral ligament ruptures of the ankle, or with delayed primary repair or secondary stabilization in the case of chronic lateral ankle instability.

Subluxing Peroneal Tenoplasty and Retinaculoplasty

Peroneal retinaculoplasty is performed under general or local anesthesia with intravenous sedation. A curvilinear incision is made approximately 1 cm inferior to the peroneal tendons as they turn behind and beneath the fibular malleolus. Care is taken to avoid damage to the sural nerve or lesser saphenous vein during deepening of the incision. Using careful blunt dissection, a full-thickness cutaneous/subcutaneous flap is reflected, exposing the obliquely oriented fibers of the deep fascia. The superior peroneal retinaculum normally presents as a well-defined thickening of the deep fascial layer, extending from the fibular malleolus to the posterolateral superior portion of the os calcis.

In cases of acute subluxation of the peroneal tendons, direct repair of the superior peroneal retinaculum may be accomplished using 2-0 absorbable sutures. If a small avulsion fracture is identified on the fibular malleolus, it may be excised or repaired depending on its size. Chronic peroneal tendon subluxation in which there is insufficient superior retinaculum remaining requires retinaculoplasty.[81] This may be performed by raising a rectangular periosteal flap from the lateral surface of the fibular malleolus, transposing it over the tendons and sheath posterior to the back margin of the fibula, and attaching the repair with drill holes in the fibula.

The Ellis Jones Achilles tenoretinaculoplasty is an excellent procedure that utilizes a small 2-inch medial strip of the Achilles tendon passed anteriorly over the peroneal tendons and attached to the lateral fibular corner with drill holes.[82]

Transfer of the calcaneal fibular ligament has become popular and is easy to perform. There are many modifications of this operation, but it is most conveniently performed by moving the fibular attachment of the ligament over the peroneal tendons and attaching it to the fibular apex with a screw and spiked washer.[83–85]

Likewise, there are several bone operations available for consideration. They fall into two categories: (1) fibular suclus operations, which deepen the groove by burring or decompression and collapse of the deep surface, maintaining the retrofibular gliding mechanism[86]; and (2) posterior sliding fibular segment osteotomies, creating a checkrein against overriding tendons.[87,88] These procedures all require screw fixation of the sliding fibular segment.

Rehabilitation is dependent on whether the procedure was osteotomy or soft tissue repair, but both concepts will require immobilization for a period of at least 4 to 7 weeks. Cast braces are encouraged to allow early physiotherapy at 7 to 9 days postoperatively.

Os Peroneum

Painful os peroneum diagnosed in combination with chronic peroneal tendinitis requires excision of the ossicle. This procedure may be performed by itself or in conjunction with other surgical procedures on the peroneal tendons. A linear longitudinal incision approximately 3 cm long is made over the peroneus longus at the level of the lateral aspect of the cuboid. The incision is then deepened, avoiding neurovascular structures. Blunt dissection is then used to identify the peroneal tendon sheath, which is incised, allowing for identification of the peroneus longus tendon. The os peroneum is usually found lateral or deep to the peroneus longus, participating in a syndesmosis or synchondrosis at the cuboid.[89] It is excised, with care taken to avoid interruption of any of the fibers of the peroneus longus. The wound is then flushed, closed in layers, and dressed. The patient is then allowed to ambulate in a surgical shoe. Range-of-motion exercises are encouraged. Physical therapy may be needed during the postoperative recuperative period to control edema, and a gradual return-to-activity program is begun approximately 3 weeks postoperatively or as indicated by any concurrent procedures performed.

Peroneal Tendon Attrition

Longitudinal fissuring of the peroneus brevis was first described in 1924 by Meyers.[90] Subsequently, Sobel and associates have done considerable work defining this condition and its role in chronic lateral ankle pain.[91,92] Peroneal tendon attrition can also involve the peroneus longus, with pain and also an ankle instability syndrome with tenosynovitis.[93–95] It is best diagnosed with MRI or contrast tenography. The midportion of the peroneus brevis longitudinal tear is usually located over the apex of the fibular malleolus, progressing distally. Fraying of the tendon also can occur as part of tendon attrition syndrome. It is believed the tear occurs from chronic pressure and trapping of the peroneus brevis tendon between the tensed peroneus longus externally and the calcaneofibular ligament deeper. Considerable tenosynovitis is usually associated with this condition.

Once the longitudinal defect establishes itself, it will not self-repair because tension from the peroneus longus against the brevis and the fibular apex forces the peroneus longus to ride into the longitudinal rent. Repair is with excision of the degenerative rent and tubing of the remaining tendon. Grafting may be necessary if the degeneration is extensive; a graft can be taken from the plantaris or even a more proximal hemisection of the peroneus longus. Synovectomy of the involved sheath is accomplished with the tenoplasty, with careful attention directed to the repair of the retinaculum. Peroneus longus attrition is less common and occurs most commonly at the apex of the fibular malleolus, but can occur proximally on occasion.[93]

Posterior Tibial Tendinopathy and Associated Conditions

The posterior tibial tendon is commonly subject to repetitive overuse injury resulting in chronic posterior tibial tendinosis. This form of progressive degeneration, which can develop under mechanical conditions such as hyperpronation syndrome, has come to be known as posterior tibial tendon dysfunction (PTTD). It is often an ongoing condition that runs a spectrum from early swelling and pain to ultimate rupture. Like Achilles tendinosis, changes in athlete training habits, and in particular improper training, result in an overuse syndrome with progressive degeneration. The incidence of of posterior tibial tendinopathy has increased with such sports as aerobics and tennis and with the participation of senior citizens in fitness programs.

The posterior tibial tendon is encased in its own tendon sheath, passing posterior to the medial malleolus and then through the tarsal tunnel before dividing into various slips with multiple insertions. The most important insertion is that of the navicular tuberosity. The tendon sheath can become inflamed, producing pain, swelling, and tenosynovitis of the posterior tibial tendon along its course. The development of this condition often coincides with strenuous athletic activity, but it can occur in all major age groups. Rheumatoid patients on steroid supplementation are known to have a propensity for this condition, along with patients with all seronegative arthropathies. The condition frequently responds to conservative treatment and oral anti-inflammatory agents if diagnosed and treated in its early stage of development. The presence of an os tibiale externum or accessory navicular may predispose to complaints of posterior tibial tendinitis, especially following eversion-type injuries. Pain is obvious near the tuberosity insertion, and there is usually swelling. Radiographs can usually define the condition well. CT, MRI, sonography, and contrast tenography may be necessary for more defined imaging at the insertion and, in particular, more proximal along its course behind the medial malleolus (Fig. 26-22). These studies will allow the determination of the dysfunctional area of the tendon or the character of the junction of an accessory navicular.

The cause of PTTD is not known but is believed to be multifactoral, with an overuse syndrome that ultimately results in progressive degeneration and attenuation with

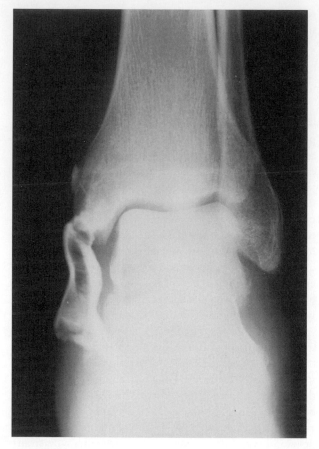

Figure 26-22 Contrast tenogram demonstrating late-stage posterior tibial tendon dsyfunction and chronic rupture.

partial or total rupture when the load reaches threshold. Suspicion remains that the zone of hypovascularity between the malleolus and the navicular tuberosity is one of the major contributing factors in the development of PTTD.[96] This is also the most frequent site of the degeneration. An underlying biomechanical fault is often detected, such as a hypermobile first ray, unstable medial longitudinal arch, and/or functional calcaneal valgus. This is often associated with a flexible forefoot valgus deformity. The intrinsic tortuous course of the tendon predisposes it to significant friction around the malleolar pulley, not unlike the peroneus brevis, which also can develop attrition and attenuation for similar reasons laterally. Unilateral complaints may be secondary to a limb length discrepancy with asymmetric pronation, producing compensation as a result of sports-specific demands. An example would be the excessive pronatory force on the back leg during the follow-through portion of a golf swing. Another example would be the inside leg of a track runner who always runs in one direction—counterclockwise, for example, on an unbanked track.

Whenever there has been injury to the posterior tibial tendon, the stage for PTTD is set. The clinician should also be cognizant of the development of unilateral "spontaneous flatfoot" unrelated to injury, with pain and swelling along the medial arch (Fig. 26-23). This is more prevalent in senior citizens involved in golf, exercise walking, aerobics, or bowling as activities. Loss of advantage of the posterior tibial tendon, or even mild disruption or stretching, allows for considerable valgus collapse of the medial architecture and arch.[97] The posterior tibial muscle is the most powerful stabilizer of the arch. Dysfunction and attenuation result in dramatic loss of stability, with a vicious cycle of events that becomes progressive. Active inversion and plantar flexion of the foot against resistance by the examiner usually reproduces the patient's pain, as would passive eversion and abduction of the forefoot. Clinical abduction of the midfoot develops, with the so-called too-many-toes sign when the deformity is viewed from behind. PTTD will not allow ipsilateral single-leg heel rise hindfoot inversion response when the patient is asked to rise up on the toes. This entity has become well recognized, and an astute clinician will be able to diagnose PTTD with a thorough examination and radiographs. In more subtle cases, sonography or MRI may be necessary in the early stages before deformity develops.

Various classification schemes have been published, and they all share common features of staging. The condition is characterized in three and sometimes four stages. All

Figure 26-23 Stage 4 late PTTD with unilateral equinovalgus.

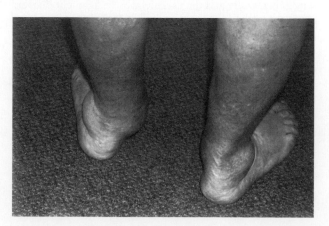

stages manifest one or more symptoms, with swelling, pain, progressive tendon degeneration with attenuation, and ultimately total rupture with progressive equinovalgus deformity.[98-101]

Conservative treatment can be beneficial in the early stage of development, but it is uncertain if this will arrest the process. Biomechanical orthotic control (to prevent chronic hyperpronation), rest, ice, and oral anti-inflammatory agents can be of value. Physical therapy modalities may be used to supplement treatment, especially when crepitation within the tendon sheath is palpable. Intrasheath steroid injections will produce immediate improvement in the symptoms. However necrosis with degenerative rupture can develop with steroid injections, so they should be avoided.[100] The athlete is kept off strenuous activity until the inflammatory phase subsides. Conservative treatment and orthotic bracing are provided in the interim. Below-knee cast bracing is helpful and may be employed for 3 to 4 weeks or longer as necessary in resistant cases.

Surgical intervention is considered when the condition is not responsive to conservative care as noted earlier. If pain and persistent swelling are present and nonresponsive to conservative care, debridement is indicated along with tendon repair of defect-specific conditions as encountered, particularly in stage 1. The posterior tibial tendon can have fiber attenuation and renting similar to the Achilles and peroneals. The obvious areas are debrided and the tendon repaired or tubed. Z-plasty shortening is recommended, along with tenosynovectomy as indicated (Fig 26-24A& B). Depending on the magnitude of encountered degeneration and the stage of the PTTD, other augmentations may be necessary, such as flexor digitorum longus transfer with side-to-side anastomosis and transfer into the navicular along with partial translocation of the tibialis anterior into the navicular (Fig 26-25). This has been noted to improve the pain of the condition, but it fails to resolve any existing valgus deformity.

Once structural deformity has set in (stages 2 through 4), bone operations will always be required if the surgeon's objective is architectural reconstruction. Procedures selected depend on objectives, which vary from patient to patient depending on age, activity level, and stage of PTTD. Calcaneal osteotomy is emerging as an ideal choice for early-stage flexible deformity. The osteotomy may be thalamic/body or cervical for lateral column elongation, or both. Open lateral wedge osteotomy with humeral head allograft is an excellent, easy solution for either lateral column lengthening or varus-producing thalmic body osteot-

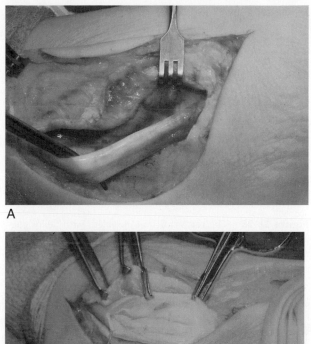

A

B

Figure 26-24 (**A**) Intraoperative findings of stage 3 PTTD, with attenuation and longitudinal rent with synovitis. This patient required lateral column lengthening and medial arch augmentation. (**B**) Attenuation, renting, and central rupture in stage 3 PTTD in preparation for flexor digitorum augmentation.

omy.[102] Medialization osteotomy is a good option and has the advantage of not requiring a bone graft/implant, but the procedure requires internal fixation. Adjunctive procedures should be done in conjunction,such as Young navicular suspensions (tibialis anterior translocation into a keyhole slot of the navicular), open wedge dorsal cuneiform osteotomy, flexor digitorum longus augmentation to the navicular, and into-talus transfer of the peroneus brevis tendon. For more severe deformity, talonavicular arthrodesis has emerged as the procedure of choice. Lateral column lengthening with interposition bone graft arthrodesis at the calcaneocuboid joint can be considered as well, with medial column augmentation procedures previously mentioned. For rigid established deformity, triple arthrodesis

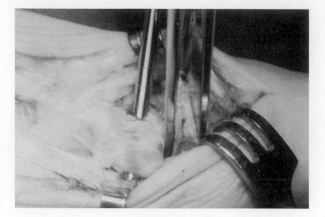

Figure 26-25 The reconstruction complete with flexor augmentation, tubing repair of the posterior tibial tendon, and split translocation of the tibialis anterior into the navicular and midfoot plantar wedge resectional arthrodesis.

remains the ultimate salvage.[103] It is certain that the athlete who develops progressive PTTD will likely have a shortened career in competitive athletics, unless early interventional surgery is undertaken and the process arrested with proper biomechanical and surgical control.

Os Tibiale Externum and Navicular Fractures

Pain in the region of the navicular tuberosity is a common finding in atheletic and active individuals. The tuberosity region is the most common site of traction avulsion fractures, which develop from aggressive torque generated by the major portion of the posterior tibial insertion and forced eversion of the foot. Three types of accessory navicular states have been described: (1) a sesamoid in the distal insertional region of the tendon, (2) a syndesmosis or synchondrosis, and (3) a "cornuate" navicular following fusion of the accessory bone.[104] The tibionavicular slip of the deltoid ligament also participates in this traction mechanism. The fragment is usually small (less than 5 mm) but can be large enough to require osteosynthesis. The larger the fragment, the more likely there is significant disruption of the tibialis posterior insertion and thus the need for surgical repair.

Accessory navicular (os tibiale externum) is probably the most common accessory bone of the foot. It can be disrupted with minor trauma, causing considerable pain that can be chronic, located in the arch. However, trauma is not necessary for this accessory ossicle to become painful. Hyperpronation and athletic overuse can transform this accessory bone into a painful problem.[105] Dorsal chip fractures at the talar interface represent nearly 50 percent of all fractures of the navicular and occur from forceful inversion, plantar flexion, and traction transmitted by the dorsal talonavicular ligament. Diagnosis is easily accomplished with medial oblique and standard view radiographs. Finally, stress fracture of the navicular occurs uncommonly and can be an occult form of "idiopathic" midfoot and arch pain in active and athletic patients. It is difficult to diagnose and requires a high index of suspicion in a competitive athlete to differentiate it from other overuse syndromes causing strain to the midfoot region. CT, bone scans, and MRI are the best modalities to make the diagnosis, because standard radiographs usually fail to reveal this fracture.

Nonsurgical treatment can be undertaken for all of the above injuries or conditions. The extent and duration of treatment is determined by the patient's objectives, age, activity, and performance level. Essentially, rest, physical therapy, immobilization, anti-inflammatory agents, and orthotics are the options. Small tuberosity avulsion fractures can often be managed in this manner. Larger fragments ultimately require repair with either excision of the fragment and tendon repair into the main body of the navicular or actual osteosynthesis of the large fragment. Accessory navicular can also be repaired by debriding the fibrous interface and using internal fixation, if the ossicle is large enough. Otherwise, a standard Kidner operation is performed with excision of the ossicle and tendon advancement. The objective ultimately focuses on restoration of the torque capacity of the tibialis posterior tendon with solid union of the tendon–bone interface. This is what ultimately eliminates the pain in the arch for these patients.

Dorsal chip traction fractures usually can be managed nonsurgically, but, if they remain painful, simple excision should be undertaken. The various medial arch-splitting incisions all work well for these procedures. Tendon repair at the navicular tuberosity interface is best accomplished with any of the currently available bone anchor systems or spiked A-O 8.0-mm washer and 4.0-mm screw. Stress fractures may require transverse percutaneous lag screw fixation introduced under image control. Appropriate immobilization is accomplished postoperatively, with early rehabilitation using a cast brace. The outcome of these injuries and problems can be very successful even for competitive athletes if early intervention is provided, which will reduce total down time.

MODIFIED KIDNER PROCEDURE

The modified Kidner is classically performed for a painful or partially avulsed os tibiale externum (os navicularis). The procedure may be performed under local anesthesia with or without intravenous sedation, using an ankle tourniquet for hemostasis, or under general anesthesia with a thigh tourniquet. With the patient in the supine position, an arch-splitting incision 4 to 5 cm in length is placed over the accessory navicular and talonavicular joint. The deep fascia is incised longitudinally between the anterior and posterior tibial tendons. The deep fascia is then reflected from the medial surface of the accessory bone, preserving the attachment of posterior tibial tendon to the remainder of the navicular.

In some cases, the accessory ossicle can be immediately appreciated. Simple "sliver" medial resection will uncover the junction of the accessory bone and the main body of the navicular, making clear the boundary and extent of the ossicle. It is carefully shelled out of its cradle in the tendinous and fibrous attachments of the posterior tibial tendon with sharp dissection, removing its fibrous attachments to the main body of the navicular. The foot should be supinated during resection of the ossicle, displacing the talar head laterally and protecting it from the osteotome. The posterior tibial tendon is then imbedded into the raw bone defect at the interface of the main navicular body with advancement and implantation with bone anchors, osteosuture, or spiked washer and screw (Fig. 26-26A & B). This advancement reinforces the posterior tibial tendon and shortens it under physiologic tension. The Kidner procedure as originally described often results in progressive flatfoot because of insufficient repair and tension in the posterior tibial tendon. Bone anchors and spiked washer–screw repair is much more solid, allowing appropriate physiologic tension at the repair site. The surgeon should understand that the Kidner operation will not suffice as a flatfoot operation. It should be used only for repair of a symptomatic os tibiale externum. This repair can be augmented with a slip from the tibialis anterior tendon if desired, but this is not normally necessary if the tibialis posterior repair site is solid.[106]

Postoperative care is the usual cast bracing or even below-knee casting for about 4 weeks with the foot and ankle in neutral position. Physiotherapy is initiated beginning with gentle range of motion within the limits of soft

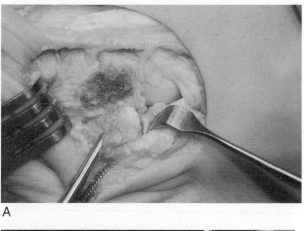

A

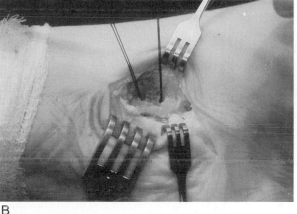

B

Figure 26-26 (**A**) Resection of the os tibiale externum and medial navicular tuberosity. (**B**) "Osteosuture" drill holes for advancement/plication of tibialis posterior insertion distally.

tissue tension to prevent stiffening of the ankle joint following 3 to 4 weeks of casting. Full recovery usually takes approximately 3 months following surgery but may take up to 6 months. Appropriate biomechanical foot orthoses should be used when indicated.

TOTAL TENDON RUPTURES

Acute tendon failure represents abrupt discontinuity of the tendon structure from tensile overload. In the nonathletic population, many tendon ruptures can be adequately treated by casting or cast bracing. The demands and objectives of the athlete are different, however, and tendon rupture in an athlete requires immediate operative repair. The two most frequently encountered tendon ruptures are of the Achilles and posterior tibial. In uncertain cases, MRI or sonography can be used to confirm the diagnosis with a high degree of accuracy. Clinical diagnosis is usually easy and accurate as well. Acute ruptures of the plantaris, tibialis anterior, peroneus longus, and flexor hallucis longus are all uncommon and also manifest obvious motor power defects associated with the loss of the specific muscle.

Acute Achilles Tendon Rupture

Total disruption of the Achilles tendon can occur from a variety of mechanisms, such as laceration or spontaneous rupture secondary to tendinosis degeneration and blunt trauma. In the athletic setting the ruptures encountered are all subcutaneous, probably from aging-related spontaneous degeneration, which is well known to occur after age 40. The integrity of the skin and subcutaneous covering of the tendon is not disrupted in these cases. The main mechanism of injury appears to be either a forceful eccentric contraction of the Achilles tendon or blunt trauma during this state in an athletic performance of some other aggressive physical activity. The athlete will recognize the problem immediately; often there is an audible "pop" and weakness sometimes causing a fall or other injury concurrently.

The patient will present with inability to plantar-flex the foot adequately at the ankle joint. Off weight bearing, some plantar flexion may be evident if the deep posterior tibial musculature is not involved. Both long flexors, the posterior tibial muscle and the peroneals, will produce some degree of active plantar flexion. The patient will not be able to perform a toe rise on the injured side, and there is usually a visible and palpable defect about 2.5 cm proximal to the insertion. Thompson's test[107–110] is classic for clinical diagnosis of the condition and involves squeezing the calf with no observable plantar flexion of the ankle. MRI or sonography can be used if the diagnosis is uncertain or the rupture subtotal with residual retained function.[77] Radiographs are necessary to rule out avulsion beak fracture.

Beak avulsion fractures are repaired by open reduction and internal screw fixation. Total rupture without avulsion fracture is repaired by percutaneous or open techniques depending on surgeon preference and other patient parameters, such as age, skin quality, anticipated level of performance, and general health considerations. Careful history and physical examination will help determine if prior tendinosis was present and thus direct the surgeon toward either open or closed treatment techniques. Open conventional repair with local augmentation is recommended, particularly if there is a history of tendinosis and the athlete is competitive. Percutaneous "open repair" can also be performed easily and carries a very low surgical risk. It may be a primary consideration while reserving conventional open repairs and plastics for those patients with re-rupture or chronic tendinosis with degeneration. Nonsurgical repairs with casting or bracing can produce a very satisfactory result in low-activity-level patients or even noncompetitive older athletes but requires about 10 weeks of casting, starting in gravity equinus and gradually moving to neutral. The literature has been very encouraging in this regard, with several studies questioning the validity of open repair after cost and surgical risk are considered. The incidence of re-rupture following closed treatment is clearly higher (about 17 percent compared to 2 percent for surgery), but the question continues to beg, does this justify the cost and risks of surgery? Individual consideration factors continue to guide surgeon preference of treatment in this condition.

PERCUTANEOUS REPAIR

The percutaneous repair may be carried out from the initial time of injury up to 7 to 10 days postrupture (Fig. 26-27A–E). Following this period, results are less than optimal because of retraction, organization of the clot, and atrophy. Percutaneous repair is performed in the prone position.[107] Anesthesia is usually local, with infiltration over the posterior aspect of the Achilles tendon and the calf. Tourniquet control is not necessary. The disrupted ends and defect in the Achilles tendon are identified by palpation. Several parapercutaneous skin incisions (about 1 cm long) are prepared medially and laterally at the borders of the Achilles tendon, 2 to 3 cm proximal and distal to the defect, as well as a third pair of percutaneous incisions at the level of the defect. Subcutaneous tissues are bluntly dissected down to the level of the tendon. At the level of the defect, blunt dissection is carried down to the tendon defect to permit evacuation of the hematoma. Beginning at the medial proximal incision, a 2-0 Tev-dek suture on a Keith needle is passed through the central portion of the Achilles tendon from medial to lateral, exiting the lateral distal aspect of the tendon at the proximal portion of the rupture. It is then retracted through the central lateral incision. The identical manuever is carried out with a suture beginning at the lateral proximal incision, angling 45 degrees and exiting at the proximal aspect of the rupture at

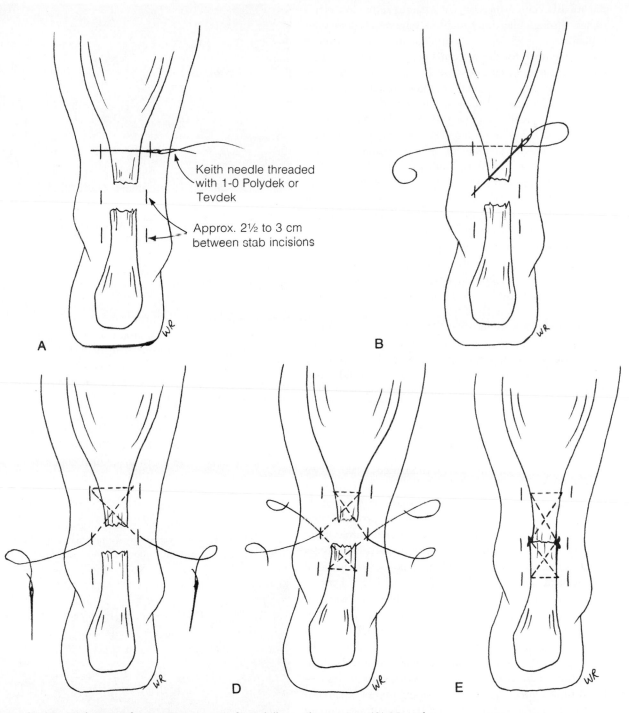

Figure 26-27 Technique of percutaneous repair for Achilles tendon rupture. (**A**) Note the six small stab incisions parallel to the tendon on the medial and lateral sides. (**B,C**) Stitching technique. (**D**) Both suture strands are in place. (**E**) Finished repair. Stab incisions can be closed with a single interrupted suture or sterile strips. (*Figure continues.*)

the medial central incision. A separate suture needle is passed through the distal incision transversely and then angled again at 45 degrees, exiting at the tendon rupture site as described for the proximal portion. The sutures at the medial and lateral aspect of the central incision over the defect are then tightened down and buried. The percutaneous incisions are then closed as desired.

The patient is placed into a well-padded fiberglass posterior molded splint or cast brace with the ankle plantar flexed moderately but not in full-gravity equinus. Rehabilitation is initiated 7 to 10 days following skin healing. The patient is then placed on regular physical therapy and allowed to dorsiflex and plantar flex the foot gently within the tolerance of the repair. Adjunctive physical therapy with EGS, ultrasound, or both can be carried out. Gentle range of motion enhances healing, whereas excessive range of motion may interrupt the new capillaries and disrupt healing. Early rehabilitation lessens the degree of ankle stiffness postoperatively and aids in alignment of the collagen fibers that bridge the defect.

Three weeks postoperatively, the patient is placed in a 90-degree cast brace hinged for continued range-of-motion exercises. Weight bearing is allowed in the cast brace early, at 3 weeks or sooner, if the repair site is solid. Total bracing protection is variable but usually lasts about 8 weeks for percutaneous repair.

OPEN REPAIR AND PLASTICS

Open repair is performed with the patient in the prone position. Under general anesthesia with thigh tourniquet hemostasis, a posterolateral incision is made near the Achilles tendon extending 2 cm centimeters proximal and distal to the defect. The incision is deepened through the subcutaneous tissue to the level of the rupture. Hematoma is evacuated, the tissue is debrided, and the defect identified and evaluated (Fig. 26-27F). Longitudinal internal tenotomy incisions are made in the torn ends of the tendon if there is any evidence of tendinosis. These pathologic sites are further debrided if encountered, preserving the tendon fibers. The tendon is then repaired using heavy nonabsorbable suture in criss-cross fashion similar to that of Bunnel. Longitudinal internal tenotomy incisions used for inspection of the central aspect of the tendon are not repaired if they are required. This allows for migration of surrounding tissue progenitors into the internal portion of the tendon to develop metaplasia.

If the defect site is necrotic with considerable fraying, debridement is performed along with local tissue augmen-

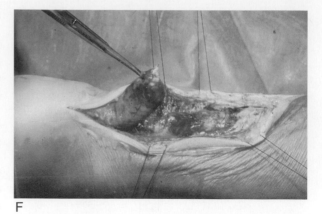

F

Figure 26-27 (*Continued*) (**F**) Acute rupture of Achilles tendon at the "watershed."

tation.[108-110] The skin approach will be considerably longer in order to gain access to local tissue for augmentation. This is also true in chronic untreated ruptures where the tendon cannot be reapproximated at surgery. There are a number of plantaris and gastrocnemius aponeurotic plastics available for consideration under these circumstances[111-114] (Fig. 26-28). In late neglected rupture, tendon transfer augmentation with either the flexor digitorum or hallucis longus, or the peroneus brevis, will be required.[81,115] Alloplastic grafts have been used as well, with good results in some studies, but there is not enough long-term study of these grafts to make firm conclusions.

Postoperative rehabilitation remains aggressive, with

Figure 26-28 Debridement of distal degeneration with gastrocnemius aponeurotic recession advancement and direct bone implantation using spiked washers and A-O screws.

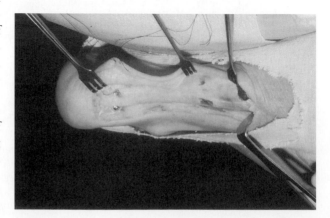

cast bracing and early gentle range-of-motion exercises at 7 to 10 days.[116] This regimen is increased gradually in intensity and magnitude, with full weight bearing in a brace almost immediately after surgery as tolerated if the repair site is deemed solid. A progressive return-to-activity program is initiated as soon as feasible. The athlete is forewarned that the prognosis is less favorable should tendinosis be found but is certainly more favorable than if surgery had not been undertaken. It may take anywhere from 6 to 24 months to gain complete use of the Achilles tendon with return to previous level of activity, and heel lifts may be necessary postoperatively.[117]

Acute Total Posterior Tibial Tendon Rupture

The biomechanics of acute rupture of the posterior tibial tendon are generated from tensile overload resulting from forced eversion or abduction. Like other acute ruptures, eccentric overload is often a factor. Pre-existing chronic degenerative tendinosis is usually an antecedent factor as well. Interestingly, the rupture is often not acutely painful and the patient recollects an audible "pop" at the time of the incident. There is obvious swelling, and pain is present between the malleolar sulcus and the navicular insertion, with a bulge at the pathologic site. Ultrasound diagnosis is a quick, inexpensive method of verification and has good accuracy.[118] A classification system has good devised that categorizes posterior tibial tendon ruptures based on location.[97,119] Type I occurs at the insertion of the navicular tuberosity, type II occurs between the level of the navicular tuberosity and the medial malleolus, type III occurs around the level of the medial malleolus, and type IV occurs proximal to the medial malleolus. The patient is unable to achieve active plantar flexion with inversion even in the absence of applied resistance. Passive eversion of the foot may or may not be painful depending on the age of the rupture.

Acute rupture is an indication for surgery in most patients and always in athletes if they wish to continue performance. The rupture is often associated with tendinosis and degeneration, and some form of local tissue augmentation is required to complete the reconstruction. Flexor digitorum longus augmentation is the most common because the graft is locally available in the surgical site, although one can use plantaris grafts and hemisections of peroneus longus as well. Neglected rupture of the posterior tibial tendon will demonstrate obvious arch collapse and equino-

valgus if the rupture has persisted for some time. This is a much more complex problem that requires bone surgery for definitive stabilization. Talonavicular arthrodesis is dependable if the deformity has minimal or no arthrosis in the remaining tarsal complex; however, it will end the career of the athlete. If end-stage equinovalgus has intervened, only triple arthrodesis can salvage the situation. A variety of calcaneal osteotomies can be used for reinforcement of tendon augmentation and local reconstruction of the posterior tibial tendon, if adequate tissue quality remains. Arthrodesis concepts in late management of this condition have now become established. Lateral column distraction lengthening arthrodesis with interposition grafting has been described as an alternative to triple arthrodesis and can be used in conjunction with medial column soft tissue reconstructions if the remaining tarsus is free of arthrosis.

Postoperative rehabilitation is specific depending on whether soft tissue or bone surgery was performed. It follows the standards in each category, allowing proper time for tendon and ligament healing, which usually requires about 4 weeks and 8 to 12 weeks for osteotomy and arthrodesis in the tarsal complex, respectively. Physical therapy specific to each type of surgery is also applied for the necessary periods until swelling and activity levels can be resumed. These are all major surgical interventions, and athletic careers are usually ended or altered irreparably.

Flexor Hallucis Longus Rupture Tendinopathy (Dancer's Tendonitis)

Rupture of the flexor hallucis longus tendon is rare, with a paucity of reported cases.[120] The two most common sites of athletic rupture are posterior to the ankle and at the base of the proximal phalanx. Recently three cases of longitudinal tear have been reported under the master knot of Henry.[121] Dancers commonly report tendinopathy around the region of the ankle, especially behind the ankle, resembling Achilles tendinitis or a painful accessory bone at the os trigonum region. "En pointe" classical ballet places incredible demand on this tendon to accomplish the maneuver.[122] Repetitive loading in this manner is believed to give rise to tendinosis nodules that restrain excursion through this tight tunnel, resulting in a trigger hallux and pain at the site of tunnel entry.[123] A fusiform thickening characteristic of other tendinopathies can be found the region behind the ankle joint as the tendon passes through the tight fibro-osseous tunnel behind the talus along the medial wall of the os calis to the sustentaculum tali.[124] Surgical decompression is about the only treatment that will allow these patients to return to their activity—and even then only guardedly. At times the muscle fibers can extend into the fibro-osseous canal, contributing to teno-synovitis with pain and swelling.[125] Decompression con-sists of laciniate ligament release in conjunction with re-lease of the fibro-osseous tunnel and repair of tendinosis nodules encountered in the tendon. Small ossicles can be found occasionally in this area and need to be carefully excised. Professional dancers need to be warned that oper-ation could end their career; however, the procedure does produce relief of the pain.

Tibialis Anterior Rupture

Aggressive eccentric muscle activity can result in acute failure of the tibialis anterior tendon. The rupture is often associated with the aging process or chronic tendinosis. The failure site is usually just proximal to the anatomic inser-tion and often retracts proximally to the level of the ankle or even lower leg, making retrieval and repair difficult, par-ticularly if left untreated for a few weeks. Drop foot is ob-vious, with tenderness over the front of the ankle and a nota-ble bulge. Pull-out wire reinforcement of the repair site and interposition tendon grafting from the peroneus longus may be required for proper restoration of continuity, especially if considerable tendinosis degeneration is present at the rup-ture interval and if retraction has occurred (Fig. 26-29A & B). Care must be taken to also repair the cruciate ligaments and synovial sheath as delicately as possible, and begin gentle rehabilitation within 2 weeks following the repair to pre-vent binding down and loss of function.

Peroneal Tendon Ruptures

Rupture of the peroneals is less common than rupture of the other extrinsic tendons of the foot. Nonetheless, aggressive athletic activity can result in a tension failure of either of these power tendons. The peroneus longus is the most difficult to repair because the rupture often occurs at the cuboid sulcus, and repair at this interval is not easy because of poor access to the distal stump. Rupture results in pain at the area along with inability to evert and plantar flex the foot and first ray segment. Peroneus brevis rupture will result in weakness of hindfoot eversion, and the rup-ture site usually presents between the fibular malleolus and the fifth metatarsal styloid process. Repair is much easier

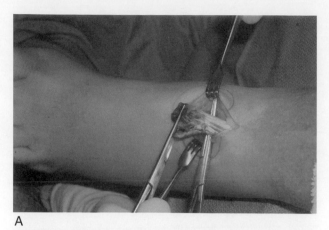

A

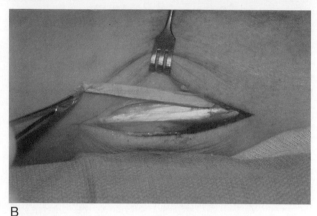

B

Figure 26-29 (**A**) Acute rupture of tibialis anterior with proxi-mal retraction into the lower leg. (**B**) Peroneus longus hemisec-tion interposition graft for repair.

than for the peroneus longus because the location allows better surgical access. Pull-out wires can be considered for reinforcement at the anastomosis repair sites if needed. Rehabilitation should always be started based on the integ-rity of the anastomosis repair site, but usually can begin about 2 weeks postoperatively. Rupture of these major tendons always requires repair when diagnosed early enough. The result of neglected rupture of these tendons with late diagnosis will be a foot and ankle deformity asso-ciated with loss of either or both of these muscles.

HALLUX VALGUS, HALLUX LIMITUS, AND RELATED FOREFOOT DEFORMITIES

Hallux valgus and forefoot deformities are more signifi-cant problems in the athlete compared to the nonathlete. These conditions can limit athletic performance as the result of pain and instability at the first metatarsal–phalangeal joint, along with digital deformities and plantar metatarsalgia with keratomas and bursitis. Biomechanical orthotic control of excessive pronatory forces in midstance and propulsion is essential for these patients, as is properly fitted athletic foot gear. Lesser digital deformities, such as hammertoes with flexible or rigid deformity, can also cause painful shoe gear impingement and bursitis along with companion plantar keratomas and metatarsalgia. Surgical repair of these conditions is indicated when pain and functional impairment develops and there is failure to respond to conservative care, orthoses, and proper shoe gear.

The basic underlying factor predisposing to the development of forefoot deformities is the same in the athlete as the nonathlete, only magnified because of their intense level of performance. The hypermobile first ray allows for progressive metatarsus primus varus and functional first ray instability with elevation as it moves about its triplanar axis of motion—dorsiflexion, adduction, and inversion. The unstable first metatarsal–cuneiform articulation is responsible for most of the abnormal movement of the first metatarsal; however, the navicular–cuneiform articulation also participates in the instability process, especially sagittal and frontal plane excursion. These abnormal motions initiate a predictable chain of events resulting in instability of the medial column, the first metatarsal–phalangeal joint, and the entire forefoot and tarsal complex. Plantar keratoma propulsive lesions may develop at the second metatarsal site as a result of the abnormal weight transfer caused by first ray and medial column biomechanical imbalance. Additional plantar keratomas can develop in response to altered forefoot mechanics and result in hammertoes and contracture of the metatarsophalangeal joints. These deformities may be rigid or flexible and can be very painful to the athlete.

Functional weight-bearing radiographic views are necessary for proper evaluation of these deformities. The quality and character of the first metatarsal–phalangeal joint is evaluated, with an assessment of joint congruency and degenerative joint changes. Assessment of the intermetatarsal angle is critical. Apparent sesamoid position may be evaluated using an anterior–posterior (AP) view; however, a plantar axial view is invaluable. Additional general radiographic observations should be made, such as the length of the first metatarsal and proximal phalanx; lesser metatarsal length, width, and declination; and phalangeal deformities. These considerations are all profiled against the general architecture and "foot type" of the athlete. A good biomechanical examination is important preoperatively, along with clinical gait analysis, in order to assess the functional capacity of the athletic patient.

Careful discussion must be undertaken with athletes to help them understand that considerable recovery can be required at times before return to competitive performance. Surgical repair of any of these conditions will ultimately depend on the severity of the deformity, the amount of interference with competition, and inadequate response to conservative treatment.

Conservative Treatment

Conservative treatment of symptomatic forefoot deformities begins with a good history and physical examination. At times, an adventitious bursa at the dorsomedial aspect of the first metatarsal–phalangeal joint may be acutely inflamed and respond to conservative treatment such as a soluble steroid injection, local applications of ice, and physiotherapy. Lesser digital deformities and contractures can be palliated as needed with orthodigital appliances, pads, and intrabursal injections of soluble steroids if painful digital bursitis develops. The patient's foot gear, including hose and shoes, is evaluated for possible contributory forces that may be present and modified as necessary.

Medium- or long-distance runners may require a varus forefoot runner's wedge, which is added to permit stability and propulsion. Medial wedging or canting of neutral orthotics compensates for limb length discrepancy in the foot as well as the functional varus seen in running. When orthotics are necessary for everyday activity, in conventional walking shoes, perpendicular-to 2-degree varus rearfoot control is used. For exercise walking, a full-length orthosis is preferred. For standing or dress shoes, an orthotic ending behind the metatarsal heads is satisfactory. For women's dress shoes, a cobra-type orthosis is preferred because it has decreased bulk and provides only medial column support.

Hallux Valgus and Bunions

Symptomatic hallux valgus with bunion can interfere with athletic function, resulting in subthreshold performance. Surgical considerations depend on the severity of deformity and amount of interference with competition. Surgical procedures fall into two main categories: soft tissue and major bone procedures with osteotomy or arthrodesis. When practical, unilateral surgical correction of hallux valgus or bunion deformity is preferred. At times, however, bilateral procedures are carried out at the request of the patient. When bilateral surgery is carried out, the recuperative phase will be more prolonged. When deformity is severe enough to warrant osteotomy with osteosynthesis or abrasion chondroarthroplasty, bilateral procedures may be impractical. The athlete must understand the time frame involved in recovery, the schedule for return to activity, and the prospects for continued performance following recuperation.

SOFT TISSUE BUNIONECTOMIES

Generally, soft tissue procedures such as the Silver, Hiss, or McBride procedures are indicated in less severe deformities with no fixed structural articular adaptive deformity. Soft tissue bunion procedures resolve the primary problem of the bunion with a painful bursitis and realign the dynamic structures about the first metatarsal-phalangeal joint. When the deformity is determined to be "soft tissue" and passively reducible, a modified McBride or Silver operation can be considered. These procedures incorporate a dynamic medial capsular repair using a portion of the abductor hallucis in the capsulorrhaphy. This type of dynamic repair is a modification of the Hiss operation.[126-130]

Contraindications for soft tissue correction include (1) a tract-bound joint with restricted, painful, or arthritic motion; and (2) an intermetatarsal angle greater than 12 degrees, unless the first metatarsal-cuneiform articulation is very flexible. Severe medial column instability at the cuneiform-metatarsal joint will require a Lapidus fusion to stabilize the column and ray. Soft tissue correction may be performed as an isolated procedure in the absence of excessive fixed metatarsus primus varus deformity and fixed tract-bound metatarsophalangeal deformity.

Operative Technique

The skin incision can be medial plantar curvilinear or dorsal, depending on the surgeon's preference. A full-thickness dermal subcutaneous flap is reflected down to the level of the first metatarsal-phalangeal joint capsule. Vital structures encountered are mobilized or protected, attempting to maintain these structures in their soft tissue fascial plane. The dorsomedial neurovascular bundle is preserved within the subcutaneous dermal flap when the lower medial approach is used. A longitudinal elliptical lenticular capsulotomy is then performed in the first metatarsal-phalangeal joint on its medial aspect. This capsular incision is extended distally over the midmedial aspect of the base of the proximal phalanx. The soft tissue is freed

from this portion and redundant bone is excised to allow for a capsulodesis distally over the base of the proximal phalanx to effect an increased lever arm of the capsular repair, thereby reducing the hallux valgus deformity. The dorsomedial prominence of the first metatarsal head is then resected with power instrumentation or an osteotome. The integrity of the plantar tibial-sesamoid groove is preserved. If the dorsal approach is used, minimal dissection lateral release can be performed through in the interspace by rectifying the hallux and tensing the lateral structures. The blade is delivered through the lateral joint capsule and along the lateral base of the hallux, slightly rotating the base of the phalanx medially to sever the adductor hallucis tendon. The intra-articular medial approach a utilizes a "through-the-joint release" from medial to lateral. A fibular sesamoidectomy is not performed. The articulations between the sesamoids and their respective facets are inspected. If erosion or arthritis is present, an abrasion arthroplasty is carried out by abrading the arthritic surface down to bleeding bone. Small perforations are placed into the subchondral surface using a 0.035-inch K-wire. If necessary, a new sesamoid groove can be carefully made with a criss-cross burr.

Extensor hallucis longus tendon lengthening is avoided, as is disruption of the hood apparatus. At times the extensor hallucis brevis is a deforming force contributing to abduction deformity, and tenotomy may be performed. Medial capsular closure is achieved with the hallux maintained in a slightly plantar-flexed and rectus position using 2-0 absorbable "oblique load sutures" directed in a plantar distal to proximal dorsal direction. Alternatively, capsular correction may be performed using a criss-crossing figure-eight 2-0 absorbable suture technique. This maintains transverse plane positioning of the hallux and also derotates the sesamoid apparatus and maintains reduction of the intermetatarsal angle. Congruency of the sesamoids and the metatarsal head undersurface is re-established with this manuever. Following capsular closure, it is important to evaluate range of motion and hallux position, making certain there is no functional restriction produced from the operation. Primary closure is achieved per surgeon preference. These operations may be combined with other adjunctive procedures aimed at reducing a flexible or fixed metatarsus primus varus deformity, such as distal or proximal osteotomy or Lapidus resectional arthrodesis.

Postoperatively, the patient is allowed to ambulate in a surgical shoe and standard postoperative care is instituted. Transverse plane splintage of the hallux is recommended for 6 to 8 weeks during the capsulodesis period. Early aggressive sagittal plane motion of the hallux is encouraged. Athletes typically begin a return-to-activity program at approximately 6 to 8 weeks postoperatively. Orthotics are used postoperatively to help control deforming pronatory forces. If combined with other surgical procedures, the postoperative course is modified accordingly.

Lapidus Arthrodesis Procedure

Resectional angular arthrodesis of the first metatarsal–cuneiform articulation is indicated in the presence of an uncontrollable hypermobile first ray located at the first metatarsal–cuneiform joint.[131] High intermetatarsal angular deformity (19 degrees or more), functional instability, and arthrosis define the major indications for this procedure. Arthroplastic or soft tissue capsule tendon balance concepts can also be combined as necessary to address the pathology at the first metatarsal–phalangeal joint.

Execution of the Lapidus fusion requires precision and planning. The operation inherently has the ability to address a high intermetatarsal angle and any elevational instability at the site of the arthrodesis. Appropriate wedge resection must be accomplished to resolve all deformity, including elevatus or plantar flexion deformity of the first ray segment. Interpositional bone grafts from the os calcis are useful and, at times, make the operation easier, reduce shortening of the segment, and result in a distraction–compression fusion. Increased stability of the first ray enhances the long-term prognosis of other procedures, such as arthroplastic repairs, proximal articular set angle (PASA) altering, or decompression osteotomies around the first metatarsal–phalangeal joint.

A dorsomedial longitudinal incision approximately 4 cm in length is placed medial to the tendon of the extensor hallucis longus. As the approach is developed proximally, care is taken to avoid laceration of the tibialis anterior along the dorsomedial aspect of the first metatarsal–cuneiform joint. The incision is deepened through the subcutaneous tissue to the joint capsule once the tibialis anterior has been tagged and protected. The dissection is carried deeply now through the joint capsule, debriding the capsule and associated soft tissue across the top of the joint in preparation for corrective wedge arthrectomy.

Power bone saw instrumentation facilitates arthrectomy with good precision. Appropriate biplanar wedge resection is accomplished, addressing the deformity. Elevatus and increased intermetatarsal deformity of the first metatarsal is resolved with a wedge arthrectomy, resecting more bone plantar laterally. In the presence of a plantar-flexed first metatarsal, the base is directed dorsolaterally. Corrective resection should be achieved at the expense of the cuneiform to preserve the attachment of the peroneus longus at the plantar lateral tubercle of the base of the first metatarsal. An appropriate wedge-shaped cancellous block graft from the back of the os calcis can facilitate this procedure and produce distraction–compression that works well.

Positioning is important and must be carefully checked with temporary transfixation. The foot is loaded, and the position of the first metatarsal head relative to the lesser metatarsals is evaluated. Definitive osteosynthesis is then delivered once the correction is deemed appropriate. Fixation is experience and preference related but is most stable with interfragmentary axial compression screws. Cannulated 3.5- and 4.0-mm cancellous screw systems have facilitated the fixation maneuver (Fig 26-30). Power driven staples can also be acceptable depending on bone quality. Pin fixation is an option but requires criss-cross orientation to lock the site in a stable fashion. The distal metatarsophalangeal correction is then undertaken as necessary with indicated procedures, which at times might also include a capital or phalangeal osteotomy.

Aftercare includes non-weight-bearing status for the first 4 weeks. A removable cast brace can be used during this period to allow rehabilitation and range-of-motion therapy at the first metatarsal–phalangeal repair site if rigid osteosynthesis has been employed. Eight weeks of brace or cast protection is required to ensure solid arthrodesis.

PROXIMAL OSTEOTOMIES OF THE FIRST METATARSAL

Proximal basal osteotomies are best reserved for rigid deformities with high intermetatarsal angle deformity exceeding 15 degrees in younger athletic patients. This parameter has changed to about 18 degrees with the evolution of various shaft osteoplasties in recent years. A stable cuneiform-metatarsal joint should be present.[132,133] The proximal metaphyseal and junctional cortical location allows a variety of geometric configurations to be utilized with good healing potential and increased stability; these include classic lateral closing wedge osteotomy, rotational crescentic or wedge osteotomy with its various plantar ledge modifications, modified A-O Juvara oblique wedge osteotomy, and medial to lateral V osteotomy. These osteotomy concepts all require solid osteosynthesis because of the long lever arm and inherent instability at the osteotomy site.[134] The base osteotomies may be combined with a Reverdin-Green or any distal cervical or head osteotomy to address an abducted PASA facet deformity if present.

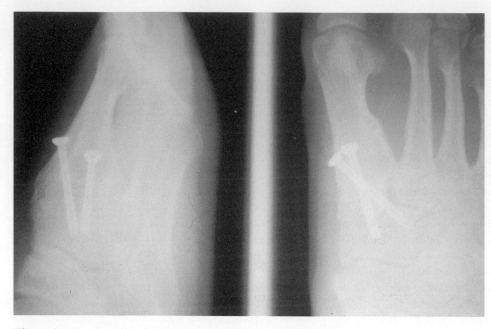

Figure 26-30 Cannulated 4.0 ACE lag screws for Lapidus fusion.

Operative Technique

The skin incision is similar to that for the Lapidus operation previously discussed but slightly less proximal. It is placed medial to the tendon of the extensor hallucis longus over the base and proximal third of the first metatarsal. The distal bunion joint surgery can be performed with a linear extension or a separate incision based on surgeon perference. Dissection should be directly to the metaphyseal flare of the bone, protecting the vital structures. The periosteum at the base of the first metatarsal is incised dorsally or obliquely and elevated depending on which type of osteoplasty will be performed.

The proper execution axis is determined; it depends on the deformity and orientation of the apex of the osteotomy. Movement of the first metatarsal will be determined by the execution axis of the osteotomy. Care is always taken to avoid disruption of the medial hinge if a wedge osteotomy is to be performed. The first metatarsal can be moved in various directions depending on the execution axis of the basal osteotomy. Pure transverse plane correction will require that the osteotomy be cut perpendicular to the weight-bearing surface as opposed to perpendicular to the long axis of the first metatarsal if a dorsal wedge–type repair is being performed. When the apex of the osteotomy is placed perpendicular to the long axis of the first metatarsal, an unwanted component of elevation of the first metatarsal head will be induced upon closure of the osteotomy site.

The geometry of the osteotomy may be defined by first driving an axis osteoguide K-wire through the medial aspect of the base of the first metatarsal, directed appropriately. This creates a failsafe hole. The distal segment may then be visualized as rotating around this imaginary hinge, permitting determination of the proper orientation of the apex before osteotomy. When the apex pin axis is angulated appropriately, the desired osteotomy is performed. Commercial osteotomy axis guides are available for wedge corrections if the surgeon desires. The surgeon is not confined to wedge osteotomy, however, and has several choices in the proximal osteotomy category. Classic lateral wedge closing[135] and the modified oblique A-O Juvara osteotomy require careful attention to the orientation axis of the bone incisions[136] (Fig. 26-31A & B). Modification of the crescentic osteotomy with an ancillary plantar transverse ledge cut is a recent innovation that allows top-to-bottom screw fixation. Medial-to-lateral Kotzenberg V osteotomy[137] has re-emerged with good outcome results.[138,139] Compression screw fixation has become popular and does facilitate rigidity and exact positioning of these precise forms of bone surgery. More than one-point fixation may be desired depending on the osteotomy geometry. The 3.5- and 4.0-mm cannulated systems have made

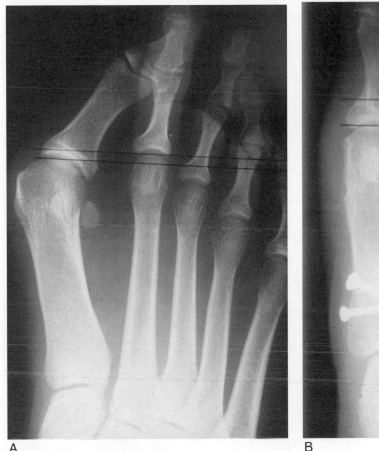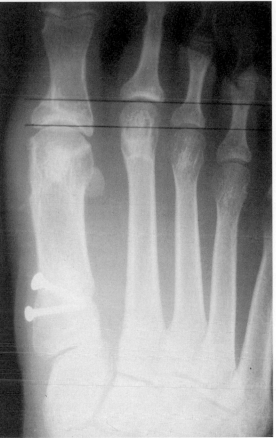

A   B

Figure 26-31   (**A**) High intermetatarsal angle structural hallux valgus. (**B**) Postoperative modified Juvara A-O osteotomy with double screw fixation and Aiken phalangeal osteotomy.

fixation of these sophisticated osteotomies more precise and convenient. The distal "bunionectomy" is the standard "soft tissue procedure" described earlier or an ancillary osteotomy as required. Loading the foot at the completion of the operation, without bandaging, is imperative to verify correction. Reversal of correction can occur with proximal osteotomy, in particular if fibular sesamoidectomy has been accomplished. This is rarely recommended unless the ossicle is arthritic or a source of impingement preventing reduction of the deformity distally.

Non-weight bearing for 6 weeks postoperatively is recommended to avoid elevatus in these proximal procedures. Cast bracing is facilitative for rehabilitation, or a cut-out fiberglass cast can allow range-of-motion therapy at the distal joint region. Progression of bone union is gauged radiographically, and the athlete typically begins a return-to-activity program at approximately 10 weeks postoperatively.

JUNCTIONAL CORTICAL METAPHYSEAL AND SHAFT OSTEOTOMY FOR HALLUX VALGUS

Hallux valgus repair with distal osteotomy has emerged as the favored procedure in most cases of symptomatic bunion deformity with an increased intermetatarsal angle. The cancellous distal head and metaphysis region has enjoyed considerable popularity as a result of the good vascular arcade and healing potential. Precision bone surgery with osteoplastic techniques using small compression screws has dramatically changed traditional concepts of bunion surgery.[140] Compression osteosynthesis has allowed an entire new realm of procedures previously not feasible. Cortical and "junctional bone" osteoplastic surgery has emerged, decreasing the indications for proximal osteotomy procedures. "Junctional bone" is defined as transitional bone between a cortical shaft segment and the spongiosa metaphyseal segment. This anatomic region is now subject to a variety of new operations with great versatility. The result has been excellent correction with more rapid rehabilitation and fewer complications common to the proximal osteotomy.

The new frontier of "rigid fixation bunionectomies" is represented by a number of modified older procedures that have re-emerged, along with some entirely new concepts and osteoplasties.[141–144] The Austin osteotomy remains the gold standard of distal osteotomy bunionectomies. This procedure has been modified by several surgeons using alternate bone incisions, small screw fixation, and currently absorbable pins and screws. The short Scarf Z-plasty is easy and very stable with two 2.0-mm screws (Fig. 26-32A & B). The basic underlying concept of all distal translational osteotomies involves shifting the capital fragment laterally, approximating the first and second metatarsal heads. This reduces the intermetatarsal angle and thus improves the alignment of the first ray segment. Multiplanar correction can be achieved with various modifications. The so-called distal osteotomies all fall into the category of all procedures that are no longer considered proximal basal osteotomies. They are classified as (1) distal capital osteotomies, (2) cervical neck osteotomies, and (3) shaft or "junctional bone" osteotomies.[140] The last category has received considerable recent attention in the literature and present-day surgical practice.

Distal osteotomy bunionectomies are indicated in low or intermediate intermetatarsal angle deformities. Structural bone and articular adaptation often has already occurred in the joint. Clinically, this may be detected by the presence of a tract-bound joint that resists passive reduction to a more rectus position. The main features of the deformity are (1) low or intermediate intermetatarsal angle deformity (10 to 15 degrees);(2) PASA abnormalities with or without intermetatarsal angle enlargement;(3) metatarsus primus elevatus; and (4) abduction of the hallux with or without rotation.

Loss of joint congruency occurs with combined structural and flexible deformities. All of the "distal osteotomies" have the capacity to restore partially or entirely the structural and soft tissue components of the deformity. Some procedures offer advantages over others, and the choice is often related to surgeon preference and experience. The lateral translational procedures are all based on

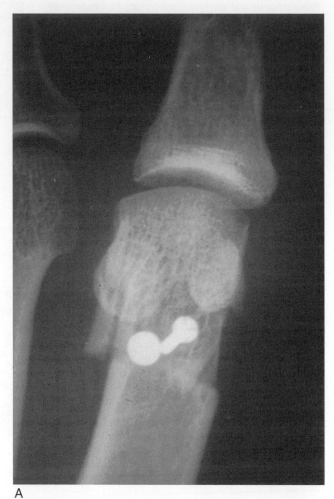

A

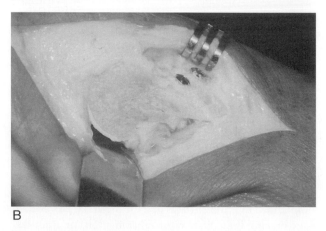

B

Figure 26-32 (**A**) Short Scarf Z sans serif-plasty with double 2.0-mm screw fixation. (**B**) The intraoperative view.

the concept of lateral bone mass shift, and thus the metatarsal width and mass is a consideration.

The classic procedure in the first category of "distal capital osteotomy" would be the Reverdin and its most common modification, incorporating a plantar shelf (Reverdin- Green -Laird). This concept essentially resolves PASA problems and is performed in the cancellous area of the head just immediately posterior to the joint cartilage. It can address low intermetatarsal angle deformity. The second category is cervical osteotomy, represented by the classic Austin V osteotomy with a 60-degree orientation of the osteotomy legs. There are numerous modifications of this osteotomy with altered orientation of the legs or double V wedge removal incorporating a PASA correction as well. The Mitchell osteotomy has been a classic procedure favored by many orthopedists. Other similar procedures are the Hohmann osteotomy, Wilson oblique osteotomy, and Turan osteotomy.[145,146] The third category is "shaft osteoplastics," represented by the "offset V osteotomy," Ludloff, Mau, and Scarf Z-plasty. These are known as "compromise osteotomies" because they are designed to shift an intermediate amount of bone mass laterally to correct intermediate-level intermetatarsal angle deformity, up to 17 degrees. All of these procedures share the ability to accept instrumentation and osteosynthesis for improved stability and postoperative rehabilitation with earlier return to function.

Technique for Reverdin Green-Laird Hallux Valgus Osteotomy

The surgeon must decide on the objectives based on the patient complaints and components of the hallux valgus deformity. Reverdin osteotomy and its modifications are best managed with a dorsal approach medial to the extensor hallucis longus tendon. The approach is carried down to the capsular apparatus, which is developed dorsomedially and then incised with minimal dissection to maintain vascular integrity to the small capital fragment postosteotomy. The medial eminence is removed in typical fashion, avoiding staking the head, and a wedge osteotomy is performed with a medial base through the cancellous portion of the head just behind the cartilage cap. This is the original Reverdin procedure. This maneuver corrects PASA and realigns the joint orientation to a rectus position, allowing some correction of intermetarsal angle if the deformity is somewhat flexible. Indicated soft tissue procedures are performed in conjunction to maintain the correction. Lateral intermetatarsal space entry should be avoided when

performing this osteotomy, if possible, because of the small remaining vascular arcade supply to the thin capital fragment.

The distal medially based wedge L modification of Green incorporates a proximal plantar ledge osteotomy, avoiding the sesamoid apparatus; this modification works well when indicated.[147,148] It has the additional feature of potential lateralization to help reduce an intermetatarsal angle deformity.[148] The osteotomy site is somewhat difficult to fixate because the distal segment is thin. A percutaneous K-wire pin can be delivered through the dorsolateral cartilage, exiting the arch region; this works well as long as the pin is recessed under the cartilage cap. Resorbable pins also have application in this procedure. Capsular work can be modified to meet the situation with oblique load sutures, inverted L or Washington Monument type.

Aftercare depends on inherent stability developed at the time of operation, but usually can be started within a few days following operation. Healing time for athletic return averages about 6 weeks, with full return at about 8 weeks.

Cervical Procedures—Austin and Modifications

The translational V osteotomy of Austin remains the gold standard for distal reconstructions, as indicated earlier. The skin approach is generally dorsal; however, a medial approach can be used if desired. Capsular approaches are also dependent on associated soft tissue correction objectives and can be any of the traditional flaps, oblique load suturing, or inverted L. An osteoguide pin is helpful to assist in proper orientation of the osteotomy displacement pattern, with attention directed to slight plantar depression with lateral displacement. The bone incisions have classically been at a 60-degree orientation. This allows maximum intrinsic stability and excellent union potential because of the vascular arcade that supplies this region in the cancellous metaphysis. Incisional skin approach and capsular dissection can be as desired based on other hallux valgus procedures. Fixation has previously been most common with a K-wire; however, small screws and resorbable pins have proved very effective.[149]

This osteotomy has been modified numerous times. The most common modification is probably the long dorsal wing, first described by Lewis and Feffer in 1981[150] and subsequently adopted by Kalish with the addition of two 2.7-mm lag screws. Vogler developed another modification in 1979 that has a longer dorsal arm, extending 75 percent of the shaft with an apex at the periphery of the

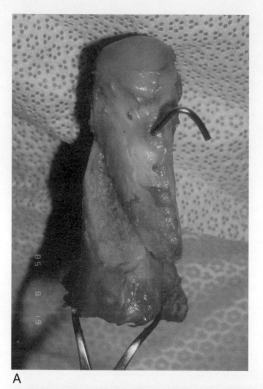

A

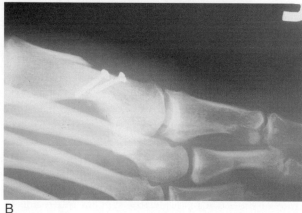

B

Figure 26-33 Offset V sans serif osteotomy shaft osteoplasty. (**A**) Dorsal view. (**B**) Medial view.

imaginary circle of the head of the metatarsal[151] (Fig. 26-33A & B).

Youngswick Modification of the Austin Osteotomy The Youngswick procedure is an important contribution to hallux valgus repair inasmuch as slight plantar flexion of the capital fragment is easily accomplished.[152] This modification employs a double osteotomy on the dor-

sal side of the V removing 1 to 2 mm of bone, which produces an obligatory depression of the capital fragment when impacted and fixated. Some laxity is created with this modification, which also decompresses the joint. Some site instability results following this modification; however, fixation easily overcomes minor problem and can be resorbable if desired. The procedure is otherwise identical to the Austin procedure.

This osteotomy is very stable and heals well. It remains the hallmark procedure for hallux valgus correction in both the athlete and nonathlete. Return to aggressive performance is similar to that with the Reverdin operation, taking about 8 weeks or longer depending on severity of the deformity and healing patterns.

Mitchell and Hohmann Osteotomies

The Mitchell[153] and Hohmann[154] osteotomies are also cervical osteotomies but are not performed nearly as often as the Austin-type repairs. These osteotomies are inherently unstable and take longer to heal because of their bone incisions and location slightly more proximal in cortical bone. Wu has published a modification of the Mitchell bunionectomy using a Herbert screw.[155] Turan has published a procedure resembling a modified Wilson osteotomy with screw fixation as well; however, the medial eminance is not resected.[146]

Rigid fixation is important if these osteotomies are considered, because of their inherent instability. Rehabilitation and return-to-activity time are longer for these procedures. These operations are not used in the athletic population with any frequency for these reasons.

Shaft Osteoplastics and Junctional Osteotomies

Technological advances in osteosynthesis and improved understanding of bone healing have heralded a new era of skeletal surgery. This is true with hallux valgus surgery as well. Athletes with intermediate deformity previously required basal osteotomies, with the inherent prolonged recuperation and rehabilitation. Osteoplastic procedures in the "junctional bone" region where the cortex meets the metaphysis have widened the parameters of indication for nonbasal proximal osteotomy.[140] Deformity of moderate degree (up to 17 to 18 degrees) can successful be managed by these new osteoplastics with rigid internal fixation. These procedures can address all the significant components of the deformity simultaneously.

The procedures most representative in this category are

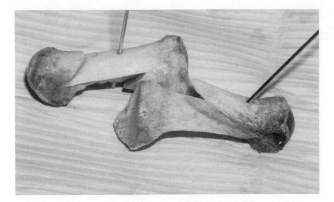

Figure 26-34 Comparison of morphology—the "offset sans serif V" osteotomy and the Scarf Z sans serif-plasty.

the Scarf Z-plasty and the offset V osteotomy (Fig. 26-34). Both of these osteotomies are intrinsically stable and manifest long, broad bone surfaces for improved healing with compression osteosynthesis screws. They can address PASA problems with a swivel maneuver as well. The offset V osteotomy has its apex at the periphery of the imaginary circle of the head of the first metatarsal and a very long cortical dorsal wing, extending at least 75 percent of the length of the first metatarsal. Lateral translation can be over 50 percent without difficulty in healing. Fixation is with one or two 2.7-mm or 2.0-mm screws. The Scarf Z-plasty is the most inherently stable of all osteoplastics currently available in the management of hallux valgus, and can also achieve at least 50 percent lateralization. It has proven to be one of the premier procedures for management of structural hallux valgus in long-term follow-up study.[157,158] It can be performed in a short or long Z configuration depending on the magnitude of deformity. The long-Z configuration has the additional advantage of considerable lateral rotation of the distal segment to further reduce high intermetatarsal angle deformities (above 18 degrees.[158] Fixation can be with 3.5-2.7-, and 2.0-mm screws or even buried K-wires cut flush with the bone surface. Fixation selection depends on bone mass and thickness of the metatarsal. Two screws or pins must be used in the long-Z configuration for fixation in this osteotomy. Two smaller 2.0-mm screws can be used for the short-Z configuration as well.

Rehabilitation is very rapid with these latter two osteotomies, in particular with the Z osteotomy, which is now the most favored osteotomy repair for the athlete with symptomatic bunion and hallux valgus deformity. Return

to competition with proper rehabilitation can be as early as 5 to 6 weeks. Return to nonathletic activity in shoe gear can be achieved, remarkably, in 2 weeks.

NONPROSTHETIC ARTHROPLASTY OF THE FIRST METATARSAL–PHALANGEAL JOINT IN ASSOCIATION WITH HALLUX VALGUS

Arthroplasty of the first metatarsal–phalangeal joint is a general category of operations including abrasion arthroplasty, various realignment osteotomies, and Keller arthroplasty with or without hemi- or total joint prosthesis. These procedures are the most common concepts in the category of arthroplasty that are employed mainly for bunion deformity with joint degeneration and pain. Allogeneic rib cartilage implants are in use on an investigational basis; these implants are shaped like a "stemmed hemi-implant" for the base of the proximal phalanx, acting as a "spacer" for interposition.

For the older athlete (50+years) who has symptomatic hallux valgus with joint destruction and fails to respond to conservative treatment, a Keller bunionectomy is effective if performed well. This operation also decompresses the ray, allowing reduction of an enlarged intermetatarsal angle. It is essential to free the sesamoid apparatus completely so that it may retract proximally postoperatively. Failure to do so could result in chronic postoperative pain, stiffness, and functional limitation. This is performed by a Villadot suture, which anastomoses the flexor hallucis longus with the intersesamoidal ligament. In effect, this accomplishes a tenodesis between the long flexor and the base of the proximal phalanx and also prevents retraction of the sesamoids. Temporary axial Steinman pin transfixation is useful across the metatarsophalangeal joint for temporary maintenance of correction while arthrofibrosis develops in the resected joint interval, which also helps prevent retraction of the hallux. The fixation is removed at 3 weeks. Active range-of-motion exercises are then initiated. Postoperatively, this results in better hallux purchase and decreased incidence of lesser metatarsalgia.

The Regnauld "autogenous implant" is an alternative consideration for the athlete with hallux valgus with severe joint destruction and phalangeal osteoproliferation.[159] It offers an alternative to more apropulsion-producing operations such as the Keller, but has a longer recovery period. Fixation is recommended and best accomplished with buried K-wires cut flush with the bone. Early rehabilitation is possible when the bone implant is stable. Good joint decompression is produced with this operation, and it can easily be performed in conjunction with distal or proximal metatarsal osteotomies as indicated for an enlarged inter-metatarsal angle deformity.

Indications for arthroplasty procedures include bunions with degenerative arthrosis, phalangeal component osteo-proliferation, metatarsus primus varus, arthritic sesamoids, progressive metabolic seropositive arthritic disease, or se-ronegative arthritic disease, such as psoriatic arthritis. Abra-sion chondroarthroplasty of the first metatarsal–phalangeal joint is indicated in mild to moderate hallux valgus/limitus in the presence of degenerative or osteochondral lesions of the first metatarsal–phalangeal joint. Osteotomy correc-tion can be performed in conjunction with capsule ten-don-balancing procedures similar to those described under soft tissue correction of hallux valgus (Fig. 26-35A & B).

PROSTHESIS ARTHROPLASTY OF THE FIRST METATARSAL– PHALANGEAL JOINT

Hallux valgus with significant subluxation of the first metatarsal–phalangeal joint and arthritic deformity pre-sents a difficult dilemma. Unfortunately, none of the cur-rently available endoprosthetic devices is acceptable for the competitive athlete. Arthroprostheses of the first metatar-sal–phalangeal joint continue to evolve but still fall short of proper performance for athletic use. Procedures de-signed to stabilize the first ray and reduce the intermetatar-sal angle, combined with an autogenous arthroplasty, have a much more favorable prognosis than endoprostheses. The exception might be an elderly noncompetitive indi-vidual with low functional demand.

AKIN OSTEOTOMY

Angulational osteotomy of the proximal phalanx of the hallux is indicated in the presence of interphalangeus ab-ductus or as an adjunctive procedure, used in combination with soft tissue or osseous repair of hallux valgus. Phalan-geal osteotomy can be accomplished proximally or distally depending on the level of deformity. Additionally, it can be performed with conventional transverse wedge resec-tion or long oblique bone incision to also resolve valgus rotation.[160] Creation of a rectus hallux by way of phalan-geal osteotomy should be avoided because of the difficulty encountered postoperatively when a rectus hallux is forced into a shoe toebox. Ideally, there should be approximately 10 degrees of hallux abductus.

A medial longitudinal incision is made at the level of the proximal phalanx, and periosteum is reflected dorsally,

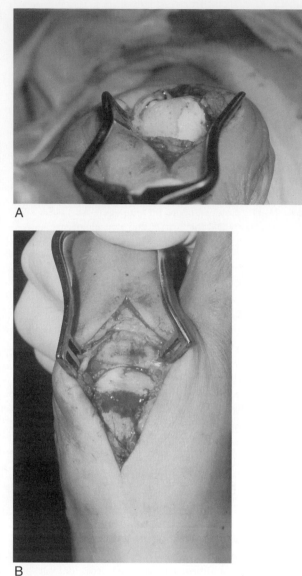

A

B

Figure 26-35 (**A**) Abrasion chondroplasty of first metatar-sal–phalangeal joint. (**B**) Abrasion chondroplasty with de-compression head osteotomy.

medially, and plantarly. Oscillating bone saws produce the finest osteotomies in the phalanx region. Wedge correc-tion can be traditional medial transverse closing or oblique wedge closing.[161] The oblique closing wedge can take either of two configurations depending on phalanx mor-phology: proximal lateral hinged, which is favored because of the cancellous apex region, or distal lateral cortical hinged. The wedge resection is always medially based. The lateral hinge is left intact and the osteotomy greenstick closed. Fixation is accomplished with a 0.045-inch K-wire driven obliquely across the osteotomy site if transverse. Effective resorbable osteosynthesis with poly-L-lactic acid mini staples has also been described.[162] Oblique osteotomies require preferably two buried K-wires. Threaded K-wires work well for this fixation maneuver and rarely migrate when buried and cut flush with the bone. Occasionally there is a large medial prominence at the base of the proximal phalanx; this may be resected with an oscillating saw, taking care to reattach the abductor hallucis tendon with drill holes and osteosuture. Closure is according to surgeon preference.

Standard postoperative care is used in accordance with adjunctive procedures performed. External K-wires are retrieved 3 to 4 weeks postoperatively. Buried K-wires cut flush with the bone usually do not require removal, unless they migrate; threaded K-wires usually avoid this problem. Use of 2.7- or 2.0-mm screws works well in the oblique phalangeal osteotomies but may require delivery of two devices. The athlete is advised of the need for possible future removal if they become symptomatic.

BUNIONECTOMY REHABILITATION PROGRAMS AND RETURN TO ACTIVITY

Six weeks postoperatively, a progressive return-to-activity program is instituted with most distal osteotomies. When abrasion arthroplastics have been carried out, early passive and active range of motion at postoperative day 2 can promote cartilage regeneration. Patients must remain non-weight bearing at the level of the first metatarsal–phalangeal joint and metatarsal sesamoid articulation for about 2 to 3 weeks for nonosteotomy joint repair and 6 weeks for proximal basal osteotomy. Ambulation may be permitted immediately in a protective forefoot fiberglass slipper splint with the shaft osteoplastics, and even earlier with the cervical osteotomies of the Austin variety.

Hallux Limitus and Rigidus

Hallux rigidus and limitus is defined as a mild to severe limitation of range of motion at the first metatarsal–phalangeal joint.[163,164] The first metatarsal should be able to dorsiflex and plantar flex about 0.5 cm in each direction, for a total range of 1.0 cm of motion. Two forms of hallux rigidus exist, with varying degrees of pain—structural and functional.[163–165] Hallux rigidus is more commonly iden-

tified with structural degenerative radiographic derangement that impairs joint motion, leading to ankylosis.[166] Functional hallux limitus exists only in the loaded state, indicating less fixation of the deformity, with passive range of motion improving off-loading. The concept of these two biomechanically distinct entities has advanced our treatment approach to this complex condition. It is believed that the condition usually begins as a biomechanical "functional" condition that progresses with structural changes and fixation of the deformity. The post-traumatic form progresses to later stages of the disease process faster because the causative factors are different.

An abnormally long first metatarsal may also be implicated in the development of hallux limitus if it is unable to plantar-flex actively against the long lever arm of ground reaction force at the first metatarsal head. Any condition that interferes with the ability of the metatarsal head to glide along the dorsal aspect of the sesamoid apparatus will also result in a hallux limitus or rigidus. These conditions include dystrophic or degenerated sesamoids with arthritic articulating surfaces with the head of the first metatarsal, or frank ankylosis of the sesamoid apparatus to the plantar surface of the metatarsal head. Post-traumatic deformity of the first metatarsal–phalangeal joint is a less common but important source of limited and painful motion. When trauma is involved, radiographic changes are usually present that define this condition as hallux rigidus.

At times, compensation for a hallux limitus or rigidus deformity will be seen with hyperextension of the hallux interphalangeal joint to allow for relatively normal closed kinetic chain ankle joint plantar flexion, or with external rotation of the lower extremity, thereby shortening the lever arm of the foot in gait and reducing toe-off demand. When the foot is able to compensate for a limitus or rigidus at the interphalangeal joint, a plantar lesion may be evident beneath the interphalangeal joint. This situation is accentuated if an osseous or cartilaginous sesamoid is present deep to the long flexor tendon.

The quality and amount of motion at the first metatarsal–phalangeal joint is evaluated in both dorsiflexion and plantar flexion. Weight-bearing examination and open kinetic chain non-weight-bearing examination is important to qualify the nature of the abnormality. The sesamoid apparatus is palpated for tenderness, and thorough radiographic assessment is performed, including axial sesamoid views to evaluate the cristae and metatarsal–sesamoid facet joint. Gait analysis may demonstrate a functional first ray instability with collapse of the medial column with hindfoot eversion. Radiographic osteoproliferation may be noted at the dorsal aspect of the first metatarsal–phalangeal joint, especially at the metatarsal component of the joint as well as the cuneiform–metatarsal unit. This is best viewed laterally. The first metatarsal is often noted to be more dorsally positioned in relation to the second metatarsal, with a "dorsal bunion bump." Alternatively, the proximal phalanx is often flexed. Dorsal jamming of the first metatarsal–phalangeal joint during closed kinetic chain hallux dorsiflexion may be demonstrated and evaluated radiographically, using a weight-bearing stress lateral view with the patient maximally dorsiflexing the first metatarsal–phalangeal joint in closed kinetic chain motion.

Classification schemes have helped surgeons understand the natural progression and surgical approach to this problem.[167,168] Current staging classifications by Regnauld and Drago define three stages of progression, while Kravitz defines four grades that are sequential in development.[169] The classifications are essentially alike and progressive for treatment protocol determination. Grade 1 is known as "pre–hallux limitus" and is entirely functional, related to the biomechanical abnormality of hyperpronation syndrome causing unlocking and metatarsus primus elevatus with minimal to no pain. There are no radiographic changes present other than slight subchondral sclerosis. Grade 2 develops dorsolateral joint pain with decrease in motion and some loss of joint space. Joint flaring may begin with metatarsal head flattening and more dense sclerosis subchondrally. Grade 3 usually demonstrates clinical and radiographic dorsal bunion prominence, considerable propulsive-phase gait pain, and joint fragments or loose bodies. Subchondral bone cysts may be present, as well as interphalangeal joint hyperextension, metatarsalgia beneath the second metatarsal, and inflammatory arthritis with periarticular proliferations. Grade 4 manifests profound ankylosis and joint destruction. The amount of pain present is determined by the amount of motion that remains and the severity of the inflammatory process generated. The sesamoids are usually fused; the joint has a trumpet appearance with extensive osteoproliferation and sesamoidal ankylosis.

CONSERVATIVE CARE

When an athlete presents with painful hallux limitus or rigidus deformity, initial conservative treatment is begun. Staging of the abnormality will assist in defining the best treatment. This may include NSAIDs, intra-articular steroid injections, appropriate physiotherapy modalities, and/or manipulation or range of motion and biomechanical orthotic control when indicated. These options are con-

fined in particular to grade 1 dyfunction. When such conservative measures fail to alleviate the patient's symptomatology, surgical intervention is recommended.

SURGERY

Operative treatment of hallux limitus or rigidus is based on the classification scheme.[169] Grade 1 impairment most often is treated conservatively, as indicated above. Nonetheless, some cases of grade 1 dysfunction are refractory to conservative care, and decompression osteotomy or depression first metatarsal osteotomy could be required. Because there are no real distal metatarsophalangeal joint changes evident, joint surgery at this level is not really indicated other than possible head decompression.

Grade 2 dysfunction demonstrates early structural joint changes, and cheilectomy dorsal "cleanup procedures" are the premier procedures. If obvious structural metatarsal abnormality exists, such as excessive length pattern or elevatus, shortening or depression osteotomy is indicated. Additionally, cheilectomy should also incorporate chondroplasty when required, with multiple subchondral perforations using a 0.035-inch K-wire in denuded areas of the joint, which is inevitably the dorsal 50 percent. Occasionally, excessive phalangeal hallux length is problematic, and osteoplastic shortening of the phalanx is indicated. Phalangeal basal elevational wedge osteotomy, such as the Bonney-Kessel, is adjunctive because it reduces the amount of metatarsophalangeal dorsiflexion normally required.

Grade 3 dysfunction demonstrates considerable joint derangement and pain. Cheilectomy is incorporated as part of other reconstructive procedures. The primary objective in grade 3 disease is joint laxity, which is produced primarily by decompression osteotomies. Basic to this concept is the salvageability of the joint with sesamoidal arthrolysis and plantar degloving. There are numerous metatarsal osteotomy modifications to choose from based on surgeon preference and severity of the disease process. The most common modifications are those of the dorsal Watermann head decompression osteotomy. Some procedures employ only metatarsal head decompression without depression of the metatarsal base, such as the dorsal Weil oblique decompression with a distal plantar apex and dorsal proximal wedge resection. Phalangeal component decompression can be achieved with the Regnauld enclavement operation, which is a unique contribution.[170] Numerous other modifications employ concurrent depression of the capital segment, including the Hohmann osteotomy, sagittal plane

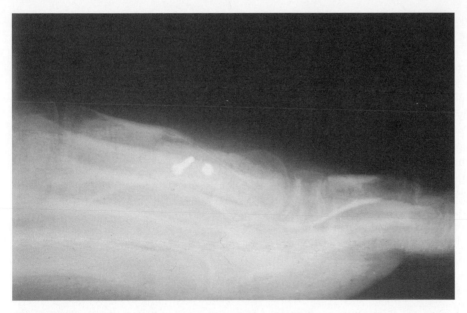

Figure 26-36 Sagittal plane Z sans serif-depression osteotomy for hallux limitus combined with Bonney-Kessel wedge osteotomy in phalanx.

Z osteotomy (Fig. 26-36), Youngswick modification of the Austin osteotomy , sagittal plane cervical V depression osteotomy, and basal wedge osteotomies such as the sagittal plane Juvara or even plantar-flexory Lambrinudi. Resectional plantar-flexory arthrectomy fusion is necessary at times if elevatus is extreme. Metatarsal decompression and depression are important concepts in grade 3 disease and form the basis of salvage in conjunction with cheilectomy and chondroplasty with drilling. New advances in osteosynthesis with cannulated screws and small plates make these options realistic and effective.

Grade 4 disease is end stage; the options are few and usually clear. Osteoproliferation is extensive, as is alteration of joint morphology. More aggressive surgery is required and the functional outcome is less effective. This has a critical effect on the athlete, and often career-ending surgery is required. Joint-destructive arthroplasties such as the Keller, with long flexor tenodesis to the plantar base of the phalanx, are often necessary. Pain relief is usually the main objective, although functional restoration is always a corollary desire. The Regnauld enclavement operation may have a role in grade 4 disease depending on the joint morphology. The joint destruction is total in this stage, and little remains to do other than total joint ablative procedures or arthrodesis. Older noncompetitive weekend athletes (60+ years) might benefit from a total joint pros-

thesis. The Valente dorsal wedge arthrectomy can produce a good pseudoarthrosis and pain relief with functional motion. Arthrodesis is the ultimate ablation and may be necessary if septic arthrosis is present, or some other form of major disaster occurs, such as a failed cemented or silicone prosthesis.

OPERATIVE TECHNIQUES

Cheilectomy and Abrasion Chondroarthroplasty

The mainstay of procedures for hallux rigidus with osteoproliferation and degenerative pain is the dorsal cheilectomy.[166] A dorsum longitudinal approach is best, medial to the extensor hallucis longus tendon. Dissection is carried directly down to the dorsum of the joint, staying medial to the extensor apparatus. This procedure can be performed with minimal tissue stripping. Capsular entry immediately demonstrates the osteoproliferative bone and degenerated cartilage. Loose bodies are often found in the dorsal pouch and extravasate upon capsular incision. The joint is placed through its range of motion and the plantar half of the joint carefully inspected, especially the sesamoidal apparatus. The dorsal half will manifest degenerative change often down to bare bone. The hypertrophic bone on the dorsum of the metatarsal is resected generously. Opposing phalangeal component proliferation is likewise resected, with a wedge resection across the top of the phalanx. This is done by protecting the metatarsal head and axial distraction and flexion of the phalanx, using a bone saw carefully. Following appropriate ostectomy on either side of the joint, sesamoidolysis is carried out with a McGlamry elevator, degloving the bottom of the first metatarsal if the sesamoids show restriction. Any degenerative sites on the upper half of the metatarsal head are carefully perforated with a 0.035-inch K-wire several times through subchondral bone. Marginal osteophytes are appropriately removed with a rongeur or bone saw medially and laterally if present. A layered closure is performed, usually capsule, subcutaneous tissue, and then skin. A small amount of soluble steroid may be instilled at closure to reduce pain and swelling.

Arthroplasty with Metatarsal Head Decompression Osteotomy or Shaft Osteotomy

Cheilectomy remains the first step in this reconstruction as well. Following dorsal resection of the osteoproliferative bone, osteotomy is facilitated by the flat cancellous surface that remains. Standard Watermann dorsal wedge resection can be performed at this juncture, and associated procedures such as subchondral drilling employed as necessary. If no plantar displacement is desired, the Weil modification can be performed with a long oblique dorsal proximal wedge resection with the distal apex near the distal plantar portion of the head. The decision to plantar flex the capital fragment is usually a good idea. The Watermann-Green distal L modification uses a plantar shelf osteotomy and dorsal medial-to-lateral wafer resection, causing some shortening.[171] Increased joint volume space results, as well as some depression of the capital fragment. Osteosynthesis is required for these osteotomies. K-wires cut flush with the bone work well; small screws can also be used. If the plantar shelf osteotomy extends far enough proximally, two 2.0-mm screws can be delivered from the dorsum. Resorbable pins can also be used for this osteotomy. Most surgeons fail to remove a wide enough dorsal wedge in this osteotomy, and they perform it too proximally. The effect is inadequate decompression and actual head elevation, making the functional limitation even worse after union has occurred.

If more significant head depression is necessary to accommodate the deformity, then a more proximal cervical osteotomy, proximal to the sesamoids, is necessary, such as the Hohmann, sagittal shaft Z osteotomy or sagittal V neck osteotomy. The Hohmann requires rigid screw fixation because of its inherent instability. The Youngswick modification of the Austin osteotomy can be used to achieve some plantar flexion in conjunction with joint arthroplasty, but its depression ability is limited.

Proximal Osteotomies for Hallux Limitus/Rigidus

Proximal depression osteotomies are used when the magnitude of deformity is too great to address distally. At times, a plantar wedge arthrectomy arthrodesis will be required at the metatarsal–cuneiform joint if arthrosis is present. All proximal osteotomy procedures can be combined with distal concepts discussed previously, including osteotomy and arthroplasty. Opening first metatarsal base wedge osteotomies are not recommended. They are not intrinsically stable and heal slowly.

Dorsal open wedge osteotomy of the medial cuneiform (Cotton osteotomy[172] just distal to the midpoint of the cuneiform works well. An autogenous or freeze-dried bone implant incorporates quickly and has excellent stability because it is placed under compression. The site is intrinsically stable because it is a distraction–compression osteotomy and no fixation is required. Considerable ray depression can be achieved with this proximal osteotomy, and care should be taken to avoid excessive plantar displacement.

Sagittal plane plantar closing base wedge osteotomy perpendicular to the first metatarsal is time honored and still works well[173] (Fig. 26-37). It requires fixation by pins, screws, or staples. Cresentic rotation osteotomy accomplishes the same task and also requires rigid internal fixation because of its instability. These osteotomies must be approached through a medial incision at the metatarsal–cuneiform region, with care taken to avoid lacerating the tibialis anterior tendon insertion.

A-O Oblique Plantar Closing Wedge Osteotomy in Hallux Rigidus A medial skin approach is used similarly to that in the traditional plantar closing wedge osteotomy, about 4 cm in length. It is placed superior to the abductor hallucis muscle belly and along the proximal shaft and metaphysis of the first metatarsal. A periosteal elevator is used to reflect periosteal soft tissue from the base of the first metatarsal along the medial, plantar, and dorsal aspects. A sagittal bone saw is then used to osteotomize the appropriate oblique wedge of bone from the base of the first metatarsal. The apex is directed dorsalproximally and the wedge base directed plantar distally. Care is taken to preserve the

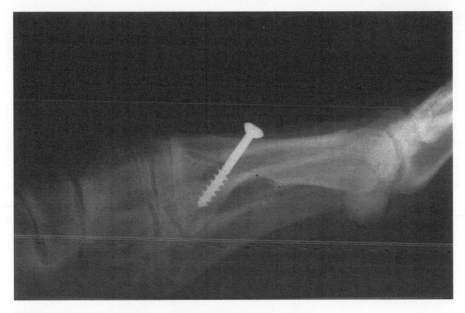

Figure 26-37   Sagittal plane depression osteotomy.

dorsal cortical hinge. The amount of wedge resected is determined to be adequate by evaluating the level of the first metatarsal in relationship to the level of the lesser met atarsals with the foot loaded and the osteotomy site clamped. Osteosynthesis is undertaken with small screws, either 2.7 or 3.5 mm, with lag technique. It is important to avoid overaggressive countersinking of the screws.

Postoperatively, the patient is maintained in a below-knee cast brace or fiberglass cast, non-weight bearing for 6 weeks. Weight bearing is not allowed on the first ray until there is radiographic evidence of union at the osteotomy site. The screw may be left in place or retrieved subsequently if necessary.

Sagittal Plane Osteotomies   Sagittal plane shaft Z osteotomy is an excellent method of rotational depression of the distal segment or direct translational depression. It is particularly useful in iatrogenic elevatus.[174] Osteosynthesis is facilitated by the long flat surfaces, and 2.7-or 2.0-mm screws are used from medial to lateral. If rotational correction is used with the Z sans serif osteotomy, a small dorsal spike will remain that must be remodeled. Cervical sagittal plane V osteotomy is probably the easiest of these procedures, and depression can be achieved by rotating the distal fragment or direct plantar translation of the fragment. Fixation is easiest with buried K-wires cut flush with the bone or left percutaneous for 4 weeks. Closure is standard for all these procedures.

Cutout fiberglass slipper cast protection may be necessary for these osteotomies, depending on the weight of the patient and the anticipated activity level. Cast bracing can be used as well and allows the advantage of total removability for rehabilitation and therapy. Return to activity is over a 6 to 10-week period of time while therapy is taking place. Standard physiotherapy may be used along with standard postoperative care. Orthotics are used postoperatively when indicated.

Bonney-Kessel Osteotomy as an Adjunct in Hallux Limitus

Painful hallux limitus in the absence of significant metatarsus elevatus deformity and normal first metatarsal length forms the basis for Bonney-Kessel osteotomy.[164] This dorsal closing wedge osteotomy is performed at the metaphyseal expansion of the base of the phalanx. This procedure is very good if there is excessive length of the proximal phalanx. Minimal intra-articular degenerative changes should be present to indicate this procedure, along with a functional residual range of retained plantar-flexory motion. It is performed in conjunction with other cheilectomy arthroplasty or chondroplasty maneuvers. This procedure does not generally increase the overall range of motion beyond what might be accomplished by simply performing a dorsal cheilectomy. It alters the arc of rotation more favorably for the remaining viable cartilage on the head of the metatarsal. It can be an effective alternative to arthrodesis in the adult.[175]

The procedure is approached similarly to others described for exposure of the first metatarsal–phalangeal joint. If a dorsal osteophytic rim is present at the base of the phalanx, it may be resected at this time, and small osteochondral defects abraded. A power oscillating bone saw is used to create a dorsal-to-plantar wedge-shaped osteotomy in the metaphysis, maintaining the plantar cortex. The amount of wedge of bone removed is dependent on how much dorsal displacement of the range of motion is required, but generally is more than first imagined. The osteotomy may be fixed with one or two K-wires either buried or percutaneous or with monofilament loop wire. Sagittal plane A-O–type osteotomies are available for consideration as well. These have their apex on the proximal plantar aspect of the phalangeal metaphysis, with the wedge resection taken dorsal distal. Closure is via 2.0-mm screws driven dorsal plantar with lag technique. The wound is flushed and closed in layers.

Postoperatively, the patient is allowed weight bearing in a wooden-soled surgical shoe or cutout fiberglass foot cast. This is left in place for approximately 4 weeks, performing gentle joint movement at the site of the cut-away slipper cast. Fixation is removed at approximately 4 weeks if protruding K-wires are used postoperatively and a return-to-activity program initiated.

Keller and Valente Arthroplasties

When degenerative joint disease exceeds 25 percent of the joint volumn with osteoproliferation, the surgeon is faced with the decision of performing a Keller arthroplasty.[176,177] The decision is also based on anticipated functional activity and the magnitude of periarticular proliferation. If the joint disease is mainly metatarsal dominant, a Stone-type arthroplasty can be considered. If the joint disease is phalangeal dominant, then a Keller arthroplasty is considered. If severe ankylosis is present with dual-component osteoproliferation, a Valente "dorsal V" arthrectomy is performed.[178] (Fig. 26-38) This is a particularly good operation, with rapid recovery, relief of pain, and good functional salvage. Sesamoidolysis can be done with any of these procedures, but arthrofibrosis usually recurs. Assuming the sesamoids are still functional, it is important to allow them to retract proximally when performing these resection procedures, except with the Valente arthrectomy. The Keller arthroplasty must be stabilized for several weeks to allow solid arthrofibrosis and fibrous tissue infiltrate to help maintain the arthroplastic interval. It is known that a functional fibrous cartilage tissue disk forms in this interval that mimics hyaline cartilage and is similar to a joint.[179] Stabilization is most easily accomplished with an axial Steinman pin maintained in position for about 3 weeks. The long flexor is always attached to the plantar

Figure 26-38 Valente V sans serif arthrectomy arthroplasty.

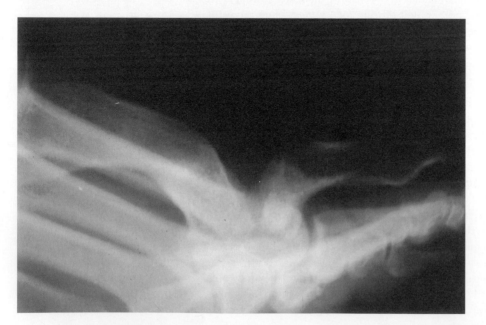

phalanx with osteosuture and drill holes to maintain some hallux purchase. Layered closure is accomplished.

Postoperatively, the patient is allowed weight bearing in a surgical shoe immediately, with rehabilitation for swelling and gradual return to activity as tolerated.

Regnauld Enclavement Decompression Autogenous Arthroplasty

Perhaps the most unique arthroplastic reconstruction is that of Bernard Regnauld.[170] His operation was first described in 1968 and went essentially unobserved until the late 1980s, when podiatric surgeons began using it. The procedure is essentially an "autogenous osteocartilaginous hemi-implant" prosthesis fashioned from the phalangeal base. The underlying concept again is joint decompression—this time on the phalangeal side of the joint. It is particularly useful in cases with a long phalanx and grade 3 or 4 disease. Modifications have include reversal of the stem with invagination of the far phalanx into the proximal metaphysis—just the opposite of the procedure originally described.[159]

A standard dorsal approach medial to the extensor tendon is used and dissection carried out essentially like a Keller arthroplasty. The phalanx is osteotomized for just slightly less than the proximal 50 percent and removed in toto from the wound. The complete removal and degloving of the segment is the concept that helps decompress the joint. In situ fashioning of the autogenous implant has also been described. It is fashioned into a "hemiprosthesis" with a distal stem of cancellous bone that is invaginated into the reamed remaining phalanx. The reverse orientation is also acceptable.[180] Fixation should be accomplished with two smooth or threaded 0.035-inch K-wires, which can be buried or external. Box loop monofilament wire can also be used in this fixation. The metatarsal head is degloved and remodeled as necessary with sesamoidolysis. Layered closure follows, and early range of motion and therapy are instituted postoperatively. Serial radiographs will demonstrate gradual incorporation of the autoimplant over a 3-month period. Return to activity is based on graft union and tolerence. This operation can be combined with proximal depression osteotomies if the elevatus deformity is severe enough to warrant same.

Hallux Interphalangeal Sesamoiditis

Hallux limitus or rigidus compensates for the loss of motion at the metatarsophalangeal joint by hyperextension at the hallux interphalangeal joint.[181] Interphalangeal cap-

sulitis and sesamoiditis can occur as part of this compensation mechanism, especially following fusion of the metatarsophalangeal joint. A painful keratoma can be present with bursitis. This area is often tender to palpation.[182]

Radiographically, the presence of an ossified sesamoid on the plantar aspect of the interphalangeal joint will usually be noted. A cartilaginous sesamoid may also be present at this same site but without radiographic evidence.

Surgical excision is recommended when the lesion is painful and nonresponsive to nonsurgical care. The symptoms of a bone ossicle and cartilage ossicle are identical; however, the accessory is usually larger and more painful when ossified. The surgical procedure produces excellent relief of symptoms with minimum down time. It can be performed through a 3-cm medial plantar longitudinal incision or direct midline plantar flexor tendon–splitting approach, or even a dorsal Z approach with the transverse leg over the joint.[183] The long flexor tendon is identified, and the accessory ossicle is proximally situated between the long flexor tendon and the plantar aspect of the interphalangeal joint. After the accessory ossicle is identified, it is excised, taking care to preserve the integrity of the flexor hallucis longus. When the plantar skin lesion is particularly keratotic, it may be ellipsed with the skin approach. Care is taken to avoid creation of an excessively wide ellipse, which would make closure difficult.

Postoperative care allows ambulation in a wooden postoperative shoe. Standard postoperative management and physiotherapy are followed as indicated. Patients typically begin a return-to-activity program approximately 3 to 4 weeks postoperatively.

Hammertoe Deformities

Hammertoe deformities are a common cause of pain and disability in the athletic population. Digital contractures lead to dorsal or distal keratotic lesions, or both, that interfere with shoe fitting and severely hinder both athletic and everyday performance. Digital contractures may be related to an imbalance among the dorsal, plantar, and/or intrinsic muscle groups, and are more commonly seen with generalized ligamentous laxity, cavus deformity, and hypermobile pes planovalgus. There is a strong familial tendency. Improperly fitting foot gear can aggravate or accelerate an existing tendency toward development of digital contractures. Generalized or isolated instability of the metatarsophalangeal joints, as in various seropositive and seronegative variant arthritides, often leads to the development of hammertoe deformity.

The most commonly seen isolated hammertoe deformities are those of the varus–rotated fifth toe, followed by those of the second toe. The third and fourth digits are also involved with generalized digital contractures, but less so as isolated hammertoes. Hallux hammertoe deformity is less common than deformity of lesser digits, but often presents in association with pes cavus deformities.

BIOMECHANICS

Hammertoes usually begin as flexible deformities and are the expression of periarticular functional imbalance of the extrinsic or intrinsic musculature, or both, inserting into the digits. This can occur in hyperpronation syndromes that alter the biomechanical orientation of the long flexors or that compromise the mechanical advantage of the lumbricales and quadratus plantae.[184] There is a delicate balance between all intrinsic and extrinsic tendon function, with a unique harmony. Any disturbance of this balance ultimately results in deformity. Three main pathomechanical scenarios result in the development of hammertoe syndrome: (1) flexor stabilization in stance phase, (2) extensor substitution in swing phase, and (3) flexor substitution as compensation for weak posterior group musculature.[185] A weak triceps surae can lead to interphalangeal flexion contracture of the toes as a result of extended and excessive phasic activity of the long flexors to assist in heel-off. The associated closed kinetic chain extension at the metatarsophalangeal joints allows for the development of gradual secondary extensor contracture. Acquired or congenital equinus results in compensatory extended and excessive phasic activity of the long extensors during swing phase, to assist in toe clearance.

The concept of flexor and extensor "substitution syndromes" engages and helps initiate the deforming process. With time, shortening and contracture develop at the plantar aspect of the proximal interphalangeal joint, with dorsal contracture of the extensor apparatus at the metatarsophalangeal joint. Valgus foot architecture with midfoot abduction generates flexor stabilization, providing stance-phase advantage of the long flexors over the interossei. The quadratus plantae subsequently loses its ability to rectify the digital alignment in stance phase. There is extension contracture at the metatarsophalangeal joint with flexion contracture at the interphalangeal joint. The progression of deformity from flexible to rigid follows the same general pattern described for the lesser digits.

Hammertoe deformities are more prevalent in persons with long, slender toes as a result of muscular imbalance associated with an increased lever arm that helps maintain contracture, in addition to deformity secondary to lack of toebox room in the shoe. Persistent deformity results in adaptive shortening of the digital neurovascular structures and skin. Gradually, the reducibility of the contracture is lost, and the deformity becomes increasingly rigid.[185]

Hallux hammertoe deformity is encountered most commonly in conjunction with a rigid plantar-flexed first ray, medial cavovarus deformity, or total forefoot equinus deformity. It may coexist with lesser digital deformity.[186]

HAMMERTOE CLASSIFICATION

Various terminologies have been used to define lesser digital deformities.[184] When extensor contracture is present at the metatarsophalangeal joint with flexion contracture of the proximal interphalangeal joint, the term *hammertoe* is most often applied. The distal interphalangeal joint is commonly normal or in hyperextension. When there is normal alignment of the metatarsophalangeal joint and proximal interphalangeal joint with flexion contracture at the distal interphalangeal joint, the term *mallet toe* is used. The term *clawtoe* has been used variably to describe a condition in which there is generalized digital contracture of all the lesser toes or isolated digital contractures of the lesser toes with extensor contracture of the metatarsophalangeal joints and flexion contracture of both the interphalangeal joints.[182,187–189]

Less common are congenital overriding or underriding hammertoes, especially the fifth. Interdigital clavus and "soft corns" in the fourth-fifth toe web space can be very painful and disabling, resulting in recurrent infection. Brachymetarsia of the fourth metatarsal, a congenital malformation, produces a dorsally subluxed fourth toe with plantar cleft. It may coexist with hammertoes of lesser digits. Ilizarov distraction histiogenesis has become the state-of-the-art corrective procedure for this difficult problem.

Lesser digital contractures with lateral and dorsal subluxation of the metatarsophalangeal joints are often seen in conjunction with hallux valgus deformity when the hallux places a lateral subluxating force on the second toe. The alternative deformity of second digital "crossover toe" can develop as well, depending on the anatomic integrity of the flexor plate. The patient's only complaint may be a painful subluxed second toe. Surgical repair might include correction of the hallux valgus if severe enough, in addition to the adjacent hammertoe. The second digital deformity, commonly referred to as "crossover deformity," has generated considerable confusion in the surgical community and requires a different approach for lasting correction.

TREATMENT

When an athlete initially presents with complaints of painful hammertoe deformities, conservative treatment is undertaken. This may include the use of biomechanical orthotic control or shoe modifications or padding when indicated. If the deformity is not severe and still flexible, biomechanical orthotic control can be helpful in controlling digital contracture secondary to excessive pronatory force. Rigid digital contracture with or without painful hyperkeratotic lesions usually requires surgical correction for adequate relief.

Soft Tissue Release and Repair of Lesser Digital Contracture

Reducible mild to moderate flexion contracture at the proximal or distal interphalangeal joint, or both, with a reducible mild extensor contracture at the metatarsophalangeal joint will usually respond to soft tissue releases.[182,187,188] The presence of advanced or nonreducible deformities or marked instability at the metatarsophalangeal joint is a contraindication to soft tissue arthrolysis and an indication for bone procedures. Percutaneous tenotomies and interphalangeal joint capsulotomies may be performed through microincisions using ophthalmic blades for both flexor and extensor mechanisms. The toe may then be manipulated appropriately to reduce contractures. No skin sutures are required, and the postoperative dressings are applied in a splintage manner with corrected alignment. Percutaneous 0.035-inch K-wires may be used to maintain reduction if the deformity is semirigid.

The patient is allowed to ambulate in a wooden postoperative shoe, and the standard postoperative course is followed. Healing is usually quite rapid from this procedure, and athletes typically begin a return-to-activity program 2 to 4 weeks later without fixation and 1 week later if splintage pinning is used. Postoperative orthotic control is indicated, and splinting of the toes in correct alignment during athletic activity for the first 6 to 8 weeks following discontinuance of dressings helps maintain correction and permit proper healing.

Clinical experience with soft tissue correction of hammertoes indicates it has limited long-term success. This is especially so with correction of multiple toes on the same foot. Often in 4 to 5 years, contractures recur secondary to ill-fitting dress shoes or to uncontrollable biomechanical forces, causing recurrent dynamic instability within the toes and metatarsophalangeal joints. The patient should advised of possible recurrence and the need for more extensive surgery later.

Interphalangeal Arthroplasty and Arthrodesis

Arthroplasty of the lesser digital interphalangeal joints is perhaps the most common surgical procedure for correction of rigid hammertoe deformity.[182,187,188] The procedure is performed through two converging longitudinal semi-elliptical incisions or a linear longitudinal approach. Distal mallet toes are best managed with two semi-elliptical transverse incisions that encompass all or part of the associated clavus on the dorsum of the toe. The wedge skin incisions are carefully placed to avoid injury to the peripheral neurovascular bundles (Fig. 26-39). The resulting wedge of skin is then excised, exposing the extensor apparatus underlying the proximal interphalangeal joint. A dorsal transverse arthrotomy is made, entering the distal interphalangeal joint in one deep incision. The head of the proximal phalanx is then freed of soft tissue attachment and resected with an oscillating bone saw. It is essential to remove an appropriate amount of bone to reduce the deformity. Excessive resection can result in a flail toe or even a hyperextension deformity if stance-phase flexor substitution is present and not controlled with an orthotic. Inadequate resection will fail to resolve the deformity.

Proximal interphalangeal arthroplasty can be managed with either two semi-elliptical transverse incisions or a longitudinal midline approach, or even serpentine incisions. This is a matter of surgeon preference. The dissection is

Figure 26-39 Distal interphalangeal mallet toe arthroplasty.

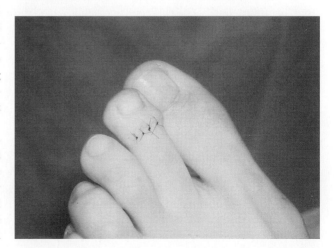

carried deeply to the joint and a transverse arthrotomy performed with delivery of the head of the phalanx into the operative site, freeing periarticular tissue. The bone is resected perpendicular to the long axis of the proximal phalanx. Long flexor tendon anastomosis can be performed on the bottom of the resection site of the proximal phalanx for a tenodesis effect to allow greater flexor stabilization postoperatively.[190,191] A small drill hole with osteosuture may be required for this maneuver.

Arthrodesis is performed through the same skin approaches. The opposing sides of the deformed joint are resected with an oscillating bone saw to achieve smooth cancellous "tabletop" surfaces for approximation. V preparation of the fusion surfaces can also be used, invaginating the proximal phalanx into the companion middle phalanx defect. This is a modification of the peg-in-hole technique.[192] Fixation is usually with a 0.045-inch K-wire, but resorbable medullary pins can also be used.[193] Peg-in-hole fusion is also an excellent technique and can be performed with the advantage of more stability with a higher rate of fusion. K-wire fixation is necessary as well for this modification. Metatarsophalangeal joint arthrolysis is performed with release of the plantar plate using a McGlamry elevator to complete the joint release. The ray site may be further stabilized by delivering the pin across the metatarsophalangeal joint and maintaining pinning for 3 to 4 weeks. Transmetatarsal fixation requires rigid surgical shoe splintage for the entire period of time; otherwise the pin can break at the metatarsal joint, making retrieval very difficult. The pin can be buried distally for simple removal under local anesthesia or left external, with daily pin care. Redundant extensor tendon is resected and then repaired with 4-0 absorbable suture. Skin is approximated with 5-0 nylon. Casting is usually not required for lesser digial fusions or arthroplastic repairs. Protective splinting of the toes with the use of 1/4-inch athletic tape may be used for an additional 4 to 6 weeks after removal of the pins, with gradual return-to-activity program. Recovery is usually uneventful. Orthotics are used postoperatively when indicated.

INTERDIGITAL CLAVUS

This is a very painful impingement syndrome often encountered in athletes and most common in the fourth web space. Juxtapositioning of the head of the fifth proximal phalanx and the lateral condyle of the base of the fourth toe produces this painful condition. A burning bursitis is often present as well. Symptomatic management involves padding and occasional short-acting intrabursal steroid injections for the competitive athlete. If the condition is persistent, only surgical arthroplasty at the head of the proximal phalanx of the fifth toe and lateral condylectomy of the base of the fourth toe will resolve the condition permanently.[194] Minimal incision ostectomy of a discrete focused clavus bone impingement can be considered if it does not extend around the entire web space. When a bone impingement clavus forms at the medial or lateral metaphyseal expansions in other digits, it is managed with selective ostectomy, either percutaneously or with a small incisional open resection. The distal lateral aspect of the fifth toe is a common location for this form of impingement, and simple ostectomy is very effective. This results in very rapid recovery for an athlete. If the lesion is web positioned, the more involved procedure is necessary, usually on adjacent sides of the lesion and associated phalangeal segments, for permanent resolution.

SEVERE LESSER DIGITAL DEFORMITY WITH DORSAL METATARSAL LUXATION

Severe lesser digital contracture can occur with complete dorsal subluxation of the metatarsophalangeal joint and a dorsal pseudofacet on the metatarsal head.[187,188] At times, the dorsal subluxation may be partial and reducible passively. This provides a good indication for selective Jones suspension of a lesser metatarsal in conjunction with the digital repair or fusion. The associated metatarsal head may be depressed with a plantar keratoma. A rigid dorsal luxation deformity with pseudofacet is uncommon in the active athletic population but can develop. It occurs almost exclusively at the second metatarsal–phalangeal joint and to a lesser degree the third and fourth.

Surgical correction is focused at reducing the digital and metatarsophalangeal joint contracture with preservation of the weight-bearing function of the metatarsal. This can be accomplished by reducing the length pattern of the ray starting within the deformed digit and progressing proximally. A progressive release will ultimately define what is required for total reduction. Digital fusion is usually necessary, followed by proximal soft tissue arthrolysis at the metatarsophalangeal joint. The best option at this point is either a partial metatarsal head arthroplasty with transmetatarsal fixation or shortening osteoplasty of the metatarsal bone to gain further relaxation within the ray. If dorsal luxation has been present for an extended period of time, degenerative arthrosis will be present and partial head arthroplasty would be indicated. Shortening osteoplasty can be accomplished most precisely and easily with the modification described by Lauf using a dorsal offset V neck osteotomy and small bone osteosynthesis 2.0-mm screws.[195] The distal Z step-down osteotomy can work nicely as well, fixated with two 2.0-mm screws. Postoperative care follows the protocol for metatarsal osteotomy, with protected weight bearing the first 4 weeks followed by physical therapy and gradual return to activity.

HALLUX HAMMERTOE DEFORMITY

Isolated flexion contracture at the hallux interphalangeal joint is encountered occasionally and is more frequently found in association with pes cavus.[186,196] Marked contracture of the extensor hallucis longus tendon produces bowing prominently viewed at the dorsal aspect of the metatarsophalangeal joint. This is a form of extensor substitution that often makes the deformity progressive. Radiographs are taken to rule out arthritis at the first metatarsal–phalangeal joint and to evaluate the flexion contracture at the interphalangeal joint. The reducibility of the deformity at both the interphalangeal and metatarsophalangeal joint must be made to determine the most effective treatment.

This deformity can be encountered following excision of both hallucial sesamoids and with injudicious elongation of the extensor hallucis long tendon during hallux valgus surgery. It also occurs following Akin osteotomies that gap at the plantar aspect and heal in malunion.

Compression Interphalangeal Fusion With Jones Suspension

Arthrodesis of the hallux interphalangeal joint can be accomplished with a variety of skin approaches. Semi-elliptical transverse provides good exposure if there is no ancillary surgery required at the metatarsophalangeal level. Otherwise, a lazy-S or Z incision with the transverse leg across the joint will work well also. A direct midline longitudinal incision provides more generous access to the associated companion deformity at the metatarsophalangeal joint, however, and is the most commonly indicated approach. A power oscillating bone saw is used for joint resection adequate to correct the deformity. All articular cartilage and subchondral bone on either side of the joint are removed and mechanical alignment achieved to determine reduction and correction. Associated transverse plane deformity can be resolved at the same time with the appropriate wedge resection at the fusion site. Osteosynthesis is best accomplished with regular or cannulated 4.0-or 3.5-

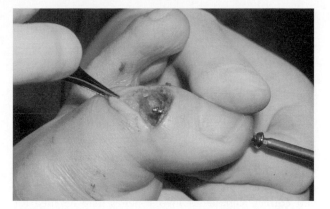

Figure 26–40 Hallux interphalangeal compression arthrodesis with lag screw fixation.

mm lag screws (Fig. 26-40); the threads should engage the dense bone near the phalangeal base if possible. Cannulation systems are much easier, and often no overdrilling is necessary. Tapping the proximal phalanx is not recommended. The alignment is checked and final compression delivered, taking care to evaluate axial rotation of the digit. If imbalance and flexible deformity remain at the metatarsophalangeal joint, then the extensor tendon is stripped proximally and mobilized and a Jones suspension performed, passing the long extensor through a trephine hole in the metatarsal head. The longitudinal incision easily allows this common adjunctive procedure. After the Jones suspension and hallux fusion, the ray segment should lie flat upon plantar loading (pushup test).[187] Closure is usually in two layers with suture of choice.

It is necessary to evaluate the metatarsophalangeal joint to be certain screw penetration has not occurred. Imaging or radiography must be done if there is doubt. A rigid cast shoe or boot will be satisfactory, or a cast brace can also be used for 4 weeks. If the screw head is prominent later following consolidation, simple retrieval is performed in the office.

Hallux Arthroplasty

In pediatric athletes with open epiphyses, hallux hammertoe may be treated by a simple arthroplastic procedure. The head of the proximal phalanx of the great toe is resected with an oscillating bone saw. The toe is then reduced in anatomic position and the long flexor tendon anastomosed to the distal resection stump by osteosuture and drill holes. This produces good flexor stabilization to prevent recurrence. Further stabilization of the site is achieved with a 0.045-inch K-wire in axial fashion. Associated contracture at the metatarsophalangeal joint is managed with dorsal capsulotomy and Jones extensor tendon suspension through the metatarsal neck. If Jones suspension has been performed, casting for 4 weeks is maintained.

Hallux hammertoe in conjunction with an arthritic first metatarsal–phalangeal joint may be treated by a combination of a Keller or Valente resection arthroplasty followed by manual reduction of the hallux hammertoe with fixation using a 0.062-inch K-wire through the interphalangeal joint and across the metatarsophalangeal joint to maintain correct alignment. Two K-wires may be used for additional correction and to prevent rotatory instability at the metatarsophalangeal joint. These pins are left intact for 4 weeks. Adjunct soft tissue lengthening procedures are used as necessary.

Lesser Metatarsal Deformities

Common lesser metatarsal deformities in the athlete occur in the central second through fourth metatarsals; splayed fifth metatarsals also occur. A plantar-flexed lesser metatarsal results in a painful hyperkeratotic plantar skin lesion and often accompanies a digital contracture or hammertoe. The first and fifth metatarsals display the greatest amount of intrinsic triplane motion, with the second metatarsal demonstrating the most rigid position, making it least adaptable to biomechanical changes in the engineering function of the foot. It is important to differentiate a plantar keratoma beneath the second metatarsal head secondary to a plantar-flexed second metatarsal from a similar lesion secondary to an elevated or hypermobile first metatarsal. A relatively long lesser metatarsal can also result in a similar lesion, commonly referred to as a propulsive-phase lesion.

The patient may present with a severe intractable plantar keratoma beneath a lesser metatarsal with obvious flexion prominence detectable by palpation and visual examination. Keratoma lesions occur between adjacent metatarsals at times, making identification of the culprit segment difficult. Careful examination, axial metatarsal head radiographs, and thorough gait assessment can ultimately define which metatarsal is contributory. This problem is often encountered in a very mobile splay foot deformity in which the metatarsals have transverse plane as well as a fore-and-aft excursion beneath the surface of the skin with loading. A weight-bearing 90-degree AP radiograph, using a lesion marker with the patient's shoes on, may define the

involved metatarsal. A sub–fifth metatarsal head keratoma may be secondary to a plantar-flexed fifth metatarsal and forefoot varus deformity, rearfoot varus deformity, ankle varus, or tibial varum. Global multiple hyperkeratotic lesions beneath the lesser metatarsal heads may be companion expressions of pes cavus or gastrocnemius–soleus or ankle equinus. Atrophy of the plantar fat pad in the older athlete can also result in this type of painful lesion. A hyperkeratotic lesion on the lateral aspect of the fifth metatarsal head (tailor's bunion) may be secondary to a lateral prominent fifth metatarsal head or to splaying of the fifth metatarsal segment and high fourth and fifth intermetatarsal angle. This deformity can cause considerable problems in rigid confining boots, athletic shoe gear, or ski boots. A hypertrophic fifth metatarsal styloid process can cause similar symptoms and pain.

LESSER METATARSAL OSTEOTOMIES

Distal Metatarsal Osteotomy

Surgical treatment of a plantar-flexed or elongated lesser metatarsal is achieved through a variety distal metaphyseal osteotomies. More thorough understanding of forefoot biomechanics and improved osteosynthesis technology has provided surgeons with better and more reliable choices for osteotomy. Careful preoperative evaluation and execution is crucial to the success of these procedures.[197] The most common osteotomies are (1) dorsal transverse or V osteotomy through and through; (2) tilt-up neck osteotomies with dorsal base wedges that are oriented transverse to the bone; (3) oblique dorsal wedges extending distal dorsal with a plantar proximal apex; (4) asymmetric V osteotomy allowing dorsal rotation, shortening, or both; and (5) sagittal Z osteotomy for rotation or step-down shortening.

These operations are all approached dorsally over the metatarsal neck with an incision about 3 cm in length. If side-by-side double metatarsal osteotomy is to be performed, the approach should be positioned between the two metatarsal necks and shafts and slightly longer. Dissection is carried directly to the neck of the metatarsal, protecting the extensor tendon, and subperiosteal dissection is carried out. Bone stripping is kept to a minimum and done only to the extent required to execute the osteotomy and fixation. Transverse through-and-through osteotomy, known as a percutaneous metaphyseal osteotomy, is the most original and involves simple transection of the neck transversely with a bone saw or forceps. V osteotomy, still probably the most common distal metatarsal osteotomy, has a distal apex just behind the region of the plantar condyles. This can be modified to resect a wedge and transform the procedure into a tilt-up procedure with a V orientation or even a V shortening full-thickness wedge resection. Fixation in the past was not common; however, osteosynthesis has evolved to the point that it has also become common but not mandatory, depending on the situation.

Tilt-up wedge osteotomies are done with a bone saw, removing perhaps 1 to 2 mm of bone dorsally and fixing the site with box wire or a K-wire. The oblique wedge osteotomy requires fixation; and a 2.0-mm screw is effective for this procedure. Countersinking is required to avoid shattering the dorsal cortex and loosing compression. Asymmetric V dorsal osteotomy is through and through but involves small section removal from the short "asymmetric leg" distally to allow proximal shortening. Two small screws, usually 2.0 mm, are used in the second metatarsal and perhaps two 1.5-mm screws in the third through fifth metatarsals. K-wires are alternative fixatives; either buried and cut flush with the bone or percutaneous. Threaded pins can be used for these procedures and buried. Z osteotomy requires a midline longitudinal bone incision and two subsequent exit incisions at either end of the longitudinal cut. Sections of bone can be removed at either end for shortening. Alternatively, this osteotomy can be rotated for either plantar flexion or dorsiflexion. Interfragmentary small bone screw fixation is required—usually two 2.0-mm screws. Excessive elevation or shortening of the metatarsal may result in transfer lesions to adjacent metatarsals; therefore, elevation and shortening must be carefully assessed.[187,188] If two metatarsals are clinically prominent with only one painful plantar lesion, consideration should focus on double osteotomy, or even selective plantar condylectomy, to prevent transfer stress and metatarsalgia.

Guarded weight bearing is permitted in a postoperative shoe or cast brace. Union is normally uneventful. If percutaneous fixation was used, the K-wire is removed 4 weeks postoperatively. A gradual return-to-activity program is undertaken with physiotherapy. Postoperative orthotics are used when indicated.

Metatarsal Base Osteotomy

Proximal osteotomy is uncommonly performed in the athlete because distal osteotomy has more rapid recovery and is more versatile in addressing the various biomechanical problems of the forefoot. Metatarsal base osteotomy is indicated in athletes who manifest global forefoot equinus and cavus foot problems with a Lisfranc apex of deformity. The osteotomies can be singular or multiple, as in the forefoot, and can take the form of dorsal transverse wedge osteotomy or dorsal oblique A-O–type osteotomy with a plantar apex. These osteotomies all require osteosynthesis, usually with K-wires or small screws as well. Recovery is longer and complications of transfer lesions can be higher because of the longer lever arm, so careful patient selection is the key to success if proximal osteotomy is selected over a distal procedure. Casting is recommended for about 3 to 4 weeks and return to activity is prolonged up to 7 to 8 weeks with this operation. Orthotics are used as necessary to control associated problems and imbalances.

PLANTAR CONDYLECTOMY

Athletes with isolated painful plantar keratomas under the metatarsals without excessive length respond well to plantar condylectomy. This under utilized procedure does not alter the length of the metatarsal and has less chance of transfer lesions with much more rapid recovery.[198] Plantar condylectomy is preferred with singular metatarsalgia in association with clinical prominence on either side of the involved metatarsal. The transfer lesions move laterally, and therefore the most favorable sites for this procedure are the second and third metatarsals; however, it can be effectively performed on the fourth metatarsal as well. Athletes with atrophic plantar fat pads form another class of candidates for this procedure.

A dorsal longitudinal skin incision is made over the involved metatarsophalangeal joint. The approach is carried deeply, protecting the extensor tendons, and proceeds to the dorsal capsule, which is incised longitudinally. A self-retaining retractor is helpful in spreading the tissue. The metatarsal head is mobilized by releasing the collateral ligaments, and a McGlamry elevator is introduced under the metatarsal head, releasing the plantar plate. An osteotome or sagittal bone saw is used to resect the bottom third of the metatarsal head that contains the condyle. The osteotome or elevator is delivered proximally and the instrument lifted dorsally, extruding the resected condyle from the wound depth. Care is taken to protect the dorsal articular surface; the McGlamry elevator accomplishes this maneuver well.[198] Closure is in layers. Clinical reduction of the plantar prominence is apparent immediately. Postsurgical care is immediate weight bearing in a surgical shoe and return to regular shoes in about 2 weeks. Return to running and athletics, at about 3 to 4 weeks, is more rapid than with most other bone surgical procedures on the foot.

CROSSOVER SECOND TOE DEFORMITY

Crossover deformity has become more recognized as a distinct entity in the past several years. It is characterized by adduction deformity of the second toe and abduction of the third toe; this results in a spreading syndrome in stance. It can occur in the absence of hallux valgus but often presents as a companion deformity as well. It produces a painful hammertoe—usually the second digit. Often the toe will lie on top of the hallux. This can be particularly troublesome for an athlete. The biomechanics and etiology of this condition are poorly understood but believed to be dysfunction of the metatarsal plantar plate with long flexor malalignment, often associated with trauma or degenerative or inflammatory joint disease causing imbalance of the intrinsic musculature periarticularly at the metatarsophalangeal joint.[197,199–202]

Soft tissue operations are described but do not hold up well, especially in severe deformities with juxtapositioned second and third metatarsal heads. This deformity requires a medialization osteotomy of the second metatarsal head as well as soft tissue release at the medial aspect of the metatarsophalangeal joint. Osteosynthesis is necessary and can be achieved with a 2.0-mm screw, small L plate, or K-wires. The osteotomy can be transverse behind the plantar condyles, with simple medial displacement, or oblique from distal dorsal to plantar proximal, also with medial displacement.[197] Thin metatarsal neck anatomy sometimes makes it easier to perform the osteotomy at the base, with a long oblique wedge removed medially. The apex of this osteotomy is entirely metaphyseal, at the proximal lateral corner of the base, directed distal medial. Adequate wedge resection must be accomplished for transverse plane medialization of the metatarsal. All of these osteotomies centralize the dysfunctional flexor mechanism, restoring the dynamic balance around the joint. Fixation is easier in this region because of a longer osteotomy surface available for delivery of two 2.0-mm screws.

Cast bracing is recommended for 3 to 4 weeks with these osteotomies. The customary return-to-activity schedule is undertaken with appropriate therapy individualized. A digital fusion might be necessary within the toe itself if a rigid deformity is manifest. Otherwise, soft tissue release along the metatarsophalangeal joint might suffice, along with a metatarsal osteotomy, either distal or proximal.

FIFTH METATARSAL DEFORMITIES

The axis of the fifth metatarsal runs in a plantar-proximal-lateral to dorsal-distal-medial direction, allowing for eversion and abduction with dorsiflexion and inversion and adduction with plantar flexion. This is a pronation and supination axis. The so-called bowed fifth metatarsal is actually a pronated fifth metatarsal. It results in the clinical entity of tailor's bunion.[203] The apparent lateral bowing or concavity is a radiographic positional observation secondary to eversion and abduction of the ray.[204] The amount of splaying of the fifth metatarsal may be mild or severe and is defined by the lateral deviation angle. It is also assessed by the fourth intermetatarsal angle and the space between the fourth and fifth metatarsal heads.[204–207]

Symptomatic lesions typically associated with abnormal fifth metatarsal biomechanics may be plantar, lateral, or plantar lateral. The most common sites are plantar lateral and lateral with the tailor's bunion deformity. Painful adventitious bursas can form at these sites. Osteotomies designed to correct these sites depend on the biomechanical expression of the deformity.

Tailor's Bunion and Plantar Keratoma Neck Osteotomies

Severity of deformity with bowing and rotation determines whether or not a distal osteotomy will be effective in reducing the deformity of tailor's bunion. It is important to evaluate whether adequate reduction of the fifth metatarsal deformity can be achieved with a distal osteotomy.[203] Factors to be considered are the transverse plane separation of the fourth and fifth metatarsal heads, the width of the distal metaphysis of the fifth metatarsal, and the level at which deviation deformity of the metatarsal is greatest. If satisfactory reapproximation of the fourth and fifth metatarsals cannot be achieved with a distal osteotomy while allowing for adequate bone contact at the osteotomy site, attention must be focused proximally in the metaphysis.

Mild splaying of the fifth metatarsal demonstrating a low lateral metatarsal deviation angle can be resolved with an oblique sliding osteotomy at the neck,[208] approached through a dorsolateral incision. Other osteotomies for consideration are the transverse V[209] medial closing wedge and Hohmann displacement type.[203,210] The incision is centered over the dorsolateral aspect of the fifth metatarsal neck and carefully deepened down to the level of the metatarsal. Care is taken to avoid the lateral dorsal cutaneous nerve. The fourth dorsal interosseous muscle is usually encountered in the fourth interspace, and the distal aspect of the abductor digiti quinti is usually encountered laterally. Subperiosteal dissection is used to expose the bone in the vicinity of the osteotomy. An oscillating bone saw is used to create an oblique through-and-through osteotomy directed distal laterally to medial proximally. "Medialization" is accomplished and the lateral prominence remaining on the proximal side of the osteotomy remodeled. The osteotomy may be fixed using a 0.062-inch K-wire or a 2.0-mm screw delivered proximal laterally to distal medially into the displaced fragment.[211] (Fig. 26-41). The obliquity of the osteotomy facilitates internal fixation. A plantar keratoma can be addressed with the same osteotomy, incorporating slight elevation and fixation with a K-wire or small screw, without lateral transposition of the fifth metatarsal head. A dorsal V osteotomy also works well for this, with or without fixation. The wound is then closed in layers.

Ambulation is allowed in a wooden postoperative surgical shoe or plaster or fiberglass foot cast. Pin fixation is

Figure 26-41 Sliding "Sponsel" oblique neck osteotomy with medialization and 2.0-mm screw fixation.

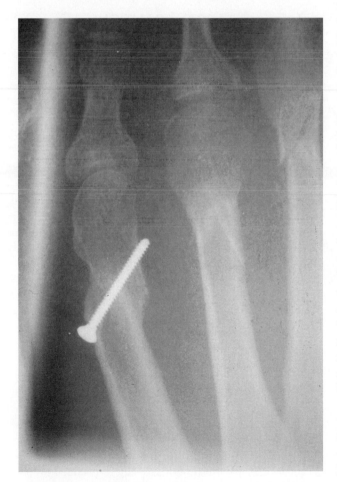

removed 4 to 6 weeks postoperatively following radiographic evidence of progression of union. At this point, a return-to-activity program is begun. Postoperative physiotherapy may be begun 7 to 9 days after surgery if necessary, and postoperative orthotics are used when indicated. Healing is usually uneventful. The lesion responds well to such surgical correction.

Base Wedge Osteotomy of the Fifth Metatarsal

When a painful tailor's bunion deformity is associated with more significant splaying of the fifth metatarsal, a proximal base wedge osteotomy is necessary.[203] The fifth metatarsal base is approached through a dorsolateral longitudinal incision, approximately 3.5 to 4 cm in length and centered over the proximal metaphysis. The insertion of the peroneus tertius will be identified as the surgical site is deepened, and its broad, fan-shaped aponeurosis is reflected laterally. The placement of the osteotomy depends on the location of the skin lesion. Tailor's bunion with no plantar lesion is managed with a transverse plane reduction of the intermetatarsal angle. This may be achieved with an obliquely placed medial closing basal wedge osteotomy, preserving a vertical lateral cortical hinge fixed with K wires or small screws. In order to produce purely transverse plane excursion of the fifth metatarsal, the apex must be perpendicular to the weight-bearing surface with the foot in a loaded position.

With a power oscillating bone saw, a dorsal-to-plantar osteotomy is then performed and then the fifth metatarsal proximal metaphysis is directed obliquely from proximal lateral to distal medial. An appropriately sized long oblique wedge of bone is removed, and the axis K-wire removed. The osteotomy is then manually reduced and the correction of the deformity assessed. Additional passes of the saw blade may be used to feather the site if necessary. Reduction of the osteotomy may be maintained with a bone clamp, and osteosynthesis performed as noted earlier. The wedge can be modified in orientation to accommodate some sagittal plane correction as well if there is a concurrent plantar keratoma with the tailor's bunion. If K-wires are used, they are retrieved at 3 to 4 weeks; they can also be buried, cut flush with the bone, and left in situ.

Ambulation is permitted in a below-knee fiberglass walking cast or removable cast brace. Therapy can begin at 7 to 9 days postoperatively if the brace is used or the cast bivalved. Immobilization is discontinued 6 weeks postoperatively following radiographic evidence of progression to union. Following final cast removal, a progressive return-to-activity program is begun. Postoperative orthotics are used when indicated. If necessary, internal screw fixation may be removed at a later date through a small percutaneous incision.

Fifth Metatarsal "Bunionette" Ostectomy

An athlete may present with a painful hyperkeratotic lesion or inflamed adventitious bursa, or both, overlying the lateral aspect of the fifth metatarsal head in the absence of a lateral displacement or deviation of the fifth metatarsal. This may be secondary to a prominent or hypertrophied fifth metatarsal head or base of the fifth proximal phalanx. This situation usually presents a problem in athletes who must wear very rigid, nonyielding athletic foot gear, such as ski boots or cycling shoes. It may also result in a painful lesion or adventitious bursitis overlying a prominent or enlarged styloid process of the fifth metatarsal. Such deformities may require surgical intervention to reduce the bony prominence, allowing for foot gear to be worn without ensuing pain or disability.

A partial ostectomy of the fifth metatarsal head is approached through a dorsolateral longitudinal incision centered over the bony prominence. The incision is deepened through the subcutaneous tissues, and the capsular tissues of the fifth metatarsal–phalangeal joint are identified. The lateral cutaneous nerves are avoided. Dissection is continued in the plane between the capsule and subcutaneous tissue laterally. A dorsolateral linear longitudinal capsular incision is formed, and capsular structures are reflected off the lateral aspect of the fifth metatarsal head. The lateral prominence of the fifth metatarsal head is resected with an oscillating saw. An associated prominence at the lateral aspect of the base of the proximal phalangeal flare is resected in similar fashion if problematic. Layered closure is performed and a postoperative compression dressing is applied. The patient is allowed ambulation in a postoperative surgical shoe. A standard postoperative course is followed, with physiotherapy as necessary. A progressive return-to-activity program is begun approximately 3 weeks postoperatively.

Reduction of Hypertrophic Styloid Process of the Fifth Metatarsal

Partial ostectomy of the styloid process of the fifth metatarsal is indicated for painful chronic impingement with bursitis, unresponsive to padding and shoe gear modifica-

tions. Ostectomy is managed with a linear longitudinal dorsolateral incision overlying the styloid process. The incision is carefully deepened through the subcutaneous tissues, avoiding the lateral dorsal cutaneous nerve or associated tendon insertions in the region. The prominent lateral aspect of the styloid process is identified and resection performed following subperiosteal dissection. An oscillating bone saw or a crescentic oscillating saw blade works well, allowing the surgeon to "scoop out" the prominent portion of symptomatic bone. If any tendon attachment is avulsed during the resection, simple osteosuture is employed to reattach it. The surgeon needs to observe minimal resection to avoid weakening the "Jones juncture," which could predispose to a pathologic fracture later. The patient is allowed ambulation in a wooden-soled postoperative shoe, and a standard postoperative course is followed. Healing is normally uneventful, and a return-to-activity program is normally begun 3 weeks postoperatively.

TARSAL COALITION

Tarsal coalition occurs in the athletic population with the same frequency as in the nonathletic population: 0.5 to 1 percent. Diagnosis of this condition often occurs earlier in athletes, particularly ballet dancers, because of the mechanical demands imposed on their tarsal complex.[212] The condition is characterized by a lack of segmentation between two normally distinct and separate tarsal bones during mesenchymal differentiation. Tarsal coalition can be characterized as a complete osseous bridge, known as a synostosis or a partial or incomplete coalition, characterized by a fibrous or cartilaginous union[213] termed *syndesmosis* and *synchondrosis,* respectively. Coalition results in limitation of joint motion with subsequent dysfunction at the subtalar or midtarsal joint complex.[214,215] The limitation of motion is more pronounced with a synostosis compared to a flexible syndesmosis. Progression of the ossifying process can occur from a partial syndesmotic coalition to a synostosis, with progressive decrease in range of motion and, most notably, regional pain sometimes extending into the leg.[216]

Functional mechanical demands on the foot and ankle in the presence of tarsal coalition often result in pain in the peritalar joints. The classic location of the pain, however, is in the sinus tarsi, resulting in the clinical syndrome of sinus tarsitis, and also medially, in particular with medial facet bridging. Peroneal musculature splinting can occur in an effort to limit painful motion, usually in maximal pronation, and is present about 29 percent of the time. This splinting mechanism has been termed peroneal spastic flatfoot.[217] Tarsal tunnel syndrome is present with medial coalitions about 24 percent of the time.[216] Chronic tarsal joint dsyfunction usually results in progressive degenerative joint changes, especially at the talonavicular and subtalar joints.[218] Ultimately, coalitions can lead to a pan-arthrodial ball-and-socket ankle joint as a form of compensation for loss of tarsal joint motion. This problem is typically asymptomatic.[219]

Anatomic Sites of Coalition

The most commonly diagnosed tarsal coalition is the calcaneonavicular bar. Medial talocalcaneal coalition is diagnosed to a lesser degree, in particular the isolated medial facet lesion. Interestingly, the talocalcaneal coalition has a slightly higher statistical occurrence rate of about 48 percent, compared to 43.6 percent for the talocalcaneal coalition.[220] This is due largely to the higher index of difficulty in diagnosing the talocalcaneal coalition, which often requires more sophisticated imaging, such as CT or MRI (Fig. 26-42). Calcaneonavicular coalition is easy to detect on standard radiographic views, especially the lateral oblique.[221] Even partially ossified calcaneonavicular bridges can be suggested with standard films. Other coalitions, such as the talonavicular and calcaneocuboid, are quite rare and usually are not as symptomatic as the talocalcaneal or calcaneonavicular bars.[222]

The calcaneonavicular coalition extends from the anterior beak region of the os calcis to the lateral extent of the

Figure 26-42 Talocalcaneal coalition viewed by frontal plane CT scan.

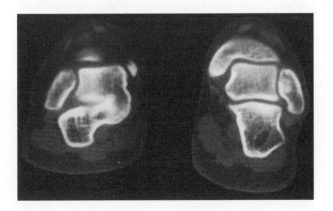

navicular, giving rise to the so-called anteater nose on lateral view x-rays. It is usually the full thickness from top to bottom on the lateral navicular aspect. It is not uncommon to have a small fibrous union component in the midarea, with the remaining mass well ossified. This behaves identically to a full ossified bar, however. The talocalcaneal bridges are most common at the medial sustentacular facet, but also develop through the entire posterior facet, the most posterior aspect of the posterior facet around the posterior process, and, even more rarely, the anterior facet. The medial sustentacular bars can often be palpated at examination and can give rise to clinical tarsal tunnel syndrome as part of the symptom complex. Tarsal tunnel syndrome might even be the first symptom of the lesion. This can be misinterpreted in the athlete as an overuse syndrome.

The condition is bilateral about 50 percent of the time, with equal male–female distribution. Pain, rigid flatfoot deformity, and subsequent talar beaking are common findings in this condition. It is genetically predetermined as an autosomal unifactoral disorder.[223]

Acquired coalitions can be post-traumatic, particularly in the subtalar joint, with arthrofibrosis resultant from calcaneal fracture. Calcaneonavicular synfibrosis can occur secondary to a midtarsal joint injury. These are uncommon occurrences but must be assessed in cases of occult peritalar pain with symptoms discussed earlier.

Diagnosis

The patient usually presents with a history of pain in the foot or ankle with swelling, limitation of motion, or both. A history of ankle sprains or some other minor injury event may be present. Motion of the major tarsal complex is limited and painful during examination. Often there is point tenderness to palpation in the region of the sinus tarsi, especially in the presence of a calcaneonavicular bar or medially over a sustentacular bar, occasionally with signs of tarsal tunnel syndrome.[216] The peroneal musculature may be in spasm, with a taut bowing of the peroneal tendons visible on the lateral aspect of the foot and ankle about 30 percent of the time. The foot usually appears quite pronated in gait and a limp may be present. Valgus deformity does not necessarily occur in tarsal coalition, although it is very common. There are some coalition cases reported in pes cavus and clubfoot, although rarely.[224,225]

Imaging studies progress from standard conventional for calcaneonavicular bars to special radiographic views such as the posterior axial tangential ski jump views of Harris and Beath for talocalcaneal bars. Calcaneonavicular coalitions are best imaged on the lateral oblique and lateral views. Talocalcaneal bars are evaluated by lateral and axial views. Lateral radiographs demonstrate several characteristic changes, such as talar beaking or "anteater nose" on the front of the os calcis, especially in calcaneonavicular coalitions. CT evaluation is the gold standard for mature coalitions and MRI for juvenile developing lesions prior to radiographic markers. Thus diagnosis is by combined clinical examination and imaging studies.

Conservative Treatment

Treatment will depend on the age of encounter, severity of symptoms, and desired athletic performance level. Conservative management is always initiated using physical therapy, including gentle range-of-motion attempts, local anesthetic and corticosteroid combination injections, oral anti-inflammatory agents, and orthotics. Following injections, some improvement of symptoms can be obtained with below-knee casting or cast bracing for 6 weeks, especially if peroneal reflex spasm is present. Manipulation is not recommended and may disrupt the coalition site, further aggravating the problem.[226]

When conservative treatment has failed to alleviate symptoms, or the deformity interferes with athletic performance, surgery can be considered. Surgical concepts for tarsal coalition have been evolving, and a variety of approaches are available, depending on the clinical situation and radiographic presentation.

Operative Techniques

Operative treatment of tarsal coalition is undertaken in response to pain and interference with performance.[227] The type of operation will further depend on the type of coalition, age of encounter, and the character of the coalition. Resection of the coalition can be considered in younger age groups up to 14 years, particularly if there are no secondary radiographic arthritic changes in the subtalar or midtarsal joint complex. Cartilaginous bars with no other articular changes are best suited for resections. Younger is better insofar as age at resection is concerned. The exception is a total posterior facet coalitions these, if painful, will require completion of the subtalar fusion if not already complete or triple arthrodesis if more distal midfoot pain presents. Isolated medial facet sustentacular bars in young patients can be excised with a subtalar joint arthroplasty. Anterior facet and extreme posterior bridge bars can likewise be excised with a form of arthroplasty.[228]

Few patients have normal function after coalition resection, and most retain some degree of gait abnormality, pain, and deformity. Excision of a cartilaginous calcaneonavicular midtarsal bar carries a better prognosis than does excision of a subtalar coalition because it is primarily extra-articular. Most juvenile coalition resection patients will have improved function and improved performance, but few have total relief of their symptoms or resolution of any pre-existing deformity. Clearly, the younger resection patients perform better than older patients, because of intervening development of compensatory arthrosis. Adolescent athletes can do quite well with resection if operation is performed early. Most can return to competitive performance.[229,230]

CALCANEONAVICULAR COALITION RESECTION—BADGLEY INTERPOSITION ARTHROPLASTY

Midfoot calcaneonavicular coalition is best approached via the lateral oblique Ollier sinus tarsi incision, 5 cm in length, protecting the intermediate dorsal cutaneous nerve at the superior extent of the incision and the peroneal tendons and sural nerve at the inferior portion.[231] The inferior extensor retinaculum is then incised and the origin of the extensor digitorus brevis muscle belly reflected off the floor of the os calcis and sinus tarsi, creating a distally based flap. A periosteal elevator facilitates complete exposure of the bar. Following complete definition, double osteotomy is performed.[231,232] Care is exercised to avoid damage to the lateral talar head or the calcaneocuboid joint. Sufficient bone or chondral tissue is resected to permit freer movement of the tarsal complex. The void is filled with the mobilized proximal portion of the extensor digitorum brevis muscle, maintained by resorbable pullout suture in the arch. This is the classic Badgley extensor digitorum brevis interposition arthroplasty operation.[232] When excising the coalition, it is important to resect adequate bone plantar medially and not merely create a dorsal lateral wedge with a plantar medial apex.[227] The wound is then closed in layers, and a Jones compression dressing with a posterior molded splint is applied.

Between 5 and 9 days postoperatively, physiotherapy may be initiated, including aggressive range-of-motion exercises, and ambulation is allowed in a postoperative wooden-soled shoe. A standard postoperative course is followed, using a progressive return-to-activity program 3 to

4 weeks postoperatively and orthotic control as needed. Athletes have responded very well to this operation when done early.

MEDIAL AND POSTERIOR TALOCALCANEAL COALITION RESECTION

Resection of the medial talocalcaneal coalition is performed under general anesthesia in the supine position, with a thigh tourniquet for hemostasis. Tarsal coalition is approached through a posteromedial inferior curvilinear incision about 6 cm in length, extending from just behind the medial malleolus distally to the level of the talar head. The incision is carefully deepened down to the level of the deep fascia and laciniate ligament, which is incised, and the tarsal tunnel is entered, protecting the neurovascular structures. This exposure allows a good view of the medial aspect of the subtalar joint and the coalition, which is readily identifiable, or the back of the posterior facet region if involved. The coalition is assessed and the extent of the required resection evaluated.

The coalition is resected with an oscillating bone saw or osteotome to permit free range of motion of the subtalar joint. When resecting sustentacular coalitions, the bottom side of the middle sustentacular facet is preserved as best as possible to maintain a supporting surface of the calcaneus. Preserving the sustentaculum tali prevents dislocation of the contents of the tarsal canal, specifically the flexor hallucis longus tendon, and supplies adequate medial support to the talar head and neck. The coalition is typically present posterior to the spring ligament, which normally does not require detachment. Interposition of tissues or material is not necessary.[216] Occasionally, the extreme posterior corner of the posterior facet will have a coalition. This coalition is more difficult to access and resect, but this can be accomplished if it comprises only a small portion of the back of the facet. CT imaging is necessary for this abnormality.

The contents of the neurovascular bundle are allowed to return to their normal anatomic position. At this time, the tourniquet may be deflated to ensure the viability of the medial neurovascular bundle. All bleeders are carefully ligated with a loose closure, neglecting repair of the laciniate ligament in order to prevent postoperative tarsal tunnel syndrome. A Jones compression dressing is applied with a posterior splint. The patient is allowed ambulation, nonweight bearing, with crutches. Five to 7 days postoperatively, a below-knee removable weight-bearing cast is applied, and physiotherapy may be begun. A standard post-operative course is followed, and aggressive range of motion is encouraged. A progressive return-to-activity program is begun approximately 4 to 8 weeks postoperatively, and orthotic control is used as needed.

Adjunctive Surgery for Tarsal Coalition

Resection of coalition segments can be combined with other operative procedures, most notably calcaneal osteotomies. The most common ancillary procedures are varus-producing heel osteotomies to help realign the weight-bearing trajectory of the hindfoot, ankle, and leg.[102] This can be accomplished with medial tuber displacement osteotomies or open wedge osteotomies (Fig. 26-43) Calcaneal osteotomy can be considered without resection of the coalition as well, to make the patient more comfortable with improved loading. For the athlete, resection of a coalition in the face of structural deformity will not restore alignment, and a concurrent calcaneal varus osteotomy is recommended. Displacement osteotomy requires osteosynthesis and open wedge osteotomy requires a lateral wall wedge bone implant. The decision to perform ancillary calcaneal osteotomy is based on severity of concurrent hindfoot valgus deformity with the coalition.[233] These operations are performed through a lateral wall approach with direct dissection technique to the bone and thick single-layer closure. If pre-existing subtalar joint disease is present, subtalar joint fusion might be a better choice. A talocalcaneal coalition that manifests a significant amount of union may also require completion of the fusion process. If alignment is satisfactory, the surgeon need only complete the

Figure 26-43 Varization heel osteotomy with lateral open wedge osteotomy using lyopholized femur shaft section.

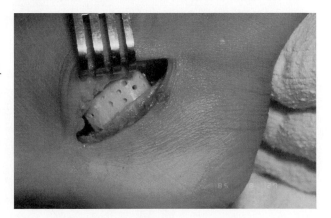

"coalition" into a more solid fusion. If the midtarsal joint is free of radiographic changes, solitary subtalar fusion can be considered. If changes present at the talonavicular joint as well, then triple arthrodesis is the premier salvage procedure.[103,234,235]

OS TRIGONUM/POSTERIOR TALAR SHELF: POSTERIOR IMPINGEMENT SYNDROME OF THE ANKLE

The os trigonum accessory bone at the back of the lateral tubercle of the talus can often become painful in competitive performance athletes, producing a posterior impingement syndrome.[236] The posterior process of the talus normally forms as a secondary center of ossification that fuses to the main body of the talus. This usually occurs by 12 years of age. The posterior process is made up of the medial tubercle and the larger lateral tubercle, which together form a groove for the flexor hallucis longus tendon. At times, the lateral tubercle of the posterior process is quite prominent and subject to injury from sudden violence. A severe plantar-flexion position or force directed to the foot can result in impingement of the lateral process of the posterior tubercle of the talus between the tibia and calcaneus, resulting in fracture.[236–238] In some cases, the secondary center of ossification does not fuse with the main portion of the body of the talus, and the lateral tubercle of the posterior process exists as a separate supernumerary bone known as the os trigonum. This ossicle may participate in a fibrous or cartilaginous union with the main portion of the talus, and therefore is subject to injury, resulting in rupture of the fibrous or fibrocartilaginous union similar to that seen with os tibiale externum. Injury to a prominent posterior talar process or os trigonum may result in subsequent degenerative changes at the posterior subtalar joint line.

The typical clinical presentation is ankle pain localized to the posterior aspect of the joint in the triangle anterior to the Achilles tendon.[238] Swelling may be evident in this region. There is pain with range of motion of the ankle joint. As a result of the close approximation between the posterior process of the talus or the os trigonum, if present, and the tendon of the flexor hallucis longus, passive range of motion of the hallux by the examiner may often reproduce the posterior ankle pain. This is often a very useful diagnostic aid in cases that are suggestive by history and radiographically but that present with more vague clinical features.

Injury to the posterior shelf of the talus may be associated with other injuries to the foot or ankle, such as lateral collateral ligamentous rupture in the case of a plantar flexion–inversion injury or a posterior malleolar fracture in the case of a severe plantar-flexory injury. Flexor hallucis longus tendinitis will often accompany the posterior talar process injury. Ballet dancers who go on full pointe are particularly prone to this type of injury.

Radiographically, a standard lateral projection of the foot may demonstrate frank fracture of the posterior process of the talus. Posterior impingement syndrome may be demonstrated with a maximally plantar-flexed lateral projection radiograph. It may be difficult to differentiate from an os trigonum, although the irregularity of the separation between the fractured process of the talus is often distinct as compared with the smooth cortical surface of the accessory ossicle. Contralateral radiographs may be important to distinguish a fractured posterolateral process of the talus from a normal os trigonum. A true os trigonum, traumatically separated from the main body of the talus, may show no distinct radiographic features. The diagnosis is supported mainly on a clinical basis by history and examination. Radiographs are examined for possible associated osseous injury, and CT is used for more definition as well. Bone scans have limited use and are not ordinarily recommended.

Conservative treatment of injury to the posterior talar shelf or os trigonum may involve the use of cast or posterior splint immobilization with physiotherapy modalities, oral NSAIDs, and steroid injections. In cases resistant to conservative treatment, surgery is required. Any associated injuries are treated as indicated.

Surgical Excision

The traditional approach to the posterior talar shelf has involved the use of a lateral longitudinal linear incision with the patient in a prone position. A medial retromalleolar approach is more direct and affords excellent exposure with reduced likelihood of damage to the flexor hallucis longus tendon or neurovascular bundle.[238] A medial incision is made posterior to the neurovascular bundle and anterior to the Achilles tendon at the medial aspect of the rearfoot. The incision is approximately 3.5 cm in length and is centered over the junction between the posterior talar shelf and the superior surface of the os calcis. This incisional placement avoids damage to the medial neurovascular structures. The incision is carefully deepened, exposing the adipose tissue anterior to the Achilles tendon. The tendon of the flexor hallucis longus is identified at the junction of the posterior talar shelf and the superior surface of the os calcis. The os trigonum or fractured posterolateral process of the talus is located here. The flexor hallucis longus tendon is retracted, exposing the injured posterior talar shelf, allowing for excision of the fragment or accessory ossicle. An osteotome and mallet may be needed to separate the injured fragment or ossicle completely from the main body of the talus. It is retrieved either medially or laterally depending on the surgeon's level of comfort with the procedure. Medial ossicle excision allows direct view of the neurovascular bundle, whereas lateral excision does not. Occasionally there are low muscle fibers coming off the flexor hallucis longus; these must be debrided gently to avoid forced intrusion into the unrelenting fibro-osseous tunnel, causing impingement pain. Fibro-osseous tunnel decompression may be necessary in recalcitrant cases.

The standard postoperative course is followed, using a below-knee Jones compression dressing, which is removed approximately 5 days postoperatively and transformed into a removable cast brace. Rehabilitation is instituted approximately 1 week postoperatively, and the cast brace protection discontinued 3 to 4 weeks postoperatively. A progressive return-to-activity program is initiated.

INJURIES TO THE ANKLE

Anterior Impingement Exostosis of the Ankle

Anterior impingement exostosis of the ankle is a relatively common condition clinically characterized by tenderness and limitation of ankle joint dorsiflexion.[239,240] Radiographs will manifest lipping and spur formation at the anterior frontier of the ankle joint.[26] Stress lateral radiographs demonstrate an abutment of the two major companion components of the ankle. The talar neck and tibial rim lipping occurs at the attachment points of the anterior ankle joint capsule. It may form as the result of excessive traction or impingement of the anterior ankle, or both. As the deformity progresses, ankle joint dorsiflexion becomes increasingly restricted. The condition has been noted in a variety of athletic activities, including football, track, soccer, and ballet. It has been termed footballer's or lineman's ankle in the past.[240]

Certain biomechanical foot types, such as forefoot equi-

nus or medial or lateral cavus deformities, can predispose to formation of anterior impingement exostosis. Fixed equinus of the forefoot on the rearfoot results in compensation at the ankle joint, reducing available dorsiflexion. Anterior compression impingement of the ankle joint is more likely with athletic activity, resulting in eventual pathologic bony alteration at the dorsal aspect of the talar neck, trochlear surface, and anterior tibial frontier. Associated conditions may coexist, such as lateral ankle instability and osteochondral defects of the talus, fibula, or tibia. Medial and lateral gutter defects of the ankle occur with loose bodies or calcifications within these compartments. Chronic ankle capsulitis and synovitis are frequent findings, resulting in swelling and arthropathy about the ankle. Type II ATTS may be a coexisting finding that occurs secondary to nerve compression from underlying osteoproliferation on the talar neck or tibial rim. The superficial peroneal nerve at the level of the ankle is less commonly impinged with this lesion.

The high demand placed on the ankle joint as a result of athletic participation often requires surgery for this condition.

ANTERIOR ANKLE ARTHROPLASTY

Anterior frontier ankle arthroplasty is best performed in the supine position under general anesthesia with tourniquet control. Anterolateral arthrotomy is the most convenient approach for this arthroplasty. It is quick and safe, elevating the vital structures in one thick subcapsular layer. Visualization is achieved from malleolus to malleolus, allowing access to the gutters for synovectomy and loose body debridement (Fig. 26-44A & B). A double incisional approach is sometimes utilized depending on the extent of disease in the gutters. When anterior tarsal tunnel or superficial peroneal nerve compression occurs in conjunction with anterior ankle osteoproliferation, the joint decompression and arthroplasty usually spontaneously decompress the involved nerves. When osteoproliferation is not extensive, arthroscopic decompression arthroplasty can be effectively performed.[241,242]

Double Incisional Approach

A double anteromedial and anterolateral incisional approach of the ankle joint can be used for dual gutter debridement if the joint disease and osteoproliferation are extensive. The lateral incision is placed at the level of the anterior ankle joint line in the interval between the fibular malleolus and peroneus tertius tendon. This incisional

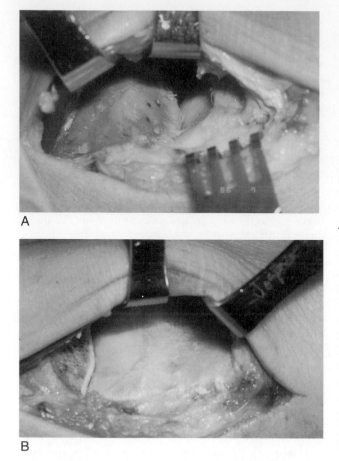

Figure 26-44 (**A**) Anterior frontier impingement arthropathy of the ankle. (**B**) Anterior frontier arthroplasty of both joint segments.

placement avoids the sural nerve and intermediate dorsal cutaneous nerve, although they are searched for to avoid incidental damage. The incision is carried directly to the joint capsule, which is elevated with a thin elevator in a thick layer. The lateral capsular incision is parallel and superior to the course of the anterior talofibular ligament to avoid accidental transection of this structure. The medial incision, located at the level of the anterior ankle joint line at the medial gutter interval between the medial malleolus and the tibialis anterior tendon, is approached in a similar fashion. Both incisions are approximately 3 to 4 cm in length. The greater saphenous vein and saphenous nerve are identified and carefully retracted. The medial incision is carried through the retinacular fibers and the tibialis anterior is retracted laterally. The anteromedial ankle joint capsule is then incised and elevated in a similar fashion. The

medial–lateral approachs are joined subperiosteally and subcapularly with a ribbon retractor to protect the anterior neurovascular structures.

Synovectomy and debridement are undertaken as indicated along the entire anterior frontier and malleolar gutters, carefully avoiding the central neurovascular bundle, which is often bound down in the arthrofibrosis and synovitis tissue. The necessary resections are performed carefully, protecting the talar dome. The talar neck and anterior trochlea are also debrided and sculpted. This is best accomplished with curved osteotomes or gouges. Frequently, a fibrocartilaginous soft tissue lesion will be encountered that extends transversely across the anterior aspect of the ankle joint. This meniscoid-type lesion can be seen arthroscopically and contributes to the pain sydrome in chronic posttraumatic conditions, but is most commonly enountered in the lateral gutter. The dorsal talar neck is carefully regrooved, and the anterior tibial rim is carefully remodeled. The talar dome, as well as the articular surfaces of the medial and lateral gutters, are carefully inspected for any residual debris or pathology, such as osteochondral defects. If present, they are treated by saucerization and drilling of the subchondral bone to enhance fibrocartilaginous infiltration. The joint is then placed through its range of motion to evaluate its function. Thorough lavage is accomplished to toilet any remaining debris from the site, and a layered closure is performed. Arthroplasty may be combined with other procedures, such as delayed primary ligamentous repair or secondary stabilization of a chronically unstable ankle.

A Jones compressive dressing is applied and range of motion initiated at 3 to 5 days postoperatively. A below-knee cast brace is useful to continue rehabilitation, with a quiescent period during the first week to allow soft tissue healing. If excision of an anterior impingement arthroplasty was combined with other procedures, the postoperative course is modified appropriately.

Acute Ankle Sprain Syndrome

Soft tissue ankle sprains are very common inversion mechanisms and comprise about 15 percent of all sports injuries.[243] The lateral ligamentous complex is involved about 85 percent of the time.[244]

In the general population, this same injury accounts for about 10 percent of all emergency room presentations. Sprains are typically classified as grade I through III and are mechanically induced by foot inversion and internal rotation of the leg.[243,245] Grade I is generally agreed to represent a small amount of macroscopic tearing (about 20 percent), slight elastic stretching with swelling, and tenderness without functional loss of integrity. Grade II presents the next sequence of the injury process, with partial ligament substance tear (about 50 percent), greater pain, and swelling with some functional deficit. Grade III demonstrates total disruption of the ligament continuity, with significant functional instability with pain and swelling over the lateral ankle complex.

The anatomy of the lateral ankle complex consists of three major ligaments—the anterior talofibular, calcaneofibular, and posterior talofibular ligaments. The anterior talofibular ligament is a blended portion of the capsule considered intra-articular. The posterior talofibular ligament is distinctively intra-articular. The calcaneofibular ligament has a very intimate relationship with the deep surface of the peroneal tendon sheath as well that can cause extravasation from the ankle and capsule into this sheath. Injury to the medial ankle ligamentous structures, represented mainly by the deltoid, is rarely solitary, without fracture elsewhere in the ankle complex. Additionally, the anterior syndesmosis is an important ligament structure that is more often injured in external rotatory traumas that result in early-stage fractures.

DIAGNOSIS AND EVALUATION

It is very difficult to differentiate grade II injury from grade III injury clinically. Brostrom confirmed this impression in 1965 when he investigated 43 ankles surgically and found that clinical point tenderness was not an adequate index of severity of ligament rupture.[246] Grade II injuries can be accurately assessed clinically about 25 percent of the time, and grade III injuries 100 percent of the time. MRI can bring this accuracy index to 60 percent for grade II injury, with the additional advantage of identifying associated injuries or chronic conditions such as tenosynovitis of the posterior tibial tendon and peroneal tenosynovitis.[243] MRI is also extremely sensitive for anterior talofibular rupture (diagnosed 100 percent of the time), as well as demonstrating healing postinjury.[247] Thus clinical examination is believed to underestimate actual ligament damage in 75 percent of grade II injuries. This often results in undertreatment unless the surgeon is aware of this tendency. Additionally, perceptual and proprioceptive dysfunction has been clearly demonstrated 1 year following ankle sprain, indicating a failure of the afferent sensory reflex response, further contributing to a feeling of clinical instability.[248,249]

MRI is not recommended routinely for evaluation of ankle sprains. It is a tool available for consideration in difficult assessment situations that have great impact, such as in highly competitive professional athletes who require exact determination of their injury in order to provide precise treatment and rehabilitation.[250] Expense factors and availability are other obvious considerations. Clearly, grade II injury is the most vulnerable to misdiagnosis, and the clinician might best err on the side of overaggressive care if this level of disruption is suspected and not confirmed with the sensitive index of MRI.

Clinical testing with frontal plane and sagittal plane stress testing remains the most common clinical method of assessment, in conjunction with careful examination and observation.[251] The anterior drawer sign often will have a positive "suction sign" or clicking sound as the anterior tibia rides over the talar dome during provocation testing.[247] A good examiner can often predict ligamentous instability with examination merely by these clinical signs and sounds of momentary luxation. Radiographic confirmation is accomplished for verification.

Contrast arthrography is inexpensive, readily available and easily performed by the experienced examiner. Although it has the slight disadvantage of being semi-invasive, it remains very helpful. This is especially true in the case of an athlete who presents 1 to 2 days following a severe rupture or sprain with an ankle that is so swollen that it cannot be effectively clinically evaluated. It is important to determine whether there has been capsular and double ligament grade III disruption of the lateral collateral ligament complex. Also, small avulsion fractures occur commonly at the anterior fibular malleolar apex and represent an acute or chronic injury with disruption of the anterior talofibular or calcaneofibular ligament. This ossicle rarely consolidates because of ligament traction and bathing in synovial fluid. It must be differentiated from subfibular accessory bone in chronic states. Double-contrast arthrograms using contrast agent, air, and a local anesthetic, and tenograms, may reveal a capsular tear as well as dye extravasation into the peroneal sheath anterior and lateral to the ankle. This pattern suggests a double ligamentous rupture, and definitive treatment can be instituted. The capsular tear may seal 5 to 7 days postinjury, resulting in a false-negative contrast study.

TREATMENT

The question of surgical versus nonsurgical ligament repair still remains controversial. Some studies demonstrate equivocal long-term outcomes following conservative treatment compared with surgery.[252] Surgery is most often selected for highly competitive or Olympic-level athletes with grade III double ruptures of the anterior talofibular and calcaneofibular ligaments.[251] Most surgeons agree that single-ligament rupture should be managed nonsurgically with functional rehabilitation, using splinting, strapping, physiotherapy, and oral anti-inflammatory medications. More confusion exists with grade II double ligament rupture, with both surgical and nonsurgical options recommended and available for consideration.

When there is doubt, nonsurgical care can be undertaken, with the realization that the pathology has been properly identified. Several studies have demonstrated a lack of sensitivity in defining single-versus double-ligament rupture, and this becomes an important question in management. Contrast studies using arthrography, tenography, ultrasound, and MRI can all help in the diagnosis and required decision making.[253] Nonsurgical management of double-ligament rupture should include functional below-knee cast bracing with concurrent gentle rehabilitation for at least 5 to 6 weeks. Gradual return to activity and training can be undertaken at that time.

It is important to bear in mind that all ligament ruptures can be managed with functional treatment by cast bracing and rehabilitation and result in a satisfactory outcome. Surgery remains the most precise method of restoration, however, and is recommended in the competitive athlete with documented severe grade III rupture of the lateral complex. Peroneal strengthening with active rehabilitation focuses on restoration of proprioceptive responses and reclaimation of the peroneal reflex splinting mechanism. Primary repair has had extensive review in the literature and has its advocates as well as adversaries. The athlete's competitive level of performance, age, and desire all merge to create a protocol that usually will help define when operation is indicated.

Small avulsion fractures occasionally occur at the anterior malleolar fibular styloid. If this presents as an acute injury, it requires excision with osteosuture repair of the anterior talofibular ligament or calcaneofibular ligament. When chronic and painful, these ossicles can be removed arthroscopically and a small arthroscopic staple delivered, plicating the anterior talofibular ligament.[254]

Primary Repair of Acute Lateral Ankle Ligamentous Rupture

Primary repair is best performed under general anesthesia with the patient in a supine position under pneumatic thigh tourniquet control. An anterolateral curvilinear skin incision is made over the ankle joint. The incision begins at the level of the tibiofibular synosmosis anterior to the fibula, extending distally as it curves posteriorly and under the lateral malleolus, terminating behind the tip of the malleolus. Dissection follows the hematoma and is continued down through the capsule, producing a full-thickness skin and subcutaneous flap.[255] The ankle compartment is inspected for visible mechanical instability, osteochondral defects, and other debris and then pressure lavaged to wash out occult material. Care is taken to avoid the superficial peroneal nerve dorsally, as well as the sural nerve and lesser saphenous vein at the distal extent of the incision. The distal aspect of the incision should not extend below the level of the peroneal tendons.

The tendons are retracted inferiorly and the calcaneofibular ligament inspected. It is repaired with 2-0 Vicryl if necessary. Occasionally, avulsion fragments from the fibular apex or calcaneal tubercle produce the ligament failure, and this must be repaired with osteosuture, bone anchors, or spiked A-O washers and screws. The anterior talofibular ligament and capsule are imbricated in one thick layer with 2-0 Vicryl, often including a portion of the local retinaculum. The correct neutral position of the ankle is achieved while performing these repairs. Layered closure is completed and a posterior splint applied. Rehabilitation begins within 2 days postoperatively with range of motion and other conventional modalities to reduce edema. A below-knee cast brace is used during rehabilitation, with gradual return to activity over the next 3 to 4 weeks.

Chronic Lateral Ankle Instability With Recurrent Ankle Sprains

Chronic lateral ankle instability with recurrent sprain is a common problem that can have devastating effects on the competitive success of an athlete. It is estimated to develop in approximately 20 percent of sprain mechanisms regardless of treatment.[256–258] It is more common in undertreated bad ankle sprains, general ligamentous laxity, and structural aberrations of hindfoot varus giving rise to biomechanical imbalance in gait and athletics. The chronic lateral ankle instability syndrome predisposes the athlete to repetitive injury, chronic pain and swelling, and impaired functional stability of the ankle. This in turn creates a psychological fear of reinjury, imparing maximum performance as well as causing loss of training time. Impaired athletic performance, disability in performing activities of daily living, and the occupational interference produce a significant economic toll on an athlete. It has become increasingly clear that more aggressive treatment for athletic ankle sprains is required other than simple icing and Ace bandage wrapping.

DIAGNOSIS

The athlete often complains of a sensation of a weakness of the ankles or a fear that they will "give out." Lateral or anterolateral pain and swelling are usually evident with weight bearing. Thorough examination is necessary to properly assess these athletes. Ancillary injury and companion fractures occur with ankle sprain syndromes and can help identify the primary problem. Examples of such injuries are avulsion fractures of the styloid process and fracture of the fifth metatarsal, anterior superior process of the calcaneus, lateral malleolus, and medial malleolus. Initial scout films are taken to rule out fracture. These studies should include the standard three views of the ankle plus a medial oblique view of the foot.

If fracture has been ruled out, it is important to assess the degree of ligamentous injury by provocation testing of the ankle. A TELOS device may be useful for clinical research or in order to achieve quantified standardized results when performing inversion and anterior drawer sign tests of the ankle.[251] Uniform and reliable outcome can usually be obtained when the same clinician consistently performs the manual stress test. Such results are comparable to those obtained from more technological methods such as the TELOS apparatus. When the TELOS device is used to aid in performing stress radiography of the ankle, a force of 15 to 25 kiloponds has been found sufficient to demonstrate ligamentous instability of the anterior talofibular or calcaneofibular ligament, or both. As noted earlier, more recently MRI has emerged as the ultimate assessment tool, albeit expensive. In the normal clinical setting these modalities are not usually available, and the surgeon must use his or her best judgment and knowledge of the condition to make conclusions for diagnosis and treatment.

An anterior drawer test is carried out with the examiner pushing down on the anterior aspect of the ankle, over the tibia, with the calcaneus stabilized on a raised rubber block. The foot is in a plantar-flexed position during this examination. In addition, it is helpful to plantar-flex the knee slightly, releasing tension from the gastrocnemius–soleus complex. This manuever will further facilitate demonstration of anterior dislocation of the ankle. The anterior drawer test can be assessed using the so-called concentric circle displacement of the talus and tibial profiles or actual measured distance from the back of the tibia to the back of the corresponding point on the talar dome.

The inversion stress test is carried out with the examiner inverting the hindfoot while simultaneously internally rotating the tibia approximately 18 degrees. An AP view of the ankle is obtained while the examiner exerts a strong inversion force to open up the lateral aspect of the ankle joint. This affords a mortise view of the ankle to facilitate measurement of lateral gapping of the ankle joint. It is essential to exert the inversion force against the calcaneus as opposed to the midfoot or forefoot area. The foot is maintained at 90 degrees' neutral position in relationship to the tibia on the sagittal plane during the inversion stress test. The amount of varus tilt and anterior displacement of the talus in the ankle mortise can then be compared to that on the contralateral side.

Considerable controversy remains regarding the assessment of inversion stress radiographs. It has been suggested that up to 23 degrees of talar tilt may be considered normal, whereas others have indicated 5 to 10 degrees' discrepancy between the injured and uninjured sides represents a single or double lateral ligamentous rupture. Comparative stress tests on both extremities must be performed. Ligamentous laxity of 10 to 15 degrees of talar tilt can occur on the uninvolved side. The diagnosis is further complicated in the presence of bilateral chronic lateral instability of the ankle.[259]

An experienced surgeon can achieve a good clinical impression of chronic luxation by feel in the form of the "click test" and "suction sign" prior to provocation radiographic confirmation. By maintaining the patient in a comfortable and relaxed position, it is often possible to obtain valid stress examinations even on an acutely injured ankle. Occasionally, it is best to sedate the patient and perform a common peroneal block when pain is severe and splinting is obvious. Anterior displacement of the talus on the anterior drawer stress radiograph of 3 mm or greater indicates significant damage with rupture of the anterior talofibular ligament.[251] The anterior suction sign and click sound are often noted with the anterior talar luxation during testing.

The anterior drawer sign is a more consistent predictable finding indicative of rupture of the anterior collateral ligament. Frontal plane talar tilt is less reliable inasmuch as there is almost no agreement on what amount of "lateral gap" is indicative of rupture. If 5 or more degrees of talar tilt are apparent on the injured side and coexist with a positive anterior drawer test, the patient most likely has disruption of the anterior lateral collateral ligament. Clinically, this must be correlated with palpable pain over the anterior and middle collateral ligaments, as well as a feeling of giving way with the anterior stress test. Characterization of instability using numerical values in degrees for the anterior and inversion stress tests is done for clinical correlations only. These values do not provide a definitive diagnosis, nor do they dictate whether surgery is appropriate.

Chronic lateral instability of the ankle unmanageable with orthotics or ankle braces is an indication for surgical stabilization. Persistent injury and instability will predispose the patient to repetitive microtrauma and progressive arthrosis and internal derangement.

SURGICAL ANKLE STABILIZATION

Surgical stabilization of the chronically unstable ankle depends on the severity of symptoms and the type of instability present. Often, double-ligament reconstruction is necessary because of anterolateral rotatory instability. Descriptions of over 50 operations for this condition have been published, some focusing on the anterior talofibular ligament, some the calcaneofibular ligament, and others both.[260,261] The controversy resolves around single-versus double-ligament reconstruction via anatomic reconstructions versus tenodesis checkrein blocks.[262,263] The consideration of tenodesis versus local tissue augmentation is not so difficult inasmuch as this is determined based on availability of local tissue at the reconstruction site at the time of operation.[246] The Brostrom operation is most popular in this regard, with periosteal augmentation flaps often mobilized distalward from the anterolateral portion of the fibula on top of the Brostrom repair site (Fig. 26-45). Also,

Figure 26–45 Modified Brostrom repair with ligamentoperiosteal flap turned downward from fibula and fixated into talar neck with spiked washer and screw. Other local retinacular tissues are also imbricated at this site for reinforcement.

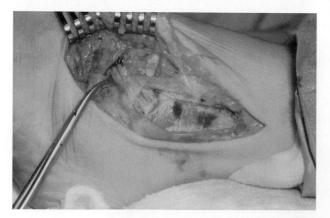

local tissue retinaculoplasty is used in conjunction with the Brostrom plastic.

If the pathology is single-ligament dissipation and instability, then single-ligament reconstruction is performed as noted above. Westlin (personal communication, Malmo General University Hospital, Malmo, Sweden) has performed a large series of extensor digitorum brevis muscle transpositions mobilizing the origin from the floor of the sinus tarsi to the anterolateral aspect of the fibula, fixed with osteosuture. This has worked well for single-ligament anterofibular instability with poor local tissue for Brostrom or retinaculoplastic repair. The osteoperiosteal flap can also be mobilized directly inferiorly to augment the calcaneofibular ligament.[262,264] Double-ligament reconstruction requires the anatomic repairs of Chrisman-Snook and variants.[265] Bauer has modified this operation with a free hemisection graft of peroneus longus, attaching the graft to the three points of anatomic insertion using spiked washers and screws.[263] Interestingly, the study of Thermann and colleagues[262] indicates very little difference in outcome with single checkrein procedures such as the Evans[266] versus the more anatomic reconstruction of Chrisman-Snook.[265] It is clear that the Evans peroneus brevis tenodesis is sufficient in the majority of clinical lateral ankle instability syndromes based on this study. However, when evidence confirms double-ligament anterolateral instability, and in particular a subtalar joint instability contribution, a full anatomic restoration directly crossing the subtalar joint is most optimum.

It is critical that structural contributions to the instability syndrome, such as hindfoot varus, be resolved through calcaneal osteotomy or other such operations to correct this component prior to reliance on soft tissue ligamentoplasty. Most of these operations utilize a lateral retrofibular skin approach, beginning behind the fibula proximally and extending toward the calcaneocuboid joint. This allows access to the peroneal tendons for mobilization or hemisection grafting if desired. It also permits good exposure of the fibula and sinus tarsi region or talar neck or body for anastomosis attachments in these regions. Two or three mini-incisional percutaneous modifications can be used as well with less dissection (Fig. 26-46). Fibular attachment sites are best created with a Michelle trephine, which creates a bone plug used to press fit the tendodesis site mechanically, making suture unnecessary. Spiked washers and A-O screws are convenient quick forms of attachment, as are any of the currently available bone anchor systems. Good results have been reported with arthro-

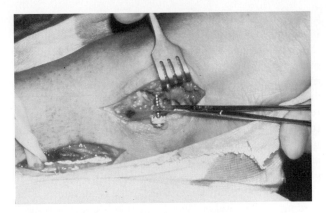

Figure 26-46 Mini-incisional ankle stablization with peroneus brevis tenodesis and screw fixation into talar neck after passing through trephine defect in fibular malleolus.

scopic stapling and plication of the anterior talofibular ligament in specific indications.[267,268]

Anterior, Lateral, and Meniscoid Impingement of the Ankle

The athlete may present with a complaint of anterolateral ankle pain that is chronic and persistent in nature and not necessarily related to any recent traumatic event. The patient often has a subjective feeling of instability or a fear of the ankle giving way. Usually there is recollection of a serious sprained ankle previously. There may or may not be a history of repeated inversion-type injuries. Nonetheless, the ankle can manifest pain medially as well as anterolaterally and is subjectively unstable. Cartilage damage and medial pain have been demonstrated in a high number of supination ankle sprains.[269]

Examination will disclose tenderness to palpation near the anterolateral talar dome or lateral gutter, especially as the examiner palpates this area. Range-of-motion and provocation testing will often reveal some degree of anterolateral rotatory instability of the ankle. This is generally detected manually with an audible and palpable click test and suction sign. Contrast study may disclose the presence of a meniscoid lesion in the lateral gutter.[270] This is the result of chronic soft tissue interposition and repetitive impingement with hyalinization. This lesion can be quite painful and present as a subjective instability syndrome. The meniscoid lesion appears as a pearly gray, rubbery, fibrous mass at the anterolateral gutter of the ankle. There is usually surrounding chronic synovitis. This is an internal

derangement syndrome, and often there is no position of comfort when such lesions are present.

DELAYED PRIMARY REPAIR

Delayed primary repair is carried out by repairing the damaged anterior talofibular and calcaneofibular ligaments, with resection of degenerative or atrophic segments of capsule and ligaments.[271] The capsule and ligaments are repaired with absorbable suture of choice and osteosuture into the bone site if necessary. The calcaneofibular ligament is repaired by excising any damaged or insufficient portion of the ligament and resuturing the ends of the ligament under moderate tension with the foot dorsiflexed and the heel perpendicular to the eventual weight-bearing plane.[271] Fibular malleolar osteoperiosteal flaps can be generated as well and mobilized inferiorly for augmentation. The anterior talofibular ligament is repaired in a similar manner, also using fibular periosteal flaps as needed. The superior peroneal retinaculum is then repaired as well if necessary, and portions of this tissue are used for local augmentation grafting. The Westlin extensor digitorum brevis myoplasty can also be used for this type of augmentation. The wound is then closed in layers. A postoperative Jones compression dressing with a posterior splint maintaining the foot and ankle in neutral position is used to help control initial postoperative edema.

Five to 7 days postoperatively, at the time of the initial dressing change, the splint is transformed to a cast brace. Physical therapy is started 7 to 9 days postoperatively and includes gentle range of motion within the limits of stable repair. This limits postoperative adhesions and stiffness of the ankle and is helpful postoperatively, if delayed primary repair was combined with excision of an osteochondral defect. The cast brace is discontinued at 4 to 6 weeks postoperatively and rehabilitation continued. Exercises are utilized to enhance strength, flexibility, proprioception, and balance. Approximately 2 months postoperatively, a progressive return-to-activity program is begun. The patient is instructed to use a stirrup brace or double upright laceup ankle brace for a period of 4 months following initial rehabilitation to improve proprioception and to provide for some lateral support.

Athletic Ankle Fracture

Athletic ankle fracture is governed by the same pathomechanics of ankle traumatology as in the nonathlete. The primary tissue failure and progression of injury are determined by the position of the foot at the time of mechanical overloading and the direction of the imposed force on the "planted" foot. Athletic maneuvers magnify this scenario as a result of peak forces generated during athletic events. The pronated foot tethers the deltoid ligament, delivering an initial traction load to the medial malleolus. The supinated foot transmits a traction load to the fibular malleolus via the lateral collateral ligaments. The imposed loads delivered are either sustained by these tissues or cause failure.[272] The ligament and bone failure that occurs pursues a defined pathway that is predictable based on foot position, direction of imposed load, and magnitude of the load. The loading force can be medially directed, causing a pure frontal plane inversion of the talus within the ankle mortise; laterally directed, causing pure frontal plane eversion; or torsional, resulting in a helical force that translates into transverse plane external rotatory motion of the talus/foot in the ankle mortise.

These pure uniplanar loading modes define the pathomechanical classification scheme proposed by Lauge-Hansen.[273–275] This is a very useful fracture classification because it defines not only the progression of failure but also the anticipated osseous and soft tissue pathology associated with these mechanisms of injury. The alternate A-O Danis-Weber scheme is based on the level of fibular fracture and designed essentially as an operative classification, and does not directly imply the disruption pattern of the peritalar ligamentous complex.[276–282]

CLASSIFICATION

The four classic Lauge-Hansen categories of ankle fracture include supination–adduction (SA), pronation–abduction (PA), supination–external rotation (SE), and pronation–external rotation (PE).[273–275] It is very important to recognize that "eversion," as described by Lauge-Hansen, refers to external rotation of the foot (with the foot being used as a lever) on the "fixated" leg in the laboratory setting. This scenario delivers the opposite force system, in which the foot is fixed on the supporting surface and the leg internally rotates in conjunction with other imposed foot positions noted earlier. The external rotatory load is responsible for the most severe ankle fractures, syndesmotic failures, and dislocations in the Lauge-Hansen classification system. Internal rotatory leg forces on the foot are commonly associated with severe "lateral ankle sprains." A ligament lesion is the mechanical equivalent of a fracture site in the scheme. Obviously, these lesions pursue alternate physiologic healing patterns characteristic of the specific tissue.

The Danis-Weber classification scheme of ankle fracture is the other main classification in use.[276–279] This much-simplified scheme directs surgical management and is based on the level of fibular fracture and associated syndesmotic involvement. Type A fibular fractures are generally transverse at or below the level of the syndesmosis. They do not result in syndesmotic disruption. This would correspond to the Lauge-Hansen SA stage I injuries. Type B fractures are spiral/oblique and initiate at the level of the syndesmosis and extend proximally (Fig. 26-47). They exhibit partial syndesmotic disruption inasmuch as the fracture pattern actually perforates the lower fibers of the syndesmosis. This heterogeneous category would include Lauge-Hansen SE and most PA injury patterns. Type C fractures can be short and oblique in appearance or long helical fibular shaft fractures above the level of the syndesmosis, and imply complete syndesmotic disruption. They corresponds primarily to Lauge-Hansen PE injuries and generally are the most unstable of all injury patterns because of extensive associated ligamentous disruption.

The Danis-Weber scheme affords a scale of increasing instability of injury based on the level of fibular fracture; it ignores associated medial ankle disruption, which has a profound bearing on resultant biomechanical stability,

Figure 26-47 Type B Danis-Weber low supination external rotation fracture with associated stage 4 medial malleolar fracture as well.

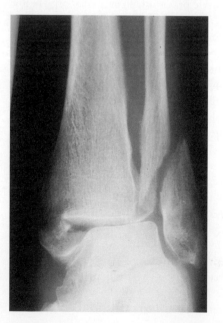

especially in type B injury. Because the type B category may constitute up to 90 percent of all malleolar fractures, this failure to discriminate may adversely skew the results of outcome-based studies that utilize this fracture classification system.[280] The detrimental effect of these injuries relates to functional incongruity of the talus relative to the tibial plafond, with resultant deminished surface contact and increases in peak pressure concentration.[281] This may lead to an accelerated arthrosis over time.

EVALUATION

Ankle fracture diagnosis is usually made based on the history and physical examination with radiographs. Physical examination should begin with visual assessment to include neurovascular integrity, obvious dislocation, distention, ecchymosis, color changes, and any compromise of the integument that transforms the injury into an "open fracture." Early reduction in the emergency department with sedation is an important management feature for dislocated ankle fractures, which are usually rotatory with posterior malleolar fractures.[283,284] Gentle manipulative assessment based on the patient's comfort level is important in order to evaluate the integrity of myotendinous, ligamentous, and bone segments. Unstable injuries often manifest crepitus on palpation at the fracture site, accompanied by nonphysiologic motion patterns. The "fibular compression test" is highly diagnostic in confirming high neck fibular fracture or, for that matter, fracture anywhere along the continuity of the fibula. This is performed by placing both hands around the lateral leg, compressing the fibula against the tibia. As the site of fracture is approached, significant pain is elicited at the level of fracture.

Radiologic studies are ordered based on the findings of the physical examination. Standard protocol includes AP, lateral, and mortise views and any additional special projections deemed helpful to better visualize areas of suspected pathology.[285-288] Malleolar fractures with greater than 2 mm of displacement warrant closed or open reduction to restore anatomic alignment.[280] Careful scrutiny of all articular surfaces for evidence of occult avulsion or osteochondral involvement is mandatory. The presence on plain radiographs of an ankle effusion of 13 mm or greater in total capsular distention has a positive predictive value of 82 percent for occult fracture and is a reasonable threshold to prompt additional imaging, including CT.[289] Trends in "managed care" have reviewed selective radiologic and imaging studies as a means to reduce costs. Implementation of the Ottawa Ankle Rules with utilization of two (AP

and mortise) instead of three standard views has been determined to be effective and may save health care dollars with minor impact on the accuracy of diagnosis.[290,291]

MANAGEMENT

The most common athletic fracture is the type B Danis-Weber low spiral oblique lateral malleolar fracture (Lauge-Hansen SE-2 injury).[292] This fracture might comprise as many as 90 percent of athletic ankle fractures.[293] Athletic fractures occur in highly active states of performance, which implies a supinated stable foot posture at the moment of morbid loading. Several studies have demonstrated simple immobilization to be sufficient treatment for this fracture if displacement is 2 mm or less. Isolated fracture of the medial malleolus is uncommon without significant associated soft tissue injury or associated fibular fracture. In general, ankle fractures with no or less than 1 to 2 mm displacement usually can be managed with closed reduction and snug casting. Later stage injuries with multiple fractures and ligament failures will require open reduction and internal fixation ORIF. This includes the mid- to late-stage rotatory injuries such as the SE and PE mechanisms with bimalleolar fracture.

Posterior antiglide plate fixation of the fibula has become standard for type B fractures (Fig. 26-48), along with medial malleolar fixation using either tension banding wires or two lag screws. End-stage PE fractures will require tibiofibular transfixation with one or two 3.5-mm "position screws" and three cortical purchases two in the fibula and one in the tibial cortex.[294] Alternate simple fixation can also be achieved with the Swedish "semirigid tech

Figure 26-48 Weber posterior fibular antiglide plate application for type B ankle fracture.

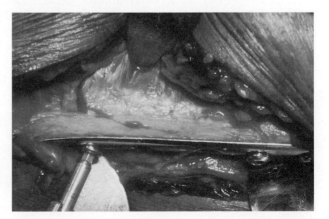

nique" of Palmer pins in the medial malleolus and Wiberg malleable syndesmotic staples with circlage wire for the fibular fracture for SE injuries.[295] This is an easy and fast method of ORIF with an element of dynamization, as opposed to the rigidity of the A-O system (Fig. 26-49). Biodegradable screws and pins are increasingly common and have been widely investigated in Scandinavia, demonstrating acceptable clinical outcomes when utilized in malleolar fractures.[296–307]

Polyglycolide and polylactide are the two nonmetallic fixatives currently utilized. Although these fixatives do not provide the mechanical stability or interfragmental compression achieved with metallic fixatives, they have demonstrated satisfactory stability in selected malleolar fractures and may represent the future.

OPERATIVE TECHNIQUE

Type B spiral low oblique fibular fracture is approached with a lateral incision, usually about 5 inches, slightly posterior to the fibula. It should extend above the proximal level of the fracture and curve slightly forward under the malleolus. The incision follows the hematoma down to the fracture site, which is debrided and lavaged. The site is reduced by reversing the mechanism using pronation and some dorsiflexion. The fracture is clamped and the posterior plate applied with no contouring. The lower end of the plate will sometimes require slight bending to cup the inferior malleolus, but this is not mandatory. The proximal screw in the plate is drilled first to help stabilize the plate on the bone, a screw is placed in the hole just proximal and then to the fracture site. As the second screw is tightened, the plate will flex and conform to the back of the fibula with a spring action, loading the plate and locking the sharp posterior spike of the fracture in its bed[308] (see Fig. 26-48). It is not necessary to place screws distal to the fracture site, although if desired an interfragmental screw can be placed across the fracture through the inferior plate holes, allowing the plate to act as a washer. The syndesmosis is always checked. If necessary, a few sutures are placed to repair any disruption that is present. This is uncommon because the syndesmosis is almost always intact in this injury. A bone hook test can be used to verify sydesmotic integrity proximally.

If the medial malleolus is fractured, this is approached next, with an anteromedial incision curving below the malleolus. This incision allows at least three surfaces of the fracture to be viewed at reduction.[309] If the anterior colliculus is fractured, tension banding is often indicated

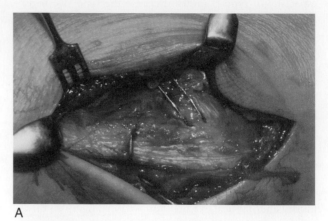

A

B

Figure 26-49 (**A**) Cedell Swedish semirigid fixation of type B fracture with double malleable syndesmotic staples and fibular circlage wire more proximal. (**B**) The radiographic appearance.

because of the small size of the fragment.[310,311] The joint is always inspected prior to the reductions and lavaged to remove loose debris or hematoma. Cartilage avulsions should be looked for routinely. They are common on the medial side of the joint interval. If the medial fracture is higher, near the joint line or above, lag screws might be more convenient; however, tension banding can also be used. Palmer pins are another option that works well for medial malleolar fractures and provides quick, stable osteosynthesis.

REHABILITION AND POSTOPERATIVE CARE

Typical casting immobilization is about 6 to 8 weeks for malleolar fractures. Malposition is frequent with closed reduction, and healing may be prolonged, with persistent swelling until complete consolidation has occurred. The period of functional rehabilitation following cast removal generally correlates with the length of immobilization and is dependent on the fracture type. Exercises to encourage range of motion, muscle strengthening, and proprioception may be required in addition to gait training under the supervision of a therapist to shorten the recovery period.[312] This is especially beneficial in injuries with major articular involvement to encourage restoration of a smooth bearing surface. However, clinical studies have shown initial improvement in joint mobility with equivocal outcome at about 1 year when comparing functional rehabilitation with complete immobilization for the fracture healing period.[313–316]

Ankle fracture is a complex subject, and the reader is referred to appropriate texts for more thorough discussion and understanding of this injury and associated surgery.

Sinus Tarsi Sydrome

Pain in the sinus tarsi with a feeling of instability in the hindfoot has become more recognized as a chronic condition. O'Connnor first described this entity in 1958 and it went unnoticed for about 20 years.[317] It occurs post-traumatically most commonly but is also seen in inflammatory diseases.[318,319] It is believed that inflammatory tissue extends from the posterior subtalar joint cavity into the anterior sinus tarsi region in these situations. The majority, however, are related to ankle sprain sydnromes and ultimately are the residual of same with chronic sinus tarsitis pain. The structures involved in this "syndrome" are the cervical ligament, talocalcaneal ligament, and interosseous

ligament.[320] These structures primarily stabilize the hindfoot and subtalar joint. In the past, these structures were not able to be imaged well; however, MRI has provided clear recognition of the anatomy of the sinus tarsi region and associated pathology. Section of these ligaments does not produce extreme subtalar joint instability, and thus objective evidence of instability from compromise of these structures is not easy to demonstrate clinically. This condition is often the unnoticed part of a bad ankle sprain syndrome.

MRI has provided greater insight into this condition. Alteration of the normal fat signal intensity occurs with replacement by infiltrate and fibrosis, as noted on pathology examination. Disruption of the interosseous and cervical ligaments is usually apparent on the MRI, often as total absence and alternative tissue replacement.[321] Proprioceptors are believed to be damaged in this region, hence the clinical sensation of instability. Sinus tarsi syndrome occurs in association with chronic valgus foot architecture syndrome, especially posterior tibial tendon dysfunction. In these situations, it is clear the lateral talar process is jamming into the calcaneal notch as a result of chronic hyperpronation contributing to the inflammatory cycle. Response to enucleation of the sinus tarsi is poor when severe hyperpronation exists because the condition is secondary.

CONSERVATIVE TREATMENT AND SURGERY

Local anesthetic–steroid infiltrates are diagnostic as well as therapeutic for extended periods of time. Anti-inflammatory agents, physical therapy, and immobilization with cast bracing all can be attempted. Athletes manifest this condition in conjunction with chronic hyperpronation syndromes as well as post-traumatic ankle sprains, as noted earlier. When symptoms are chronic and unresponsive, soft tissue decompression of the sinus tarsi is indicated by excising "Hoke's tonsil," as this tissue has become known. This is accomplished by excising the superficial portions of the sinus tarsi and scar tissue along with the leading synovial fringe of the posterior subtalar joint cavity.[322] Outcomes for this procedure have been excellent, and recovery with full return to activity can be anticipated.[251] Portions of the inferior retinaculum may also be involved and require some excision as well.

Rehabilitation is active mobilization with physical therapy. Down time is usually about 5 weeks with this procedure. A gradual return-to-activity schedule is pursued.

Common Athletic Avulsion and Overuse Fractures

Small avulsion ankle fractures are often seen in athletes that can give a false impression of a minor injury. Common are the fibular apex avulsions of the lateral collateral ligaments, avulsions of the anterior portion of the medial malleolar colliculus, and the Wagstaff avulsion of the sydesmostic fibular tubercle and its tibial counterpart, the tubercle of Chaput.[277] The lateral fibular "fleck fracture" is indicative of superior retinacular compromise. Although they are small fragments, these portions of bone have important characteristics that guides surgical management decisions. At times, these avulsions require primary repair along with investigation of the soft tissue ruptures associated with them.

The Jones fracture at the metaphyseal–diaphyseal junction of the fifth metatarsal is a common overuse syndrome often incapacitating an athlete. It should be differentiated from the fifth metatarsal styloid avulsion traction fracture, which has a different biomechanical origin and different methodology of treatment. Much has been written on this overuse flexural fracture, and it is now more clear that this fracture should be subjected to early osteosynthesis in the athlete, with axial lag screwing. Nonsurgical management of this injury has a high incidence of delayed or nonunion and refracture. Cannulated screws have facilitated internal fixation of this injury, making surgery the optimum mode of care for this fracture, occasionally combined with inlay bone grafting. Styloid avulsion fractures, in comparison, are usually managed with cast bracing if distraction of the fracture segment is not significant.

Other avulsion fractures of importance in the athlete are the dorsal navicular avulsion fracture, navicular tuberosity traction fracture, navicular stress fracture, cuboid stress fracture, and medial calcaneal tuberosity avulsion fracture. Most of these injuries are traction overload injuries mediated by associated ligaments or tendons. Traction in the dorsal navicular–cuneiform ligaments during forced plantar-flexion mechanics results in the dorsal navicular fracture. Direct impacts to this region can also produce this same injury. Surgery is only required if chronic pain persists, and is confined to simple excision of the small fragment. Navicular tuberosity avulsion fractures result from forceful deceleration pull of the posterior tibial tendon or spring ligament traction. If a significant portion of the tuberosity is pulled off, surgical repair is indicated to maintain the integrity of the posterior tibial tendon. This can be done with a small lag screw and spiked washer if the frag-

ment is large enough, or tension band wire. Cast bracing is required for about 3 to 4 weeks to allow consolidation of the segment.

Navicular and cuboid stress fractures result in chronic pain in the associated anatomic region and can be demonstrated on bone scan imaging or CT if chronic occult pain presents. Surgery is rarely considered in these overuse injuries, and only after failure of functional cast bracing and demonstrated inability to heal the site. Prolonged athletic disability can result from these injuries, often in part as a result of delay in diagnosis because these fractures are not always detected on standard radiographs. Calcaneal medial tuberosity avulsion fractures can occur from heavy impact on a pronated foot and are managed with cast bracing and heal well. The tendo Achillis posterior avulsion fracture at the posterior beak of the os calcis will require internal fixation with lag screws to maintain the integrity of the tendo Achillis.

BIOMECHANICAL CONDITIONS OF THE FOOT

Cavus Foot

A cavus foot is a multisegmental deformity characterized by a rigid equinus of the forefoot on the hindfoot.[323,324] The equinus may be global, involving the entire forefoot, or confined to a specific ray segment, such as lateral column cavus, medial cavus, or rigid plantar-flexed first ray. Global forefoot equinus demonstrates a uniform planar attitude compared with the rearfoot when the ankle is in neutral position. The plane of the first through fifth metatarsals, however, lies plantar to the transverse plane of the rearfoot (Fig. 26-50). This type of foot compensates at the ankle joint with dorsiflexion in order to maintain the forefoot and the rearfoot on a level weight-bearing surface simultaneously.[323,324] There is no measurable foot compensation at either the subtalar or midtarsal joint complex, assuming no other deformity. This is a sagittal plane deformity.[325] Weight-bearing radiographs will demonstrate an increased calcaneal pitch angle, as well as an increase in the declination angle of the metatarsals and cuboid when viewed on a lateral profile. The talus will demonstrate maximal dorsiflexion in the ankle mortis on the lateral view, with limited potential for further excursion because it has reached its end range.

Examination may reveal limitation of ankle dorsiflexion; however, this is accommodative to the forefoot equinus,

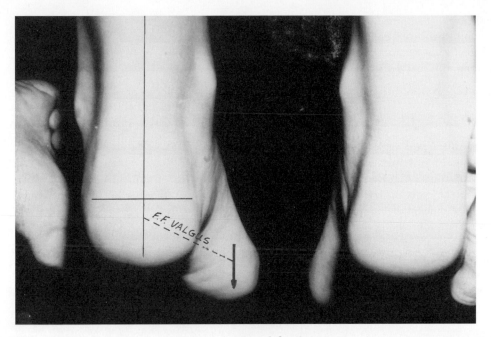

Figure 26-50 Compensated rigid forefoot valgus deformity.

with subsequent compensatory ankle dorsiflexion. This concept known is as pseudoequinus.[326] Adequate dorsiflexion of the rearfoot about the ankle joint axis of motion is present; however, the equinus of the forefoot on the rearfoot places a demand for additional ankle joint dorsiflexion beyond the normal limits. Clearly, in this deformity there is no real equinus of the triceps surae. Achilles tendon lengthening is not ordinarily indicated in this condition.[327,328] Pseudoequinus may result in additional clinical and radiographic findings, such as anterior impingement exostosis of the ankle.

LATERAL CAVUS

A lateral cavus is characterized by a rigid equinus of the lateral column on the rearfoot without medial column equinus. During the off-weight-bearing examination, when the subtalar joint is placed into neutral position and the midtarsal joint is maximally pronated by dorsiflexing and abducting the lateral column, plantar flexion of the lateral column may be visualized. Instead of the normal straight sagittal contour of the lateral border of the foot, some degree of concavity will be seen, the severity of which is related to the extent of deformity. Examination of the medial column is unremarkable and, overall, there is an apparent forefoot varus secondary to the lateral column deformity.

In this foot type, the plane of the lesser metatarsals at the lateral column is below the level of the rearfoot, whereas the medial column lesser metatarsals are on a plane level with that of the rearfoot. A flexible plantar-flexed position of the first metatarsal may be evident, and must be distinguished from a rigid deformity. On weight bearing, this foot assumes the position of calcaneal valgus secondary to compensation of both the ankle and subtalar joints. Dorsiflexion of the ankle joint occurs to bring the plane of the lateral column to a level equal to that of the rearfoot, while compensation of the subtalar joint occurs in order to bring the medial column down to the level of the ground.[329]

Radiographically, increased calcaneal pitch angle, as well as increased declination of the lateral column, will be evident, as well as dorsal rotation of the talus in the ankle mortise. Subtalar joint compensatory pronation will be evident as an anterior break of the cyma line secondary to anterior talar displacement on the calcaneus.

MEDIAL CAVUS

A medial cavus deformity is characterized by a normal relationship of the lateral column to the rearfoot, with rigid plantar flexion of the medial column. This is especially evident at the level of the first metatarsal and sometimes, to a lesser extent, at the second and third metatarsals. During non-weight-bearing examination, the normal straight lateral border will be evident, with the medial column of the foot displaced below the plane of the rearfoot and the lateral column. On weight bearing, this foot demonstrates no ankle joint compensation yet compensates at the subtalar joint in the direction of supination to permit the entire forefoot and rearfoot to purchase the supporting surface simultaneously.[329]

Radiographically, a normal calcaneal pitch angle as well as normal declination of the fifth and fourth metatarsals is evident, with an increase in the declination angle of the first metatarsal. A posterior break in the cyma line is viewed laterally secondary to posterior talar glide on the calcaneus during compensatory supination. This foot will not demonstrate the pseudoequinus seen in a total forefoot equinus or plantar-flexed lateral column. Calcaneal pitch is controlled by the lateral column, whereas subtalar joint position is controlled by the relationship between the medial and lateral columns of the foot (S. D. Smith, personal communication).

Cavus foot classification and terminology is confusing, and represents different perspectives in evaluation and surgical concepts of correction. Alternate characterizations include anterior cavus, posterior cavus, local cavus, and global cavus. These subtypes can be further divided into rigid, semirigid, and flexible deformity. These subtypes all convey the complex personality of this deformity and its compensation mechanisms. Flexible or semiflexible cavus foot involves compensation at the midtarsal joint complex. A true cavus foot is characterized by a rigid equinus of the forefoot on the rearfoot, and compensatory mechanisms involve the ankle or subtalar joints, or both, primarily[330] (Fig. 26-51). The flexible or semiflexible cavus foot is not truly a cavus foot at all inasmuch as compensation is occurring at the midtarsal joint. In reality, this is a type of flatfoot that starts with a high arch off weight bearing.

Cavus deformity may be either congenital or acquired. Neuromuscular and higher central neurologic lesions are well recognized causative factors in the development of pes cavus.[331] Cavus deformity is also a component of congenital clubfoot. When no definitive neurologic or neuromuscular lesion can be isolated, cavus deformity is labeled "idiopathic."[332] Generally, when assessing cavus deformity as it relates to the athlete, the deformity is more often characterized as idiopathic, with single-component or column involvement, and less severe in character. A discussion of the full scope of cavus deformity and associated surgery is beyond the scope of this chapter, and the reader is referred to appropriate texts for more information.

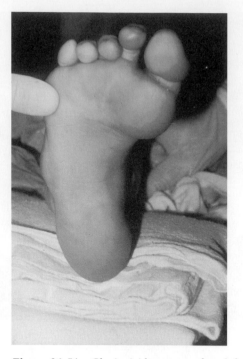

Figure 26-51 Classic rigid cavovarus foot deformity. Note rearfoot varus, forefoot valgus, and lateral column luxation at fifth metatarsal–cuboid joint.

ATHLETIC MANIFESTATIONS

The presence of a compensatory-type cavus deformity will lead to numerous mechanical problems: painful propulsive keratotic skin lesions (especially beneath the fifth metatarsal region), hammertoes, anterior ankle impingement pain and exostosis, anterior tarsal tunnel syndrome, interdigital neuroma, stress fracture, plantar fasciitis, retrocalcaneal bursitis and exostosis, and Achilles tendinitis. Structural heel varus deformity in a cavus foot will simulate clinical chronic lateral ankle instability. Medial cavus deformity can result in similar symptoms as a result of supinatory compensation at the subtalar joint in the absence of calcaneal deformity.

Severe cavus deformity is not common in the mature adult athlete, because the patient with this foot type will normally present with significant limitations long before attaining skeletal or "athletic" maturity. Surgical considerations in cavus deformity are most common in a developing athlete with future promise (e.g., the high school athlete), with symptomatic cavus foot and associated sequelae that are unresponsive to conservative treatment such as orthotic control. It is important for both the surgeon and the patient to realize that the surgical correction of cavus deformity does impose risks, as well as possible long-term rehabilitation postoperatively. Staging of procedures is often appropriate, allowing time for bone and soft tissue adaptation to occur before addressing additional components of the deformity.

CAVUS FOOT SURGERY IN THE ATHLETE

Staging operative procedures in the athlete is a wise decision. This allows time for the soft tissue and skeletal components to adapt in order that a more accurate evaluation of the effect of a surgical procedure can be made. Often, digital contractures will spontaneously reduce after correction of cavus deformity. If spontaneous reduction fails to occur, other soft tissue procedures are available, such as a Hibbs midfoot suspension extensor digitorum longus transfer to the midfoot to eliminate painful extensor substitution, which contributes to symptomatic hammertoe syndrome[333] (Fig. 26-52). Rigid hammertoes will require interphalangeal arthrodesis.[334] In any event, up to 6 to 12 months of postoperative rehabilitation should be anticipated following major tarsal osseous correction of cavus deformity before a level of competitiveness may be regained in the athlete. The high-caliber high school athlete with tremendous future potential who is suffering from a complex and disabling condition such as pes cavus deformity often can afford the length of down time, considering that the alternative may mean loss of future competitive ability. This point must be clearly understood by the younger athlete and the parents.

There are a variety of cavus foot presentations with associated deformities that may require surgical intervention. The most common cavus deformity responsive to surgery is rearfoot varus, plantar contracture, and plantar-flexed first metatarsal with hallux hammertoe. There may be associated contractures of the lesser metatarsophalangeal joints as well as other digital contractures. Indicated surgery could include plantar release, elevational dorsal wedge osteotomy of the first metatarsal base, and a Dwyer calcaneal osteotomy. Adjunctive bone and soft tissue procedures on the lesser digits and metatarsophalangeal joints is deferred. Spontaneous resolution or significant improvement of these other companion deformities can occur following the major surgical procedures.

Modified Jones suspension with compression arthrodesis of the interphalangeal joint of the great toe is necessary for severe and rigid deformities with extensor hallucis longus

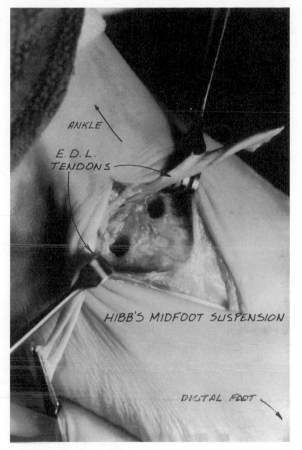

Figure 26-52 Hibbs midfoot suspension to eliminate extensor substitution contributing to dynamic hammertoes.

substitution in gait or running.[335] The first ray segment must demonstrate reducibility for this combination to be effective.[336] The entire forefoot can be tested for reducibility with the "push-up test." Otherwise, elevational base metatarsal osteotomy will be required, with compression fusion of the interphalangeal hallux joint. Soft tissue tendon balancing procedures are helpful at the lesser metatarsophalangeal joints, including lesser metatarsal Jones-type suspensions with digital soft tissue releases if the deformities are flexible.[337]

HINDFOOT VARUS DEFORMITY

Varus deformity of the rearfoot can result result in a calcaneus unable evert to the perpendicular position with maximum rearfoot pronation.[338] This foot functions around an inverted heel position, which is even more problematic for an athlete than for a nonathlete because of ultimate impact forces at heel contact with weight trajectory shift proximal into the ankle and knee as well. Most athletes cannot tolerate this malalignment syndrome unless it is within the bounds of compensability, which are narrow. The deformity is generally bilateral but may present unilaterally following congenital or acquired conditions, such as trauma. It may present as one component of cavovarus deformity, which produces varus deformity of the hindfoot from compensation mechanisms in the midtarsal joint or the medial column. It is important to investigate and rule out various neuromuscular disorders capable of producing such deformity. A major neurologic or neuromuscular defect is generally not anticipated in the athletic population; however, it does occur. "Idiopathic cavus" may well represent occult neuromuscular disease imbalance of extrinsic or intrinsic musculature.[331,339]

Evaluation of rearfoot varus deformity requires elimination of the forefoot influence on the position of the rearfoot. A rigid plantar-flexed first ray will result in secondary hindfoot varus compensation. The rearfoot is isolated from the forefoot by having the patient stand on a book or block, such that the first ray is not supported. If deformity persists during the block test, a structural heel varus is present as a separate deformity[340,341] (Fig. 26-53A & B).

Hindfoot varus deformity predisposes the athlete to repeated inversion ankle injuries and even eventual chronic lateral ankle instability. It is imperative to recognize the heel varus as the mechanical source of the imbalance and perform a lateral wedge valgus-producing heel osteotomy to shift the mechanical balance medially.[101] This alone is usually sufficient to restore balance. If secondary ligamentous insufficiency has developed from chronic sprains, then soft tissue stabilization tenodesis or ligamentoplasty will be required in conjunction with the heel osteotomy. Calcaneal osteotomy is contraindicated when the heel varus deformity is positional and mainly compensational. The pathologic source in the forefoot must be corrected in order to resolve the positional imbalance in the hindfoot complex.[102,339]

Figure 26-53 (**A**) Structural cavovarus with predominant midfoot and forefoot problem deformity and hindfoot varus as a form of compensation when viewed posteriorly. (**B**) Coleman lateral block test neutralizes the medial column deformity component and also reduces the heel varus, which was compensatory in A.

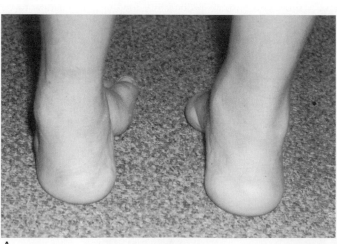

A

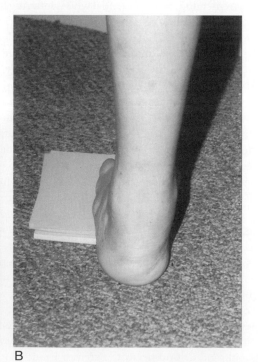

B

Valgus-Producing Calcaneal Osteotomy

A varus deformity of the heel is best managed with a Dwyer-type lateral closing wedge osteotomy.[342-344] General anesthesia is preferred, with the patient in a lateral or lateral recumbent position exposing the lateral wall of the heel. Tourniquet control provides good visualization to execute the procedure and avoid injury to the sural nerve in the operative site. The approach is a posteroinferior curvilinear incision placed over the lateral wall of the os calcis. The proximal portion of the incision begins behind the lateral malleolus just proximal to the superior posterior surface of the calcaneus and courses distally to the calcaneocuboid joint region. The sural nerve is tagged and protected and a deeper bold incision is made down to the bone immediately behind and parallel to the peroneal tendons. The periosteum is elevated superiorly and inferiorly along the expanse of the bone, including the peroneal tendons in the superior skin flap. The sural nerve may run either above or below the primary skin approach depending on the severity of the deformity and the exact positioning of the incision. The lateral wall of the os calcis is viewed and landmarks are identified.

The osteotomy is carried from immediately behind the subtalar joint superiorly to the area just behind the calcaneocuboid joint inferiorly and is relatively parallel to the peroneal tendons. The osteotomy is carried to but not through the medial cortex, which serves as a stabilizing hinge. The typical wedge resection measures about 5 to 10 mm to effect correction (Fig 26-54). Occasionally, the osteotomy must be feathered with the bone saw blade to weaken it medially and allow tight osteotomy closure. A plantar Steindler myofascial release is often performed concurrently through the inferior portion of the incision. The plantar release can help facilitate resolution of some of the forefoot equinus deformity if present.[345,346] Valgus heel osteotomy does not increase the overall range of motion, but it allows a vertical heel position, displacing the available range of motion in the direction of eversion. Full subtalar joint pronation will now allow the calcaneus to evert past the perpendicular, and the heel-to-leg relationship will now be less inverted when the subtalar joint is in neutral position. Excellent fixation is achieved using two or three power-driven staples, percutaneous Steinman pins, or lag screws.

The Dwyer-type osteotomy can be modified with slight proximal displacement to accommodate some compensated equinus, axial valgus rotation of the tuber, or alterna-

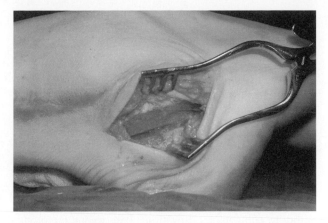

Figure 26-54 Dwyer "valgus-producing" lateral wedge osteotomy.

tive bone incisions involving an L configuration. The surgeon must decide on any additional subtle correction required by these maneuvers.

Calcaneal osteotomy may be performed in a cavovarus-type foot with varus deformity of the rearfoot and an abnormally high calcaneal pitch angle secondary to forefoot equinus. Additional procedures aimed at reduction of the forefoot equinus should be performed concurrently, along with Steindler myofascial plantar release. Valgus heel osteotomy in the presence of an unresolved rigid medial column plantar flexion or rigid forefoot equinus deformity would exacerbate the pseudoequinus and is contraindicated.

Layered closure is performed, and a below-knee compression dressing applied with the foot maintained at 90 degrees in a non-weight-bearing posterior splint or cast brace. Physiotherapy is initiated 7 to 9 days postoperatively. Partial weight bearing in a cast brace with crutches is permitted, progressing to full weight bearing at about 4 weeks. The osteotomy unites quickly, especially with solid fixation, in about 6 to 8 weeks, and the cast is usually removed at 6 to 8 weeks. Progressive rehabilitation and a return-to-activity program is initiated. Postoperative orthotics are used if necessary.

RIGID PLANTAR-FLEXED FIRST METATARSAL

Excessive rigid plantar flexion of the first metatarsal results in keratoma beneath the first metatarsal head, bursitis, sesamoiditis, and/or a fractured sesamoid usually accompanied by a cocked hallux deformity. Subtalar joint varus compensation is required for a rigid plantar-flexed first metatarsal. Splaying of the fifth metatarsal may be evident with tailor's bunion formation, and the athlete may be more apt to develop ankle sprains, lateral ankle instability, or retrocalcaneal exostosis. A rigid plantar-flexed first ray is a form of medial cavus deformity and may coexist with other components of forefoot equinus on the rearfoot or varus deformity of the calcaneus.

Rigid plantar-flexed first metatarsal responds poorly to conservative treatment. Treatment is individualized, depending on the type and degree of deformity and the resultant disability of the athlete. Surgery is often necessary for this condition in the athlete because there is limited ability to compensate. Elevational base wedge osteotomy is the appropriate procedure, with an osteosynthesis screw, loop wire, or K-wire.[133] Flexible medial cavus or nonrigid plantar flexion of the first metatarsal in conjunction with hallux hammertoe deformity is treated by a soft tissue correction using a modified Jones tenosuspension as indicted earlier. If the hallux is not hammered, a tenodesis at the interphalangeal joint can be satisfactory; however, a fusion is more dependable over the long term and does not interfere with athletic function if the metatarsophalangeal joint is functional.

First Metatarsal Dorsal Base Wedge Osteotomy

A dorsolinear approach to the dorsal aspect of the first metatarsal base is carried out through a 3.5- to 4-cm linear longitudinal incision medial to the extensor hallucis longus tendon. The deep fascia is incised in line with the skin incision, and the extensor hallucis longus tendon is identified and retracted laterally. The first metatarsal–cuneiform articulation and the periosteum overlying the dorsal aspect of the first metatarsal base are identified. A linear longitudinal dorsal periosteal incision is performed at the metaphysis of the first metatarsal, and periosteal soft tissues are reflected medially and laterally. Careful subperiosteal elevation is performed in the first interspace to avoid any embarrassment of the deep planter artery. A dorsal-to-plantar transverse wedge-shaped osteotomy is performed approximately 1 cm distal to the first metatarsal–cuneiform joint, preserving the plantar cortex of the first metatarsal.[347] This wedge is fashioned with its base dorsal and apex plantar. A sufficient portion of bone is removed in order to reduce the rigid plantar-flexed deformity of the first metatarsal. Iatrogenic metatarsus primus elevatus deformity can be produced with excessive wedge resection and should be avoided. The wedge resection should be sufficient to allow the first metatarsal to be elevated to the level of the plane of the lesser metatarsals or just slightly beyond. Fixation is by surgeon preference and can be crossed K-wires, screws, or power staples, depending on osteotomy orientation. The wound is then closed in layers and a compressed dressing is applied.

Partial weight bearing with crutch assistance is allowed in a below-knee cast for 2 to 3 weeks. The foot is protected for an additional 2 to 3 weeks in a full weight-bearing cast brace. Total casting rquirement is 4 to 6 weeks. Physiotherapy can be started approximately 1 week postoperatively. Consolidation of this osteotomy is rapid and certain. External percutaneous K-wires are retrieved at about 4 weeks. The postoperative course is modified appropriately if any additional procedures were performed concurrently.

MIDFOOT OSTEOTOMY

Lesser tarsus Cole midfoot osteotomy is occasionally indicated for severe forms of cavus in an athlete that fail to compensate adequately or interfere with performance.[329,348–350] This can be a debilitating procedure and should be carried out only when the deformity fails to compensate or conservative measures prove insufficient. It is often the best method to manage painful rigid global metatarsalgia problems with keratoma formation and midfoot apex deformity.[351] Patients who require this osteotomy usually have neuromuscular disease or congenital deformity, and their athletic performance is impaired early in life. Other forms of lesser tarsal cavus osteotomy, such as the Japas and Saunders procedures, are not recommended.[350,352]

COLE MIDFOOT OSTEOTOMY

Lesser tarsal wedge closing osteotomy is best performed with two incisions—one dorsomedial over the navicular-cuneiform joints, about 4 cm long, and one dorsolateral over the cuboid, measuring about 3 cm.[350,353] These two approaches are connected subperiosteally with a sharp elevator and retracted with a 1-inch Penrose drain. The neurovascular bundle is elevated in the soft tissue isthmus between the two incisions. The exposure readily allows a good view of the cuboid and cuneiforms when viewed either medially or laterally. Dorsal wedge osteotomy is started medially with a plantar apex, removing a wedge at least 1.5 cm in width. The osteotomy of the cuboid is performed through the lateral approach. An oscillating bone saw conveniently performs this maneuver. Care is

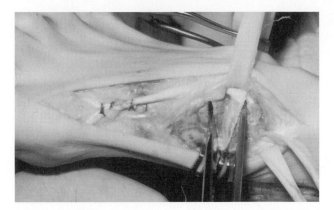

Figure 26-55 Cole midfoot osteotomy combined with Jones suspension for rigid cavus foot. Dwyer osteotomy is also done in this foot type.

taken to avoid penetrating too far laterally from the medial approach; otherwise, the fourth and fifth metatarsal base joints can be entered. Adequate viewing is available with these two approaches, with a minimum of soft tissue dissection (Fig. 26-55). The osteotomy site is closed with plantar forefoot dorsiflexion pressure and fixed with multiple power-driven staples both medially and laterally. This allows rapid fixation with good stability. The plantar osteotomy site and ligaments should be kept intact in order to produce a tension band effect on the bottom side of the osteotomy at closure. Layered closure is performed with posterior splinting for the first 4 days followed by casting. This osteotomy is very stable and can be ambulated upon by the second postoperative week.

Cole midfoot osteotomy approaches the deformity at its apex, which is the optimum location for osteotomy.[350] It provides dramatic reduction of deformity and is the only complete transverse osteotomy through the entire midfoot that is recommended. It is the optimum method of correction with the least amount of surgery and is most preferred. Lesser tarsal osteotomy can be combined with other procedures, such as valgus-producing calcaneal osteotomy and first metatarsal osteotomy. This is more comprehensive surgery and requires more extensive recovery.

Postoperative rehabilitation is started 7 to 9 days postoperatively and the posterior splint transformed to a cast brace during this same period. The osteotomy consolidates in 6 to 8 weeks. The postoperative course and physiotherapy regimen may be modified according to additional procedures.

The biomechanical consequences of major midfoot sur-

gical intervention must be anticipated. Both the surgeon and the patient must be willing and prepared to accept a possible prolonged period of postoperative rehabilitation or postoperative complications such as swelling and some numbness as a result of sensory impairment.

Flexible Flatfoot Deformity and Associated Compensation Conditions

The term *flatfoot* is a generic clinical description defining a foot with a depressed or absent medial longitudinal arch. This description is of limited value and fails to convey the real problem related to this deformity. Medial column tarsal instability is determined easily both visually and clinically at examination. Not all arches are created equal, and some patients can manifest a decreased medial longitudinal architecture and be "within normal limits." It becomes more difficult to define the point of "pathologic hyperpronation," but it is usually clear to an experienced clinician when "normal" has been exceeded. Additionally, these patient begin to experience associated symptoms: leg fatigue, knee pain, and forefoot static problems such as hammertoes, neuromas, metatarsalgia, plantar fasciitis, and progressive hallux valgus, especially if the source is compensated equinus contributing to the hypermobile flatfoot.[354] The term *flexible flatfoot* is used to describe reducible collapse and hyperpronation of the tarsal joints of the foot with loss of stability and locking. These patients become symptomatic usually as skeletal maturity is approached because of loss of plasticity of their osseocartilaginous tissues.

BIOMECHANICS AND CLINICAL PRESENTATION

Closed kinetic chain pronation of the subtalar joint results in eversion of the calcaneus with plantar flexion, adduction, and anterior displacement of the talus on the calcaneus.[355] The midtarsal joint complex is then unlocked, permitting exaggerated mobility of the forefoot on the rearfoot in the direction of pronation.[356] The tension-banding mechanism of the plantar myofascial mechanism becomes dysfunctional (Fig. 26-56).[357,358] Persistent flatfoot results in compensated equinus that is very destructive to continued function or growth in an immature foot.

Conditions with ligamentous laxity or skeletal abnormalities, such as forefoot varus deformities, may be underlying etiologic factors in flatfoot. There is often a strong familial history. The juvenile athletic patient with severe

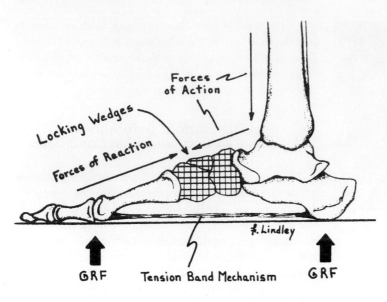

Figure 26-56 The stabilization mechanism of the tarsal complex. Locking is based on instrinsic stability produced by induced compression through wedge segments and a functional tension banding mechanism of the plantar fascia.

flexible flatfoot deformity may or may not complain of pain. Careful history, including interview of the parents, is important in order to determine subtle subjective complaints such as clumsiness during walking, running, or other athletic activities. Abnormal shoegear wear is evident if evaluated. It is interestig to note that surgeons often fail to examine the shoes of their patients. Subluxation of the subtalar joint in the direction of pronation results predominantly in a frontal plane deformity with excessive heel valgus, talonavicular ptosis, and clinical collapse of the medial column. Sagittal plane deformity results in a slightly everted heel position of less than 6 degrees with significant collapse of the medial column secondary to navicular–cuneiform breach. Transverse plane deformity exists when there is abduction of the forefoot on the rearfoot at the midtarsal joint with less than 6 degrees of eversion of the heel and collapse of the medial column. Cuboid abduction deformity is usually present as well, especially in transverse plane compensated flatfoot. These deformities are passively reducible and distinct entities separate from rigid flatfoot deformities, such as vertical talus, tarsal coalition, or peroneal spastic flatfoot.

Accurate radiographic analysis is essential in the evaluation process and includes the use of standard weight-bearing views in the angle and base of gait. Planal dominance of the deformity will assist the surgeon in proper treatment, whether it be conservative or surgical.[359] Neutral-position weight-bearing films might also be helpful. CT scans or MRI may be indicated in suspected coalition abnormalities in the preadolescent group. The full scope of this complex entity is beyond the intent of this chapter, and the reader is referred to specialized texts regarding same.

CONSERVATIVE TREATMENT

Appropriate treatment for symptomatic flexible flatfoot deformity requires careful consideration of the level and major plane of the deformity. Tarsal stabilization with functional orthotics is indicated in all stages of reducible deformity. Heel stabilizers or other biomechanical orthotic devices may be effective in allowing the foot to readapt to a more functionally efficient state if treatment is initiated early enough in the immature foot. Between the age of 6 and the adolescent growth spurt, in the moderately severe hyperpronated foot, initial conservative treatment using orthotics can still be initiated with good functional outcome and improved performance.[360] Mild to moderately severe flexible flatfoot deformity in the young athletic patient near or at the adolescent growth spurt should also be stabilized with a functional orthotic. Operative intervention is considered when functional control is insufficient and impairment of performance is noted. Secondary symptoms are often present that focus attention on the severity of the deformity and need for further treatment.

SURGICAL PROCEDURES

Surgical reconstructive procedures for severe collapsing flexible flatfoot and other forms of painful compensated flatfoot have historically been controversial in the literature. Foot and ankle surgeons are becoming more aware

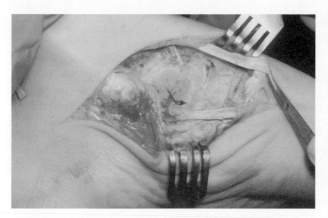

Figure 26-57   Medial column stabilization with tibialis anterior translocation into navicular (navicular suspension) and open wedge (Cotton) dorsal opening osteotomy of medial cuneiform with tibial bone implant.

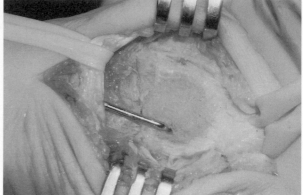

Figure 26-59   Medial column arthrodesis at navicular-cuneiform joint with arthritis or rigid medial column deformity.

of the value of surgical intervention in specific situations, and the number of publications and modifications of various operations continues to increase. Patients with severe subluxatory deformity between the age of 6 and the adolescent growth spurt can be considered for limited surgical intervention. These procedures usually fall into the category of soft tissue repairs such as percutaneous tendo Achillis lengthening or selective gastrocnemius aponeurotic recession for equinus release with medial column tension banding using tibialis anterior translocation. Young navicular suspension or Cotton-type medial cuneiform dorsal open wedge osteotomy[102,172,361,362] (Fig. 26-57) or

Figure 26-58   Varus-producing open wedge calcaneal osteotomy with humeral head allograft.

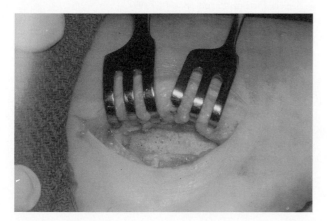

cervical and lateral open wedge calcaneal osteotomy[363–366] (Fig. 26-58) and tuber medialization osteotomy[367,368] are emerging as very effective limited surgical procedures with maximum benefit in carefully selected cases of symptomatic flatfoot in all age groups. Medialization osteotomy requires screw or K-wire fixation to maintain the displacement correction.

Lesser tarsal medial column midfoot arthrodesis is performed less commonly in athletes, but does have a role if pain is severe enough with nonreducible deformity or arthritic changes (Fig. 26-59). These are usually fusions at the navicular–cuneiform joints using operations such as Miller and Hoke-type fusions with sagittal plane compensation or breach.[369,370] Arthrodesis will disable an athlete longer, but, if the sagittal plane arch pain, deformity, and disability are severe enough to disrupt continued performance, fusion at this level will be required. Recovery will be prolonged—as much as 5 to 7 months compared with soft tissue medial column navicular tenosuspensions.

REFERENCES

1. Suppan RJ, Ritchlin JD: A non-disabling surgical procedure for ingrown toenail. J Am Podiatry Assoc 52:900, 1962
2. Yale JF: Phenol-alcohol technique for correction of ingrown toenail. J Am Podiatry Assoc 64:46, 1974
3. Cangiolosi CP, Schnall SJ: Comparison of the phenol-alcohol and Suppan nail technique: Curr Podiatry 30:25, 1981
4. Landon GC et al: Subungual exostosis. J Bone Joint Surg Am 61:256 1979
5. Miller-Breslow A, Dorfman HD: Dupuytren's (subungual) exostosis. Am J Surg Pathol 12:368, 1988

6. Greger G, Catanzariti AR: Osteochondroma: review of the literature and case report. J Foot Surg 31:298, 1992

7. Burns AE, Stewart WP: Morton's neuroma. J Am Podiatry Assoc 72:135, 1982

8. Miller SJ: Surgical technique for resection of Morton's neuroma. J Am Podiatry Assoc 71:181, 1981

9. Mann RA, Reynolds JLC: Interdigital neuroma—critical clinical analysis. Foot Ankle 3:238, 1983

10. Jarde O, Trinquier JL, Pleyber A et al: Intermetatarsal neuroma—surgery—metatarsalgia. Rev Chir Orthop 81:142, 1995.

11. Bernedetti RS, Baxter DE, Davis PF: Clinical results of simultaneous adjacent interdigital neurectomy in the foot. Foot Ankle Int 17:264, 1996

12. Mulder JD: The causative mechanism in Morton's metatarsalgia. J Bone Joint Surg [Br] 33:94, 1951

13. Subotnick SJ: Medial plantar digital proper nerve syndrome (Joplin's neuroma)—typical presentation. J Foot Surg 21:166, 1982

14. Wilson S, Kuwada GT: Retrospective study of the use of plantar transverse incision versus a dorsal incision for excision of neuroma. J Foot Ankle Surg 34:537, 1995

15. Dereymaeker G, Schroven I, Steenwerckx A, Stuer P: Results of excision of the interdigital nerve in the treatment of Morton's metatarsalgia. Acta Orthop Belg 62:22, 1996

16. Nelms BA, Bishop JO, Tullos HS: Surgical treatment of recurrent Morton's neuroma. Orthopedics 7:1708, 1984

17. Banks A, Vito G, Giorgini TL: Recurrent intermetarsal neuroma: a follow up study. J Am Podiatr Med Assoc 86:299, 1996

18. Malay DS, McGlamry ED, Nava CA Jr: Entrapment neuropathies of the lower extremity. p. 668. In McGlamry ED (ed): Comprehensive Textbook of Foot Surgery. Vol. 2. Williams & Wilkins, Baltimore, 1987

19. Mann RA: The tarsal tunnel syndrome. Orthop Clin North Am 5:109, 1974

20. DiGiacomo MA, Bernstein AL, Scurran B, Karlin JM: Electrodiagnosis of the tarsal tunnel syndrome. J Am Podiatry Assoc 70:94, 1980

21. Stern DS, Joyce MTL: Tarsal tunnel syndrome: a review of 15 surgical procedures. J Foot Surg 28:290, 1989

22. Orner GE: Physical diagnosis of peripheral nerve injuries. Orthop Clin North Am 12:207, 1981

23. Heimkes B, Posel P, Stotz S, Wolf K: The proximal and sital tarsal tunnel syndromes. Int Orthop 11:193, 1987

24. Goodman CR, Kehr LE: Bilateral tarsal tunnel syndrome. J Am Podiatry Assoc 73:256, 1983

25. Zahari DT, Ly P: Recurrent tarsal tunnel syndrome. J Foot Surg 31:385, 1992

26. Vogler, HW, Stienstra J, Montgomery F, Kipp, L: Anterior ankle impingement arthropathy: the role of anterolateral arthrotomy and arthroscopy. Clin Podiatr Med Surg 11:425, 1994

27. Herrik R, Herrik F: Rupture of the plantar fascia in middle aged tennis player: a case report. Am J Sports Med 11:95, 1983

28. McElgun T, Cavaliere R: Sequential bilateral rupture of plantar fascia in a tennis player. Sports Med 84:137, 1994

29. Pai V: Rupture of the plantar fascia. J Foot Ankle Surg 35:39, 1996

30. Rolf C, Gunter P, Ericsater J, Turan I: Plantar fascia rupture: diagnosis and treatment. J Foot Ankle Surg 36:112, 1997

31. Leach R, Jones R, Silva T: Rupture of the plantar fascia in athletes. J Bone Joint Surg Am 60:537, 1978

32. Poux D, Chirstel P, Demarais Y et al: Les ruptures de laponevrose plaintare. J Traumatol Sport 6:77, 1989

33. Christel P, Rigal F, Poux D et al: Surgical treatment of rupture of the plantar fascia. Rev Chir Orthop 79:218, 1993

34. Mitchetti ML, Jacobs SA: Calcaneal heel spurs: etiology, treatment and a new surgical approach. J Foot Surg 22:234, 1983

35. Baxter DE, Thigpen CM: Heel pain: operative results. Foot Ankle 5:16, 1984

36. Gill LH, Kiebzak GM: Outcome of nonsurgical treatment for plantar fasciitis. Foot Ankle Int 17:527, 1996

37. Kitaoka HB, Luo ZP, An KN: Mechanical behavior of the foot and ankle after plantar fascia release in the unstable foot. Foot Ankle Int 18:8, 1997

38. Tountas AA, Fornasier VL: Operative treatment of subcalcaneal pain. Clin Orthop Rel Res 332:170, 1996

39. Sammarco GJ, Helfrey RB: Surgical treatment of recalcitrant plantar fasciitis. Foot Ankle Int 17:520, 1996

40. Teitz CC, Garrett W, Miniaci A et al: Tendon problems in athletic individuals. J Bone Joint Surg Am 79:138, 1997

41. Vogler H, Bauer G: Contrast studies of the foot and ankle. p. 439. In Weissman SD (ed): Radiology of the Foot. Williams & Wilkins, Baltimore, 1989

42. Astrom M, Rausing A: Chronic Achilles tendinopathy. Clin Orthop Rel Res 316:151, 1995

43. Movin T, Gad A, Reinholt FP, Rolf C: Tendon pathology in long standing achillodynia: biospy findings in 40 patients. Acta Orthop Scand 68:170, 1997

44. Arner O, Lindholm A, Orell SR: Histologic changes in the subcutaneous rupture of the Achilles tendon. Acta Chir Scand 116:484, 1958/59

45. Lagergren C, Linholm A: Vascular distribution in the Achilles tendon: an angiographic and microangiographic study. Acta Chir Scand 116:491, 1958/1959

46. Burry HC, Pool CJ: Central degeneration of the Achilles tendon. Rheumatol Rehabil 12:177, 1973

47. Nelen G, Martens M, Burssens A: Surgical treatment of chronic Achilles tendinitis. Am J Sports Med 17:754, 1989

48. Schepsis AA, Leach RE: Surgical management of Achilles tendinitis. Am J Sports Med 15:308, 1987

49. Williams JG: Achilles tendon lesions in sport. Sports Med 3:114, 1986

50. Astrom M, Gentz CF, Nilsson P et al: Imaging in chronic Achilles tendinopathy: a comparison of ultrasonography, magnetic resonance imaging and surgical findings in 27 histologically verified cases. Skeletal Radiol 25:615, 1996

51. Martii H, Kvist H, Matti UK et al: Chronic Achilles paratenonitis: an immunohistologic study of fibronectin and fibrinogen. Am J Sports Med 16:616, 1988

52. James SL, Bates BT, Osternig RL: Injuries to runners. Am J Sports Med 6:40, 1978

53. Subotnick SI, Roth WE: Achilles tendinopathy. p. 293. In Jay R (ed): Current Therapy in Podiatric Surgery. CV Mosby Co., St. Louis, 1988

54. Subotnick SI, Sisney P: Treatment of Achilles tendinopathy in the athlete. J Am Podiatr Med Assoc 76:10, 1986

55. Sarrafian SK: Anatomy of the Foot and Ankle: Descriptive, Topographical, Functional. JB Lippincott Co., Philadelphia, 1983

56. Kvist MH, Lehto MU, Jarvinen M, Kvist HT: Chronic achilles paratenonitis: an immunohistologic study of fibronectin and fibrinogen. Am J Sport Med 16:616, 1988

57. Kvist H, Kvist M: The operative treatment of chronic calcaneal paratenonitis. J Bone Joint Surg [Br] 62:353, 1980

58. Kvist M, Jozsa J, Kvist H: Chronic Achilles parateonitis in athletes: a histological and histochemical study. Pathology 19:1, 1987

59. Schepsis AA, Leach RE: Surgical management of Achilles tendonitis. Am J Sports Med 15:308, 1987

60. Cummins JE, Anson JB, Carr WB et al: The structure of the calcaneal tendon (of Achilles) in relation to orthopaedic surgery with additional observations on the plantaris muscle. Surg Gynecol Obstet 83:107, 1946

61. White JW: Torsion of the Achilles tendon: its surgical significance. Arch Surg 46:784, 1943

62. Husson JL, deKorvin B, Polard JL et al: Achilles tendon—chronic—MRI. Acta Orthop Belg 60:408, 1994

63. Chaudhani VP, Bradley YC: Achilles tendon and miscellaneous tendon lesions. Magn Reson Imaging Clin North Am 2:89, 1994

64. Leadbetter WB, Mooar PA, Lane GJ, Lee SJ: The surgical treatment of tendinitis: clinical rationale and biologic basis. Clin Sports Med 11:679, 1992

65. Testa V, Maffulii N, Capasso G, Bifulco G: Percutaneous longitudinal tenotomy in chronic Achilles tendonitis. Bull Hosp Joint Dis 54:241, 1966

66. Morris KL, Giacopelli JA, Granoff D: Classification of radiopaque lesions of the tendo Achilles. J Foot Surg 29:533, 1990

67. Fowler A, Phillip JF: Abnormality of the calcaneus as a cause of painful heel: its diagnosis and operative treatment. Br J Surg 32:494, 1945

68. Ruch JA: Haglund's disease. J Am Podiatry Assoc 64:1000, 1979

69. Malay DS, Duggar G: Heel surgery. p. 264. In McGlamry ED (ed) : Comprehensive Textbook of Foot Surgery. Vol. 1. Williams Wilkins, Baltimore, 1987

70. Schepsis AA, Wagner C, Leach RE: Surgical management of Achilles tendon overuse injuries: a long term follow-up study. Am J Sports Med 22:611, 1994

71. Saxena A: Surgery for chronic Achilles tendon problems. J Foot Ankle Surg 34:294, 1996

72. Chao W, Deland JT, Bates JE, Kenneally SM: Achilles tendon insertion: an in vitro anatomic study. Foot Ankle Int 18:81, 1997

73. Hoerr NL, Pyle DI, Francis CC: Radiographic Atlas of Skeletal Development of the Foot and Ankle: A Standard of Reference. Charles C Thomas, Springfield, IL, 1962

74. Johnson RE: Podiatric radiology. p. 231. In Levy L, Hetherington VJ eds: Principles and Practice of Podiatric Medicine. Churchill Livingstone, New York, 1990

75. Subotnick SE: Podiatric Sports Medicine. Futura, Mount Kisco, NY, 1975

76. Jones DC, James SL: Partial calcaneal osteotomy for retrocalcaneal bursitis. Am J Sports Med 12:72, 1984

77. Haygood TM: Magnetic resonance imaging of the musculoskeletal system. Part 7: The Ankle. Clin Orthop Rel Res 336.318, 1997

78. Hatch DJ: Chronic stenosing peroneal tenosynovitis. The Lower Extremity 1:197, 1994

79. Newell SE, Woodle A: Cuboid syndrome. Physician Sports Med 9:71, 1981

80. Boberg J, Kalish SA, Banks AS: Ankle conditions. p. 508. In McGlamry ED (ed): Comprehensive Textbook of Foot Surgery. Vol. 1. Williams & Wilkins, Baltimore, 1987

81. Vogler HW, Bauer GR: Myotenoplastic maneuvers about the foot and ankle. p. 220. In Jay R (ed): Current Therapy in Podiatric Surgery. CV Mosby Co., St. Louis, 1988

82. Jones E: Operative treatment of the chronic dislocation of the peroneal tendons. J Bone Joint Surg 14:574, 1932

83. Rudolphy VJ, Poll RG: The long term result of the "Leidenplasty" for dislocating peroneal tendons, abstracted. Acta Orthop Scand Suppl 262:59, 1994

84. Platzgummer H: On a simple procedure for the operative therapy of habitual peroneal tendon luxation. Arch Orthop Unfallchir 61:144, 1967

85. Pozo JL, Jackson AM: A rerouting operation for dislocation of peroneal tendons: operative technique and case report. Foot Ankle 5:42, 1984

86. Slatis P, Santavirta S, Sandlein J: Surgical treatment of chronic dislocation of the peroneal tendons. Br J Sports Med 22:16, 1988

87. DuVries HL: Surgery of the Foot. p. 253. St. Louis, Mosby—Year Book, 1959

88. Kelly RE: An operation for the chronic dislocation of the peroneal tendons. Br J Surg 7:502, 1920.

89. Sarrafian SK: Anatomy of the Foot and Ankle. JB Lippincott Co., Philadelphia, 1983

90. Meyers AW: Further evidences of attrition in the human body. Am J Anat 34:241, 1924

91. Sobel M, Bohme, WO, Levy ME: Longitudinal attrition of the peroneus brevis tendon in the fibular groove: an anatomic study. Foot Ankle 11:124, 1990

92. Sobel M, Bohme WO, Markisz JA: Cadaver correlation of peroneal tendon changes with magnetic resonance imaging. Foot Ankle 11:384, 1991

93. Khoury NJ, El-Khoury GY, Saltzman CL, Kathol MH: Peroneus longus and brevis tendon tears: MR imaging evaluation. Radiology 200:833, 1996

94. Anderson E: Stenosing peroneal tenosynovitis symptomatically simulating ankle instability. Am J Sports Med 15:258, 1987

95. Yao L, Cracchiolo A, Seeger LL: MR findings in peroneal tendonopathy. J Comput Assist Tomogr 19:460, 1995

96. Frey C, Sheriff M, Greenidge N: Vascularity of the posterior tibial tendon. J Bone Joint Surg Am 72:884, 1990

97. Jahss MH: Spontaneous rupture of the tibialis posterior tendon: clinical findings, tenographic studies and a new technique of repair. Foot Ankle 3:158, 1982

98. Meuller TJ: Acquired flatfoot secondary to tibialis posterior dsyfunction: biomechanical aspect. J Foot Surg 30:2, 1991

99. Hutchinson BL, O'Rourke EM: Tibialis posterior tendon dysfunction and peroneal tendon subluxation. Clin Podiatr Med Surg 12:703, 1995

100. Myerson M: Adult acquired flatfoot deformity. J Bone Joint Surg Am 78:780, 1996

101. Johnson K, Strom DE: Tibialis posterior tendon dysfunction. Clin Orthop Rel Res 239:196, 1989

102. Vogler H, Bojsen-Moller F, Montgomery F, Kipp L: The biomechanical role of calcaneal osteotomy in varus and valgus hindfoot deformities. The Lower Extremity 2:63, 1995

103. Vogler H: Triple arthrodesis as salvage for end stage flatfoot. Clin Podiatr Med Surg 6:591, 1989

104. Sella EJ, Lawson JP, Ogden JA: The accessory navicular synchondrosis. Clin Orthop Rel Res 209:280, 1986

105. Dobas DC, Pietrocarlo TA: Accessory navicular in a skier: a case report. J Am Podiatry Assoc 67:126, 1977

106. Smith TF, Murrell J, Jones RH: Flatfoot: Kidner procedure. p. 242. In Jay R (ed): Current Therapy in Podiatric Surgery. CV Mosby Co., St. Louis, 1988

107. Ma GW, Griffith TG: Percutaneous repair of acute closed ruptured Achilles tendon: a new technique. Clin Orthop 128:247, 1977

108. Kuwada GT: Classification of tendo Achilles rupture with consideration of surgical repair techniques. J Foot Surg 29:361, 1990

109. Kuwada GT: Critical analysis of tendo Achilles repair using Achilles tendon rupture classification system and repair. J Foot Ankle Surg 32:611, 1993

110. Kuwada GT: Diagnosis and treatment of Achilles tendon rupture. Clin Podiatr Med Surg 12:633, 1995

111. Parker RG, Repinecz M: Neglected rupture of the Achilles tendon: treatment by modified Strayer gastrocnemius recession. J Am Podiatry Assoc 69:548, 1979

112. Schuberth JM, Dockery GL, McBride RE: Recurrent rupture of the tendo Achilles: repair by free tendinous autograft. J Am Podiatry Assoc 74:157, 1984

113. Lindholm A: A new method of operation in subcutaneous rupture of the Achilles tendon. Acta Chir Scand 117:261, 1959

114. Bosworth D: Repair of defects in the tendo Achillis. J Bone Joint Surg Am 38:111, 1956

115. Teuffer AP: Traumatic rupture of the Achilles tendon: reconstruction by transplant and graft using the lateral peroneus brevis. Orthop Clin North Am 5:89, 1974

116. Mortenson NH, Skov O, Jensen PE: Early mobilization of operatively treated Achilles tendon ruptures—a clinical and radiographic study, abstracted. Acta Orthop Scand Suppl 253:64, 1993

117. Eggan P, Marti RK: A functional period after repair of Achilles tendon ruptures, abstracted. Acta Orthop Scand Suppl 256:74, 1994

118. Hsu TC, Wang CL, Wang TG, Chiang IP: Ultrasonic examination of the posterior tibial tendon. Foot Ankle Int 18:34, 1997

119. Funk DA, Cass JR, Johnson KA: Acquired adult flatfoot secondary to posterior tibial tendon pathology. J Bone Joint Surg Am 68:95, 1986

120. Krackow KA: Acute rupture of flexor hallucis longus. Clin Orthop Rel Res 150:261, 1980

121. Boruta PM, Beauperthuy GD: Partial tear of the flexor hallucis longus at the knot of Henry: presentation of three cases. Foot Ankle Int 18:243, 1997

122. Hamilton WG: Tendonitis about the ankle joint in classical ballet dancers. Am J Sports Med 5:84, 1977

123. Inokuchi S, Usami N: Closed complete rupture of the flexor hallucis longus tendon at the groove of the talus. Foot Ankle Int 18:47, 1997

124. Sammarco GJ, Miller EH: Partial rupture of flexor hallucis longus tendon in classical ballet dancers. J Bone Joint Surg Am 61:149, 1979

125. Theodore GH, Kolettis GJ, Micheli LJ: Tenosynovitis of the flexor hallucis longus in a long distance runner. Med Sci Sports Exerc 28:277, 1996

126. McBride E: A conservative operation for bunions. J Bone Joint Surg 10:735, 1928

127. Hiss MJ: Hallux valgus: its cause and simplified treatment. Am J Surg 11:51, 1931

128. McBride ED: The McBride bunion hallux valgus operation. J Bone Joint Surg Am 49:1675, 1967

129. Butler WE: Modifications of the McBride procedure for correction of hallux abductovalgus. J Am Podiatry Assoc 64:585, 1974

130. Pressman M, Stano G, Krantz M, Novicki D: Correction

of hallux valgus with positionally increased intermetatarsal angle. J Am Podiatr Med Assoc 76:611, 1986

131. Cantanzaritti AR: First metatarsal-cuneiform arthrodesis. p. 171. In Marcinko D (ed): Comprehensive Textbook of Hallux Valgus Reconstruction. Mosby–Year Book, St. Louis, 1992

132. Schuberth J, Reilly C, Gudas C: The closing wedge osteotomy. J Am Podiatry Assoc 74:13, 1984

133. Henel C, Lindholm J: First metatarsal wedge osteotomies. J Am Podiatry Assoc 72:550, 1982

134. Landsman A, Vogler HW: An assessment of oblique based wedge osteotomy stability in the first metatarsal using different modes of internal fixation. J Foot Surg 31:211, 1992

135. Loison M: Note sur le traitement chirurgicale du hallux valgus d'apres l'etude radiographique de la deformation. Bull Mem Soc Chir 27:528, 1901

136. Juvara E: Nouveau procede pour la cure radicale du "hallux valgus." Presse Med 40:395, 1919

137. Schotte M: Zur operativen korrektur des hallux valgus in sinne Ludloffs. Klin Wochenschr 50:23, 1929

138. Markbreiter LA, Thompsen F: Proximal metatarsal osteotomy in hallux valgus correction: a comparison of crescentic and chevron procedures. Foot Ankle Int 18:71, 1997

139. Easley ME, Kiebzak GM, Davis WH, Anderson RB: Prospective, randomized comparison of proximal crescentic and proximal chevron osteotomies for correction of hallux valgus deformity. Foot Ankle Int 17:307, 1996

140. Vogler HW: Shaft osteotomies in hallux valgus reduction. Clin Podiatr Med Surg 6:47, 1989

141. Ludloff K: Die beseitigung des hallux valgus durch die schraege planto-dorsale osteotomie des metatarsus I. Arch Klin Chir 110:364, 1918

142. Saxena A, McCammon D: The Ludloff osteotomy: a critical analysis. J Foot Ankle Surg 36:100, 1997

143. Meyer M: Eine neue modifikation der hallux valgus operation. Zentralbl Chir 53:3215, 1926

144. Mau C, Lauber HT: Die operative behandlung des hallux valgus (Nachuntersuchungen). Dtsch Z Chir 197:363, 1926

145. Wilson JN: Oblique displacement osteotomy for hallux valgus. J Bone Joint Surg [Br] 45:552, 1963

146. Lindgren U, Turan I: A new operation for hallux valgus. Clin Orthop Rel Res 175:179, 1983

147. Todd WF: Osteotomies for the first metatarsal head: Reverdin, Reverdin modifications, Peabody, Mitchell and Drato. p. 170. In Gerbert J (ed): Textbook of Bunion Surgery. Futura, Mt. Kisco, NY, 1981

148. Laird PO, Silvers SH, Somdahl J: Two Reverdin-Laird osteotomy modifications for correction of hallux abducto valgus. J Am Podiatr Med Assoc 78:403, 1988

149. Landsman A, Hanft J, Yoo C et al: Stabilization of a distal first metatarsal osteotomy with absorbable internal fixation. The lower Extremity 1:37, 1994

150. Lewis RJ, Feffer HL: Modified Chevron osteotomy of the first metatarsal. Clin Orthop Rel Res 157:105, 1981

151. Vogler HW: The "off-set V osteotomy" in hallux valgus reduction. In Jay R (ed): Current Therapy in Podiatric Surgery. p. 158. BC Decker, Toronto, 1988

152. Youngswick F: Modification of the Austin bunionectomy for treatment of metatarsal primus equinus associated with hallux limitus. J Foot Surg 21:114, 1982

153. Hawkins FB, Mitchell CL, Hedrick D: Correction of hallux valgus by metatarsal osteotomy. J Bone Joint Surg 27:387, 1945

154. Hohman G: Symptomatische oder physiologische Behandlung des Hallux Dolgis. Munch Med Ohnschr 33:1042, 1921

155. Wu KK: Wu's bunionectomy: a clinical analysis of 150 personal cases. J Foot Surg 31:288, 1992

156. Schoen NS, Zygmunt K, Gudas C: Z-bunionectomy: retrospective long term study. J Foot Ankle Surg 35:312, 1996

157. Kramer J, Barry LD, Helfman DN et al: The modified Scarf bunionectomy. J Foot Surg 31:360, 1992

158. Duke H: Rotational Scarf (Z) osteotomy bunionectomy for correction of high intermetatarsal angles. J Am Podiatr Med Assoc 82:352, 1992

159. Regnauld B: The Foot: Pathology, Etiology, Semiology, Clinical investigation and Therapy. p. 271. Springer-Verlag, New York, 1986

160. Schwartz N, Hurley JP: Derotational Akin osteotomy: further modifications. J Foot Surg 26:419, 1987

161. Springer KR: The role of the Akin osteotomy in the surgical management of hallux abducto valgus. Clin Podiatr Med Surg 6:115, 1989

162. Barca F, Busa R: Resorbable poly-L-lactic acid mini staples for the fixation of Akin osteotomies. J Foot Ankle Surg 36:106, 1997

163. Bingold AC, Collins DH: Hallux rigidus. J Bone Joint Surg [Br] 32:214, 1950

164. Davies GF: Plantarflexory base wedge osteotomy in the treatment of functional and structural metatarsus primus elevatus. Clin Podiatr Med Surg 6:93, 1989

165. Kessel L, Bonney G: Hallux rigidus in the adolescent. J Bone Joint Surg [Br] 40:668, 1958

166. Geldwert JJ, Rock GD, McGrath MP, Mancuso JE: Cheilectomy: still a useful technique for grade 1 and grade II hallux limitus/rigidus. J Foot Surg 31:154, 1992

167. Drago JJ, Olaff L, Jacobs AM: A comprehensive review of hallux limitus. J Foot Surg 23:213, 1984

168. Regnauld B: The Foot: Pathology, Etiology, Semiology, Clinical Investigation and Therapy. p. 344. Springer-Verlag, New York, 1986

169. Kravitz SR, LaPorta G, Lawton JH: KL progressive staging classification of hallux limitus and hallux rigidus. The Lower Extremity 1(1):55, 1994

170. Regnauld B: Technique personnelle de la cure chirurgicale de l'hallux valgus. Ann Podol 6:395, 1968

171. Feldman KA: The Green-Watermann procedure: geomet-

ric analysis and preoperative radiographic template technique. J Foot Surg 31:182, 1992

172. Cotton FJ: Foot statics and surgery. Trans N Engl Surg Soc 18:181, 1935

173. Lambrinudi C: Metatarsus primus elevatus. Proc R Soc Med 31:1273, 1938

174. Cicchinelli LD, Camasta C, McGlamry ED: Iatrogenic metatarsus primus elevatus: etiology, evaluation and surgical management. J Am Podiatr Med Assoc 87:165, 1997

175. Southgate JJ, Urry SR: Hallux rigidus: the long term results of dorsal wedge osteotomy and arthrodesis in adults. J Foot Ankle Surg 36:136, 1997

176. Ganley J, Lynch F, Darrigan R: Keller bunionectomy with fascia and tendon graft. J Am Podiatr Med Assoc 76:602, 1986

177. Fuson S: Modification of the Keller operation for increased functional capacity. J Foot Surg 21:292, 1982

178. Saxena A: Valenti procedure. J Foot Ankle Surg 35:178, 1995

179. dePalma L, Tulli A, Sabetta SP: Histological study of the phalangeal articular side following Keller procedure for hallux valgus. J Foot Surg 31:355, 1992

180. Hanft JR, Kashuk KB, Toney M, Schabler J: Modifications of the Regnauld osteochondral autogenous graft for correction of hallux limitus/valgus: a 2 year review. J Foot Surg 31:116, 1992

181. Roukis TS, Hurless JS: The hallucal interphalangeal sesamoid. J Foot Ankle Surg 35:303, 1996

182. Mann RA (ed): Surgery of the Foot. CV Mosby Co. St. Louis, 1986

183. Yu G, Nagle CJ: Hallux interphalangeal joint sesamoidectomy. J Am Podiatr Med Assoc 86:105, 1996

184. Green D, Brekke M: Anatomy, biomechanics and pathomechanics of lesser digital deformities. Clin Podiatr Med Surg 13:179, 1996

185. Green DR, Ruch JA, McGlamry ED: Correction of equinus related forefoot deformities. J Am Podiatry Assoc 66:768, 1976

186. de Palma L, Colonna E, Travasi M: The modified Jones procedure for pes cavovarus with claw hallux. J Foot Ankle Surg 36:279, 1997

187. Kelikian H: Hallux Valgus, Allied Deformities of the Forefoot and Metatarsalgia. p. 305. WB Saunders Co. Philadelphia, 1965

188. Jimenez AL, McGlamry ED, Green DR: Lesser ray deformities. p. 57. In McGlamry ED (ed): Comprehensive Textbook of Foot Surgery. Vol. 1. Williams & Wilkins, Baltimore, 1987

189. Grumbine NA, King GA: Clawfoot deformity. Clin Podiatr Med Surg 13:221, 1996

190. Marcinko DE, Lazerson A, Dollard MD, Schwartz, N: Flexor digitorum longus tendon transfer for correction of hammer digit syndrome. J Am Podiatry Assoc 74:216, 1984

191. Kravitz S, Fenice JV, Maehrer M, Kline R: Long flexor tenodesis for cock-up hammer deformity. The Lower Extremity 2:275, 1995

192. Kimmel HM, Garrow S: A comparison of end-to-end versus "V" arthrodesis procedures for correction of digital deformities. Clin Podiatr Med Surg 13:239, 1996

193. Giovinco JD: End-to-end arthrodesis with absorbable pin and suture fixation. Clin Podiatr Med Surg 13:251, 1996

194. Zeringue GN, et al: Evaluation and management of the web corn involving the fourth interdigital space. J Am Podiatr Med Assoc 76:210, 1986

195. Lauf E, Weinraub GM: Asymmetric "V" osteotomy: a predictable surgical approach for central metatarsalgia. J Foot Ankle Surg 35:550, 1996

196. Woodhaus LE: A 3-year follow up study of hammer digit syndrome of the hallux. J Am Podiatry Assoc 64:955, 1974

197. Johnson JB, Price TW: Crossover second toe deformity: etiology and treatment. J Foot Surg 28:417, 1989

198. DuVries HL: New approach to the treatment of intractable verrucae plantaris (plantar wart). JAMA 152:1202, 1953

199. Goforth WP, Urteaga AJ: Displacement osteotomy for the treatment of digital transverse plane deformities. Clin Podiatr Med Surg 13:279, 1996

200. Bogy LT, Vranes R, Goforth WP et al: Correction of overlapping second toe deformity: long term results including a 7 year follow-up. J Foot Surg 31:319, 1992

201. Collins B, Collins W: Surgical correction of transverse plane deformities at the lesser metatarsal phalangeal joints. J Foot Surg 23:159, 1984

202. Coughlin MJ: Crossover second toe deformity. Foot Ankle 8:29, 1987

203. Fallet L: Pathology of the fifth ray, including the tailor's bunion deformity. Clin Podiatr Med Surg 7:689, 1990

204. Fallet L, Buckholz JM: Analysis of tailor's bunions by radiographic and anatomical display. J Am Podiatry Assoc 70:597, 1980

205. Giannestra NJ: Foot Disorders—Medical and Surgical Management. 2nd ed. Lea & Febiger, Philadelphia, 1973

206. Davies H: Metatarsus quintus valgus. Br Med J 1:664, 1949

207. Gerbert J, Sgarlato TE, Subotnick ST: Preliminary study of closing base wedge osteotomy of 5th metatarsal for correction of tailor's bunion deformity. J Am Podiatry Assoc 62:212, 1972

208. Sponsel KH: Bunionette correction by metatarsal osteotomy: preliminary report. Orthop Clin North Am 7:809, 1976

209. Throckmorton JK, Bradlee N: Transverse V sliding osteotomy: a new surgical procedure for correction of tailor's bunion deformity. J Foot Surg 18:117, 1978

210. Hohmann G: Fuss und Bien. p. 145. JF Bergmann, Munich, 1951

211. Catanzariti AR, Friedman C, Distazio J: Oblique osteotomy of the fifth metatarsal: a five year review. J Foot Surg 27:316, 1988

212. Synder RB, Lipscomb AB, Johnston RK: The relationship of tarsal coalitions to ankle sprains in athletes. Am J Sports Med 9:313, 1981

213. Downey MS: Tarsal coalitions: a surgical classification. J Am Podiatr Med Assoc 81:187, 1991

214. Pachuda NM, Laday SD, Jay RM: Tarsal coalition: etiology, diagnosis and treatment. J Foot Surg 29:474, 1990

215. Buckholz JM: Peroneal spastic flatfoot. In McGlamry ED (ed): Fundamentals of Foot Surgery. p. 337. Williams & Wilkins, Baltimore, 1987

216. Takakura Y, Sugimoto K, Tankaka Y, Tamai S: Symptomatic talocalcaneal coalition. Clin Orthop Rel Res 269:249, 1991

217. Harris RI, Beath T: Etiology of peroneal spastic flatfoot. J Bone Joint Surg [Br] 30:624, 1948

218. Cowell HR, Elener V: Rigid painful flatfoot secondary to tarsal coalition. Clin Orthop 177:54, 1983

219. Bettin D, Karbowski A, Schwering L: Congenital ball and socket anomaly of the ankle. J Pediatr Orthop 16:492, 1996

220. Sormont DM, Peterson HA: The relative incidence of tarsal coalition. Clin Orthop 181:28, 1983

221. Perlman MD, Wertheimer SJ: Tarsal coalitions. J Foot Surg 25:58, 1986

222. Pontious J, Hillstrom HJ, Monahan T, Connelly S: Talonavicular coalition: objective gait analysis. J Am Podiatr Med Assoc 83:379, 1993

223. Plotkin S: Case presentation of calcaneonavicular coalition in monozygotic twins. J Am Podiatr Med Assoc 86:433, 1996

224. Spero CR, Simon GS, Tornetta P: Clubfoot and tarsal coalition. J Pediatr Orthop 14:372, 1994

225. Stuecker RD, Bennett JT: Tarsal coalition presenting as a pes cavo-varus deformity: report of three cases and review of the literature. Foot Ankle 14:540, 1993

226. Mosier KM, Asher M: Tarsal coalitions and peroneal spastic flatfoot: a review. J Bone Joint Surg Am 66:976, 1984

227. Cohen AH, Laughner TE, Pupp G: Calcaneonavicular bar resection: a retrospective review. J Am Podiatr Med Assoc 83:10, 1993

228. Kitaoka HB, Wikenhesier MA, Shaughenssy WJ: Gait abnormalities following resection of talocalcaneal coalition. J Bone Joint Surg Am 79:369, 1997

229. Morgan RC, Crawford AH: Surgical management of tarsal coalition in adolescent athletes. Foot Ankle 7:183, 1986

230. Elkus RA: Tarsal coalition in the young athlete. Am J Sports Med 14:477, 1986

231. Cowell HR: Extensor brevis arthroplasty. J Bone Joint Surg Am 52:820, 1970

232. Badgley CE: Coalition of the calcaneus and the navicular. Arch Surg 15:75, 1927

233. Cain TJ, Heyman S: Peroneal spastic flatfoot: its treatment by osteotomy of the os calcis. J Bone Joint Surg [Br] 60:527, 1978

234. Vogler H: Triple arthrodesis as salvage for end stage flatfoot. Clin Podiatr Med Surg 6:591, 1989

235. Vogler HW: Arthrodesis in foot and ankle surgery: the history, concept, techniques, failure and salvage. Foot Ankle 9:161, 1997

236. Stibbe AB, vanDijk CN, Marti RM: The os trigonum syndrome, abstracted. Acta Orthop Scand Suppl 262:59, 1994

237. Hamilton WG: Stenosing tenosynovitis of the flexor hallucis longus tendon and posterior impingement upon the os trigonum in ballet dancers. Foot Ankle 3:74, 1982

238. Hamilton WG, Geppert MJ, Thompson FM: Pain in the posterior aspect of the ankle in dancers. J Bone Joint Surg Am 78:1491, 1996

239. Gessini L, Jandolo B, Pietrangeli A: The anterior tarsal tunnel syndrome. J Bone Joint Surg Am 66:786, 1984

240. Subotnick S: Anterior impingement exostosis of the ankle. J Am Podiatry Assoc 66:958, 1976

241. Scholten D, van Dijk CN: Arthroscopic treatment of the anterior impingement syndrome of the ankle abstracted. Acta Orthop Scand Suppl 262:57, 1994

242. Lundeen RO: Manual of Ankle and Foot Arthroscopy. P. 87. Churchill Livingstone, New York, 1992

243. Frey C, Bell J, Teresi L et al: A comparison of MRI and clinical examination of acute lateral ankle sprains. Foot Ankle Int 17:533, 1996

244. Mesgarzadeh M, Schneck CD, Tehranzadeh J et al: Magnetic resonance imaging of the ankle ligaments. Magn Reson Imaging Clin North Am 2:39, 1994

245. Balduini FC, Tezlaff J: Historical perspectives on injuries of the of the ankle. Clin Sports Med 1:3, 1982

246. Brostrom L: Sprained ankles. Acta Chir Scand 130:560, 1965

247. DeSimoni C, Wetz HH, Zanetti M et al: Clinical examination and magnetic resonance imaging in the assessment of ankle sprains treated with an orthosis. Foot Ankle Int 17:177, 1996

248. Bullock-Saxton JE: Sensory changes associated with severe ankle sprain. Scand J Rehab Med 27:161, 1995

249. Freeman MA: The etiology and prevention of functional instability of the foot. J Bone Joint Surg [Br] 47:678, 1965

250. Cardone BW, Erickson SJ, Hartog SJ, Carrera GF: MRI of injury to the lateral collateral ligamentous complex of the ankle. J Comput Assist Tomogr 17:102, 1993

251. Kuwada GT: Current concepts in the diagnosis and treatment of ankle sprains. Clin Podiatr Med Surg 12:653, 1995

252. Munk B, Christense KH, Lind T: Treatment of ruptured lateral ankle ligaments: a 9-13 year follow up, abstracted. Acta Orthop Scand Suppl 253:64, 1992

253. Raatokainen T, Putkonen M, Puranen J: Arthrography, clinical examination and stress radiograph in the diagnosis of acute injury of the lateral ankle ligaments. Am J Sports Med 20:2, 1992

254. Hasegawa A, Kimura M, Tomizawa S, Shirakura K: Sepa-

rated ossicles of the lateral malleolus. Clin Orthop Rel Res 330:157, 1996

255. Anderson KJ, LeCrocq JF: Operative treatment of injury to the fibular collateral ligament of the ankle. J Bone Joint Surg Am 36:825, 1964

256. Rijke AM, Jones B, Vierhut PA: Injury to the lateral ankle ligaments of athletes: a post traumatic follow-up. Am J Sports Med 16:256, 1988

257. Moller-Larsen F, Wethelund JO, Jurik AG et al: Comparison of three different treatments for ruptured lateral ankle ligaments. Acta Orthop Scand 59:564, 1988

258. Colville MD: Reconstruction of the lateral ankle ligaments. J Bone Joint Surg Am 76:1092, 1994

259. Fordyce AJW, Horn CV: Normal talar tile angle. Clin Orthop 140:37, 1979

260. Larsen E: Static or dynamic repair of lateral instability. Clin Orthop Rel Res 257:184, 1988

261. Gillespie HS, Boucher P: Watson-Jones repair of lateral instability of the ankle. J Bone Joint Surg Am 53:920, 1971

262. Thermann H, Zwipp H, Tscherne H: Treatment algorithm of chronic ankle and subtalar instability. Foot Ankle Int 18: 163, 1997

263. Bauer GR: New method for reconstruction in lateral ankle instability. J Am Podiatr Med Assoc 85:459, 1995

264. Zwipp H: Treatment of chronic two plane instability of the ankle joint: syndesmoplasty versus periosteal flap versus tenodesis. J Foot Surg 29:33, 1990

265. Chrisman OD, Snook GA: Reconstruction of lateral ligament tears of the ankle. J Bone Joint Surg Am 51:904, 1969

266. Evans DL: Recurent instability of the ankle: a method of surgical treatment. Proc R Soc Lond 446:333, 1953

267. Lundeen RO, Hawkins RB: Arthrosopic lateral ankle stabilization. J Am Podiatr Med Assoc 75:372, 1985

268. Hawkins RB: Arthroscopic repair for chronic lateral ankle instability. P. 155. In Guhl JF ed: Foot and Ankle Arthroscopy. Slack, Thorofare, NJ, 1993

269. van Dijk CN: Study of the cause of pain on the medial side of the ankle joint after supination injury, abstracted. Acta Orthop Scand suppl 253:10, 1993

270. Wolin I, Glassman F, Sideman S et al: Internal derangement of the talofibular component of the ankle. Surg Gynecol Obstet 91:193, 1950

271. Gould N, Selligson D, Gassman J: Early and late repair of lateral ligament of ankle. Foot Ankle 1:84, 1980

272. Vogler HW: Basic concepts of bioengineering in osteosynthesis, bone performance and bone failure—an introduction. Clin Podiatr Med Surg 2:161, 1985

273. Lauge-Hansen N: Fractures of the ankle II: combined experimental-surgical and experimental-roentgenologic investigations. Arch Surg 60:957, 1950

274. Lauge-Hansen N: Fractures of the ankle IV: clinical use of genetic reduction. Arch Surg 64:488, 1952

275. Lauge-Hansen N: Fracture of the ankle III: genetic roent-genologic diagnosis of fractures of the ankle. Am J Roentgenol 71:456, 1954

276. Lindsjo U: Classification of ankle fractures: the Lauge-Hansen or AO system? Clin Orthop 199:12, 1985

277. Muller ME, Allgower M, Schneider R, Willenegger H: Manual of Internal Fixation. 3rd ed. Springer-Verlag, New York, 1991

278. Danis R: Theorie et Pratique de l'Osteosynthese. p. 142. Masson, Paris, 1949

279. Weber BG: Klassifikation und operations indikation der oberen spruggelenks. p. 51. Verleg Hans Huber, Bern, 1966

280. Bauer M, Bergstrom B, Hemborg A et al: Malleolar fractures: nonoperative versus operative treatment. A controlled study. Clin Orthop 199:17, 1985

281. Michelson JK: Current concepts review: fractures about the ankle. J Bone Joint Surg Am 77:142, 1995

282. Destot E: Traumatismes du Pied et Rayons X Malleoles, Astragale, Calcaneum, Avant-pied. Masson, Paris, 1911

283. Harper MC: Talar shift: the stabilizing role of the medial, lateral, and posterior ankle structures. Clin Orthop 257: 177, 1990

284. Raasch WG, Ldarkin JJ, Draganich LF: Assessment of the posterior malleolus as a restraint to posterior subluxation of the ankle. J Bone Joint Surg Am 74:1201, 1992

285. Michelson JD, Magid D, Ney DR et al: Examination of the pathologic anatomy of ankle fractures. J Trauma 32:65, 1992

286. Sclafani SJA: Ligamentous injury of the lower tibiofibular syndesmosis: radiographic evidence. Radiology 156:21, 1985

287. Sarkisian JS, Cody GW: Closed treatment of ankle fractures: a new criterion for evaluation—a review of 250 cases. J Trauma 16:323, 1976

288. Phillips WA, Schwartz HS, Keller CS et al: A prospective, randomized study of the management of severe ankle fractures. J Bone Joint Surg Am 67:67, 1985

289. Clark TWI, Janzen DL, Ho K et al: Detection of radiographically occult ankle fractures following acute trauma: positive predictive value of an ankle effusion. Am J Roentgenol 164:1185, 1995

290. Anis AH, Stiell IG, Stewart DG et al: Cost-effectiveness analysis of the Ottawa Ankle Rules. Ann Emerg Med 26: 422, 1995

291. Vangsness CT, Carter V, Hunt T et al: Radiographic diagnosis of ankle fractures: are three views necessary? Foot Ankle Int 15:172, 1994

292. Harper MC: The short oblique fracture of the distal fibula without medial injury: an assessment of displacement. Foot Ankle Int 16:181, 1995

293. Harper MC: An anatomic study of the short oblique fracture of the distal fibula and ankle stability. Foot Ankle 4: 23, 1983

294. Parfenchuck TA, Frix JM, Bertrand SL et al: Clinical use of

a syndesmosis screw in stage IV pronation-external rotation ankle fractures. Orthop Rev, suppl. 23, 1994

295. Cedell CA: Supination-outward rotation injuries of the ankle: a clinical and roentgenological study with special reference to the operative treatment, abstracted. Acta Orthop Scand Suppl 110, 1967

296. Ahl T, Dalen N, Lundberg A et al: Biodegradable fixation of ankle fractures. Acta Orthop Scand 65:166, 1994

297. Bostman O, Hirvensalo E, Vainionpaa S et al: Int Orthop 14:1, 1990

298. Frokjaer J, Moller BN: Biodegradable fixation of ankle fractures: complications in a prospective study of 25 cases. Acta Orthop Scand 63:434, 1992

299. Bostman O, Partio E, Hirvensalo E et al: Foreign-body reactions to polyglycolide screws. Acta Orthop Scand 63: 173, 1992

300. Partio EK, Bostman O, Hirvensalo E et al: Self-reinforced absorbable screws in the fixation of displaced ankle fractures: a prospective clinical study of 152 patients. J Orthop Trauma 6:209, 1992

301. Bostman OM: Intense granulomatous inflammatory lesions associated with absorbable internal fixation devices made of polyglycolide in ankle fractures. Clin Orthop 278:193, 1992

302. Dijkema ARA, van der Elst M, Breederveld RS et al: Surgical treatment of fracture-dislocations of the ankle joint with biodegradable implants: a prospective randomized study. J Trauma 34:82, 1993

303. Bostman OM: Oteolytic changes accompanying degradation of absorbable fracture fixation implants. J Bone Joint Surg [Br] 73:679, 1991

304. Liu Y, Rong G: Absorbable SR-PGA implant in orthopaedics: preliminary results of treatment of fractures. Chung Hua Wai Ko Tasa Chih 33:51, 1995

305. Pihlajamaki H, Bostman O, Hirvensalo E et al: A biodegradable expansion plug for the fixation of fractures of the medial malleolus. Ann Chir Gynaecol 83:49, 1994

306. Bostman OM, Pihlajamaki HK, Partio EK et al: Clinical biocompatibility and degradation of polylevolactide screws in the ankle. Clin Orthop 320:101, 1995

307. Bucholz RW, Henry S, Henley MB: Fixation with bioabsorbable screws for the treatment of fractures of the ankle. J Bone Joint Surg Am 76:319, 1994

308. Vogler HW: The Weber posterior anti-glide fibular plate for Type B ankle fracture. p. 627. In Scurran B (ed): Traumatology of the Foot and Ankle. Williams & Wilkins, New York, 1989

309. Pankovich AM, Shivaram MS: Anatomical basis of variability in injuries of the medial malleolus and the deltoid ligament: clinical studies. Acta Orthop Scand 50:225, 1979

310. Skie MC, Ebraheim NA, Woldenberg L et al: Fracture of the anterior colliculus. J Trauma 38:642, 1995

311. Skie MC, Woldenberg L, Ebraheim NA et al: Assessment

of collicular fracture of the medial malleolus. Foot Ankle 10:118, 1989

312. Segal D, Wiss D, Whitelaw G: Functional bracing and rehabilitation of ankle fractures. Clin Orthop 199:39, 1985

313. Hedstrom M, Ahl T, Dalen N: Early postoperative ankle exercise: a study of postoperative lateral malleolar fractures. Clin Orthop 300:193, 1994

314. Ahl T, Dalen N, Lundberg A et al: Early mobilization of operated on ankle fractures. Acta Orthop Scand 64:95, 1993

315. Tropp H, Norlin R: Ankle performance after ankle fracture: a randomized study of early mobilization. Foot Ankle Int 16:79, 1995

316. Godsiff SP, Trakru S, Kefer G et al: A comparative study of early motion and immediate plaster splintage and internal fixation of unstable fractures of the ankle. Injury 24:529, 1993

317. O'Connor D: Sinus tarsi syndrome: a clinical entity. J Bone Joint Surg Am 40:720, 1958

318. Claustre J, Simon L, Allieu Y: Le syndrome du tarse existe-t-il? Rheumatologie 31:19, 1979

319. Kjaersgaard-Anderson P, Soballe K, Anderson K et al: Sinus tarsi syndrome: presentation of seven cases and review of the literature. J Foot Surg 28: 3, 1989

320. Taillard W, Meyer JM, Garcia J et al: The sinus tarsi syndrome. Int Orthop 5:117, 1981

321. Beltran J: Sinus tarsi syndrome. Magn Reson Imaging Clin North Am 2:59, 1994

322. Fried A, Dobbs B: Sinsus tarsi synovectomy. J Am Podiatr Med Assoc 75:445, 1985

323. Smith TF, Pitts T, Green D: Pes cavus. p. 731. In McGlamry ED (ed): Comprehensive Textbook of Foot Surgery. Vol. I. 2nd ed. Williams & Wilkins, Baltimore, 1992

324. Green DR, Ruch JA, McGlamry ED: Correction of equinus related forefoot deformities. J Am Podiatry Assoc 66: 768, 1976

325. Gudas C: Mechanism and reconstruction of pes cavus. J Foot Surg 16:1, 1977

326. Whitney AK, Green DR: Pseudoequinus. J Am Podiatry Assoc 72:365, 1982

327. Brockway A: Surgical correction of talipes cavus deformities. J Bone Joint Surg 22:81, 1940

328. Alnik I: Operative treatment of pes cavus. Acta Orthop Scand 23:137, 1954

329. Green DR, Lepow GM, Smith TF: Pes cavus. p. 287. In McGlamry ED (ed): Comprehensive Text of Foot Surgery. Vol. I. Williams & Wilkins, Baltimore, 1987

330. Volger, HW: The biomechanical and surgical reconstruction of talipes equinovalgus and cavovarus deformations. Acta Orthop Traumatol Turica 29:342, 1995

331. Vogler H: Surgical management of neuromuscular deformities of the foot and ankle in children and adolescents. Clin Podiatr Med Surg 4:175, 1987

332. Brewerton DA, Sandifer PH, Sweetnam DR: "Idiopathic" pes cavus: an investigation into its aetiology. Br Med J 2: 659, 1963

333. Hibbs R: An operation for "claw foot." JAMA 73:183, 1919

334. Lambrinudi C: An operation for claw-toes. Proc R Soc Med 21:239, 1927

335. Jones R: The soldier's foot and the treatment of common deformities of the foot. Part II: claw foot. Br Med J 1:749, 1916

336. Kelikian H: Deformities of the lesser toes. p. 283. In Hallux Valgus and Allied Deformities of the Forefoot and Metatarsalgia. WB Saunders Co., Philadelphia, 1965

337. Heyman CH: The operative treatment of claw foot. J Bone Joint Surg 14:335, 1932

338. Root ML, Orien WP, Weed JH: Normal and Abnormal Function of the Foot, Vol. II. Clinical Biomechanics Corp., Los Angeles, 1977

339. Silver CM, Simon SD, Spindall E et al: Calcaneal osteotomy in varus and valgus deformities of the foot in cerebral palsy. J Bone Joint Surg Am 49:232, 1967

340. Coleman SS: Complex Foot Deformities in Children. pp. 147, 167. Lea & Febiger, Philadelphia, 1983

341. Coleman SS, Chestnut WJ: A simple test for hindfoot flexibility in the cavovarus foot. Clin Orthop Rel Res 123:60, 1977

342. Dwyer FC: Osteotomy of the calcaneum for pes cavus. J Bone Joint Surg [Br] 41:80, 1959

343. Dwyer FC: The treatment of relapsed clubfoot by insertion of a wedge into the calcaneum. J Bone Joint Surg [Br] 45:67, 1963

344. Dwyer FC: The present status of the problem of pes cavus. Clin Orthop Rel Res 106:254, 1975

345. Steindler A: Operative treatment of pes cavus. Surg Gynecol Obstet 24:612, 1917

346. Steindler A: Stripping of the os calcis. Am J Orthop Surg 2:8, 1920

347. Stephens R: Dorsal wedge operation for metatarsal equinus. J Bone Joint Surg 5:485, 1923

348. Cole WH: The treatment of claw-foot. J Bone Joint Surg 22:895,1940

349. Brockway A: Surgical correction of talipes cavus deformities. J Bone Joint Surg 22:81, 1940

350. Jappas LM: Surgical treatment of pes cavus by tarsal V-osteotomy. J Bone Joint Surg (Am) 50:927, 1968

351. Leal LO, Notari MA: Cole osteotomy: Navicular-cuneiform arthrodesis-transcuboidal osteotomy. Clin Podiatr Med Surg 8:637, 1991

352. Saunders JT: Etiology and treatment of clawfoot. Arch Surg 30:179, 1935

353. Vogler HW: Paralytic deformities of the foot & ankle—surgical management. p. 531. In Marcinko DE (ed): Therapeutics of the Foot & Ankle. Williams & Wilkins, Baltimore, 1992

354. Subotnick SI: Equinus deformity as it affects the forefoot. J Am Podiatry Assoc 61:423, 1971

355. Root ML, Weed JH, Sgarlato TE: Axis of motion of the subtalar joint. J Am Podiatry Assoc 56:149, 1966

356. Vogler HW: Biomechanics of talipes equinovalgus. J Am Podiatr Med Assoc 77:21, 1987

357. Hicks JH: The function of the plantar aponeurosis. J Anat 85:414, 1951

358. Hicks JH: The mechanics of the foot. II. The plantar aponeurosis and the arch. J Anat 88:25, 1954

359. Green DR, Carol A: Planal dominence. J Am Podiatry Assoc 74:98, 1984

360. Franco AH: Pes cavus and pes planus. Phys Ther 67:688, 1987

361. Young CS: Operative treatment of pes planus. Surg Gynecol Obstet 68:1099, 1939

362. Kraus W: The operative treatment of juvenile flatfeet and abducted feet. Am Digest Foreign Orthop Lit First Q 32, 1971

363. Mosca VS: Calcaneal lengthening for valgus deformity of the hindfoot: results in children who had severe, symptomatic flatfoot and skewfoot. J Bone Joint Surg 77:500, 1995

364. Jacobs AM, Oloff LM, Visser HJ: Calcaneal osteotomy in the management of flexible and non flexible flatfoot deformity: a preliminary report. J Foot Surg 20:57, 1981

365. Evans D: Calcaneo-valgus deformity. J Bone Joint Surg [Br] 57:270, 1975

366. Dollard MD, Marcinko D, Lazerson A, Elleby D: The Evans calcaneal osteotomy for correction of flexible flatfoot sydrome. J Foot Surg 23:291, 1984

367. Koman LA, Mooney JF, Goodman A: Management of valgus hindfoot deformity in pediatric cerebral palsy patients by medial displacement. J Pediatr Orthop 13:180, 1993

368. Koustogiannis E: Treatment of mobile flatfoot by displacement osteotomy of the calcaneus. J Bone Joint Surg [Br] 53:96, 1971

369. Miller OL: A plastic flatfoot operation. J Bone Joint Surg 9:84, 1927

370. Hoke M: An operation for the correction of extremely relaxed flatfoot. J Bone Joint Surg 13:773, 1931

27

Arthroscopy and Endoscopy

RICHARD O. LUNDEEN
PATRICK A. DeHEER

[The ankle joint] is not suitable for arthroscopy.

M. S. Burman, October 1931

The ankle has long been the subject of investigation by physicians intrigued by its function and pathology. Its biomechanical secrets have been unlocked by investigators such as Barnett and Napier,[1] Close,[2] and Isman and Inman.[3] Diagnostically, arthrography, computed tomography (CT) scanning, and magnetic resonance imaging (MRI) have been well accepted and used following suspected traumatic and nontraumatic ligamentous and osseous injuries, often in conjunction with stress and plain-film radiographs. In addition, the classification and mechanisms of injury of ankle fractures[5,6] have been a controversial but well-documented subject of interest in the podiatric and orthopedic literature. Unfortunately, there has been a lack of investigation to aid in the diagnosis and identification of pathology in patients who are neither subject to chronic lateral ankle instability nor victims of trauma. Advances in techniques of endoscopic examination and specialization of the equipment needed to perform such tasks have enabled surgeons to bridge the gap between routine diagnostic and treatment modalities and open arthrotomy of the afflicted joint.

With the development of this technology, applications for its use have been expanded to include the performance of procedures that have traditionally been performed by making an incision and directly visualizing the operative site. In a movement that parallels the trend from open toward laparoscopic cholecystectomy, routine procedures for common problems in the foot are not under the do-

main of the knife but rather becoming arthroscopic surgical procedures. As with the introduction of knee arthroscopy, these procedures are at the forefront of discussions both didactic and philosophical as to their efficacy as well as the potential for abuse. The most prominent procedure being performed arthroscopically is, of course, the endoscopic plantar fasciotomy. As technology and surgeons' skills advance, such discussions are left to the righteous and politicians as additional procedures evolve, including endoscopic decompression for interdigital neuromas, arthroscopic ankle and subtalar joint fusions, and arthroscopic resection of the os trigonum, or Stidia's process, and of Haglund's deformity and retrocalcaneal bursae.

HISTORICAL PERSPECTIVE

Ever since the knee joint was first examined with a cystoscope in 1918, surgeons with the foresight to realize the significance of intra-articular examination without performing an open arthrotomy have attempted to refine the instrumentation and technique of arthroscopy. This has been accomplished to the extent that arthroscopic instruments have been developed that permit diagnostic and operative procedures in the hip, shoulder, elbow, interphalangeal joints, temporomandibular joints, and essentially any body cavity.

Endoscopy is a combined work of Greek origin: *endon*, meaning "within," and *skopein*, meaning "to see." Takagi of Tokyo first coined the word "arthroscopy" during the 1900s. It too, is Greek in origin and combines *arthron*, meaning "joint," and *skopein*, "to see." Endoscopy dates back in the recorded literature to 1806, when Dr. Phillip Bozzini[7] reported on the use of an instrument consisting of a hollow silver tube with illumination provided by a beeswax candle. He reported to the Vinenna Conference of Medicine on his use of this instrument in several body cavities and the interior of osteomyelitic bone. Takagi first used a cystoscope in a knee in 1918. Soon after, he developed a 7.3-mm instrument that he called an arthroscope. In Switzerland, Bircher[8] reported on an arthroendoscopic examination of the knee in 1921. He was the first to report on arthroscopic examination of a meniscus, using a combination of nitrogen and oxygen gas to distend the knee joint.

Burman,[9] at the Hospital for Joint Diseases in New York City, reported on the use of a 4.0-mm arthroscope in 1931, after examining 19 cadaver knees and other joints, in his classic paper. It was his observation that the ankle joint was not suitable for arthroscopic examination due to its small size and the fact that he was unable to insert a fine-gauge needle into a cadaver ankle joint. He admitted, that with improvements, arthroscopic access to the ankle joint might be possible. Burman later reported on the arthroscopic examination of the elbow, ankle, and shoulder, in addition to the knee. Several years after Burman's original paper, Takagi[10] published a manuscript on the routine methodology for arthroscopic examination of the ankle joint.

With the advent of World War II, further development of the arthroscope stopped. It was not until after the war that Watanabe, a protege of Takagi, began further developing arthroscopic instrumentation. In 1957 he published his classic book, "Atlas of Arthroscopy."[11] Watanabe, in 1960, presented his No. 21 arthroscope, which quickly became the standard for arthroscopic examination of the knee and provided the basis for further development of current arthroscopes. Arthroscopy in North America remained at a standstill until R. W. Jackson returned to Canada after studying under Watanabe in Tokyo. Jackson was successful in establishing arthroscopy as the routine method of examination of the knee joint in the United States,[12] along with Dandy,[13] O'Connor,[14] and Johnson,[15] among others.

The first North American course in arthroscopy was held in Philadelphia in 1972. The International Arthroscopy Associated was founded in 1975, with Watanabe serving as its president. Since then, many seminars have been held on arthroscopy, but they have primarily been limited to the knee. In 1983, the first course was held that exclusively dealt with foot and ankle arthroscopy, under the direction of one of the authors (R. O. L.). Articles dealing with ankle arthroscopy began to appear in the 1980s, first by Drez et al.[16] then by Heller and Vogler,[17] and by numerous other authors in the following years. As techniques were expounded upon, results were reported and indications and criteria established for routine ankle procedures. Diagnostic ankle arthroscopy evolved into the performance of surgical procedures, making synovectomy, debridement, and the resection of avulsion and transchondral fractures primary reasons to perform ankle arthroscopy. In 1983, Hawkins utilized Lanny Johnsons' staple to plicate the anterior talofibular ligament in order to perform a lateral ankle stabilization.[18] At the time, arthroscopic lateral ankle stabilization seemed incredible, but it soon set the tone for future developments, proving that almost anything that can be performed by open arthrotomy can be performed with arthroscopic assistance. Just when lateral ankle stabilizations performed through the arthroscope were being digested, a little-known case report by Schneider in 1983[19] became available, demonstrating the use of an arthroscope to perform an ankle fusion. Reports of the use of this procedure did not appear in literature until 1989.

If the ankle could be fused arthroscopically, other joints could also be treated in a similar manner. Such was the case with the subtalar joint, the fusion of which was reported in 1994.[20] Arthroscopic treatment of other subtalar and rearfoot pathologies appeared in the literature. Such was the case in the reporting of the arthroscopic resection of an os trigonum and Stieda's process[21] and the use of the arthroscope in treating a retrocalcaneal bursa.[22]

In perhaps the most controversial use of arthroscopy since it was first used in the knee, Barrett and Day[23] reported on an endoscopic plantar fasciotomy for the treatment of chronic fascitis and heel-spur syndrome. Sparking a debate that is currently raging today, a spinoff technique was used for the endoscopic decompression of interdigital neuroma.[24]

CONTRAINDICATIONS AND COMPLICATIONS OF ARTHROSCOPY

Although arthroscopy is a minimally invasive and atraumatic procedure, it is not without potential complications and its own contraindications to surgery. Advances in arthroscopic equipment and technology have resulted in many contraindications no longer being considered absolute, and others no longer considered contraindications. A septic joint had been listed as a contraindication, but the early work of Takagi and Watanabe was on knees with septic arthritis due to tuberculosis. In a septic joint, arthroscopy is used to evaluate, irrigate, and drain the joint. Local cellulitis or systemic infection are contraindications for arthroscopy, as well as any other elective surgery. Anklylosed or severely arthritic joints with altered normal anatomy have been considered contraindications, but this is no longer necessarily true. With the alternative treatments for these types of joints being open arthrotomy, joint fusion, or replacement, arthroscopy becomes a viable option. In a severely abnormal joint, it is important to weigh the cost versus benefit of an arthroscopy. Many times arthroscopy will not be the definitive treatment, yet may give the patient several pain-free years until a more definitive but sometimes disabling procedure is indicated.

Many of the common complications associated with arthroscopy are often the result of controllable factors, such as poor technique, inexperience, lack of trained assistance, overzealous manipulation of the lower extremity or arthroscopic equipment, improper instrument selection, iatrogenic contamination, and improper patient selection. The potential complications associated with any surgical procedure also apply to arthroscopy. These specific complications associated with arthroscopy are best categorized as preoperative, perioperative, and postoperative. The main preoperative complication associated with arthroscopy involves the use of a leg holder. Leg holders provide stability to the lower extremity during the procedure, but improper placement of the leg holder near the fibular head can result in damage to the common peroneal nerve and a subsequent drop foot.

Most complications occur during the perioperative period, and several postoperative complications can be directly related to perioperative events. Most perioperative complications are related to the arthroscopic portals. Vital structure damage, joint entry difficulties, and instrument breakage may result with improper portal placement or technique. Each portal is associated with one or more vital structures that potentially may be damaged. The anteromedial portal of the ankle joint is in close proximity to the great saphenous vein and saphenous nerve. Superficially, the medial dorsal cutaneous nerve is located in the general area of the anterior central portal. Deeper, the dorsalis pedis artery and deep peroneal nerve are in this region. The most commonly damaged vital structure associated with portal placement is the lateral dorsal cutaneous nerve, which is located in the vicinity of the anterolateral portal.

The posteromedial portal, which is often not used, overlies the tarsal tunnel and its vital structures. The posterolateral portal is located near the sural nerve and small saphenous vein. The anterior subtalar joint portals are located over the sinus tarsi, with branches of the intermediate dorsal cutaneous nerve traversing this area. The metatarsophalangeal joints are approached with portals placed on either side of the long extensor tendon directly over the specific joint. The dorsal digital vital structures must be avoided when making portals to the metatarsophalangeal joints. Avoidance of portal complications is accomplished by prevention. Knowledge of the anatomy associated with each portal is of the utmost importance. Skin incisions should be made through the skin only, and not into the deeper structures. A mosquito hemostat is then used to bluntly dissect to the capsule. Finally, sharp trocars should be replaced with blunt obturators for cannula insertion.

Joint distention is another common perioperative complication. Overdistention can cause the joint capsule to rupture, leading to extravasation of fluid into the surrounding tissues and subsequent loss of distention. If extravasation is evident perioperatively, a compression bandage should be applied to prevent further fluid migration. Nerve damage can also result from overdistention.

Mechanical joint distractors have been associated with many of the ankle arthroscopy complications. Common associated complications are ligament damage, pin breakage, bone infection, sinus tract infection, fractures, and technical difficulties. With the use of this instrument declining, many of the previously reported complications are no longer prevalent.

Cannula insertion can also cause neurovascular or articular damage. This is best prevented by avoiding the use of trocars. Iatrogenic articular lesions are termed "skid marks." Partial-thickness lesions do not usually require treatment, but full-thickness lesions must be abraded. This type of lesion can also be caused by the tip of the arthroscope. Compressive damage to the articular surface from the arthroscope can occur when examining the medial and lateral gutter, or the posterior ankle joint through the sagittal groove of the talus. Another common iatrogenic cause of articular damage is power equipment. Abraders are more aggressive than shavers and therefore more likely to cause articular damage.

Due to the small stature of the arthroscopic equipment, instrument breakage may occur. It is important to check the ends of instruments for any possible breakage. If instrument breakage does occur, and it is not noted intraoperatively, postoperative radiographs will reveal the interarticular foreign body. Interarticular foreign bodies can be retrieved manually or by the use of a magnetized rod.

Poor joint visualization is a common perioperative complication. One of the most common causes of poor visualization is fogging of the arthroscope. This usually occurs during the sterilization process while soaking the equipment in activated glutaraldehyde. Fogging can be prevented by sterilizing the equipment instead of soaking. If the equipment is used several times during the day, then soaking is required or special arthroscopic sterilizers can be used. Fogging is best treated by removing the eyepiece from the arthroscope and wiping both sides clean. Defogging solutions are also available if the problem is recurrent.

Scratching of the protective lens cover can also lead to poor visualization. This usually occurs due to improper handling of instrumentation, especially power equipment. If significant damage occurs, replacement of the arthroscope is required. Clouding produces poor visual qualities similar to fogging, and is due to separation of the protective lens cover from the lens system. Moisture then may enter the lens system. This often occurs with manipulation of the arthroscope and secondary contact between the lens cover and articular surfaces or other operative equipment. The initial treatment for clouding is similar to that for fogging. If this does not resolve the condition, then replacement of the arthroscope is required. Poor picture quality may also be attributed to any of the other components of the arthroscopic system. Therefore, it is important to be familiar with these components and any potential complications that may alter picture quality.

The instrumentation used for arthroscopic lateral ankle stabilization has several potential inherent complications. This system consists of an insertor/distractor and 5.5-mm staples. Complications such as inadvertent insertion into articular surfaces, insufficient plication of the anterior talofibular ligament, fracture of the bone, and unstable staple placement have been reported. Proper training prior to attempting the use of this system is therefore imperative.

Other potential perioperative complications that can affect visualization are redouts and whiteouts. Redouts are the result of intra-articular bleeding, usually due to poor hemostasis. This can be controlled by maintaining joint distention at proper levels, and by appropriate tourniquet use. If the problem persists, epinephrine injected into the joint will help decrease the bleeding. Whiteouts are associated with improper light intensity resulting in extreme brightness of the picture. Automatic light sources commonly used today prevent whiteouts from occurring. If this problem arises, light intensity should be decreased.

Postoperative infection rates for arthroscopy are similar to those of any other surgical procedure. Common factors that affect infection rate include surgical trauma, procedure length, and intraoperative sterility. Factors unique to arthroscopy that may also affect the infection rate include hemarthrosis, fluid extravasation, or the presence of synovial fistulas. Prophylactic antibiotic usage is not recommended unless a concurrent open procedure accompanies an arthroscopy. Postoperative arthroscopic infection should be treated in a manner similar to standard postoperative infection protocols.

Many of the postoperative neurovascular complications are the results of arthroscopic portal placement or instrument insertion. Use of proper technique is of the utmost importance in avoiding these complications. Postoperative treatment for neurologic complications includes immobilization, steroid injection, physical therapy, oral anti-inflammatory medications, and possibly secondary surgical intervention. Pain directly associated with portal sites postoperatively is most often attributable to surgical trauma or neurovascular damage. The treatment for painful portals includes surgical silicone gel placed directly over the portal site, local steroid injections, anti-inflammatory medication, and physical therapy.

Postoperative hemarthrosis can lead to permanent cartilage damage due to enzymatic degradation and pressure. This is one of the more potentially severe complications of foot and ankle arthroscopy. Hemarthrosis may occur with synovectomies, abrasion arthroplasties, or intraoperative damage to a vascular structure. Proper technique and thorough knowledge of local anatomy are key to preventing intraoperative damage to vascular structures. Appropriate intraoperative hemostasis is also important in preventing postoperative hemarthrosis. Postoperative measures that can help prevent hemarthrosis formation include leaving one portal open for drainage, applying a firm postoperative compressive dressing, and ice and elevation. The use of a cast brace to limit motion at the ankle joint is also beneficial postoperatively. Aspiration, exsanguination, and lavage in conjunction with ice, elevation, and compression are used to treat postoperative hematomas. If this does not result in a significant decrease in pain and edema, a repeat arthroscopy is then indicated. Longstanding hemarthrosis leads to adhesive capsulitis and fibrosis. This is usually best treated with a repeat arthroscopy, the timing of which is dependent upon the pain. Persistent pain after surgery may occur with any surgical procedure, and treatment following arthroscopy should parallel the standard protocol for this complication. If the pain persists, examination of the area with repeat postoperative radiographs or specialized studies, such as MRI or CT scan, may reveal an intraoperative foreign body or another bony pathology that had not been previously diagnosed.

ARTHROSCOPIC TECHNIQUE

The ankle can be approached from both its anterior and posterior aspects. For anterior approaches, the patient is placed supine on the surgical table and, once positioned, a leg holder is attached to the table and placed over the distal one-third of the tibia. A tourniquet is used and applied to the midthigh when a general anesthetic is used or around the ankle with a local. Once the limb is exsanguinated by elevation for 3 minutes or by use of an Esmark bandage, it is placed in the holder and secured. A pillow or rolled sheets can be placed under the knee for support. When using the leg holder, one must be careful to roll the hip and knee inward to allow the ankle to be maintained in its desired position in the frontal plane. The holder should also be placed well below the fibular head to avoid damage to the common peroneal nerve. If operative procedures are being performed on both extremities, it may be easier to attempt arthroscopy without using the leg holder. An assistant may be used to maintain the ankle position.

The patient's foot is prepped using standard aseptic technique with an appropriate surgical scrub up to the level well above the malleoli. The foot and ankle are exsanguinated and the tourniquet inflated. The leg can then be inserted into the leg holder and secured in that position. The patient is then draped in the usual manner; plastic-lined drapes designed especially for arthroscopy are preferable. If necessary, arthroscopy drapes can be cut with scissors to allow access to the contralateral extremity.

Anesthesia for both diagnostic and surgical arthroscopy of the foot and ankle may be general, regional, or local. General anesthesia is recommended while learning arthroscopic technique or with the anxious patient. The use of a thigh tourniquet necessitates an anesthetic other than local due to the resultant pain.

Diagnostic and operative arthroscopies lasting approximately 1.5 hours can be performed under local anesthetic using an ankle tourniquet with or without a leg holder. Using a 10-ml syringe of 2 percent lidocaine with epinephrine, a wheal is raised in the subcutaneous tissue over each anticipated portal of entry. The needle is then directed into the joint and the anesthetic solution is injected until resistance is felt. As distention of the joint occurs, there may be slight concurrent dorsiflexion of the foot on the leg. Slight hallux plantar flexion may also be noted. The surgeon should closely observe the joint during distention to prevent infiltration of subcutaneous tissue. Uneven distention is suggestive of decreased capsular elasticity, thereby limiting the space inside the joint and making visualization more difficult. Once the joint has been distended, a #15 blade may be used to perform a stab incision, following the skin lines, at the desired portal of entry. Patient tolerance to local anesthetic administered in this manner is excellent, allowing office arthroscopy if properly equipped. The only pain felt is a slight burning when making a subcutaneous wheal. As the joint is being distended, there may be an occasional dull pain at the posterior aspect of the ankle.

When using general anesthetic, we prefer to make portal incisions prior to joint distention because of better visualization of topographic anatomy. For distention, an 18-gauge needle on a syringe with a minimum of 20 ml of normal saline or lactated Ringer's solution (preferred) is injected through the anticipated portal for joint distention. We prefer using the anteromedial portal because it allows almost subcutaneous access to the joint and directs the needle away from the cartilage. The average adult ankle requires approximately 10 to 15 ml of fluid for full distention. When distending a joint, it is important that the solution enter the joint capsule and not the subcutaneous tissue; therefore, continuous palpation of joint margins is recommended.

After skin incision and adequate joint distention, a curved hemostat is inserted through the incision to spread the soft tissue and retract any vital structures. Traditionally a trocar has been placed within the cannula and, with the palm of the hand, twisted in order to pierce the capsular structures, where a release of resistance will be felt. An obturator is then inserted and used to manipulate the cannula into its desired position in the joint. Oftentimes only the blunt obturator is used within the cannula after careful blunt dissection of soft tissues has been performed. This decreases the risk of scoring the articular cartilage upon piercing the joint capsule or neurologic damage, especially when using an anterior central portal, because of the proximity of the neurovascular bundle. With the obturator removed, the arthroscopic camera can be placed within the cannula and ingress as well as egress lines can be established.

Adequate ingress and egress of solution through the joint is mandatory to provide adequate visualization for operative or diagnostic procedures. Normally ingress is maintained through a port with a turncock on the cannula that contains the arthroscope. This system allows constant flow around the lens, keeping it clear of debris. Traditionally the pressure of the fluid is maintained with gravity by placing two 1,000-ml bags of lactated Ringer's elevated on an IV pole. Arthroscopy tubing is used to allow the lactated Ringer's to flow directly into the cannula. Infusion pump systems are often used, making for a more consistent and controllable infusion of fluid. Other newer systems are available. The basis of these systems is two separate pumps that allow independent flow and pressure control. This is accomplished by controlling flow through the joint with the outflow pump and regulating pressure with the inflow pump. These self-contained units should include all the tubing and "hookups" needed to run lactated Ringer's. The egress flow can be achieved with a second portal and cannula, or the arthroscope shaving equipment can be attached to a suction unit, or the shaver can be directly attached to the outflow of the pump systems. It is important that outflow not exceed inflow, preventing low joint pressure and loss of visibility, when using any system.

Once an ingress or egress line, or both, has been established and the arthroscope is properly positioned within the cannula, joint visualization should begin. The surgeon must now identify a familiar structure to be orientated anatomically. This may be difficult with adhesive capsulitis or hypertrophic synovitis, but can be aided with gentle ankle dorsiflexion and plantar flexion. Once the anatomic location within the joint has been established, scanning of the joint can commence.

The posterior aspect of the joint can be approached from the supine, lateral recumbent, or prone position. When the patient is supine, the foot and ankle is prepped and draped similar to when the patient is prone. The prone approach is not used as much because most pathology is located in the anterior pouch of the ankle or can be assessed through supine positions.

In the supine position, lax joints may allow passage of the arthroscope by manual distraction of the ankle and passage of the arthroscope through the sagittal groove of the talus into the posterior pouch. An ankle distractor can also be used to allow posterior joint access. When the patient is in a lateral recumbent position, two stacked portals behind the peroneal tendons are made at the level of the posterior joint line. One portal is used for scope placement and the other used for the shaver.

When the patient is positioned prone, the posterior joint pouch can be entered as described for the anterior pouch or can be entered extra-articularly. Here an obturator is used to make a channel to the capsule and the arthroscope is placed in that position behind the joint. A shaver is then placed in an adjacent portal and triangulated into visualization. A rent is then made in the capsule, allowing access into the joint, and further debridement can continue until the entire posterior aspect of the joint is visualized.

PRINCIPLES OF ARTHROSCOPY

Arthroscopy is a technically demanding procedure that carries a high learning curve, but, as in all arts and sciences, the procedure can be broken down into several basic components. When experiencing difficulty in a procedure, one must step back and review the basics. These basic facts are that an arthroscope can only do three things: piston, sweep, and rotate. By combining these actions, one can also triangulate. The surgeon should not attempt to demand anything else from the arthroscope because it will not be able to respond.

The type of arthroscope used is dependent on the needs and skills of the surgeon and the type of instruments available in the marketplace. Most scopes are approximately 4.0 mm in diameter, with an optics length from the eyepiece of the instrument to its tip of 4 to 6 inches. All are compatible with video monitoring and recording systems and contain a side arm for the insertion of the light guide. All arthroscopes are placed into a joint through a cannula that contains at least one side arm with a stopcock for ingressing or egressing fluids. The ends of all arthroscopes have a cover lens and contain a "tip cut" that determines the direction of visualization. A tip cut that is perpendicular to the long axis of the arthroscope that will give 0 degrees' deflection of the image. Because the ability to manipulate the arthroscope within a joint is dependent on the field of vision present and inherent within the arthroscope, most instruments do not have a 0-degree tip cut because this will allow visualization strictly in a straight ahead position. If the tip cut is angled any number of degrees, by rotating the arthroscope the field of vision can then be manipulated to be increased by a factor of the angulation. Therefore, most arthroscopes have a tip cut of 25 to 30 degrees. This allows the instrument to be rotated and the field of vision increased in the direction of the angulation. The direction of angulation is either a fore or aft obliquity depending on the manufacturer. Fore-oblique scopes have a tip cut that is angled in a direction in front of the light guide attachment to the arthroscope, whereas with aft-oblique scopes the tip cut is angled directly in a direction behind the attachment for the light guide.

Rotation is one of the most important functions of an arthroscope, and is dependent on the angulation of the tip cut. As a 25-degree oblique arthroscope is rotated, a large field of vision can be attained. Unfortunately, as the arthroscope is rotated, the visual image presented on the monitor is similarly rotated. This necessitates concurrent repositioning of the camera to an upright position as needed. By rotating the arthroscope, one is able to utilize one single portal for observation of the joint being inspected.

Pistoning is a function of the optical system of the arthroscope. All arthroscopes magnify to some extent. This magnification is a function of the position of the tip of the instrument relative to the object being viewed. Therefore, the further the tip of the instrument is away from an object, the greater will be its field of vision, and therefore the object will appear less magnified. Conversely, the closer the tip of the instrument is to the object being viewed, the more the field of vision will be decreased and the greater the magnification of the object will be. By pistoning the tip of the arthroscope further away from the object, one will change the field of vision as well as the magnification of the object.

Sweeping is the third function of an arthroscope. By sweeping the tip of the arthroscope from side to side or up and down, the field of vision of the arthroscope will be redirected. Because the portal in which the arthroscope is placed acts as a fulcrum at the level of the skin, the tip of the arthroscope will be anywhere from 1.0 to 2.0 cm away. By sweeping in various directions, large changes to the field of vision can be achieved. Even slight motions yield significant changes. Therefore, small, deliberate motions are necessary in order to stay within the desired area of the joint.

Triangulation is a method by which an object is placed by the operator into the field of view of the arthroscope. By combining rotation, pistoning, and sweeping, the surgeon can guide the arthroscope to any anatomic area of the ankle or foot from a carefully placed portal. Once the tip of the arthroscope is in the desired anatomic area, an adjacent portal is used to introduce the object toward the operator by placing it in the field of view of the arthroscope. This is accomplished by first placing the arthroscope in the desired position and then directing it toward the object to be triangulated. The object is then placed into an adjacent portal and carefully introduced in the direction of the tip of the arthroscope, compensating for the distance between the skin and actual position of the tip of the instrument. The object is then manipulated until it is in the field of vision or it can be felt to be touching the arthroscope

and can then be guided carefully into the field of vision. This is a technique that is done "blind" and therefore requires skills that are gained with experience. Care must be taken to avoid inadvertent damage to the articular surfaces or vital structures when attempting to triangulate. Surgeons must remember, when triangulating arthroscopic burs or blades, not to operate those instruments until they are directly visualized through the arthroscope. Inadvertent shaving, abrading, or cutting with a knife greatly increases the complications of the procedure, directly affecting outcome.

ARTHROSCOPIC COMPARTMENTS OF THE ANKLE AND PORTALS OF ENTRY

The ankle can be divided into three anterior (Fig. 27-1) and two posterior (Figs. 27-2 and 27-3) compartments, with access to each being achieved through anatomically corresponding portals of entry. Structures from adjacent portals may also be visualized because overlap will occur. The anterior compartment (Fig. 27-4) is larger and contains most of the pathology contributing to or resulting from chronic ankle pain.

The anterior central compartment is approached through a portal located along the ankle joint line at the point just lateral to the extensor hallucis longus tendon. The dorsalis pedis artery and neurovascular bundle lie just lateral to this point, and must be identified by palpating the arterial pulse and avoided. On entering the ankle from this portal, one may be able to visualize the anterior synovial wall. The distal anterior lip of the tibia, the tibial plafond, and the synovial reflection at the tibia and on the talar neck are easily examined. Also visible is the central concave trochlear portion of the talus. Plantar flexion of the foot facilitates visualization of the talar dome, and dorsiflexion of the foot permits the visualization of the talar neck and synovial reflection.

The anterolateral compartment can be examined through a portal placed just lateral to the peroneus tertius tendon along the ankle joint line. Care must be taken to avoid the intermediate dorsal cutaneous nerve, which can be located in the area just above the dorsal aspect of the depression overlying the sinus tarsi, lateral to the talar head. This approach permits visualization of the anterolateral synovial wall and its attachment to the fibular malleolus, the anterior talofibular ligament and fibers thereof, the dorsolateral trochlear surface of the talus, and the lateral talar dome. The interval between the lateral aspect of the talar

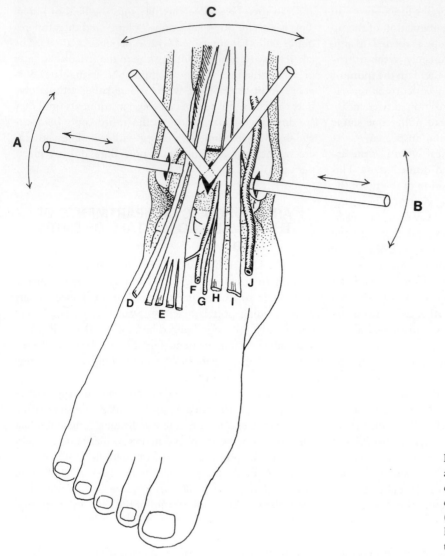

Figure 27-1 Anterior ankle portals. A, anterolateral; B, anteromedial; C, anterocentral; D, peroneus tertius; E, extensor digitorum longus; F, anterior tibial artery (dorsalis pedis); G, deep peroneal nerve; H, extensor hallucis longus; I, tibialis anterior tendon; J, greater saphenous vein.

dome and the fibular malleolus is termed the lateral gutter, above which is the lateral interval consists of the space between the lateral edge of the tibia, the medial aspect of the fibula, and the dorsolateral aspect of the talar dome. The described space within the lateral interval is the tibiofibular synovial recess, which is bound superiorly by the interosseous ligament. Contained within this recess is an outpocketing of synovium, the tibiofibular synovial fringe (Fig. 27-5). This is a normal arthroscopic finding; it can become thicker, denser, and hypertrophied in response to inflammatory changes but this does not necessarily make it a pathologic entity. Resection of this structure should

only be done when it obliterates access to the posterior aspect of the joint. In the posterior aspect of the lateral interval, the posterior synovial wall may be visible. At the inferior aspect of the lateral gutter, the fibular malleolus can be visualized along with the fibers of the anterior talofibular ligament coursing anterior and medial to the trochlear surface of the talus.

The anteromedial portal is placed along the ankle joint line at the junction of the tibia and medial malleolus and the medial aspect of the talar dome. It lays just medial to the tibialis anterior tendon. The anteromedial portal permits visualization of the anteromedial synovial wall and

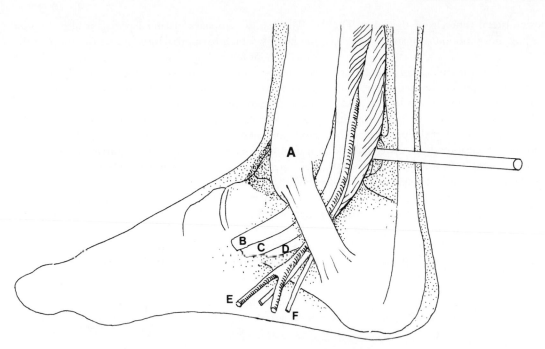

Figure 27-2 Posteromedial ankle portal. A, tibial malleolus; B, tibialis posterior tendon; C, flexor digitorum longus tendon; D, flexor hallucis longus; E, posterior tibial artery and branches; F, tibial nerve and branches.

its attachment of the medial malleolus, and the deep fibers of the deltoid ligament may be observed. The interval between the medial malleolus and the medial surface of the talar dome is called the "medial gutter." Dorsal to the medial gutter is a rounded portion of the tibia that continues to form the medial malleolus. We have termed this

Figure 27-3 Posterolateral ankle portal. A, fibular malleolus; B, peroneal tendons; C, lesser saphenous vein; D, sural nerve.

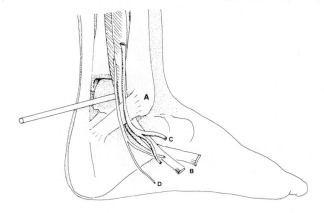

the "medial bend." The dorsomedial aspect of the trochlear surface of the talus can also be identified.

The posteromedial compartment lays along the posterior margins of the ankle joint, with a portal of entry best placed just medial to the Achilles tendon. The posterior tibial artery and neurovascular bundle must be identified and the portal of entry made between it and the tendo Achillis. It may be difficult to palpate the joint at this location. This approach permits visualization of the posteromedial synovial wall, the posteromedial articular surface of the talus, and the posterior surface of the tibial malleolus. At the posterior aspect of the articular surface of the tibia, one may observe the deep portion of the posterior tibiofibular ligament forming a labrium to deepen the tibial articular surface.

The posterolateral compartment is inspected through a portal located at a point along the levels of the posterior joint line lateral to the Achilles tendon. Care must be taken to avoid the sural nerve, which runs posterior to the peroneal tendons. The small saphenous vein must also be avoided. This approach reveals a view of the posterolateral synovial wall, the posterolateral articular surface of the talus, the posteromedial articular surface of the fibular malleolus, and the posterolateral tubercle of the talus. The deep portion of the posterior tibiofibular ligament may be seen as well.

The posterior aspect of the ankle can also be approached with the patient in the lateral recumbent position, exposing the lateral surface of the lower leg and ankle. Two stacked portals are made, 1.5 to 2.0 cm apart, with the inferior portal being at the level of the posterior joint line, directly behind the peroneal tendons. Care must be exercised to avoid the lesser saphenous vein and sural nerve. This is best accomplished by making a small cutdown incision through the skin and then, by using a smaller curved hemostat, bluntly dissecting a tunnel to the posterior capsule at the level of the joint line. Both portals are prepared in this manner, and the arthroscopic cannula is placed by using its obturator in the superior portal. Operative instruments are then passed through the inferior portal.

The use of two stacked lateral portals is also the best method by which to approach the posterior aspect of the subtalar joint for pathology in that area, particularly in the resection of Steida's process (enlarged posterolateral talar process) or an os trigonum. In this instance, a similar technique is used, the same vital structures are avoided, and portals are placed inferior to those used for accessing the ankle joint. Here, the inferior portal is placed at the level of or just above the posterosuperior surface of the calcaneus, with the superior portal being placed 1.5 to 2.0 cm above.

The anterior aspect of the subtalar joint is similarly best approached through two stacked portals in the sinus tarsi. When arthroscoping this area of the joint, the inferior portal is placed just anterior to the lateral articular process at or slightly above the level of the calcaneal sulcus. The superior portal is then placed directly above by 1.5 to

Figure 27-4 Normal arthroscopic anatomy of the anterior aspect of the ankle.

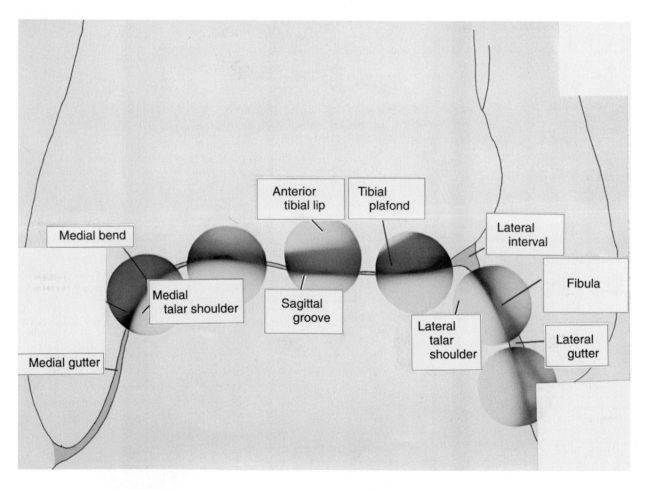

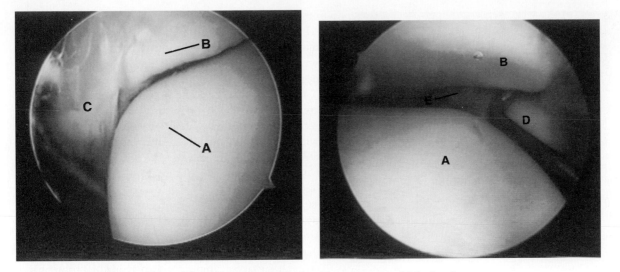

Figure 27-5 The lateral interval of the ankle. A, lateral talar shoulder; B, anterior tibial tubercle; C, anterior inferior tibiofibular ligament; D, fibula; E, tibiofibular synovial fringe and the tibiofibular synovial recess.

2.0 cm. Again, the arthroscope is placed in a manner similar to that described for accessing the posterior aspect of the joint, and operative instruments are placed in the inferior portal.

Metatarsophalangeal joints are also accessible arthroscopically and accessed in similar manners. When approaching these joints, a medial and lateral superior portal is used and placed on either side of the long extensor tendon at the level of the joint line medial or lateral to the long extensor tendon. Care must be taken to avoid the neurovascular bundle; therefore, the cutdown incision should be placed between the tendon and the anticipated location of these vital structures. Blunt dissection is used to create a channel in the subcutaneous tissue, allowing any vital structures to be reflected.

Through the portals discussed above, access can be gained to virtually every joint described. Specialty portals can be placed at the inferior aspect of the medial and lateral gutters of the ankle (or any other arthroscoped joint) in order to assist in the resection of avulsion fractures or loose bodies, or for the performance of other procedures. In these cases, portals are best made by directing the arthroscope into the desired position in the joint and, by transillumination of the cutaneous structures, marking the exact location of the portal on the skin. This also assists in avoiding vital structures because the veins are silhouetted by the light.

Use of ankle distractors to forcibly open the joint, transmalleolar approaches, and trans-Achilles tendon approaches are all virtually unnecessary except in rare instances. Physicians properly trained in foot and ankle arthroscopy techniques will avoid their use because they are rarely needed and increase the complication rate of the procedure.

ARTHROSCOPIC PATHOLOGY

Arthroscopic pathology can be generalized or joint specific. Generalized pathologies are classified as soft tissue, cartilaginous, or osseous.

Soft Tissue Pathology

Soft tissue pathologies are often referred to as "impingement syndromes." Hypertrophy of normal synovium due to inflammation causes a soft tissue buildup within the joint; with motion, the capsule compresses this hypertrophic soft tissue lining against the articular surfaces. Pain results from alteration of the capsular and ligamentous structures that comprise the articular nerve supply. Impingement syndromes can be the sole cause of joint pain or associated with other pathologies. Activity-related joint

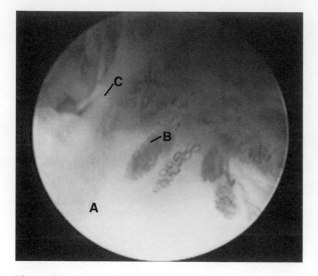

Figure 27-6 Acute hypertrophic synovium. A, talus; B, injected vessels of a hypertrophic synovial villus; C, hyalinized synovium that is not acute in nature.

pain, without other obvious articular pathology, is a leading indication of impingement syndromes.

Synovium covers all intra-articular structures except the cartilaginous surfaces, and lines the capsule. The capsule is divided into intimal and subintimal layers. The intimal layer is highly vascular and cellular, while the subintimal layer is mostly fibrous and acts as supportive tissue. The subintimal layer is consistent with the periosteum. The function of the synovial membrane is to act as a filtering system and produce synovial fluid. Synovium may be folded, to expand and contract with joint motion. These folds are called synovial plica, but they are not usually visible in the ankle.

Arthroscopically, normal synovial villi are small and not independently visible. Abnormal synovial villi elongate, appearing as long, transparent, fingerlike projections with a central red "injected" vessel (Fig. 27-6). These abnormal villi can produce a fibrin exudate, which can cloud the joint. Continued inflammation leads to villous necrosis, which gives an opaque appearance to the tips of the villi (Fig. 27-7). The necrotic tips can flake off into the joint, further clouding it.

Synovitis can occur as a single pathologic process of the joint or the result of inflammation associated with another pathology. Synovitis is divided into acute and chronic forms. Acute synovitis presents with transparent, hypertrophic villi with a central red injected vessel. With more in-

tense inflammation or with trauma, the central injected vessel can rupture, with the villi filling with blood. This is termed "hemorrhagic synovitis." Chronic synovitis appears with opaque villi, with frayed tips of various lengths from degeneration. Synovial pileup is another form of synovitis. This occurs with continued inflammation resulting in increased amounts of synovitis that "piles up" into the joint recesses. This synovial pileup may then become impinged with joint movement. The treatment for any type of symptomatic synovitis consists of arthroscopic synovectomy.

Fibrous bands are another form of soft tissue pathology that occur when fibrin exudate from hypertrophic synovitis aggregates to form masses, which then become hyalinized by being compressed between the capsule and articular surfaces. They appear as thin and whispy bands that vary in shape and are loosely attached to degenerated articular surfaces. There are two types of fibrous bands that can be identified arthroscopically. The small, loosely attached bands are not considered pathologic and do not require treatment. The thick, firm, cordlike bands are considered pathologic. These are attached to one or both ends of degenerated articular surfaces or hypertrophic synovium (Fig. 27-8). These structures must be resectioned with a shaver or punch. Large lesions may also be resected from their attachment site, grasped, and pulled from the joint.

Meniscoid bodies are a form of traumatically induced synovial pileup that becomes hyalinized. Their appearance is similar to osteochondral bodies, but differ in that they are attached firmly to the synovium (Fig. 27-9). These soft

Figure 27-7 Chronic hypertrophic synovitis. A, lateral talar shoulder; B, opaque frayed chronic villus projections; C, anterior tibial tubercle.

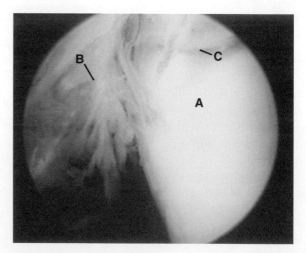

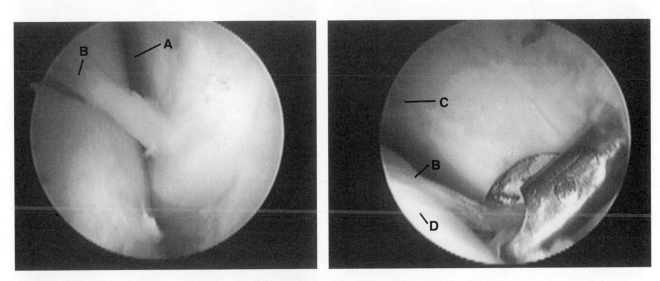

Figure 27-8 Pathologic fibrous band attaching to the fibula laterally and coursing medially over the lateral talar shoulder. A, lateral gutter; B, fibrous band; C, lateral shoulder of the talus.

Figure 27-9 Meniscoid bodies. A, talus; B, fibula; C, anterior talofibular ligament.

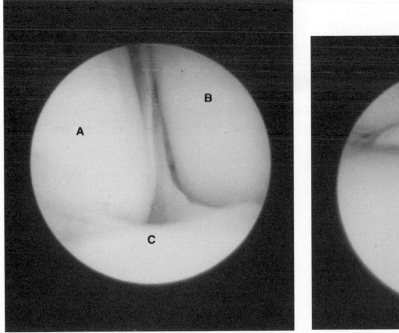

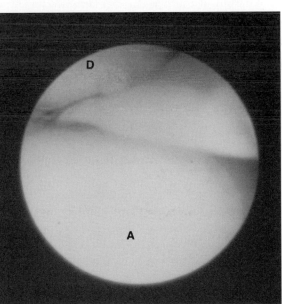

tissue lesions are considered pathologic. Meniscoid bodies can usually be resected with a synovial shaver. If the lesion is large, it must be sharply incised from its synovial attachment and then removed with a grasper.

Adhesive capsulitis results from trauma to the capsule or severe arthrosis, which results in fibrosis and loss of elasticity of the capsule. The alteration of the capsular structure is the primary cause of pain, as well as soft tissue impingement between the articular surfaces. Arthroscopically, the joint will be difficult to enter due to capsular inelasticity and severe hypertrophic synovitis. It is usually easier to enter this type of joint horizontally rather than vertically, placing the arthroscope in the medial or lateral portal instead of the central portal. Another technique that is helpful to gain joint entry is to shave an entry into the joint. This is done by using the obturator to palpate the joint surface. The arthroscope is then introduced into the area. Through a separate portal, a synovial shaver is then introduced. The tip of the synovial shaver is located by triangulation. The shaver is turned toward the joint, and a rent is made in the synovium to visualize the joint (Fig. 27-10). A joint space is created by resecting the hypertrophic synovium and capsule. If the synovial shaver is not effective in resecting the adhesive capsulitis, a suction punch is recommended. During resection of adhesive capsulitis, care must be taken to avoid iatrogenically induced damage to the articular surface. Another factor to consider when treating adhesive capsulitis is postoperative hematoma. This can occur with the significant soft tissue resection that is required for adequate treatment. To help prevent this postoperative complication, one of the portals should be left open for drainage, the extremity should be elevated and iced for 2 to 3 days postoperatively, and a firm postoperative compressive dressing should be applied.

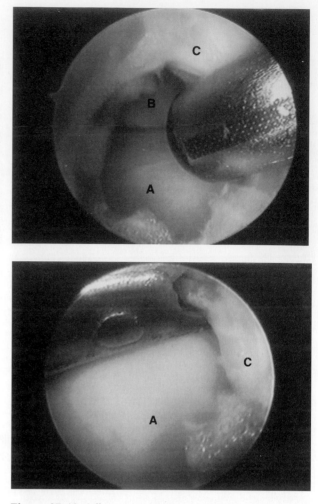

Figure 27-10 Adhesive capsulitis in the anterior aspect of the ankle. A, talus; B, anterior tibial lip; C, adhesive capsule.

Cartilaginous Lesions

Cartilage is firm yet pliable. Normally cartilage will depress with pressure, and then return to its original shape when the pressure is removed. Cartilage is able to withstand compressive and tensile forces. Collagen fibrils provide resistance to tensile forces, while glycoprotein resists compression. The glycoprotein aggregates to form a viscous gel that attaches to the collagen fibrils to resist compression. Cartilage appears opaque and white, and is usually between 2.0 and 3.0 mm thick in the ankle joint. The metatarsophalangeal joint articular cartilage is considerably less thick. Cartilage lacks any blood or nerve supply.

It is bounded by subchondral bone via a lock-and-key mechanism between the zone of calcified cartilage and the subchondral bone plate. Just above the zone of calcified cartilage is the zone of noncalcified cartilage, which stains as a basophilic line with hematoxylin and eosin. This is termed the "tidemark." It is the level where the vascular supply to the cartilage ends, and is an important arthroscopic landmark for abrasion arthroplasty.

Cartilage is divided into three layers: deep, tangential, and superficial (Fig. 27-11). The deepest layer is a thick, vertical layer of collagen-forming fibril arches. The intermediate tangential layer consists of a mesh arrangement between the arches of deep vertical fibrils. The superficial layer consists of horizontal superficial fibrils. This superficial layer is covered by a membrane termed the "lamina splendens," which provides a protective barrier to the cartilage matrix and is attached to the periosteum. Breakdown of any of these layers constitutes a cartilaginous lesion that is pathologic depending on the extent of matrix exposure and loss.

Cartilaginous lesions include subchondral erosions, chondromalacia, and chondral lesions. *Subchondral erosions* result from hypertrophy of synovium. As the synovium accumulates over cartilaginous surfaces, nourishment of the chondrocyte is reduced, leading to cell death. In addition, as synovium hypertrophies, enzymes are released to the joint, especially to areas in direct contact with the piled-up synovium, resulting in enzymatic degradation of the cartilaginous surface. These lesions appear as exposed subchondral bone or subchondral bone covered with a thin layer of loose fibrous or reactive fibrous tissue (Fig. 27-12). Reactive fibrous tissue is often hemorrhagic and considered to be pathologic. These erosions are treated by resection with a curette, abrader, or shaver. Nonreactive tissue covering a subchondral erosion is not considered to be pathologic, but does indicate inflammatory and degenerative changes. This type of lesion is best treated by flushing the joint and performing light debridement with a probe or shaver. Uncovered exposed subchondral bone is also considered pathologic, but does not require treatment unless complicated by fracture or further degenerative changes. These lesions are commonly seen at any joint margin, particularly the anterior tibial lip and anterior aspects of the medial and lateral malleoli.

Chondromalacia results from a degenerative process within the cartilage itself. In general terms, chondromalacia means softening of the cartilage. This is a commonly encountered pathologic process seen arthroscopically. Chondromalacia is classified by two systems that are important in determining the type of arthroscopic treatment and postoperative prognosis.

The Collins classification system is used to describe gross chondromalacic changes.[25] A grade 1 lesion presents as softening and fraying of the cartilaginous surface. These lesions are usually not symptomatic. Grade 2 lesions also exhibit softening and fraying of the cartilaginous surface, but additionally present with fissuring of the cartilage to the level of the subchondral bone. Mild arthritic changes within the joint are associated with grade 2 lesions. Grade 3 lesions present with extensive fraying and fissuring of the cartilage with small areas of exposed subchondral bone. There are usually significant arthritic changes associated with grade 3 lesions, including asymmetric joint space narrowing with limited range of motion. Grade 4 lesions present as large areas of cartilage loss to the level of the subchondral bone. This type of lesion is associated with significant arthritic changes both clinically and radiographically.

The Goodfellow classification system consists of superficial and basal degenerations, which are further subdivided into four categories each.[26] The Goodfellow classification is more useful for the arthroscopist because it views the chondromalacic changes on a microscopic level, dividing them into two types: superficial and basal (Fig. 27-13). Superficial chondromalacia presents as an erosion of the superficial layer with disruption of the lamina splendens. The matrix elements are then exposed to abnormal forces, which leads to increased degeneration of the cartilaginous

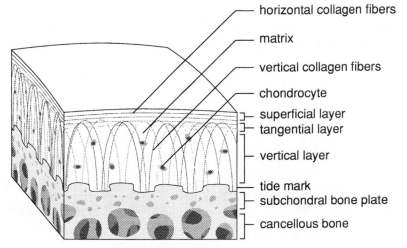

Figure 27-11 The layers of normal cartilage. (From Lundeen RD: Manual of Ankle and Foot Arthroscopy. Churchill Livingstone, New York, 1992, with permission).

horizontal collagen fibers

matrix

vertical collagen fibers

chondrocyte

superficial layer
tangential layer

vertical layer

tide mark
subchondral bone plate
cancellous bone

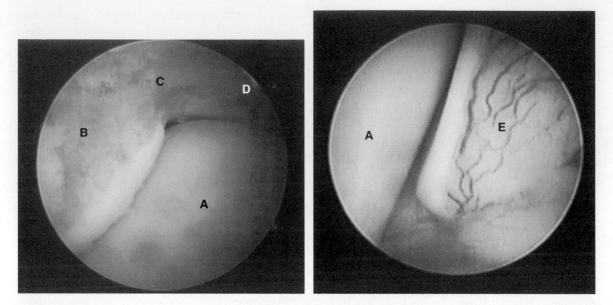

Figure 27-12 Subchondral erosions. A, talus; B, anterior tibial lip; C, medial bend; D, medial malleolus; E, fibula.

surfaces. Type 2 lesions are deeper than type 1, with exposed tangential fibers. Type 3 lesions show deeper degeneration, exposing matrix elements and fissuring to the level of the subchondral bone. Type 4 lesions have exposed deep matrix elements and subchondral bone, forming a more generalized lesion. Basal chondromalacic type 1 lesions present as softening of the cartilaginous surface, with separation of the tangential and deep fibers. Type 2 basal lesions present as a blister formation occurring in the superficial layer. The superficial layer remains intact, and the matrix elements become more disorganized than in type 1 lesions. Type 3 basal chondromalacic lesions present as ruptured layers of cartilage with exposed matrix elements. Type 4 basal lesions are a continuation of the type 3 lesion with exposure of subchondral bone.

Before treating chondromalacia, it is important to have a thorough understanding of the above-mentioned classification systems, as well as cartilage anatomy and physiology. Other factors important in deciding whether or not to treat chondromalacia include the patient's preoperative symp-

Figure 27-13 Goodfellow's classification of chondromalacia. (From Lundeen RD: Manual of Ankle and Foot Arthroscopy. Churchill Livingstone, New York, 1992, with permission.)

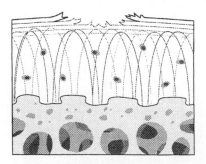

Superficial Degeneration

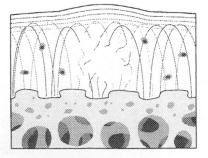

Basal Degeneration

toms, the joint condition, and the condition of the patient. Small areas of fibrillated cartilage are best treated by chondroplasty. This consists of debridement of affected areas to help reduce irritation and friction within the joint, but promotes no healing of the defect. If significant amounts of subchondral bone are exposed, an abrasion arthroplasty is indicated. Abrasion arthroplasties are performed by abrading subchondral bone to the level of the tidemark in order to promote revascularization of the area to initiate fibrocartilage repair. An abrasion arthroplasty is usually performed if the lesion is less than 1 cm in diameter, but careful evaluation must be made concerning the lesion and the overall joint appearance. With significant arthritic changes and large lesions, only a light debridement is recommended, with resection of any osteophytic lesions and flushing of the joint. This form of treatment can provide significant relief of preoperative symptoms without the long rehabilitation time of a large abrasion arthroplasty. This is the most common form of treatment for type 3 and 4 chondromalacic lesions. Overly aggressive abrasion arthroplasty or resection of hypertrophic marginal osseous linings only mobilizes the joint and increases amounts of exposed cancellous bone, leading to a disastrous postoperative result.

Chondral lesions are difficult to diagnose preoperatively, and therefore the classification system devised by Bauer and Jackson is best utilized for mapping out the postoperative treatment and prognosis.[27] Occasionally, chondral lesions can be detected preoperatively with the use of MRI scans. Chondral lesions are grouped into six types, with types I through IV having a traumatic etiology and types V and VI occurring from degenerative changes within the joint. Type I chondral lesions present as a linear crack in the cartilage. Type II lesions appear as stellate lesions. Type III chondral lesions present as a cartilaginous flap. If the cartilaginous flap is avulsed, exposing subchondral bone, this is a type IV lesion. Type IV and V lesions are degenerative in nature and more consistent with chondromalacia. Type V lesions appear as fibrillated cartilage with little exposure of the subchondral bone. Type VI lesions show exposed subchondral bone with surrounding areas of cartilaginous fibrillation.

Chondral lesions are differentiated from subchondral lesions in that, in chondral lesions, the subchondral bone is not involved with the lesion. However, secondary degenerative, sclerotic, or cystic changes may occur in the subchondral areas as the disease process progresses. Traumatic chondral lesion types I through IV are treated by resection of the chondral defect with an abrasion arthroplasty to

promote revascularization. Type V lesions, like chondromalacia, are treated with a chondroplasty via synovial shaver or abrader. This is only a superficial debridement of the area and does not promote revascularization. Type VI lesions, similar to extensive chondromalacic lesions, are best treated by debridement of the joint via synovectomy, flushing, and removal of any loose bodies. Superficial debridement of the area may also be beneficial. Extensive abrasion arthroplasty is usually not warranted.

Osseous Lesions

Most osseous lesions are joint specific. The two common forms of generalized joint osseous lesions are osteochondral bodies and subchondral bone cysts.

OSTEOCHONDRAL BODIES

Osteochondral bodies are small, round, loose bodies within a joint or attached to the synovium. These lesions are usually covered with a cartilaginous type of tissue. They vary in size, may be single or multiple, and may be associated with chondromatosis or chronic synovitis. In chronic hypertrophic synovitis, the necrotic tips of the synovial villi can flake off into the joint, aggregate, and then become hyalinized, possibly turning into osteochondral bodies.

Small osteochondral bodies are readily visible arthroscopically, but oftentimes cannot be seen radiographically. These smaller lesions are often freely mobile within the joint and easily grasped for removal. Larger lesions may be visible radiographically, but often are not visible arthroscopically because they are engulfed by hypertrophic synovium. To remove these lesions, a synovial shaver is used to resect all hypertrophic synovium around the lesion. It is possible to resect the osteochondral body with the synovial shaver while performing the synovectomy. The area should be thoroughly probed to feel for any remaining masses. If the lesion is not resected with a synovial shaver, once the synovectomy has been completed, the lesion may be sharply dissected away from any synovial attachments and removed with a grasper.

Meniscoid bodies can appear similar to osteochondral bodies, except they are shaped to the contour of the articular surfaces and are firmly attached to synovium. This is in contrast to osteochondral bodies, which tend to be round and loosely or not attached to the synovium.

Large flat osteochondral bodies, especially when located in the lateral aspect of the ankle joint, may represent a stage IV transchondral fracture. When this type of lesion is identified arthroscopically and removed, the anterolateral aspect of the talar dome should be thoroughly inspected for any signs of an osteochondral fracture. If a lesion is identified on the talar dome, it should be treated by abrasion arthroplasty or drilling.

SUBCHONDRAL BONE CYSTS

Subchondral bone cysts are often diagnosed incidentally or with the use of CT or MRI scans. These lesions often are not evident on plain radiographs. Subchondral bone cysts, by definition, do not involve the cartilaginous surface, but extend to the subchondral and cancellous bone. Because the cartilaginous surface is intact, visualization of the lesion is difficult arthroscopically unless its location can be determined by corresponding radiographic studies.

By correlating preoperative radiologic studies to identify location of the lesion, and with the use of a probe to inspect the area for softened areas of cartilage, the lesion can be delineated. Once the lesion is isolated, the softened cartilage is punched through with a probe to completely dissect its boundaries. A curette or abrader is then used to debride the cartilaginous tissue and the cystic lesion itself. With large cystic lesions, access for debridement may be limited. Therefore, an open arthrotomy may be indicated if complete access to the cystic lesion is not possible arthroscopically.

AVULSION FRACTURES

Avulsion fractures are a common injury in the ankle occurring at ligamentous attachment sites, or joint margins. Most can be treated arthroscopically. Occasionally a small arthrotomy incision for fragment excision is required. Small lesions are resected, while larger lesions are fixated when acute injury is involved.

These fractures are associated with significant amounts of hypertrophic synovitis. If the lesion is chronic, fibrous tissue and scar tissue may encompass the fracture fragment. This makes arthroscopic visualization difficult, mandating a thorough debridement and synovectomy to identify the fracture. If the fracture is to be excised, it must be freed from all soft tissue attachments by sharp dissection. This is usually accomplished with a banana blade. The fragment is grasped and removed using a twisting and pulling motion. The fragment should remain under direct observation until it is through the portal. If the avulsion fracture is from the distal tip of the fibula, the anterior talofibular ligament should be examined for instability. If instability is present, it should also be treated concurrently. Avulsion

fractures from the anterior tibiofibular or deltoid ligaments do not usually result in instability and can be simply excised. Larger acute avulsion fractures are best fixated with cannulated screws and closed-reduced under arthroscopic visualization, with open arthrotomy when necessary.

MEDIAL IMPINGEMENT LESIONS

Medial impingement lesions occur with inversion injuries resulting in damage to the tibial plafond and medial bend by compression from the medial talar shoulder.[28] Type A lesions consist of cartilage degeneration and often subchondral bone erosion. Type B lesions present as blistering of the cartilage at the medial bend due to basal degeneration. Oftentimes the lesion will be covered with fibrous tissue or hypertrophic synovium. Type A and B lesions are usually more indicative of repetitive inversion sprains, and may not be distinct pathology. These lesions are treated with debridement of any overlying soft tissue and resection of the medial impingement lesions with a curette, shaver, or abrader.

Type C lesions extend through the subchondral bone into the tibial plafond (Fig. 27-14). The lesion is covered with intense reactive fibrous tissue that is often hemorrhagic. These lesions are triangular in shape with a central posterior apical fibrous plug, which helps delineate the extent of the lesion. Treatment is by resection with a curette, abrader, or both. Type C lesions can be pathologic entities or associated with posteromedial transchondral talar dome fracture.

TRANSCHONDRAL FRACTURES

Transchondral talar dome fractures have been classified into four stages by Berndt and Harty based on their location and appearance.[29] These fractures are located on the posteromedial or anterolateral shoulders of the talar dome. Anterolateral lesions result from excessive inversion and dorsiflexion of the foot, while posteromedial lesions occur by inversion and plantar flexion. Anterolateral lesions are usually wafer shaped and shallow, because of shearing forces. Posteromedial lesions are deep and cup shaped, due to shearing with torsional impaction.

Stage I fractures are due to compression and present as a softened area of cartilage. Acute lesions are difficult to diagnose. Often the diagnosis is not made until the lesions further degenerate at which point radiographs show cystic changes and subchondral sclerosis. If a patient has chronic ankle pain with a history of trauma that does not respond to conservative treatment, a CT or MRI scan can be uti-

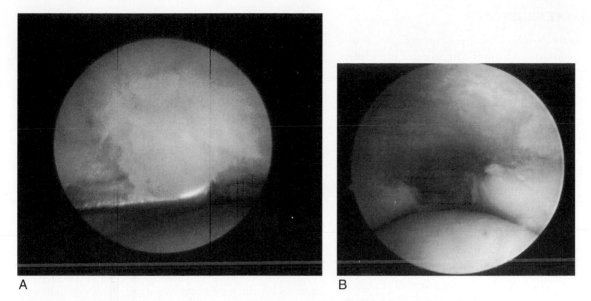

A   B

Figure 27-14 A type 3 medial impingement lesion at the medial bend of the tibia shown with a probe piercing the softened lesion (**A**) and following resection (**B**). Note the triangular nature of the lesion and how its apex extends proximally onto the tibial plafond.

lized to diagnose these fractures when plain films are negative. Stage I fractures are treated by abrasion arthroplasty or drilling.

Stage II fractures consist of a partially detached fragment of subchondral bone and cartilage. These lesions can sometimes be detected radiographically if large enough. They are easily identified arthroscopically by the fracture line. Older stage II fractures are treated by completely freeing the fragment, excision, and abrasion of the defect. Acute lesions usually respond to conservative treatment.

Stage III fractures are completely detached but remain within their subchondral bone crater. These are usually evident radiographically and easily seen arthroscopically. Treatment involves in toto removal of the fracture after it has been freed with a probe or curette. The crater and margins can then be abraded, especially if sclerosis is present. Resection of these lesions is done only when the bone has failed to heal after acute onset.

Stage IV fractures are stage III lesions that are outside the subchondral bone crater. Treatment consists of arthroscopic removal of the fragment and abrasion of the defect left from avulsion of the fragment. Acute stage IV lesions can be reduced arthroscopically and fixated with absorbable pins.

Anterolateral lesions are the most common location for transchondral fractures. This location also provides better accessibility for arthroscopic treatment. However, this does not mean posteromedial fractures cannot be treated arthroscopically. Posteromedial fractures have a high correlation with type C medial impingement lesions. Upon resection of the medial impingement lesion, the posteromedial fracture can be seen and approached anteriorly (Fig. 27-14). The obliquity of the arthroscope is used to adequately visualize the fracture site in the resected medial impingement lesion. An abrader, curette, or grasper is then passed through the resected impingement lesion and the fracture site is treated. After the fracture has been resected, the base of the lesion is debrided to bleeding subchondral bone. This can be checked by applying suction via a cannula, which promotes bleeding. If significant sclerosis is present, a 0.045-inch Kirschner wire is used to drill the fracture base.

ANTERIOR TIBIAL LIP FRACTURES

Fractures of the tibial lip can occur anteriorly or posteriorly. Posterior fractures are larger and usually associated with other areas of involvement. This type of fracture occurs with plantarflexion ankle injuries. These fractures are best approached from the posterior aspect of the ankle joint, and usually require fixation when large. Small, isolated posterior fractures can be treated by excision.

IMPINGEMENT EXOSTOSES

Impingement exostoses usually occur off the anterior tibial lip, but in arthritic joints can arise off the malleal. When identified, associated joint symptomatology must be evaluated. This is done by putting the ankle joint through its range of motion and looking for corresponding degenerative changes on the talar dome. Often significant hypertrophic synovitis is located in the area of these lesions. Treatment consists of resection of the impingement exostoses by abrasion or with a small osteotome and mallet. Soft tissue changes and talar dome lesions are also treated concurrently.

SUBTALAR JOINT

Most of the arthroscopic pathologies associated with the subtalar joint are generalized; the most common is sinus tarsi syndrome. This condition responds well to arthroscopic soft tissue debridement of the sinus tarsi contents. Specific osseous pathologies to the subtalar joint include avulsion fractures, lateral talar process fractures, and loose bodies. Arthroscopic resection of these lesions allows for increased mobility and decreased disability postoperatively, when compared to open arthrotomy.

METATARSOPHALANGEAL JOINTS

Specific pathologic processes that occur around the first metatarsophalangeal joint include central osteochondral lesions of the first metatarsal head, gouty arthritis, pathologic bone cysts within the proximal phalanx of the hallux, and turf toe. Osteochondral lesions located at the central aspect of the first metatarsal head are usually post-traumatic and are often apparent radiographically. The central aspect of the first metatarsal head must be probed to delineate areas of softened cartilage. An abrasion arthroplasty is then performed, and any hypertrophic synovium is treated concurrently.

Gouty arthritis has a high predilection for the first metatarsophalangeal joint and can be treated arthroscopically, provided no significant arthritic changes have occurred within the joint. The joint is best treated by arthroscopic synovectomy and flushing to remove any sodium urate crystals.

Cystic lesions within the base of the proximal phalanx of the hallux are often the result of trauma. These lesions are evident radiographically and can be further evaluated with CT scans. This type of lesion can also be treated arthroscopically via an abrasion arthroplasty and removal of the contents within the subchondral bone cyst.

Turf toe that is unresponsive to conservative therapy can be treated arthroscopically. Arthroscopic treatment generally consists of synovectomy, general debridement, and flushing of the joint. During the procedure, the corresponding aspects of the metatarsophalangeal joint should be examined for any cartilaginous or osteochondral defects.

Specific pathologies associated with the lesser metatarsophalangeal joints are limited to Freiberg's infarction or chronic synovitis/capsulitis. Once significant arthritic changes have occurred within the joint, arthroscopic intervention becomes a less viable treatment choice. Gaining access to a severely arthritic joint can become prohibitive to an arthroscopic procedure. Additionally, resection of hypertrophic soft tissues and debridement of the marginal osteophytes tends to increase motion of the joint, which may result in increased symptomatology. Arthroscopy of the lesser metatarsophalangeal joint is an excellent treatment in a younger Freiberg's patient, with only minimal arthritic changes. The joint is treated by synovectomy, debridement, and generalized flushing of the area.

DIAGNOSTIC ARTHROSCOPY

The diagnostic reliability of arthroscopy is extremely high. In correlating arthroscopy with arthrography and open arthrotomy, Huang et al.[30] found arthroscopic diagnosis confirmed in 96 percent of cases. DeHaven and Collins[31] determined the accuracy of arthroscopic diagnosis to be correct in 95 to 98 percent of cases "in competent and experienced hands." The advantage of arthroscopy is that it affords direct visualization of cartilaginous surfaces and synovial structures. We have also noticed a surprising and occasionally dramatic relief of preoperative symptoms following diagnostic arthroscopic examinations in our patients. Watanabi et al.[11] noted this therapeutic value and attributed it to washing of the joint space in a process called "articular pumping," which he credited to Mikki in 1948. In this procedure, the joint is distended with saline to a high pressure for 6 seconds. The pressure is then reduced and held at that level for 12 seconds. The process is repeated three or four times, and the fluid is withdrawn from the joint cavity. Watanabi observed the length of the effects from this procedure to be shorter than those from arthroscopy, and described studies in what he termed "joint profusion," in which larger volumes of saline are used to irrigate a joint.

In reviewing his arthroscopic procedures, Jackson[32] states that 25 percent of all diagnostic arthroscopy cases are therapeutic, with symptomatic relief derived from the noninterventional therapeutic benefits. He goes on to state that these benefits include joint lavage, which accounts for approximately 21 percent of the benefits, and breakdown of adhesions, contributing to about 4 percent of the therapeutic benefits. Diagnostic arthroscopy is currently performed for two reasons; for intra-articular evaluation and preoperative treatment planning, and for its therapeutic benefits.

To maximize the therapeutic benefits of diagnostic arthroscopy, certain drugs can be washed through the joint for added therapeutic effect. At the end of the procedure, a 22-ml, mixture of fluid is injected into the joint, with manual compression maintaining the fluid intra-articularly for several seconds, and then excess fluid is manually removed by external compression. This fluid consists of 14 ml of 1/2 percent bupivacaine plain, 4 ml of dexamethasone phosphate, and 2 ml of Duramorph (Elkins-Sinn, Inc., Division of A.H. Robbins Co., Cherry Hill, NJ). The bupivacaine effectively anesthetizes the joint for 10 to 12 hours and the dexamethasone decreases inflammatory response for 24 to 48 hours. Adding the Duramorph, which is a synthetic morphine, enhances the effects of the bupivacaine and dexamethasone and greatly diminishes pain in the first 5 to 7 days. In addition, saline is avoided as an irrigating solution because Ringer's lactate has proven to be less detrimental to chondrocyte metabolism, as shown by Reagan et al.[33]

In order to evaluate results of diagnostic foot and ankle arthroscopy, 70 cases were reviewed. All were performed before the availability of miniaturized power instrumenta

tion. Sixty-six arthroscopic inspections were done in the ankle joint (Table 27-1), 13 of which resulted in subsequent open arthrotomy (Table 27-2). Seven joints other than the ankle were examined (Table 27-3), two of which were followed by open arthrotomy. Ankle pathologies that responded most dramatically to diagnostic arthroscopy were those diagnosed as having fibrous adhesions, fibrosis, or both; hypertrophic and hemorrhagic synovitis; and specific and nonspecific abnormalities of the cartilage (chondropathies). These also were the most frequent diagnoses encountered. Cases of degenerative joint disease responded well, but relief of symptoms was short lived, lasting only approximately 6 months. The chondral and/or osteochondral bodies encountered in the series were unusually large in either number or size, necessitating removal by open arthrotomy. In this series, some chondral bodies were removed by aspiration through an egress cannula or with a small pituitary rongeur. Many small loose bodies can be contained within the hypertrophic synovial tissue and are therefore difficult to visualize, one reason so few strictly diagnostic arthroscopies are performed currently. Another reason is that, if the moderator of the inflammatory process, which is the synovium, can be resected by synovectomy, then the therapeutic benefits of the procedure will be greatly enhanced.

In this series, only one transchondral fracture fragment was amenable to arthroscopic removal; the other two cases required open arthrotomy. Post-traumatic hemarthrosis was effectively treated by irrigation and joint lavage follow-

Table 27-1 Review of Diagnostic Ankle Arthroscopy and the Influence of Arthroscopic Procedure on Complaints[a]

Diagnosis	Results				
	Excellent	Good	Fair	Unimproved	Total
Fibrosis/fibrous adhesions	13	2	0	2	17
Synovitis (hypertrophic and hemorrhagic)	12	2	0	2	16
Chondropathy					
Chondromalacia	7	0	0	1	8
Osteochondral defect	0	1[b]	0	0	1
Articular fissuring	1	0	0	0	1
Ankle instability[b]	5	0	0	0	5
Degenerative joint disease	3	0	0	1	4
Loose bodies	3	3[b]	0	1	7
Transchondral fracture	0	1	0	2[b]	3
Hemarthrosis	1	1	0	0	2
Gouty tophaceous deposit	2[b]	0	0	0	2
TOTAL	47	6	0	10	66

[a] Include pain, swelling, stiffness, and other complaints.
[b] See Table 27-2.

Table 27-2 Open Ankle Arthrotomy Following Diagnostic Arthroscopy

Diagnosis	Procedure	Results				
		Excellent	Good	Fair	Unimproved	Total
Ankle instability	Lateral stabilization	5				5
Loose bodies	Removal	3				3
Tophaceous gout	Tophi removal	2				2
Osteochondral defect	Curettage and drilling			1		1
Transchondral fracture	Curettage and drilling		1	1		2
TOTAL		10	1	2	0	13

ing visualization of the collateral ankle ligaments and cartilaginous surfaces.

In gouty patients, uric acid crystals that remained in solution within the joint could be removed by irrigation. Gouty deposits visible at the synovial reflection radiographically were invariably embedded in fibrous tissue, necessitating open arthrotomy for removal. In two cases, the gouty deposits were found at the synovial reflection at the talar neck, causing an impingement on dorsiflexion resulting in synovitis, synovial hypertrophy, and fibrosis. In evaluating ankles that were opened subsequent to arthroscopy, those undergoing stabilization or removal of loose bodies and uric acid deposits responded well. By contrast, open arthrotomy for chondropathy and transchondral fractures resulted in the persistence of preoperative symptoms. The joints of the foot are more difficult to arthroscope because of the strong collateral ligamentous structures, narrow joint spaces, and small capsular pouches. Nonetheless, arthroscopic evaluation of these joints has been both a challenge and a benefit in treatment planning. Reviewing seven cases, all but one required some type of operative procedure. This was the inspection of a calcaneonavicular synchondrosis that benefited from the lysis of adhesions and irrigation of the surgical site.

As mentioned, strict diagnostic arthroscopy alone with-

Table 27-3 Review of Diagnostic Arthroscopy of the Foot

Joint	Diagnosis	Procedure	Results				
			Excellent	Good	Fair	Improved	Total
First metatarsophalangeal	Gouty arthritis	Total joint replacement	1				1
First metatarsophalangeal	Severe fibrosis and hypertrophic synovitis	Arthroscopy with medial capsular release		1			1
Calcaneocuboid	Postoperative staple in cuboid with synovial hypertrophy and adhesive capsulitis	Removal of staple	1				1
Talonavicular	Post-traumatic hemorrhagic synovitis with partial avulsion of posterior tibial tendon	Arthroscopy with stapling		1			1
Subtalar	Prolonged sinus tarsi pain following arthroereisis	Arthroscopy with casting		1			1
Calcaneonavicular	Calcaneonavicular synchondrosis	Arthroscopy	1				1
Talonavicular	Osteochondral body with severe synovial hypertrophy	Open arthrotomy	1				1
TOTAL			4	3	0	0	7

out any type of further operative intervention is rarely performed. This is due to the readily available hand and motorized instrumentation. Also, as a matter of cost effectiveness, if greater therapeutic outcome can be achieved through greater intervention at the same sitting, the overall cost will be dramatically reduced.

OPERATIVE ARTHROSCOPY OF THE FOOT AND ANKLE

With the advent of the arthroscope and diagnostic arthroscopy, it was only a matter of time before surgeons began contemplating surgical procedures under arthroscopic control. Geist,[34] in 1926, wrote of the possibility of arthroscopic synovial biopsy, but nothing appeared in the literature until Watanabi[35] credited himself with the first arthroscopic meniscectomy. The first documented clinical study was not reported until 1978, when Dandy[36] presented his experience with partial meniscectomy. In the years to follow and escalating to the present, reports have documented additional operative procedures that can be performed arthroscopically. Such surgery includes partial synovectomy, synovial biopsy, removal of chondral and osteochondral bodies, excision of transchondral fractures, cartilaginous shavings, resection of fibrous bands, and stabilization procedure and fusions.

Many of the operative procedures performed on the foot and ankle are mechanical in nature in that they require physical probing, grasping of a lesion, or debridement. Specific procedures that actually represent specific techniques include the following: abrasion arthroplasty, chondroplasty, synovectomy, ligamentous stapling, ankle and subtalar joint fusion, anterior approaches to posteromedial transchondral fractures, resection of the os trigonum, plantar fasciotomy, and the treatment of Morton's neuroma and Haglund's deformity. The basis behind each of these arthroscopic and endoscopic procedures is discussed.

Abrasion Arthroplasty

Johnson, in 1979, introduced the technique of arthroscopic abrasion arthroplasty of the knee. Subsequently, the technique has been carried out successfully in the shoulder, elbow, hip, and ankle. Full-thickness articular lesions with exposure of underlying bone can be abraded with a high-speed bur.

It has been shown histologically that dead osteons on the surface are devoid of any blood supply. For reasons that are not well understood, such osteoarthritic lesions are typically accompanied by pain at night and while resting. The pain is often relieved by aspirin or other anti-inflammatory medications.

Johnson[37] observed arthroscopically that chondromalacic defects in the patella filled in with fibrocartilage and healed following intra-articular debridement, and that a profuse vascularity exists 1.0 mm below exposed sclerotic subchondral bone in degenerative arthritis. By carrying out a gentle arthroscopic debridement or abrasion of such exposed bone lesions, down to a depth of about 1.0 mm, the underlying capillary blood vessels are exposed. If the patient pursues a diligent program of active range-of-motion exercises and non-weight-bearing partial activity over an 8-week period, a layer of fibrocartilage is formed. Histologically, this tissue appears as an intermediate type of tissue that is more vascular and more cellular than hyaline cartilage of a normal joint, but not as cellular and disorganized in appearance as fibrous tissue. Typically, the chondrocytes are small and round and more numerous than in hyaline cartilage. This tissue is not normal cartilage, but clinical results indicate that it relieves pain, presumably by a resurfacing phenomenon. Some modification of lifestyle is often necessary to prevent further breakdown and development of symptoms in a weight-bearing joint that is admittedly incongruous to start with, usually due to some initial trauma.

The primary application of abrasion arthroplasty in ankle arthroscopy is to treat anteromedial and posteromedial transchondral fractures. These lesions are variably covered with a fibrous plug within the defect of the lesion or by degenerated cartilage and subchondral bone. Probing and curetting can resect this tissue from the lesions, but applying abrasion arthroplasty techniques to trim the sides of the lesion, debride sclerotic bone at the base of the lesion, especially in posteromedial lesions, and revascularize the defect has vastly improved the outcomes in the long-term treatment of transchondral fractures.

In the past, simple curettage or drilling of the defects was performed in order to debride the lesions and attempt a revascularization process. The main advantage of abrasion arthroplasty in these instances is the ability to provide a more structured environment for the enhancement of neochondrogenesis in the reparative process involved in the healing of the defect. Therefore, a more mature hyaline cartilage-like covering will be produced.

Chondroplasty

By definition, chondroplasty means remodeling of a cartilaginous surface. This procedure does not affect cartilage healing because it does not evoke an inflammatory response, because cartilage is not debrided below the zone of calcified and noncalcified cartilage, or the "tidemark." Chondroplasty is a means whereby irregular portions of cartilage can be trimmed. Because there is no effect on the initiation of the healing process, it is questionable whether chondroplasty performs any real function other than a means to trim loose edges and give the appearance of a cleaner, better debrided joint. Care must be exercised not to damage any healthy cartilage in the areas in which the chondroplasty is being performed because these areas will not be able to heal either.

Chondroplasty can be performed by simple use of a curette or an abrader or, most commonly, with the use of a full-radius shaver. Aggressive chondroplasty serves no goal other than to destroy cartilaginous surfaces. If a healing process is to be evoked, an abrasion arthroplasty or subchondral drilling must be concurrently performed.

Synovectomy

Synovectomy is perhaps the most common procedure performed in joint arthroscopy because the synovium is the mediator of the inflammatory process. Any condition that irritates the intra- or even periarticular structures will create a synovial response. The synovium, being the most vascular portion of the diarthrodial joint, is the first to respond within several hours after the initiation of a disease process. Synovium, which is usually microscopic and not visible to the naked eye, consists of a one- or two-cell-thick layer arranged in a series of folds in order to allow for extension and flexion of the capsular and articular structures. With the magnification of the arthroscope, synovium appears as a coarse, off-white lining of the interior portions of capsular structures. Synovial reflections, which are the areas between the synovium and the hyaline articular cartilaginous portions of the joint, are lined with periosteum, which is similarly lined with synovium. Intra-articular ligaments such as the anterior talofibular and anterior inferior talofibular ligaments in the anterior aspect of the ankle are lined with synovium. Only the hyaline cartilage is spared of synovial covering. This is true only in normal joints. With degeneration, fibrillation of cartilage, and exposure of subchondral bone, synovium will hypertrophy onto the abnormal articular surfaces.

As a means of increasing the surface area of the synovium, cells are arranged in villous or fingerlike structures. Each villi has a central vessel supplying it. This helps serve the primary function of the synovium, which is to filter

substances from within the joint as well as to produce synovial fluid. The folds that occur in the synovium allow expansion and contraction of the capsule during joint motion. With inflammation, the villous processes elongate, appearing as highly visible, thin, transparent, fingerlike projections with a central red vessel. This vessel, when red and appearing irritated, is termed to be "injected" when seen arthroscopically. The more acute the inflammatory process, the longer and more slender the synovial villi. The central vessel makes a tortuous course through the midportion of the villi, giving it a very characteristic appearance.

With continued inflammation, the villi become extremely long and the tips degenerate, giving them a cloudy appearance. This eventually begins to engulf the entire villous formation. Continued inflammation causes necrosis of the tips of the villi, resulting in a particulate exudate that is commonly seen in the joint upon initial entrance arthroscopically. Common to inflammation of the acutely inflamed villous formation is the excretion of a fibrin exudate. This also can be seen oftentimes clogging the joint upon initial entrance.

Eventually the villous tips continue to necrose, becoming very irregular and jagged in appearance and accumulating within the joint in its various pouches in masses. Acute inflammation is readily recognizable because it is red and hemorrhagic in nature, whereas chronic inflammation is indicative of frayed, opaque, off-whitish appearing villous formations or masses within the joint pouches in the greatest areas of the inflammatory process.

Synovectomy refers to the excision of the normal or abnormal synovium or both. When synovium can be visualized through the arthroscope, it is abnormal and represents hypertrophy of the structure. An experienced arthroscopist learns to "read" the synovium, judging from its appearance whether it is acute or chronic in nature and from which part of the joint the greatest amount of inflammation arises. In this manner the experienced surgeon can delineate which component of the disease process seen within the joint is the most irritating to the joint, and thereby determine the primary etiology of the pathology that is visualized.

The most common instrument used to perform a synovectomy is a 3.5- or 4.0-mm full-radius shaver. Other shavers are available but generally in small joint arthroscopy are not necessary. By utilizing various speeds at which the shaver blade turns, by varying levels of suction as well as amounts of fluid being ingressed into the joint, and by manipulating the forward and reverse or oscillating modes of the shaver, the synovectomy procedure is performed.

Synovium that is compressed between the joint surfaces and the capsular structures often forms thickened masses of compacted synovial tissue and becomes "hyalinized." These masses usually can be resected by the full-radius shaver but, if too thick or fibrous, a suction punch may be required for their resection. Punches in general do not work well for synovectomy due to its "gummy" nature. In cases where severe hypertrophic synovitis exists or it is more fibrous in nature, a larger diameter blade can aid in speeding its resection.

The reader must be cautioned that there are areas of normal synovial tissue within the ankle. These are primarily located in the tibiofibular synovial fringe, which is contained between the tibia and fibula in the lateral interval posterior to the anterior inferior talofibular ligament within the tibiofibular synovial recess. It is characteristically thicker and "gummier" in appearance and texture than normal hypertrophic synovium. Because it is a normal structure, it should not be resected, as often is done by the inexperienced surgeon. There are times at which inflammation of the tibiofibular fringe can cause it to become hypertrophied, but this is rare and responds to gentle debridement with a shaver. Some authors refer to this as a lateral impingement lesion,[38,39] but under most circumstances it is a normal structure that should not be resected.

Arthroscopic Stapling Procedures

Stapling of the anterior talofibular ligament to control rotational instability of the talus was first described by R. L. Hawkins (personal communication, 1985). He was familiar with the arthroscopic stapling repair of avulsions of the anterior cruciate ligament from the anterior wall of the intercondylar notch of the femur, avulsions from the lateral wall of the intercondylar notch, and advancement of the glenohumeral ligament and subscapularis tendon into the scapular neck for arthroscopic treatment of recurrent anterior dislocation or subluxation of the shoulder. Subsequently, a 5.5-mm staple for use with the ligamentous and capsular repair system manufactured by Instrument Makar (Instrument Makar, Inc., Okeunos, MI). has been used in the treatment of chronic anterolateral instability of the ankle.[18]

Many patients with a history of recurrent inversion injuries of the ankle discover a feeling of looseness of the ankle. Those who are more severely affected may have a positive anterior drawer test in which the examiner's hand can slide the entire foot forward in relation to the tibia while stabilizing the lower leg with the opposite hand. Many of the patients will also have increased talar tilt evidenced radiographically. When inversion stress is applied to the ankle, the talus appears to tilt out from beneath the lateral portion of the tibia. A positive response to this test is usually quite subtle, unless the calcaneofibular ligament is torn in addition to the anterior talofibular ligament.

Johnson and Markoff[40] carried out a biomechanical study on cadaver ankles, confirming the importance of the anterior talofibular ligament as a stabilizer of the ankle. They reported results similar to those of previous investigations concerning the ligament's providing increased rotational stability of the talus but, more importantly, they established its role in contributing to the stabilization of the ankle in varying degrees of plantarflexion. Also noted was the increased risk of damage to the other ankle ligaments following resection of the anterior talofibular ligament.

Diagnostic arthroscopy of patients with chronic lateral instability of the ankle has revealed a relative laxity or ballooning of the entire lateral capsule and anterior talofibular ligament when viewed from the anterolateral portal. Hypertrophic or hemorrhagic synovitis or both are often present along with articular cartilage defects seen at the medial aspect of the joint, where the corner of the talus impinges the tibia at the medial aspect of the plafond during subluxation. Loose bodies and osteochondral or chondral lesions are also infrequently visualized.

The concept behind any ankle-stabilizing procedure is to limit internal rotation, plantarflexion, and adduction of the talus; of these supinatory components, the limitation of internal talar rotation is the most important. Arthroscopic stapling for chronic ankle instability achieves this by a shortening or tightening of the lateral capsule and the anterior talofibular ligament (Fig. 27-15). The procedure was originally described as follows. The vertical surface of the talus is abraded just distal to its lateral articular surface. The abrasion is done with a small abrading bur, usually less than 4.0 mm. Enough bone is abraded so as to remove enough surface articular cartilage until bleeding cancellous bone appears. The arthroscopic staple is then inserted through an accessory anterolateral portal so that both capsule and anterior talofibular ligament (which are contiguous structures) can be advanced and stapled securely into the prepared talus (Fig. 27-16).

An alternative site for stapling is on the anterior border of the fibula at the level of the insertion of the anterior

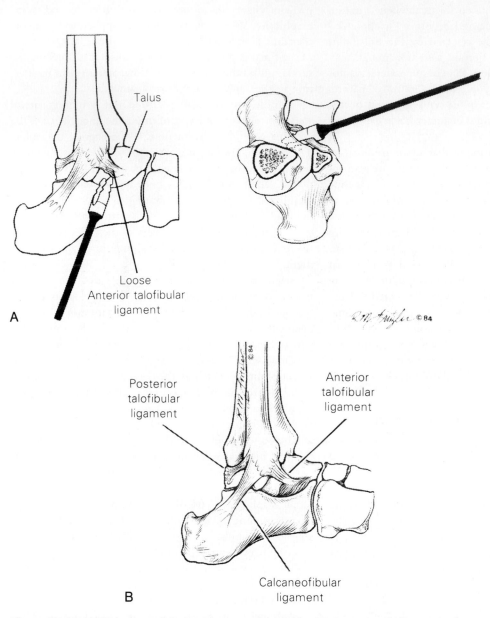

Figure 27-15 (**A**) Ligaments of the lateral aspect of the ankle. (**B**) Loosening (ballooning) of the anterior talofibular ligament and stabilization by advancement and "reefing" of the ligament and capsule through arthroscopic stapling.

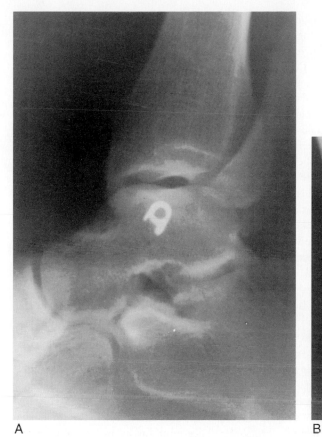

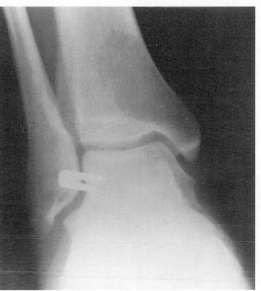

A   B

Figure 27-16 Lateral (**A**) and anteroposterior (**B**) ankle radiographs showing placement of the arthroscopic staple. The anterior talofibular ligament and capsule are interposed between the staple and talus, giving the effect of a lack of penetration by the staple.

talofibular ligament. With lateral ankle instability, this ligament appears to almost "peel" laterally off the anterior border of the lower portion of the fibular malleolus, leaving an osteochondral defect (lesion) in its place. This is often covered with synovium or a reactive fibrous tissue under which is degenerated subchondral bone. The osteochondral lesion is located between the normal hyaline articular surface of the medial surface of the fibula, the attachment of the anterior inferior tibiofibular ligament above, and the anterior talofibular ligament below. When these lesions are debrided, a quality cancellous bone defect remains. This makes a perfect location for placing the two tines of the arthroscopic staple from an inferior lateral accessory portal. In addition, this method eliminates the need to abrade a portion of normal cartilage and subchondral bone off the lateral trochlear surface of the talus and utilizes an abnormal entity, the osteochondral lesion of the fibula, as a location to effect the capsulorrhaphy.

As an alternative to stapling, Motek II (Johnson & Johnson, Norwood, MA) surgical anchors can be substituted. In these instances, two anchors are placed into the abraded portion of the talus or debrided area of the anterior border of the fibula. Each anchor has two polyester sutures. The capsule and ligament are sutured into the bed of the cancellous bone by tying the sutures between the two anchors. The use of Motek anchors is technically more difficult and does not appear to give a consistently secure capsulorrhaphy, but eliminates the need for future removal of the staple. Arthroscopic staples are removed if they become symptomatic in the postoperative period following complete healing of the surgical site.

It is interesting to note that Markoff and Johnson's theories do persist in practice. Because of the importance of the anterior talofibular ligament in the rotational stability of the ankle, mere plication and capsulorrhaphy not only affects the anterior drawer sign of the talus, which would be expected, but also can have a profound effect on the degree of talar tilt. All too often surgeons think in planes similar to radiographic projections. Therefore, it is often declared that an abnormal talar tilt infers damage to both the anterior talofibular and calcaneofibular ligaments, whereas, if the talar tilt is normal and the anterior drawer sign is abnormal, only damage to the anterior talofibular ligament exists. If this were the case, then capsulorrhaphy of the anterior talofibular ligament would not affect the talar tilt when an abnormal talar tilt was present. Obviously this is not the case, and physicians must rethink the biomechanical aspects of ankle instability and realize the importance of the anterior talofibular ligament in providing rotational stability to the talus. It must be remembered that inversion ankle sprains are triplanar motions consisting of plantar flexion, adduction, and inversion of the talus, all consistent with supination. It is not a one-planar abnormality and therefore should not be thought of in that way. It is for this reason that plication of the anterior talofibular ligament can effectively stabilize the ankle without primary repair of the calcaneofibular ligament in certain cases.

Obviously gross amounts of instability, especially in the presence of a cavus foot type and supinated rearfoot in the stance phase of gait, may require a more aggressive repair of the lateral ankle structures or the rearfoot. These cases must be evaluated independently and procedures selected at the discretion of the surgeon according to foot type, pathology present, and experience in which procedures have worked best in that surgeon's hands for a specific condition.

Ankle and Subtalar Joint Fusion

Fusion of the ankle or subtalar joint is a continuance of the aggressiveness and theory of abrasion arthroplasty. The basis of abrasion arthroplasty is to debride the cartilage and subchondral bone approximately 1.0 mm below the junction of the two in order to gain access to the tidemark, which is an eosinophilic staining area representing the junction between the zones of calcified and noncalcified cartilage, which is the level of vascularity in the subchondral bone plate. By debriding the entire joint surfaces in this manner, the subchondral bone is denuded to its level of vascularity so that, when the joint surfaces are approximated, fixated, and immobilized, the osseous structures can unite and effect a fusion.

Through the normal anterior and posterior arthroscopic portals, the entire ankle and subtalar joint can be abraded in order to create a fusion. The joint is then immobilized by various means similar to those that would be utilized for open procedures. Cannulated screws are usually used, but other methods of fixation can be used with fluoroscopy, such as an external fixator.

In the ankle, two or three 6.5-mm cannulated screws are often used. Most commonly, one is placed between the medial malleolus and the talus coursing from the posteromedial aspect of the medial malleolus distally and anteriorly into the talus. A second anterolateral screw is placed from the anterolateral aspect of the tibial plafond above the anterior tibial tubercle, coursing medially, distally, and posteriorly. A third screw can be placed horizontally through the fibula into the talus in order to compress the fibula against the lateral trochlear surface of the talus with or without a (percutaneous) fibular osteotomy. The subtalar joint is most frequently fixated with a 6.5-mm cannulated screw from the anterior aspect of the talar neck interiorly and proximally across the abraded portion of the posterior talar facet, or in the calcaneal sulcus of the sinus tarsi into the calcaneal tuberosity.

Because the ankle joint is large, the tibial plafond, medial and lateral malleolar articular surfaces, and trochlear surface and dome of the talus are easily visualized. Unfortunately, the subtalar joint consists of three smaller joints, the largest and most accessible of which is the posterior facet. This can usually be abraded through two stacked portals in the sinus tarsi as traditionally described. Occasionally a posterolateral portal must be utilized in order to introduce the abrader to denude cartilage at the posterior downward-sloping portion of the joint. The anterior subtalar facet is usually left intact, but the middle facet should be abraded. This is accomplished with the use of a synovial resector, clearing the contents of the sinus tarsi at its inferior aspect in the calcaneal sulcus. The structure is followed laterally until the articular margins of the middle facet can be identified; then the abrader is introduced through the inferior portal and, utilizing the normal compression between the joint surfaces, it is resected. The abrader is placed at the middle of the adjacent joint structures and both sides of the joint are simultaneously debrided. Once the middle and posterior facets are thoroughly resected, the cannulated screw is inserted with the use of fluoroscopy into the talar neck and calcaneus (Fig. 27-17). Direct visualization to ensure adequate compression of the posterior facet can be accomplished both with the arthroscope and by fluoroscopy.

Arthroscopic fusion of the ankle and subtalar joints, when indicated, can be very effective, but should only be used in joints without significant ankylosis that are arthroscope accessible. Significant varus or valgus deformities must not be present, and the patient must have adequate bone stock and healing capabilities and be compliant to allow the use

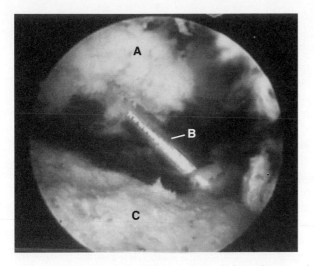

Figure 27-17 Abraded posterior calcaneal facet showing the talar articular surface (A), shaft of a 6.5-mm cancellous screw used for fixation (B), and calcaneal articular surface (C).

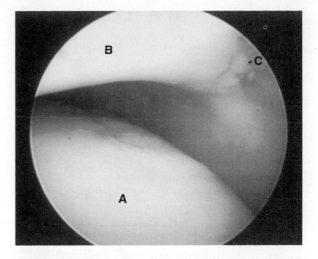

Figure 27-18 A posteromedial transchondral talar dome fracture. A, medial talar shoulder; B, anterior tibial lip; C, medial impingement lesion.

of this method. In addition, an ankle distractor can be used if needed.

Anterior Approach to Posteromedial Transchondral Fractures

Transchondral fractures of the talar dome are routinely resected and treated with abrasion arthroplasty. Posteromedial transchondral lesions are located posteriorly on the talar dome at the level of the medial talar shoulder, making them difficult to access by open arthrotomy or by arthroscopy.

Lundeen has described a technique whereby a characteristic lesion at the medial bend of the tibial plafond is identified and has described this as a medial impingement lesion.[28] This lesion occurs from the abutment of the medial talar shoulder on the adjacent portion of the tibial plafond when the foot is plantarflexed and inverted. Because of the mechanism of injury, almost all posteromedial transchondral fractures are associated with medial impingement lesions (Fig. 27-18). These lesions must be resected, and, in doing so, a natural defect is made allowing access to the posterior talar dome lesion.

When a medial impingement lesion is identified, it is curetted, abraded, or both, creating a channel onto the tibial plafond posteriorly whereby access and visualization of the fracture at the posterior portion of the talus is possible. Similarly, through an adjacent portal an abrader, cu-

rette, probe, or other instrument can be triangulated to the lesion, allowing for its inspection and resection.

Resection of the Os Trigonum and Steida's Process

Routine access to the posterior aspect of the subtalar joint allows visualization of the posterior joint line of the posterior calcaneal facet of the subtalar joint. Following synovectomy, the lateral talar process is identified. An enlarged lateral aspect of the joint margin (Steida's process) is resected when symptomatic with a small osteotome and mallet under direct visualization and removed from the joint. In cases where the lateral process of the talus is completely or incompletely separated (os trigonum), it is identified arthroscopically and freed up with a small osteotome so it can be removed from the joint (Fig. 27-19).

Traditional open arthrotomy of the posterior aspect of the subtalar joint is often difficult because the lateral talar process is deep and hard to access from the usual lateral approach. Arthroscopic resection provides an exceptional way to atraumatically resect these lesions but can be difficult, requiring an expert arthroscopist or subsequent open arthrotomy.

Plantar Fasciotomy

Arthroendoscopic plantar fasciotomy has become a common topic of discussion among many orthopedists and most podiatrists. This is because heel pain is one

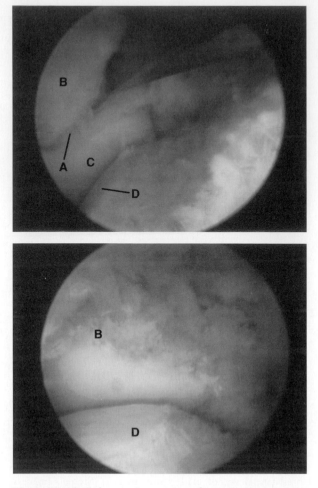

Figure 27-19 Arthroscopic resection of a symptomatic os trigonum (A), fibrous tissue separating the os trigonum (B), and lateral process of a talus (C). The talus (D) is shown below.

of the primary reasons podiatric patients seek medical help. Due to the high number of persons complaining of heel pain, the threat of overutilization of surgery abounds, because the vast majority of heel pain patients can become asymptomatic through conventional, conservative treatment.

Traditionally, heel spur surgery has been risky and in the past not a procedure a surgeon or patient readily consented to perform or to have done. Typical recoveries from heel spur surgery required 8 to 12 weeks, and patients were constantly reminded of the guarded prognosis of the procedure and the fact that oftentimes it did not work even when the conservative care, including anti-inflammatory medications, shoe modifications, and

foot orthoses, were continued. A recent alternative, described originally by Barrett and Day,[23] offers a seemingly uncomplicated, innovative, and predictable procedure, endoscopic plantar fasciotomy, for alleviation of heel pain.

Arthroscopy by orthopedic surgeons and podiatric physicians has long been a procedure scrutinized for overutilization. However, the number one reason a patient seeks help from a podiatrist in this country is heel pain. When heel pain is combined with arthroscopy, as with laser surgery, a new promotional mechanism is created, opening itself up for overutilization. Many podiatric physicians have recently been employing a modified percutaneous plantar fasciotomy with or without the resection of a calcaneal spur in the treatment of infracalcaneal spurs. This carries less morbidity than the performance of a large open fasciotomy and calcaneal spur resection because it is less traumatic and offers an alternative to endoscopic procedures.

Traditional heel spur surgery is often met with prolonged disability or untoward results consisting of continued heel pain, lateral midfoot jamming, destabilization of the arch, or entrapment syndromes, particularly of the medial calcaneal branches of the posterior tibial nerve. Endoscopic plantar fasciotomy avoids most of these pitfalls when performed properly, greatly diminishing the morbidity and complication rate of the procedure.

Endoscopic plantar fasciotomy requires a purist view of biomechanics and surgical application. Hicks[41] was perhaps the first proponent of the biomechanical importance of the plantar fascia when he described its "windlass effect." The fascia's ability to act as a windlass or a destressing mechanism between the anterior and posterior aspects of the arch makes it a structure that is commonly tethered due to patient weight, abnormal pronation, or a decreased elasticity of the plantar fascia secondary to the aging process. Anything that places increased tension on the plantar fascia can create inflammation along its body or particularly at its insertion. The highest concentration of stress appears to be at the medial tubercle of the calcaneus. The plantar fascia is divided into three bands, the medial of which is the largest and thickest due to increased stress demanded by the medial arch and the amount of motion inherent in it. The central band is thinner and wider, whereas the lateral band is very thin and oftentimes rudimentary compared to the other two bands.

Traditional plantar fasciotomy involves resection of the plantar fascia from the tubercles of the calcaneus. It is difficult to determine how much of the plantar fascia or the muscular insertions of the first or second layer of plantar musculature is being resected. When being done by feel (percutaneously), the tendency is to overrelease not only the plantar fascia but the associated plantar intrinsic musculature that arises from the calcaneal tuberosities. In addition, the presence of a calcaneal spur is all too tempting, and therefore, when present, it is usually rasped or resected with an osteotome, a rongeur, or some other type of instrument.

Podiatric physicians are all too aware of problems that can occur with overzealous resection of the plantar fascia or resection of the calcaneal spur. Not only does the arch lose its stability, but resection of the spur can create a stress riser, precipitating a calcaneal fracture. A stress riser is not even needed to produce such a fracture because isolated release of the plantar fascia can provide a similar result due to the loss of its windlass effect. With the tendo Achillis creating a constant tension on the posterior aspect of the calcaneus, a loss of its antagonist, the plantar fascia, places excess stress on its inferior surface, possibly leading to fracture. When a stress riser created by the resection of a calcaneal spur is added, the chance of a fracture occurring increases dramatically.

In performing an endoscopic plantar fasciotomy, a slotted cannula is placed approximately 1.5 to 2.0 cm in front of the medial tubercle of the calcaneus at the level of the medial band of the plantar fascia. The cannula is directed perpendicular to the long axis of the foot under the plantar fascia by using a fascial elevator to clear a channel; then, by incising the lateral aspect of the foot, the cannula and the obturator used for its passage are exited laterally. The obturator is removed, the cannula is cleared of moisture and fat with cotton-tipped applicators, and a 4.0-mm, 25- or 30-degree arthroscope is inserted. The plantar fascia is then probed, identifying the medial extent or investment of the fascia under the abductor hallucis muscle. The medial band of the fascia is then probed laterally until a fatty area is identified and the intermuscular septum is visualized between the abductor hallucis and flexor digitorum muscles. A retro cutting knife is inserted through the lateral opening of the cannula and the medial band of plantar fascia is transected from its medial investment to the intermuscular septum with the fascia under tension by fully dorsiflexing the foot. When released adequately, the medial fascial ends will separate, revealing the belly of the flexor digitorum brevis muscle (Fig. 27-20). Instratek (Spring, TX) makes a marked cannula providing landmarks to assist in assuring that only the medial band is incised.

Once the muscle is visible, no further resection should be performed, and the arthroscopic instruments can be removed and the cannula irrigated. The cannula is then removed and its portals sutured. The plantar fascia must not be resected more than the amount required to release the medial band of the plantar fascia. This procedure will not yield consistent results if the middle or lateral bands are released or if a spur is resected.

By performing endoscopic plantar fasciotomy by the technique described and by adequately treating these patients preoperatively with conservative methods, assuring that their plantar heel pain is in fact mechanical in nature and not due to systemic disease such as rheumatoid arthritis, the results are predictable and consistent. Occasional central band pulling or mild aching in the lateral tarsus may occur after the surgery, but will resolve with conservative care or with time as the plantar fascia reforms and restabilizes the arch. Orthotic devices may not be needed after surgery, but because they are often prescribed preoperatively, patients are urged to continue wearing them to prevent other problems. Time will tell the outcome of endoscopic plantar fasciotomy, but it appears that the revolution started by ankle arthroscopy has finally met its match in terms of the deliverance of a unique new procedure destined to revolutionize yet another aspect of podiatric medicine and surgery.

Endoscopic Decompression for Intermetatarsal Neuroma

The traditional surgical treatment for intermetatarsal neuromas has been the resection of the involved plantar intermetatarsal nerve. This is perhaps the only nerve in the human body that is resected as its initial and primary surgical procedure. Because most benign nerve conditions represent compression or entrapment syndromes, proponents of the endoscopic decompression of the intermetatarsal nerve (EDIN) technique are finding that this is in fact the case with Morton's or intermetatarsal neuromas.

The performance of this procedure requires the use of Instratek instrumentation. This set, especially designed for the EDIN procedure, consists of a metatarsal spreader, banana-shaped obturator or fascial elevator, small probe, knife handle, and small slotted cannula. Disposable instruments are also needed that consist of swabs to clear the cannula, a ruler to mark the placement of the incision on

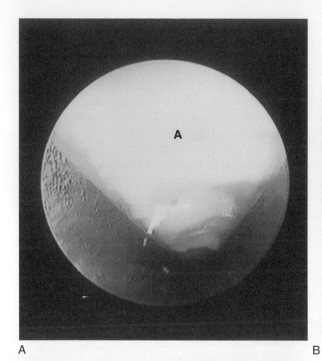

A

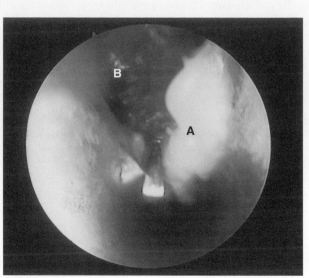

B

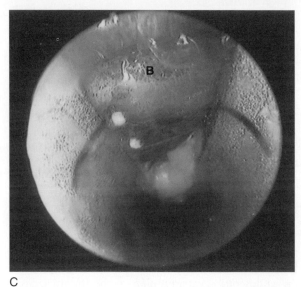

C

Figure 27–20 Endoscopic plantar fasciotomy. (**A**) Plantar fascia as it appears in the slotted cannula. (**B**) The fascia being resected by a triangular knife blade, exposing the belly of the abductor hallucis muscle. (**C**) The fully resected medial band of the plantar fascia showing the belly of the abductor hallucis muscle and the fat plug overlying the intermuscular septum. The marks on the cannula give the approximate location of the intermuscular septum to prevent overaggressive resection of the central or lateral bands of the plantar fascia.

the plantar aspect of the foot, and triangular cutting blades that attach to the nondisposable handle. Also needed is a 2.4-mm, 30-degree Stryker arthroscope, a camera, and a light source.

When performing the EDIN procedure, any type of local or general anesthetic can be utilized. Patients are placed supine on the operating table and the foot is prepped

and draped in the usual manner as for any other foot procedure. With a marking pen, the metatarsal head adjacent to the intermetatarsal nerve being released is marked both dorsally and plantarly. The plastic ruler that is part of the disposable EDIN procedure kit is then placed on the plantar aspect of the foot so that its distal markings are in the web space between the toes and its proximal marking is placed directly in line with the space marked between the plantar aspect of the metatarsal heads. The proximal portion is marked, which is where the cannula will exit the foot. A small stab incision is then made at this plantar mark, in between the toes in the web space, and dorsally at the level of the metatarsal necks where the they had been previously marked. The curved obturator (fascial elevator) is then inserted into the web space incision and a plane is freed directly under the intermetatarsal ligament (which is palpated by feel), between the metatarsal heads, and out the plantar incision. The metatarsal retractor is then inserted dorsally into the incision between the metatarsal heads and the instrument is spread to resistance.

The obturator used for placement of the cannula is inserted and the cannula is placed in the web space incision through the channel made by the fascial elevator under the intermetatarsal ligament and out the plantar incision. The proximal end of the cannula is marked so that the slotted portion can be placed superiorly against the intermetatarsal ligament. The swabs are then used to clear the the cannula of fluid and fat, and the 30-degree arthroscope is inserted into the cannula from between the toes, with its obliquity placed upward so as to look toward the slot in the cannula and the intermetatarsal ligament. Initially upon entering into the cannula, one can see the skin followed by a fatty area proximal to which is the intermetatarsal ligament. By using the probe, the confines of this ligament can be palpated. Once the ligament can be visualized, the knife used for its release is entered proximally from the plantar aspect of the foot into view through the arthroscope (Fig. 27-21).

Making sure that tension is placed on the intermetatarsal ligament with the metatarsal spreader, the EDIN knife is used to incise the intermetatarsal ligament in its entirety, making sure to get the proximal and distal portions. Proximally, the transverse head of the abductor hallucis muscle can be visualized, oftentimes in association with the lumbricales tendon. A full release requires complete transection both proximally and distally of the intermetatarsal ligament, taking care not to incise any venous structures that may be around it, especially at the distal portion of the cannula between the skin and the ligament. Care must also be taken not to incise the muscle belly or lumbricales tendon. Once the ligament is transected, the spreader is

Figure 27-21 Endoscopic decompression for intermetatarsal neuroma. The anterior aspect of the intermetatarsal ligament (**A**) is visualized in the spotted cannula and, when resected, exposes the belly of the transverse head of the abductor hallucis muscle proximally (**B**).

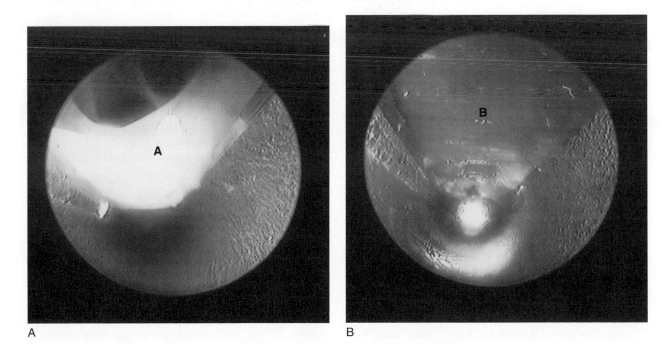

A   B

used to further separate the metatarsals until one can ensure that a complete release has been performed. At this point the metatarsal should move freely when the spreader is opened and closed.

Once the release is thought to be complete, the cannula is flushed with the small bulb syringe included in the disposable kit and removed. The fascial elevator is then placed back into the web space incision and the area between the metatarsal heads at the level of the ligamentous release is probed in order to ensure that no fibers of the intermetatarsal ligament persist. This can be done with the metatarsal spreader in place or with it removed. If some fibers can be palpated, then the spreader must be reinserted, the cannula reinserted with its obturator, and the arthroscope reinserted and the area between the metatarsals probed to find any remaining portions of the intermetatarsal ligament. If any portion remains, it is usually the part of the intermetatarsal ligament that forms in the intermuscular septum at the distal border of the abductor hallucis muscle. When visualized, the knife is reinserted and these areas fully released. Again the intermetatarsal space is probed with the fascial elevator to assure a clean resection. When this is accomplished, all instrumentation is removed and the three portals sutured with an appropriate material, such as 4-0 nylon.

When performing this procedure, care must be exercised to prevent placement of the cannula above the intermetatarsal ligament or at a level below the ligament and underlying fatty tissue, placing it dangerously close to the intermetatarsal nerve or its digital branches.

Postoperative care is similar to that for a traditional neuroma procedure, where a mild compression dressing is applied to the forefoot. Ambulation is allowed within 24 to 48 hours and ice is used initially to decrease the edema. The patient is seen postoperatively anywhere from 3 to 10 days following the surgery and, if edema persists or pain is present, a mild compression dressing is reapplied. If the patient is relatively asymptomatic at that time, a removable compression dressing is applied to the forefoot and the patient is allowed to work into an oversized pair of shoes.

Most patients seem to do well, especially when just one interspace has been operated on. Surgery on more interspaces, or bilaterally, usually requires additional time in dressings to support and compress the foot as needed. It seems that, by releasing the intermetatarsal ligament and mobilizing the forefoot, postoperative discomfort and edema can tend to linger for a while, especially compared to the recovery from an endoscopic plantar fasciotomy procedure, where only a partial release of the plantar fascia

is performed, preventing increased mobilization of the foot.

Complications of the EDIN procedure are similar to those of the traditional neuroma surgery. Although numbness may occur, it is usually transient and related to the edema created by the procedure releasing the intermetatarsal ligament. Numbness may occur if the plantar intermetatarsal nerve or its digital branches are resected during the ligamentous release. Other problems include instability of the digits by inadvertent transection of the lumbricales tendon, hematoma from resection of a vessel during the release, or entrapment neuropathy of the intermetatarsal nerve or its digital branches from excess bleeding, scar formation, or by partial resection of the plantar intermetatarsal nerve or its branches. The ultimate complication, of course, is that the procedure does not work. In these cases either an inadequate release was performed or the patient's condition was misdiagnosed. If a true degenerative process of the nerve has occurred, resection of the nerve may be necessary.

Overall, the results of the EDIN procedure have been encouraging and very rewarding. It is not to be used in the presence of stump or amputation neuromas or with entrapment neuropathies resulting from open neurectomy procedures. Failed EDIN procedures are usually the result of inadequate resection of the intermetatarsal ligament or inadvertent partial or complete transection of the intermetatarsal nerve, or from excessive bleeding that results in entrapment neuropathy. Treatment of these conditions requires open resection of the intermetatarsal nerve.

Endoscopic Resection of Haglund's Deformity and Retrocalcaneal Bursae

Endoscopy can also be used to resect the posterosuperior prominence of the calcaneus and an associated retrocalcaneal bursa adjacent to the calcaneus and the tendo Achillis above its insertion. Traction exostoses that are at the insertion of the tendo Achillis, calcification within the substance of the tendo Achillis, or so-called pump bumps at the posterosuperior lateral surface of the calcaneus must be approached by traditional open procedures.

When pain at the posterior aspect of the heel can be attributed to a Haglund's deformity, which is a prominence of the posterosuperior aspect of the calcaneus or hyperostosis in that area with an associated retrocalcaneal bursitis above the insertion of the tendo Achillis, endoscopy can be utilized. In these cases a standard 4-mm, 30-degree oblique arthroscope is used with appropriate camera and light source. The patient is placed in the prone position with foot overhanging the table and anesthetic of choice utilized. The foot is then draped in the usual manner for a rearfoot surgery.

The posterosuperior aspect of the calcaneus is approached by two portals placed adjacent to the anterior border of the lateral aspect of the tendo Achillis just above the posterosuperior surface of the calcaneus. A small longitudinal cutdown incision is made and a curved mosquito hemostat is used to retract soft tissue adjacent to the portals. An arthroscope is then placed in either the heel or lateral portal by first using the obturator to place the cannula into the space between the superior aspect of the calcaneus and the tendo Achillis above its insertion. Once this can be palpated, the obturator is removed and the arthroscope inserted. Ingress of fluid for distention is then achieved through the cannula. An obturator is then used to create a channel through the opposing portal to allow the percutaneous passage of a 3.5-mm full-radius shaver. Once visualized, the space between the tendo Achillis and calcaneus is freed of fat, synovitis, or bursal tissue.

Once an adequate space has been created, visualization of the posterior and superior portion of the calcaneus can be identified, as well as the longitudinal fibers of the tendo Achillis and the point of its insertion into the middle one-third of the calcaneus (Fig. 27-22). Thorough synovectomy and resection of soft tissue or bursal material is important, and this space must be thoroughly shaved to assure adequate resection of inflammatory tissue. Visualization of the posterosuperior aspect of the calcaneus includes observation of the smooth fibrocartilaginous aspect of the calcaneus that comes into contact with the adjacent tendo Achillis. It is this osseous structure, a Haglund's deformity, that is to be resected. Through the portal by which the shaver was passed, a 4.5-mm or smaller bur (abrader) is inserted. Once visualized, the posterosuperior surface of the calcaneus is abraded away from the tendo Achillis toward the subtalar joint at approximately a 45-degree angle. This could also be accomplished through the use of small osteotomes and the area could then be filed with a small rasp or with the use of the abrader. In either case the posterosuperior surface of the calcaneus must be resected away from the tendo Achillis to prevent impingement of the two structures and interposing tissue (Fig. 27-23). Once adequately resected, the area is thoroughly flushed, arthroscopic instruments are removed, and the portals then sutured with an appropriate material.

Postoperatively, an above-ankle compression wrap is

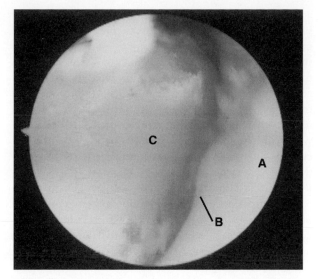

Figure 27-22 Arthroscopic Haglund's resection with visualization of the tendo Achillis, the articular surface between the posterior aspect of the calcaneus and the tendo Achillis (B), and the posterosuperior surface of the calcaneus (C), or the Haglund's deformity.

Figure 27-23 The Haglund's deformity is being resected from an opposite portal with an osteotome, shown resecting the posterosuperior surface of the calcaneus away from the tendo Achillis (A).

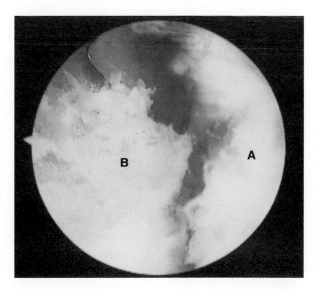

applied and oftentimes a cast brace is used. Postoperative instructions are then given similar to those for a traditional procedure for resection of Haglund's deformity. Normally the operated foot is immobilized for 3 to 4 weeks and then the patient is eased out of the cast brace into the removable compression wrap and eased into a shoe. Postoperative recovery is significantly shorter with arthroscopy than with more traditional open procedures, but still requires 3 to 5 weeks until a majority of the discomfort subsides. The chance of wound dehiscence is minimal, and range of motion of the subtalar or ankle joint is not affected. In addition, the traditional "chasing the bump" problem, where overzealous resection of the posterior and superior surface of the calcaneus occurs, is prevented because only the portion of the calcaneus that comes into contact with the tendo Achillis is resected.

REHABILITATION IN ANKLE AND FOOT ARTHROSCOPY

One of the advantages of arthroscopy is the minimum amount of tissue disruption, allowing a decreased period of immobilization and enabling faster recovery from surgical procedures when compared to more traditional open procedures. Nonetheless, tissue must still heal biologically.

The surgeon must take care not to give patients unrealistic expectations concerning recovery. As the number as well as the type of procedures available by arthroscopy increases, so will the challenge of tailoring specific rehabilitation programs for the patient and the procedure. Because of this, it is important to consider the principles outlined here.

Initially, arthroscopic procedures involve the creation of an incision and the disruption of periarticular tissues, resulting in a potential for bleeding. This must be prevented as much as possible by proper perioperative technique, as discussed earlier. A postoperative modality that will also assist to reduce hemostasis as well as edema is cold therapy. The vasoconstrictive properties of cold therapy not only will reduce acute swelling and effusion but also have an anesthetic property. Traditional ice bags served this purpose, but several companies have developed cold therapy systems that will provide constant cooling and compression with a prefabricated boot that can be incorporated into the postoperative dressing. These cold systems have been tolerated by the patients very well, and decreased pain medication use has been documented.

Also secondary to periarticular disruption is resultant muscular inhibition and resistance to ankle joint motion. The surgeon must base the immediate postoperative rehabilitation upon the surgery performed as well as the patient. With routine ankle arthroscopy procedures, partial immobilization (splint or flexible cast and surgical shoe) is used, along with cold therapy, elevation, and active as well as passive range-of-motion exercises. If more advanced techniques such as lateral ankle stabilization have been performed, there is a greater need for immobilization (below-knee cast), with corresponding decreased range-of-motion work. Alternatively, if the goal is to promote fibrocartilaginous growth to fill a resected defect, active range of motion will be encouraged to a greater extent at an earlier time. Active range of motion can be as simple as allowing the patient limited ambulation or partial weight bearing postoperatively. Passive range of motion has become popular with the increased availability of continuous passive motion devices specifically designed for the ankle. Nonsteroidal anti-inflammatory drugs can also aid in reducing inflammation in the initial postoperative phase of rehabilitation.

As pain and edema decrease, strength and motion can be encouraged through isometric exercises and increased ambulation as well as weight bearing. A mild compressive dressing can now replace bulky cold therapy devices and compression dressings. The goal during this period is to maintain muscle tone and at the same time to retrain eccentric and concentric muscle groups. Care must be taken to avoid increasing activities too quickly, resulting in hematoma and delaying rehabilitation. Useful activities include stationary bicycling, swimming and ankle dorsiflexion/plantar flexion with towel assist.

Pain will subside with later healing, but joint effusion persists along with muscle weakness. Although the weakness is much less than that observed following knee arthroscopy, it is important to initiate functional activities to improve proprioception and flexibility and to maintain muscle and joint motion. Helpful exercises include figure-eight running, unilateral leg press, unilateral trampoline balance drills, BAPS board, or jumping rope.

During later period of rehabilitation, the emphasis changes to progressive resistance exercises throughout the full range of motion. There should be no joint effusion or pain on motion. Running can be initiated, graduating into jumping. Full motion must be encouraged along with attempting to build confidence in the patient.

The progression that patients pass through with this scheme depends on the expected level of activity they are to return to, as well as the amount of swelling, pain, and lack of joint motion present both preoperatively and postoperatively. In cases of more involved pathology, such as severe osteoarthritis, an ankle or foot orthosis or both may be used along with appropriate medication and lifestyle modification.

ACKNOWLEDGMENTS

We wish to thank Richard Hawkins, M.D., for his contribution to the section on ankle stabilization, and Michael J. Baker, D.P.M., for his contributions on technique and rehabilitation.

REFERENCES

1. Barnett CH, Napier JR: The axis of rotation at the ankle joint in man: its influence upon the form of the talus and the mobility of the fibula. J Anat 86:1, 1952
2. Close JR: Some applications of the functional anatomy of the ankle joint. J Bone Joint Surg [Am] 38:761, 1956
3. Isman RE, Inman VT. Anthropometric studies of the human foot and ankle (Biomechanics Laboratory, Technical Report 58) University of California, San Francisco and Berkeley, San Francisco, 1968
4. Gordon RB: Arthography of the ankle joint. J Bone Joint Surg [Am] 52:1623, 1970
5. Lange-Hansen N: Fractures of the ankle. II. Combined experimental-surgical and experimental-roentgenologic investigations. Arch Surg 60:957, 1950
6. Weber BG: Die Verletzungen des oberen Sprunggelenkes. 2nd ed. Huber, Bern, 1972
7. Bozzini P: Lichtleiter, eine Erfindung zur Anschauung innerer Theile und Krankheiten nebst der Abbildung. J Pract Arzn Wund Berl 24:107, 1806
8. Bircher E: Die arthoendoskopie. Zentralbl Chir 48:1460, 1921
9. Burman MS: Arthroscopy or direct visualization of joints: an experimental cadaver study. J Bone Joint Surg 13:669, 1931
10. Takagi K: The arthroscope. J Jpn Orthop Assoc 14:359, 1939
11. Watanabe M, Takeda S, Ikeuchi H: Atlas of Arthroscopy. Igaku-Shoin, Tokyo, 1957
12. Jackson RW, Abe I: The role of arthroscopy in the management of disorders of the knee: an analysis of 200 consecutive examinations. J Bone Joint Surg [Br] 54:310, 1972
13. Jackson RW, Dandy DJ: Arthroscopy of the Knee. Grune & Stratton, New York, 1976
14. O'Connor RL: Arthroscopy. JB Lippincott, Philadelphia, 1977
15. Johnson LL: Diagnostic Arthroscopy of the Knee: The Knee Joint. Excerpta Medica, Amsterdam, 1974
16. Drez D, Guhl JF, Gollehan DL: Ankle arthroscopy—technique and indications. Clin Sports Med 1:35, 1982
17. Heller AS, Vogler HW: Ankle joint arthroscopy. J Foot Surg 21:23, 1982
18. Hawkins R: Arthroscopic lateral ankle stabilization. Presented at Arthroscopy for the Podiatric Surgeon, Indianapolis, December 1983
19. Schneider A: Arthroscopic ankle fusion—a case report. Presented at the annual AANA Meeting, New Orleans, 1983
20. Lundeen RO: Arthroscopic fusions of the ankle and subtalar joint. Clin Podiatr Med Surg 2:395, 1994
21. Lundeen RO: Arthroscopic resection of the os trigonium and Steida's process. Poster presented at the annual meeting of the American College of Foot and Ankle Surgeons, 1993
22. Zimmer TJ: Arthroscopic surgery of the foot. p. 174. In Guhl JF (ed): Foot and Ankle Arthroscopy. 2nd ed. Slack, Thorofare, NJ, 1993
23. Barrett SL, Day SV: Endoscopic plantar fasciotomy for chronic plantar fascitis/heel spur syndrome: surgical technique; early clinical results. J Foot Surg 30:568, 1992
24. Barrett SL, Pignetti TT: Endoscopic decompression for Morton's neuroma: preliminary study with cadaveric specimens; early clinical results, J Foot Ankle Surg, 33:503, 1994
25. Collins DH: The Pathology of Articular and Spinal Diseases. p. 74. Edward Arnold Publishing Co., London, 1949
26. Goodfellow J, Hungerford DS: Patello-femoral joint mechanics and pathology. 2. Chondromalacia patella. J Bone Joint Surg [Br] 58:29, 1976
27. Bauer M, Jackson RW: Chondral lesions of the femoral condyles: a system of arthroscopic classification. Arthroscopy 4: 99, 1988
28. Lundeen RO: Medial impingement lesions of the tibial plafond. J Foot Surg 26:37, 1987
29. Berndt AL, Harty M: Transchondral fractures (osteochondritis dissecans) of the talus. J Bone Joint Surg 41:988, 1959
30. Huang T, Rodney RW, Bormadel R, Ray RD: Correlation of arthroscopy with other diagnostic modalities. Orthop Clin North Am 10:523, 1979
31. DeHaven KE, Collins RH: Diagnosis of internal derangement of the knee: the role of arthroscopy. J Bone Joint Surg [Am] 57:902, 1975
32. Jackson RW: The current role of arthroscopy in the management of knee problems. Orthop Trans 6:469, 1982
33. Reagan BF, McInery VR, Treadwell BU: Irrigating solutions for arthroscopy—a metabolic study. J Bone Joint Surg, [Am] 65:5, 1983
34. Geist ES: Arthroscopy: preliminary report. J Minn 46:306, 1926
35. Watanabe M: Arthroscope: present and future. Surg Ther 26(7):73, 1972
36. Dandy DJ: Early results of closed partial meniscectomy. Br Med J 1:1099, 1978
37. Johnson LL: Healing of human articular cartilage: an arthroscopic view. Orthop Trans 5:400, 1981

38. Ferkel RD, Weiss RA: Correlative surgical anatomy. p. 88. In Guhl JF (ed): Foot and Ankle Arthroscopy, 2nd ed. Slack, Thorofare, NJ, 1993

39. Japour C, Vohra P, Giorgini R, Subel E: Ankle arthroplasty: follow-up of 33 ankles—effect of physical therapy and obesity. J Foot Ankle Surg 35:203, 1996

40. Johnson EE, Markoff KL: The contribution of the anterior talofibular ligament to ankle laxity. J Bone Joint Surg [Am] 65:81, 1983

41. Hicks JH: The mechanics of the foot: the plantar aponeurosis and the arch. J Anat 88:25, 1954

42. Lundeen RD: Manual of Ankle and Foot Arthroscopy. Churchill Livingstone, New York, 1992

V

Podiatric Considerations of Specific Sports

28

The Mechanics of Dance and Dance-Related Injuries

STEVEN KRAVITZ
CARLA MURGIA

Dance as an athletic activity uses unique body positions and specific movements on a repetitive basis that are not common to other sport and movement forms. Pointe stance (standing on the toes), as done in classical ballet, is an obvious example. However, the reader should be aware of other body positions or postures, such as flat back, hinges, contractions, spiral releases, forced arch, demi-pointe, and plié, that the dancer controls and sustains while he or she develops movement phrases. The quality of the movement, which is dependent on the creative decisions of the choreographer and artistic director, may be dynamic and high impact, quick and abrupt, or any other unique combination. Thus, dance as an athletic activity has an implied set of biomechanical circumstances unique to this art form and a set of injuries related to these mechanics common to it but not common in other forms of athletic activity. The lower torso, inferior extremity, and foot, as the distal end of the weight-bearing chain, are significantly affected by these biomechanical principles. The physician responsible for the dancer patient should maintain a high level of suspicion of poor mechanical function in a patient presenting with a history of recurrent injury. A basic understanding of the mechanical relationships produced through dance can be extremely helpful in the short-term and long-term management of these remarkable athletes.

BIOMECHANICS OF BODY POSITIONS IN DANCE

Turn-Out

Ballet, jazz, and to some degree, modern dance use turn-out stance. It is based on five classical ballet positions that require the feet to be placed 180 degrees away from each other, heel facing heel and toes facing in opposite directions (Fig. 28-1). The 180-degree aesthetic is more rigorously adhered to in classical ballet; however, the stance is common to most concert dance forms. Ideally, this stance is to be accomplished by applying the required lateral rotation solely through the hip. However, many dancers are unable to attain enough hip rotation to produce the desired foot position. Dancers sometimes create the illusion of the desired foot position by tilting the pelvis forward, by laterally rotating the tibia at the knee, or by applying an abductory force to the pedal segment. This allows the dancer to approximate the ideal classical 180-degree line of the right to the left foot. The pelvic tilt produces excessive compressive forces on the posterior aspect of the vertebral bodies and discs of the lumbar spine and results in subsequent lumbar strain. The rotation at the knee produces excessive strain of the soft tissues at the medial aspect of the knee. The abduction placed on the foot leads to subtalar and midtarsal joint (oblique axis) pronation. The two

645

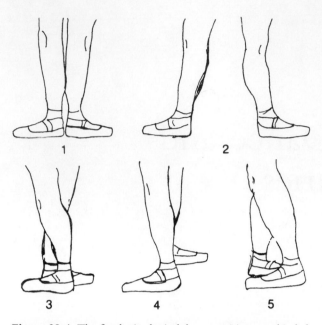

Figure 28-1 The five basic classical dance positions used in ballet: positions 1, 2, 3, 4, and 5. (From Kravitz SR, Hubert S, Ruziskey JA, Murgia CJ: Biomechanical analysis of maximal pedal stress during ballet stance. J Am Podiatr Med Assoc 77: 484, 1987, with permission.)

joints are triplanar in movement; therefore, the required abduction cannot occur without simultaneous eversion and dorsiflexion at both articular interfaces. A dancer who is excessively pronated and/or who has a mediocre skill level often produces the appearance of a collapsed longitudinal arch structure. This rolled-in appearance has been termed by dancers as "rolling in at the ankle," a phrase commonly seen in dance literature.

We have found evidence in independent research that would suggest that a highly skilled dancer can cause pedal abduction without the expected frontal plane calcaneal eversion component.[1] The baseline study reports on approximately 20 dancers and demonstrates statistically significant findings for this small group. More research is needed in this area; the physician should be aware, however, that motion is triplanar in both the midtarsal and subtalar joints; thus movement reflective of these articulations should be assessed, to whatever extent possible, in all three body planes.

There are several possible explanations for greater than expected movement in the transverse plane, while having less than the anticipated movement in the frontal plane. It may be that the highly skilled dancer uses enough intrinsic

and extrinsic pedal musculature to stabilize the first ray in the sagittal plane, decreasing the usual occurrence of developmental hypermobility and subsequent dorsiflexion. This would result in a relative supinatory force on the rearfoot (subtalar joint axis), providing the visual appearance of a stable arch structure and tending to decrease subtalar pronation. Another explanation would assume that a natural selection process exists favoring the dancer with an oblique midtarsal joint axis angled more acutely with the transverse plane than average. This would yield greater forefoot abduction and would thus enable the dancer to excel more easily in forms where the aesthetic emphasis is placed on the open line of 180 degrees. Both of the preceding concepts would allow for larger amounts of pedal abduction with a decreased calcaneal eversion component. The phenomenon of foot abduction, while maintaining an apparently stable calcaneal stance position, appears to be particularly more common for the highly skilled professional ballerina and is not usually seen in jazz dancers and modern dancers, nor is it usually seen in ballet dancers who are less skilled.

In summary, the forced turn-out position occurs when a dancer places the feet on the supporting surface in an externally rotated position relative to each other, beyond what can be attained solely through external rotation at the hip. This consequently produces excessive strain at the medial aspect of the knee and a pronatory reaction to the foot, which are common etiologies of multiple overuse syndromes. Sports medicine practitioner be highly suspicious of this mechanism with a history of recurrent or migratory injuries.

Pointe, Demi-pointe, and Forced Arch Stance

Pointe stance is a position in which the dancer stands on the toes, as in classical ballet. It is performed using specially constructed pointe shoes that are neutral (i.e., have no right or left). The pointe shoe contains a rigid shank and toebox. The toebox extends from the distal aspect of the shoe to the area corresponding to the metatarsal heads of the intended foot. The dancer must often mold the shoe to his or her foot to attain comfort. It is not unusual for the professional dancer to wear out a new pair or several pair of shoes in a single performance. Footwear often accounts for a significant portion of a dance company's budget.

Demi-pointe stance is a position in which the dancer

stands on the metatarsal heads while the ankle is fully plantar flexed and the metatarsophalangeal joints are maximally dorsiflexed. Forced arch stance is a position in which the dancer stands on the metatarsal heads while the ankle is fully plantar flexed, the metatarsophalangeal joints are maximally dorsiflexed, and the knee is flexed. Because pointe, demi-pointe, and forced arch positions require the ankle to be fully plantar flexed, the narrow portion of the posterior talar dome becomes the primary articulating area within the ankle mortise. Stability in these positions is highly dependent on maintaining a rectus pedal structure and requires significant development of the tibialis posterior and other supinators as well as the peroneus brevis, to help maintain a rigid lateral column. Deviation from rectus leads to relative inversion or eversion of the rearfoot on the forefoot. This is called "sickling in" or "sickling out" and is indicative of poor muscular development and/or technique. The dancer with a weak lateral column will often maintain the sickled position, even when not weight bearing. The forefoot must be locked on the rearfoot at the midtarsal joint to maintain the straight-line appearance of the foot. This sickled appearance is not only aesthetically unappealing to the dancer's or choreographer's eye, but leads to ankle and foot sprain as well as strain to the myotendinous structures. Exercise programs to develop the appropriate musculature are an essential component of the treatment regimen used in treating this "weak foot" as reflected in pointe, demi-pointe, or forced arch stance.

Pedal weight distribution *en pointe* through visual inspection of the ballerina leads to the conclusion that possibly most of the weight-bearing force is applied to the distal aspect of the digits. However, many dancers report that a significant portion of weight is often applied to the medial aspect of the first metatarsal head, as the dancer "leans into the toebox." Research by Kravitz[2] presented to the 1984 Summer Olympic Scientific Congress supports the sensation reported by these dancers. Electrodynographic interpretation of ballerinas in *relevé* (two-pointe stance) and *passé* (one-pointe stance) shows considerable pressure produced on the medial aspect of the first metatarsal head and the medial as well as lateral aspects of the hallux interphalangeal joint, indicating the necessity for the second toe to act as a buttress, stabilizing the hallux from abductory migration. The data indicated that maximum force was exerted at these sites during the periods of transition from flat to demi-point and pointe. Further analysis of photographs of ballet dancers supports the impression that the medial aspect of the foot bears most of the weight. The dancer often tends to move the forefoot in a lateral direction from the rearfoot longitudinal axis. When the foot is flat on the floor, such a movement would be described as abduction of the forefoot. The motion occurs in the transverse plane around the oblique axis of the midtarsal joint as the plantar aspect of the foot is parallel to the supporting surface.

A foot in pointe, demi-pointe, or forced arch stance performs the movement described previously with the plantar aspect of the foot in the frontal plane rather than the usual orientation (i.e., parallel to the supporting surface). For this reason, the lateral movement of the forefoot (relative to the longitudinal axis of the rearfoot) is best described as eversion rather than abduction. The movement of the forefoot allows the medial aspect of the first metatarsal head and the medial aspect of the hallux to become areas of significant weight bearing. This mechanism of action would not be possible without the appropriate construction of the toebox, such as the one found in the classical ballet pointe shoe.

The mechanism of action is exacerbated when the dancer performs the passé (one-pointe stance). To maintain balance during passé, the dancer places the total body center of gravity over the base of support, which requires adduction of the lower extremity toward the midline of the body. Thus this stance produces larger amounts of the previously described forefoot eversion. In this stance the medial aspect of one foot, which becomes the primary weight-bearing area, is placed in closer proximity to the floor. In fact, electrodynographic studies reveal that more force is exerted on the medial aspects of the first metatarsal and hallux in passé than in relevé (two-pointe stance). One would expect this occurrence, because one-pointe stance puts total body weight on one foot, whereas in two-pointe stance the weight is distributed between the two feet.

Plié and Its Reaction to Forced Turn-Out

Plié is a flexed-knee position. A dancer may perform grand plié (full knee flexion) or demi-plié (knee flexion with the heels in contact with the floor). The flexibility of the posterior soft tissue structures of the leg determines the amount of knee flexion that occurs during demi-plié. Grand plié is most often used as part of the warmup. Demi-plié is used throughout most movement sequences as a preparation or force production phase for many movements and as a landing or force reduction phase when completing movements, such as leaps, jumps, or turns. The demi-plié is also an integral part of preparation and conclusion in the execution of various lifts. A flexed knee will permit transverse plane movement at the articular interface, producing an expected 10 to 15 degrees of tibial rotation relative to the femur in these athletes. When the dancer tilts the pelvis forward and "cheats" or forces turn-out at the knee, the lateral torque placed distal to the hip may be fully, or at least partially, absorbed by the femoral tibial articulation. However, as the dancer extends the knee from the flexed position, the externally rotated tibia is no longer able to maintain the transverse plane orientation. The leg segment is forced to internally rotate relative to the femur as extension proceeds. The mechanism of straightening the knee from a flexed position, while in a forced turn-out stance, has been termed "screwing the knee." As the dancer proceeds through the force production phase of the plié in preparation for airborne skills, the magnitude of the forces is large. A study conducted with force plates revealed that, although highly skilled dancers spent less time in the plié preparation, the magnitude of the forces were much larger than those generated by less skilled dancers.[3] Thus the combination of screwing the knee while generating large forces at the knee has been considered as a primary factor initiating inflammatory response to the joint. Dancer's knee (often thought of as a form of patellar chondromalacia), synovitis, capsulitis, tendinitis, and other factors predisposing the performer to early degenerative changes have all been implicated.

One should note that, as the dancer straightens the knee in the previously described fashion, the leg will not only rotate internally relative to the thigh, but will also do so with respect to the foot, which is planted firmly on the supporting surface. The talus, locked in the ankle mortise, follows the leg and adducts in the transverse plane. Inferior support for the talus, such as the spring ligament, is no longer in an appropriate position to stabilize the bone as it adducts and simultaneously plantar flexes. The result is subtalar joint pronation, unlocking of the lateral column, and subsequent hypermobility of the first ray. The overly pronated foot has been well documented as being highly correlated with subsequent overuse injury in many athletes. Our experience demonstrates similar findings with dancers.

Pelvic Reaction to Forced Turn-Out

To attain more pedal abduction during turn-out stance (Fig. 28-2), the dancer may tilt the anterior aspect of the pelvis forward and inferiorly, while the posterior pelvis moves backward and superiorly in a reciprocal fashion.

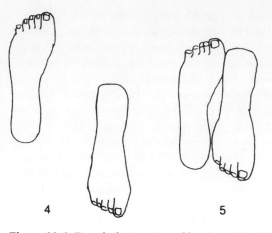

Figure 28-2 Dorsal-plantar views of fourth position (4) and fifth position (5), showing turn-out stance. (From Kravitz SR, Hubert S, Ruziskey JA, Murgia CJ: Biomechanical analysis of maximal pedal stress during ballet stance. J Am Podiatr Med Assoc 77: 484, 1987, with permission.)

The net result produces flexion at the hip joint and increased lumbar lordosis. Rather than the thigh moving anteriorly to produce hip flexion, it is the pelvis that flexes posteriorly on the thigh. Relative to the articular portions of the hip, however, the movement is the same—that is, flexion. Flexion of this joint often relaxes such tissues as the iliofemoral or pubocapsular ligaments, permitting increased external rotation at the hip. While this anterior pelvic tilt provides a method for "cheating," it often leads to problems associated with lumbar lordosis, such as vertebral body and disc compression and muscular spasm. Dancers often refer to the appearance as swayback and lament the subsequent loss of abdominal strength and "support of the pelvic floor."

ASSESSMENT OF TURN-OUT AND EXAMINATION OF THE DANCER

The well-trained dancer has usually been taught at a young age that "rolling in at the ankle can lead to foot and knee injury." In addition, the hypermobile pronated foot is not pleasing in appearance to those of the dance world. The pronated subtalar joint leading to lateral column instability, loss of an appropriate fulcrum for the peroneus longus, and the subsequent production of first ray hypermobility is the mechanism responsible for the "rolled in at the ankle" reference. It is not uncommon for these athletes to attempt to stabilize the appearance of an arch to their feet by supplying significant load to the subtalar supinators. Thus, forced turn-out is not always easy to recognize through gross visual inspection.

Assessment of turn-out is best made through measuring transverse plane motion and orientation of the lower extremity. We attempt to gain a general understanding of the inherent mechanical factors through measuring hip external rotation, with the joint extended and the patient in a supine dorsal recumbent position. This is then added to the measured malleolar torsion. The sum minus 10 degrees gives the "theoretical maximum turn-out," which is compared with the clinically measured pedal abduction normally used by the dancer to attain the first classical position. A longitudinal bisection of the second ray, relative to the midsagittal plane bisection of the body, provides the coordinates for the first position measurement. The measurement is made on three separate stances, and the average of these is used for the comparative analysis; however, the deviation of each stance attempt should be no more than a few degrees from the calculated average, assuming that the patient is performing the first position with expected consistency. The possibility of a forced turn-out stance is suggested when the clinically determined first position measurement exceeds the theoretical maximum turn-out calculation.

The therapeutic management of the dancer includes educating the patient toward an understanding of the mechanical factors involved with his or her performance. A recommendation to decrease the stance abduction slightly, as indicated by the previously described evaluational process, can be helpful in decreasing the overuse injury pattern.

Dancers have extraordinary control over their body movement, possessing an extremely developed kinesthetic awareness, muscular strength, flexibility, and coordination. In addition, dancers use mental imagery to learn and perfect skills, as well as to convey the message of the choreographer. The combination of these physical and mental skills and techniques can be incorporated as an integral part of the long-term treatment regimen for the dancer hindered by improper technique, including relatively small degrees of pedal hypermobility. We have found it helpful for the dancer to imagine the foot as a tripod. This image incorporates the heel, fifth metatarsal head, and first metatarsal head as primary centers of weight bearing when standing flat on the floor, in one of the five classical dance positions. Exercise programs designed to strengthen extrinsic and intrinsic pedal musculature, coupled with the described type of imagery, are helpful in decreasing the tendency to de-

velop forced pronatory reactions. These techniques, combined with a basic understanding of the mechanical factors, allow the patient to appreciate the need to maintain appropriate body orientation, and the necessity to not force the turn-out through foot pronatory abduction.

The assessment of external hip rotation in both the extended and flexed positions is beneficial in differentiating soft tissue from osseous limitations of this vital movement. Tightness of such structures as the pubocapsular or iliofemoral ligaments can be appreciated through decreased hip movement. The well-schooled, skilled dancer will often demonstrate equal ranges of motion in both flexed and extended positions of the hip. High-caliber performers usually start their training at a young age, when the tissues are most responsive to gradual slow stretching. A dancer of less skill who is plagued by nonosseous restriction, however, should still be encouraged that slow static stretching can positively augment a limitation of hip transverse plane excursion.

OVERUSE INJURIES

A set of specific injuries relative to dance movements are commonly seen in dancers but are not seen in other types of athletic patients. These pathologies are related to the mechanical demands placed on the lower extremity to produce the previously described movements.

Fractures and Stress Fractures

Although major fractures that result from a single-event trauma are rare in dance, they can occur as a result of applied compression, tension, shearing, torsion, and bending forces. The most common single event producing deleterious forces is landing from a jump or leap. The occurrence of spontaneous fractures can be minimized by learning and practicing proper mechanics and by taking class and performing on resilient floors. Some have suggested that dancers wear appropriate shoes; however, this is not necessarily an option because of the aesthetic demands of the dance form and/or choreographer; as an example, modern dance is quite often performed barefoot.

Dancers do not perform single-plane movements, but rather employ movements that require a combination of twisting and turning while producing or absorbing force. In addition, because of the repetitive nature of the rehearsal environment, particular body parts of dancers are often subject to chronic fatigue. This produces the ideal environment for agonist and antagonist muscles to misfire or fire out of sequence or timing and develop stress-related injury patterns.

STRESS FRACTURES AT THE BASE OF THE METATARSALS

This injury pattern is commonly found in the dancer. Fatigue fractures (as these injuries are sometimes called) most often occur midshaft or at the anatomic neck of the metatarsal in other forms of athletics. The different location of this injury in the dancing population appears to be related to the turnout stance. This is especially true when the position is forced. The reactive first ray hypermobility allows for the anticipated transfer of weight from the first to the second metatarsal. However, the vector of force applied is one of abduction, as well as the usual sagittal plane dorsiflexion load common to most athletic activity. In fact, primarily sagittal plane loading to the relatively thin second metatarsal is common in any circumstance that approximates the biomechanics of the normal gait or running cycle, when associated with an unstable medial column. It is the abducted pedal position that, when accompanied by first ray hypermobility, adds a transverse plane, abductory-directed load to the second metatarsal. It would appear that the applied force reaches maximum tension and compression (on opposite sides of the metatarsal) near its base, where it is rigidly embraced by the attaching ligaments and surrounding osseous structures. Thus, the physician should be aware of augmentation of this stress-related injury relative to its anatomic location in dance, as opposed to sports-related activity.

Diagnosis can be confirmed by pinpoint pain over bone and pain at the suspected fracture site through the application of a dorsiflexion force to the plantar aspect of the metatarsal head. Tenderness should be noted at the base area of the metatarsal with this pressure applied. Applying a tuning fork or brief passing of a low-dose ultrasound head over the suspected stress fracture may at times produce tenderness or a sharp pain as well.

The immediate treatment for this condition is rest and the augmentation of weight bearing through the use of a felt metatarsal balance pad (with a depression or punchout for the second metatarsal head). Long-term therapy, especially if the patient presented with a recurrent history of injury, requires biomechanical assessment for turn-out and appropriate adjustment of the dance pedal position. Orthotic use with a temporary Morton's extension may also be a helpful adjunct.

TIBIAL STRESS FRACTURES

These fractures may occur in the midshaft of the tibia and, in our experience, can be slow in healing. Cutaneous electrical stimulation has been used adjunctively with rest. Long-term management is often facilitated by the use of exercise programs to build well-toned muscle bulk on the legs. Experience would suggest that the soft tissue acts as a shock-absorbing structure, decreasing stress loads applied to the bone. This impression has previously been substantiated in the medical literature. Such muscular development has been helpful, because recurrence of this injury is a common complaint without enhancing the body's capacity to dissipate the stress load produced on the dance floor. Biomechanical analysis of forced turn-out, as well as pointe stance and the presence of sickling, should also be considered.

Intermetatarsal Space Neuroma

This neuroma is actually located between the proximal phalangeal bases and thus, in a sense, it is incorrectly named. The lesion is relatively common, especially in ballet, probably because of the pointe stance and the compression produced because of the rigidity of the toebox as the dancer rises *en pointe*. Treatment is similar to that of any other patient, consisting of such therapeutic approaches as physical medicine, padding, orthotics, steroid injection, and surgical excision. The dancer should be treated symptomatically during the performing period of the year. Surgical excision should be considered for the dancer whose performance capability has been affected by chronic or recurrent symptoms, when conservative measures have proved ineffective. The patient can return to barre exercises after the 21st post-operative day, gradually increasing the load to the operated foot. After suture removal but before 21 days, the dancer may opt to do such exercises using the good foot as the support extremity and the surgical foot as the non-weight-bearing working leg. Water barre exercises, that is, using a swimming pool with the water line at barre height, or using even deeper water, are an excellent means of allowing the dancer to rise to the pointe position with decreased load to the operated foot. Stress can be gradually increased, in a controlled manner, as the dancer moves toward more shallow water until full weight-bearing load is able to be assumed. Return to full dance activity in approximately 8 weeks is expected. The subject should be cautioned that increased load must be achieved in a gradual manner; too much too soon may produce hemorrhage or other damage to the surgical site.

Intermetatarsal aneurysm has been described in the literature. We suspect that the mechanical factors producing the relative increased frequency of neuroma are possibly associated with aneurysm in this anatomic location, as described by Sammarco and Miller.[4,5]

Tendinitis

Muscle strain and myositis often result from dancing barefoot or on nonresilient surfaces for long hours. The mechanics of push-off, when dancers propel themselves, as well as those of landing from a leap or jump, place extraordinary demands on the flexor muscles of the foot, particularly the flexor hallucis longus. Dancers who force the turn-out and provate the foot create excessive strain on the flexor hallucis longus, which must now act to aid the supination of the foot as well as apply plator-flexory load to the hallux.

FLEXOR HALLUCIS LONGUS TENDINITIS

Inflammation of the flexor hallucis longus tendon structure will cause tenderness in the posterior ankle, or just inferior to the medial mallcolus, as the tendon courses through the talar posterior tubercles and the tarsal tunnel. The syndrome is more commonly seen in the latter anatomic location. Chronicity and continued strain can lead to stenosis of this structure, producing a "trigger toe,"[5,6] which snaps the hallux into an attitude of plantar flexion or dorsiflexion as the stenosis is pulled through either side of the tarsal tunnel. Surgical release of the tendon stenosis may be necessary when this condition develops. Prior to the development of the described tendon hypertrophy, physical medicine in the form of ultrasound and hydrotherapy, along with rest and possible adjunctive oral anti-inflammatory medication, may be beneficial. A short duration of rigid immobilization followed by active exercise programs using full range of motion with gradual progressive resistance has been useful for treatment in the acute state.

It is not uncommon to be able to palpate an asymptomatic crepitus along the laciniate ligament, as the hallux is dorsiflexed and plantar flexed in a reciprocal fashion. We do not treat the condition unless it is symptomatic.

The strain produced on the great toe flexor tendon is related to the amount of work required by the muscular

structure to oppose hallux hyperextension *en pointe*. Ankle dorsiflexion to the end range of motion, with simultaneous hallux dorsiflexion, will usually evoke a symptomatic response; the use of an object to resist hallux plantar flexion, starting from various degrees of digital dorsiflexion, will often produce similar patient reactions. Both clinical situations place the tendon under significant tension.

Inflammation of the Achilles tendon will cause pain distally toward and/or at its insertion. It is the result of the repetitive sudden overstretching of the structure associated with the plié preparation followed by forceful concentric tension of the push-off, which is then followed by the forceful eccentric tension of the posterior muscle complex when completing many movements. Often the dancer will "dance through" the pain, which permits the weakened structure to progress from microscopic tears to a full-blown rupture. Although this occurrence is not frequent, it can develop from the more common chronic condition that develops following one or more acute tendinitis episodes. If the Achilles tendon is thick and elastic, the dancer may alternatively develop tendon inflammation and multiple tears at random sites in one or both heads of the gastrocnemius. Both conditions should be treated immediately to eliminate the devastating consequences of a complete tendon rupture.

Plantar Fasciitis

Inflammation of the plantar fascia is a common problem among dancers. It can be the result of repetitive jumping and landing or, more commonly, the result of long hours of training and practice barefoot or in shoes that lack longitudinal arch support. (All dance shoes have little or no longitudinal arch support). Dancing through this type of injury often becomes a chronic problem, and leads to other compensatory injuries, such as shin splints, hamstring strain, and hip and low back pain. The injury is best treated with rest, ice, and an appropriate tape support of the longitudinal arch. Dancers may avoid the dreaded down time associated with most injuries by adhering to a limited rehearsal schedule with the appropriate arch strapping. Orthotics for walking activity may be helpful.

Talar Compression Syndrome

Pain in the posterior ankle, especially when related to maximal plantar flexion of the joint, as occurs in pointe stance, is the chief complaint in talar compression syndrome. Fingertip pressure applied to the posterior talar tubercle area, and/or maximal active or passive extension of the joint, are clinical methods of evoking a symptomatic response. This is in direct contrast to flexor hallucis longus tendinitis, which typically uses ankle and hallux dorsiflexion as diagnostic indicators.

The dancer who presents with talar compression syndrome may express a sensation of limited ankle plantar flexion and may thus feel unstable in pointe stance. The syndrome is caused by compression of the posterior talus during maximum ankle plantar flexion and has three basic etiologies. The first of these is an enlarged posterior talar process that impinges on the posterior distal tibia at the end range of extension. The process may fracture, requiring immobilization. We have used short leg casting for 3 weeks, followed by a second 3-week period during which the cast is bivalved, allowing for non–weight-bearing exercises in all directions except plantar flexion. The exercises are tailored simply for mild range of motion, decreasing ankle stiffness, and associated cast disease.

A second etiology is an os trigonum,[7] which also becomes entrapped and compressed on the posterior inferior tibia during end range of ankle extension. Finally, a third, less common, etiology is related to a decrease in the trough of the posterosuperior shelf of the calcaneus. In this instance, the posterior talar tubercle becomes impinged on the calcaneus inferior to it during the same motion described. Diagnosis may be more difficult and requires lateral ankle plantar-flexion stress radiographs to assist in defining the pathology. Bilateral views for comparison are suggested to assist in attaining accurate assessment.

Treatment of the acute condition requires rest, physical therapy, oral anti-inflammatory agents, and so forth. We do not use steroid infiltration in the proximity of the flexor hallucis longus tendon because the previously described excessive strain placed on it during pointe stance. Surgical excision for a displaced nonhealing fracture of the posterior talar process may be necessary. The literature describes removal of this fragment[8,9] as well as excision of an enlarged posterior talar process[9] through either a medial or a lateral approach. We prefer the lateral approach for fragment excision and have found casting and conservative treatment to be successful for the dancer patient with nondisplaced fracture.

Long-term treatment to prevent recurrence of the syndrome may necessitate biomechanical analysis of ankle range of motion. The dancer should be instructed as to where end range of motion occurs and should be made aware that attempting to move beyond this limit will risk

redevelopment of this syndrome. Furthermore, chronic inflammatory response in this or any joint can potentially lead to early degenerative changes.

It is interesting to note that several performers with limb length discrepancy developed the described syndrome while attempting to overextend the foot and ankle of the short side in an attempt to gain length of the entire extremity and adjust for the unequal limb length. Full biomechanical assessment can provide vital information for this and all recurrent overuse injuries. Demi-pointe and pointe analysis for sickling, knuckling down,[10] digital hyperextension, and other indicators of muscle weakness and/or poor technique should be part of the overall biomechanical evaluation.

Anterior Tibiotalar Impingement Syndrome

Tenderness in the anterior aspect of the ankle elicited by joint dorsiflexion is the presenting complaint in anterior tibiotalar impingement syndrome. Our experience indicates that 15 degrees of dorsiflexion with the knee extended or flexed is desirable in decreasing the possibility of developing various overuse injuries. This is an important factor for differentiating anterior tibiotalar impingement syndrome from ankle equinus. Most podiatric literature defines equinus of this joint as less than 10 degrees of dorsiflexion motion.[11] However, the dancer may easily surpass this measurement and still present with pain at the anterior ankle structure because of the amount of dorsiflexion motion often required while performing dance activity. Thus motion of anatomic areas that meets the standards often regarded as defining normalcy under typical ambulatory conditions may produce limitation of movement under the excessive requirements for dance activity.

The etiology of this impingement syndrome may be related to an exostosis on the dorsal talar neck, providing osseous blockage of excessive dorsiflexion attitude. Another etiology is related to a wide anterior talar dome leading to impingement of the articular aspect of the medial malleolus. The diagnosis here is difficult and may be assisted through bone scan technique.

Treatment is usually of a conservative nature, incorporating RICE (rest, ice, compression, and elevation), oral anti-inflammatory agents, ultrasound, and other physical medicine modalities. Educating the patient toward knowledge of anatomic end range of motion is necessary in preventing recurrence. This is extremely important with regard to etiology of a wide anterior dome. Impingement on the medial malleolus could be extremely destructive if allowed to remain in a chronic state of inflammation.

Patellar Subluxation and Chondromalacia

At some point during a career, a dancer may experience nonspecific knee joint pain. The physician may find that the dancer responds to pressure placed on the anterior surface of the patella. Upon further examination, the physician finds that the patella does not ride firmly in the intertubercular groove, but slides easily from medial to lateral and vice versa. Although repeated trauma to the knee may cause the softening and subsequent tearing of the hyaline cartilage on the posterior articular surface of the patella, a large Q angle and muscular imbalance of the quadriceps group are quite often the cause of the pathology. If the intertubercular groove is shallow, the Q angle is large, and the vastus lateralis is strong, a dancer may experience patellar subluxation, particularly when the mechanism of landing requires the quadriceps group to be in eccentric tension. Female dancers, particularly those who force the turnout, are most susceptible to this type of injury. Following ice and rest, the dancer should begin a progressively aggressive quadriceps strengthening program. Occasionally pieces of articular cartilage slough off and create the classic "joint mice" condition. This occurrence causes significant inflammation, pain, and swelling. Although rest and decreased weight bearing permit the dancer to maintain some degree of activity, surgery may be the only option to resolve this chronic and debilitating situation.

Snapping and Subluxating Hip

Quite often dancers complain of the sensation of a snap occurring in the hip. This is usually the result of the greater trochanter of the femur rotating laterally under the iliotibial band. The sensation may be felt on the support leg, when the dancer balances on one leg. In this case the tensor fascia lata and the gluteus medius are maximally tensed to stabilize the pelvis relative to the thigh. Occasionally the dancer will experience the snapping sensation in the "gesture leg." In this case the dancer abducts the laterally rotated non-weight-bearing leg in the frontal plane. If the lateral rotation is not complete, the snapping or popping sensation is produced as the greater trochanter moves into position. Occasionally the iliofemoral ligament may produce a hip click as it moves over the femoral head during

hip abduction, particularly in dancers with narrow hips, who have limited range in external rotation and unlimited range in abduction. Although pain is seldom associated with any of the previously mentioned situations, degeneration of the greater trochanter may result if the snapping or clicking hip is experienced over an extended period of time. The problem is sometimes alleviated when the dancer embarks on a program that stretches the medial rotators and strengthens the lateral rotators and abductors of the hip. However, caution should be exercised when the dancer attempts to increase the range of lateral rotation.

Another common problem among dancers, particularly female dancers who have overstretched the iliofemoral and pubofemoral ligaments and hip joint capsule in an effort to increase turn-out, is the complaint that the hip "goes out." As in the case of patellar subluxation, continual hip subluxation results in degeneration and subsequent arthritic conditions.

Shin Splints

One of the most common problems experienced by dancers is a dull ache in the vicinity of the anterior inferior shin. It is sometimes unclear if the problem originates at the anterior or posterior tibial muscles or at the tibia in the form of stress fractures. It is certain that the problem most often occurs at the beginning of conditioning, when dancers commence the performance of new and unfamiliar movements, or on new floor surfaces. The pain becomes more intense after activity has ceased, and is usually associated with inadequate fitness for the new activity or fatigue. The occurrence of shin splints is greater in dancers who force the turn-out and pronate the foot or have a naturally pronated foot type. Prophylactic conditioning of the leg—that is maintaining muscular balance of the leg and stretching the anterior and posterior tibial muscles before and after activity—is helpful. However, appropriate taping and/or physical medicine is required for the dancer who is plagued with this condition.

Sprains

Sprains seldom occur in dancers; when they do, the most common sites are the knees, ankles, and toes. As previously mentioned, dancers rotate the tibia in an effort to create the illusion of greater turn-out. The rotation produces excessive torsion forces at the knee, particularly at the medial collateral ligament. The dancer with a weakened medial collateral ligament may experience a sprain of the structure when performing a ballistic movement, such as a jump or a leap. Although the occurrence is infrequent, caution should be exercised in the dancer with medial knee pain.

Toe sprains are common, particularly in barefoot dancers. The dancer can usually continue modified activity by taping the involved second, third, or fourth toe to an adjacent toe and wearing a sneaker or similar shoe for support and protection during the rehearsal phase. A sprain of the great toe is treated by tape support of the distal interphalangeal and metatarsophalangeal joints in a crossover fashion.

Ankle sprains are common in activities that require the ankle to be placed in a plantar-flexed position during performance or participation.[12] The narrow aspect of the talar dome lying within the ankle mortise is said to provide an increased aspect of instability to the joint complex. Inversion sprains are the most common. However, pointe stance requires maintenance of plantar flexion of the joint to its end range of motion and requires it to be held statically, often for relatively long periods of time. This peculiar aspect of ballet coupled with the fact that the plantar-flexed ankle is more common in this athletic pursuit than in most others (gymnasts often presents with a similar joint attitude) produces anterior ankle strain and sprain. Strain refers to the development of anterior ankle extensor tendinitis.[13] The ankle capsular and ligamentous structures are frequently sprained when the ballerina performs "over pointe," a position in which the ankle is overextended, tending to allow the dancer to fall forward off the dorsal and anterior aspects of the foot and ankle. Finally, the practitioner presented with a history of chronic anterior lateral ankle pain should suspect a sinus tarsi syndrome and should differentiate this from sprain of the anterior talofibular ligament.[14] Treatment and diagnosis of these injuries is similar to that in any highly competitive athlete, except with regard to location of some of the injury patterns as described herein.

SUMMARY

This chapter presents basic concepts regarding the biomechanics and related injury pattern of dance. Emphasis has been placed on ballet, jazz and modern dance, all of which use the five classical dance positions. Other dance forms (e.g., ballroom, tap) have not been discussed; however, they use similar mechanical aspects to the extent that their performance incorporates the basic movements addressed herein.

When immobilization becomes necessary, the other body parts can often be exercised. This helps maintain overall body conditioning, decreasing the recovery time required to return to full dance activity. Techniques described include using the injured leg as the working (non-weight-bearing) leg during barre exercises, as well as exercising in a swimming pool (water barre) to add weight gradually.

The physician should be aware of the motivational factors involved when dealing with the personality of the artistic dancer. These patients are highly motivated toward their chosen profession. Competition is prevalent; therefore, the practitioner must attempt to treat the dancer in a manner that requires the shortest period of "down time"—the period during which the dancer is unable to perform because of injury. This not only requires accurate diagnosis and treatment but necessitates the ability to understand the movements of the activity and the relationship of these movements to re-injury as well. Decreasing the possibility of injury development, while assisting the patient to reach peak performance level, is best accomplished through appreciation of the biomechanical factors involved in the competitive world of dance performance.

REFERENCES

1. Kravitz SR, Hubert S, Ruziskey JA, Murgia CJ: Biomechanical analysis of maximal pedal stress during ballet stance. J Am Podiatr Med Assoc 77:484, 1987

2. Kravitz SR, Murgia CM, Huber S, Saltreck KR: Biomechanical implications of dance injuries. p. 43. In: The 1984 Olympic Scientific Congress Proceedings—The Dancer as Athlete, Vol. 8. Human Kinetics Pub., Champaign, IL, 1985

3. Murgia CM: Selected biomechanical variables associated with three dance leaps. Doctoral dissertation, Temple University, 1995

4. Sammarco GJ, Miller EH: Forefoot conditions in dancers. Foot Ankle 3:85, 1982

5. Sammarco GJ, Miller EH: Partial rupture of the flexor hallucis longus tendon in classical ballet dancers. J Bone Joint Surg [Am] 61:149, 1979

6. Hamilton WG: Stenosing tenosynovitis of the flexor hallucis longus tendon and posterior impingement upon the os trigonum in ballet dancers. Foot Ankle 3:74, 1982

7. Quirk R: Talar compression syndrome in dancers. Foot Ankle, 3:65, 1982

8. Hamilton WG: The dancer's ankle. Emergency Med 14:42, 1982

9. Howse AJ: Posterior block of the ankle joint in dancers. Foot Ankle 3:81, 1982

10. Kravitz SR, Fink K, Huber S et al: Osseous changes in the

second ray of classical ballet dancers. J Am Podiatr Med Assoc 75:346, 1985

11. Kleiger B: Anterior tibiotalar impingement syndromes in dancers. Foot Ankle 3:60, 1982
12. Hamilton WG: Sprained ankles in ballet dancers. Foot Ankle 3:99, 1982
13. Hamilton WG: Tendonitis about the ankle joint in classical ballet dancers. Am J Sports Med 5:84, 1977
14. Meyer JM, Lagier R: Post traumatic sinus tarsi syndrome. Acta Orthop Scand 48:121, 1977

SUGGESTED READINGS

Ende LS, Wickstrom J: Ballet injuries. Physician Sports Med 10: 100, 1982

Hardaker WT, Margello S, Goldner L: Foot and ankle injuries in theatrical dancers. Foot Ankle 6:59, 1985

Howse AJ: Disorders of the great toe in dancers. Clin Sports Med 2:499, 1983

Kravitz SR, Huber S, Murgia C et al: Biomechanical study of bunion deformity and stress produced in classical ballet. J Am Podiatr Med Assoc 75:338, 1985

Kravitz SR: Dance medicine. Clin Podiatry 1:417, 1984

Root ML, Orien WP, Weed JH: Clinical Biomechanics, Vol. II. Clinical Biomechanics Corp, Los Angeles, 1977

Saunders JB, Inman VT, Eberhart HD: Major determinants in normal and pathologic gait. J Bone Joint Surg 35:543, 1953

Washington EL: Musculoskeletal injuries in theatrical dancers: site, frequency, and severity. Am J Sports Med 6:75, 1978

29

Step/Bench Aerobic Dance and Its Potential for Injuries of the Lower Extremity

JEFFREY A. ROSS

In the past 20 years, aerobic dance has become one of the most popular forms of exercise activity in America. With its popularity increasing yearly among participants, this form of "exercise dance" has evolved from its rudimentary form of high-impact aerobic dance, which incurred a multitude of lower extremity injuries, to a safer form of low-impact dance. By reducing the impact to the lower extremities, this also helped to reduce the number of injuries seen by the sports medicine specialist. During the initial years of aerobic dance, participants worked out on a combination of thin carpet and padding over hard concrete floor. Exercise physiologists and medical specialists quickly saw the need for change in the surface, and designed high-tech air-suspended wooden floor surfaces. This contributed to a significant reduction in the trauma to the lower extremity, leading to an immediate decline in the number of injuries seen. However, with the advent of step/bench aerobics, once again injuries were observed to increase.

Over the years, aerobics instructors as well as the aerobic dance participants themselves have become well informed and better trained. Health magazine articles, a certifying course for the instructors, improved aerobic and cross-trainer shoe design, better supervision, and the interaction of the sports medicine community and awareness of aerobic dance have all become integral component of the sport. Due to this interaction between instructors, trainers, and sports medicine specialists, there has been a marked decrease in the number of injuries seen by the foot and lower extremity specialist.

Approximately 10 years ago, aerobic dance evolved into a new form utilizing a platform, referred to as either "step" or "bench" aerobics. The purpose of this new dance exercise was to allow participants an alternative to a standard high-impact or low-impact workout, one that was designed to reduce impact forces to the lower extremity as in the low-impact workout. Simultaneously, it would also allow virtually the same, if not greater, cardiovascular benefits as did the high-impact workout. Developed by Reebok, the "step" also incorporates circuit training, with a series of specific exercises performed at consecutively arranged stations. Interval training has also been incorporated into the dance routines to improve conditioning and stamina. Once again, aerobic dance instructors found themselves becoming choreographers, now having to master their way around a "step" that is just 43 inches long by 16 inches wide by a minimum of 4 inches high (see Box). In the beginning years, many instructors felt that increased step height translated into a harder, more vigorous workout. However, now many are questioning the advantages of increased height, and vary their elevations in one-, two-, or three-step increments.

With the addition of new equipment to the dance studio, a new vocabulary to direct the dance steps was also

657

THE STEP

Features and Benefits

Adjustable height—3-in-1 step adjusts from 4 to 6 to 8 inches

Platform inclines/declines—works as a weight bench

Made of polyethylene—durable and stable

Grid platform surface—nonslip, shock-absorbing for safety

Rubber floor pads for traction and stability

Technical Specifications

Material—durable high-density polyethylene

Weight—Platform: approximately 8 pounds; blocks: 2 pounds each

Load capacity—500 pounds

Dimensions—43″ long × 16″ wide × 4″ high

Safety—The platform and support blocks have four rubber pads on the bottom that provide excellent traction on any flat, dry floor

---

developed. Terms such as those listed below (see Box) were added to the dance lexicon. Unaware novices would not know if they were participating in an exercise class, or if they were auditioning for the chorus in a Broadway play. The intricacies of these movements to music, with an instructor barking instructions, have a definite learning curve, and for the participants the early stages of a routine can be quite frustrating.

TERMINOLOGY

Helicopter move (half-hop turn)

Inner thigh

Diagonal lunge

Power knees

Leg extensions

Over the top

Straddle the bench

Double-knee with jog

Jack and jump

Karate and squat

Shoes have always been an important factor since the inception of aerobic dance. Early in the development of the sport, aerobic shoes were not much more than a court shoe with a slightly raised heel. However, over the years, technological advances in design have led to a much more stable and performance-oriented aerobic shoe. Today, aerobic shoes, known as "cross-trainers," appear to have become standard equipment, particularly among the dance instructors. With running incorporated in the routines in addition to the lateral movement and impact off the bench, the cross-trainers have proven to be quite invaluable.

Step/bench "aerobicizers" feel that this variation is a challenging, intricate, enjoyable, and yet safe form of aerobic dance exercise. As with any other new trend, not enough is known about the sport until years of experience and clinical observation data have been collected. With the explosion of step/bench aerobic participants, the number of dance-related injuries presented to many clinical practices has increased. What at first appeared to be an improvement over high-impact aerobics only proved that injuries can occur even in the safest of organized exercise programs. What is necessary to understand are the etiologies as well as the mechanisms of these injuries. This pertinent information would help to correlate the interactions between participants, instructors, equipment, and the sport itself.

The most important factor in the prevention of step/bench aerobic injuries is the instructors themselves. When several instructors were asked to comment and give specific observations concerning injuries and their prevention, most agreed "that technique was very important in the avoidance of injuries, and that repetition was dangerous." It has been shown that, if during a routine a step were to be performed too quickly (over 128 beats per minute), then the participants cannot secure their entire foot on the bench. That can cause a foot to "hang" over the edge, resulting in strain or pulling of the Achilles tendon, posterior tibial tendon, or peroneal tendons. In addition, it could lead to strain of the long plantar fascia, or intrinsic plantar musculature of the foot. This can result in an overuse tendinitis of any one of these structures. By stepping ballistically off the step, this can also lead to a significant impact overuse injury, such as sesamoiditis, stress fracture, or neuroma development. It was the consensus of the instructors that stepping too far back from the bench could lead to a hyperextension and traction of the Achilles tendon, eventually developing a chronic Achilles tendinitis or calcinosis.

Instructors adamantly agreed that close observation was imperative. By not being totally mindful of participants' foot placement on the bench and knee alignment in relationship to the lower leg, overstriking the floor from the bench could occur, resulting in overuse knee injuries or shin splints. Keeping an eye on the class can reduce the number of injuries just through correction of the participants' technique and body positioning.

Older instructors who have been teaching for 10 years or more concurred that, by having taken the proper certified training courses and having "matured" to a particular teaching level, they were then able to teach a much safer class and help to avoid the many pitfalls that may lead to these overuse injuries. Older instructors also agreed to the fact that younger instructors who have not experienced injuries themselves often teach a much more demanding class. It has been shown that participants who have just begun the step/bench aerobic routine would encounter injuries more frequently than their "seasoned" counterparts. One instructor, when questioned, responded that "When an instructor teaches too hard, the class perceives it as the 'best', but concomitantly it could also be the most dangerous." This instructor trainer also noted that, "the instructors who have not taught for over 10 years do not understand the particular injuries, or have the experience to avoid the actions that could cause many of these injuries to occur." There are a number of factors that can help lower the incidence of these injuries: certified instructors, carefully selected music, smooth choreography, and cueing to the beat of the music, as well as the participants taking the class. Surveying the class before the initial workout can help determine any pre-existing overuse injuries or potential for any new injuries to occur. The instructors want their classes to be safe, but yet they want their class participants to be excited about class and have a physically demanding workout. Their dilemma is to choose between a safe and efficient workout, and an aggressive and challenging one that might lead to the occurrence of an overuse injury.

Prevention of injuries is always a concern of sports medicine specialists; however, when aerobicizers train to such high levels that they ignore the potential for injury, then a need for concern is apparent. When questioned about level of intensity of their classes, one instructor responded, "some people in the step/bench classes feel that if they do not get out of bed sore and stiff, then it wasn't a great workout the day before, and something is wrong." There is obviously something drastically wrong in that reasoning, so it is imperative for the sports medicine specialist to understand the psychological dynamics of the participants. Many of these individuals may have physical or psycholog-

ical disorders (i.e., amenorrhea, anorexia nervosa, osteoporosis) that can lead to serious repercussions when they take up aerobic dance. Examples such as severe weight loss and stress fractures should be an alert signal to the sports medicine specialist.

As many instructors have become more experienced, they have then advanced to the next level and have now begun to "step to safety." Many of these instructors themselves have suffered from a multitude of injuries, and are now attempting to avoid further or recurrent injury. Some of these instructors have begun by lowering the step, or gone to just the bench alone (without blocks) in order to reduce knee or Achilles tendon strain as well as plantar fascia traction, while offering the same cadiovascular workout. These instructors who have learned through experience and injury have become successful with less pizazz, but simultaneously offer good safe workouts.

As a result of this investigation, a preliminary survey consisting of 329 participants was conducted, with 153 claiming that they has suffered some discomfort or pain due to step/bench aerobics, whereas 163 denied any complaints. Of those who were injured, 43 claimed that they had sought treatment by a foot specialist. When questioned about their aerobic shoes, 105 claimed that they had some problem with their shoes (i.e., blisters, improper fit, not enough support, cutting off circulation, irritation), while 197 denied any problems. The most common sites for the incidence of injury were the (1) knee, (2) calf, (3) Achilles tendon, (4) foot, and (5) shin. Greater numbers are necessary in order to determine trends and specific etiologies.

The instructors who were interviewed provided several tips for participants to help prevent such problems:

1. Keep the knees slightly bent, never locking the knee.
2. Bring the foot all the way up to the bench, so that the heel is not hanging off.
3. Keep the knee over the ankle (creates less strain on the knee).
4. Push off with the heel (not with the knee) with either squats or lunges.
5. Keep the head up and the chest tall (to prevent lower back strain).
6. Avoid stepping too far away from the bench.
7. Avoid stepping balistically off the step.
8. Keep your pace; avoid stepping too quickly.
9. Do not be afraid to lower the bench to a lower level in order to avoid injury.

They also offered tips useful to aerobic dance instructors:

1. Class size is important to allow the instructor to observe and correct.
2. Keep the pace of the step at 128 beats per minute; exceeding this pace will not allow the whole foot to rest on the bench.
3. Technique is very important in order to prevent injuries.
4. Excessive repetition of steps can be dangerous.
5. Stay under three platforms; hyperextension of the knee could occur with more.

6. Stetching and warmup is crucial to avoiding injuries.

Step and bench aerobic dance can be a very enjoyable and simultaneously a vigorous workout. By knowing the simple rules, and with proper instructor supervision, serious injuries can be avoided. Videotapes with carefully designed instruction can also aid in the prevention of unnecessary injuries. Via the use of step/bench participant surveys, enlightenment and health care participation of the sports medicine foot specialist can begin. Understanding the mechanics of the sport, the terminology, and the biomechanics of the individual participant can help to elucidate what types of injuries may occur, and how they can be prevented.

30

Skiing Injuries/ Cross-Country Skiing

ROBERT M. PARKS

THE EVOLUTION OF CROSS-COUNTRY SKIING

To fully appreciate cross-country skiing as it is practiced today, with its variety of techniques and applications, it is of great importance to understand how the sport has evolved into its present form. Winter enthusiasts acknowledge that the words "cross-country skiing" conjure up a spectrum of images that range from telemark skiing to Lycra-clad cross-country freestyle racers. Similar misconceptions stifling cross-country skiing's growth range from views that "walking on skis can't be much fun" to the idea that only an elite few possess the physical stamina to enjoy the sport.

The popularity of cross-country skiing varies greatly from country to country. It should be no surprise that the sport has a large following in those regions that have an abundance of snowfall. In many countries of the world, cross-country skiing has a heritage that dates back as far as 4,000 years, when it was used primarily as a mode of transportation. In 1994 the world was witness to the popularity of cross-country skiing in Norway during the Olympic games in Lillehammer. Scandinavian spectators braved the cold for days to get a glimpse of their nation's Nordic heroes. It is ludicrous to think that cross-country skiing in the United States will attain the popularity that it enjoys in Scandinavian countries any time soon, but indices project that it has tremendous growth potential over its present status in the United States.

When comparing the expense of downhill and cross-country skiing, many believe that the former is pricing itself out of reach of many Americans and therefore limiting its potential for growth. Although not inexpensive, cross-country skiing is beginning to fill an ever-larger niche for those who desire winter ski activities but do not wish to mortgage their houses to pursue those activities.

The lack of U.S. success in international cross country ski racing, compared to downhill, has also hindered its growth in this country. In the early 1980s many saw the success of U.S. cross-country skier Bill Koch as a possible turning point for cross-country skiing popularity in the United States. Many thought his visibility in winning the World Cup in 1982 and the silver medal in the 1976 Olympics and his role in revolutionizing cross-country skiing by popularizing the marathon skate technique as pivotal. Unfortunately, United States has had very little success in international competition since that time, and Bill Koch was never elevated to the popularity of such sports heroes as Frank Shorter, who caused such a boom in the sport of running.

Cross-country skiing is likely to be the beneficiary of two very popular sports activities now being enjoyed by millions in the United States: rollerblading and the indoor cross-country ski trainer. Despite the clear potential for bodily injury, rollerblading has become a favorite pastime for children and adults alike. The rhythmical skating motion that simulates roller skating and ice-skating is bound to have some eventual spillover into ski skating, which

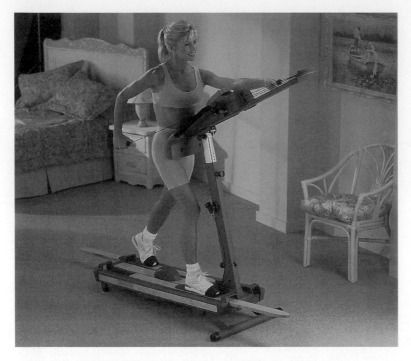

Figure 30-1 Research shows that a program of balanced fitness improves women's muscular strength, endurance, and cardiovascular fitness. NordicTrack, which simulates the motions of cross-country skiing, works major muscles with low impact. (Courtesy of Nordic Track Corporation, with permission.)

uses the same motion but uses the upper body as well to overcome the increased resistance of snow versus asphalt. Research indicates that cross-country skiers, by using both arms and legs over an extended period of time, are often able to achieve fitness levels unparalleled by those in any other aerobic sport.[1] Indoor cross-country skiing machines have emerged to provide a workout similar to that of cross-country skiing, and have become extremely popular in recent years (Fig. 30-1). Exercise enthusiasts find the dynamics of cross-country ski machines to be enjoyable and fluid in motion. Reports indicate that exercisers prefer this type of exercise equipment to stationary bikes and treadmills. It is not difficult to extrapolate that this indoor machine's popularity will potentiate a spillover effect into cross-country skiing.

VARIATIONS IN CROSS-COUNTRY SKIING

Most skiers, being more familiar with downhill than cross-country skiing, do not realize that downhill skiing as we know it today is a recent development and divergence from cross-country. It has only been since the advent of power-driven ski lifts that skiers with a downhill preference no longer needed equipment characteristics necessary for skiing uphill. Boots for downhill skiing no longer needed to flex and bend along the sole, and the ski boot's heel could be fixed solidly to the ski to optimize the transmission of force, allowing the skier to turn with more ease. Downhill skis have also evolved from a double camber that allows the tip and tail to bend as the midsection grips the snow to a single camber for better steering ability. Ski weight for downhill skis became less of a concern, and the skis' torsional strength was enhanced, which again optimized turning ability.

In cross-country skiing it has long been realized that a lighter weight and narrow ski will ski faster, but at the expense of control, especially on ungroomed terrain. Conversely, wider skis to a point will enhance stability for ungroomed or downhill terrain. The same principle holds true for cross-country ski boots. Lighter weight boots are good for speed but offer little in warmth and control for backcountry skiing. It has only been since the development of fiberglass, graphite, and other similar stiff but lightweight materials that cross-country equipment has evolved into an endless array of possibilities. Today, cross-country skiing can be subdivided by virtue of technique and equipment into racing freestyle, racing classic (typically, equipment weight is inversely proportional to the cost), light touring, backcountry, mountaineering, and telemark. Specific equipment requirements may vary depending on skier weight, ability, and preference for flat, uphill, or downhill terrain.

ACUTE SKI INJURIES

Injuries and injury patterns seen in cross-country skiing tend to differ greatly depending on the specific technique of cross-country skiing being used. Acute injuries that may occur in mountaineering or telemark skiing vary greatly from those of racing or light touring primarily as a result of boot, binding, and ski requirements as well as the propensity for these skiers to reach greater skiing velocities on downhill slopes. Studies have found that 88 percent of all acute cross-country injuries occurred on downhill terrain, whereas only 12 percent had occurred on flat or uphill terrain.[2] Injury patterns in cross-country versus downhill skiing have also shown that the age profile of injured cross-country skiers exceeds that of the downhill skier[3] (Fig. 30-2). Logical speculation would suggest that the type and magnitude of acute trauma sustained in the cross-country skier would be more severe in older age groups.

Studies have also surprisingly found that acutely injured cross-country skiers tend to be more seriously injured than their downhill counterparts.[4,5] These findings might partially be explained by the fact that many, if not most, of the less severe cross-country injuries go unreported. Cross-country skiers are able to ski anywhere that snow is found, so even injuries requiring medical care will be diffusely scattered throughout the medical community and not sequestered around ski areas. This fact makes the accurate tabulation of cross-country ski injury patterns very difficult to obtain. The limited ability to evacuate injured cross-country skiers in remote mountainous terrain makes it paramount that cross-country skiers have some basic knowledge of first aid and that they always try to ski in groups. Other statistics correlating to the geographically unrestricted nature of cross-country skiing indicate that cross-country skiers are more susceptible to acute upper body injuries when compared to downhill skiers.[2,5–7] Certainly, for the cross-country skier, unregulated terrain and other unsuspected dangers exist that downhill skiers are not subjected to on groomed and patrolled terrain.

Despite the fact that many cross-country skiers prefer sparsely populated areas to ski, Nordic ski centers are becoming more popular. These areas, where cross-country skiers can enjoy the advantages of machine-groomed terrain, have made it possible to tabulate from rather large skier studies the overall incidence of injury for cross-country skiing. Two of the larger studies[2,4] have determined the incidence of injury for cross-country skiing to be approximately 0.49 to 0.72 injuries per 1,000 skier days, as compared to downhill skiing, which approximates 2.0 to 3.5 injuries per 1,000 skier days.

Figure 30-2 Percentage distribution of age groups of injured cross-country skiers in relation to injured alpine skiers. (From Steinbruck K: Frequency and etiology of injury in cross-country skiing. J Sports Sci 5:187–196, 1987, with permission.)

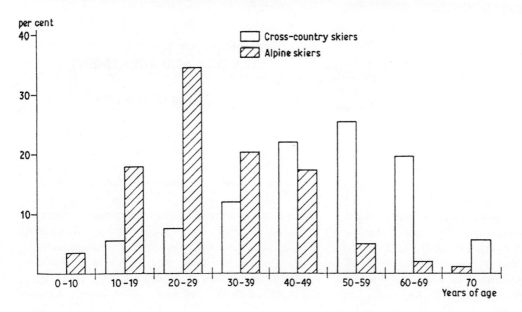

Studies have shown that 49 percent of all acute injuries in cross-country skiing occur within the lower extremities.[2] The etiology and care of these injuries, do not have biomechanical implications as they relate to specific techniques. These topics are not discussed further in this chapter, however, two points should be made regarding acute injuries to the knee and ankle. It is evident that acute injuries to the knee joint, typically including the medial collateral and anterior cruciate ligaments, seem to be inversely proportional to the support and stability of the cross-country ski boot and binding. Mountaineering and telemark boots and bindings transfer torque into the knee joint when a typical ski entrapment fall occurs in much the same way as does downhill equipment. Cross-country ski boots that offer intermediate support and stability subject the ankle to sprains and fractures in much the same fashion as downhill equipment did before modern-day boots. Increasing rates of knee and ankle injuries have encouraged some binding manufacturers to introduce release-type bindings for backcountry and telemark-type skiing. At this writing, cross-country bindings with release features are quite primitive when compared to their downhill counterpart.

OVERUSE CROSS-COUNTRY SKI INJURIES

Nontraumatic injuries, or those that occur insidiously, account for the largest percentage of cross-country ski injuries that will present in a clinical setting for nonemergent care. This fact should come as no surprise since cross-country skiing is a noncontact, aerobic-type sport that vigorously uses both upper and lower extremities repetitively for long periods of time. One study[8] found that 72 percent of all overuse cross-country ski injuries occurred at or below the level of the knee. Orava et al. also found that 60 percent of these injuries were either precipitated or exacerbated by nonskiing activities. Competitive cross-country skiers and those who push the physiologic limits in seeking aerobic fitness by training for long hours clearly subject themselves to a much greater risk of injury. Comparative studies have shown, however, that overuse cross-country ski injuries occur at only one-fourth the rate of injuries seen in running and jogging.[8] Data collected by the Swedish National Cross-Country Ski Team during the 1983 and 1984 seasons found that 75 percent of all injuries sustained were overuse injuries, compared to 25 percent traumatic injuries.[8] Other studies confirm the fact that younger and more competitive cross-country skiers run an increased risk of overuse injury.[9]

When looking at factors that influence the incidence of overuse injuries of cross-country skiing, one must go back to the fact that very few sports involve exertional moments of force on so many parts of the body. This occurs as the skier attempts to propel body weight and equipment against the sum total of "drag" derived from the interface of ski–snow friction, gravity, and wind resistance. One might think that the cross-country skier is spared the increased ground reaction forces of running sports. Studies have shown that cross-country skiers using diagonal stride can easily achieve vertical compressive forces (not percussive in nature, however) during the kick phase that achieve 1.6 times body weight.[10]

Many overuse injuries that occur in cross-country skiing involve muscles and tendons responsible for forward sagittal plane movement. The traditional cross-country skier and especially freestyle skier is also subjected to injuries that occur from rotatory torque of the lower extremity and back that occurs on the transverse plane. The diagonal stride in cross-country skiing maintains the skier's foot position in a constant forward direction while the foot is essentially fixed to the forward-moving ski (Fig. 30-3). The asynchronous pendulum-like motion of both the upper and lower extremities over the skis imparts a degree of transverse rotational torque as the skier maneuvers over the skis. The lower extremities and backs of freestyle cross-country skiers are subjected to very high degrees of transverse plane torque. With skis placed obliquely to the line of forward progression, the body moves rhythmically from side to side, never staying aligned over one ski for more than a fraction of a second (Fig. 30-4).

SPECIFIC OVERUSE INJURIES: ETIOLOGY AND TREATMENT

Tendinitis of the Hip

Tendon strains and soreness around the hips are seen with some consistency in cross-country skiers. Cross-country skiing is unique compared to downhill skiing, in which skis are held more statically in a natural body stance position. In cross-country, whether it be classical technique, in which the extremities are flexing and extending, or skating, in which they are also abducting and adducting, the hips and muscles that govern this function are never at rest. Probably the most critical factor in cross-country skiing that potentiates injury more so than in running is the weight of the skis and boots, which must be retrieved

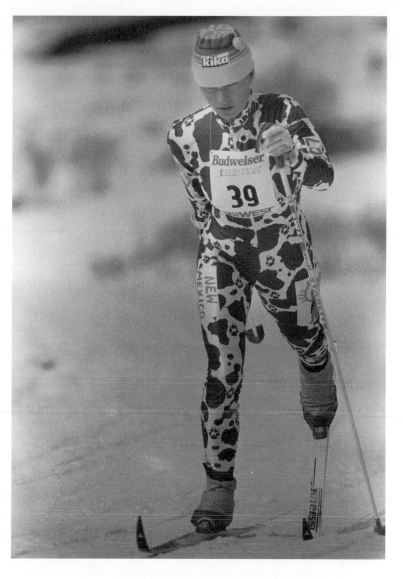

Figure 30-3 Freestyle cross-country skiing (Ivana Radlova). (Copyright by David M. Benyak; all rights reserved.)

at the end of each stride. This repetitious reversal of motion while under load at the hip may precipitate tendon inflammation. Diagonal striders should make certain their skis do not slip when aggressively skiing flat terrain or when climbing, because the hip joint will be thrust into hyperextension, causing strains of the adductors and hip flexors. Freestyle skiers are particularly vulnerable to soft tissue strains of the hip because this technique requires continued hip abduction and external-internal rotation. Actively kicking and thereafter retrieving the gliding ski seems to be the critical function of this technique. In addition to the strains previously mentioned, skaters are prone to gluteal strains around the greater trochanter and inflammation of the tensor fascia lata.

Hip injury prevention includes proper preseason conditioning and stretching. Skiers should restrict the duration of early-season skiing and avoid consecutive skiing days to allow for sufficient body adaptation.

Medial Knee Strain

Strain to the pes anserinus and other soft tissue structures on the medial aspect of the knee occurs commonly with cross-country skiing. I would suspect that this is the most

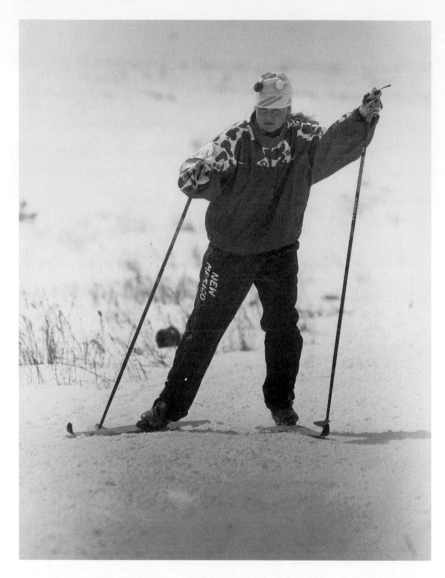

Figure 30-4 Skate in cross-country skiing (Pernilla Graun). (Copyright by David M. Benyak; all rights reserved.)

common overuse injury to the knee in which the act of skiing is the primary etiology, and not other coexisting sports activities. Skiers with prior histories of injuries to the knee joint and medial knee will run an increased risk of injury. Medial knee pain may occur with both classical and freestyle techniques, with the later being more common. Pain potentiated by the classical technique depends on the terrain being skied and occurs most frequently early in the season in less skilled skiers. As will be seen, terrain, snow conditions, lack of preseason conditioning, and skier ability are common denominators for almost all overuse injuries. These factors should be kept in mind for the practitioner to address when taking an injured skier's history.

When one analyzes a less proficient cross-country skier from either the front or the back, even when skiing machine-groomed terrain, it will likely be noticed that a degree of functional genu valgum exists in both limbs. I refer to this suboptimal body alignment (which is also seen in some downhill skiers) as one of the beginning skier's self-preservation techniques. This technique and others, such as sitting back on the skis, are used in hopes of preventing falls, but almost always result in greatly decreasing skiing efficiency. If one imagines a skier's body mass centered over both limbs held in a valgus alignment, it becomes clear that falls to the outside of one's skis become less likely. This positioning, however, puts a valgus stress on the knee much like that which would occur in a runner who is knock-kneed, and results in a tractional force on all medial knee structures. A skier holding the limbs in this position statically would be bad enough, but considering the dynamics of each limb during diagonal striding and the component of rotational torque that enters the knee, it can be appreciated that injury could ensue. I try to make inexperienced skiers aware that, to commit their body weight over one ski and actuate an efficient kick during diagonal stride, they will have a tendency to fall to the outside of their skis from time to time.

Freestyle skiers, and again inexperienced ones, are even more prone to medial knee strain. Beginning skaters will have difficulty properly aligning and commiting their body weight over the gliding ski, resulting in a knee valgus alignment. This alignment results in constant or premature in side edging of the gliding ski and an abbreviated glide phase. In this scenario the hips do not align rhythmically with the gliding ski and are squared more toward the line of forward progression. This puts a tremendous valgus stress on the knees. Coaches and physicians should realize that skiers who exhibit excessive valgus positioning as a result of poor technique, as described earlier, will also assume a maximally pronated foot when that extremity is subjected to body weight. Although it may be helpful to examine the feet to rule out abnormal foot mechanics, it should be understood that improvement in technique is of paramount importance. I specifically recall in the mid-1980s, when the skating boom first began, that an abundance of skiers were incorrectly faulting compensatory pronation for their inability to ski more efficiently. It was found that foot beds and foot orthoses did little to correct this problem, and only through proper instruction and experience did they become more proficient skiers.

When treating overuse medial knee pain in cross-country skiers, it is important to moderate activities as necessary and logically strengthen the knee using standard protocol for knee rehabilitation. Skiers may need to be guided in regard to technique modification and be placed on less challenging or groomed terrain. Ski boots with good support, specific for their intended purpose, and a lighter weight ski should all be considered.

Patellofemoral Syndrome

Overuse injuries to the patellofemoral joint are not frequently caused solely by cross-country skiing. However, cross-country skiing, and particularly the classical technique, does possess risk factors that can contribute to patellofemoral pain. Repetitive flexion and extension of the knee coupled with the possibility of patellofemoral malalignment resulting from either abnormal structure or function can lead to injury. Ground reaction forces imparted upon each lower extremity, however, seldom exceed body weight, and in fact weight distribution is occasionally balanced equally by both limbs (double poling, gliding, and single kick–double pole). With the variety of terrain and techniques available to cross-country skiers, the load transmitted to the patellofemoral joint is done so in a variety of subtle variations. This would be contrasted with running or cycling, wherein knee function is mechanically repetitious. Backcountry skiers who carry heavy packs for overnight trips should be aware that they incur a significantly greater risk of developing patellofemoral pain and should see that they prepare physically for such endeavors.

In my practice, individuals using indoor ski machines seem to develop more patellofemoral pain than their outdoor counterparts. This is likely due to the greater frequency with which these machines might be used and the fact that lower limb mechanics in performing the ski stride are more repetitious in their motion than those of outdoor skiing.

Anterior Compartment Syndrome

Skiing-induced anterior compartment syndrome of the leg was one of the first notable injuries believed to be unique to the technique of skating or freestyle skiing.[11] This injury was seldom seen with the classical technique. When performing the diagonal stride in classical cross-country skiing, the ski is never lifted off the snow, with the possible exception of the end stage of the kick phase (this is a result of an active kick and does not change the mechanics of ski retrieval back into its forward position). The forward advancement of each ski into its glide position uses primarily the hip flexors and little active leg function.

In skating, the ski glides out obliquely with respect to the line of forward progression. When approaching the end of the glide phase, the hip turns away from the gliding ski, the ski initiates an edge, and the foot actively plantar flexes against the ski to effect an active kick. As the kicking limb extends and the body mass moves away from the kicking ski, the ski must be actively lifted from the snow back to its starting position under the body. The ankle must dorsiflex from its plantar-flexed kick position to at least a 90-degree foot–leg angle to lift the ski tip off the snow. As the extremity recoils, the foot–leg angle must remain near 90 degrees until the ski is replaced on the snow. The repetitive use of the tibialis anterior muscle to perform these functions may result in inflammation or hyperemia within the anterior leg compartment.

A number of issues regarding equipment modifications for the freestyle skier emerged very rapidly to make ski retrieval more efficient and to lessen the likelihood of developing anterior compartment syndrome. The evolution of ski equipment for the freestyle skier over the last 10 years has included stiffer boots and bindings to keep the boot in closer proximity to the ski. This helps prevent tip drop during ski retrieval. Shorter and lighter skis have also been developed to help the skater develop and maintain a faster cadence. Skiers and coaches have also experimented with binding placement by moving the binding forward on the ski by 1 to 2 cm. This modification is reasonable if found to be necessary because of anterior leg pain, but should not be done at the expense of overall ski performance. Freestyle skiers with shoe sizes larger than size 12 may want to advance their binding placement further forward than what is typically designated by the ski and binding specifications. This will place the center of body mass more appropriately over the skis' running surface and will improve skiing efficiency.

The majority of anterior compartment syndromes seen today involve inexperienced or early-season freestyle skiers who have yet to develop sufficient strength in the anterior leg musculature. A high cadence rate and variable snow conditions can also precipitate this condition's onset. Individuals with a prior history of exercise-induced anterior compartment syndrome brought on by other sports should be aware that they run a high risk of exacerbating their symptoms with freestyle skiing, and precautionary measures should be addressed. Beginning freestyle skiers should consider using the ultra-short freestyle skis until they have developed sufficient skiing skills.

Symptoms of anterior compartment syndrome are identical to those seen in runners. Generalized pain will be present over the leg's anterior compartment. Symptoms are typically only present when the athlete is involved in vigorous and repetitive activity such as running or freestyle skiing. Examination should include strength and flexibility testing for the calf and anterior leg musculature. Dysequilibrium between the anterior and posterior compartments of the leg is frequently seen with congenital or acquired contractures of the gastrocnemius–soleus complex. Skiers should be advised to warm up adequately and, when racing, should be advised to start more slowly. An aggressive

daily stretching program for the calves as well as a prudent strengthening program for the anterior musculature should be advised. Chronic cases of anterior compartment syndrome should undergo compartmental pressure testing while running on a treadmill. Recalcitrant cases are often amenable to surgical releases of the fascial compartment.[12]

Peroneal Tendinitis

Cross-country skiers are prone to medial and particularly lateral tendinitis about the ankle. This tendency is due to the freedom of movement that exists between the cross-country ski boot and binding as well as the limited amount of ankle support that some cross-country ski boots afford. Skiers wearing lightweight or low-cut boots or those skiing with this boot design on irregular terrain may be prone to develop peroneal tendinitis.

With either skating or classical skiing techniques, unconscious firing of the peroneal tendons is often done by inexperienced skiers to evert the heel and pronate the subtalar joint. This maneuver throws body weight toward the inside edge of the skis and has the same effect as the knee valgus position previously discussed. This position is assumed in an attempt to prevent a fall, but is done so at the expense of balanced weight distribution on the skis, which in turn reduces glide efficiency. Excessive use of this muscle group in beginning skiers can also be attributed to excessive skier anxiety or tension within the legs, as is true with any technique-oriented sport. Proper instruction should see that body alignment is properly placed over the skis so unnecessary muscle splinting within the ankle will not occur.

Beginning skaters may be prone to peroneal tendon overuse in much the same way as ballet dancers. When a dancer assumes a demi-plié, the externally positioned feet should occur as a result of "opening the hips" and not as a result of foot pronation. If the freestyle skier's hips and knees are not aligned over the gliding ski, the knee will internally rotate with respect to the gliding ski and the resulting torque will pronate the foot. The peroneal tendons will therefore be forced to contract in an attempt to stabilize the foot and limb and maximize glide length.

Therapists and coaches should look critically at equipment and technique issues when peroneal tendinitis presents, but should not forget to check the skier's feet for problems of intrinsic instability. A thorough biomechanical exam should include forefoot-to-rearfoot relationships, subtalar joint neutral position, gait analysis, static stance, and a single-foot balance test. The balance test should not show excessive interplay between the tibialis posterior and peroneal musculature, and heel alignment should be maintained at or near vertical. If mechanical foot pathology is of potential concern, varus canting, arch supports, and, when necessary, custom foot orthoses should bring dramatic results. Custom orthotic devices made primarily for cross-country skiing need to be aimed at achieving maximum control, much like the control needed for downhill skiers. Skier tolerance to a highly controlling orthotic device is usually quite good. Orthotic devices should be fabricated to the same bulk limitations that would be appropriate for a pair of soccer shoes, because cross-country ski boots should fit snugly and are often confining. All other therapeutic measures used in the treatment of peroneal tendinitis would be similar to those used in any good sports-oriented regimen.

Retrocalcaneal Bursitis and Achilles Tendinitis

Inflammation of the Achilles tendon or posterior heel is only occasionally seen in cross-country skiing. Achilles tendinitis will more frequently be seen in classical rather than freestyle skiing. The active kick and plantar flexion of the ankle through a large range of motion performed in the classical technique is likely the dominant cause. In freestyle skiing the kick is applied obliquely instead of vertically and, if using a top-of-the-line skating boot, ankle range of motion is restricted and better supported. When eliciting a history from skiers with Achilles or retrocalcaneal pain, many will be discovered to have developed the injury in cross-training sports or will have had an episode of hindfoot pain some time in the past.

Unlike running activities, which result in an abrupt heel contact, the heel and Achilles tendon are not subjected to any impact forces with cross-country skiing. It is only the mechanics of active plantar flexion against forefoot resistance during the kick phase that may result in injury.

Older cross-country skiers who develop posterior heel pain should undergo radiologic examination to rule out the possibility of a coexisting calcaneal step deformity or the presence of a posterior heel spur. These individuals may be particularly prone to develop posterior heel symptoms when attempting to ski and should be made aware of the fact that their condition may become chronic or recurrent in nature. Skiers with posterior heel pain should be sure that the heel counter of their boot fits comfortably against

the heel. If an area of excessive pressure exists, the boot should either be modified or replaced. Skiers with Achilles tendon or heel pain should either alternate skiing techniques or cut back from skiing as necessary to allow adequate healing to take place. Appropriate therapeutic measures, including physical therapy as well as stretching and strengthening of the Achilles tendon, should all be suggested as indicated by the stage of injury that exists. Recalcitrant injuries to both the Achilles and posterior heel may require surgical intervention if all conservative measures of treatment have been exhausted.

Plantar Fasciitis and Heel-Spur Syndrome

Plantar fasciitis is one of the most common injuries to occur in the foot. This injury can, in fact, be brought on by any number of seemingly benign activities, such as prolonged standing or a change in shoe gear. It is therefore difficult to pinpoint one activity, such as cross-country skiing, as the sole precipitating cause. In middle-aged or older individuals, it appears that fasciitis occurs not so much as a result of the type of physical activity, but more so the magnitude. There are some features unique to cross-country skiing, however, that may be implicated in the development of plantar fasciitis and warrant consideration.

The freedom of movement of the foot inside many cross-country ski boots, and the boot's torsional instability, require the foot to work more actively to initiate edge control and balance. The cross-country ski boot's freedom of movement within the binding system also demands more intrinsic activity within the foot. Attempting to edge a ski on sloped terrain can become tiring and potentially strain the plantar aspect of the foot. Beginning skiers who lack sufficient proprioceptive balance can also strain the foot by overutilizing the small intrinsic muscles of the arch. In comparison, downhill skiers transmit forces through their limbs and feet much more efficiently because their feet are firmly held within the confines of a rigid ski boot.

Practitioners treating individuals with plantar fasciitis must elicit a detailed history, including all activities that might be implicated in the evolution of fascial pain. If it is thought that the skier's level of fitness should have otherwise tolerated the physical demands of the sport, then equipment and particularly the boots should be examined. As is true with any properly fit shoe, the ball of the foot should work harmoniously with the boot. If the boot is either too large or too small, the foot will not flex with the inherent flex point of the boot, and fascial strain may result. The stiffness of the binding should also be examined to see that the qualities of binding function suit the intended use. Most light touring bindings are designed to flex at the toe-binding interface as opposed to older designs where the toebox itself was required to bend. Much of the foot's flexion, necessary during the kick phase, is therefore taken up within the binding and not entirely within the boot. This feature is quite helpful for those with tendencies toward fasciitis, but more importantly for those with forefoot pathology.

Forefoot Deformities

Cross-country skiers may be subjected to a host of possible forefoot aches and pains. Downhill skiers, by comparison, are usually prone to only those injuries that would be attributed to the noncompliance of the boot's plastic shell. These complaints frequently involve problems related to irritation on either the first or fifth metatarsal heads. In addition to this set of circumstances, cross-country skiers are subjected to stresses that arise from the foot's repetitive flexion inside the boot.

As discussed with plantar fasciitis, an improperly fit cross-country ski boot can be responsible for a number of foot maladies. With the diagonal stride, a boot that is too short may bind across the metatarsal shafts as the boot's normal flex occurs proximal to the metatarsal heads. Certainly the toes would be forced too far forward in the toebox of the boot, creating pressure problems for the toes and nails. If the boot is too long, the foot will not be able to efficiently flex the boot because the force applied through the ball of the foot will be proximal to the boot's natural flex point.

Arthritic deformities of the metatarsal heads and particularly the first metatarsophalangeal joint will become aggravated by the classical skiing technique. I have examined a number of cases where cross-country skiing was the first sport to precipitate symptoms in a previously asymptomatic joint, although radiographs displayed a well-established deformity. Skiers with hallux limitus or similar deformities should gravitate toward stiffer boots and use only those bindings that offer flexion characteristics.

Sesamoiditis is another forefoot complaint that should be treated by instituting boot modifications. Actively kicking off of a foot that is pronated or whose weight is medially displaced can subject the tibial sesamoid to excessive forces, creating inflammation and subsequent pain. Free-style skiers also subject the sesamoids to strain at the end of the kick phase. In this instance, the skater's ski is on an inside edge and body weight is medially displaced as the knee internally rotates away from the kicking ski. Cross-country skiers with sesamoid pain should be treated with a dancer's pad to accommodate the first metatarsal head or should have an appropriate arch support or custom orthotic device placed in their boots.

Digital and Nail Injuries

Cross-country injuries to the toes and toenails occur at a higher frequency than those seen in downhill skiers. In the downhill ski boot, the foot is statically held within the confines of the boot and the toes actually recede back as the skier bends forward. In cross-country skiing, the foot moves more actively in the boot as the boot flexes with each stride. As previously stated, boots should fit snugly, but adequate room must be allowed for thick socks. The flex of the boot should match the anatomic flex of the foot. Skiers with contracted digits should cover prominent toes with moleskin or other suitable covering. Toenails should be trimmed closely before each outing to prevent trauma and subungual hematomas.

Cross-country skiers should guard themselves against the possibility of blistering and frostbite. If wearing two pairs of socks, those made of a synthetic material should always be put on *under* cotton or wool socks to allow for wicking of perspiration away from the foot. This will better insulate the foot from the cold and prevent blistering. Skiers should also be instructed to stay on their skis as much as possible because the ski functions as an insulator. Boot covers should always be available if extremely cold temperatures are anticipated.

CONCLUSION

Although injury data for cross-country skiers are limited, a consensus of authors support the fact that this sport is considerably safer than downhill skiing. Cross-country skiing injuries specific to the lower extremities are found with near-equal frequency to those occurring in the upper extremities. The majority of injuries seen in cross-country skiing are classified as nontraumatic or overuse in nature, although it should be realized that many of these injuries go unreported or are attributable to multiple sports. Traumatic injuries are becoming more common as freestyle techniques and lighter weight equipment have resulted in significantly faster skiing velocities. Injury patterns when comparing classical versus freestyle technique vary widely. I am not aware of any studies that have specifically compared injury patterns for these two techniques of cross-country skiing. Personal experience would indicate that freestyle skiing may result in more frequent injuries to the hips and upper extremities when compared to the classical techniques.

In Alpine Skiing

Jeffrey A. Ross
Steven I. Subotnick

Alpine or downhill skiing is a complex skill that requires controlled pronation, setting the foot, ankle, and lower extremity on the inside ski edge. Pronation sets the inside edge of the downhill (control) ski, and allows for the skier to lean inward against that ski, which holds a skidless arc throughout the turn. While balanced on a beam of flexible composite $2\frac{1}{2}$ inches wide, the skier drives the shin forward against the stiff boot cuff and swings the hips to the opposite direction. The ski rolls onto its sharp steel edge and bites the snow, creating a carved arc across the hill. The lateral g-forces build as the skier carves around the turn. The skier leans farther inward to counter those forces, keeping the center of gravity exactly in line with the combined centrifugal and gravitational forces. Variations of lower extremity biomechanics, on all three body planes, can markedly affect the skier's ability to create controlled turns, and as a result may predispose the skier to injury if the abnormality is serious enough. These variable factors may include structural biomechanical deformity, functional deformity, or dynamic imbalances of muscles. Flexibility, strength, and proper range of motion of the lower extremity provide the needed elements to function normally in this demanding activity. Decreased range of motion as seen in pre-existing injuries, which may predispose to biomechanical imbalances, can significantly alter a skier's ability to ski safely and efficiently. Weak muscle groups, decreased range of motion of important joints, and poor flexibility have clearly been associated with increased muscular effort, resulting in fatigue. Fatigue has been shown to be one of the main factors in the incidence of downhill skiing injuries.

Witherell[13] tested more than 1,000 racers and recreational skiers in 1971. He found that four of five were unable to stand perfectly flat on the undersurfaces of their skis in a straight running position and, consequently, rode on the outside edges excessively. Using high-speed photography, Subotnick[14] found that 80 percent of 30 skiers studied failed to have proper edge control as a result of various biomechanical abnormalities of the lower extremity and, in fact, could not ski parallel. These skiers instead contorted their bodies in attempts to compensate for biomechanical abnormalities while borrowing pronatory forces from other joints, usually the hip and knee. In Subotnick's study, most of the skiers responded favorably to a combination of cants and/or foot orthoses. Many skiers overcame fatigue, poor style, and poor edge control by using orthoses in their ski boots. Ross[15] reported on how the Electrodynogram (EDG) could provide documentation of the skier's foot and leg function in relationship to snow (ground) surface, boot, and foot bed. The skier's performance was plotted on a time–pressure curve, which helped determine which particular areas of the foot bore normal versus abnormal amounts of weight, as well as which portion of the foot and ankle were functioning either too long or too short in the ski (gait) cycle. The EDG helped to determine that forces are transmitted from both the forefoot and the rearfoot, which is essential in up- and downweighting and in the completion of proper turns. Abnormalities such as excessive foot pronation, shortened heel contact, and excessive propulsive phase on the toes, with extreme forward lean of the boot and asymmetry between the two feet, were seen, all affecting the skiers' effectiveness and performance. Many skiers overcame some of these lower extremity abnormalities, including fatigue, poor skiing style, poor edge control, and foot imbalances, by using various orthotic controls in their ski boots. Ross and Cohen[16] reported that custom insoles for mild foot and lower leg imbalances, as well as prescription orthoses for the more severe rearfoot and forefoot abnormalities, could be very valuable in helping to provide proper foot bed balance, and to improve ski performance and efficiency. It is now commonplace for custom ski-boot fitters to provide their clients with some form of foot orthoses. Today, with easy-to-customize liners and removable full-length soft support systems within them, custom insoles or prescription orthoses may be substituted for the pre-existing footbed. Various cants and heel and forefoot wedges can be added to the footbeds to attain neutral foot control within the boot. In spite of these advances in technology, the sports medicine foot specialist is often consulted to evaluate the effectiveness of the various foot control devices placed in boots or to make recommendations for additional control and/or boot modification.

The sports physician should have a basic knowledge of boot design and skiing performance, as well as a working relationship with a boot shop and fitter. With the benefit of these two experts' guidance, skiers can ski more comfortably and efficiently. The sports physician can determine foot type and potential for problems and pinpoint existing biomechanical and physiologic defects. He or she can diagnose bony deformities, fatigue areas of the foot, biomechanical imbalances, areas of friction and irritation, poor circulation, nerve entrapments, and metabolic disorders. All are factors in proper boot selection. Drawing on this medical information, the boot fitter can decide if the skier will require a volume boot, designed for wide, high-arched feet; a narrow, shallow heel pocket; or a thin, thick, or adaptable liner.

When an unbalanced foot is placed in a ski boot, the action of tightly buckling down can accentuate or aggravate the biomechanical imbalances within the lower extremity, which can then lead to an overuse injury or trauma. It is beneficial for the sports physician to be aware of those biomechanical abnormalities and variations of the lower extremity, and how those factors can intercede in alpine skiing. Today's boots have many characteristics that provide excellent comfort and adaptability. Many boots fit a broad range of foot types, and in many ways the inner lining and foot bed are beginning to resemble those of a running shoe. However, because of the variety of foot abnormalities, such as bunions, tailor's bunions, and hammertoes, specific boot modification to provide for comfort and enhanced performance is essential.

BIOMECHANICAL DEFORMITIES THAT AFFECT SKIING

Biomechanical variables that affect gait also influence the complex motions involved with downhill skiing. Skiing is a sport that depends heavily upon ski edge control. It relies on transverse plane motions of the lower extremity that are translated into frontal plane motions in the form of pronation and supination. In addition to the transverse and frontal plane motions, there is also sagittal plane motion, which acts in a forward lean position to absorb shock on varying terrains.

The foot is a dynamic structure even when held fairly rigid in a ski boot. Any semblance of irregularity in the foot will have a negative effect on boot comfort and performance. It has been shown that 2 to 5 degrees of pronation is ideal for putting a ski on edge without locking the foot to the point where there is no margin for error.[17] When the foot is allowed to be in neutral position, all the joints function efficiently and allow for controlled skiing movement. If improperly aligned, an overly pronated foot collapses excessively medially on each turn, resulting in overedging. A supinated subtalar joint has the opposite implication; it places weight primarily on the outside edge of the ski, and the knee has to drive exceedingly inward in order to put the inside of the ski on edge. Because of these excessive rearfoot imbalances, a skier may not be able to edge properly at all. This can create a situation where the foot is operating less efficiently, resulting in greater fatigue and inefficient power transference.

During a ski turn, a combination of downweighting and upweighting takes place as the skier transfers weight from one ski to another, or more specifically from the downhill control ski to the uphill ski as it assumes a downhill position (Figs. 30-5 and 30-6). In transferring weight, the skier moves from a position of pronation on the control downhill ski to pronation on the new control uphill ski. This maneuver is accomplished by unweighting the downhill ski while rotating and supinating the downhill lower extremity to change direction. Weight is then rapidly transferred to the new downhill ski, with rotation and pronation of the new downhill lower extremity, while rotating and supinating the new uphill extremity. This can be summarized very simply by stating that skiing is a series of linked turns that help to control the direction and speed of descent down a ski slope. The carved turn is composed of three fundamental components: pivoting (turning), edging, and pressuring the ski. Pivoting into a new direction occurs when unweighting reduces the pressure applied to the ski tips and tails. After unweighting is completed, edging acts by decelerating the speed and direction of the skis. The function of edging is accomplished by the induction of ankle eversion. Additional edging is provided by progressive knee and hip flexion, together with valgus positioning of the knee. Meanwhile, the upper body continues to face downhill independent of the lower legs. This separation of the upper and lower extremities is referred to as *counter-rotation*.

Maintaining the center of gravity over the skis by optimum body positioning is the key. This is referred to as *angulation*, and can be characterized by variable factors such as the degree of ankle joint dorsiflexion and eversion, flexion of the knee and hip, and lateral bending of the waist, with upper body counter-rotation. This will help maintain body weight over the downhill ski.

It is clearly understood that lower leg alignment is an important factor in skier comfort, safety, and performance.[14,18,19] It is important to understand the mechanics

Figure 30-5 Turning with the downhill knee tucked and behind. (From Subotnick SI: Appendix 3: The biomechanical basis of skiing. In Subotnick SI (ed): Podiatric Sports Medicine. Futura, Mt. Kisco, NY, 1975, with permission.)

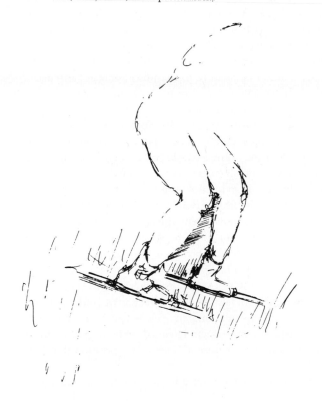

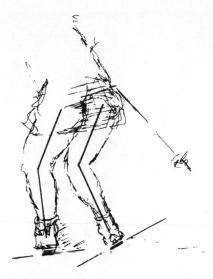

Figure 30-6 Effect on the edges of turning with the downhill knee tucked and behind. (From Subotnick SI: Appendix 3: The biomechanical basis of skiing. In Subotnick SI (ed): Podiatric Sports Medicine. Futura, Mt. Kisco, NY, 1975, with permission.)

of how and why a ski turns in order to appreciate the significance of the leg–boot–ski interface and ways in which abnormal biomechanics can affect this relationship.[20] To accomplish maximum alignment of the knee and lower leg, the tibia must be in line with the rearfoot and forefoot and perpendicular to the snow.

Obviously, this complex, coordinated pattern of movement is affected by lower extremity biomechanical deformities. The complex structure of the lower extremity, the multiple degrees of freedom present in the lower extremity joints, and the variations that might produce abnormal shoe wear, postural fatigue, foot deformity, and/or an overuse injury may be compounded when combined with widely varying snow conditions and rapid changes in terrain. The ski acts analogously to an extended foot. It multiplies the forces transmitted through the lower extremity because of the increased lever arm and surface area. The skier needs to maintain a center of gravity over the skis, and yet have the ability to reduce speed or change direction instantly. The kinesthetic relation between the foot, boot, ski, and snow is critical. Thus small degrees of imbalance become significant because they can affect the skier's posture and his or her ability to distribute weight, initiate turns, and develop edge control.

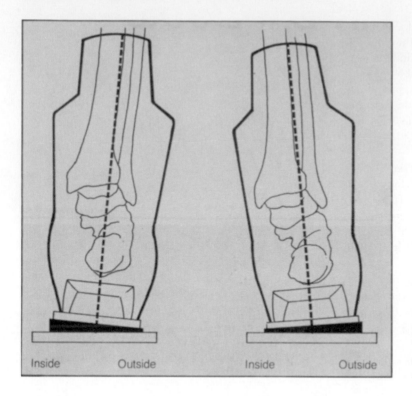

Inside Outside   Inside Outside

Figure 30-7 (A) Tibial varum and cant. **(B)** Tibial valgum and cant. (From Subotnick SI: Foot orthoses in ski boots. Physician Sports Med 10: 61, 1982, with permission.)

Tibial Varum

Tibial varum (Fig. 30-7) is a result of an uncompensated varus deformity of the tibia, which transmits instantaneously to the ski–snow interface and causes the skier to ride excessively on the outside edge of the ski. When a skier has more than 8 to 10 degrees of tibial varum deformity, he or she will have a great deal of difficulty initiating a parallel turn without "catching" the outside edge. In order to accomplish a successful turn, the skier will have to roll the legs back and forth, jump, or "stem" in order to unlock the outside edge. Outside ski edging is often associated with tips being crossed, which eventually leads to sudden falls. In cases of uncompensated tibial varum, it is difficult for the skier to continue to ride a "flat" ski, particularly in the tuck position (Fig. 30-8).

When the skier uses all the pronatory motion at the subtalar and midtarsal joints in order to flatten the foot to the ground, the lower leg may need to be pronated further by internal rotation and increased valgus at the knee, in order to ski effectively. This can result in additional strain and fatigue, which can lead to a "wandering" ski and poor edge control. With the foot maximally pronated in the boot, abnormal boot pressure occurs along the lateral mal-

leolus, which has a tendency to migrate posteriorly when the foot is maximally pronated and dorsiflexed. In addition, strain along the medial longitudinal arch (abductor hallucis, medial band plantar fascia), as well as the gastrocnemius–soleus musculature of the posterior leg, particularly the Achilles tendon, may result from functioning in this extended pronatory position.

Most current overlap high-performance boots provide a boot cuff adjustment to accommodate varying degrees of tibial varum and create a flat ski surface. The nonadjustable boots have a preset angle predetermined for the average skier; thus the individual skier is unable to adjust for varying degree of the tibial varum seen in the lower extremity. It should be noted that men typically have a greater degree of tibial varum than women. As a result, the cuff angle found on men's boots allows for this variance.

Correction of tibial varum can easily be accomplished by aligning the skier's leg to his or her normal skiing position, with the ankles dorsiflexed, feet apart, and knees and hips flexed. When standing in a relaxed position, with both feet together, most skiers have a higher degree of tibial varum than in their normal skier stance position (Fig. 30-9).

The simplest, most reliable method to treat excessive

tibial varum is to use a full-length, canted, in-boot foot orthosis. The canted wedges used in the past to control excessive tibial varum have been replaced by full-length foot orthoses since 1985. External plastic cants placed between the boot and the ski were effective in controlling tibial varum but led to overcontrol as well as catching of the outside edge. They also proved somewhat cumbersome, were expensive to install, were nonadjustable, and could interfere with effective binding release capability. In contrast, full-length foot orthoses have the advantage of providing for total foot contact within the boot, correcting for biomechanical imbalances within the foot, and providing comfort as well as reliable, effective edge control[21] Today, with the improved design changes in boots, canting is only utilized in extreme tibial varum conditions or in the case of limb length discrepancies.

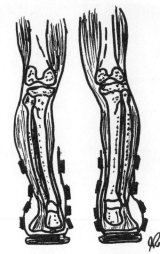

Figure 30-9 Tibial varum measurement. The skier is standing in the bent-knee functional skiing position. With the inner boot removed, note the close approximation of the lateral aspects of the lower legs, and the gaps in the boots medially. Before correcting this malalignment, an orthotic must be placed on the base board of the boot.

Figure 30-8 Uncompensated tibial varum, with inadequate boot control, leading to difficulty in riding a "flat" ski in the tuck position. Note the tendency for the skier to ride on the outside edge.

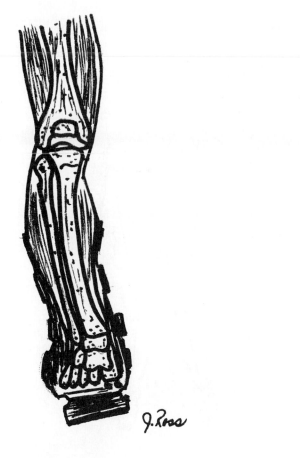

Correction of tibial varum is accomplished by aligning the boot cuff with the skier standing on his or her foot bed with the inner boot liner removed, and standing with the knees flexed and apart, assuming the skier's position. By dropping a plumb bob down from the center of the knee, the boot fitter or sports physician can measure the angle of deviation of the boot's shaft. The boot cuff is then aligned by placing a wedge under the boot, thus moving the skier's knee between the first and second metatarsal. This method, referred to as *leveling*, is used to align the boot cuff parallel to the long axis of the lower leg. A second method, *filling in*, has the skier stand on a device such as the Neuman Canting Machine or the P.K. device. The machine allows for the boot's sole to tilt medially or laterally, in order for the skier's knee to be aligned between the first and second metatarsal. In both cases, after proper canting, the boot rests at an angle slightly less than 90 degrees on the ski (Fig. 30-10).

Tibial Valgum

Tibial valgum, or genu valgum of the knees, results in an excessive inside ski edging, which results in a decrease in uphill ski control and catching an edge on flat terrain.

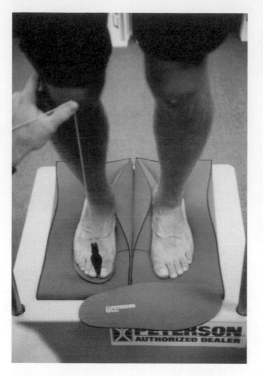

Figure 30–10 The Neuman Canting Machine.

This lower leg abnormality is not seen as often as tibial varum. Tibial valgum is often associated with coxa vara–genu valgum at the knee, pronated feet, and excessive anteversion. Correction of excessive foot pronation decreases the amount of coxa vara–genu valgum and brings the tibia to a more perpendicular position, thereby eliminating the need for cants.

In most instances the use of an orthosis is sufficient. However, when excessive tibial valgum is present, as was the case in tibial varum, and a foot orthosis is not able to control the improper knee–lower leg alignment, a cant may be necessary to correct the remaining malalignment. This will help to prevent excessive internal femoral rotation and valgus stress at the knee, which ultimately can result in patellar tracking and patellofemoral joint syndrome pain. Excessive tibial valgum can also lead to increased medial collateral ligament strain of the knee, and even result in increased injury during a fall.

Subtalar Varus

Rearfoot varus as compared to tibial varum may not be evident in the skier's static position, but rather appears only when he or she is engaged in dynamic skiing. Rearfoot varus is associated with pronatory compensation and leads to the same problems encountered with tibial varum (Fig. 30–11). In the case of a perfect foot, the rearfoot and forefoot are perfectly aligned and perpendicular to the long axis of the tibia. With the foot weight bearing in the boot, the subtalar varus foot will assume a pronated position, characterized by ankle eversion, abduction, and dorsiflexion.[22] Skiers who have a predisposition to pronation could be subject to increased instability, particularly if compounded by a marked tibial varum angle.

Excessive pronation in the skier as a result of excessive subtalar varus may be seen with collapse of the longitudinal arch, particularly when the overlap buckles of the boot are tightened. With the need for ankle eversion, an increased amount of pressure will be focused on the inside edge of the ski and the medial column of the foot. When the skier is unable to compensate for this excessive pronation and tibial rotation, he or she will be forced to push the medial aspect of the knee excessively in order to maintain control of the ski edge. It is clear that the higher degree of subtalar varus will translate into a greater medial knee pressure and

Figure 30–11 Compensation for varus subtalar joint with internal rotation. (From Subotnick SI: Appendix 3: The biomechanical basis of skiing. In Subotnick SI (ed): Podiatric Sports Medicine. Futura, Mt. Kisco, NY, 1975, with permission.)

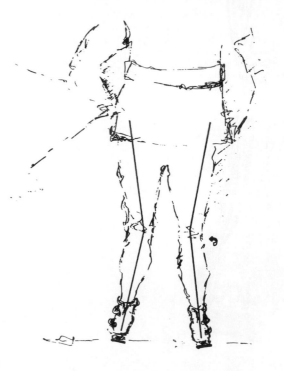

increased pressure to the medial column of the foot. In addition, skiers with excessive pronation will have difficulty with technique, and will present with a number of clinical entities.

One of those clinical entities is cramping. As a result of excessive pronation, and in an attempt to stabilize the foot in the boot, skiers will commonly adjust their buckles and tighten down on them exceedingly. It may indeed give the skier a "tighter fit"; however, it will usually push down on the dorsal arch and compress the longitudinal arch. This excessive tightening of the boot may lead to compromised circulation to the foot, which can lead to a cramped and cold foot. In addition, this may also cause undue amounts of pressure on protruding bony areas of the foot (i.e., bunions, tailor's bunions, hammertoes) and retrocalcaneal heel areas.

In order to compensate for subtalar varus and rearfoot imbalance, a medial varus rearfoot posting is utilized. This will provide stability for the subtalar and midtarsal joints by creating support for both the heel and the longitudinal arch. The forefoot balancing is considered separately. With this full-length orthosis, the amount of valgus movement and medial boot pressure is drastically reduced, thus providing more efficient skiing style and improved edge control. In addition, the medial wedge rearfoot posting will help to eliminate pressure points, particularly overlying the medial malleolus and navicular.

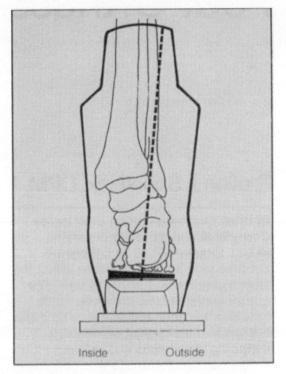

Figure 30-12 Forefoot varum controlled with an in-shoe post. (From Subotnick SI: Foot orthoses in ski boots. Physician Sports Med 10:61, 1982, with permission.)

Forefoot Varum

Forefoot varum can create problems similar to those seen in subtalar varus (see Fig. 30-7). To compensate for this forefoot imbalance, the foot must evert, thus reducing the available pronation necessary for efficient edging. When excessive forefoot pronation occurs, this may cause arch fatigue and/or cramping. In addition, other common complaints are strain of the medial band of the plantar fascia, which can result in plantar fasciitis or an abductor myositis. To compound the problem with excessive forefoot pronation, the forefoot abducts on the rearfoot, creating a transverse plane deformity; consequently, a tailor's bunion deformity or fifth digit hammertoe condition may be aggravated. As a result of this forefoot imbalance, associated pathology of the hallux nail may occur as a result of abnormal rotation. The nail may strike the upper part of the ski boot, resulting in a subungual hematoma, or strike the adjacent second digit and create an ingrown toenail.

Proper forefoot varus control in skiing is obtained using a full-length orthosis (Fig. 30-12). An orthosis to the metatarsal heads is not sufficient because forefoot posting is required, which may be uncomfortable under the distal edge of the device. The device can be made from an in-boot casting. This cast is posted or balanced to provide for appropriate rearfoot and forefoot neutral control when the skier assumes the functional downhill skiing position with the feet parallel. A vertical plumb bob line is dropped from the midpoint of the patella, and should drop to the vicinity of the second metatarsal. Occasionally, if the forefoot correction is inadequate, thin wedges may be necessary under the medial forefoot of the orthosis. If the skier feels the additional stability, then there was inadequate forefoot posting. Conversely, if the forefoot is overcorrected, the vertical line will fall more laterally, and the skier will feel a tilting of both the foot and the knees to the outside of the boot. It is imperative not to overuse rearfoot posts inasmuch as they may cause the heel to ride too high in the boot, causing a boot fit problem and/or irritation at the posterior aspect of the heel. Overcorrection of the rearfoot will lead to problems with outside edge control.

In skiing, particular attention should be focused on edge control, as with multidirectional sports, in that the sports practitioner should never overcorrect in the direction of varus.

Forefoot Valgum

Another entity that can have an influence on skiing technique and forefoot complaints is a forefoot valgus. This condition is usually secondary to a plantar-flexed first ray or a total forefoot cavus deformity. It may also be associated with a cocked hallux hammertoe, which can cause irritation of both the hallux interphalangeal joint and the hallux nail. This requires ski-boot toebox modification to allow for appropriate room. Another condition that can develop in a compressed ski boot is sesamoiditis. Because of the plantar-flexed first ray and squeezing of the forefoot shell, compression of the sesamoid apparatus can occur. This will cause pain on every occasion when the skier downweights and applies pressure to the first metatarsal head. In addition, lateral pressure from the boot can cause irritation on a prominent styloid process of the fifth metatarsal base. A forefoot valgus will produce a greater tendency to lateral strains of the foot, ankle, leg, and knee. This is in contradistinction to forefoot varus and/or tibial varum, which cause medial strain. Approximately 20 to 25 percent of the population has a forefoot valgus or cavus foot. Because of the cavus foot type, and the peroneal spasm occurring during skiing, a calcanocuboid joint syndrome with peroneal tendinitis also may occur.

Compensation for forefoot valgus or cavus foot occurs by inversion of the foot. This creates external rotation of the leg with excessive lateral ski and boot pressure. This biomechanical deformity is corrected with a full-length, in-boot, semiflexible orthosis, balancing the lateral aspect of the forefoot while accommodating the plantar-flexed first metatarsal. A forefoot valgus post is utilized for balancing of the first metatarsal ray, and to prevent undue amounts of pressure beneath the metatarsal head and sesamoid apparatus. In addition, the pressure points where the ski boot overlies bony prominences are treated with boot modification by either the boot technician or the sports physician. A heat gun together with a hydraulic pressure ball are used to soften and "blow out the shell" of the toebox of the boot, permitting formation of accommodative pockets for bony prominences.

A high-arched foot with pain secondary to dorsal arch boot pressure may be treated by moving the buckles on the boot, choosing a larger volume boot, or selecting a rear-entry boot. A dorsal exostosis of the first metatarsal–cuneiform joint in the cavus foot is similarly treated by moving buckles or by modifying the exterior shell of the boot to this bony prominence. In addition, one can remove the insole and utilize an orthosis or rearfoot/forefoot wedge. A heel lift, adding foam to "float" the bump, is also very helpful. Failure to accommodate for the high-arched foot or bony prominences may lead to nerve compression, tendinitis, or bursitis.

Transverse Plane Asymmetry

Transverse plane asymmetry may be caused by soft tissue and/or bony restrictions in the hip joints. Excessive anteversion is demonstrated by greater internal rotation of one leg and foot than the other. Internal tibial torsion, demonstrated by an in-toed gait, can cause excessive strain of the internal hip rotator muscles as well as an imbalance, making parallel skiing quite difficult. This transverse plane motion of the foot/boot can enhance crossing of the ski tips. Skiers are advised to participate in a preseason stretching and conditioning program in order to increase external rotation at the hip joint. Ballet, roller skating, and ice skating will help to develop these muscle groups, particularly in younger skiers. Excessive pronation is also associated with excessive internal rotation of the lower extremities, as well as metatarsus adductus, and can be treated with a prescription orthosis.

Winter and Lafferty[23] noted that internal tibial torsion is a functional disadvantage of the would-be parallel skier because compensating for it by external rotation of the feet can result in excessive weight over the outside ski edge. Another method of compensation for this condition is to hop turn or stem from ski to ski. The parallel skiing method is difficult to perform because the sagittal axis of the body lies medial to the foot, resulting in overpronation of the foot and loss of inside edge control.

Limb Length Discrepancies

Anatomic limb length discrepancies are a result of the overgrowth or undergrowth of long bones. Functional limb length discrepancies develop from a malpositioning of the various joints of the lower extremity. In some cases a shortening or overpowering of a muscle group(s) of one limb over the contralateral side may cause a functional limb length discrepancy. Another example is that of a foot that is more pronated than the other, creating a functional limb length discrepancy as well as a lateral pelvic tilt. In this case the skier will typically abduct and pronate the foot on the short leg side, thereby losing inside edge control and thus making it difficult to turn in the direction of the long leg.

Limb length discrepancy is usually not a problem on steep terrain or in mogul situations. However, when skiing on flat terrain, an unevenness of the two limbs can develop into a dangerous situation. Skiers with limb length imbalance of the lower extremity who had no difficulty with steep challenging terrain may be at greater risk at the end of this difficult run when they relax, having reached easy flat terrain. Often the skier will inadvertently catch an inside edge in this scenario, when he or she least expects it.

Keeping in mind that using a heel lift for skiing or other sports when only a functional limb length discrepancy is present may cause unilateral weakness of the involved extremity, it is recommended that cases where an anatomic difference of 3/8 inch or more is present be the only time that a heel lift is utilized for the shorter leg. In cases where both an anatomic and a functional limb length abnormality is present, it is usually necessary to add functional orthoses to the heel lift, as well as other appropriate care of the spine or feet. Ski boots can usually accommodate a heel lift fabricated onto an in-boot orthosis up to 1/4 inch. A lift over 1/4 inch is placed as a wedge within the midsole of the boot. In general, the full deficiency is corrected at the rearfoot, one-half at the metatarsal head level and one-fourth at the toe level. The same formula is used for other multidirectional sports, including running sports. An example of this formula would be a 1-inch lift at the heel of a ski boot with a 1/2-inch lift under the metatarsal heads and a 1/4-inch lift under the toes. An in-boot orthosis with a 1/4-inch heel lift would have a 1/8-inch lift under the ball of the foot with a 1/16-inch lift under the toes. This allows for a better forward lean position of the lower leg shin in the boot and a more natural skiing style.

Ski Boots

Ski boots have always been the center of attention concerning comfort, fit, and performance. The standard phrase for years among skiers has been, "My boots are killing me!" Quite often we have heard the common complaint that ski boots were cold, tight, and irritating, and that skiers could not wait to loosen them or to take them off completely.

After years of technological advances, ski boots now fit better, feel better, and perform better. Designing a ski boot that has all of these characteristics has become a challenge to the manufacturers and boot fitters (technicians). In fact, fitting a boot has become such a science that specialty boot-fitting shops have sprung up at ski resorts nationwide. The reason, simply, is that the human foot is not the same for everyone. Because of its dynamic nature, foot morphology changes subtly every few years. A foot that appeared normal 10 years ago may now have developed a bunion, hammertoe, or plantar-flexed metatarsal with callus formation. These are all new considerations to factor into when determining the right boot for the skier.

This is where the experts come in. Providing skiers with the best boot it takes a knowledgeable ski-boot fitter and a sports medicine physician who understand boot design and skiing performance, and who can solve imbalances of the lower extremity and accommodate for bony prominences. It is imperative that the sports physician have a working relationship with the boot shop and fitter. With the benefit of these two experts' knowledge and under their guidance, skiers can now ski much more comfortably rather than in the pain to which they were accustomed.

Performance is another important consideration in the design and selection of a ski boot. Now that forward-entry, traditional design, and mid-entry boots have become more comfortable and provide much better performance, ski boot companies have placed more emphasis on performance than convenience. Since its introduction in the 1970s, the rear-entry boot design has just about become extinct in the racing performance category. Even the traditional rear-entry companies have gone to an overlap high-performance design. Now, most companies have expanded the overlap design from the performance level to the all-terrain boot level. Overlap ski boot designs continue to make their impact on the boot market. The mid-entry hybrids that had become popular over recent years have seen that appeal wane. The rear-entry boots continue to see their appeal and demand plummet.

Rear-entry boots, which became an overnight success in the 1980s, had a number of advantages over the traditional overlap forward-entry design. The single most important feature was the ease of entry and exit. Because of the boot's one-piece construction, the skier was able to achieve a better, more uniform tightening or loosening of the boot. The next most important characteristic was warmth. Since 1985, the "heat for the feet" designs by Lange, Caber, and Raichle have incorporated a battery pack in the back of the boot, which produced enough current to supply a printed-circuit heater with a couple of minutes of power whenever the toes began to tingle or feel numb. A third advantage of the rear-entry boot was the ease of fit, better known as the "pillow fit." Compared to the conventional overlapping shell, which closes around the foot, usually with a three-, four-, or five-buckle system, the rear-entry one-piece unit has more room and fewer "pressure points" because there is more air space between the shell and foot.

Ski boots have become biomechanically sophisticated. There are many adjustable features, taking into account the biomechanics of skiing and the individual biomechanical requirements of the skier. Some of these features are internal versus external canting systems, adjustable "spoilers" or shaft angle adjustments, boot flex, forward lean, internal/external heaters, and custom heat-moldable liners made of ethyl vinyl acetate (EVA). Side cuts continue to gain attention by providing a soft overflex, particularly on the outside part of the boot (Fig. 30-13). For those skiers whose feet get cold easily, a rear-positioned "heater" may be necessary. Heater coils travel from the shaft of the boot down below the foot bed and provide much-needed heat to the ball of the foot and the toe area.

Figure 30-13 Ski boot with side cuts.

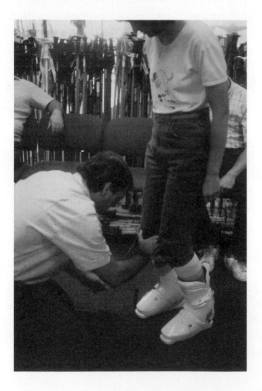

Boot measuring has also improved in the last decade. The Salomon rear-entry was the first boot that measured the foot by volume, based on a measurement of instep girth (HIP, or heel, Instep, perimeter) combined with foot length. By using a volume fit, one can assume that the foot will be drawn closer to the shell as the boot is tightened. This provides a more sensitive contact between boot and ski, thus improving performance.

Ski boots are made of a plastic shell that does not bend. In general, the more expensive the boot, the stiffer it is. However, more expensive boots usually have more adjustable features, such as an adjustable lean, double-plane adjustable canting, and forward lean tension adjustment. The rearboot, when preferable, eliminates buckles over the dorsum of the foot and particular a high instep, while providing for a comfortable, snug fit of the foot within the boot. Tradition forward entry overlap designs allow for more adjustments over the dorsum of the foot and fit close to the foot anatomically.

Beginning (novice) and recreational skiers of average or below-average ability often make the mistake of buying ski boots that are more expensive and stiffer than necessary. These boots accentuate forward lean and are too stiff for novices. Determining boot flex depends on the skier's ability and strength. Adjusting the boot's flex changes the amount of motion of the foot in the boot, as well as its flexibility and strength. To determine how much flex in the boot is correct, there are several factors to be considered: (1) what type of terrain and snow conditions are encountered, (2) how much energy and response is needed, and (3) the amount of leverage to the ski that is needed. The amount of flex is strictly an individual consideration.

The forward lean adjustment affects comfort as well as performance. In rear-entry boots, the forward lean is established by the front cuff. In the conventional forward entry boot, it is the opposite. Forward lean also affects the leverage to the ski. This in turn affects positioning in the turn, radius of the turn, pressure anteriorly, and energy and glide. Again, snow conditions can also determine how much forward lean is needed. By changing the forward lean angle, one can reduce or even eliminate the anterior shin discomfort that, in a ski survey conducted by Ross,[24] proved to be the most common skier's complaint about boots. Another important point is that attempting longer radius turns takes more energy from the tip of the ski to the tails, which requires more forward lean angle in the boot. A shorter radius turn does not require as much energy in the ski; therefore, the skier will be in a more upright position, thus requiring less forward lean. Stiffer boots with increased forward lean are more appropriate for advanced to expert skiers, who have developed skiing techniques comparable to the sophistication of their boots.

A stiff ski boot, particularly in the overlap performance designs, does not permit normal compensatory motion within the midtarsal and subtalar joints of the foot, and places additional stress upon the knee and hip. When this boot design is used, an orthosis can provide for neutral foot control within the ski boot if imbalances are present. Because every foot is different, custom-made semiflexible thermoplastic orthoses provide the best results. These devices are full length with a sulcus ridge, to increase the proprioception of the toes while allowing for accommodation of metatarsal heads plantarly (Fig. 30-14).

Most ski boots have removable foot beds that may be replaced with custom-made orthoses. Two of the pioneering orthoses in the skiing field, Peterson and Superfeet, use a semi-weight-bearing molding process, seeking neutral position. The Peterson approach uses a knee stabilizer apparatus built into the platform to accurately align the knee over the foot for complete lower body correction. Knee angulation is the key to performance skiing, and proper

Figure 30-14 Ski boot with semirigid orthosis.

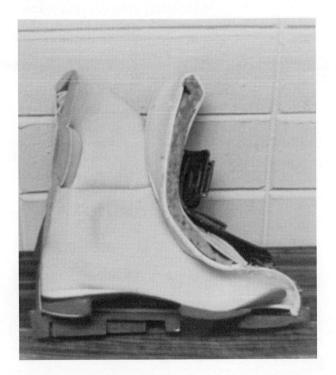

knee–foot alignment (relationship) is just as important as seeking subtalar joint neutral position. The Peterson device is similar to an impression-made sporthotic (skithotic)-type device. The Superfeet orthotic, as is the Peterson, is made at the ski shop or at the ski area, and is composed of a single-density, rigid yet flexible Birkenstock cork, covered with a moisture-protective nylon. The traditional orthosis tends to function better in a ski boot when made from an in-boot cast, with the skier assuming a neutral ski stance position. The difference between a prescription orthosis and a custom insole is the amount of correction and stability in the rearfoot, subtalar joint, midtarsal joint, and forefoot. This control of excessive supination/pronation and locking of the midtarsal joint (stability) will result in better edging and increased performance.

Problem Areas in Boots

As Killham noted, there are various sections to the ski boot that are referred to as "zones of fit"[25]:

Zone One: The Foot Bed—The foot must be balanced well on a good foot bed, whether it be the boot's bed or an extrinsic orthosis. Without this proper balance or "alignment," edging problems or cramping of the foot could occur. Rearfoot or forefoot (wedging) can correct these imbalances.

Zone Two: The Tongue—The tongue fills the void between the leg and foot in the anterior portion of the boot. It should apply an even amount of pressure over the shin and instep, while it pushes the foot down into the boot and back against the heel. Without the ability for the instep to move up and forward, the heel will be unable to lift upward.

Zone Three: The Hindfoot—The shape and volume of the sides of the shell control lateral ankle motion and edging. Without proper hold and contact between boot and ankle, there will be too much side-to-side motion. An EVA heat-set foam liner or silicon-injected foam versus the flow boot, would fill the void better and prevent this excessive motion.

Zone Four: The Shaft—Proper fit and contact provides better edging and control. When the knees are driven forward with flex, the better the fit, the less distortion will be seen.

Zone Five: The Forefoot—Forefoot balance is a must, particularly in cases of forefoot varus.

The variety of clinical conditions that can produce problems in skiing, have many possible solutions related to each of the zones of fit. For example, a loose forefoot could be the result of a narrow foot; one should check for excessive pronation or a sock that needs to be thicker. A compressed foot may be due to a wide foot, bunion formation, or possibly an interdigital (metatarsal) neuroma. Shell modification, a thinner sock, or forefoot balancing (orthosis) could solve this problem. A tailor's bunion or enlarged fifth metatarsal resulting from forefoot supination could cause pain and compression. A forefoot varus wedge, orthosis, foam remodeling, and possible boot modification are the cure. For numbness or burning in the forefoot resulting from a high "instep," or plantar-flexed first or fifth metatarsal (sesamoiditis), a custom insole or orthotic device is necessary. A painful foot flexing angle can be seen in the case of a hypertrophied or overactive anterior tibial or extensor hallucis longus tendon overlying the anterior ankle. Other causes might be the front cable, a high instep, or setting the flex too tightly. Adding foam, correcting the flex setting, or remove foam from the tendon areas are various possible solutions. A dorsal metatarsal–cuneiform exostosis may result from excessive bone growth and/or chronic irritation, as well as a hypermobile first ray. To correct for this problem, the insole is removed and an orthosis or rearfoot/forefoot varus wedge is inserted. Also, a heel lift and foam to "float" the bump are added and the exterior shell is heated and modified.

A painful medial/lateral malleolus can result from either too narrow or too wide (prominent ankle bones) an ankle. For a narrow ankle, a donut and foam sides can be added to the inner boot and a varus wedge shim (horseshoe) to the heel. For the large ankle, grinding and slitting the inner boot is helpful. The prominent navicular is due to excessive pronation and malposition of the posterior tibial tendon. An orthotic device or custom insole with a proper rearfoot varus wedge is essential. Adding foam to the inner boot to floating the bump and grinding with padding will help. A Haglund's deformity, or retrocalcaneal exostosis, is due to a varus heel, supinated subtalar joint, and irritation posteriorly. A rearfoot varus wedge, orthosis, foam (sheet), and a cut out (moon) around the prominent area are indicated. A painful boot top at the upper and lower shin is due to poor leg alignment and improper pressure distribution. A sharp anterior tibial tendon is occasionally seen. To help resolve this problem, one must change the forward lean of the boot, add a heel lift, create a tunnel for the tibia, and check for tightness of the buckles or lower leg cable. Pain in the posterior boot top calf region is seen

with a large calf girth or lower calf muscle. Adding a heel lift, cutting away foam from the back spoiler pad, and sometimes taking away from the front inner boot will help. Pressure from the lateral boot top is due to a tibial varum, uneven pressure (buckle or cable) distribution, or a pronounced peroneal tendon. Readjusting the lateral cant and adding a rearfoot varus wedge and a lateral wedge shim with a sheet of foam will help to alleviate this pain.

With the advent of forward lean angles, the boot spoiler has been responsible for the rise in anterior cruciate ligament tears, pushing the number of (an incidence that had been consistently 20 percent is currently up to 24 percent). Ankle injuries have nearly disappeared; however, an improperly fitted boot or design can still result in an ankle injury. Tibial spiral fractures have been reduced significantly, but old or incompatible equipment can result in this injury. A properly fitted and well-designed boot can reduce rotational injuries to the lower leg.

A boot that fits too snugly or cramps down on the posterior calf muscles can cause decreased blood flow, and may result in frostbite or numb toes. By definition, frostbite is the result of thermal trauma to a part of the body caused by excessive or prolonged exposure to severe cold. If the exposure is sufficiently severe, and with duration, actual freezing of the tissues may be produced. Because the extremities have little muscle mass and low resting heat production, they have a lower mean resting skin temperature, unlike skin covering areas of high resting heat production, which have high skin temperatures. Therefore, the extremities will more easily suffer cold injury.

Casting for In-Boot Ski Orthoses

When casting for ski orthoses, an in-boot cast allows for functional orthosis fabrication. After application of the plaster, a plastic bag is placed over the foot, which is then placed within the boot. The leg and foot are held in a neutral position while the skier applies moderate downward pressure. This ensures a proper fit of the orthosis within the boot and offers control necessary when the athlete is in a neutral position (Fig. 30-15). This forward lean with the casting technique also enables the medial longitudinal arch and medial plantar fascia to depress the plaster cast material, allowing for intrinsic accommodation during fabrication of the orthosis to ensure that the skier patient will not develop medial pressure, resulting in a medial plantar fasciitis, from the orthosis.

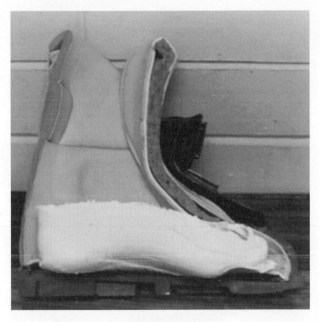

Figure 30-15 Ski boot with negative cast.

Cants

A cant is a wedge of plastic with a low coefficient of friction that fits between the bottom of the boot and the ski. Whereas cants were popular during the 1970s, their popularity dwindled during the 1980s, but they have seen a resurgence in the form of boot soles with 1-,2-,3-, or 4-degree positive or negative cants or in the Dalebout, an interchangeable canted sole that snaps onto the bottom of the boots. Many ski coaches prefer that their ski racers use in-boot orthoses and slightly overcompensate for mild varus imbalances in the legs and feet. Cants are also less popular because of the adjustable canting found within many ski boots. Only two boot companies use sole canting, whereas many skiers use cuff adjustment systems. Several types of cuff adjustment systems that move the cuff, or part of the cuff, medially or laterally are available.[26] It has been shown that cuff adjustment systems that move the rear and front cuffs provide for more correction than do the systems that move only one cuff. It is important to move the cuff properly to follow the lower extremity outline, providing a shorter distance for the skier's leg to move in order to get on edge. Skier's who have formed a bad habit of compensating for their malalignment will be forced to push the knees inward, thus developing a more knock-kneed attitude in order to get their skis on the inside edge.

The internal cant mechanism corrects for abnormalities of the lateral angle of the skier's leg. This type of adjustment permits the skier to keep the skis flat when in neutral stance. An example of this adjustment would be the "spoiler" or shaft angle adjustment (Fig. 30-16). The spoiler can be adjusted to one of any three positions: 2.5 degrees, 4.0 degrees, and 5.5 degrees of lateral cant. If a skier is having difficulty with edging and obtaining a flat ski surface, then the sports physician or ski shop boot technician should do one of the following:

1. Determine if the foot is in neutral position. If the skier has difficulty getting on the inside edge, a rearfoot varus wedge orthosis or supportive foot bed will help.
2. If the skier is catching the outside edge, increase the lateral cant setting.
3. If the skier is catching the inside edge, decrease the lateral cant setting.

An important factor to understand is that there is a two-vector relationship involved. The first vector is for correcting alignment. The hip-to-knee–knee-to-ski relationship should be 90 degrees, and is corrected with the cuff shaft adjustment. The second vector is the sole of the foot–ski relationship, corrected by orthosis or external canting wedge. Jackson Hogan of Ski Salomon boot company claims, "canting off the sole of the boot is more efficient than canting the shaft. This results in an efficiency in mo-

Figure 30-16 "Spoiler" or shaft angle adjustment.

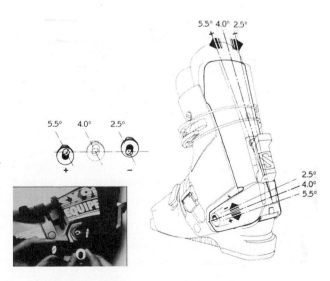

tion." It should be noted that 13 of the top 15 World Cup skiers in 1986-87 had their boots canted on the high side in relationship to the outside.

With the decrease in popularity of cants, there is a corresponding increase in the popularity of custom-made full-length orthoses for skiing. However, it should be understood that ski orthoses are designed for that sport, and, if they are used for other sports, problems may develop. Ski orthoses may provide excessive, ineffective control during running and may be inappropriate for multidirectional sports.

Witherell[13] identified several problems that may need a cant or orthosis:

1. Excessive wear of the outside edges of the heels of shoes
2. Inequality in ski edging when comparing the uphill with the downhill ski when standing across the hill
3. Inability to break the stemming habit, no matter how many lessons a skier has had
4. If the skier has to initiate a turn with a hop
5. When the skier leans excessively on the inside of a turn or depends too much on the outside ski
6. If there is a great difficulty in holding the heel on ice, despite excellent skis and boots
7. If a skier turns in one direction better than the other

The electronic cant machines of the 1970s and 1980s have been replaced by the highly technical and knowledgeable ski boot fitters. Many of these fitters have taken courses given by experts in the fields of biomechanics, anatomy, and boot design. Ski boot companies sponsor workshops before the ski season, in order to familiarize technicians with the design changes for the coming year. Sports podiatrists have contributed greatly to this education and sharing of information, which has created a meaningful relationship between the two specialties. This in turn has resulted in better service to the skiers.

One of the most reliable methods of determining the thickness of the cant or the amount of medial wedge on the ski orthosis is through the use of the goniometer to measure the amount of tibial varum present with the skier in a neutral parallel downhill position. Skiers should be measured with ski boots on and off, with knees slightly flexed in a normal parallel position and the boots buckled to normal tightness, standing on a firm surface. The amount of motion in a boot can then be evaluated. The neutral position is first evaluated barefooted, then later with the boot on. The actual varum deformity in the lower third of the leg is measured as shown in Figure 30-17. The

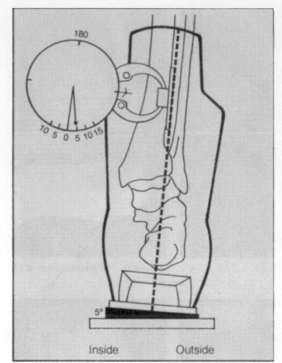

Figure 30-17 Measurement of tibial varum to determine the degree of cant needed. (From Subotnick SI: Foot orthoses in ski boots. Physician Sports Med 10:61, 1982, with permission.)

degree of deformity corresponds to the necessary degree of thickness of cant or the amount of varus wedge on the orthosis. This is easily translated by measuring the width of the ski, then determining the degree of varus control necessary. If the skier decides that a cant is needed, normally a commercially available #1 cant is used for tibial varum of 5 to 6 degrees, a #2 for 6 to 7 degrees, a #3 for 8 to 9 degrees, and a #4 for 9 to 10 degrees. It is always better to undercant because overcanting leads to excessive outside edge position.

COMPUTERIZED GAIT ANALYSIS IN SKIING

Computerized gait analysis utilizing the Electrodynogram by Langer can provide a documentation of the nature of the function between the foot and lower extremity in the ski boot. It also measures the intensity and duration of forces that occur throughout the feet. By using the computer readout of these measurements, the sports physician can determine the function in the boot and recommend stretching, changing inner soles, boot modification, or orthosis therapy. In severe cases where surgical intervention may be required, this information can help make that determination.

The computerized gait analysis adds a significant new dimension to skier evaluation, whereas before radiographic analysis and visualization were our only means of diagnosing a foot or leg problem. Today the EDG or updated F-Scan can literally put our eyes inside the skier's boot and on top of the skier's skis. The computer analysis can provide a documentation of the skier's foot and leg function in relation to snow (ground) surface, boot, and foot. We can plot the skier's performance on a time–pressure curve, then determine which particular areas of the foot bear normal versus abnormal amounts of weight, as well as which portions of the foot and ankle are functioning for either too long or too short a time in the ski (gait) cycle. This valuable information can be used to predict what types of problems a skier may encounter in the future, either with boot performance or with comfort.

On a skiing simulator and with the use of the gait analyzer, we can focus on the forces that are transmitted both from the rearfoot and the forefoot regions, which can be translated into up- and down-weighting and completion of turns. The resulting data can determine how a skier carries his or her body weight on specific areas of the foot, within the boot on the foot plate. Cases where elongated pronation and supination take place can be easily seen. When the heel is not making contact with the foot bed for a sufficient time, as in the case of tight hamstrings, gastrocnemius–soleus equinus, short Achilles tendon, or ankle block, once again computer analysis will detect this condition. In addition, we can predict if the skier is spending too much time propulsing on the toes and exhibiting excessive forward lean in the boot. A limb length difference can also be revealed with computer analysis.

The obvious benefactors of this information are the advanced intermediate or expert skier, racer, and professional. Improved performance and skiing technique are all benefits of this investigation. Correlations and integrations of the influences of the upper body to the lower extremity are constantly being discovered.

TREATMENT AND PREVENTION OF OVERUSE INJURY

Traumatic injuries to the lower extremities are a common problem faced in this risky sport. Knees have replaced ankles as the more common site involved. Increased boot cuff height has nearly eliminated ankle injuries and made boot-top tibia and fibula fractures a more typical injury, particularly in twisting, torquing falls. Failure of the ski bindings to release is the usual etiology behind knee and lower extremity injuries. The National Ski Patrol as well as ski shops technicians strongly recommend a binding release check before the ski season and again during the course of the season. Equipment checks of boots, skis, and bindings are essential to avoid unwarranted injuries. Worn-out ski boots and skis with poor camber as well as defective edges can decrease effective skiing technique and promote injury. Improperly fitted boots and poor biomechanics are all problems that be addressed by the boot technician and sports physician in preventing injury.

Most alpine ski injuries, however, occur as a result of fatigue. Improper preseason conditioning and poor muscle preparation are two other major reasons why skiers injure themselves. Lack of proper stretching and flexibility exercises is also a contributing factor. Muscle groups that are weak should be strengthened, and the skier should begin a properly guided strength and conditioning program. Opposing muscles groups that are weak or too tight need to be strengthened or stretched properly, to avoid overpowering of stronger muscle groups.

Initial treatment in all overuse injuries, particularly in downhill skiing, is the elimination or reduction of inflammation, or altering the underlying cause of the inflammation. The first steps are to apply cold to the injured part to help reduce the swelling and inflammation, rest the extremity until the pain has been reduced, apply compression to reduce the swelling, and elevate of the body part to reduce the fluid flow to the extremity. Better known as RICE, this initial treatment can greatly help to reduce pain, swelling, and long-term effects of the injury. Such immediate treatment can help avoid a delayed or permanent injury. In some cases immobilization may be necessary to put the injured part at rest. Physical therapy modalities, including nerve stimulation, whirlpool, ultrasound, iontophoresis, fluidotherapy, acupressure massage, and joint restoration, are all key elements in the rehabilitation of the injured skier. Prevention, however, is the key in reducing these overuse injuries.

CONCLUSION

Technical advances in research and development by the ski and ski boot companies have afforded the downhill skier a more comfortable and safer ski experience. The sports physician must be cognizant of the various problems that skiers face, whether biomechanical imbalances leading to poor ski technique or performance problems related to foot or boot-fit discomfort. Skier's complaints must be addressed with an understanding of lower extremity biomechanics related to skiing, boot design, and boot-fitting difficulties, as well as the interrelationship between a ski orthosis and the boot in which in rests. It is important for the sports practitioner to understand that catching edges, difficulty initiating and completing turns, crossing tips or tails, and pressure points and cramping from boots may all be symptoms of an underlying biomechanical condition. Each year boots and equipment change, and it is imperative that the sports physician keep abreast of new designs and technology. In many cases boot modifications will be necessary, and ski shop owners and their boot technicians will welcome the sports physician's experience, expertise, and assistance. The skier with foot problems should always present to the sports physician's office with the ski boots, as do runners with their running shoes.

A Comparison of Alpine and Cross-Country Skiing
JEFFREY A. ROSS

The obvious reasons for the popularity of cross-country skiing in the United States is that, as the fitness craze has taken root, Americans have discovered another exercise activity for participants of all ages that provides some of the best cardiovascular activities available. According to Elson,[27] 1 hour of cross-country skiing is equivalent to 2 hours of downhill skiing, 2–12 hours of tennis, or 4 hours of cycling at 5.5 mph. This endurance sport is an excellent means by which upper as well as lower body development can be achieved. Only swimming accomplishes as much of an even development of the muscular groups with aerobic effects. This sport can be used as a safe cross-training activity for runners, particularly in cases where underdeveloped anterior muscle groups (quadriceps and anterior tibial muscles) are surpassed by overdeveloped posterior groups (hamstrings and gastrocnemius–soleus). One can participate in cross-country skiing for a fraction of the cost of downhill skiing, and can participate almost anywhere. As in Europe, cross-country skiing is used as a means of transportation in addition to its exercise benefits. When runners are unable to participate in their sport because of inclement weather conditions, ski touring can provide the same exercise advantages, and concomitantly work those muscle groups in a much more even fashion. Many skiers have begun to cross-country ski as an alternative or adjunct to traditional downhill skiing.

Unlike Alpine skiing, cross-country skiing has a different technique, as well as application. In downhill skiing, the heel and lower leg are locked in a rigid boot, lending control to the foot's rearfoot complex. In addition, the skis rarely deviate from directly underneath the body's center of mass, and the downhill position is such that a close parallel location of the skis is a constant. In downhill skiing the body's center of mass is located directly over the rearfoot complex (subtalar joint) and, with properly aligned joint compressional forces, rearfoot neutrality is maintained.

In comparison, cross-country skiing involves a heel that is repeatedly lifted from the ski surface and lowered again, allowing for skier imbalance. The classical technique for cross-country skiing is what is commonly referred to as a swing kick and glide. Utilizing the poles to create upper body stability and propulsion, the heel is kicked upward to maintain the forward motion, with a forefoot propulsion on the ski. A smooth alternating gliding motion is accomplished with a technique known as the diagonal stride. By alternating the opposite arm and leg forward, a ski gait is created similar to walking and jogging.[28] Analogous to running, as the pace increases, the forward lean of the body over the skis will increase. This will then produce a swing-phase ski that, as it touches the snow, will slide forward in a motion known as the "glide." The opposite-sided ski, known also as the stance phase ski, will press down into the snow under full pressure, thus creating a stable platform in which a plant and push-off will occur.

The velocity of the diagonal stride is affected by three factors: stride length, stride rate, and horizontal skier velocity. Stride length pertains to how far a cross-country skier can kick and then glide. According to Duoos-Asche, the stride length is one of the most important factors in increased skier velocity. The number of kicks and glides performed in a certain time frame, also known as the stride rate, also has a bearing on the velocity, but to a lesser degree than the stride length. The horizontal skier velocity is the total forward velocity achieved from stride length and stride rate. Among racers and those cross-country skiers who want to achieve maximum energy efficiency, achieving the greatest stride length and stride rate is the key.

Cross-country skis are quite different than downhill skis, with mid-ski widths of the average downhill ski approximately 2 ½ inches, whereas cross-country racing skis typically measure 1 ¾ inches in width. Considering the tremendous irregularities in snow terrain, the cross-country skier is in many respects like the ice skater, balancing on a single blade but not having the advantage of the ankle support seen with ice skates. The tenuous stability of the cross-country skier and greater potential for biomechanical imbalance allow the sports physician to have a significant impact on the skier's ability and performance.[29]

The ski equipment for cross-country skiing is exceptionally different. For the telemarker and backcountry skier, a ski that is comparable to the downhill ski is essential. These particular skis are much heavier than the traditional "in-track" cross-country skis. In addition, they have a metal edge to facillitate downhill performance, compared to the non-metallic-edged cross-country version. The weight in the tips of touring skis is much lighter, and the stiffness is much less. Moving toward the tour racing skis, the skis and tips become even lighter and the flexibility in the tips becomes even greater.

Cross-country boots are an intermediary between backcountry and racing boots in both design and support. There are the high-top styles that keep snow off the ankles in fresh powder, and there are the classical racing boots, which are cut much lower and are significantly lighter. Compared to traditional downhill ski boots, the touring boot has much less support yet much more freedom of movement. The touring skier does not need the stability for exaggerated turns, since cross-country skiing is a fairly unidirectional sport with moderate curves encountered. As a result of this flexibility, and lack of stability, the boot will accentuate the skier's biomechanical imbalances and, as a result, create malalignment of the lower extremity over the skis.

Biomechanical considerations for the cross-country skier are very similar to those for the downhill skier. Once again, proper alignment with the patellas focused directly over the skis in a bent-knee skiing position is essential. Bulky, rigid orthoses in cross-county boots are not recommended. Rather, a more flexible, lighter orthosis is preferred. Often a simpler way to accomplish these goals is to utilize wedges under the rear or forefoot. Often cutting away part of the insole of the boot will help to accommodate an orthosis with a forefoot extension. With respect to the cross-country boot, thinking thin is truly best.

Snowboarding
JEFFREY A. ROSS

This new variation of downhill skiing has made a big impact on the sport, and in the industry. This exciting winter sport, in which the snowboarder slaloms down a slope standing sideways on the board, resembles a cross between skiing and a skateboarding. Over the past 20 years, more ski areas now have provisions for snowboarders, and, with that, the concern for increased injury has become the new focus.

This winter version of skateboarding surfing has its risks, as does downhill skiing. It is not uncommon for snowboarders to fall quite often as a result of the exaggerated uphill edging that is required in this sport. Most injuries in this sport result from the falls that occurred, as well as striking obstacles or colliding with other skiers/boarders on the mountain.

According to Ganong et al.,[30] snowboarders sustain a wide variety of injuries: 44 percent upper extremity; 43 percent lower extremity; 12 percent head, spine, or torso; and 4 percent miscellaneous. The most common injury sites that Ganong et al. reported were the wrist (trauma and fractures), followed by the knee (sprains and ankle fractures). Upper extremity injuries frequently occur as a result of the forces transmitted to the upper extremity as the snowboarder falls with both legs fastened to the board. Without the independence of individual leg movement, the chance for recovery is much less than in downhill skiing.

Unlike downhill skiing, which involves the integration of foot, knee, and hip motion, snowboarding concentrates its energy on the hips and knees, because short pivoting turns are the norm. In adolescents, excessive hip rotation can be a source of irritation within the acetabulum. Impaction injury of the hip secondary to high snowboard jumping can lead to a potential avascular necrosis of the femoral head. Biomechanical balancing is just as important in snowboarding boots as it is in ski boots. With riding the board edge being as important as it is in this sport, it is essential that the foot be as neutral on the midsection of the board as possible.

Snowboarders wear a variety of boots; the most popular and earliest styles is the soft variety, with the full hard shell and half-shell being more recent designs. Typically, as with the evolution of the downhill ski boot, the soft boot will allow for a greater number of injuries compared to the other two. The soft boot injuries are predominantly seen in the ankles, whereas the more rigid full shell boots protect the ankles yet allow for more forces to be transmitted to the knees. This will result in more frequent knee injuries.

As the sport develops more interest, advanced technology will direct new shell designs with improved binding systems. With improved equipment, and biomechanical considerations, snowboarders will discover improved performance in a safer sport.

REFERENCES

Cross-Country Skiing

1. MacDougall JD, Hughson R, Sutton JR et al: The energy cost of cross-country skiing among elite competitors. Med Sci Sports Exerc 11:270, 1979
2. Boyle JJ, Johnson RJ, Pope MH et al: Cross-country skiing injuries. p. 411. In Johnson RJ, Mote CD Jr (eds): Skiing Trauma and Safety. Fifth International Symposium, ASTM STP 860. American Society for Testing and Materials, Philadelphia, 1985
3. Steinbruck K: Frequency and etiology of injury in cross-country skiing. J Sports Sci 5:187–196, 1987
4. Sherry E, Asquith J: Nordic (cross-country) skiing injuries in Australia. Med J Aust 146:245, 1987
5. Boyle JJ, Johnson RJ, Pope MH: Cross-country ski injuries: a prospective study. Iowa Orthop J 1:41, 1982
6. Westlin NE: Injuries in long distance, cross-country and downhill skiing. Orthop Clin North Am 7:558, 1976
7. Hemborg A, Edlund G, Gedda S: Skidskador: Jämtlands län 1977-en översikt. Läkartidningen 29:116, 1982
8. Orava S, Jaroma H, Hulkko A: Overuse injuries in cross-country skiing. Br J Sports Med 19:158, 1985
9. Orava S: Exertion injuries due to sports and physical exercise. Dissertation, Kokkola
10. Pierce J, Pope M, Renstrom P et al: Force during measurements in cross-country skiing. Int J Biomech 3:382, 1987
11. Parks RM: Biomechanics and technique analysis of classic and freestyle Nordic skiing. Clin Podiatr Med Surg 3:679, 1986
12. Gertsch P, Borqeat A, Wälli T: New cross-country skiing technique and compartment syndrome. Am J Sports Med 15:612, 1987

Alpine Skiing

13. Witherell W: If you can't ski parallel, cant. Skiing, January, 1977
14. Subotnick SI: Foot orthoses in ski boots. Physician Sports Med 10:61, 1982
15. Ross JA: Computerized gait analysis in skiing: The Electrodynogram and its use in the ski industry. Ski, 1985
16. Ross JA, Cohen S: If the boot fits you probably have a custom insole. Ski Oct: 184, 1984
17. Ross JA, Wernick J: Foot biomechanics in skiing: clinical study. Presentation at American Academy of Podiatric Sports Medicine, 1981
18. Trevino SG, Alvarez R: The spectrum of lower leg injuries in skiing. Clin Sports Med 1:263, 1982
19. Witherell W: How the Racers Ski. WW Norton, New York, 1972
20. Macintyre JG, Matheson GO: Clinical biomechanics of skiing. Can Fam Physician 34:107–114, 1988
21. Subotnick SI: The biomechanical basis of skiing: a preliminary report. 64, 1974
22. Jones SL, Bates BT, Osternig LR: Injuries to runners. Am J Sports Med 6:40, 1978
23. Winter WC Jr, Lafferty JF: The skiing sequelae of tibial torsion. Orthop Clin North Am 7:331, 1976

24. Ross JA: Ski boot pain survey, Ski Magazine, 1978–1980. Ski
25. Killham D: Ski Boot Technical Manual.
26. Lipton L: Correcting skier stance. Podiatry Today, Dec: 77, 1991

A Comparison of Alpine and Cross-Country Skiing

27. Elson PR: Ski bound? Ski Canada's 1978 Guide to Cross Country Skiing. 2nd ed.
28. Parks RM: Podiatric Sports Medicine Care for the Cross Country Skier. Presentation at American Academy of Podiatric Sports Medicine. Phoenix, AZ, May 1989
29. Palamarchuk H: Cross-country skiing. p 615. In Subotnick SI (ed): Sports Medicine of the Lower Extremity. Churchill Livingstone, New York, 1989

Snowboarding

30. Ganong RB, Heneveld EH, Beranek SR, Fry P: Snowboarding injuries: a report on 415 patients. Physician Sports Med 20:114, 1992

31

Basketball Injuries

PAUL M. TAYLOR
GARY GORDON
MICHAEL K. LOWE

Basketball is one of the most physically demanding sports; as a result, participants are subject to numerous injuries. In addition to the extensive running activity, basketball requires jumping, cutting, and periods of rapid acceleration. Although intended as a noncontact sport, there is obviously strenuous contact between players and occasionally between players and the floor.

The basketball player is subjected to stress in almost all parts of the body. The feet, ankles, and knees must absorb tremendous impact shock; the muscles and tendons are under constant loading forces; and the lower back is stressed by the hyperextension that occurs with shooting and rebounding. The shoulders also must endure stress through their full range of motion while passing, reaching for loose balls, and rebounding, and the body itself is subjected to contusions from elbows and collisions with other players.

Since the basketball player is subjected to this type of stress, it is not surprising that the incidence of injuries is high among these athletes. Persons responsible for their medical care must be able to recognize these potential injuries, assist with strengthening and stretching programs to prevent these injuries, treat the injuries as they occur, and help establish rehabilitation programs for rapid recovery from any injuries.

ACUTE AND OVERUSE INJURIES

Two basic types of injuries can occur: acute injuries and overuse injuries. Acute injuries are the sudden type of injury; the athlete is immediately aware that an injury has occurred. These are usually the more forceful type of injury, such as an ankle sprain or tendon rupture. The acute type of injury is generally obvious; it will require immediate treatment and will usually require that the athlete discontinue participation in the game. The overuse injury or overuse syndrome is a more subtle type of injury. It will develop more gradually and is caused by a low-grade stress, applied with many repetitions over a long period. Examples of the overuse injuries are patellar tendinitis or sesamoiditis, plantar fasciitis, and shin splints.

These types of injuries will require different treatment plans and will affect the level of participation of the athlete differently. The acute injury may require complete rest, whereas the overuse injury can be treated while the athlete continues to play or only reduces the level of activity. Occasionally, the type of injury may overlap. An overuse injury may develop into an acute injury, such as an Achilles tendinitis progressing to an Achilles tendon rupture. This is why it is important to recognize the different types of injuries and to establish an appropriate treatment plan.

BASIC TREATMENT PLAN

Whenever a basketball player sustains any type of injury, a basic treatment plan should be established that will protect the athlete from further injury, permit return to activity as soon as possible, and prevent the injury from recurring. The basic treatment plan can be divided into three

BASIC TREATMENT PLAN

1. Immediate treatment
   a. Diagnose the injury
   b. RICE (rest, ice, compression, elevation)
2. Continuing treatment
   a. Medication (pain, anti-inflammatory agents)
   b. Physical therapy and rehabilitation
3. Correction of any biomechanical problems
   a. Internal imbalance (muscle or structural)
   b. External imbalance (shoes, playing surface)

steps (see Box): (1) immediate treatment, (2) continuing treatment, and (3) correction of any biomechanical problems.

Immediate treatment consists of RICE (rest, ice, compression, and elevation). The amount of rest will vary depending on the degree of the injury. Ice can be used immediately after an acute injury to reduce swelling and pain or, with an overuse injury, after activity, again to reduce the swelling. Compression can range from a simple elastic bandage to a splint to immobilize an area after an acute injury. Elevating an injured area will also help minimize swelling. The amount of swelling should be controlled after an injury to reduce the time needed for recovery and rehabilitation.

The continuing treatment stage consists of steps to reduce pain and swelling and to rehabilitate the injured part to prevent future injury. The use of oral anti-inflammatory agents, ranging from aspirin to nonsteroidal anti-inflammatory drugs (NSAIDs), is indicated at this time. Physical therapy should be initiated with the goal of reducing any residual swelling, increasing range of motion, and strengthening the injured part.

The last step in the basic treatment plan is to correct any biomechanical imbalances. This would involve both internal and external factors. Internal factors include structural problems within the body, such as excessive pronation, a pes cavus foot type, or a tibia varum. It also includes muscle imbalances that occur in athletes when the demands of a particular sport create overdevelopment of certain muscle groups. External factors include shoes and playing surfaces. This basic approach to treating an injured athlete should be considered for each injury and then modified to meet the needs of the individual athlete.

The basic treatment plan will also have to be modified depending on the level of the player. A professional basket-

ball player will obviously require more intensive treatment then the casual or weekend athlete. A treatment plan for the casual athlete will emphasize longer periods of rest and a more gradual return to activity. The college or professional player will need to reduce the rest time and ensure a more rapid return to activity. This is accomplished through a more aggressive treatment plan. College or professional players will have a trainer and doctor available immediately to evaluate an injury and start treatment. They will also have access to physical therapy and a rehabilitation program on a two- or three-times-a-day basis. This would not be practical for the casual athlete, who also must go to work on a daily basis.

COMMON BASKETBALL INJURIES
(see Box)

Toenails

Toenail injuries are common in basketball players. The constant starting and stopping causes the foot to slide forward in the shoe, jamming the nails against the front of the shoe; the players also frequently have their toes stepped on during a game. As a result, such injuries as subungual hematomas, ingrown toenails, and onychauxic nails may occur. Since these athletes use public shower rooms, onychomycosis is also common. Treatment for these nail problems requires immediate relief and allowing the athlete to continue to play. Definitive surgical procedures should be delayed until the end of the season. Subungual hematomas should be treated by drilling the nail plate to establish drainage and applying an antibiotic cream and a light compression dressing. Opening the front of the skin where

COMMON BASKETBALL INJURIES

Toenails (subungual hematoma, onychomycosis, ingrown nails, onychauxic nails)

Blisters

Stress fractures

Plantar fasciitis/heel spurs/heel bursitis

Ankle sprains

Knee injuries

Muscle pulls and tears

Tendinitis

the skin swells is less traumatic than nail drilling. An ingrown nail should have the offending corner removed and then be treated with warm soaks and topical antibiotic. An onychauxic or onychomycotic nail should be treated by grinding down the nail, and the mycotic nail should be treated with a topical antifungal agent.

Blisters

Blisters are usually a problem only during the start of the season. Treatment should include draining the blister but leaving the roof of the blister in place, and applying an antiseptic solution and a protective dressing. Specialized dressings such as Second Skin can be used for persons with more sensitive skin who have recurring problems. Insoles that reduce shear, such as Spenco or Sorbothane, are helpful. In severe cases, these materials can be used over a soft orthotic device for maximum protection. Those who are prone to blisters should apply Vaseline to the skin before putting on their socks.

Stress Fractures

The repetitive stress that occurs in basketball is responsible for a high incidence of stress fractures. These fractures occur most commonly in the metatarsals and tibia but are also seen in the tarsal bones and fibula. On rare occasions, a stress fracture may develop in the femur or patella. Initial treatment requires rest and immobilization. In most cases, this will result in healing in 4 to 6 weeks. When resuming play, the athlete may wear a soft insert with a buildup to redistribute the weight away from the metatarsal for 4 to 8 weeks. This reduces the stress to the fractured metatarsal.

Some fractures will develop a delayed healing or a nonunion. When this occurs, it may be necessary to correct the nonunion surgically by removing any fibrocartilagenous material from the fracture site and placing a bone graft across the fracture. A fracture at the base of the fifth metatarsal, just distal to the joint (Jones fracture), has a high incidence of nonunion. When this type of injury occurs in the higher level athlete, consideration should be given to immediate screw fixation and immobilization.

Plantar Fasciitis–Heel-Spur Syndrome–Heel Bursitis

Basketball players frequently suffer pain on the bottom of the heel. This may be due to a plantar fasciitis, heel-spur syndrome, or a heel bursitis. Regardless of the specific

diagnosis, the initial treatment is generally the same. The foot is strapped with a low-dye strap before playing, ice is applied after playing, oral anti-inflammatory agents are started, and soft orthotic devices are fabricated. Physical therapy consisting of whirlpool and ultrasound is also helpful. If symptoms do not improve, cortisone injections may be needed, followed by 3 to 4 days of complete rest. Severe cases sometimes require cast immobilization, and only rarely is surgery necessary to release the plantar fascia or excise the plantar heel spur.

Ankle Sprains

Ankle sprains may be one of the most common injuries in basketball. The extent of the injury should be evaluated carefully in order to determine the appropriate treatment plan. At the time of the injury, the RICE principles should be applied. The degree of the sprain should then be established. A mild sprain will result in only mild pain and swelling, and the tenderness will be localized to the anterior talofibular ligament. A moderate sprain will involve more extensive ligament disruption, with greater pain and swelling. Ecchymosis may be present over the foot and ankle. There will be pain over the anterior talofibular and the calcaneofibular ligaments. A severe sprain will indicate damage to all the lateral ankle ligaments and possibly an avulsion fracture of the lateral malleolus. With moderate or severe ankle sprains, the potential for injury to surrounding tissues exists. The ankle should be inspected for peroneal tendon injury, subtalar joint involvement, os trigonum fracture, avulsion fracture at the base of the fifth metatarsal or the head of the fibula, and peroneal nerve injury.

The extent of treatment for ankle sprains will depend on the degree of injury. A mild sprain may only require RICE and 2 to 3 days of rest. A moderate sprain will require longer immobilization with strapping or a soft cast for 2 to 3 weeks and physical therapy and a period of rehabilitation. A severe sprain requires 6 weeks of cast immobilization with an initial 2 to 3 weeks of non-weight bearing. An extensive rehabilitation program should follow the immobilization. With a severe sprain, especially if there is a positive anterior draw sign and excessive talar tilt on stress radiographic views, primary surgical repair of the ligaments has been recommended.

An ankle sprain can be a very debilitating injury and should never be dismissed as "only a sprain."

Knee Injuries

The knee in basketball is subject to both acute and overuse injuries. Jumping, sudden changes in direction, and colliding with another player can all result in an acute injury to the knee. This may involve meniscal injuries, sprain of the collateral ligaments, or even rupture of the cruciate ligaments. Treatment for these injuries may range from immobilization and rest for knee sprain to surgical correction of cruciate ligament injuries.

Overuse injuries of the knee may include tendinitis of any of the tendons around the knee, bursitis or synovitis, and fluid buildup within the knee. In basketball, "jumper's knee" (which is a patella tendinitis) is common. Treatment for the overuse injuries should follow the basic treatment plan, with reduction in the level of activity, ice after activity, anti-inflammatory agents, bracing or strapping of the knee, physical therapy, and rehabilitation to strengthen muscles around the knee.

Muscle Pulls and Muscle Tears

Muscle pulls and tears are common in basketball. These injuries can range from a mild muscle pull that will not limit play to a complete muscle rupture that can be debilitating. The initial treatment for a muscle pull is RICE to stop the bleeding and reduce any swelling. Once bleeding and swelling have been controlled, heat and gentle range of motion is started to avoid adhesions. The injured muscle must be strengthened. This will prevent further damage and compensation by other muscle groups.

One potential complication of muscle injuries is myositis ossificans, wherein calcifications may develop in the muscle belly. This becomes a chronic problem and is difficult to treat. A rupture of a muscle belly is a serious injury and may require surgical correction and months of rehabilitation before the player can return.

Tendinitis

Inflammation can occur in almost any tendon in the lower extremity of a basketball player. Commonly, the Achilles and patellar tendons are affected. The peroneal, posterior tibial, and biceps femoris and the tendons of the hamstring muscles may also be affected. Tendinitis injuries are generally overuse injuries, and the basic treatment plan should be initiated.

PREVENTION OF INJURIES

Since basketball players are subject to so many potential injuries, a primary concern should be prevention of these injuries. Steps to prevent injuries should involve training, technique, equipment, and stretching and strengthening programs.

The training program and proper technique can be considered together. During training camp, the emphasis for injury prevention should be on conditioning, gradual warmup, stretching, developing aerobic and anaerobic fitness, and a cooldown period. Conditioning should actually begin long before training camp starts. An off-season conditioning program should include maintaining aerobic fitness as well as a strengthening program. Although basketball emphasizes speed and agility, as the quality of players improves, strength is becoming more important. A strengthening program will improve the athletes' performance and very likely will help reduce the potential for injury.

Stretching exercises should be done before each practice and game. A tight muscle will have less ability to give under a forceful stretch and will be more susceptible to a muscle pull or tear. Also, gentle stretching will gradually warm the muscle before playing and reduce injury potential. Players with tight muscle groups who have been subject to previous injuries should be instructed in stretching exercises for those specific muscle groups. This stretching should be done at a separate time, in addition to the stretching done before playing.

Proper technique should be taught at a young age. Once improper techniques are learned, it is much more difficult to break these bad habits. Techniques to avoid injuries include awareness of foot position for better balance, using both legs for rebounding, and avoiding reliance on the dominant leg. Players should be taught positioning for rebounding to avoid hyperextending the back. They should also be able to anticipate where and how they will land after jumping, to avoid landing in an unbalanced position where falling or twisting ankles or knees is likely. Proper training and technique are the shared responsibility of the coach, trainer, and team doctor.

Because ankle sprains are a common injury in basketball, strapping is frequently used as a preventive measure to help protect the ankle. A combination of a high-top shoe and strapping is the best method of preventing ankle sprains or reducing their severity. There are many acceptable methods for strapping an ankle, which usually include a combination of figure-eight strapping with ankle locks and stirrups. Although taping may be the best method, it is also expensive. The team that has a limited budget should consider using one of the reusable ankle wraps or braces. Strapping can also be used to treat other injuries, such as plantar fasciitis, muscle pulls, or any joint sprain.

Orthotic devices are used frequently in basketball players to treat or prevent injuries. The particular type of device will depend on the injury, the foot type, patient's age, and the level of play. The younger player, at the high school or early college level, will respond well to a semirigid device with a soft top cover that will provide good control. As players get older and more experienced, they are more resistant to a device that will change the function or "the feel" of the foot. For this type of athlete, a softer type of orthotic device, such as Plastizote or leather, will be better accepted. The athlete with a pes cavus foot type will also do better with the softer type device, which may not provide as much control but will provide more shock absorption. For the more serious basketball player, it may be worth considering a soft orthotic device to replace the existing insole in the shoe, in order to provide maximum protection to the feet and all the structures of the lower extremity. In casting and fabricating an orthotic device for a basketball player, it must be recognized that the player requires a greater range of motion and generally must be allowed more pronation than in other sports. Therefore, the casting should be done in a semi-weight-bearing position. In order to reduce the potential for ankle sprains, the rearfoot should not be posted in varus, unless there is a specific reason. Any rearfoot post should be at 0 degrees. Orthotic devices can be used to treat or prevent a number of problems for the basketball player. The type of device and the amount of posting must be carefully evaluated, since the functional demands of basketball are different from those in many other sports.

PROFESSIONAL BASKETBALL PERSPECTIVE

National Basketball Association (NBA) players' longevity is determined by both talent and injury, but oftentimes neither is in the control of the player. Those players who play the longest in the NBA have a synergistic combination of talent and ability to stay away from career-ending injuries. The result of a 1991 NBA Career Longevity Study NBA Career Longevity Database were provided to NBA teams, trainers, and team physicians. It provided a baseline of the "standard" NBA player.

The average number of years played by position certainly was related to the amount of mileage the player would encounter in his position:

Center	8.8 years
Forward	7.8 years
Guard	7.3 years

Those players who had fewer injuries per year were also the players to have the longest career longevity:

Played 1–5 years:	1.5 injuries per year
Played 6–7 years:	1.3 injuries per year
Played 8–10 years:	1.2 injuries per year
Played 13–20 years:	0.9 injuries per year

Certainly, one can readily see from these numbers that injury prevention to the professional player is of great value both to the player and to the team organization, which has invested heavily in his career. Some injuries are not as preventable as others. Even some of the acute injuries can be influenced by wise preparation of player conditioning, strength and flexibility, shoe gear selection and timely replacement of the shoes, and use of orthotics to help in functional weight distribution of foot and ground reaction forces.

Examples of how preventative medical care can be of great value include the following:

1. The return to activity of the athlete from nonseason strengthening to a competitive level of participation requires a certain level of stress changes to bone in response to the amount of stress and time of work done to bone physiology. Wolf's law dictates that bone will adapt to external forces applied to it, but only at a certain rate. When these forces exceed the ability of bone to adapt, then negative changes begin to occur within the bone structure. This creates an eventual stress fracture. This can be decreased by keeping a certain level of weight-bearing loading available to the athlete during off-season training in expectation of returning to seasonal full-contact workouts.

2. Of the fractures that occur in the NBA, the metatarsal stress fracture is the most frequent. Tibia stress fracture is second, followed by navicular stress fracture. This is truly an overuse injury. It is an injury on which preventative medicine can have a great impact fiscally and competitively (especially when viewed in light of the amount of money the NBA player is paid per game and that the team will not receive his services for the 3 to 6 weeks minimum required for the stress fracture to heal).

a. Those players who have structural need of orthotic accommodation will dramatically allow for sharing of ground reactive forces to the foot weight-bearing structure. Players frequently enter the NBA having already had several stress fractures during their college career. The college level requires much less activity as will the NBA each year, both in longevity of season and games played per season. 41.5% of the players in the NBA use some type of orthosis. The most frequently used device is that of a semirigid plastic in 34% of those players who use an orthotic. A shock-absorptive combination of leather materials are next most frequently used, followed by heat-formed shock-absorptive materials.

b. The use of proper shoe gear has a strong relationship to the performance and stability of foot function within the shoe. Those shoes that complement foot requirements for stability, flexibility, and shock absorption can greatly aid in the dissemination of stress to foot structure. Those participating in medical care of the athletes should have an influence in the choices of shoe gear used by the athlete. This is certainly tempered by professional shoe contracts with large shoe companies and the professional athlete.

3. The amount of stress applied to the shoe gear before replacement with a new shoe also has a profound influence upon protecting the athlete. The sports medicine practitioner readily recognizes the need of timely replacement of running shoes to prevent and treat existing injuries. Most runners are encouraged to replace shoe gear every 350 to 500 miles depending upon the size of the runner and his or her running environment. The same should be true of the basketball player. The average runner will spend about 66 hours in running to accumulate 500 miles on a pair of shoes (8 min/mile pace times 500 miles). The average high school or collegiate athlete will work out easily 72 h/mo. Basketball shoes are now all made of the same types of materials, that is, ethyl viny acetate or polyurethane midsole and a harder outer sole material. These materials all have a fatigue factor that greatly influences function of the foot and stress delivered to bone and soft tissue structures. Players in the NBA will rarely use a pair of basketball shoes for longer than 7 to 10 days before replacing it with a new pair of shoes.

A positive secondary by-product of frequent shoe change is that of a protective influence of shoe gear on foot and ankle stability in response to external forces. As the shoe is worn over hours of use, the leather uppers slowly begin to stretch in response to the rotational forces applied. Also, the midsole material slowly deforms or compresses in response to repetitive ballistic starting and stopping of play. As these external changes to the shoe continue, the rotational movement of the foot with in the shoe slowly increases in range of motion. Therefore, with newer shoe usage there will be fewer inversion injuries as compared to injuries due to the lack of support from worn and stretched shoe gear materials that lack the integrity to decelerate foot rotational movement beyond normal positioning.

The NBA players choose a wide variety of shoe gear styles to play in. Sixty-eight percent of the players utilize a high-top shoe, 15 percent utilize a three-quarter-top shoe, and only 10 percent will use a low-top basketball shoe for regular play.

Even with all of this care and attention, the inversion injury is still a prevalent injury in the NBA. In the 1990–91 season, 289 incidences of ankle sprain were recorded in 167 subjects (NBA Career Longevity Database). It should be noted that no ankle surgery was done on any of those subjects. The ability to rehabilitate the injured ankle is the norm rather than the exception, even at the level of play required of an NBA participant.

Once the injury has been treated for the initial inflammatory changes of tissue damage, support of the structure is important to allow for return to activity. Proprioceptive deficits are frequent postinjury findings of ankle inversion injuries. The player must have a return of strength and proprioception or his ability to perform highly ballistic movement with that ankle becomes unlikely. Second, without strength and proprioception, the rate of re-injury to the athlete is significant.

32

Soccer Injuries

NICHOLAS M. ROMANSKY

Soccer is certainly the most popular sport in the world, with an estimated 60 million players in 150 countries, as registered with the International Federation of Football Association (FIFA).[1,2] American competitive soccer has grown steadily in the last decade at all levels, including the youth leagues and high school and college teams. The Soccer Industry Council of America has found that, in 1990, there were 16 million soccer participants in the United States, and 75 percent of these participants were under the age of 18.[3] Soccer has ranked third in the total number of participants under the age of 18, and is second only to basketball for the total number of participants under the age of 12.[3] The Soccer Industry Council of America has also reported that the number of National Collegiate Athletics Association (NCAA) member institutions sponsoring men's and women's soccer has increased from 178 and 0, respectively, in 1970, to 243 and 93 teams, respectively, in 1990.[3] With this steady growth in soccer's popularity, the incidence of soccer injuries has also increased. However, when compared to American football, youth soccer players sustained two to five times fewer injuries.[4] Although interest in soccer has grown, there have been only a few epidemiology studies done.

This chapter is designed to provide a foundation for the understanding of soccer injuries, which have produced a corresponding need for athletic trainers, physicians, and other concerned health care professionals to develop a knowledge of this relatively new American sport and its unique scope of injury. The most common soccer injuries seen from the elementary school level through the World Cup Soccer level and their treatment are described, and information on prevention and rehabilitation is provided.

FOOT

Apophysitis

Apophysitis is commonly seen in the calcaneus and fifth metatarsal base.[5,6] It can be seen in other growth plates in the foot and ankle, but is less common in these areas.[7] Apophysitis is an inflammation of the growth plate usually created by traction placed on the growth plate from attachment of a tendon or muscle. In the calcaneus, the clinical signs most noted include: compression tenderness of the growth plate on direct palpation and pain upon ambulation. Local heat may accompany these symptoms. Treatment includes stretching for the tight posterior group of the hamstring and calf muscles; a Neoprene 3/8-inch heel lift, which is decreased by 1/8 inch to level over a 3-week period; a Tuli's heel cup or Silipos Viscoheel; and oral prescription and over-the-counter nonsteroidal anti-inflammatory medications. Proper training shoes become very important to the injured player. A turf shoe with a harder and higher heel counter should be used. For more severe cases, partial or complete rest may be instituted along with the above-mentioned remedies. Rarely, fiberglass cast immobilization is required.

Dorsal Foot Contusions

Dorsal foot contusions, where a bruise occurs on top of the foot from a collision with an opposing player or by striking the ball very hard, can occur at all levels of play. A Silipos gel pad or a felt pad should be used for compression and shock absorption when playing. In addition, a foam tongue pad can be used. Oral anti-inflammatory medications, ultrasound, and electrical stimulation are the modalities of choice.

Plantar Fasciitis

Plantar fasciitis is the inflammation of the thick fibrous band of tissue on the plantar aspect of the foot, originating from the plantar aspect of the calcaneus and inserting into the plantar metatarsal heads with extensions to all five toes. This is characterized by first-step pain, in the morning or after getting up to walk from a sitting position. Commonly the area of plantar fasciitis is caused by fatigue after prolonged playing or training sessions. This is complicated by the lack of an arch support in the common molded cleat or from a flat-molded shoe. Plantar fasciitis may become a prolonged problem. Low-dye tape strapping, oral anti-inflammatory medications, oral steroids, local physical therapy treatments, and over-the-counter or prescription orthotic devices, may be used in treatment. The player is further told to wear sneakers and not go barefooted. Slow static stretching is critical, especially if ankle dorsiflexion is limited. A tennis or golf ball may be used to massage the foot by rolling the ball under the foot against the floor.

Common Foot Problems

Common podiatric foot problems, such as ingrown toenails, blisters, and athlete's foot, are encountered at all levels of soccer play. It is imperative that nail care is performed properly, cutting the nails straight across. However, if the soft tissue borders are hypertrophic, the nail borders should be trimmed back on a diagonal direction or be rounded off. This should be done by the team doctor and not the player to ensure that the entire nail spicule is removed. It is possible that a simple surgical procedure such as a phenol and alcohol nail border removal can be done. Blister and callus formations are treated locally with debridement and the use of Silvadene cream for ruptured blisters. Painful toenails due to contusions or stepping injuries may be padded by using a Silipos (Silipos USA, New York, NY) digital gel pad/sleeve. This tends to work better than the typical tube foam.

Stress Fractures

Stress fractures are commonly seen in the lesser metatarsals.[7-10] This can be seen in the youngest and most inexperienced players through to elite, world class athletes. Com-

monly the fifth metatarsal fracture is seen due to the actual poor biomechanical design of soccer shoes, prolonged playing, and overuse syndrome. Rest, cast immobilization, or open reduction–internal fixation with screw or plate fixation may have to be considered. Specifically, the Jones fracture at the base of the fifth metatarsal, which is more diaphyseal, is due to overuse. In addition, the typical base avulsion fracture is due to forceful traction on the peroneus brevis tendon at its attachment at the fifth metatarsal base.

LEG

Quadriceps Contusions

Quardriceps contusions are frequently seen due to an opponent's knee colliding with the player's thigh. This commonly causes an acute hematoma in the midcentral aspect of the quadriceps muscle. The player should be escorted off the field, and the knee held in maximum flexion with ice and compression. Oral anti-inflammatories are started immediately, and the patient is kept in this hyperflexed position throughout the night. In the morning, a warm whirlpool and hydroculator pack is used with range-of-motion exercises and stationary bicycling. Therapy should continue with a Neoprene compression sleeve 24 hr/day. The chief concern with quadriceps contusion is the possibility that myositis ossificans. This can occur due to calcification of the hematoma. Radiographs may be required, and, rarely, surgical excision is needed. With time, this problem resolves with very aggressive, active physical therapy.

Strains

Strains of the hamstring and quardricep tendon are frequent. This occurs because players have well-developed quadriceps and hamstring muscles which are continually contracted. A soft tissue/bone growth differential during the growing years may create players with chronically tight muscle groups, leading to strains and partial tears.[11] At the origin or insertion, these strains may become chronic for an entire season. It is imperative that stretching and local physical therapy be instituted as soon as possible after the player makes the initial complaint. Massage, ultrasound, electrical stimulation, and stretching become the mainstays of treatment. On occasion, a radiograph or magnetic resonance imaging (MRI) may be done to rule out a partial or complete tear or avulsion fracture at the origin or insertion.

Shin Splints

Shin splints are an inflammation of the tibialis anterior or posterior muscles with soleus involvement. Sharpey's fibers become torn away from the tibia, usually in the lower to middle third of the leg. Most commonly, this painful inflammation is seen with sudden increased frequency and intensity of training with overall poor training habits. The training surface and worn or poor shoe gear commonly contribute to this painful syndrome. Tight musculature, growth, and flatfoot causing abnormal biomechanical forces can also be part of the overall shin splint picture. The collapsible flatfoot seen in the stance position should be controlled with an over-the-counter arch support or a custom orthotic device. Prescription full length orthotics work especially well. Full-length soccer orthotics work especially well. Acute symptoms are treated with the usual physical therapy modalities and with the use of a Neoprene sleeve to compress the lower leg 24 hr/day. Oral anti-inflammatories, as well as stretching and proper training habits, should be instituted. The player should stay off surfaces of either extreme, such as concrete or sand and should also avoid hills. Training should be done in running sneakers or turf shoes.

Prolonged acute shin splint syndrome may lead to tibial stress fractures, necessitating radiographs and a three-phase bone scan for diagnosis. If a tibial stress fracture is encountered, then the lower leg Air Cast with anterior panel brace is used for 6 weeks, with non-weight-bearing training allowed until the acute symptoms subside in 2 to 4 weeks. Oral steroids using the Medrol Dosepak may be used for the acute and chronic shin splint syndrome when no tibial stress fracture is present.

Compartment Syndrome

Compartment syndrome commonly occurs when the pressure in the affected leg is 30 mm Hg greater than in the unaffected side. Pressure in the leg increases with activity, causing any of the five signs of compartment syndrome: pulselessness, paresthesia, paralysis, pain, and pallor. The slit catheter test can be performed with relative ease using the Stryker Catheter Kit. A fasciotomy may have to be done in one or all three of the lower leg compartments. Early diagnostic testing may include radiographs, MRI, and a three-phase bone scan.

ANKLE

Capsulitis

Capsulitis of the ankle joint is a common injury which is caused by poor field conditions, a direct blow injury, or aggravation of the ankle capsule due to a previous ligament injury. At all levels of play, fields not properly maintained can create inflammation in either the medial or lateral gutters of the ankle joint. Palpable tenderness is most commonly elicited in the lateral gutter. On occasion, localized swelling is seen. The player feels sharp pain on range of motion and on cutting. Radiographs should be taken to rule out any type of internal derangement of the ankle. This internal synovitis is usually self-limiting. Local physical therapy modalities and shoes with a strong rear foot counter resolve this problem. Oral anti-inflammatory medication, tape strapping, and sometimes prescription orthotic devices with a deep heel cup assist in the resolution of the acute problem. On occasion, chronic synovitis will require arthroscopy for resection of the hypertrophic synovium. Following stress radiographic evaluation, a lateral ankle stabilization procedure may be required if the primary cause of the capsulitis is ankle instability.

Strains and Sprains

Strains and sprains of the ankle commonly occur in both the inversion and the eversion type. Aggressive early therapy with active and passive range-of-motion exercises, local physical therapy, and use of tape strapping or an Air Cast is suggested.[12] The degree of partial or complete rupture determines whether surgery is indicated. Usually aggressive therapy and strengthening of the extrinsic muscles and soft tissue resolve this problem. Frequently, synovitis can occur in the ankle joint, requiring the above-mentioned treatment plan. In more severe ankle sprains or poorly responding cases, an osteochondral lesion of the talus may be present. Spurring of the inferior tibia or fibula or walls of the talus may occur, causing a painful ankle joint, especially with cutting. Steroid injection therapy, oral anti-inflammatory medication, and physical therapy modalities such as ultrasound and electrical stimulation are helpful. Arthroscopic evaluation and treatment may be required.

Os Trigonum Syndrome

The os trigonum syndrome, or fracture of the lateral process of the calcaneus, is sometimes seen with a strong plantar-flexory motion as the player strikes the ground when attempting to hit the ball or when an opponent and the player collide for a 50/50 ball. The lateral process of the talus gets caught between the posterior tibial malleolus and calcaneus, causing a partial to complete fracture of the lateral process. Comparative lateral standing radiographs should be taken. A three-phase bone scan or MRI may be indicated to rule out this fracture. In a small percentage of patients, a detached process is present, and it must be determined if this is a growth plate abnormality due to lack of fusion or if the player has a history of a previous injury. Usually injection therapy resolves this problem; however, surgical excision may be needed to remove this small bone fragment. Care should be taken when this procedure is done to inspect the flexor hallucis longus tendon to see if an injury has occurred to the tendon as it slides through this area.

Achilles Tendinitis

Achilles tendinitis can be an acute or chronic problem. Overuse and lack of stretching are common causes of this painful injury. The typical flat soccer shoe causes and aggravates this lesion.[13,14] Thickening of the tendon, crepitus, or pinpoint tenderness proximally 4 cm above the Achilles tendon insertion are common clinical signs. The use of local physical therapy modalities, such as ultrasound, electrical stimulation, contrast baths, and a noncompressible Neoprene heel lift are used. The 3/8-inch heel lift is initially used for 10 days; then the height of the lift is decreased by 1/8 inch every 10 days until, after 1 month's time, no heel lift is used. It is possible that a partial tear may be present, and MRI evaluation may be indicated. Training should include the use of a turf shoe or running sneaker as much as possible since the heel in the shoe is usually higher than the typical flat soccer shoe. Oral anti-inflammatory medications and oral steroids may be used to decrease the inflammation in the tendon. The use of injection therapy is absolutely contraindicated.

KNEE

Ligament Injuries

Anterior cruciate ligament injury requires radiographic and MRI evaluation, and surgical intervention with early physical therapy. With aggressive physical therapy, the player can be back at a competitive level in 4 to 7 months. Medial collateral ligament strains and sprains are very common occurrences at all levels of play. Palpable tenderness and discomfort on kicking is present. This is commonly seen with improper biomechanics of kicking, a direct blow injury, or poor quadriceps development. Local care includes active and passive range-of-motion exercises, physical therapy modalities, and strengthening of the quadriceps and ligament structures about the knee. Oral anti-inflammatory medications, Neoprene sleeve use, and stationary bicycling all help in the acute and chronic resolution of the strain or sprain.

Meniscus Tears

Meniscus tears occur with poor field conditions, cutting, and collision with an opponent player. Surgical intervention through arthroscopy may be required.

Patellofemoral Syndrome

Patellofemoral syndrome encompasses a variety of diagnoses.[15] Runner's knee or chondromalacia are only two of the common ailments included in this syndrome. Types of pain include burning and dull or sharp pain during or after activity. The pain usually increases while going down stairs, during prolonged sitting, or when getting up from a seated position. The player may exhibit crepitus, tight hamstrings, increased Q angle (females), and palpable tenderness and pain behind the patella surface. Treatment to alter the patellar tracking includes exercises to strengthen the quadriceps muscles, bracing, and shoe orthotics to control abnormal pronation. At times, operative intervention is required to release the lateral retinaculum and resect friable cartilage.

This syndrome is commonly seen in female players with increased femoral anteversion, genu valgum, or foot pronation. Tight hamstrings, poor quadriceps strength, and a tall female athlete all contribute to this problem. This is commonly the female athlete who also encounters shin splints. A women's wider pelvis makes her a more likely candidate for genu valgum and increased Q angle.

Patellofemoral stress syndrome, and specifically chondromalacia treatment, has two objectives[15]: to reduce inflammation and to improve the alignment between the patella and femur. Chondromalacia may be seen with the overuse syndrome as well. Surgery may be performed with arthroscopic evaluation to remove the fibrillated cartilage. Full kicking motion and forceful long kicking should be discontinued until all pain and symptoms have resolved for both the patellofemoral stress syndrome and the chondromalacia. Orthotic devices can be very helpful for long-term control of symptoms and overall alignment.

HIP

Contusions, bursitis, and hip flexor complex syndrome comprise most of the abnormalities seen at this joint level. Groin pain may be acute or chronic and may originate from the hip, the groin itself, the lower abdomen, or the lumbosacral region.[2,16–18] This is very common due to collisions and slide tackling, especially when playing on hard or artificial surfaces. Diagnostic testing should include radiographs, bone scan, or MRI evaluation. Conservative treatment to relieve pain and inflammation, including the use of anti-inflammatory medications, ultrasound, and electrical stimulation, in conjunction with rest and stretching, usually benefits most players. If in fact the origin of pain and disability is from the groin area, then surgical repair/release may be indicated.[18]

LUMBOSACRUM

Lumbosacral injuries include strains of the lumbosacral spine. Conservative treatment with rest, stretching, physical therapy, and oral medications, such as anti-inflammatory medications and muscle relaxants, benefits most players. Sciatica or radicular pain may occur with the tall athlete or after a specific injury during a collision. Abdominal development and proper mechanics of kicking usually decrease the chance of recurrence. A thorough examination with diagnostic procedures (radiography) will detect the most common causes of the lumbosacral spine and sacroilium injuries.

PREVENTION

Soccer injuries can be significantly decreased with adequate coaching and supervision, during properly designed training sessions.[19] Changes in shoe design are critical in the occurrence, the frequency, and the amount of significant injuries. Preseason training should start slowly. Specific programs should be given for each individual player based on his or her weaknesses. It is beneficial to have a massage therapist, physical therapist, and aerobics instructor. Preseason ballet instruction, especially for stretching, is very beneficial. Getting away from the "American football" mentality of overaggressive, three-a-day training sessions will significantly decrease injuries. Separating fitness sessions from tactical and technical sessions will help the physical and mental status of the player, decreasing the occurrence of injuries.

Whether preseason or in season, running shoes should be used during training sessions, as much as possible. The frequency, intensity, time, surface, and shoes used in training sessions should be properly managed with each player. A change in any two of these variables will lead to overuse syndrome. For the younger athlete, up to age 8, it is suggested that sneakers or turf shoes be used since all brands of molded or stud cleats have too flat a sole. Many times the heel counter of the shoe is not adequately built with height or hardness. Until better design of the soccer cleat is undertaken, the same injury patterns will continue. The use of prescription orthotic devices has certainly helped in the prevention and treatment of lower extremity injuries. Until the significance of designing a better soccer cleat is understood and produced for all age levels of play, the same injury patterns will continue.

REHABILITATION

Aggressive, injury-specific physical therapy is the mainstay of treatment of a player with an injured body part. This is especially true for the postsurgical player. Even those players with immobilization for a short time can experience deconditioning of minor and major muscle groups that can lead to chronic problems. The role of the sports physician and athletic trainer has grown significantly, with increasing emphasis on early dynamic splinting and bracing instead of casting and immobilization. Even with the most complex and significant soft tissue or bone injury, knowing when to treat aggressively or conservatively is paramount for returning the patient to optimal playing capacity. Athletes should not be allowed to return to play until there is no functional disability as measured by range of motion, strength of injured area, and ability to perform sport-specific maneuvers, such as figure-eights and cutting for ankle injuries, and 30- to 50-yard dashes for general lower extremities injuries. Additionally, pain, soft tissue swelling, and tenderness of injured area should be minimal prior to a player's return. The athlete's desire to return to play should also be considered. If the player does not want to play, then further evaluation and therapy may be required.

Initial treatment of on-the-field trauma, regardless of type or severity, centers around reducing swelling and pain. This usually entails one or more of the RICE modalities (rest, ice, compression, and elevation). RICE should be initiated as soon as possible, preferably on the field or in the emergency department while awaiting further evaluation.

SUMMARY

Minor lower extremity injuries are most commonly encountered in soccer. Proper immediate evaluation must be completed by the coach, trainer, and physician so minor injuries do not become chronic problems for the athlete. Suggestions for injury prevention include correct training habits, provision of optimal equipment, prophylactic ankle taping, controlled rehabilitation, exclusion of players with chronic joint instability, disciplined play in the game and practice situation, well-trained/well-educated health care professionals, biomechanically stable/functional shoe gear/design, and optimum playing field conditions.

ACKNOWLEDGMENTS

A special heartfelt thanks to Lisa M. Hanson for her writing and editing contributions. Ms. Hanson is a freelance technical writer in the Philadelphia, Pennsylvania, area.

REFERENCES

1. Ekstrand J, Gillquist J: Soccer injuries and their mechanisms: a prospective study. Med Sci Sports 15:267, 1983
2. Engstrom B, Johansson C, Tornkvist H: Soccer injuries among elite female players. Am J Sports Med 19:372, 1991
3. Soccer Industry Council of America: Data presented at the U.S. Soccer World Cup Symposium on Sportsmedicine, Orlando, FL, 1994. In Garrett WE (ed): Sportsmedicine Book. Baltimore, Williams & Wilkins, 1996
4. Pritchett JW: Cost of high school soccer injuries. Am J Sports Med 9:64, 1981
5. Backous DD et al: Soccer injuries and their relation to physical maturity. Sports Med 142:839, 1988
6. Nilsson S, Roaas A: Soccer injuries in adolescents. Am J Sports Med 6:358, 1978
7. Matheson GO et al: Stress fractures in athletes. Am J Sports Med 15:46, 1987
8. Mandelbaum BR: The Medical Field. Soccer Division, Nike, Inc., Beaverton, OR, 1995
9. Stanitski CL, McMaster JH, Scranton PE et al: On the nature of stress fractures. J Sports Med 6:391, 1978
10. Wilson ES, Katz FN: Stress fractures: an analysis of 250 consecutive cases. Radiology 92:481, 1969
11. Ekstrand J, Gillquist J: The frequency of muscle tightness and injuries in soccer players. Am J Sports Med 10:75, 1982
12. Birrer RB, Cartwright TJ, Denton JR: Primary treatment of ankle trauma. Physician Sports Med 22:33, 1994
13. Clarke TE, Frederick EC, Cooper LB: Effects of shoe cushioning upon ground reaction forces in running. Int J Sports Med 4:247, 1983
14. Clement DB, Taunton JE, Smart GW: Achilles tendinitis and peritendinitis: etiology and treatment. Am J Sports Med 12:179, 1984
15. Hunter-Griffin L: The patellofemoral stress syndrome. Your Patient & Fitness 3(2):9, 1990
16. Ackermark C, Johansson C: Tenotomy of the adductor longus tendon in the treatment of chronic groin pain in athletes. Am J Sports Med 20:640, 1992
17. Renstrom P, Peterson L: Groin injuries in athletes. Br J Sports Med 14:30, 1980
18. Taylor DC, Meyers WC, Moylan JA et al: Abdominal musculature abnormalities as a cause of groin pain in athletes: inguinal hernias and pubalgia. Am J Sports Med 19:239, 1991
19. Ekstrand J, Gillquist J: The avoidability of soccer injuries. Int J Sports Med 4:124, 1983

SUGGESTED READINGS

Albert M: Descriptive three year data study of outdoor and indoor professional soccer injuries. Ath Train 18:218, 1983
Baxter DE: The Foot and Ankle in Sport. Mosby-Year Book, St. Louis, 1995
Ekstrand J, Gillquist J et al: Incidence of soccer injuries and their relation to training and team success. Am J Sports Med 11:63, 1983
Jones BH, Bovee MW et al: Intrinsic risk factors for exercise-related injuries among male and female Army trainees. Am J Sports Med 21:705, 1993
Martire JR: The role of nuclear medicine bone scans in evaluating pain in athletic injuries. Clin Sports Med 6:713, 1987
Poulson TD, Freund KG et al: Injuries in high-skilled and low-skilled soccer: a prospective study. Br J Sports Med 25:151, 1991
Prather JL, Nusynowitz ML, Snowdy HA et al: Scintigraphic findings in stress fractures. J Bone Joint Surg [Am] 59:869, 1977
Smodlaka VN: Groin pain in soccer players. Physician Sports Med 8:57, 1980
Subotnick SI, Sisney P: Treatment of Achilles tendonopathy in the athlete. J Am Podiatr Med Assoc 76:552, 1986
Sullivan JA, Gross RH et al: Evaluation of injuries in youth soccer. Am J Sports Med 8:325, 1980
Torg JS, Pavlov H, Torg E: Overuse injuries in sport: the foot. Clin Sports Med 6:291, 1987

33

Cross-Training and Associated Injuries

PAMELA SISNEY

HISTORY OF CROSS-TRAINING

The organized sport of cross training began with the triathlon in 1978, when a few servicemen stationed in Hawaii, bored with marathoning, decided to attempt the "ultimate" endurance event. They decided that it would consist of a 2-mile swim in the ocean, followed by a 112-mile bike ride, followed by a marathon. Since its inception with only a few athletes, cross-training has grown to a worldwide sport with millions of participants and an Olympic berth as of 2000. The original event, the Ironman Triathlon held in Hawaii, which includes the original distances, attracts worldwide competition, with participants qualifying in their home country for admission. Not all triathlons are as grueling as the Ironman event, with most triathletes participating in shorter events. These may consist of a 0.5-mile swim, a 25-mile bike, and a 10-km (10K) run. The biathlon has gained more acceptance and participation as cross-training has progressed and triathlons have waned. The growth in multisport competition appears to be in the biathlon and duathlon (run, bike, run) area, or in "geographic" multisport competition (canoe, bike, run or snowshoe, kayak, run, etc.). Internationally, triathlons are growing rapidly, but in the United States, participation has decreased due to lack of interest by younger people or insurance/cost issues. With over 1 million participants in 1992 in multisport racing, injuries associated with this activity become more common in the sports medicine practice. Since the multisport competition consists of consecutive activities, practitioners see the typical injuries of each sport plus injuries characteristic of multisport competition, usually due to overuse.

Multisport events take a surprisingly low toll on the body. This is attributed to the low intensity of training in each event, which involves no sprinting or all-out performance. The ultimate goal is efficiency. Research in the area is just beginning. It appears that the most common injuries are of the overuse type, with athletes complaining of tendonitis, bursitis, and muscle strains. Injuries also seem to be more frequent in athletes with little experience, since they often use inappropriate equipment or training methods. An individual must be counseled about the sport and appropriate equipment for future injury prevention, in addition to solving the acute need.

BASIC COMPONENTS OF A TRIATHLON

A triathlon begins when the athlete enters the water (the swim or canoe is usually first) and ends when the person crosses the finish line of the run. The transition time between events is as short as possible. The athletes first swim or canoe an open water course, then run from the exit of the event to a transition area where their bikes are, and where they put on bike shoes and clothing as quickly as possible. They then ride the course, come back to the same transition area, put on running shoes, run the course, and cross the finish line. A typical short event will take around 2 to 2.5 hours for the winner. An event such as the Ironman will take 8 to 10 hours to complete. It is important to learn from patients the level of competition they are involved in. Very little standardization exists, so anything is possible.

ANATOMY-RELATED INJURIES AND THEIR PREVENTION

A general description of the anatomy involved in each sport is a basis for understanding the general injuries, the injuries particular to each sport, and the prevention of these injuries.

Swimming

Swimming usually involves interval-type work in a pool situation as training, although competition is usually in an open body of water. Athletes should be able to swim at least 1 mile in the pool prior to competition. The anatomy involved in swimming includes the neck, shoulder, and back musculature, particularly the rotator cuff. This includes the subscapularis, supraspinatus, infraspinatus, and teres minor muscles. Swimming also involves the deltoid, the latissimus dorsi, the pectorals, and the quadriceps and gastrocnemius muscles in the leg.

The most common area of the anatomy that is injured in swimming is the shoulder area. The lower extremity is rarely injured in swimming, hence the use of swimming as rehabilitation for sports that principally use the lower extremity. However, stretching should be concentrated on the quadriceps and gastrocnemius tendons to ensure flexibility.

Cycling

Cycling training involves riding the bicycle many training miles, usually a minimum of 50 to 100 miles per week. The anatomy involved includes the lower back, the quadriceps muscle of the upper leg, the gastrocnemius muscle of the lower leg, and the buttocks musculature. The most common problems with cycling are knee pain and neck and back strain.

The lower back is at risk for pain in cycling due to the bent-over position. Any back pain should be checked appropriately for differentiation from structural causes, ruptured discs, and nerve impingement. Simple strains of

thoracic or lumbosacral paravertebral muscles can often be alleviated by shifting position, moving the seat forward (or backward) on its mount, or varying the length of the handlebar stem. The quadriceps provides the power in cycling and is also the area most often injured in a bicycle crash, usually with contusions. These injuries should be treated with ice, massage, and immobilization of the muscle to prevent myositis ossificans. Cycling builds up the vastus medialis of the quadriceps group, which is seldom injured. A complete tear will result in a void and a change in coutour but little functional defect. The strength of the quadriceps is important in preventing knee pain, the most common cycling complaint. Patients can be placed on a quadriceps strengthening program via leg lifts with weights or by leg press.

The gastrocnemius–soleus muscle is another power source for both running and cycling. Tears will result in pain upon plantar-flexing of the foot. Heel lifts or non-weight bearing can be prescribed, depending on the severity of the strain. Disability can range from 1 to 10 weeks. Rehabilitation on an inclined plane of up to 20 degrees using Prostrech (San Antonio, TX) devices for passive dorsiflexion, done for at least 10 minutes two to three times a day, is a must with any gastrocnemius–soleus strain. If the pain is down at the insertion (along the Achilles tendon), disability may result, and care should be taken to treat appropriately, avoiding any chance of rupture. Achilles tendinitis treatment consists of RICE (rest, ice, compression, and elevation) initially, followed by gradual stretching. Heel lifts should be employed in all shoe gear to take stretch off the muscle. Inflammation can be further decreased with anti-inflammatory agents and physical therapy modalities. The athlete should refrain from running or cycling, or both, until the pain has stopped; a strengthening program can then be started. Complete rupture of the Achilles tendon rarely occurs in running or cycling. A defect can be felt and Thompson's test is positive: a squeezed calf muscle normally produces plantar flexion, but if the tendon is ruptured, no plantar flexion will occur.

Numbness is a common complaint in cycling, affecting the hands, feet, and buttock area. Numbness of the hands and genital area is referred to as cyclist's palsy because it is so common. Numbness in the genital region occurs because of compression of the pudendal nerves. These nerves course from the spinal cord along the sacroiliac region and over the tailbone, tracking to the genitals. Pressure on the area (more likely in males, due to less fat padding in the area) can cause paresthesia and numbness in the scrotum, penis, or both. This can be aggravated by individual anatomy that does not permit the ischial tuberosities to bear the brunt of pressure, from being down on the drops for a long period, or from an uptilted saddle. The patient should evaluate the saddle position—the distance from the handlebars—to determine whether it is too far back, forcing the saddle to rest on the nerve. This can be alleviated by moving the saddle forward or shortening the stem. The angle of the saddle should be checked; it should be straight, not up (or down), level with the top tube. If the saddle is too high, the rider has to scoot forward to reach the pedals. A variety of saddles are available, and the patient may require a wider or narrower model. Saddles come in a variety of padding thicknesses. Also available are Spenco (Spenco Products, Waco, TX) and other seat covers to add padding. Changing position can also help, as do anti-inflammatory agents.

Numbness is also a problem of the feet, particularly on longer rides in cool or cold weather. This is usually a result of traction from the toe straps across the dorsum of the foot, compressing the intermediate and medial dorsal cutaneous nerves. In cold weather (less than 55°F), blood flow is decreased to the extremities, and this, along with no movement in the foot due to efficiency on the pedal (hence the toe straps tightened down), leads to numbness. This problem can be alleviated by keeping the feet warm by moving them around within the shoes, loosening the toe straps, or wearing cover boots over the shoes (or plastic bags over the socks to conserve heat). Clip-in pedal systems (e.g., Look Pedal Systems, Descente America, New York, NY) that clamp the foot into a special pedal requiring no toe strap usually solve this problem as well.

Running

Running primarily involves the lower extremity, principally the hamstring muscles, the iliotibial band, the gastrocnemius–soleus complex, and the posterior tibialis muscles. Running also affects the knee joint and the heel area of the foot. The most common area of injury in male runners is the heel or plantar fascia; in females, the knee and shin are most often cited. In triathletes, overuse is the most frequent cause of injury; a biomechanical defect exists that causes them to be susceptible to running injuries. Overuse will affect the iliotibial band, knee joint, shins, and heels most frequently.

Canoeing/Rowing

Rowing is a power and endurance sport working on the arms, the trunk, and, depending on the boat, of the leg. Canoeing accounts for very few muscular injuries but puts a lot of demand on the cardiovascular system. It principally involves the flexor of the arm along with the pretoralis, triceps, and latissimus dorsi of the back. All the abdominal muscles are also active with the bending motion of the stroke.

GENERALIZED TRIATHLON INJURIES

The most common type of injuries encountered in triathloning include heat and cold injuries, fatigue, nutritional problems, and overuse injuries common to this sport in particular. According to Labman (unpublished results) the number of nontraumatic or overuse injuries far outweighs the number of traumatic injuries; these overuse injuries include heat and cold intolerances.[1,2]

Hyperthermia and Dehydration

The most common injury is heat stroke or hyperthermia and, along with it, dehydration.[3] Most triathlons are run in the summer and often in high humidity, and last anywhere from 2 to 9 hours. Fluid intake becomes crucial. Fluid replenishment errors, excess heat or both can sabotage all the hours of training, all the hard work, and the chances of succeeding in the race. Hyperthermia and dehydration problems can be analogous to those encountered by marathon athletes, because the time that the person is expending energy is often the same, if not longer. Heat builds up during exercise and is dissipated through perspiration. As long as water loss is replaced, the cooling process continues but, without added water, the body begins to overheat, placing severe demands on the cardiovascular system. Dehydration is the term used to describe what happens when there is not sufficient water to maintain the body's thermoregulatory system. The first signs of dehydration are thirst, quickening of the pulse, and nausea. By the time an athlete has lost 4 percent of body weight from sweating and other water losses, performance will already have diminished by 10 to 15 percent. As the situation worsens, the athlete will stop sweating, as there is no water to spare, and will begin to experience chills, hallucination, and disorientation. By then, the athlete will be staggering; in severe cases, death from heat stroke can result without proper medical treatment. The body literally cooks itself to death.

While thirst is generally an adequate gauge of water needs in a sedentary situation, it does not always serve well in competition. It takes time for water to work its way into the body—around 10 to 15 minutes for 8 ounces of water on an empty stomach. Heavy exercise tends to blunt the athlete's awareness of thirst. By the time thirst is felt, it is often too late. If the activity is continued in this condition, the body will be unable to catch up with the water needs, replacing only 50 to 60 percent of the loss. That is why it is so important to reiterate to athletes that they must drink, even if they are not thirsty. In races that take the athlete less than 2 hours to complete, fluid replacement means water. The primary concern is to avoid dehydration.

For races that last longer than 2 hours, the need for hydration is shared by the need for refueling or supplying energy for the muscles and brain to operate efficiently. Glucose is the fuel that the body needs, coming primarily from carbohydrates in foods. It is stored in the liver and muscles as glycogen. The liver is only able to store approximately 400 calories of glycogen, which can then be used to serve the needs of the body. Muscles can store 2,000 calories in the form of glycogen, but it is bound down, and the storage sites are not capable of releasing the glycogen to needier muscles or other parts of the body. When engaging in heavy exercise, the glycogen is depleted as it feeds the muscles but, by introducing glucose into the body during the exercise, the glycogen stored in the muscles is used more sparingly. During exercise, the glucose is not converted to glycogen, since there is an immediate need for it. Simple carbohydrates are converted into glucose faster than complex carbohydrates and enter the bloodstream faster, accounting for the "sugar rush." Complex carbohydrates are broken down into simple carbohydrates at a slower rate.

If the daily diet is high in complex carbohydrates, the body will have all the glycogen stores that are possible. The problem is that the body can only store enough glycogen to last through 2 hours of moderately intense exercise. When it completely runs out, the person will "hit the wall" or "bonk." These are expressions used to describe the sudden onset of fatigue, sometimes accompanied by lightheadedness, sluggishness, and a slower pace. "Bonking" is a result of hypoglycemia. When hypoglycemia results, the brain perceives the body as being tired and warns the body that the fuel is running out.

To counter this energy deficit, special fluids have been developed. These fluids contain extra carbohydrates, introduced into the system during physical activity to postpone this "running out of gas." In races that take longer than 2 hours to complete, energy replacement drinks or solid food can make the difference between a mediocre and peak performance. The problem is now to formulate an appropriate concentration of sugars and carbohydrates that will provide the muscles with the necessary fuel to continue functioning without depriving the body of the water it needs for its cooling process. Since it takes 10 to 15 minutes for a cup of plain water to be absorbed into the body from an empty stomach, if the athlete drinks something other than plain water with a concentration of carbohydrate additives that is too high, it can take 30 to 45 minutes longer for the stomach to empty. When the concentration of molecules in an energy replacement solution exceeds the level found in body fluids, it must be diluted before it can be processed. Therefore, water is automatically rerouted from the body's internal sources and sent to the stomach to accomplish dilution, leaving the person even more dehydrated. If the concentration of an energy replacement drink, or any drink other than plain water, is wrong, the athlete is subjected to both a further loss of fluids and inability to get glucose into the body. Undiluted fruit juices, soda pop, and certain energy replacement drinks can be detrimental to performance by slowing the transportation of water to the body, aggravating the chances of dehydration. The right compromise must be found. Various researchers have determined that a solution with a sugar concentration (whether sucrose, fructose, or glucose) of 2.5 percent or less will empty from the stomach almost as quickly as plain water,[4] while providing the carbohydrates and glucose needed to fuel muscles. Any drink can be easily diluted to an appropriate concentration by using some mathematics and adding water.

To deal with the slowdown of water and carbohydrate absorption, glucose polymers are now used in energy replacement drinks, such as Gatorade and Cytomax. Glucose polymers, such as maltodextrin, are large carbohydrates formed by glucose molecules linked in a chain. These are larger than simple sugar molecules, so more carbohydrate can be delivered per molecule unit, although the overall concentration of molecules remains the same. This type of energy replacement drink provides the highest possible level of carbohydrates without dramatically slowing the delivery of the critically needed water.

If the athlete gets all the electrolytes needed in a healthy diet, those ingested in a race may harm performance if they slow the delivery of the water to the body.[5] However, research shows that some athletes do develop hyponatremia. Research published in various journals cited cases of athletes who drank large quantities of fluids to prevent dehydration but who ended up in hyponatremic encephalopathy while participating in a 100-km road race.[6]

Research done by Labman at the Health Plex Center for

Human Performance Research (University of Tennessee, Knoxville) showed that, at the end of the Ironman event, 18 percent of athletes surveyed and 65 percent of athletes treated after the race were sodium chloride depleted. Current research appears to show that certain athletes do require electrolyte replacement, but that in the general population of athletes it is not a necessary factor. Therefore, athletes should be discouraged from using electrolyte replacements.

In summary, athletes should be counseled as to appropriate water and energy intake. In a race under 2 hours, water is all that is needed; 8 to 20 ounces should be consumed 30 minutes before the race starts. The athlete should then begin drinking in the transition area following the first event and take a drink every 15 minutes. For triathlons that take 2 to 4 hours to complete, an energy replacement fluid or solid food (e.g., Power Bar, Power Foods, Berkeley, CA) should be considered. Again, 8 to 20 ounces of water should be consumed before the race; after taking off on the bike, an energy replacement drink should be consumed every 30 to 45 minutes, with water intake continuing at 15-minute intervals. The athlete should establish a regular sequence of water, replacement drink, water, water, replacement drink, and so on. In races that last longer than 4 hours, the athlete will want to consume an energy-replacement drink at closer intervals, say every 20 minutes on the bike and every 30 minutes on the run. Again, drinking water should continue every 10 to 15 minutes.

Hypothermia

The other generalized injury that often results in a triathlon is hypothermia. This usually occurs early or late in the season during the swim section of the event (or during a weaker event). Hypothermia is dropping of the body's temperature, and it happens to male much more than to female athletes due to their lower percentage of body fat. Male athletes should be forewarned that hypothermia is something to be aware of and that precautions should be taken if water temperature falls below 65°F. Athletes can protect themselves with wetsuit flotation devices (if allowed) in the race and particularly by a cold-weather swimming cap made of Neoprene (wetsuit material), since most of the body's heat is lost through the head. In a winter event, layering of clothing and use of newer wicking fabrics is mandatory.

Overuse Injuries

Overuse injuries are probably the most common type of injury in a triathlon. These injuries result from overdoing training, putting undue stress and strain on particular muscles or ligamental groups. The most commonly injured areas are the knee, shoulder, and ankle, with 70 percent of injuries due solely or partly to running.

Tendinitis was the main overuse injury encountered in Labman's survey of 355 male and 11 female triathletes who competed in the October 1984 Ironman event (unpublished results). Bursitis, muscle strains, and joint inflammation made up the rest of the injuries. Most overuse injuries result in little loss of training time, with the average loss in one Labman study being 2 months for men and 1 to 2 months for women.

More research is needed to compare the specific overuse injuries of triathletes with those seen in long-distance runners and cyclists. The best form of treatment for overuse injuries is knocking down the training level or substituting some other type of training for the one that aggravates the injury. Also, using the RICE method of treatment to reduce inflammation, using an oral anti-inflammatory agent, and stretching and strengthening the abused area are helpful. Many of these overuse injuries are covered in various parts of this text.

One unusual overuse presentation that is occurring in triathlons in increasing numbers is overuse injuries to the hip. These are relatively rare in the athletic population, being reported at less than 5 percent[7] and less than 2.69 percent,[8] but are being seen increasingly in endurance athletes. Frequent injuries are sacroiliitis, pelvic and femoral neck stress fractures, and osteitis pubis. These injuries appear to affect women more than men, probably because of the difference in structural anatomy. Triathletes also tend to develop strength in particular muscle groups not used as frequently, such as the abductor muscle. An imbalance in the adductor group could lead to an increase in shear forces along the sacroiliac joints due to an increased tilt of the pelvis. This can, in turn, lead to inflammation and, with continued shear, possible stress fracture. If a patient had a concomitant limb length discrepancy, it would further increase this pelvic tilt. The patient may present with complaints of back pain and buttock or hamstring palpation of the sacroiliac area. Radiographs should be taken, and possibly a bone scan done, for further confirmation or to rule out stress fracture. A bone scan can be important to rule out a femoral neck fracture, which can be a devastating injury, and one that needs immediate referral.

(Without treatment, it can lead to displacement, avascular necrosis, and subsequent osteoarthritis.[9])

Other hip/pelvic overuse injuries to look for are osteitis pubis, an irritation of the symphysis pubis (its presence should be considered with abductor strain), gluteus medius strain/tendinitis, and trochanteric bursitis. Gluteus medius tendinitis and trochanteric bursitis are difficult to differentiate from each other, although trochanteric bursitis is usually most tender lateral to the greater trochanter, with pain on resisted hip abduction. Trochanteric bursitis can also be secondary to iliotibial band syndrome at it origin (versus normal presentation at its insertion). Treatment for all these injuries is conservative, with rest, alternating a non-weight-bearing activity (such as swimming) with the regular weight-bearing exercise regimen, local physical therapy, correction of any biomechanical abnormalities, strengthening of the affected area, anti-inflammatory agents, and icing.

OTHER INJURIES SPECIFIC TO EACH SPORT AND THEIR PREVENTION

Swimming/Canoeing

Swimming in a triathlon is usually done in an open-water situation, be it a lake, a river, or the ocean. Each particular type of body of water adds its own characteristics to the swim. In particular, the athlete should be counseled with regard to swimming in salt water. It is very important to drink even more, since the salt from the ocean water will pull fluid out of the body more rapidly. Salt water can also lead to more chafing, and can contain creatures such as jellyfish that can cause stings or other type of bites. Freshwater lakes often contain large areas of weeds, which can contain small crustacea. These should be eliminated from the skin area by washing prior to continuing in the race. This is not always possible, but is something that the swimmer should be aware of if the race is a longer one.

Swimming or canoeing probably involves the least amount of trauma to the body, while equally working the upper and lower extremities and developing aerobic and anaerobic capabilities. Injuries, with the exception of rotator cuff irritation and shoulder strains, are uncommon. Labman's study showed that only 8 percent of triathlete injuries result from swimming.[2] Lower extremity injuries are virtually nonexistent, with the exception of extensor tendonitis secondary to a plantar-flexed position of the foot with traction from the water. However, this is rare unless fins are frequently used in training.

Cycling

Knee pain is the most common injury particular to cycling. It is usually caused by chondromalacia patellae but can also include patellar tendinitis or bursitis. The patellofemoral joint is under a lot of stress in cycling. Often the rider is to blame for the knee pain in that the seat is too low or too high. If the seat is too low, the knee is flexed too much at the area of most force in the downstroke, generating excessive pressure across the patellofemoral joint. The proper saddle height can be estimated with the person sitting square on the saddle and the pedal at the bottom of the stroke (i.e., one leg at 6 o'clock and one at 12 o'clock). At this point, the knee should be flexed 10 to 20 degrees. The saddle should be on a parallel level to the top tube, not tilted up or back. The saddle should be positioned such that, if the arm is flexed at the elbow and the base of the elbow is placed against the saddle, the tips of the fingers should just meet up with the handlebars.[10] For an even more exact fit, a patient can be referred to a bicycle shop that carries the Fit Kit (New England Cycling Academy, Stowe, VT) This is a kit especially devised for fitting people to their bicycles precisely. The evaluation usually costs $30 to $50.

If a rider is using cleated shoes, cleat placement can also put excess strain on the knee. If cleats are adjusted too far inward, excessive pressure is placed on the inside of the knee. If the cleat is adjusted too far outward, excessive pressure is placed on the outside of the knee. The shoes should be adjusted such that the metatarsal heads are directly over the pedal spindle. Women require a little more inward tilt to account for their wider hips. Again, this can be accomplished with the Fit Kit.

Another cause of knee pain is pushing gears that are too high. Beginning riders usually have the notion that the bigger the gear they push, the faster they can go, resulting in a low cadence (rpm), whereas the competitive rider usually selects a gear that can be comfortably pushed between 80 and 100 rpm. When cranking along slowly in a high gear at low cadence, the rider is getting more force across the patellofemoral joint. Even when pedaling at a higher rpm, the rider is actually causing much less wear and tear to the knee joint and also increasing aerobic efficiency.

Pronation can also be a problem that leads to knee pain. This is more a problem of the elite rider. A triathlete who has a pronation problem while running also has a pronation problem while cycling that should be adjusted in both areas. This can be evaluated on a stationary trainer while watching the cyclist from the rear, looking for valgum, while the patient is pedaling. The patient can be evaluated from the front as well, making sure that the patella is facing directly forward. If the patella is tilted toward the inside, the cleat can be externally rotated. Orthotics used in a running shoe do not work well in a cycling shoe; a runner's orthotic is designed to work during heel strike and during toe-off, whereas in bicycling there is no heel strike and no stance phase. Since most cyclists strike simply in the forefoot, good results can usually be achieved with a medial wedge in the front half of the shoe, making sure that it is under both the front and back plate of the pedal, or under the cleat. Some canting can also be done underneath the cleat, although with some of the newer pedal systems it becomes impossible. If chondromalacia patellae does develop, the cause should be determined. It should be recommended that training be done on flat ground, not on any hills, and that cadence be kept between 80 and 100 rpm, with only low gears used. Icing, anti-inflammatory agents, and compression can be used for the area.

The other injuries that are common primarily to cycling are traumatic injuries, usually resulting from a fall. A person who is on a bike 4,000 to 8,000 miles per year is eventually going to fall. Patients should be reminded of the importance of wearing a helmet. They should also be counseled as to how to treat road rash (traumatic scrapes). Patients can be taught how to roll appropriately when falling off the bike. Road rash should be cleaned immediately with water, from the water bottle, to remove dirt. Infection, including tetanus, should be a consideration. The area should be kept moist; Spenco Second Skin works well with some sort of tube gauze wrapped around it. Road rash is often extremely painful, and the patient may want to use aspirin or a stronger analgesic. Again, it is important to cleanse the area well because superficial infections are common complications of these injuries.

Running

Labman's studies indicate that 70 percent of all triathlon training injuries are associated with running.[11] Unfortunately, in most triathletes, the initial response to any injury is to "run through it." Therefore, the practitioner will usually only see the patient when the pain becomes intolerable and the subject is forced to go to a physician. By then, it is usually too late for easy cures and short layoffs. It is important to make the athlete aware that some of these injuries can be prevented with early treatment.

The most common running injury in the female athlete is chondromalcia patellae. Chondromalacia means softening of the cartilage, usually cartilage around the patella. Symptoms are a dull, aching pain in the knee, which usually gets better with running, only to get worse after the run. In the beginning the pain is annoying, but gradually, with continued training, it tends to worsen. There will be pain with flexion and with extension of the knee joint when pressure is applied to the patella. Pain will be worsened by stair climbing and hill running. In the acute stage, the patient must be told that running must be avoided altogether until the initial inflammation is reduced somewhat. Treatment usually consists of orthotics and anti-inflammatory agents; if the chondromalacia is accompanied by maltracking (in which the patella is pulled too far to the lateral aspect), resulting in further abrading of the cartilage, surgery is often the only alternative. Strengthening of the quadriceps muscle often helps in chondromalacia and maltracking problems. If the quadriceps are strong, they will bear much of the brunt of the force. Weight training can be done with leg extension machines, but the patient should not be put through the full 90 degrees of leg extension, but rather only 45 degrees. This prevents future abrading of the cartilage.

The most common injury in the male athlete is plantar fasciitis, in which the patient presents with a painful heel, relating that the pain is worse in the early morning with the first step. Pain is aggravated with running, usually after the run. Plantar fasciitis can often be corrected with orthotics or heel lift, along with icing and anti-inflammatory agents. Steroid injections are also beneficial in these cases, but care must be taken to administer only a limited amount of steroids, because prolonged use can cause atrophy of the heel pad and result in a disabling condition. Surgery should only be considered in the rarest of incidents.

Another common running overuse injury is iliotibial band syndrome. The band runs from the greater trochanter down past the femoral condyle to the lateral condyle of the tibia on the outside of the knee. This is seen particularly in the beginning runner or in the very experienced runner running long distances. As the knee flexes and extends, the bursa overlying the femoral condyle becomes irritated by the clicking of the iliotibial band over it. This click can often be palpated and even heard. The patient will often relate that the pain is increased while driving, as the knee is held in the flexed position. Treatment consists of rest, ice, and stretching exercises. The stretching exercises must be done religiously and often will suffice to correct the situation. If the pain persists, a steroid injection can be used on a one-time basis.

Shin splints is a "garbage bag" term for a number of conditions that affect the anterior aspect of the tibia. The most common problem is usually periostitis, an inflammation of the periosteum as the muscles pull it away from the bone, causing inflammation. This is usually a result of too much motion within the foot, which can be corrected with orthotics. The patient will present with pain with exertion. Rest, ice, and anti-inflammatory medications often work well. In the more experienced athlete, shin pain can be a result of a compartment syndrome, wherein the lower leg muscles grow larger than their sheaths will accommodate, causing pain with exercise. This can be a medical emergency, and a careful history should be taken to rule this out. Other causes of shin pain include stress fracture, with pain occurring with impact of the foot while running. The patient will usually continue to train; the fracture line will expand and pain will eventually occur with walking and then at rest. The patient should have radiographs, bone scans, and possibly computed tomography scans done to rule out a stress fracture.

The most common tendinitis injury is to the Achilles tendon. This is seen principally in beginning runners or in runners increasing hill or track running. Other causes are stiff-soled shoes or worn-out shoes. Treatment should therefore first consist of determining the cause of the problem and correcting or stopping it. Then ice and anti-inflammatory agents are used. The athlete is advised to cut back on all hill running and fast running. A heel lift can be used in the shoe. It is important to tell the athlete that Achilles tendinitis often precedes Achilles rupture, and care should be taken to treat it appropriately.

The use of orthotics is mentioned throughout this section on running injuries. In a triathlon, the runner will usually be wearing a pair of racing flats, which are often difficult to fit with a typical orthotic. Experience has shown that a temporary orthotic fabricated by the sports physician often works best. This orthotic should be as lightweight as possible, using Plastazote or Spenco for the foot bed. A heel pad should be incorporated into it along with a varus wedge-type material running all the way to the distal end of the toes. This is important because triathletes spend a lot of time up on the toes, in a racing gait, and need control in the forefoot as well as in the midfoot.

REFERENCES

1. Murphy P: Ultrasports are in—in spite of injuries. Physician Sports Med 14:180, 1986
2. O'Toole M: Medical considerations in triathletes. AMMA Newsl, no. 4, 1986
3. Hiller WD: Dehydration and hyperthermia during triathlons. Med Sci Sports Exerc 17:219, 1985
4. Wheeler KB, Bannell JG: Intestinal water and electrolyte flux of glucose-polymer electrolyte solution. Med Sci Sports Exerc 18:436, 1986
5. Noakes TD, Goodwin N, et al: Water intoxication: a possible complication during endurance exercise. Med Sci Sports Exerc 17:370, 1985
6. Hiller D: Medical and physiological considerations in triathlons. Am J Sports Med 15:1987
7. Clement DB, et al: A survey of overuse injuries. Physician Sports Med 9:47, 1981
8. Smith R, McKenzie DC, Tauton JE, Clements DB: A survey of overuse traumatic hip and pelvic injuries in athletes. Physician Sports Med 13:131, 1985
9. Devas MD: Stress fracture of the femoral neck. J Bone Joint Surg [Br] 47:728, 1965
10. Hodges M: Bike fit. Triathlon Mag 7:38, 1986
11. Collins K, Edwards TL: Field test of the effects of carbohydrate solutions on endurance performance and selected blood serum chemistries on perceived exertion. Med Sci Sports Exerc 16:190, 1984

34

Bowling Injuries

ROBERT J. WYSOCKI

Sixty-five million people bowl, either in an organized league or casually, as a form of recreation and sport. Ages range from 5 to over 85 years. Professional touring bowlers constitute a small percentage of this group.

This chapter stresses the importance of determining the amount of force going through the foot. Bowling is generally recognized as relatively benign, and little is written about injuries or degenerative changes occurring in the lower extremity secondary to participation. Nonetheless, the need for understanding of the biomechanics of the sport involved before attempting appropriate treatment is important and is emphasized in this chapter.

The difference between the power thrust foot and the nonpower thrust foot and, specifically, the development of degenerative arthritis of the first metatarsophalangeal joint and lesser metatarsophalangeal joints that may result secondary to improper form are discussed. The excessive forces going through the first metatarsophalangeal joint may predispose to degenerative arthritis. Surgical intervention for painful arthropathy and deformity of the first metatarsophalangeal joint should take into account these forces. There is a high rate of failure of implant arthroplasty due to these excessive forces. Thus treatment should be conservative; when surgical intervention is mandatory, with stage IV degenerative arthritis of the first metatarsophalangeal joint, a distraction Keller arthroplasty would be preferred over an implant arthroplasty.

A flexible orthosis is preferred for bowling because these orthoses allow for some support but also provide for motion, especially pronation, which is necessary for appropriate performance of the sport. Shoe therapy, physical medicine, and palliation are most useful.

INJURIES

The most common acute injuries in bowling occur due to the wrenching of the sliding knee, the lower back, and the long flexors of the bowling hand. Overuse injuries of the lower extremity may include chronic plantar fasciitis, heel-spur syndrome, tibial sesamoiditis, and the development of painful arthrosis and hallux limitus of the first metatarsophalangeal joint. Excessive valgus deviation of the great toe within the bowling shoe can create ingrowing of the hallux nail borders. Bowlers who pronate excessively may complain of sinus tarsi syndrome with lateral compression below the fibular malleolus. Pre-existing conditions, such as hammertoes, hallux valgus and bunion, or tailor's bunions may be aggravated by the activities of bowling. Acute injuries respond to physical therapy and appropriate rest and rehabilitation. Chronic injuries respond to biomechanical balancing of the foot, shoe therapy, physical therapy, and padding and taping.

Although bowling shoes look similar, the soles are quite different. One sole is for sliding, the other for braking. The slide is halted when the rubber heel comes in contact with the floor. If stopping is abrupt, toenail and digital injuries occur. Subungual hemorrhages or hematomas may be secondary to jamming of the first metatarsophalangeal joint. Sticking at the foul line is common, and serious injury, including falling, may be unavoidable. An adducted or abducted sliding foot position has a pronounced effect on the foot, ankle, knee, hip, and lower back. Appropriate attention to proper form and foot function may correct overuse abnormalities of the lower extremity associated with bowling.

The braking shoe helps anchor the slide. Preferably the trailing foot stays in contact with the floor, but the forefoot is dorsiflexed, presenting the probability of injuries, most often a traumatic arthritis of the first metatarsophalangeal joint. This is induced when the foot bends against the stiff toebox. The condition is accelerated by a last "thrusting" action that occurs on the step preceding the slide. Radiographs illustrate the degenerative hypertrophic joint changes (Fig. 34-1). The degenerative joint disease may be secondary to what professionals call the power thrust. This places undue force on the first metatarsophalangeal joint.

DYNAMICS OF BOWLING

Bowling, although appearing to be a benign sport, is not without its problems. The sports medicine specialist should be aware of the preferred movement in bowling as the bowler approaches the foul line (Fig. 34-2). The walk should be smooth and gliding, because lurching or a heavy, awkward gait may predispose to injury. The body should be balanced over the feet. A plumb line continuous from the apex of the shoulder through the deeply flexed knee onto a sliding foot is evidence of good form and body balance. There should be coordination between the upper and lower extremity (Fig. 34-2B).

Few modern bowlers demonstrate this straightforward directional tracking or the light, balanced weight transmission of equipoise. When the foot does not track straight ahead within its own parameters (approximately 10 degrees abduction), balance flexion at the metatarsophalangeal joints cannot occur. The ankle (hinge action) then deviates from the direction required by movement (Fig. 34-2D). Stress results, and ultimately extrinsic compensation becomes overt. This compensation may lead to medial plantar fasciitis, ankle strain, valgus strain at the knees, and hip or back strain.

PRETEEN BOWLERS

Preteen and child bowlers often approach the foul line in a disorganized, strained, forceful, or violent manner. Gyrations, tilting, and "coming out of the plane" are evident on telecasts of such events. I believe this may be because children use adult-sized bowling balls, which place undue stress on the upper and lower extremities, causing a contorted form. These balls, although considerably lighter (approximately 7 pounds), have a circumference equiva-

lent to those of the balls used by adults. The child cannot maneuver a sphere of this size and must contort to get a relatively small body out of the way of the large ball. This may happen during the back-swing position. Dropping the shoulder, tilting the spine, twisting the feet, and flexing the elbow in place lead to poor bowling form and postural symptoms. A pattern develops that is carried forward to adult years.

These bowlers become known as "crankers." They are easily identified by a jerky movement and an abrupt and even twisting slide, with straight knees so that tremendous lift and spin can be applied to the bowling ball. This is in direct contrast to the more graceful "stroker," who emulates a rhythm and tempo desirable in the bowler with good form. It is an understatement to say that longevity will follow the stroker and certainly not the cranker, for whom injuries are more common.

HANDEDNESS: LEFT- OR RIGHT-SIDE DOMINANCE

The power thrust foot is directly related to handedness and should be of prime concern to the foot physician. Surgery performed on the thrusting foot is more likely to fail over time. In this foot, the demand is greater, the torque is greater, the vulnerability of the foot is magnified, and internal structures can weaken and even collapse (Fig. 34-1). Left- or right-footedness, like handedness, should be carefully considered in any pretreatment evaluation for bowling, golfing, or even nonathletic injuries (see Box). For example, a joint arthroplasty, with or without implant, will be more successful and enduring in the foot that has less demand placed on it. Lateral forces through the foot, abetted by external rotation of the leg, practically guarantee post-treatment or postoperative problems. Similar operations, performed bilaterally, will seldom produce the same result after a span of time; right- or left-side dominance is often the reason for this.

Such a procedure was recommended to a world-class bowler for a "very sore bunion" on his power thrusting foot—in this case the right, since he was right-handed. Slow-motion videotape showed that his delivery was powered with tremendous thrust off the medial side of his great toe, and the transmission of lateral forces (aided by his foot being in an out-toed position) was quite obvious. An implant would never hold up under such great demand. To preserve the implant, he would be forced to compromise his style to accommodate the altered joint. I advised

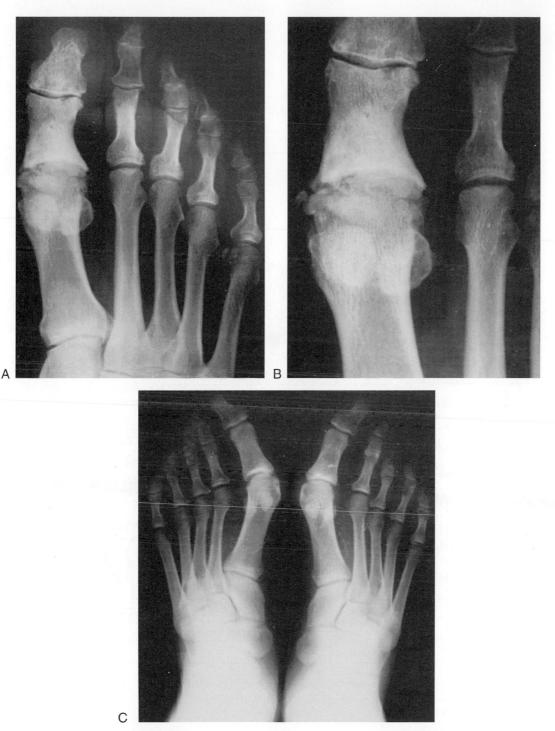

Figure 34–1 (**A&B**) Radiographs of right-handed bowler showing hallux rigidus of the power thrust foot and degenerative hypertrophic joint changes. (**C**) Radiograph of right-handed bowler with out-toed right foot thrust.

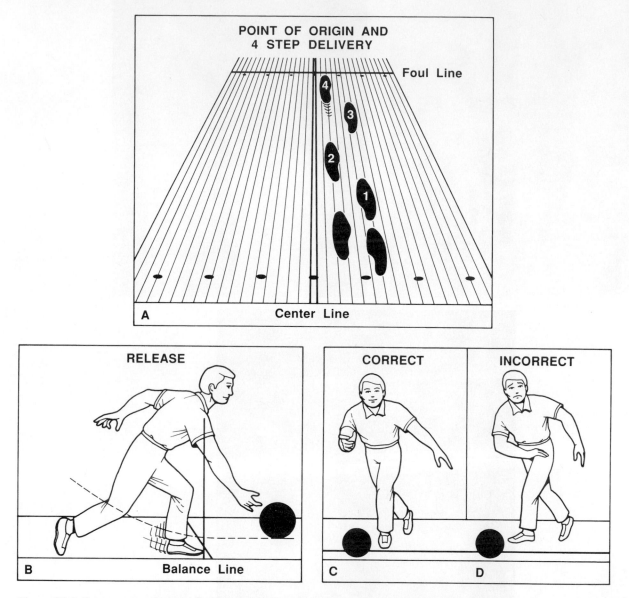

Figure 34-2 Proper approach to the foul line. (**A**) Point of origin and four-step delivery. (**B**) The shoulder–bent knee–foot arrangement should form a straight line at release. (**C**) Correct and (**D**) incorrect body alignment at release.

against the procedure. More than a few athletic careers have come to an end because this compromise interfered with the instinctual motion that made these athletes great in the first place. This type of operation is best performed at the end of an athlete's career.

TREATMENT MODALITIES

In treating bowling injuries, I prefer mechanical joint mobilization and manipulative therapy, reciprocal exercises and rehabilitation, and trigger point therapy in conjunction with standard conservative podiatric sports medicine techniques (see Box).

Mechanical Joint Dysfunction and Manipulative Therapy

Every joint in the body has a movement built into it—a certain amount of excursion between the moving parts that allows for efficient, economical function. Joints that are not used to their full range of motion lose motion over a period of time and compromise biomechanical function.

Normal excursion movement is mandatory and is a prerequisite to functional movement.

Mechanical joint dysfunction has been found to be a considerable factor in the cause of intrinsic or extrinsic musculoskeletal pain (e.g., shin splints, muscle spasm, point of maximum tenderness pain, pain at metatarsophalangeal joints, and strain and dysfunction of the midtarsal and rearfoot joints). When function becomes impaired, the ability to perform the rhythmic athletic movement so necessary for bowling is reduced. Compensation is the end result, with asymmetric function.

Symmetric functional range of motion at joints can be re-established through mobilization and manipulation, as described in the chapter on physical therapy (see Ch. 21). Once major contractions have been relieved, the patient should be put on a maintenance program and taught how to continue with a fitness program at home.

Correct biomechanical alignment of the lower extremities is established through the use of appropriate shoes and foot orthotics. Appropriate foot and leg movement for the professional bowler should be explained by the practicing physician; further coaching may be necessary from a teaching professional. Proprioception is enhanced by having patients do appropriate proprioceptive rehabilitative maneuvers (see section on proprioceptive neuromuscular rehabilitation in Ch. 21.)

It is important to emphasize to bowlers that a small amount of discomfort may progress to more severe discomfort and dysfunction in the future. In my experience, appropriate intervention at the beginning of a process has saved many bowlers from progressive severe disability.

Trigger Point Therapy

Trigger points, points of maximum tenderness causing reflex pain proximally and distally, are not uncommon in the injured athlete. The type of pain suffered may be more of an aggravation than frank acute pain. Trigger point pain appears to be secondary to overuse, fatigue, and excessive strain or abrupt stretching. When stimulated or palpated, these trigger points cause specific pain syndromes, muscle spasm, stiffness, and/or weakness. Oriental medicine considers blocked acupuncture points, or neurolymphatic points, to be responsible for trigger point pain and secondary reflex weakness and disability. Both locally and in distant target areas, trigger points should be evaluated. The more common forms of referred trigger point syndromes have been mapped anatomically. Once established, trigger points can be activated by often seemingly minor physical or emotional stresses.

Trigger points have been implicated in a variety of pain phenomena, including muscle spasm (myalgia), muscular (nonjoint) manifestations of arthritis, muscle inflammation (myositis or myofasciitis), and inflammation of the white fibrous tissue that comprises muscle sheaths and fascial layers of the whole muscle joint–tendon–ligament system (fibrositis or myofibrositis).

Trigger points are usually associated with palpable nodules of fibrous tissue. Physiologically, they form a self-sustaining cycle of pain–more spasm–more pain. This vicious circle may be interrupted at the sensory (afferent) or at the motor (efferent) point of the mechanism.

Manual trigger point compression, dry needling, or injection of an anesthetic solution will intervene at the sensory level, possibly by stimulating the brain stem production of enkephalins and endorphins. The reflex arch may also be short-cut by way of the gate control mechanism. This would be similar to using a transcutaneous electrical nerve stimulation unit or doing acupuncture or acupressure. The result, however, is a palpable softening of the tense muscle tissue, signaling muscle relaxation and pain relief, which may last for days, months, or more. Often, trigger point therapy is necessary for appropriate relaxation of soft tissue before mobilization and manipulation of contracted joints can be carried out. I prefer deep muscle massage; trigger point compression; injection with local anesthetic, vitamin B_{12}, or both; neurotherapy; and acupuncture when treating musculoskeletal injuries. Along with their considerable benefit to the bowler, these modalities also help other athletes and may be useful in post-traumatic or surgical pain with reflex spasm.

Trigger point therapy, mobilization and manipulation, and other forms of manual physical therapy are enhanced by massage, as well as electrical physical therapy modalities such as ultrasound and electrogalvanic stimulation. When swelling is present, electrogalvanic stimulation or ultrasound in an ice slush may be most beneficial. The pain cycle must be stopped, spasm relieved, and functional range of motion re-established to allow the body to heal itself.

Reciprocal Exercise

The movements of the musculoskeletal system during bowling are asymmetric. The interaction between agonist and antagonist musculature, unilateral overdevelopment (sports-specific hypertrophy), hypertonicity, and contralateral hypotonicity should be carefully observed. With asymmetric movement, prime movers overdevelop at the expense of those muscles less used. The right-handed bowler would be expected to have a stronger right arm. This same form of asymmetric overdevelopment is seen in such sports as fencing or running, with overdevelopment of the legs and relative underdevelopment of the upper extremity.

Despite the need for asymmetric motion for execution of the movements of the sport, symmetric balanced development of the muscles and joints of the lower extremity is necessary for appropriate function over the long run in sports. Thus appropriate strength, flexibility, and balance exercises should be prescribed for all athletes to maintain optimum fitness. Overuse contraction should be reversed with appropriate stretching and strengthening exercises. Dynamic imbalance must be treated appropriately, just as in the runner who overdevelops the gravity muscles at the expense of the antigravity muscles.

The range of motion of bowlers should be carefully observed before a foot orthotic is prescribed. It is generally advisable to use a soft temporary support during the initial phases of therapy, as well as rehabilitative therapy to establish dynamic balance. Once full range of motion has been re-established, more permanent orthoses may be prescribed.

SUGGESTED READINGS

Hang KF: Manual of Neural Therapy According to Hunake (Regulating Therapy with Local Anesthetics. 1st English ed.). Karl F. Hang Publishers, Heidelberg, 1984

Lawson H: Dynamic Muscular Relaxation, 1988

Meagher J, Boughton P: Sports Massage. Double Dolphin, New York, 1980

Pruden B: Myotherapy: The Trigger Point Compression Technique. Ballantine Books, New York, 1984

Rolf IP: Rolfing: The Integration of Human Structures. Harper & Row, New York, 1977

Shay A: 40 Common Errors in Bowling and How to Correct Them. Contemporary Books, Chicago, 1979

Tikker R: The Art of Joint Manipulation. Contra Costa Foot Clinic, Concord, CA, 1991

Travell JG, Simons DG: Myofascial Pain and Dysfunction. Williams & Wilkins, Baltimore, 1983

Walther DS: Applied Kinesiology. Vol 1: Basic Procedures and Muscle Testing. DC Systems, Pueblo, CO, 1981

35

Golf Injuries

AYNE F. FURMAN

The number of golfers in the United States is on the rise, with approximately 25 million players in 1997, according to the National Golf Foundation. Even though there is a level of participation similar to or higher than that found in running and aerobic dancing, the number of publications devoted to golf injuries is far less.

This chapter is intended to aid the sports medicine practitioner in understanding the demands, biomechanics, and footwear requirements of golf as they relate to the lower extremity. This understanding is intended to assist the practitioner in determining the significance that golf may have in contributing to a patient's injury or prolonging its recovery.

GOLF THE SPORT

Golf is often viewed by nonplayers as a game requiring little or no physical fitness. Actually, golf is a sport that requires considerable agility and coordination to properly and effectively swing a golf club to strike a ball in the desired direction. While the physical demands are not great, some degree of strength and aerobic conditioning is still needed to negotiate the terrain and the obstacles designed into many golf courses. In fact, a golfer who walks an 18-hole course may cover 5 miles; even if a cart is used, the walking distance may be 2 miles.

INJURIES

The majority of golf-related injuries in both amateur and professional players are of the upper extremity, primarily involving the lower back, wrist, and elbow.[1,2] Approxi-

mately 10 to 12 percent of golf injuries occur in the lower extremity.[1] The most common injuries reported, and observed by me, are plantar fasciitis,[3,4] neuromas,[4] patello-femoral syndromes,[2,3] first metatarsophalangeal joint impingement syndromes,[4] trochanteric bursitis,[2,3] and Achilles tendinitis.[2]

THE GOLF SWING

Although the time spent swinging a golf club during a round of golf is a small fraction of the total playing time, the importance of a proper golf swing to the game is paramount. Both the difficulty of achieving a satisfactory golf swing and the number of golfers striving for this precision are emphasized by the countless books and videos dedicated to this aspect of the game.

In order to effectively treat golf swing-related injuries, the sports medicine practitioner requires a basic understanding of the mechanics of the golf swing. This awareness, and an appreciation for the difficulty involved, will help the practitioner to understand how a lower extremity injury may have occurred.

The golf swing can be divided into five phases: setup, take-away, forward swing, impact, and follow-through. During setup, the golfer positions the club and body over the golf ball with the left shoulder toward the target (this assumes the golfer is right handed) (Fig. 35-1). Take-away begins as the golf club is moved back over the right shoulder. During this phase, there is a weight shift to the lateral border of the right foot, which supinates (Fig. 35-2). The forward swing begins with the golfer shifting weight to

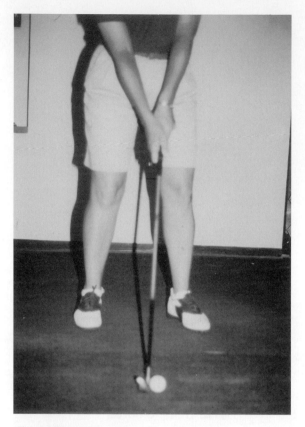

Figure 35-1 Setup.

weight in the left foot during follow-through, depending on the club being used.[6]

ETIOLOGIES OF GOLF INJURIES

There is limited information in the literature addressing the etiology of lower extremity golf injuries.[7] Epidemiologic studies that do mention lower extremity injuries generally do not consider in which part of the game the injury occurred: walking or playing (swinging the golf club). Because of the significant walking component of golf, participants are exposed to similar injuries and the same etiologic factors of injury that occur with walking.

Age can certainly be a contributing factor to golf injuries. According to the National Golf Foundation, over 40 percent of all golfers are over the age of 40. This older population of golfers are more likely to have pre-existing conditions with lessened flexibility and increased degener-

Figure 35-2 Take-away. As the body rotates, weight is shifted to the right foot.

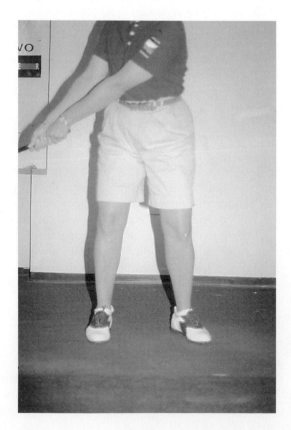

the left foot together with the forward motion of the golf club. During the forward swing phase, the right foot pronates and a valgus stress is placed on the right knee and first metatarsophalangeal joint. At impact, the golf club makes contact with the golf ball and most of the body weight has shifted to the left foot. At this time, there is continued valgus stress on the right knee and first metatarsophalangeal joint (Fig. 35-3). Follow-through is the final phase, when the golf club motion continues over the left shoulder and the body rotates to face the target. During this phase, the left foot supinates and torsional stress is placed on the right knee and hip (Fig. 35-4).

According to popular belief, golf involves symmetric foot motion. Contrary to this belief, the peak forces and the amount of pronation and supination in each foot during the golf swing are asymmetric as weight shifts from right to left.[5,6] An example of this asymmetry is found when one investigates the overall peak forces during the golf swing. These can reach 133 to 150 percent of body

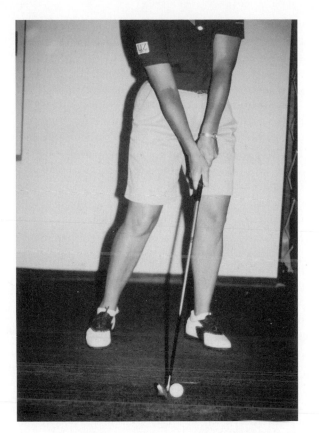

Figure 35-3 Impact. Note how medial the right knee is compared to the right foot.

ative joint disease.[8] These conditions can be aggravated during the game from the torque and rotation required for the golf swing and by walking over uneven terrain, which may include hills, sand traps, cart paths, rocks, and canted ground (Fig. 35-5).

Other etiologic factors that can be attributed to injury of the lower extremity are listed in the Box below.

GOLF SHOES

Golf shoes should assist the lower extremity to function as a base of support for the golf swing by reducing foot slippage and offering lateral stability. In addition, golf shoes should provide comfort while walking. Relatively limited research and development has gone into golf shoes when compared with golf club and golf ball designs.[9] More extensive exploration must be performed to determine the optimum design of a golf shoe for function, performance, and protection from injury.

Currently available golf shoes can be divided into three categories:

1. Traditional leather-soled shoes (Fig. 35-6). These generally have a classic cosmetic appearance, a fairly rigid sole, steel shank, and welt method of construction. The welted construction of these shoes allows them to be made in multiple widths (personal communication with FootJoy).
2. Ethyl vinyl acetate (EVA)/polyurethane (PU) midsole/outersole combination shoes (Fig. 35-7). These tend to have a more flexible forefoot than the leather-soled shoes, provide more cushioning and shock absorption, and are usually lighter than leather-soled golf shoes.

Figure 35-4 Follow-through. There is a valgus force being applied to the medial aspect of the right foot as most of the weight is shifted to the lateral border of the left foot.

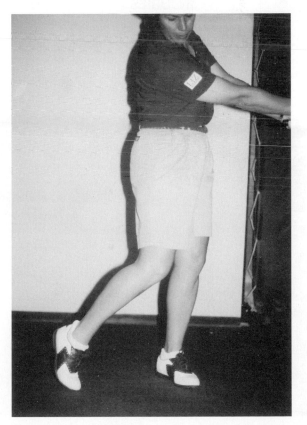

ETIOLOGIC FACTORS IN GOLF-RELATED LOWER EXTREMITY INJURY

Improper shoe gear for the golfer's foot type and playing style

Overuse/excessive practice

Poor swing technique

Inflexibility/improper warmup

Falling/slipping

Walking/hitting on uneven terrain

Golf cart accidents

3. Spikeless shoes (Fig. 35-8). These tend to be light weight and generally have the most overall shoe flexibility when compared with the other types.

TREATMENT OF GOLF-RELATED INJURIES

In addition to the normal treatment regimen the practitioner uses for a particular injury, the following modalities should be considered when appropriate:

1. *Shoe category change*: Change to a shoe design more appropriate to the patient's foot structure and injury.
2. *Changes in technique*: The golfer's technique should be assessed by a golf professional, and preferably one with some understanding of injuries. The professional's observation and assessment should correct any swing errors or possibly make recommendations to change the golfer's swing to put less stress on a particular area.
3. *Flexibility program*: A stretching program directed at the hamstrings, gastrocnemius–soleus complex, and iliotibial band should be initiated.
4. *Conditioning program*: Some form of aerobic exercise three times a week should be considered.
5. *Spike conversion*: Replace steel spikes in golf shoes with plastic cleats (i.e., Softspikes) (Fig. 35-9). These will help absorb impact during the walking portion of the game, especially while on cart paths.
6. *Spike modification*: Try removing the spike(s) that are under the painful area of the foot (i.e., metatarsal head).
7. *Modification of equipment*: Change to a pull cart instead of a carried golf bag.

ORTHOTICS

An orthotic placed in a golf shoe should ideally not restrict the needed motions of the foot during the golf swing. Therefore, golf orthotics are fabricated with a flexi-

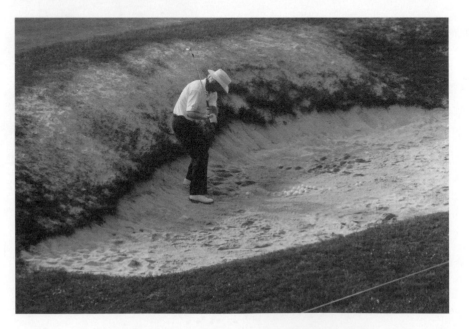

Figure 35-5 This sand trap illustrates a steep and canted playing surface of a golf course.

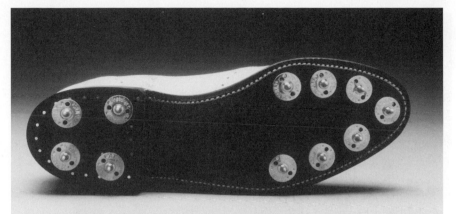

Figure 35-6 Outsole of a leather-soled golf shoe.

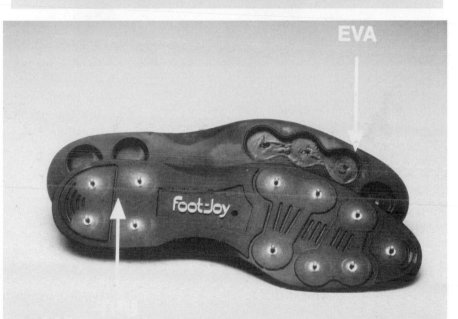

Figure 35-7 The EVA midsole and PU outsole.

Figure 35-8 The outsole of a spikeless golf shoe. There are no removable spikes.

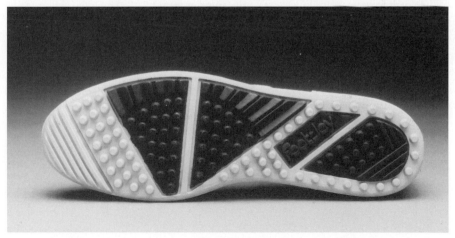

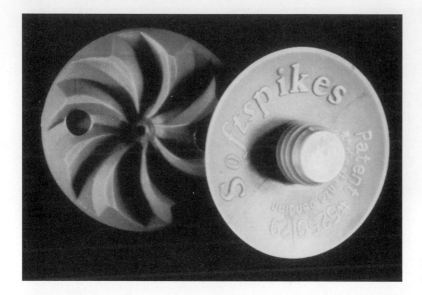

Figure 35-9 Softspikes cleats are made of PU and can replace removable steel spikes.

ble shell, provide support through the longitudinal arch, and are prescribed with a perpendicular or no rearfoot post. It is my clinical experience that, in some cases when the patient has significant subtalar or forefoot varus or walks the course, the flexible type of orthotic device (that being used during the recover from an injury) is not sufficiently therapeutic, functional, or both for the foot. For these patients, a more rigid shell should be tried with a lower durometer of posting.

CONCLUSION

The small percentage of lower extremity injuries found in golfers should not dissuade a practitioner from considering golf as the cause or contributing source of an injury when treating a patient that plays the game. With a more educated and aware approach, the patient will be better helped to recover more quickly and with less limitation of activity during the recovery period.

REFERENCES

1. McCarroll JR, Rettig AC, Shelbourne DK: Injuries in the amateur golfer. Physician Sports Med 3:18, 1990
2. Stover CN, McCarroll JR, Mallon WJ: Feeling up to Par: Medicine from Tee to Green. F.A. Davis Company, Philadelphia, 1994
3. McCarroll JR: Golf. p. 375. In Fu FH, Stone DA (eds): Sports Injuries: Mechanisms, Prevention and Treatment. Williams & Wilkins, Baltimore, 1994
4. Wysocki RJ: Bowling and golf injuries. p. 647. In Subotnick SI (ed): Sports Medicine of the Lower Extremity. Churchill Livingstone, New York, 1989
5. Johnson H: How to feel a tour pro's foot pressure. Golf Digest 2:65, 1992
6. Williams KR, Cavanagh PR: The mechanics of foot action during the golf swing and implications for shoe design. Med Sci Sports Exerc 15:247, 1983
7. Batt ME: A survey of golf injuries in amateur golfers. Br J Sports Med 26:63, 1992
8. Batt ME: Golfing injuries: An overview. Sports Med 16:64, 1993
9. McNerney JE: How golf shoes work . . . and how to choose a pair that works for you. Golf Illustrated 6:78, 1990

36

Baseball Injuries

JEFFREY F. YALE

Although the sports medicine aspects of baseball center on injuries to the throwing arm,[1-4] lower-extremity injuries include all those seen in other running sports.[5,6] Most arm injuries occur secondary to faulty foot placement. Injuries to the lower extremity may occur as a result of sliding into a base or diving after a ball, from sudden bursts of speed necessary to steal a base or to chase down a fly ball, and during training drills. Common lower extremity injuries seen in baseball include spike injuries; abrasions and contusions; hamstring, quadriceps, adductor, psoas major, and triceps surae muscle strain; ankle sprains, and meniscal tears. Play on yielding surfaces in warm weather and on hard surfaces in cold weather predisposes to Achilles tendinitis and heel-spur syndrome. Blister formation is the most common baseball player injury. The hard clay infield results in excessive inshoe friction and pressure, with resulting "hot spots" and blister formation.

The many overuse problems experienced by baseball players are usually seen during the conditioning period prior to competition. Common overuse injuries include plantar fasciitis, Achilles tendinitis, anterior and posterior shin splints, extensor hallucis longus tenosynovitis, anterior and posterior Achilles bursitis, greater trochanteric bursitis, iliotibial band, heel-spur and patellofemoral syndromes, and blisters. Biomechanical inefficiencies predisposing to overuse injury are controlled with foot orthotic devices in combination with stretching–strengthening exercise programs.

Because baseball is a running sport, running conditioning programs are incorporated into the training regimen. Motion, function, and strength are the three training factors stressed. Interval training, fartlek, and speed work enhance adaptation to stress, resulting in optimum conditioning. Inherent stance positions of the batter, catcher, umpire, and field player can often be enhanced by control of faulty foot function.[7] Proper stride, foot placement, coordinated upper and lower extremity movement, and throwing, fielding, catching, and running technique are essential in preventing baseball injuries.[8]

Various forms of a base-running drill may be used within the baseball conditioning program. The base-running drill prepares the athlete for quick starts and 90-foot sprints. Running through first base, stealing second base, taking a lead off second base, and scoring on a base hit are examples of various base-running drills. A series of these drills may be repeated four to six times, providing aerobic training specific to the sport. Sliding drills with spikes removed help prevent injury during the game. The use of breakaway bases substantially decreases the risk for or occurrence of sliding-related injuries.[8,9]

INJURIES SPECIFIC TO VARIOUS POSITIONS

The baseball team consists of a pitcher; catcher; first, second, and third basemen; shortstop; right, left, and center fielders; designated hitter; trainer; and coaches. In slow-pitch softball, there are four outfielders. The trainer is the pivotal person in regard to the medical treatment of athletes in all sports, including baseball. The trainer is the single most experienced person in detecting medical-related problems in his or her athletes. With the trainer's invaluable assistance, the podiatric physician will be better able to interpret individual mechanism of injury and assist in prevention and treatment.

Pitcher

A right-handed pitcher's stance includes the following components. The right leg must be externally rotated with the foot pointing 45 degrees laterally and the left leg and foot pointing toward the batter. The right foot must be supinated and stable. An uncompensated rearfoot varus or forefoot valgus may predispose to ankle inversion injury. In order to throw the ball with velocity, the pitcher must have all weight on the right foot while in the balanced or tucked position. With faulty technique, if the pitcher overthrows, there will be a tendency to overextend, putting adverse stretch on the right extremity hamstrings. The left foot must contact the ground with the forefoot. If overstriding occurs, with the left foot making contact with the heel, a hamstring injury may occur. The left foot should point forward toward the hitter after the ball is thrown. The left foot should be neither supinated nor pronated. If the left foot is supinated, the right knee and right throwing arm will be injured. If the left foot is pronated, an injury to the left medial knee may result.

Baseball pitchers exert significant friction and pressure on the medial aspect of the forefoot on the same side as the pitching arm. This friction and pressure may result in recurrent blisters and bleeding, the formation of hyperkeratosis or severe discomfort, or both, resulting in negative alteration of pitching style. If the usual movements of an athlete are altered, a secondary injury may occur. Alteration of the usual pitching form may predispose to secondary knee, ankle, hip, and/or upper-extremity injury.

Lower extremity biomechanics related to the pitcher may vary. Variables include length of stride, foot and toe position, body pitching angle, and relationship of the body to the pitching rubber and batter. Children should be discouraged from mimicking pitchers, to avoid the development of poor playing habits predisposing to future injury.

Batter

Foot placement is crucial to the batter, or hitter. The feet should be shoulder-width apart, with weight borne on the forefeet ("getting rhythm"). With the knees flexed 5 to 10 degrees, weight is transferred, in a right-handed batter, to the right foot. The most important biomechanical aspect of right-handed batter movement is the efficient transfer of weight from the right foot to the left foot. Batting is a sequence of coordinated muscle activity, beginning with the hip, followed by the trunk, and terminating with the arms.[10]

As the right-handed pitcher assumes the balanced position with his left rear pointing at the batter, that is the cue for the right-handed batter to begin an unlocking motion, resulting in weight transfer to the right foot, bending of the left knee, and facing the left rear toward the pitcher. The right foot must be stable relative to the ground, that is, supinated with the leg externally rotated. These motions precede the most important batting maneuver: weight transfer from the right foot to the left foot. The left foot is bearing little weight as the bat is held anticipating swing. As the bat swings forward, a pivoting motion must take place on the forefeet and at the hips, resulting in weight transfer from the right foot and leg to the left foot and leg. Both feet are now pointing toward the pitcher.

If the ball is pitched inside or outside, the feet are not moved. Movement occurs at the hips, with the umbilicus pointed toward third base when the batter is hitting an inside pitch and toward first base when hitting an outside pitch.

With the right-handed batter's left foot forward, foot balancing as on thin ice, any limitation to subtalar pronation (e.g., cavovarus, uncompensated rearfoot varus) will predispose to lateral ankle sprain. Foul balls may bounce off or directly into the medial aspect of the left foot or into the left anterior compartment. Some players wear anterior shin guards for protection. Balls fouled off the left great toe may result in subungual hematoma. The incidence of being hit with a foul ball is much greater than being hit by a pitched ball.

Catcher and Umpire

The catcher must be in a crouched position, with weight borne evenly on the forefeet in the ready position. The catcher must be able to respond to inside or outside pitches by loading and unloading each foot. Premature fatigue ensues in catchers with compensated rearfoot varus or other foot problems, predisposing to excessive subtalar pronation. Foul balls may injure the great toes, the unprotected area just above the patella, or both.

Umpires wear steel toebox safety shoes. Because the umpire is in the inside position relative to the batter with the left foot forward, he is at risk of getting hit by the ball.

First Baseman

The first baseman is prone to right leg hamstring injuries secondary to stretching while reaching for the ball while the heel of the right foot is in contact with the edge of the base. Injury to the medial heel may result when the runner steps on this area as he runs through first base.

Shortstop and Second Baseman

Injuries occur most frequently to the shortstop and second baseman during a double play. These players are susceptible to getting hit below the knee by a runner or sliding runner. The rules were changed several years ago at the high school and college school level. It is now unacceptable for the runner to cross-body block the fielder. A base runner must now slide directly into the base.

Outfielders

Outfielders sustain hamstring injuries and ankle inversion injuries from their quick field response in an effort to follow the vector of the ball. Cavovarus foot type predisposes to lateral ankle injury. Stepping in potholes, drainage areas, or on an uneven field will predispose to ankle injury as well.

The outfielder is intent on catching the ball and throwing it within the least possible time. If the ball is caught far to the left, the lower extremities are not in the ideal position for throwing the ball. This may result in injury to the throwing arm. Ideally, the ball should be caught just right of front—over and in front of the throwing shoulder—while stepping into the ball with the right foot. This will enable the fielder to throw the ball with utmost velocity and efficiency.

Base Runner

The base runner is predisposed to injury depending on foot type, range of motion, muscle strength, and flexibility. The hitter running through first base must not overstride and hit the base with the heel. This will result in hamstring injury. Also, because the lead foot and leg are extended and supinated just before heel contact, inversion on contact occurs, resulting in lateral ankle injury. When the forefoot makes initial contact with the base, a first metatarsophalangeal hyperextension injury may occur.

From a teaching standpoint, sliding into a base is called "falling." The player leads with the left foot and leg slightly off the ground, contacting the base with the heel. The right leg is flexed at the knee and tucked under the left extended leg. The "fall" is taken on the gluteal muscles, which have the most padding, hence less chance of abrasion.

BASEBALL AND ORTHOTICS

Baseball shoes should have a stable counter, deep toe-box, rigid shank, and flexible sole.[1] High-school players use rubber cleats, while college and professional baseball players use metal cleats—three cleats on the fore-foot and three on the heel. Baseball shoes are becoming lighter in weight at the expense of stable heel counters and medial longitudinal support.

Polypropylene foot orthoses have been used alone or in combination with latex shields to control adverse function and to protect the medial and dorsal aspects of the hallux in pitchers.[11] Excessive dorsiflexion of the hallux must be avoided while the latex shield impression is being taken. The latex shield encompasses the forefoot so as to avoid slippage. Talcum powder is used between the shield and foot. Creams, oils, or ointments should not be used as a separating medium. The foot, with shield in place, should fit comfortably into the appropriate baseball shoe. However, Polisner[11] found, through interview, that one major league baseball team's pitchers were reluctant to wear foot orthoses or shields.

PREVENTION OF INJURY

While it has been shown that the performance of the most elite players is superior to that of less able players even at very early ages,[12] overall conditioning through motion, function, and strength training will still minimize injury. Triceps surae, hamstring, and intrinsic foot muscle stretching flexibility exercises are of great importance. Temporary foot or shoe padding, or both, to control adverse function or to protect a part often makes the difference in a game's successful outcome. Semirigid static foot orthoses can prevent many associated overuse injuries. The incidence of "posterior shin splints" alone makes podiatric input invaluable to the baseball player, trainer, and coach. Diagnosis and treatment of specific athletic injuries is discussed in depth in other sections of this text. The reader is referred to those sections for specific treatment guidelines.

ACKNOWLEDGMENTS

I wish to express my sincerest thanks to Joseph Benanto, head baseball coach, and William E. Kaminsky, ATC, athletic trainer, Yale University, New Haven, Connecticut, for their invaluable help.

REFERENCES

1. Jobe FW, Pink M: The athlete's shoulder. J Hand Ther 7: 107, 1994

2. Magnusson SP, Gleim GW, Nicholas JA: Shoulder weakness in professional baseball pitchers. Med Sci Sports Exerc 26: 5, 1994

3. Timmerman LA, Andrews JR: Undersurface tear of the ulnar collateral ligament in baseball players: a newly recognized lesion. Am J Sports Med 22:33, 1994

4. Podesta L, Sherman MF, Bonamo JR: Distal humeral epi-
physeal separation in a young athlete: a case report. Arch Phys Med Rehabil 74:1216, 1993

5. Yale JF: Firm Footings for the Athlete (A Preventive Injury and Self-Help Guide for Those Athletes Involved in the Running Sports). Ansonia, CT, 1981

6. Yale JF: Yale's Podiatric Medicine. 3rd ed. Williams & Wilkins, Baltimore, 1987

7. Yale JF: Yale's Podiatric Medicine. 3rd ed. p. 446. Williams & Wilkins, Baltimore, 1987

8. Janda DH, Wild DE, Hensinger RN: Softball injuries: aetiology and prevention. Sports Med 13:285, 1992

9. Sliding-associated injuries in college and professional baseball 1990–1991. MMWR Morb Mortal Wkly Rep 42(12):223, 1993

10. Shaffer B, Jobe FW, Pink M, Perry J: Baseball batting: an electromyographic study. Clin Orthop 292:285, 1993

11. Polisner RI: Latex shields for major league baseball players. J Am Podiatr Med Assoc 76:590, 1986

12. Schulz R, Musa D, Staszewski J, Siegler RS: The relationship between age and major league baseball performance: implications for development. Psychol Aging 9:274, 1994

37
Tennis Injuries

JEFFREY A. ROSS

As with all court sports, tennis involves various multidirectional movements. Unlike jogging/running, which is unidirectional, tennis involves a forward–reverse as well as side-to-side motion. When combined with the service and net play, tennis can be the source of many minor as well as serious injuries. Many of the injuries can involve inflammatory processes; however, all too often we see traumatic fractures/dislocations as well as tears and rupture of ligamentous and tendon structures.

Many of the injuries encountered in tennis, as in other sports, are due to overuse syndromes. In fact, studies reveal that approximately 30 to 50 percent of all sports injuries are due to overuse.[1-3] The overuse syndrome injuries have a common etiology, a repetitive trauma that eventually interferes with a tissue's ability to repair itself.[4] This chapter presents an appreciation of those tissues and structures that are subject to injury, as well as the mechanics of repeated injury in the sport of tennis.

INFLAMMATION IN OVERUSE INJURIES

In tennis, overuse injuries may create inflammatory processes in tissues to varying degrees. Inflammation is the direct result of repetitive microtraumatic forces. The mechanisms of inflammation are regarded as a necessary component of the healing process. Acute (repair) inflammation is productive, whereas chronic inflammation can be destructive and disabling. It is imperative for the sports medicine physician to keep chronic inflammation to a minimum in order to prevent overuse injuries from becoming irreversible.

After initial vasoconstriction and hemostasis, the body creates a local vasodilation, leading to the release of capillary fluid. Prostaglandin production in inflammation causes vasodilation and produces edema. This can lead to bone resorption by stimulating osteoclastic activity. Prostaglandin activity can be inhibited by nonsteroidal anti-inflammatory drugs, which act by inhibiting prostaglandin synthesis.

Following an injury, a variety of cells with different functions migrate to the area. Neutrophils begin the breakdown of adjacent tissues; collagenase macrophages possess many proteolytic enzymes and phagocytotic cells. Lymphocytes are important in chronic inflammation; fibroblasts produce collagen and help in the reparative process of muscle, tendon, and ligament injuries.

TENDON INJURIES

Overuse injuries to tendons are quite common in tennis. Tendons are comprised of elastin and collagen, brought together in complex segments. The individual fibrils gather to form fibers, then fibers group together to form fascicles, with their intertwining producing a tendon. The tendon–muscle unit is the basis behind muscle contraction, due to its stretch. The tendon is subject to extreme and repetitive actions, particularly in sports. This continuing stretching during exercise can cause fatigue, as often seen in overuse syndrome. Because of the poor blood supply of tendons, repeated subintimal injury and delayed healing are common. The Achilles tendon is the most commonly injured in sports, according to Clancy.[5]

729

Achilles Tendinitis

Achilles tendinitis can result from a multitude of problems: biomechanical imbalances, limb length discrepancy, lack of proper stretch prior to activity, court surface, and shoe design and wear patterns.

The most common location for symptoms of Achilles tendinitis is 2 to 5 cm proximal to the insertion of the tendon into the calcaneus. This insertional area has a relatively poor blood supply. If only the tendon is involved, then it is regarded strictly as an Achilles tendinitis. However, when the sheath or paratendon is involved, then we regard this as a tenosynovitis (paratenonitis). Volk describes 42 cases of tenosynovitis of the lower extremity. He noted a crepitation at the myotendinous junction, and describes this condition as a peritendinitis crepitans. In some rarer situations a stenosing tenosynovitis of the synovial sheath can occur.

As Subotnick[6] noted, in Achilles tenosynovitis the size of the tendon sheath is increased but the underlying tendon itself has no increase. Where there is hypertrophy of the tendon sheath, crepitation may be present below the sheath in a sclerosing tendinitis. As can be expected, with chronic inflammation of the Achilles tendon, degeneration of the tendon locally can occur, causing damage and possible partial or complete rupture.

Some of the factors that may be involved in acute or chronic Achilles tendinitis are excessive pronation, limb length discrepancy, tight gastrocnemius–soleous complex, Haglund's deformity, or short Achilles tendon. The amount of heel contact during baseline-to-net play can result in pull or irritation of the Achilles tendon or tendon sheath.

The initial treatment of Achilles tendinitis is to decrease the activity, or attempt to eliminate the causative factors. Effective stretching exercises may reduce or eliminate the problem. A simple heel lift, to raise the calcaneus and take the load force off the insertion, can be helpful. A prescription orthotic device can add heel lift and reduce excessive bursal irritation (retrocalcaneal bursitis). The orthotic device can also reduce excessive pronation, with its resulting pull on the Achilles tendon.

Haglund's Deformity (Retrocalcaneal Exostosis) Bursitis

Frequently a rearfoot varus, and in many cases a forefoot varus, will result in a supinated rearfoot heel strike, causing irritation of the posterosuperior lateral border of the calcaneus by rubbing against the athletic shoe. Due to chronic irritation and formation of bursal projection, a superficial Achilles tendon bursitis or retrocalcaneal bursitis can occur. I have even seen in some patients hyperkeratotic and even intractable plantar keratoma lesions develop overlying the retrocalcaneal bursa and exostosis.

One can radiographically determine the retrocalcaneal bursal projection either by posterior calcaneal angle (Fig. 37-1) or by parallel pitch lines (Fig. 37-2). Keck and Kelly[7] observed that an increase in the parallel pitch lines, and not in abnormal posterior calcaneal angle, determined the degree of posterior heel bursitis.

I have observed that a tennis player who lands on the lateral posterior aspect of the heel either in baseline-to-net play or in the reverse may develop such a pathology. The bursal sac contains a small amount of synovium-like

Figure 37-1 Determination of the retrocalcaneal bursal projection by posterior calcaneal angle.

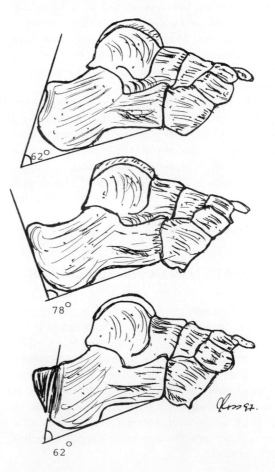

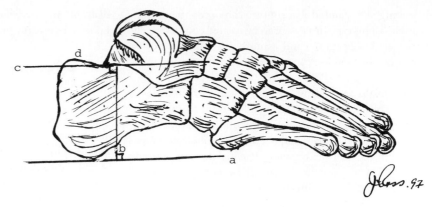

Figure 37-2 Determination of the retrocalcaneal bursal projection by parallel pitch lines.

fluid. The chronic irritation described above will cause the bursa to be inflamed, resulting in a thickening of the bursal wall, with effusion. At the posterior aspect of the calcaneus at the insertion of the Achilles tendon, calcification of the tendon can occur, also leading to inflammation of the bursa.

This bursitis and Haglund's deformity can lead to incapacitation of the tennis player, as with the runner. Conservative treatment would involve change or modification of the shoe gear, steroid injection into the bursa with complete rest, and heel lifts or prescription orthoses. It is important to augment this treatment plan with an adequate stretching program, particularly for the Achilles tendon. When conservative management has failed, surgical intervention may be necessary, with excision of the bursa alone or in combination with resection of the retrocalcaneal exostosis. It is important to ensure that adequate resection of the superoposterior (lateral) border is performed; otherwise, possible recurrence may be seen.

Spontaneous Rupture of the Achilles Tendon

In tennis, as in basketball, quick sudden starts can cause undue force in the Achilles tendon. Barfred[8] stated that the tendon is subject to injury when

1. Tension is applied quickly
2. The tendon is under tension before loading
3. The tendon is weak compared to the muscle

As mentioned earlier, a recurrent injury is a previously injured tendon can cause partial or complete rupture.

Options for treatment of Achilles tendon ruptures vary according to the individual athlete's level of involvement in the sport. Some authors believe that all Achilles tendon injuries should be conservatively treated while others believe in immediate surgical repair. There are the various procedures and criteria to consider also, all of which can be very confusing when trying to determine the proper treatment plan. I believe that, in the case of a partial tear, conservative casting in equinus is always the proper treatment. Complete ruptures, however, should be surgically repaired because of the possibility of a debilitating injury that would cause a sudden end to the player's career.

Both treatment philosophies have their complications, due to poor blood supply in the region. Surgical correction can sometimes result in wound infection of sloughing of the skin. Adhesions will result in either surgical or nonsurgical cases. In the case of conservative care, the threat of re-rupture always looms and should be an important consideration. The Cybex dynamometer can be used post-trauma to determine the decrease in endurance.

Posterior Tibial Tendinitis and Spontaneous Rupture of the Tibialis Posterior Tendon

In a tennis player who has a flexible flatfoot or pronated subtalar joint, every time the individual leaves the baseline and quickly moves forward or sideways for a shot, a rapid inverted movement takes place usually to the forefoot. This repetitive supinated subtalar motion can cause irritation to the tibialis posterior tendon. A quick and sudden movement imparted to an inflamed posterior tibial tendon can cause a spontaneous rupture. Lipsman and associates noted a case history in which this injury also occurred in golfing. They noted that rupture can occur after a teno-synovitis. This type of injury can be treated conservatively; however, better results and a more anatomically normal posterior tibial tendon can be achieved with surgical intervention.

The tibialis posterior is an important invertor and plantar flexor. The subluxation of this tendon can also have disastrous effects for the tennis player. By unlocking the midtarsal joint, excessive pronation occurs that can create a functional limb length discrepancy. Placing unusual amounts of weight and force on the medial column during arm extension and follow-through can create an unstable limb, and thus an inefficient shot.

Dislocation or Subluxing of the Peroneal Tendons

As previously mentioned, tennis involves quick starts and stops. The quick backward or side-to-side motion can be the source of chronic ankle sprains or even a peroneal dislocation. The mechanism of injury in this particular case would be a forced dorsiflexion of the mildly inverted foot, followed by a violent reflex contraction of the peroneal muscle. This sudden forceful action can cause a rupture of the peroneal retinaculum and displacement of the peroneal tendon.[9,10]

The primary action of the peroneal muscles is eversion of the foot. During tennis they act by providing the final pronation and propulsion during the run. They also act by stabilizing the ankle joint. If the peroneal tendon were in spasm, with a shallow fibular groove present, or when a partial or complete tear of the peroneal retinaculum has occurred, then a subluxation of the peroneal tendon can take place. A sudden violent plantar flexion and inversion can cause the tendon to snap forward around the lateral malleolus. If a tear of the retinaculum or the lateral collateral ligaments occurs, then dislocation or subluxation of the tendons can occur.

In the sport of tennis, not only can a forward plantar-flexed inverted foot cause this injury, but in retreating for a shot the same mechanism can occur. In fact, in "back-pedaling" the foot is probably more unstable than when moving in the forward direction. If the shot is wide also, that will add another component of directional instability.

Obviously, the acute injury can be treated surgically to obtain the optimum results. Ankle instability usually accompanies subluxation of the peroneal tendon, and the ankle mortise should be checked. Stress examination and talar tilt measurements will determine if a concomitant ankle stabilization procedure should be performed.

POSTERIOR AND ANTERIOR SHIN SPLINTS

Tennis players who actively and frequently participate in the game, particularly in singles play, may develop "shin splint syndrome." The term *shin splints* is a catch-all phrase, often used to describe posteromedial tibial pain. The conditions that we see in tennis injuries that can be lumped into the category of shin splints are as follows:

Stress fractures of the tibia

Compartment syndrome

Inflammation of the dorsiflexor tendons of the foot

Irritation of the periosteum due to tearing apart of the muscle–fascia interface

Strains of the anterior and posterior tibial tendons

This pain and tenderness located along the distal two-thirds of the medial tibial shaft can cause a debilitating condition in a tennis player.

A study conducted by Lillevedt and colleagues showed that there were significant differences among the alignments of the lower extremity of those subjects who had no shin splints, previous shin splints, and present shin splints. The etiologies of tennis-related shin splints can be grouped into various categories:

1. Court surfaces (cement, composit, clay, etc.)
2. Training methods (number of days' participation, number of sets and level of play)
3. Range of motion, flexibility and muscle function, shoe design (court shoes)
4. Alignment of the tennis player

Prost[11] and Subotnick[12] noted that excessive pronation can cause malalignment and produce symptoms consistent with shin splint syndrome.

In tennis, when approaching a forehand shot, a right hander must step into the ball with the left leg and foot and plant the right foot parallel to the net. In the study conducted by Lellivedt et al., external rotation of the femur with the hip extended and dorsiflexion of the ankle with the knee flexed were the two most common variables related to shin splint syndrome. These two mechanisms are both seen in the basic forehand return shot in tennis.

The usual treatment of such an injury would be rest and slow, progressive return to tennis activity. Taping, ultrasound, fluidotherapy, and electrotherapeutic modalities will help during the recuperative process; however, attention should be paid to the etiology. An orthotic device that prevents excessive pronation during the midstance static phase, locks the midtarsal joint, and balances the forefoot will allow for proper subtalar neutral position during the typical shot.

COMPARTMENT SYNDROMES

The compartment syndromes seen in tennis can be divided into two categories. The first involves the tennis player who has not adequately prepared, and then proceeds to play many strenuous games in rapid succession. The result can be quickly elevated intramuscle pressure, followed by rapid decrease and return to normal levels. The second type can result from a previous injury, such as a posterior tibial muscle tear or herniation, or chronic anterior tibial or peroneal tendinitis. The chronic inflammation to these tissues during quick starts and stops in tennis can cause recurrent chronic compartment syndrome. This will cause edema, increased intra-muscular pressure, and pressure on nerve trunks. This can be a chronic injury, which can reduce a tennis player's number of playing days significantly.

Mubarak et al.[13] use the wick or slit catheter technique under sterile conditions where the catheter is inserted into the involved compartment using local anesthesia. The catheter is used to monitor compartment pressures at rest and during exercise. The presence of the catheter creates an exercise environment that creates pain and eventually causes the subject to stop the exercise. Three pressures are recorded: the resting pressure, the pressure during exercise, and the pressure after exercise. Resting normal values of 0 to 8 mm Hg are seen. During exercise the pressure rises to over 50 mm Hg and just postexercise it declines to 30 mm Hg. After 5 minutes it should return to its pre-exercise levels. Levels can be monitored and, if the pressure exceeds the resting value by two times in exercise, then a recurrent compartment syndrome can occur.

According to the results obtained by Veith et al.,[14] if the tennis player continues to play "hard exertional" tennis (particularly tournament play), then the symptoms of a recurrent compartment syndrome may continue indefi-

nitely. If this is the case, then a surgical decompression of the fascial defect may be necessary. This will cause the muscle to "spread out" and reduce intracompartmental pressure. Obviously, surgical intervention would be saved for the "serious" tennis player who requires optimum dynamics in muscle performance and who suffers from recurrent compartment syndrome.

STRESS FRACTURES

As in running or aerobics, tennis sees its share of stress fractures. In service or net play there is a great deal of jumping and unilateral landing. When running to and from the net, the tennis player places incredible forces through the foot unequally.

Morris and Blickenstaff[15] used the term *fatigue fracture* in their publication because the term implies the result of mild forces or stress with eventual alteration or disruption of a material, such as bone. Therefore a stress fracture is not the result of a single occurrence, but rather an ongoing process. The end result may be fracture, but in actuality it is the product of continued applied forces on the bone creating a defect (weakness) by resorbing bone in advance of the laying down of new bone.

In tennis, metatarsal stress fractures are the most common. After such an injury, palpation of the area will usually determine the site of the fatigue fracture. As in running, the most commonly seen fractures are of the third, second, and fourth metatarsals, in descending order. On radiologic analysis, the site will most often be seen at the level of the distal third of the metatarsal shaft. Callus formation may not be seen for at least 3 weeks. The standard special procedure for early detection is the technetium-99 diphosphonate three-phase or single-phase bone scan. This can help detect a fracture within days after the injury.

The clinical signs and symptoms accompanying the stress fracture will include edema, erythema, and pinpoint tenderness when palpated. Many times pain may be elicited upon forced dorsiflexion/plantar flexion, as well as elevation/declination of the entire metatarsal ray. Percussion of the bone from a distance may elicit pain at the fracture site.

Other primary locations of potential stress fractures in the tennis player include the calcaneus, particularly when landing hard on the court from an overhead jump shot, service, or net play. Forced dorsiflexion, utilizing the same shots, can also result in a fracture of the tibial plateau or distal shaft of the tibia. When the patient presents clinically, it is important to determine from the history the exact mechanism of injury that occurred on the court. This may help differentiate a stress fracture from other injuries. Together with clinical evidence, a stress fracture may be diagnosed. My experience has always dictated that, when there is suspicion of a stress fracture, the injury should be treated as such.

Treatment varies in the tennis player according to the time when the diagnosis was made. Also, the severity of the fracture must be taken into account. If it is a fresh injury, an Unna boot (soft compression cast), with overlying elastic tape and a postoperative surgical shoe, is usually indicated. Ice, elevation, and anti-inflammatory medication are usually helpful. Follow-up repeat applications of heat (warm gentle whirlpool) and fluidotherapy (dry whirlpool) are helpful in accelerating bone healing. If the fracture is severe enough, cast immobilization and non-weight bearing may be necessary. However, if displacement is present, particularly in midshaft fractures, or if angulation takes place, then closed or open reduction with internal fixation is indicated.

Rest, immobilization, and no tennis play usually for 4 to 8 weeks postinjury is necessary. Should the tennis player return before adequate callus formation has taken place, secondary fracture could take place either at the same site or at a new location (due to fatigue). This could result in a displaced fracture, one that now requires more intervention. Tennis is an impact sport, and to allow a player early return to play postfracture could be disastrous.

FRACTURE OF THE POSTERIOR PROCESS OF THE TALUS

An injury that is not commonly seen is the fracture of the steadus process or posterior process of the talus. This injury is seen more often in ballet; however, an analysis of the motions of tennis oftentimes reveals the similarities. Tennis can demonstrate very graceful motion or a sudden violent action. When the tennis player lands in forced plantar flexion, or plantar flexion/inversion, the posterior process of the talus strikes the posterior margin of the tibia, and either a groove can develop or a fracture can occur. Turner[16] described fracture of the posterior talus due to sudden violence. When the foot is placed in equinus, the posterior process can be visualized against the tibia.

The tennis player may present with edema and ecchymosis in the posterior ankle region. Usually the area will be painful upon direct palpation. When dorsiflexing and

plantar flexing the hallux and digits (flexor hallucis longus and flexor digitorum longus), pain may be elicited at the level of the fracture site. Radiologic analysis will often reveal a fracture of the talus. The best view for diagnosis is the oblique of the rearfoot. Immobilization is commonly not very successful. With motion of the flexor tendons and poor blood supply of the talus, fusion of the fracture segment is often doomed. Therefore, surgical intervention is often indicated, with excision of the fracture segment. Postoperatively, a below-knee walking cast set at 90 degrees is indicated. Within 1 to 2 weeks the cast may be removed and early ankle mobilization instituted. Activity can be resumed within a 6- to 8-week period.

NEUROMAS

In tennis, as in aerobics and running, trauma to the heel tissues and calcaneus can frequently be seen. It is not totally uncommon to see injury to and entrapment of the medial (inferior) calcaneal nerve.[4,17] Branches of this nerve follow the tuberosity of the calcaneus. Injury to this nerve can occur from landing on hard surfaces with excessive pronation, due to its position superficial to the abductor hallucis muscle, flexor digitorum brevis muscle, and plantar aponeurosis.

With an injury to the medial calcaneal or inferior calcaneal nerve, sensory innervation to the greater part of the heel pad and superficial tissues overlying the inferior aspect of the calcaneus will be impaired. As Tranz[18] observed anatomically, its position makes the calcaneus vulnerable to pressure or inflammation in this region, which probably is a common cause of heel pain. The physician should first differentiate between the two distinct nerves. Further investigation may be performed by electromyographic and nerve conduction studies. These are proven tools in identifying the pathology of the medial and lateral plantar nerves. Thus they could be applied for such use with the inferior calcaneal nerve.

Treatment may vary according to the severity of the pain and the duration of the symptoms. Injection therapy may prove very helpful in conjunction with the modalities of ultrasound, nerve stimulation, fluidotherapy, and Accuscope.

Another type of neuroma, the intermetatarsal neuroma, is most commonly seen in the third interspace. This probably would be seen more often in female tennis players, due to dress shoe wear and flexibility. In tennis play a common etiology would be forefoot imbalance, since tennis players spend most of the time on the forefoot, particularly when guarding the baseline and rushing to the net. Initially the tennis player may only describe occasional numbness or burning, but, if left unchecked, more persistent symptoms such as shooting pain or paresthesias may present. Again, conservative measures should be attempted first, using strappings, injection therapy, physical therapy, and finally orthotic biomechanical balancing with particular concentration on the forefoot. I believe that, if these conservative measures fail after a suitable period of time, then surgical intervention should be considered. Excision may be done via traditional means, or laser eradication/ evaporation may be utilized with significant reduction in scar tissue formation.

ANKLE JOINT INJURIES

As in basketball, lateral ankle sprains can often be seen in tennis. These most often occur during net play or when the player lands in an inverted plantar-flexed position after jumping or an extended stride. As noted by Garrick,[19] ankle injuries are the most common injury seen in sports. O'Donoghue[20] notes that, since the ankle joint is functionally a hinge joint, normally permitting only dorsal and plantarflexion, it follows that injuries to the ankle are primarily due to lateral stresses that force the ankle through a range of motion it does not normally possess. This is usually the mechanism of injury seen in the lateral ankle tennis injury.

Another ankle injury is to the deltoid ligament, the mechanism being an eversion-plantar flexion and abduction sprain. If severe enough, this can even lead to fractures of the medial malleolus, as in lateral injury resulting in avulsions of the fibular apex. Although not nearly as common as the lateral ankle injury, the deltoid injury can be just as painful and debilitating.

Two immediately useful investigative tools are stress anterior films and the anterior drawer test to determine the integrity of both the medial and lateral collateral ligaments of the ankle. Checking for talar tilt may be helpful to determine if conservative cast therapy or surgical repair is necessary. Comparison of both ankles is always necessary. Another investigative tool is the arthrogram. This should be employed within 48 hours to be truly effective. The radiographic appearance or "leakage pattern" of the contrast media can determine the degree of ligamentous rupture or capsular damage. In addition, the exact location of the injury can also be determined. With rupture of the deltoid ligament, leakage of the dye will be inferior to the tip of the medial malleolus, radiating superiorly along the medial aspect of the ankle.

Computed tomography (CT) scans can be used to help define the exact nature of the injury. One of the obvious advantages of CT scans is their precise re-creation of the structures for minute injuries (e.g., osteochondritis disseans) and for comparison of the opposing ankle. Magnetic resonance imaging can pinpoint specific soft tissue injury (i.e., ligamentous, capsular, tendon) without the radiation exposure to the patient. Arthroscopic evaluation of the ankle may be used as another investigative/therapeutic tool. Excision of small bone fragments, hypertrophied synovium, chronic synovitis, osteochondral defects, or impingement syndromes may render relief from painful ankles for the tennis player.[21]

Styloid fractures of the base of the fifth metatarsal are also seen in tennis players having experienced a lateral, plantar-flexion inversion mechanism injury. Proximal fifth metatarsal fractures can be categorized into two specific types: (1) a fracture of the tuberosity, and (2) a fracture of the metatarsal shaft within 1.5 cm of the tuberosity. These fractures, depending on the extent of displacement or nondisplacement, can either be treated aggressively with surgical intervention and screw fixation for the younger competitive tennis athlete or conservatively for the nondisplaced fractures, with a non-weight-bearing plaster or fiberglass cast for 6 to 8 weeks.

PLANTAR FASCIITIS

Plantar fasciitis occurs quite often in tennis athletes. With constant starts, stops, side-to-side motions, and reverses of direction, a great deal of stress and strain can occur. A pulling at the origin of the plantar fascia located at the medial tubercle of the calcaneus occurs. With increased inflammation, a shooting pain distal to the hallux and proximally along the medial calcaneal nerve can occur. The tennis shoe, playing surface, excessive pronation level, and duration of play are all components of the typical overuse injury.[22,23]

With this particular injury, it is strongly recommended that tennis players decrease playing time significantly or cease playing completely. The biomechanics of the foot is one of the first problems to address. A major subtalar or midtarsal joint "fault" could be the culprit. The correct tennis shoe gear or a properly designed orthotic may help excessive pronation that has caused the common overuse injury. Heel cups, strapping, steroid injections, and/or homeopathic injections in conjunction with physical therapy are often very helpful in treatment of the symptoms. However, it is important to find the etiology in order to prevent recurrence of this injury during this racquet sport.

HALLUX LIMITUS/RIGIDUS, FIRST METATARSOPHALANGEAL JOINT HALLUX

Another common problem faced by younger tennis players is pain in the first metatarsophalangeal joint of the great toe. Quite often the etiology is a functional hallux limitus, hallux abductovalgus (bunion), or degeneration of the joint. This problem is often described as pain upon push-off and particularly during the explosive phase of push-off during running. This can result in joint swelling, restriction of joint motion, and destructive changes of the joint. Radiographic evidence of hyperostosis of the first metatarsal head or base of the proximal phalanx or both narrowing of the joint space, and subchondral sclerosis of the articular surface of the metatarsal head will be seen.

Conservative treatment with ice after activity, anti-inflammatory agents, therapy, and a prescription orthotic with a Morton's extension to help toe purchase can prove invaluable. A stiffer solid shoe can also help eliminate excessive motion at the first metatarsophalangeal joint. Unfortunately, surgical intervention for the tennis player with joint destruction may be necessary. Joint replacement with a hemi- or total implant may be chosen in order to restore motion and allow resumption of play. Arthrodesis of the first metatarsophalangeal joint of the hallux in 15 to 20 degrees of dorsiflexion is another alternative for relief of these symptoms.[24]

SESAMOID PROBLEMS

The sesamoid bones have long been a mysterious twosome that were first recognized by the Greeks as small round bones resembling a sesame seed, hence the term *sesamoid*.[25] However, it was the ancient Hebrews who popularized their existence.[26,27] It was believed that these bones were indestructible, and therefore, those searching for answers to the question of life after death surmised that they were the resting place of the soul.[28]

With more than 50 percent of body weight transmitted through the great toe complex, including the metatarsophalangeal joint and the tibial (medial) and fibular (lateral) sesamoids, in a high-impact sport such as tennis, joint stress can cause isolated injury directly to either or both sesamoid

bones. This can occur in either the seriously competitive tennis player or the recreational player. Various factors that may affect the sesamoid apparatus and their musculotendinous complexes and articular surfaces are the type of shoe gear, impact forces involved with foot plant, biomechanical imbalance, court surfaces, and pre-existing conditions.

In tennis, due to high ground reaction forces upon the first metatarsophalangeal joint, and the constant push-off and pronatory "pivoting" of the hallux in game play, the sesamoids act by assisting gait and provide additional flexor strength. When those forces mentioned above, measured at three times the body weight, pass through the sesamoids, the tibial sesamoid bears the brunt of this pressure, particularly during the push-off (dorsiflexion) phase. Thus it is apparent why there is such a discrepancy between injuries of the tibial versus the fibular sesamoid. A hallux abductovalgus can lead to a lateral shift of the tibial sesamoid, creating a situation of increased pressure beneath the head of the first metatarsal. With the sesamoid vulnerable to these excessive forces, subchondral erosion or even fracture of the sesamoid can occur. It is not uncommon for a tennis player with a semirigid or rigid plantar-flexed first ray to develop sesamoiditis or injury to the sesamoid apparatus.

Routine radiographs with comparison views of the contralateral foot can often determine if there is a bi- or tripartite sesamoid or fracture involved. Axial "sesamoidal" views can determine if there is deviation of the sesamoids or if the tibial sesamoid is more plantar grade, and with standing forces far beyond normal. Bone scans and CT scans can also help to determine if a fracture is present.

Preventative measures are often invaluable. Proper shoe selection can help avoid injury to the sesamoids. Court surface selection and amount of play are also important considerations. Prescription orthotics with proper forefoot measurements can be used, including a Morton's extension, dancer's pads, or both to accommodate the sesamoid apparatus.

Conservative care is always called for after diagnosis of a stress fracture to the sesamoid(s). After confirmation by radiography approximately 3 weeks after injury, casting or immobilization with a removable-cam walker is recommended. Delayed union is determined at 4 months and nonunion at 6 months. After all conservative means have been exhausted, surgical intervention excision of the nonunited fractured sesamoid is indicated. A permanent orthotic is necessary in order to prevent deterioration of the hallux and the formation of hallux abductovalgus. The orthotic will also help to prevent further injury to the remaining sesamoid, and provide for normal length of the flexor hallucis longus and brevis tendons.

DIGITAL INJURY AND NAIL PROBLEMS

With constant forefoot shear pressure, and toes hitting against the ends of tennis shoes on quick pivots and stops, injuries to the toes and nails are quite common in tennis. Blisters due to skin irritation by the shoe can often occur due to improperly fitted shoes (e.g., too long, short, narrow, or wide; insufficient toebox room); biomechanical factors (e.g., hammertoes, rotated hallux, plantar-flexed first rays); dermatologic considerations (e.g., mycotic skin infection, eczema, psoriasis); and nail disorders. Proper shoe selection and fit is critical to preventing irritation and blister formation. Proper trimming of toenails, and avoiding excessive shoe pressure, can prevent the formation of ingrown toenails.

Shoe technology has advanced tremendously, resulting in a variety of new types of tennis footwear. When selecting the proper shoe, the tennis player should consider specific court surfaces. Clay and composition courts are better played in lighter and more flexible shoes. Hard surfaces require more rigid, shock-absorbing shoes. Of course, the biomechanics of the tennis player's feet are a very important consideration. Tennis players who are overpronators or oversupinators must choose shoes that are appropriate for their foot type or condition. If a tennis player suffers from knee, foot, or ankle complaints, a prescription orthotic may have to be placed in their tennis shoes. Treatment of overuse tennis injuries with a well-designed prescribed orthotic can decrease symptoms and prevent frequent recurrences.

Tennis court surfaces are a separate factor to be considered. These surfaces can be divided into clay, composition, hard court, wood, carpet, and grass. The harder the surface, the greater the stress to the feet and lower extremities, whereas the softer courts provide less stress to the feet and knees. Older tennis players with degenerative arthritis and foot pathology should choose a surface that does not cause as much trauma to the joints and lower extremities. After injury, a soft surface is often recommended during rehabilitative stages, starting out on clay and carpet and progressing to harder surfaces as the athlete recuperates.

CONCLUSION

Tennis is a very active and often aggressive sport, complicated by frequent injury. As discussed, understanding of the mechanisms of injury on the part of the sports practitioner can often help in diagnosis and later treatment. Knowledge of lower extremity biomechanics during tennis play can be of help in order to prevent injury before it actually happens. Proper shoe selection, stretching, conditioning, flexibility, strengthening, and properly balanced lower extremities and feet can also help to reduce the incidence of injuries. Understanding the dynamics and stresses that this sport entails will aid in the diagnosis and treatment of tennis sports medicine injuries.

REFERENCES

1. Orava S: Exertion injuries due to sports and physical exercise: a clinical and statistical study of nontraumatic overuse injuries of the musculoskeletal system of athletes and keep-fit athletes. Thesis, University of Ovler, Finland, 1980.
2. Renstrom P, Johnson RJ: Overuse injuries in sports: a review. Sports Med 2:316, 1985
3. Sperryn PN, Williams JGP: Why sports injury clinics? Br Med J 5966:364, 1975
4. Herring S, Nilson K: Introduction to overuse injuries. Clin Sports Med 6, 1987
5. Clancy WG: Tendinitis and plantar fasciitis in runners. In D'Ambrosia R, Drez D (eds): Prevention and Treatment of Running Injuries. Charles B. Slack, Thorofare, NJ, 1982
6. Subotnick SI, Sisney P: Treatment of achilles tendinopathy in the athlete. J Am Podiatr Med Assoc 76:552-557, 1986
7. Keck SW, Kelly PJ: Bursitis of the posterior part of the heel. J Bone Joint Surg 47:267, 1965
8. Barfred T: Experimental rupture of the Achilles tendon: comparison of various types of experimental rupture in rats. Acta Orthop Scand 42:528, 1971
9. Frey C, Sheriff M: Tendon injuries about the ankle in athletes. Clin Sports Med 7, 1988
10. Murr S: Dislocation of the peroneal tendons with marginal fracture of the lateral malleolus. J Bone Joint Surg 43:563, 1962
11. Prost WJ: Biomechanics of the foot. Can Family Phys 25:827, 1979
12. Subotnick SI: Podiatric Sports Medicine. Futura, Mt. Kisco, NY, 1975
13. Mubarak SJ, Hargens AR, Owen CA et al: The wick catheter technique for measurement of intramuscular pressure: a new research in the clinical tool. J Bone Joint Surg [Am] 58:1016, 1976
14. Veith RG, Matsen FA, Newell SG: The current anterior compartmental syndromes. Physician Sports Med 8:80, 1980
15. Morris JM, Blickenstaff LB: Fatigue Fractures. Charles C Thomas, Springfield, IL, 1967

16. Turner WA: A secondary astragalus in the human foot. J Anat Physiol 17:82–83, 1982

17. Murphy PC, Baxter DE: Nerve entrapment of the foot and ankle in runners. Clin Sports Med 4, 1985

18. Tranz SS: Heel pain. Clin Orthop 28:169, 1963

19. Garrick JG: The frequency of injury, mechanism of injury and epidemiology of ankle sprains. Am J Sports Med 5:241–242, 1977

20. O'Donoghue DH: Impingement exotosis of the talus and tibia. J Bone Joint Surg 39A:835, 1957

21. Jaivin JS, Fercel RD: Arthroscopy of the foot and ankle. Clin Sports Med 13(4) 1994

22. Gibbs RC: Tennis toe. JAMA 228:24, 1974

23. Leach RE, Lewis T: Tennis injuries. p. 460. In Sports Injuries: Mechanics, Prevention and Treatment. Williams & Wilkins, Baltimore, 1985

24. Coughlin MJ: Arthrodesis of the first metatarsophalangeal joint as salvage for the failed Keller procedure. J Bone Joint Surg [Am] 69:68, 1987

25. Horose J: Disorders of the great toe in dancers. Clin Sports Med 3:499, 1983

26. Helal B: The great toe sesamoid bones: the less or lost souls of Ushaia. Clin Orthop 157:82, 1981

27. Jahss MD: The sesamoids of the hallux. Clin Orthop 57:88, 1981

28. McBryde AM, Anderson RB: Sesamoid problems in the athlete. Clin Sports Med 751, 1988

38

Football Injuries

JOHN E. McNERNEY

It is interesting to note that, although football is a contact sport, sports such as gymnastics and aerobic dance can have much higher per capita injury rates.[1-6] However, more acute injuries are sustained in football than most other sports.[1-6] A survey of high school football in 1980 found that the lower extremity accounted for one-third of the injuries and one-half of the total cost.[4] Sprains and strains of the knee, ankle, and back and contusions of the lower extremity accounted for nearly half of the injuries reported.[4,6] In 1996, the National Athletic Trainers Association (NATA) found that the number of injuries in high school football remained about the same from the 1980s to the present,[6] with 46 percent of the injuries occuring in the lower extremity, 14.5 percent in the knee, and 14.2 percent in the foot and ankle.

Football injuries are influenced by many factors; the surface, style of play, size, speed, and conditioning are just a few variables.[1,4-10] There is some evidence to support the claim that artificial surfaces produce more injuries than natural turf, especially when the knee, ankle, or big toe joints are considered.[7-10] The National Football League Players Association found that, although head, neck, and spinal injuries remain a prime concern because of the potential for catastrophic consequences, lower extremity injuries are more often a cause of lost playing time.[9,10]

SKIN PROBLEMS OF THE FOOT

Shoes used in football are often an aggravating factor or cause of injuries in football.[11-13] Some players fit their turf shoes or cleats too tight or snug; when this is coupled with sweat and thick socks, problems may ensue. Biomechanical abnormalities and the movements required in football can also create friction and skin shear, which lead to skin lesions.[12,13] Blisters, corns, calluses, intractable plantar keratoses (IPKs), verrucae, and tinea pedis are skin pathologies commonly seen in football. Ingrown or thickened nails are also common.[12-14]

Most skin lesions can be diagnosed clinically, but, in the case of warts or fungal infections of the nails or skin, biopsy or other lab tests can be helpful in differentiation. Radiographs may be helpful in differentiating IPKs from other hyperkeratotic lesions.[12]

Blisters should be drained and protected and the cause eliminated where possible. Spenco Second Skin or moleskin is useful.[12,13] Hyperkeratoses should be pared down, and, when a mechanical cause can be found (shoe gear, bony protrusions, skin shear, etc.), it should be corrected (i.e., change shoes; use protective padding, shock-attenuating insoles or orthotics).[12,13] Verrucae may be excised or cauterized, or cryo- or chemotherapy may be used until they resolve.[12,15] Problem nails should be trimmed and cut as necessary.[12-14] Surgical removal of ingrown or incrypted nails is often necessary.[12,13] Fungal infection of the skin or nails may respond to topical antifungals such as Lamisil or Spectazole.[12,14] I treat skin fungus for about 2 to 4 weeks and fungal nails for 6 months or more; I sometimes use oral antifungals.

NEUROLOGIC PROBLEMS IN THE FOOT AND ANKLE

The most common nerve injuries in sport are caused by entrapment or trauma (neurapraxia) to a nerve.[12] In football, nerve injury can be caused by direct trauma or trauma due to ill-fitting shoe gear.

Morton's Neuroma

This is by far the most common neurologic disorder found in athletes.[12] It has been described as an entrapment neuropathy with degenerative intraneural fibrosis.[16] Morton's neuroma is characterized by pain radiating to the third and fourth toes (although it can involve other toes). A palpable "click" may be elicited on medial and lateral compression of the foot (Mulder's sign).[12,17] Tight shoe gear and push-off in gait often exacerbate the pain, which may also radiate or burn along the entire dorsum of the foot.[12]

Diagnosis of neuromata is for the most part clinical. The history and physical (especially a positive Mulder's sign), symptoms, magnetic resonance imaging (MRI), or ultrasound may all aid in diagnosis, but radiographs are routinely negative.[12] Early-stage treatment may be simple: wider shoes, metatarsal pads, shoe inlays, or oral nonsteroidal anti-inflammatory drugs (NSAIDs).[12,18] In later stages, injection of cortisone or surgery is often necessary.[12,18] Football shoes that are tight or narrow at the ball of the foot should be discarded.

Neurapraxia of the Medial Dorsal Cutaneous Nerve

This injury is usually caused by direct trauma (being stepped on or "cleated"), or due to irriation on the dorsum of the foot from tight shoe laces or restrictive banding in the upper. It is particularly prevalent in football players with high-arched (cavus) feet, or those with a metatarsal–cuneiform exostosis (boss). It is characterized by pain and burning over the dorsomedial aspect of the foot, radiating pain to the hallux, or both. It is caused by a neurapraxia of the medial dorsocutaneous branch of the superficial peroneal nerve, or the medial branch of the saphenous nerve.[12]

The diagnosis is clinical, and by exclusion. Radiographs may show a dorsal exostosis, but other tests, including electromyography (EMGs), are generally negative.[12] Treatment is symptomatic, with lace pads or variable cleat lacing, change of shoes, NSAIDs, vitamin B_6 therapy (50 mg tid for 1 month), cortisone injection, and orthotics all helpful in certain cases.[12] Surgery to release the entrapped nerve is rarely necessary, but exostectomy of the metatarsal–cuneiform boss can sometimes be beneficial.

Tarsal Tunnel Syndrome

Compression of the posterior tibial nerve by the laciniate ligament as a result of trauma or excessive pronation may be a cause or aggravant of this condition.[12,18] It is

characterized by diffuse, erratic burning or radiating pain, or a tingling and numbness in the foot or ankle. The pain is often increased by standing, walking, or running.[18] There may be an associated Tinel's or Valliex's sign when the nerve is percussed.[12]

A positive EMG (standing EMGs are more reliable), Tinel's or Valliex's sign, and/or attenuation of pain by a posterior tibial nerve block are all helpful in diagnosis, but radiographs and MRIs are rarely useful.[12] When the etiology is pronation, orthotics may erradicate or ameliorate the pain.[12] Cortisone injections, NSAIDs, and physical therapy can be useful. In recalcitrant cases, release of the posterior tibial nerve via sectioning of the laciniate ligament is generally successful.[12,18]

BONE AND JOINT PROBLEMS OF THE FOOT AND ANKLE

Turf Toe

Dollar described new pathologies associated with artificial turf and provided mechanisms of action.[19] The injuries described were traumatic injury to the metatarsophalangeal joint and metatarsal–cuneiform joint. The term *turf toe* describes a capsular or ligamentous sprain of the metatarsophalangeal joint, but it has been expanded to include joint subluxation, dislocation, sesamoiditis, and/or joint or sesamoid fractures.[19–25] We can also use this term to describe similar injuries in the lesser metatarsals.[12,21]

Turf toe causes pain or limitation of motion in the metatarsophalangeal joint on dorsiflexion, plantar flexion or rotation; pain on palpation of the dorsal joint line, medial aspect, or sesamoid apparatus; and/or periarticular ecymosis, edema, or rubor.[19–24] In a recent survey, 45 percent of the professional football players questioned suffered from this injury.[20,22] The most common mechanisms of injury were metatarsophalangeal joint hyperextension (85 percent), hyperflexion (12 percent), or valgus stress (3 percent).[20,22] Eighty-three percent of turf toes occurred playing football on artificial turf, although this injury is seen in other sports and on other surfaces.[20–24] Flexible turf shoes have been implicated as a cause of this injury.[19–24] Sixty percent of the injured players were offensive and 32 percent played defense, and direct trauma such as being tackled or fallen on caused most injuries.[20,22]

History and clinical symptoms coupled with radiographs are generally sufficient for diagnosis. In difficult cases, MRI, computerized tomography (CT) scan, or bone scan may be helpful.[19–25] Treatment of "turf toe" starts with RICE (rest, ice, compression, and elevation), physical therapy modalities (ultrasound, electrogalvanic stimulation massage), NSAIDs, rigid outsole football shoes, orthotics (with Morton's extensions), spring steel (16- to 18-gauge) innersoles, and adhhesive "turf toe" strapping (reinforced with moleskin).[19–24] In recalcitrant cases, injection of steroid or surgery may be required.[20–25] Sequelae include loss of motion, which can predispose the player to hallux limitus or rigidus that may lead to chondromalacia or arthritis of the metatarsophalangeal joint.[20–23] Joint osteophytes, soft tissue calcification around the metatarsophalangeal joint, and hallux valgus can also occur.[20–23] Plantar metatarsophalangeal joint pain in turf toe must be differentiated from bipartite or fractured sesamoids.[20,25]

Lisfranc's Joint Injuries

Dollar described "turf joint," an injury on artificial turf that caused pain and swelling in the first metatarsal–cuneiform joint.[19] Sheilds stated that tarsometatarsal joint injuries represented "a significant, although often occult, disability injury in professional football players".[26] Injuries to the midfoot may be caused by extreme dorsiflexion, plantar flexion, or abduction through Lisfranc's articulation, and are classified as a ligamentous sprain (grade I), a partial tear (grade II), or total ligamentous disruption (grade III).[27] The injury is hallmarked by pain and swelling in the region of the first metatarsal–cuneiform articulation, pain on midfoot range of motion, and inability to bear weight or push off the affected foot.[19,26,27] It can cause significant disability, often requiring 6 to 10 weeks before the player can return to play.[26]

A history of trauma and clinical presentation are generally sufficient for diagnosis. Radiographs are often negative (although chip fracture may be seen), but diastasis of Lisfranc's joint, edema, or both may be documented.[26–28] Technetium-99, CT, or MRI scans are useful in difficult diagnostic or longstanding cases to define abnormal bony alignment or ligament disruption.[26,27]

Early treatment to control edema and pain may include RICE, NSAIDs, immobilization (Unna boot, cast, or taping), and/or limitation of weight bearing.[19,26,27] Casted biomechanical orthotics are indicated prior to return to play.[19,26,27] Surgery is rarely indicated, but recalcitrant injuries, especially those with diastasis or fracture, may require open reduction with screw or Kirschner wire fixation, or fusion, to fully resolve the injury.[26–28]

Ankle Injuries

SYMPTOMS AND ETIOLOGY

Ankle sprains are endemic to most sports. In football, ankle injuries are second only to knee injury in incidence of injury to the lower extremity.[1,4–6] While lateral ankle sprains are among the most common football injuries, injury to the tibiofibular syndemosis has the highest morbidity.[29–34] The deltoid ligament is rarely injured, but its injury can be troublesome.[29–31] Heidt noted that ankle sprains accounted for 11.4 percent of game-related injuries in the National Football League (NFL), with each team reporting an average of four sprains per season.[29] A total of 18.3 percent of NFL players had sustained a sprained ankle; most occurred on artificial turf (70 new sprains in a 10-year span).[30]

The etiology of ankle sprain is varied, but the mechanism of injury will often aid in diagnosis. The most common mechanism of injury is plantar flexion/inversion, which causes failure of the anterior talofibular ligament, followed by the calcaneofibular, posterior talofibular, and tibiofibular ligaments, in that order.[29–31] The deltoid ligament is often injured in eversion/external rotation, along with the tibiofibular ligament and the interosseous ligaments (the tibiofibular ligament may also be injured by extreme dorsiflexion of the ankle).[29–31] Pain, edema, and inability to continue play are the most prevalent symptoms.[29–31]

DIAGNOSIS

Diagnosis is generally made by history and physical exam. The mechanism of injury; history of a "snap," "pop," or "crack"; point tenderness; inability to bear weight; and the pattern of swelling are all helpful diagnostic aids.[29–31] Positive clinical signs or tests also aid in diagnosis. A positive anterior drawer sign (a "clunk" or 7 to 8 mm of distraction) is indicative of anterior talofibular ligament disruption.[29–31] Inversion stress (a laterally palpable talar head) is positive when both the anterior talofibular and calcaneofibular ligaments are disrupted.[29–31] A positive fibular squeeze test (Hopkinson's sign), or pain on external rotational stress is indicative of injury to the syndesmotic ligaments of the ankle.[29,32–34] Radiographs are often necessary for diagnosis. Anterior–posterior, lateral, and mortise views of the ankle are valuable when fracture or syndesmotic injury is suspected.[29–34] Stress views such as inversion stress or talar tilt (anterior talofibular and calcaneofibular ligaments), rotational stress (deltoid or syndesmotic ligaments), or anterior drawer stress (anterior talofibular ligaments) can help diagnose ligamentous disruption.[29–34] Other diagnostic aids, such as MRI, CT, or technetium bone scans, are helpful in difficult diagnostic situations.[29–31]

TREATMENT

Lateral Ankle Sprain or Rupture

Treatment of ankle sprains depends on the severity and location of injury.[29–31] Lateral sprains are often graded I through III. Grade I sprains show minimal edema and pain, no loss in ability to bear weight, and minimal change in the range of motion.[31] Grade II sprains have moderate edema, eccymosis, and pain, with some limitation of weight bearing and range of motion.[31] Grade III sprains have extreme edema, eccymosis, and pain, with loss in range of motion and inability to bear weight.[31] Similar gradations are used for other types of ankle sprains.

The vast majority of ankle sprains in the NFL are treated nonoperatively with early mobilization.[29,30] Early treatment of sprains focuses on control of inflammation (RICE) and functional support. Later, the ability to bear weight, proprioception, strength and flexibility, control of pain and edema, and return to play are addressed.[29–31] The athlete is allowed to bear weight with support so that motion occurs only in the noninjured planes. Casting is used with reservation since it may cause atrophy as well as loss of strength, mobility, and function, and result in delay of active rehabilitation.[29–31] Removable braces, range-of-motion walkers, ligament protectors, Unna boots, or taping are utilized to allow early mobility with protected weight bearing.[29–31]

Aggressive rehabilitation is instituted as soon as possible. Proprioceptive training is key to both proper rehabilitation and preventative therapy.[29–31] Teeter boards, proprioceptive platforms, slide boards, and modified Romberg's balance tests are utilized to regain proprioceptive ability.[29–31] Strength and flexiblity are addressed via therabands, Cybex, ankle platforms, minitrampolines, and active static or proprioceptive neuromuscular facilitative stretching.[29–31] Pain and edema are controlled via physical therapy modalities (electrogalvanic or transcutaneous stimulation, ice, etc.), or NSAIDs.[29–31] Return to play is allowed when the athlete can perform certain physical tests (i.e., walk and jog painlessly, sprint and run a figure eight with minimal pain, and propriocept and hop on the affected ankle).[29–31] Bracing, taping, foot orthotics, and high-top shoes can be used after an ankle sprain to allow more rapid return to play and protect the injured part from recurrent sprains.

Surgery for lateral ankle sprain is discouraged, and only severe grade III injuries or recurrent sprains that are debilitating to the athlete should be considered.[31,35,36] Brostrom and others have shown conclusively that postoperative results of early primary repair were no better than delayed ligamentous reconstruction in restoring the functional stability of the ankle.[31,35–37] I prefer laterally posted, casted orthotics to prevent reinjury in lateral sprains.

Deltoid Ligament Sprain or Rupture

Grade I or II injury to the deltoid ligament has a treatment protocol similar to that for lateral sprain, but often takes longer to heal. Grade III injury can be associated with fracture of the malleoli and may require closed reduction and casting, or open surgical reduction.[29–31] I find medially posted biomechanical foot orthotics extremely helpful in preventing reinjury in deltoid ligament sprains.

Tibiofibular Syndesmotic Ligament Sprain or Rupture

Injuries to the syndesmotic ankle ligaments are less common than lateral ankle sprains, but they are more disabling and require more intensive rehabilitation.[32–34] In a recent NFL study, players with lateral ankle sprains missed an average of 0.04 games, while those with syndesmotic sprains missed 1.4 games (50 percent missed 2 or more games).[32] Syndesmotic injuries required more treatment days (19.5) and more therapeutic modalities (6.9) when compared to lateral sprains (7.8 days and 5.2 modalities).[32] The presentation of this injury is also different. There is less edema and greater pain, and the pain is centered above the ankle mortise and is reproduced by external rotation of the foot and ankle rather than inversion/eversion. The player may be able to stand, walk, and even toe-off at times, but be unable to cut or pivot. Stress films may reveal an avulsion fracture or diastasis in the ankle mortise (comparative views are needed).[32–34] Technetium bone scans or MRI may help to depict the amount of soft tissue damage in the ankle mortise. Repeat radiographs may show interosseous calcification.[32,34] One must be mindful of maissoneuve (high fibular) fracture above the level of the ankle joint with this injury.[32]

Treatment is dependent on the gradation of injury. Grade I injuries (no loss of stability) are treated with RICE, aggressive therapy, taping, and ankle–foot orthoses.[34] Grade II injury (moderate instability) is treated via all the above and crutch walking until nonpainful.[34] Grade III (severe instability) or recalcitrant grade II injury may require cast immobilization or surgery.[34] I have found that, in lingering injuries, injection of lidocaine with hyaluronidase has helped to speed recovery in selected cases. In all grades, the use of adjunctive aids to reduce rotary motion in the lower leg are helpful (i.e., ankle–foot orthoses, ankle braces, foot orthoses, and taping).[32–34] Surgery is discouraged in all but the most severe cases of frank diastasis; this injury generally heals with few sequelae (no range of motion loss or instability).[32–34]

Myositis, Tendinitis, and Bursitis of the Foot, Ankle, and Lower Leg

SYMPTOMS AND ETIOLOGY

"Shin splints," plantar fasciitis, and Achilles tendinitis are all common injuries in football.[1,4,6] Pericalcaneal pain may be due to plantar fasciitis, calcaneal bursitis, Achilles tendinitis (enthesitis), stress fracture, and, in younger players, apophysitis (Sever's disease), to name a few.[1,24,38–42] Lower leg pain can be secondary to medial tibial stress syndrome, stress fracture, exertional compartment syndrome, or tendinitis of the peroneal, anterior, or posterior tibial muscles.[1,24,38–43] A major contributor to all the above injuries in football is the cleat. Many cleats have little or no stability in the heel or through the arch.[1,11] When athletes play on hard-packed dirt or grass, the cleats may not penetrate the ground, with the cleat becoming the only part of the shoe in contact with the surface. This causes distortion of the shoe through the shank and collapse of the athlete's arch when running or pivoting. The mechanical instability of the cleat alone, or in combination with abnormal biomechanics in the player, often leads to injury.

In all the above injuries, pain is the most prevalent symptom. The intensity, location, and gradation of pain is helpful in diagnosis.[38–42] Edema may or may not be present or observable.[38–42] Gait disturbances such as limping, shortened stride, or inability to pivot to one side also aid in diagnosis.[38–42]

DIAGNOSIS AND TREATMENT

Pericalcaneal Pain

Pain around the heel bone in football players is common, especially early in the season.[1] In the younger athlete (ages 8 to 13, or above), inflammation in the calcaneal apophysis (Sever's disease) is common.[24] Apophysitis is caused by traction on the plantar fascia and Achilles tendon. Pain is noted with compression of the heel bone (especially laterally). Limping or swelling in one or both heels is sometimes seen.[24,38] Concomitant findings might include a tight tendo Achillis (with or without tendinitis), abnormal foot biomechanics, a violent heel strike in gait, or the use of poorly constructed cleats.[1,24,38] Radiographs are generally negative. The apophysis can be visualized, and is sometimes fragmented, but this is not considered to be abnormal.[38]

Early treatment may include RICE, molded arch supports, aggressive calf stretching, and change of shoe gear. Cleats must have a rigid cleat plate (nonyielding under body weight), or must be distributed throughout the arch.[1] Aggressive calf stretching is imperative, and is used in lieu of heel lifts (if heel lifts are used, I discontinue use within the month to avoid further shortening in the gastrocnemius–soleus complex).[38] Later treatment includes biomechanical orthotics, NSAIDs, physical therapy, and, in rare cases, short leg walking casts.[24,38] I rarely use heel cups; they seldom work and, moreover, do nothing to restore the normal biomechanics around the calcaneus. Surgery is never indicated.

"Heel-Spur Syndrome" (Plantar Fasciitis)

The combination of plantar fasciitis, calcaneodynia (heel pain due to bursitis, periostitis, or myositis), and Achilles tendinitis is commonly referred to as "heel-spur syndrome." It is a common football injury.[1,4,6] Like apophysitis, it may be due to poor cleat selection.[1] The most salient feature is pain, which may be along the fascia, over the medial or lateral calcaneal tubercles, and/or the Achilles tendon.[1,38,40,41] Pain during or after sports, during the first steps in the morning, and when arising after sitting is common.[38,40] Radiographs may show an inferomedial calcaneal spur or, in rare instances, a stress fracture.[38] Bone scan, MRI, or blood tests may be helpful in differentiating heel-spur syndrome from other conditions (i.e., stress fracture or arthropathy). Early treatment may include RICE, molded arch supports, taping (low dye), calf stretching, NSAIDs, and cleat change.[38,40] Since abnormal biomechanics is most often the cause, foot control is essential.[38,40,41] I find flexible orthotics work better (i.e., cork and leather, Plastazote, or flexible acrylic). NSAIDs, cortisone injections, or both can be used as anti-inflammatory agents.[38,40] In recalcitrant heel pain, one must consider stress fracture, nerve entrapment (tarsal tunnel or medial calcaneal), and gout or other arthritides.[38,40,41]

The vast majority of these syndromes respond to conservative care. Surgery should be used as a last resort, and considered only when all available options have been exhausted. Despite claims to the contrary, heel spur or plantar fascial surgeries have a poor long-term prognosis.[44]

Achilles Tendinitis and Retrocalcaneal Bursitis

Football players commonly complain of pain in the posterior portion of the heel.[1] The pain may be due to Achilles tendinitis or bursitis or both in the retrocalcaneal area.[38,40–42] Football cleats may irritate the posterior part of the heel bone, especially when there is an enlarged exostosis (Haglund's deformity).[40] Constant rubbing over this area causes inflammation of the retrocalcaneal bursa and pain. Traction through the tendo Achillis may cause pain at its attachment to the heel bone (enthesitis).[38,40,42] Chronic irritation at the enthesis, or posteriorly over the heel bone, can lead to retrocalcaneal heel spurs.[38,40,42] Tendinitis of the Achilles is also seen about 1 to 2 cm above the heel bone (the narrowest portion of tendon), and at the aponeurotic junction.[38,42] The location and intensity of the pain are key in diagnosis. Swelling or thickening of the tendon may indicate a partial tear.[38,42] Retrocalcaneal edema may indicate bursitis or spurring.[38,40,42] Radiographs may show tendon calcification or bone spurs, and MRI may show rupture or edema of the tendon.[38,40,42] Pain, edema, decreased motion, and stiffness are common.[38,40,42]

Treatment includes RICE, NSAIDs, aggressive calf stretching, cleat change, and arch support or taping.[38,40,42] Later, orthotics, physical therapy (with emphasis on calf flexibility, not strength), and heel lifts are helpful.[38,40,42] For recalcitrant pain, I may consider heel cups or cortisone injection prior to surgery on retrocalcaneal spurs. Likewise, I may use heel lifts and injection of hyaluronidase in recalcitrant Achilles tendon pain prior to surgery.[33] These measures can often obviate the need for surgery and lengthy recuperation. Exostectomy of the calcaneus with generous removal of bone is usually successful if all else fails.[38,40] Paratenon stripping, removal of degenerated tendon, and/or tendo Achillis repair can be successful in selected cases.[38,42]

"Shin Splint" and Exertional Compartment Syndromes

While runners are most often victims of shin splint pain, this injury is also common in football.[1,4,6] "Shin splint syndrome" is a term applied to a group of injuries that occur in the lower leg. We can grade these injuries from 0 to 4.[38] Grades 1 and 2 are characterized by a mild or aching pain along the course of the anterior or posterior tibial or peroneal muscle or tendon during or after play.[38,39,41,43] The terms *myositis* and *tendinitis* are used to describe this injury.[38,39,41] Unresolved, the pain becomes more intense while the area of involvement decreases.[38,39,41] There may be sharp pain during or after play that is generally localized in the anterior or medial shin or lateral leg.[38,39,41] Pain may continue after sports, even when at rest. This is a grade 3 injury, and the terms *stress reaction to bone* and *medial tibial stress syndrome* are used to describe it.[38,39] Continued stress will cause a grade 4 injury, which is characterized by sharp pinpoint pain that may be constant, even with inactivity. Activity causes a marked increase in pain that may be enough to cause the player to stop activity. This end-stage injury is termed *stress fracture*.[38,39,41] The area of involvement and the degree or progression of pain are all that is generally necessary to diagnose this condition. Radiographs, technetium bone scan, or MRI may be help to confirm the diagnosis.[38,39,41] It is common to have a negative radiograph, while bone scans or MRIs are positive, in both stress reaction and stress fracture.[38,39,41] A high index of suspicion and good clinical judgment are the best diagnostic tools.

An uncommon but important cause of leg pain in sports can occur because of exertional compartment syndrome.[38,39,43] The syndrome is caused by increased intracompartmental pressure in one or more of the four osseofascial compartments in the lower leg.[33,39,43] Leg pain may be severe and debilitating, but a short rest will generally alleviate the pain.[43] There may also be paresthesias associated with this disorder.[43] Differentiation from the acute traumatic form that occurs after a direct blow to a muscle is imperative.[39,41] Traumatic compartment syndrome can lead to ischemia, muscle necrosis, and loss of function.[45] Diagnosis of exertional compartment syndrome is by history, intracompartmental pressure measurement (an elevation of 10 to 15 mm Hg in the resting pressure of a dangling leg versus the reading supine is considered positive), or both.[39] Radiographs and electromyography can aid in differentiating this condition from stress fracture or neurologic disorder.[43,45]

Treatment of lower leg pain is symptomatic. Rest, ice, NSAIDs, and calf stretching are indicated early.[38,39] Abnormal foot biomechanics are a major contributing cause of shin splint syndrome, so arch supports or orthotics are an essential part of treatment in all stages.[38,39,41] I have found the use of extended forefoot posted semiflexible or semirigid orthoses to be more effective than conventionally posted (behind the metatarsal head) orthoses. In recalcitrant cases, switching to a more stable cleat, physical therapy (with emphasis on calf muscle flexibility and not strength), and alternate training (swimming or cycling) are helpful.[1,38] It is interesting to note that stress fracture of the lower leg will recur in 30 to 40 percent of athletes who return to sport without using biomechanical foot orthoses.[46] Anecdotal evidence suggests that cushioning in shoes helps to prevent shin splints, but more recent research disputes this claim.[47] Exertional compartment syndromes are treated the same as shin splints; recalcitrant injuries are resolved via lower leg fasciotomy.[38,39,43,45]

OTHER INJURIES IN FOOTBALL

Overuse injuries of the knee, hip, and low back are common in football.[1] These injuries do not differ significantly from those seen in other sports. The reader is referred to the chapters in this book that highlight these problems. In general, overuse injuries in football will respond to more stable cleat, flexibility and/or strength exercises, arch supports or orthotics to negate abnormal biomechanics, physical therapy and judicious use of medication, regardless of location.[1] Levy and Fuerst[1] and Moore[10] among others note that pre- and postseason conditioning programs are essential in preventing injury at all levels due to the increased injury rates seen when players are fatigued.

REFERENCES

1. Levy AM, Fuerst ML: Sports Injury Handbook: Professional Advice for Amateur Athletes. p. 167. John Wiley & Sons, New York, 1993
2. Garrick JG, Requa RK: Epidemiology of women's gymnastics injuries. Am J Sports Med 8:261, 1980
3. Ritchie DH, Kelso SF, Bellucci PA: Aerobic dance injuries: a retrospective study of instructors and participants. Physician Sports Med 13:130, 1985
4. Pritchett JW: High cost of high school football injuries. Am J Sports Med 8:197, 1980
5. Meeuwisse WH, Fowler PJ: Frequency and predictability of sports injuries in intercollegiate athletes. Can J Sport Sci 13: 35, 1988
6. Welch TF: N.A.T.A. high school football injury study. N.A.T.A. News, April: 16, 1996
7. McCarthy P: Artificial turf: does it cause more injuries? Physician Sports Med 17:159, 1989
8. Keene JS, Narechania MS, Sachtjen KM, Clancy WG: Tartan turf on trial. Am J Sports Med 8:43, 1980
9. Skovron ML, Levy IM, Agel J: Living with artificial grass: a knowledge update. Part 2: epidemiology. Am J Sports Med 18:510, 1990
10. Moore M: N.F.L. players hear injuries quantified and analyzed. Physician Sports Med 10:199, 1982
11. Torg JS, Quedenfeld TC: Effect of shoe type and cleat length on the incidence and severity of knee injuries among Philadelphia high school football players. Res Q 42:203, 1971
12. McNerney JE: Sports-medicine considerations of lesser metatarsalgia. Clin Podiatr Med Surg 7:645, 1990
13. Hershman EB, Nicholas S: Management of callus, corns, nail deformity and other skin problems of the foot. Presented at the National Football League Physicians Society meeting: Sports Medicine 1994: An N.F.L. Perspective, Washington, DC, March, 1994
14. DeLauro TM, Hodge W: Dermatophytosis—a review of diagnosis and current therapy. Clin Podiatr Med Surg 3:427, 1986
15. McCarthy DJ: Therapeutic considerations in the treatment of pedal verrucae. Clin Podiatr Med Surg 3:433, 1986
16. Morton TG: A peculiar and painful affliction of the fourth metatarsal phalangeal articulation. Am J Med Sci 71:35, 1976
17. Mulder JD: The causative mechanism in Morton's metatarsalgia. J Bone Joint Surg [Br] 33:74, 1951
18. McGlamry ED (ed): Comprehensive Textbook of Foot Surgery. Vol. 2. p. 628, 678. Williams & Wilkins, Baltimore, 1987
19. Dollar JD: The introduction of new pathologies associated with athletic performance on artificial turf. p. 107. In Rinaldi RR, Sabia ML (eds): Sports Medicine 1978. Futura, Mt. Kisco, NY, 1978
20. Levy AM: Turf toe. Presented at the National Football League Physicians Society meeting: Sports Medicine 1994: An N.F.L. Perspective, Washington, DC, March, 1994
21. Clanton TO, Butler JE, Eggert A: Injuries to the metatarsophalangeal joints in athletes. Foot Ankle 7:162, 1986
22. Rodeo SA, O'Brien S, Warren RF et al: Turf-toe: an analysis of metatarsophalangeal joints sprains in professional football players. Am J Sports Med 18:280, 1990
23. Sammarco JG: How I manage turf toe. Physician Sports Med 15:113, 1988
24. Santopietro FJ: Foot and foot related injuries in the athlete. Clin Sports Med 7:563, 1988
25. Frankel JP, Harrington J: Symptomatic bipartite sesamoids. J Foot Surg 29:318, 1990
26. Shields CL: Tarsal-metatarsal joint injuries in professional football players. Presented at the National Football League Physicians Society conference, San Francisco, April, 1992
27. Scranton PE: Ankle and foot problems: Lisfranc's injuries. presented at the National Football League Physicians Society Meeting: Sports Medicine 1994: An N.F.L. Perspective Washington, DC, March, 1994

28. Resch S, Stenstrom A: The treatment of tarsometatarsal injuries. Foot Ankle 11:117, 1990

29. Heidt RS: Ankle and foot injuries. Panel Discussion at the National Football League Physicians Society conference, San Francisco, April, 1992

30. Hedit RS, Dormer SG: Lateral and medial ankle sprains. Presented at the Sports National Football Physicians Society meeting: Sports Medicine 1994: An N.F.L. Perspective Washington, DC, March, 1994

31. Balduini FC, Vegso JJ, Torg E: Management and rehabilitation of ligamentous injuries to the ankle. Sports Med 4:364, 1987

32. Markman AW: Syndesmotic ankle sprains. Presented at the National Football Physicians Society meeting: Sports Medicine 1994: An N.F.L. Perspective, Washington, DC, March, 1994

33. Hopkinson WJ, St. Pierre P, Ryan JB, Wheeler JH: Syndesmosis sprains of the ankle. Foot Ankle 10:325, 1990

34. Taylor DC, Bassett FH: Syndesmosis ankle sprains: diagnosing the injury and aiding recovery. Physician Sports Med 21:39, 1993

35. Brostrom L: Sprained ankles V: treatment and prognosis in recent ligament ruptures. Acta Chir Scand 132:537, 1966

36. Brostrom L: Sprained ankles VI: surgical treatment of "chronic" ligament ruptures. Acta Chir Scand 132:551, 1966

37. Freeman MAR: Treatment of ruptures of the lateral ligament of the ankle. J Bone Joint Surg [Br] 47:661, 1965

38. Bowyer BL, McKeag DB, McNerney JE: When a beginning runner overdoes it. Patient Care April: 54, 1994

39. Jones DC, James SL: Overuse injuries of the lower extremity. Clin Sports Med 6:273, 1987

40. Torg JS, Pavlov H, Torg E: Overuse injuries in sport: the foot. Clin Sports Med 6:291, 1987

41. Duddy RK, Duggan RJ, Visser HJ et al: Diagnosis, treatment, and rehabilitation of injuries to the lower leg. Clin Sports Med 8:861, 1986

42. Myerson MS, Biddinger K: Achilles tendon disorders: practical management strategies. Physician Sports Med 23:47, 1995

43. Edwards P, Myerson MS: Exertional compartment syndrome of the leg: steps for expedient return to activity. Physician Sports Med 24:31, 1996

44. Contompasis JP: Surgical treatment of calcaneal spurs: a three year post surgical study. J Am Podiatr Assoc 64:987, 1974

45. Abramowitz AJ, Schepsis AA: Chronic exertional compartment syndrome of the lower leg. Orthop Rev 23:219, 1994

46. Sheehan G: An overview of overuse injuries in distance runners. Ann NY Acad Sci 301:877, 1977

47. Simkin A, Leichter I, Giladi M et al: Combined effect of foot arch structure and an orthotic device on stress fractures. Foot Ankle 10:25, 1989

39

Complementary Approaches

Introduction

STEVEN I. SUBOTNICK

In 1995, over one-third of health care consumers went outside the standard medical system and paid out of pocket for services not available from their insurance providers (health maintenance organizations, preferred provider organizations, etc.) for alternative health care.[1] In the future, many health care consumers will be cared for by acupuncturists, certified massage therapists, chiropractors, homeopaths, or naturopaths along with their allopathic physician.

Modern medicine is geared for intervening at the crisis stage; little is done to prevent chronic disease, and the tools to treat chronic disease are limited. Add to this the burden of medical cost management systems trying to contain the cost of care by decreasing the physician's ability to provide appropriate care, and the disillusionment with the system among both providers and the public becomes obvious.

As complementary medicine becomes more integrated into the health care system and more patients take responsibility for their own health, physicians must be trained in wellness, prevention, fitness, and nutrition. They must also be familiar with the benefits as well as the limitations of the various complementary systems available. Patients are going to these practitioners with or without their physicians' approval. Sports medicine has always been a team approach, and the team is now expanding for the benefit of all.

Throughout the world, complementary medicine is being integrated into the mainstream. In Scotland, 25 percent of physicians have taken a course in homeopathy, and over the past 4 years, 50 percent of physicians in England have used homeopathic remedies in their offices. In 1986, the *British Medical Journal* reported that 42 percent of British physicians referred patients to homeopaths, and, in a survey of 28,000 members, 80 percent reported that they use some form of complementary medicine.[2]

Each of the alternative disciplines discussed in this chapter has its own approach, but all share a fundamental viewpoint on the nature of humans and healing that is at odds with the basic tenets of allopathic medicine. The eminent medical historian Harris L. Coulter wrote of the schism between allopathic medicine and the so-called alternative natural therapies.[3] Prior to 20th century medicine, the Empirical School, based on the idea that observation and experience lead to theory and that the body possesses an "energetic essence" or "vital force," predominated. The Rationalist School advocated by Descartes and Newton developed practices from theories, reduced components to parts, and viewed the body as essentially mechanical in nature. The division is between the vitalist (the natural alternative disciplines) and the reductionist (the allopaths).

In 1910, following publication of the Flexner Report, federal legislation limited medical practice licensure to those who graduated from allopathic institutions. This resulted in the system that has been responsible for the miraculous diagnostic, surgical, and acute-care intervention we have in this and most industrialized countries today. Despite these incredible advances, chronic disease is increasing at alarming rates, and there is not a true system of preventive medicine. Why? The Vitalist would say that the human being cannot be described by simple scientific terms. We are far more complex than the sum of our parts. The body is a self-healing organism that, given the proper support on all levels, will generally heal itself. Microbes cause disease that must be treated allopathically when toxic compromise or a weak immune system invites the microbes to multiply. Disease is the dynamic untuning of the whole being. In such cases as infection, the body's immune system can be enhanced by natural means (homeopathy, ayurveda, herbs, acu-puncture, naturopathy) and allowed to fight disease on its own, thereby developing natural active resistance and a strong immune system.

Both the allopathic and the alternative systems have their place. Our primary concern as clinicians is the total well-ness, health, and welfare of our patients, and we must provide them with the integrated health care that will meet their needs. Physicians must have a familiarity with alterna-tive medicine, and the following attempts to meet that need.

Homeopathic Medicine
STEVEN I. SUBOTNICK

Homeopathy originated in 1776 with the publication of *Essay on New Curative Principles* by Dr. Samuel Hahnem-ann.[4] Hahnemann, a German physician, was the first to introduce and systematize the use of natural remedies at very high dilutions (homeopathic potencies) that are the source of much of the controversy surrounding homeopa-thy today. Italian physicians and researchers Bellavite and Signorini[5] report that research has shown that homeopathy is effective and that its efficacy it not simply definable as a placebo effect. Their explanation of the effectiveness of homeopathy involves quantum physics and the principles of resonance and bond angle.

The fundamental principles of homeopathy are

1. The body is a self-regulated system with the innate ca-pacity to heal itself.
2. The natural healing processes of the body can be en-hanced by giving an ill person extremely dilute dosages of substances that, when given in larger dosages to a healthy person, would cause similar symptoms—the so-called law of similars.
3. A person who is ill must be treated according to the specific and unique symptoms he or she displays. The symptoms should not be suppressed because this will drive the disease deeper into the body, causing more serious chronic disease.
4. Treatment must take into account the spiritual, mental, and emotional state of the patients, as well as the physi-cal symptoms.
5. Substances used for remedies, when prepared by strictly controlled procedures, become increasingly more po-tent as they undergo specific processes of progressive succussion (activation) and dilution.

The law of similars figures in the medical and philosoph-ical systems of Hippocrates and St. Augustine, and was rediscovered by Hahnemann. A disease could be cured by administering a substance that, in a healthy subject, causes symptoms similar to those of the disease (hence Hahnem-ann's 1796 dictum "*simila, similibus, curentur*"). This is in contrast to allopathic medicine, which functions by the law of opposites, using potent drugs to suppress symptoms looking for an opposite effect, as with antipyretic, antibi-otic, or anti-inflammatory drugs. In fact *allopathic* means "other than."

The homeopathic concept of treating the patient rather than the disease is explained further by an example from Dr. Douglas M. Gibson.[6] Three patients with influenza are treated with three different remedies. The first patient presents with chills, is anxious and restless, and wants to be covered up and drink fresh water. Her eyes and nose are producing an irritating mucous, runny discharge causing reddening of the nose and upper lip. She also presents with gastrointestinal symptoms (vomiting and diarrhea). The remedy indicated for this patient is *Arsenicum album* (arsenic in homeopathic dilution). The second patient in the same epidemic feels tired and lethargic, experiences chills, and complaints of occipital headaches. He wants something warm on his back, wants to stay stock-still in bed, and cannot make any kind of physical effort. The remedy indicated in this case is *Gelsemium* (yellow jasmine). The third person has influenza with a feverish temperature, and his most striking symptom is achiness throughout the entire body, as if all the bones were broken. The remedy indicated is *Euphatorium perfoliatum* (boneset). All three patients have the same influenza virus, but each reacts differently; thus their treatments, based on the uniqueness of their symptoms, are different.

To the homeopath, a symptom like fever says very little, in that it is a very nonspecific reaction of the inflammatory process. The homeopath will take great care to analyze the types of fever and concomitant symptoms as a guide to establishing the right remedy. In my practice most patients are given homeopathic remedies. I often inject remedies for neuromas, heel spurs, arthritis, tendinitis, fibromyalgia, bursitis, chronic pain, sympathetic maintained pain, and reflex sympathetic dystrophy. There are no unwanted long-term results, as might be seen with repeated cortisone injections, and the injections are more often than not successful. Cortisone is reserved for the failures of this method, and surgery for the failure of both. Homeopathy has added a whole new dimension to my practice and my ability to serve my patients.

HOMOTOXICOLOGY

Homotoxicology was founded by Hans Reckeweg, a German physician who in 1952 began to formulate the principles of homotoxicology based on homeopathic principles. His formulations of complex remedies represent a blending of classical homeopathy with allopathic medicine. Reckeweg observed that the patients he was treating were far more toxic than those of Dr. Hahnemann, their diseases were more complex, and, because of the many allopathic medicines that these patients were given, the obstacles to treatment by classical homeopathy were greater. He recognized the need for and developed deep *nosodes*, remedies made from the diseased tissue itself. In his view, diseases are a recognizable set of symptoms and the symptoms associated with a given disease are a manifestation of the activation of the body's defense system. The living organism is a biologic flow system, with substances conducive to health supporting the flow system without disturbing the homeostasis and with toxic substances (which Reckeweg termed *homotoxins*) upsetting the equilibrium. Illness represents the body's attempt to compensate for damage caused by toxins, whether they are endogenous or exogenous. Reckeweg's system is easier than classic homeopathy for physicians to grasp in that he presents treatment protocols for allopathic disease categories. He identified the hormonal responses of excretion, reaction, and deposition, as well as the cellular phases of impregnation, degeneration, and final neoplastic breakdown. Homotoxicology relies upon stimulation of deficient enzyme systems and organs, detoxification, and drainage. Once a clear classic homeopathic remedy emerges, the single *most similar* classic remedy is given. This system is practiced widely in Germany and France by homeopathic physicians.[1]

Chinese Medicine and the Treatment of Lower Extremity Problems

DAVID R. ALLEN

The use of Chinese medicine, which includes acupuncture, moxibustion, and herbal preparations, is one of the most efficacious ways of treating sports injuries. Acupuncture has been used for the past 5,000 years in China, and its use has spread throughout Europe, America, and other parts of the world. There are various schools of acupuncture, but they all share the same basic philosophy, that of the underlying unit of the body–mind, and "seeing" the patient as whole rather than as a list of symptoms. Symptoms represent not an illness to be eradicated separate from the whole of the person, but an imbalance to be corrected. This imbalance has exceeded the natural healing powers of the body, and it needs assistance to achieve homeostasis.

Acupuncture is founded upon the recognition of a universal energy underlying all living things. This energy, called "chi," flows throughout the human body in an extensive network of channels called meridians. Acupuncture points are located along these channels, and it is here that the energy can be manipulated to achieve a balance in the body. When the flow of the energy within the meridian system is balanced, then there is good health. When it becomes disrupted and uneven, then we experience illness or pain. The goal of acupuncture, then, is to assist the body in its innate ability to heal itself.

The word *chi* has been translated as "life force," the animating force within us which supports life. Without it there is no life. Everyone is aware of the presence of chi, on some days we have a lot of energy and on others we are lethargic and run down. The proper amount, quality, distribution and flow of chi is essential for good health.

ILLNESS AND DISRUPTION OF CHI

In Chinese medicine, the injury is evaluated as to the disruption of the chi and blood. Joints are often affected because the blood and the chi are more concentrated in the joints. Chi travels into and out of the body at the joints. There can also be symptoms and signs along the course of the channel or meridian. For instance, an imbalance on the gallbladder channel can manifest as pain anywhere along the meridian, which runs from the eye, and ends at a point on the fourth toe. The signs and symptoms can also be found in the sense organ and the orifice that are associated with each meridian. In some cases the channel will connect on a deeper level to the organ itself, indicating a more severe problem. In this case leg pain could be associated with a pain or illness of the gallbladder itself.

In any injured area there will be considerable blood and chi stagnation. Chi drives the blood, so when its flow is interrupted, the blood does not move properly and thus stagnates. When the circulation of blood and chi stagnates, numbness, tingling, pain, or ache occurs in the area of stagnation.

The etiology of injuries can be thought of in the Chinese system as coming from five different causes:

1. Overuse of a limb or body part causing a stagnation of chi and blood, or causing a deficiency of chi and blood

2. Trauma and injury causing local stagnation of chi and blood

3. The invasion of external pathogenic factors (in Chinese medicine this is described as the invasion of wind, cold, or damp causing a stagnation of chi and blood and leading to pain)

4. A deeper organ problem leading to a channel problem

5. Emotional problems that can affect the channels and lead to pain and stiffness

Western medicine would embrace mechanisms 1 and 2

above, but would not necessarily acknowledge 3 through 5. This is an important contribution that Chinese medicine gives to the world, allowing us to have a more comprehensive evaluation of patients.

DIAGNOSTIC TECHNIQUES

In acupuncture, the diagnosis has three parts: to see, to feel, and to ask (also to smell and taste in some cases). The injury or illness will be defined by its modalities. For example, questions would be asked to find out if the injury is improved or worsened by hot or cold, pressure, or movement. It is important to note where the main pain is and if it radiates, whether hot or cold improves the condition, and what other factors make it better or worse. The onset, whether acute or chronic, and the length of time that the problem has persisted are also important.

In the treatment of sports injuries, it is important to make the distinction between an exterior problem affecting the meridians or channels, and an interior problem affecting the organs. Most acute sports injury problems involve exterior problems and will be confined to the channel or meridian.

A further distinction is made in sports injuries as to whether the injury is "full" or "empty." Full symptoms result from a stagnation of chi and blood. This leads to intense pain, stiffness, contractions, cramps, intense heat or cold, and intense skin color changes. Empty symptoms result from deficiency of chi and blood. This leads to dull ache, weak muscles, numbness, atrophy of muscles, and less intense temperature and skin changes.

From this examination a diagnosis is made and clear treatment principles are delineated. The examiner must evaluate the modalities of the injury or illness. How much of the patient's problem is due to an external cause, and how much is due to an internal cause? To what degree is the injury a full condition, and to what degree an empty condition? Is it hot or cold? Is the external cause overuse, trauma, or a pathogenic factor? Does this condition represent a combination of an external and an internal cause, or does an inherent weakness in the body predispose to the acute injury? Is the condition due to an internal cause only? It is important to note that the treatment will vary depending on the evaluation. For example, ice, which is used routinely in Western medicine, would be only applied in certain conditions.

ACUPUNCTURE TREATMENT

Treatment by acupuncture involves the placing of fine 34- or 36-gauge needles in various parts of the body. The depth can vary from a few millimeters to several inches depending on which part of the body is being treated. Local points near or around the injured site or more distant points from the injury can be treated. There are also points with special applications that might be used. If a body part is red and painful, a point on the opposite side of the body part may be used. Likewise, points on the opposite side of the body and the opposite limb can be used.

The treatment with needles can be somewhat complicated in that the manipulation of the needle can affect the body in different ways. The needle is manipulated with a reducing movement if there is an excess condition, or moved with a tonifying movement if there is an empty or deficient condition. If the area is cold, moxibustion (the burning of an herb on the skin) may be needed to warm the area of injury. In some cases bleeding can be used to decongest stagnated areas. Other treatments may include ice, rest, exercise, herbal plaster, herbal ligaments, and auricular or ear acupuncture.

In the Chinese system, typical Western diagnostic categories are not used; for example, Achilles tendinitis may be thought of as stagnant chi and blood in the kidney or bladder channel. However, several lower extremity injuries and conditions have been found to respond well to acupuncture. Tendinitis, tenosynovitis, chondromalacia, Achilles tendinitis, planter fasciitis, low back sprain, and sciatia are just a few of the conditions that respond well to acupuncture.

The principles of acupuncture treatment can be illustrated with a case history from my private practice.

Mr. A is a 30-year-old man who, while playing golf, felt a sudden severe pain in his right lower back. He had injured his back in the past playing sports, but had been pain free for several years. On presentation, he walked with great difficulty, bending to the right. He described the pain as beginning in the lower right lumbar area and radiating down into his buttocks, and down the back of his leg to his foot. His physical exam revealed muscle spasm in the right lumbar perispinal area, with a positive straight leg raising test. Deep tendon reflexes and sensation were intact. He was diagnosed as having an acute lumbar strain with disc protrusion at the L5–S1 disc. His pulse diagnosis showed weakness on the kidney area, indicating a chronic tendency for back injury.

His treatment began with checking his acabani balance. Because all meridians are bilateral, it is important to assess the balance between the two sides. He was found to have an imbalance with an excess of energy on the right bladder meridian. Needling at bladder 57 on the left leg corrected this. These are many different ways to treat this patient, depending on the orientation of the practitioner. In this case, bladder 64 was used bilaterally to strengthen the bladder channel, bladder 62 to clear the bladder channel, kidney 4 to support the kidneys, and bladder 23 and bladder 33 on the back. In this case, the needles were left in for 30 minutes.

Mr. A needed eight further treatments over the next 3 weeks and five additional treatments over the following 5 weeks. He was put on an exercise program to strengthen his back, which included stretching and progressive resistance exercises. He had complete resolution of his symptoms at the end of treatment.

CONCLUSION

It is important to know that, prior to acupuncture treatment, every patient goes through a complete evaluation for any presenting condition. This would include a history, a physical exam, and appropriate laboratory and radiological testing, all of which are done before treatment is initiated. Western medical doctors, as well as licensed acupuncturists, would go through this procedure.

Acupuncture in its own right and as an adjuvant to Western medicine is a wonderful tool in the right hands. I encourage all readers to delve more deeply into this amazing style of medicine.

Naturopathic Sports Medicine
DREW COLLINS

For millenia, the art, science, and philosophy of balancing the many elements of the human experience—soil, water, herb, fire, air, light, and love, the materials of our earthly existence—have framed our lives. All are tools in the hands of the healer/physician. True preventive medicine comes when, from within the safety of a therapeutic relationship, we discern the obstacle to cure. When the functions of spirit, mind, and body are flowing in harmony, diseases that could otherwise be manifest are prevented. Whether dealing with internal disease, musculoskeletal trauma, or an emotional or spiritual crisis, the naturopathic physician uses both modern and ancient ways.

Diagnosis is critical to good medicine, but the question the naturopathic physician asks is, what caused the vital force of the individual to respond with these symptoms? Even trauma, such as a sprained ankle, may be described as the result of universal forces working to achieve a perfection of balance. In the terminology of Eastern medicine, when blockage occurs in the highest vibrational body (the spirit), it then manifests increasingly at each of the lower (dense) bodies. The healer works at the higher spiritual level to draw out a response at the lower emotional, mental, and physical levels, for which the physician is responsible.

Primary care is a philosophy of eclecticism, and is truly the heart of naturopathic medical training. Naturopathic medicine builds on each physician's observations and experiences to consistently advance its usefulness to humanity. Competency is achieved in the disciplined use of modern diagnostic equipment, and laboratory test results are compiled to get a thorough overview of the Western medical diagnosis. Naturopathic physicians do not hesitate to recommend the right test at the most economic and efficient time. Then, building on ancient knowledge of the body, naturopathic physicians also use urine, saliva, blood, feces, and all manner of physiologic and pathologic discharges for diagnosis. As early proponents of hyperwavelength and microwavelength phenomena, naturopathic physicians are interested in all nonharmful diagnostic and therapeutic uses of radiation. In addition to ultrasound, plain and computerized radiography, and magnetic resonance imaging studies, a science of anatomic landmarks has emerged in which information from palpation, acupuncture, facial, and osseous landmarks is noted and recorded to enhance the equipment-related findings.

Physicians also listen to their patients using the knowledge they inherited from those before them. Listening is a nonjudgmental patient-physician union with therapeutic intent. The physician who listens will hear the real needs of the patient.

PHILOSOPHIC PRINCIPLES OF NATUROPATHIC MEDICINE

The philosophy of naturopathic medicine comes from the heart. It is in a doctor from the earliest stirrings of altruism.

Primum Non Nocere

Primum non nocere, do no harm, is the first principle taught in naturopathic medical school. Harm is a subjective concept, but the standard of maximum health and growth of body, mind, and spirit is applied to all decisions. Even excision of a body part could be considered nonharmful to the whole if it was done with the highest intent and followed by skillful rehabilitation. Informed consent goes a long way toward ensuring a favorable outcome of any minor or major surgery or physical procedure. People are more accepting of their fate if they are partners with their doctors.

Tolle Causam

As long as there has been fear of the unknown, humankind has sought the whys of calamities, pestilence, famines, plagues, and war. The philosophy of *tolle causam*, or treat the cause, reminds us to enlarge our scope when treating disease or injury. To a scientist, the cause must encompass unseen factors. The milieu is everything, and the microbe is nothing, to quote Beauchamp. Even accidents have causes that are apparent to the trained observer. The cause of repeated traumas is the need to unblock the stagnation of the subtle bodies.

Holism

We who would treat our patients holistically follow the naturopathic tenet that our existence is more than the sum of its parts. Social, economic, political, environmental, and spiritual constraints all play a role.

Vis Maticatrix Naturae

Nature's healing power acts through physical and mental mechanisms to restore health. An accumulation of experience leads the naturopathic physician to the certainty that there is an innate "wisdom" to the process of disease, and that healing occurs in long and short cycles. Many naturopathic patients learn that they must first get a little bit worse before they get better. Much of a naturopathic physician's counseling involves helping a patient understand that this style of medicine does not suppress symptoms, but rather brings them to fruition and resolution in order to detoxify the body.

A chronic state of disease exists when the body has built up waste, debris, and toxic substances. Symptoms of disease are the body's attempts to discharge accumulated waste and toxins. Naturopathic medicine assists the body in this process by shifting the chronic quiescent state of pathologic accumulation to one of acute immediate reaction, whether on the physical, mental, or emotional level. This enables the body to respond in a natural manner with the normal healing state.

The naturopathic physician's goal is to assist nature in returning the body to proper functioning, using such techniques as diet, exercise, osteopathy, acupuncture, and homeopathic medicines. Treatment is aimed at producing an acute, parasympathetically mediated state in which toxins and wastes trapped in the intracellular substance are freed through liquefaction so that they may be eliminated from the the body. All medicines should be carefully chosen to assist in the production of an acute liquefaction of all the body's toxins, spiritual, emotional, mental, and physical. Detoxification should be mediated with skillful understanding. We must always consider what the patient is capable of going through, what the support system will allow, the time available for this response, and the patient's understanding of what must be done to get the maximum benefit from treatment. A great deal of counseling, discussion, and, of course, teaching is involved with this type of medicine.

Whatever the wound, trauma, or misery, naturopathic medicines are transformational. We anticipate a return of old symptoms in following Herring's law of cure.

Docere

The Latin term *docere* (to teach) is the forerunner of our word "doctor," and naturopathic physicians take seriously the role of teacher. Sports medicine injuries, as well as sports medicine training and excellence in performance and coaching, all involve an active dialogue between client and professional. The naturopathic sports physician uses handouts, books, reading material, and information gleaned from the Internet, peer-reviewed journal articles, and international symposia, as well as the wisdom of the ancients, to bring about the individual's transformation.

THE DISCIPLINE OF NATUROPATHIC MEDICINE

History of Naturopathic Medicine

Naturopathic medicine is an eclectic field that was first organized as a discipline in a unique medical school in Europe in the late 1800s. It was brought to the United States as a combination of the "Nature Cure" sanitariums and a philosophy of living with God under the precepts of nature, using water, fasting, diet, and natural hygiene to elicit a cure. This philosophy was combined with the emerging science and therapeutics of homeopathy, so "nature" and "opathy" were joined to coin the term *naturopathy*. Benedict Lust was the primary spearhead of the American naturopathic medical movement, and became a prolific writer about, as well as a proponent of, this emerging field.

The field of naturopathic medicine continued to develop throughout the early 1900s, and then waned in popularity as its schools were closed through the lack of funding that followed the Flexner report. This report advised wealthy investors, such as Andrew Carnegie, to support only those medical schools that were aligned with universities, and promulgated the idea of the individual not being as important as the mass of humanity. Experimentation in the hospitals could therefore be connected directly to the medical schools, and research aimed at providing cure or relief to the masses legitimized the suffering or death of the individual or the experimentation on the individual as long as it occurred in the process of accumulating data for the good of the future understanding of health and disease in humankind. Thus medical schools became closely associated with medical research, and medical research became associated with studies involving large groups of people and less involved with the understanding of a single case and resolving that case to the betterment of that individual at all costs. The practice of medicine became more the use of pharmaceutical agents that had increasingly suppressive effects, particularly those that had petrochemical origins and proprietary qualities so that they could be patented and marketed exclusively under the purveyance of a particular company.

Medicine became more and more associated with getting a diagnosis and giving a medication that only one company had the right to sell, and less about teaching pa-

tients how to heal themselves. The discoveries in field hospitals during the first and second world wars changed the practice of medicine both in the United States and abroad with the development of sulfa drugs and later antibiotics. The tremendous, dramatic response to single or combined forms of these drugs took medicine in the direction of "miracle cures" and quick results without regard to other aspects of the individual. The spirit, mind, and emotions were relegated to different departments in universities and were looked on as more esoteric and not necessary for medical therapy. The body became fractionated in the eyes of the physician. With the use of chemicals such as antibiotics, there was no real need to pursue individualization of therapy because one compound fit everybody's needs and suppressed what were seen as the great killers, the infectious diseases. With the advances in emergency surgery, particularly abdominal surgery, during the world wars, surgery rose to the forefront as the dominant skill in medicine, so surgical procedures became the most advanced and surgery the most sought-after specialty to pursue.

In the 1960s and 1970s, Western medicine continued to pursue miracle drugs, although variations on antibiotics began to fail and we began to realize there was an end to this free lunch. Western medicine became bankrupt in its philosophy when we realized we needed another paradigm to understand why people were not getting healthier, but were actually getting sicker and sicker. Interest in immunology grew, but it was not until the increases in the incidence of viral superdiseases such as hepatitis and AIDS that medical professionals started talking seriously about the immune system as a force to be reckoned with. Cancer, for example, is a disease that still confuses the medical profession because you can never kill it all, irradiate it all, or cut it all out. It demands a total change of the body's milieu before the person is healed, and many survivors have delved into their mind, spirit, and emotions to achieve a cure.

The revolution of perspective that occurred in the 1960s brought a return to looking at a bigger picture—that humanity is part of a whole. The ideas of taking care of the planet and turning back to nature, cultivating one's own food, and turning away from some of the profit-oriented directions that medicine, as well as society in general, were taking led to a reawakening of interest in home health care and herbalism, and with it interest in seminars and books and popular lay press information that empowered people to treat themselves. This renewed interest in natural medicine and access to information from all over the world did not come from the medical community; in fact, the medical community has tried in every way possible to limit and destroy access to information that did not promote and sustain its own paradigm. Even the understanding of nutrition as a form of medicine and therapeutic intervention via dietary and lifestyle changes has been ridiculed for the last 30 years, despite the public's interest in it and demands for information regarding how to help themselves. So, any naturopathic medicine that is available now to the public, whether it be licensed physicians practicing naturopathy or published information about self-care, exists in spite of the efforts of the American Medical Association and the pharmaceutical industry. These groups are only now realizing that the trend toward naturopathic medicine is of great interest to the consumer public, and represents big money. Western medicine is starting to address the need for studying these precepts in medical schools.

The Profession of Naturopathic Medicine

Naturopathic medicine as a profession was renewed in the 1970s with the opening of a naturopathic medical school in Portland, Oregon, which had an extension campus in Witchita, Kansas. A 4-year doctorate degree, at first certified through the Department of Education, including student loans and available financing, was the beginning of a small but important option for people interested in a medical career. There are now four naturopathic medical schools in the United States. Their curriculum is based on a standardization by the Council of Naturopathic Medical Education, and they grant doctoral degrees to postgraduates who are schooled in all the premedical sciences. Students go through a resident program, including a clinical internship, and board specialization is now being established throughout the states. The graduates of the naturopathic medical schools are eligible to take a national board exam, and each individual state has the option of licensing these graduates.

There are now 13 states in which naturopathic medical school graduates can sit for a physicians' licensing exam; these states differ in slight degree as to the scope and range of the physician's license they bestow pending the completion of the national exam. The physicians who are licensed to perform naturopathic medicine are generally licensed to diagnose, prescribe for, and treat any condition of the human body. Sports medicine is one of the courses of training, and naturopathic physicians are in great demand

in this field for their understanding of the holism of the human condition. More and more coaches and trainers who are interested in excellence and performance are adding a naturopathic physician to their teams. With reference to sports medicine, the following therapeutic techniques are currently being taught in the naturopathic medical schools.

One of the longstanding therapeutic regimens that a naturopathic physician has at his or her disposal is physiotherapy machinery: ultrasound, interferential current, biphasic current, microamperage current, diathermy, and transcutaneous electrical stimulation, as well as electrostimulation to acupuncture needles. All of these devices can be used to bring fresh oxygenated blood to an area of healing and pump lymph and fluid containing damaged tissue out toward the organs of elimination.

Attention to the musculoskeletal system is central to sports medicine. Adjustments of spinal segments that may be misaligned as a result of trauma or prior to the trauma will definitely speed or improve the nerve impulses to the wounded area and assist healing.

Depending on the nature of the practice, the naturopathic physician may choose to address mind-body therapies, including guided imagery. For example, a person in a recent car accident may need to go back through hypnotherapy regression and relive the shock felt at the time of the accident so she can get on with her life and not be terrorized about driving in a car. Any deep subconscious fears or blocks concerning any trauma, especially recurring wounds or recurring accidents, can be addressed through guided imagery.

Depending again on the clinician and the style of practice, herbal therapies in the form of tinctures or oral supplementation with pills can assist healing. Comfrey (*Symphytum officinale*) is a fabulous herb for broken bones; it has actually been known as boneknit. The old standby arnica (homeopathic *Arnica montana*) can be used as a cream or applied as a tincture topically, although not in an open wound. Arnica is one of the first plants that would be appropriate for most traumas, especially crushing blows. Most sports injuries can benefit from arnica. *Ruta graveolens* is usually used in homeopathic potency, particularly if there is ligamentous involvement. *Rhus toxicodendron* is better for chronic swelling, especially if there is raised, serous-discharging skin involvement, but could be used for arthralgias and the "rusty hinge" sort of person who gets better once movement is restored.

Bee venom therapy is also in the domain of naturopathic physicians. The injection of cultured honeybee venom is used according to standard protocols of the various international apiary societies. The venom of live bees is premeasured in their stings, so the naturopathic physician can either hold the actual bee with a tweezers and sting the person several times in the area of trauma, which will bring a healing response from the body rapidly to that area, or buy vials of bee venom that have been harvested by apiarists and inject the venom with a very fine needle in a triad of wheals, using a 50:50 mixture of procaine to stimulate the body's immune system.

The naturopathic physician will often refer patients to sports massage therapists, reiki masters, qi gong practitioners, yoga teachers, Feldenkrais or Alexander therapists, jin shin jitsu practitioners, or a whole host of other allied professionals who can help the body to heal by various therapeutic regimens involving human touch.

The eclectic and orchestrated use of all manner of diagnosis and treatment methods is the specialty of a naturopathic physician, but particular emphasis is placed on understanding that the body is a complex combination of frequencies. The highest frequency is the spirit or soul; the lower frequencies are the emotional body and the mental body (represented along the acupuncture meridians), and then the physical body, which is the level at which sports medicine is currently practiced. In the next century, sports medical care must incorporate naturopathic techniques that encompass the complexity and multiple phases of human existence.

THE ART OF NATUROPATHIC MEDICINE

Parasympathetic Versus Sympathetic Responses

The body is regulated by two divisions of the autonomic, or self-directed, nervous system. The sympathetic nervous system operates predominately during times of stress injury, or crisis, and is designed to produce short-lived responses that keep the body from being hurt or hurt more. The parasympathetic nervous system is designed to reverse the sympathetic effects, and to promote healing and growth. The function of the sympathetic nervous system is coordinated by a nerve trunk that runs along the spinal column and is not under direct central nervous system control. Therefore, the moment a person is stressed, the sympathetic nerves can directly activate various organs to cause an immediate response to threat or injury. Under this "fight or flight" sympathomimetic response, all unnecessary systems are shut

down for short-term survival. Cortisol, secreted by the adrenal gland, is the predominant hormone produced in this response, and under its influence the body is prevented from activating its inflammatory and immune responses until the short-term survival goal is achieved. It is after that short-term reaction that the parasympathetic nervous system begins to act to return the body to its normal functional state, and to respond to injury.

Under parasympathetic dominance, the subconscious has access, glands secrete, and the immune system is stimulated to action. The parasympathetic-dominated reactions are normally cycled throughout the day and to a greater extent when we are inhaling. The temporary inflammations it produces follow the acid-base cycle in our body, and our body's connective substance goes variously from gel to solid or solid to liquid under the influence of this diurnal change from sympathetic to parasympathetic dominance. Thus the body tends under healthy conditions to have its own ebb and flow from one predominant neural state to another. When an injury occurs, the body is first locked in the sympathetic state and then switches over into the parasympathetic. The time of parasympathetic dominance is very similar to when a person is in shock after an accident. The lack of orientation to place, time, and space exhibited by a person in shock is evidence of this state of parasympathetic dominance; because the central nervous system is not in control, the person is not in a linear analytical mental mode at this point. He or she is in a healing mode that is not mental.

The parasympathetic nervous system mediates all the classic signs of inflammation: redness because the blood is red, pain because nerve sites are stretched when fluid rushes into an area, heat because blood is warm, swelling, and loss of function. These cardinal signs of inflammation are often referred to as or are mistaken for an infection, which is a similar process but with the addition of microbiologic life forms secreting their own exotoxins and stimulating the immune system further by their presence. Often people are treated for an infection when actually they just have an inflammatory process. Much of Western medicine stimulates the sympathetic mechanisms with medicines that work on adrenal or sympathomimetic receptor sites to suppress inflammation and keep white blood cells from doing their job, and in general keep down swelling or the continued destruction of tissues. However, the body was never intended to be under that sympathetic influence for very long.

Western medicine needs to discover the use of the parasympathetic state for healing. True healing is the opposite of sympathomimetic-medicated suppression. During parasympathetic-predominant fever, for example, the intracellular substance liquifies. This is known as going from gel to sol, and it usually occurs in an acidic state. The intracellular substance liquifies since it is a colloid, and, during that acute liquification, toxic substances, debris, and physiologic waste are liberated via the lymph system back through the major organs of elimination—the lungs, liver, kidneys, and skin. The body can be assisted in the healing process by further stressing it in order to encourage even fuller parasympathetic response.

The trained observer will note that many naturopathic therapies go through the cycle of stimulating the sympathetic nervous system to ensure the paradoxical response of the parasympathetic nervous system as a secondary, healing reaction. Such naturopathic remedies as manipulation, acupuncture, homeopathic injections, therapeutic discussion, and hot and cold applications have their primary effects by "challenging" the body to induce a sympathetic response, after which the body is allowed to swing back into the opposite autonomic neural state, which is the parasympathetic.

Thus much of naturopathic medicine, and this is really key, returns the patient to the parasympathetic state only after a strong swing of the pendulum to the sympathetic side so that the return swing falls further over to the parasympathetic state. These naturopathic stimulations shock the body, which is critical to the naturopathic philosophy. Naturopathic medicine often does stimulate or shock the body because of the secondary parasympathetic effect that comes after the stimulation. The art of naturopathic medicine is knowing how to skillfully and with the least amount of injury or harm produce that shock so as to get that secondary response. Often the patient is asked to encourage the parasympathetic state by resting quietly or taking time out to reflect.

Naturopathic Sports Medicine

The art of naturopathic sports medicine is revealed in the different approach to a typical sports injury—ankle sprain. Western medicine treats such an injury in a sympathetic-mediated fashion, as is seen by the use of cortisol in its synthetic form, cortisone. Many sports injuries are treated with cortisone, which reduces inflammation and allows rapid return to sports activity. As most physicians know, however, cortisone is a short-term strategy that has long-term consequences of destruction of cartilage and

other tissues, as well as lack of physiologic response over time. In addition, from the naturopathic viewpoint, the use of cortisone prevents healing by maintaining a sympathetic response state in the body. The goal of sports medicine is to find a strategy that allows actual resolution to occur, so cortisone can only be seen as a short-term, temporary solution. Naturopathic treatment of sports injuries must take the bigger approach and include the whole of the person, not just the trauma.

A person with a sprained ankle would be treated in the holistic frame of thinking by asking if this is a recurring injury. If so, there was probably some significant imbalance in energetics of the body in one limb or the other or in some part of the body, which usually can be traced by the naturopathic physician to the corresponding acupuncture meridians. The naturopathic physician then looks for point-specific wounds or blockages on the meridians and tries to use meridian therapy, working above and below the site to move the qi with either acupuncture needles, acupressure, cupping techniques, ska, scraping, injection therapy, or moxibustion.

The sprain itself would be treated aggressively, possibly even contrary to the American Red Cross guidelines of rest, elevation, icing, and compression, because naturopathic medicine holds that, with the correct use of hot and cold, you can actually increase and improve the healing time without causing any lasting damage. Thus a sprained ankle could be immediately assisted with rapid use of alternating hot and cold hydrotherapeutic compresses, always ending with cold. Hydrotherapy is one of the therapies that naturopathic physicians are exclusively trained in. Another is the use of injections of homeopathic medicines, most notably Traumeel and Zeel and Procaine Compositum (BHI Heel Company). These remedies are often used with vitamin B_{12} and/or some neuropathy solutions, such as procaine 2% or something as simple as saline. The injection techniques vary, but injections are often given at the site of damage and then above and below it along the corresponding acupuncture meridians. This is done in a fairly aggressive manner once or twice a day, even the day of the injury, and then followed up on a daily basis for at least a week.

With the injection therapy would go oral supplementation with bromelain, the 2,000 to 3,000 IU coagulating unit strength, as much as 500 mg every hour for a total dose of up to 10 g of bromelain per day, often taken between meals. At this dosage level, however, the patient can actually take bromelain around the clock and with meals to get the tissue levels up. Chondroitin sulfate, sulfur-containing amino acids, and glucosamine sulfate can be used if there is a joint or ligamentous tear. Herbal medications, such as *Calendula succus* (freshly expressed juice of the calendula flower), applied topically or in the 200c potency on a gauze pad with water, will speed the recovery of an abraded area.

In treating the whole body, the naturopathic physician would also want to make sure that the person gets the proper amount of rest. Sleep is nature's soft nurse, as Shakespeare put it. In addition, nutrition must be addressed, including higher intakes of vitamins C, E, and A, bioflavinoids, zinc, and glutathione peroxidase. A sodium-restricted diet with plenty of fresh fruits and vegetables is important, and digestion can be enhanced with hydrochloric acid taken before meals.

The healing state is not a mental state; it develops out of a stimulus or shock that may result from injury or the purposeful application of naturopathic treatments to induce it. Often patients are "stuck" in the sympathetic response state, merely exhibiting symptoms of their unhealed injury and unable to shift over into the healing parasympathetic state. A skilled naturopathic physician can help these patients resolve their injuries and complete the healing process.

Osteopathic Approach to the Athlete
HARRY D. FRIEDMAN

OSTEOPATHIC PHILOSOPHY

Osteopathic medicine has always stressed the interrelationship of the body's multisystem functions as well as the inseparable unity of the whole person.[8,9] Having its roots in the late 19th century, its founder, A. T. Still, M.D., inspired a medical reformation that combined medical knowledge with a holistic approach stimulating the body's inherent capacity for health and healing.[10,11] Having prospered within a uniquely American institution, osteopathic physicians have espoused the benefits of providing manipulative medicine as an adjunct to primary health care.[12–14] Diagnostic and therapeutic applications of osteopathic problem solving have wide-ranging benefits for clinical outcomes, cost containment, and performance enhancement.[15,16]

In the attuned athlete, feedback control mechanisms are highly sensitized, responding with precision and power to subtle changes in proprioceptive and neuromuscular demands.[17] Optimal systemwide function also requires the unimpeded supply of proper blood nutrients and disposal of metabolic waste products, coordinating symphonic function of internal physiologic processes. Peak athletic performance requires not only the proper placement and coordination of each part in relation to the whole but also necessitates a unity of the whole that enhances the function of each part. This reflects the unique capacity within each individual to inspire harmony and balance while achieving personal greatness.

In osteopathic medicine the precept that "the whole is greater than the sum of its parts" has definite applications for clinical assessment and management.[18] Manual palpatory assessment can appreciate the vitality and function of the whole as well as the individual parts. Osteopathic medicine therefore uniquely cares for both the whole person and the parts that make up that person. To accomplish this, we must carefully study the structural and functional relations of the body's inherent integrative functions, because structure and function are reciprocally related.[19] These relationships allow for the capacity to function simultaneously as an undivided whole as well as an intricately coordinated machine. Osteopathic manipulative approaches therefore can alternately evaluate the function of the whole or its component coordinated parts and provide treatment that enhances each.[20]

These integrative functions bestow upon individuals the

ability to regulate, repair, and express themselves fully and without compromise as long as basic physical and psychoemotional needs are satisfied. These needs are significant and can be appreciated more fully when viewed in light of the osteopathic concept. Proper nutrition, shelter from the elements, regular exercise, socioeconomic stability, self-respect, and love are needs that are required to function optimally. Osteopathic assessment focuses on the function of processes that reflect the satisfaction of these needs through observation, palpation, and clinical problem solving.

Specifically osteopathic assessment considers the mobile function related to

1. Whole-body, regional, and segmental structure and motor function

2. Respiratory and circulatory mechanics associated with thoracic cage and diaphragmatic function, and its relationship to optimal arterial supply and venous and lymphatic drainage

3. Reflexes and interrelationships coordinating central nervous system and autonomic nervous system functions, including balance, psychological, neuroendocrine, and immune functions

4. Three-dimensional biomechanical connective tissue configuration and associated balance and counterbalance of dynamic responses to weight-bearing stress and strain

5. The energetic capacity of the individual to respond to the complex multisystem demands of physical and psychoemotional function.

By enhancing mobile functions related to these physiologic capacities, osteopathic medicine promotes the coordinated function of body structures and the capacity of the individual to function as a vital, purposeful whole.

Osteopathic Models of Human Function

Five models of human function have been developed to provide a better understanding of the precepts of osteopathic medicine.[21] These five models are holistic man, neurologic man, circulatory man, self-regulating man, and energy-spending man. The holistic man model can be appreciated in the concept of myofascial continuity.[22,23] If we start with bone, we see that it is wrapped in the periosteum, a dense fibrous layer of connective tissue. The periosteum is then attached to fibrous connective tissues called tendons, and these tendons then become continuous with the skeletal muscle fibers, which are themselves wrapped in fascia. The relationship is repeated throughout the body in the myofascial attachment of one bone to another bone. In like fashion, every part of the body is attached to every other part, and between and through these attachments run the blood vessels, nerves, and visceral structures that make up the rest of the body. Holism lies in the fascias of the body, separating but also connecting every part of the body, relating it to the whole. Additionally, holism reflects the dynamic relationship between biologic, psychoemotional, and behavioral processes.[24,25] In real life, it is essentially this holism that allows a person to recover from a life-changing event such as paralysis, mobilizing the necessary resources of body, mind, and spirit to meet and overcome these disabling challenges.

The second model is neurologic man.[26-30] Neurologic function has clear segmental relationships that connect the upper limb to the neck and upper thoracic spine as well as the lower limb to the lumbosacral spine. Each segment of this nervous system is related to the spinal segment that runs between two vertebrae. This segment is responsible for transmitting nociceptor, mechanoreceptor, and proprioceptor impulses from the periphery and controlling motor responses in skeletal and smooth muscle. These are complex processes that involve the somatic and autonomic nervous systems as well as communication with nearby spinal segments and supersegmental pathways. Through these many interconnections, alterations in somatic structures can influence visceral structures and vice versa.[31,32] Additionally limbic system function influences and is influenced by somatic and visceral function.[33]

The third model is circulatory man; this concept involves the coordinated function of the respiratory and circulatory systems.[34] The importance of diaphragmatic function within many compartments of the body is central to the proper delivery of arterial fluids and return of venous and lymphatic waste products. The thoracic cage contains two important diaphragms, one at the inferior and the other at the superior thoracic aperture. These diaphragms possess extensive connective tissue attachments to the muscular and bony structures that they approximate. Important neurovascular and visceral structures also traverse these diaphragms. These diaphragms are connected not only by connective tissue and muscular attachments, but also through pressure gradients established within body cavities along which venous and lymphatic fluids are returned to the thoracic cage. Optimal circulatory function is dependent on these musculoskeletal and physiologic relations.

The fourth model, self-regulating man, represents the key distinction between allopathic and osteopathic medicine.[35-40] In allopathic medicine, the primary focus is on evaluating and treating disease processes using various external agents to influence internal function. This approach ignores the many host responses that are central to the individual's ability to maintain optimal health and to resist as well as recover from disease. These internal mechanisms that promote health and resist disease are related to the integrative functions of the body as well as the unifying principle of the whole.

Finally, we have the last model of energy-spending man. Osteopathic medicine has often described the musculoskeletal system as the primary machinery of health and disease, with the viscera being termed the *secondary machinery*. The concept says that the heart, lungs, intestines, and other organs provide supportive processes that provide the energy for the musculoskeletal system to carry out our daily activities. The effects of segmental and regional motor disturbances on energy-spending man are considerable.[41,42] Increased energy consumption from compensatory muscle activity and higher metabolic demands result from even the smallest injury to the lower extremity.[43,44] Multiple insults of this type are constantly challenging the energy demands of the individual, and compromise the available energy that may be required to perform other functions, such as recuperative responses to illness and stress responses to psychoemotional demands.

PRINCIPLES OF OSTEOPATHIC ASSESSMENT

Evaluation of athletic performance must consider the weight-bearing function at play during specific activities in a specific individual and at a particular moment in time. All weight-bearing activities share a basic fundamental relation to gait function that serves as a useful common starting point for evaluation. The osteopathic evaluation of gait assesses both the dynamic interplay of components making up the gait cycle and the overall unity of body movement.[45] Regional observation of body symmetry identifies both structural and functional components that influence gait. Position and relative lack or excess of movement is noted from head to toe, comparing left to right, front to back, and top to bottom. Areas of altered structure or function are recorded and compared with a similar assessment repeated after osteopathic intervention.

Assessment of whole-body function during gait requires a different focus on the entire body moving through space. This can be accomplished by using peripheral vision to look at the space surrounding the body as it participates in ambulatory movement. What draws attention are areas of relative absence of motion and their associated substituted or compensatory movements. Complex whole-body patterns of movement and countermovement can often be appreciated in three-dimensional, spiraling pathways that connect seemingly unrelated areas of the body. These connections are recorded in the areas of hypo- and hypermobility noted.

Regional testing of dynamic body movement can also be conducted, assessing both structural and functional symmetry. Regional movements are performed, observing for proper muscle firing sequencing and the balance of agonist and antagonist relations.[46-48] Specific tests might include *hip extension*, where the relative inhibition of the gluteus maximus muscle is often substituted by overstimulation of the hamstring and paraspinal muscles. Often an underlying psoas muscle hypertonicity is also present, causing a reflex inhibition of the gluteus maximus. *Hip abduction* testing observes for the function of the gluteus medius and minimus muscles, which are often inhibited by hypertonicity in the hip abductor mechanism as well as in the synergistic overactivity of the tensor fasciae latae, iliopsoas, and quadratus lumborum muscles. *Abdominal trunk* curls test the relative strength of the abdominal muscles, which can be inhibited by hypertonic paraspinal muscles and associated synergistic overdevelopment of the iliopsoas mechanism. *Shoulder abduction* can be monitored for imbalance of muscles, usually reflecting a relative inhibition of the inner scapular muscles, with reflex relationships to overstimulation in pectoralis, upper trapezius, and levator scapulae muscles. *Head flexion* can be observed for proper muscle balance between the deep neck flexors, which are usually inhibited by the overstimulated suboccipital muscles. Synergistic overstimulation is also often apparent in the sternocleidomastoid and scalene muscles, causing a relative hyperextension of the head on the neck, forward positioning of the head in the standing position, and increasing kyphosis below the level of C4. Altered movement patterns of this type contribute to uneven weight-bearing mechanics, proprioceptive dysfunction, impaired coordination and reflexes, increased energy demand and metabolic waste products, and eventually degenerative diseases and chronic pain syndromes.[49]

Observation of weight bearing during specific athletic activities requires a thorough knowledge of the normal weight-bearing movements required by that sport. Evaluation of coordinated muscle function and reflexes can be accomplished through assessment of whole-body and regional movements. Regional motion testing in the osteopathic approach focuses on areas of relative decreased mobility and compensatory areas of increased mobility.[50] The osteopathic approach only begins with these observations, and generally emphasizes segmental disturbances that interfere with the regional participation of whole-body movements and disturb the proprioceptive feedback function. For example, a rib dysfunction may interfere with the athlete's normal arm motion, which might interfere with the hand-eye coordination necessary to hit or catch a ball. Identification and subsequent treatment of this rib dysfunction would reestablish more optimal afferent feedback information and enhance hand-eye coordination.

Once an area of regional dysfunction or decreased mobility has been identified, segmental evaluation of that disturbance is performed. This involves identifying the exact location of altered tissue texture and tension as well as characterizing the altered rotary and/or translatory motion characteristics at the segment identified.[51] Additionally, areas of regional hypomobility are evaluated for tension reflected in the passive connective tissue space that connects and supports the active neuromuscular elements. Connective tissues respond to dynamic stress and strain by reorganizing to accommodate and balance forces that influence proprioceptive and neuromuscular control mechanisms.[52] This reorganization involves collagen and reticular fibers, which proliferate, causing increased stiffness in what is essentially a colloid-fluid matrix.[53,54] Optimal function of connective tissue requires a relative predominance of its fluid-gel properties over its more solid tensile properties (sol-gel matrix).[55] Dynamic fluid properties are subsequently compromised with dysfunction, causing a relative turbulence and loss of vitality of these tissues. Such connective tissue deformation is characterized by three-dimensional shortening and thickening and is perceived as a palpable tension and twist of myofascial structures. Responding to both initial and ongoing stress from postural strain and traumatic injury, connective tissue deformation easily compromises neurovascular and musculoskeletal structures. There is associated compromise of cellular and immune elements, which normally require a relative fluid predominance in the sol-gel matrix. Palpation of these mobile disturbances requires highly developed psychomotor skills that necessitate time and practice to master.

With most weight-bearing activities, the importance of the lower extremity and lumbopelvic mechanism cannot be overstated.[56,57] Disturbances in this mechanism can result from primary dysfunctions at either end of the chain or at both ends.[58] With the passage of time, however, secondary compensatory disturbances will become more primary due to persistence of the altered feedback mechanisms and changes in the connective tissue structure and function. However, it is also almost universally true that, when the primary disturbances are located and resolved, the associated compensatory neuromuscular and myofascial dysfunctions begin to resolve spontaneously. This point underlines the importance of reflex and compensatory changes between specific areas of dysfunction and more distant, seemingly unrelated areas.

OSTEOPATHIC APPROACHES TO PATIENT MANAGEMENT

Enhancing self-regulatory and self-healing mechanisms within the unified function of the whole patient is the primary focus of osteopathic treatment.[59] This can be reflected in balanced function of the active neuromuscular and passive connective tissue elements comprising the body's mobile systems.[60] Regional and segmental disturbances in neuromuscular control can be resolved through skilled observation of patient responses to the systematic application of corrective manipulative forces.

Alterations in tissue tension characterizing mobile dysfunction are monitored for their response to rotary and/or translatory motions applied by passive operator control.[61–64] Corrective forces are then brought to bear by operator or patient effort or by inherent self-regulating forces within the patient. Patient responses to manipulative forces maintain, enhance, or sometimes reverse the corrective impulses of treatment. Often these responses are associated with other areas of disturbed physiologic function. These related disturbances may involve more primary mobile dysfunctions or other physiologic mechanisms that require treatment. Such other physiologic mechanisms include viscerosomatic reflex activity, compromised respiratory still circulatory mechanics, and connective tissue dysfunction that may compromise neural, vascular, or visceral structures.[65,66]

Corrective forces can be direct or indirect. Direct technique engages and overcomes the restrictive barrier and lengthens tight muscles and fascia. Indirect techniques move away from the restrictive barrier toward greater tissue relaxation and spontaneous release characterized by reduced afferent feedback and recovery of the dynamic physiologic midline.[67,68] Both direct and indirect principles stimulate the inherent restorative capacity in the patient by reestablishing dynamic fluid and tissue balance related to whole-body vitality. Manipulative procedures can require patient activity (i.e., muscle contraction) or can be passive, the forces being introduced by the operator with or without impulse. Additionally, inherent forces within the patient can be utilized to influence manipulative procedures, including respiratory motion, connective tissue creep, and hysteresis, and the patient's inherent capacity for health and healing.[69–71]

Lower extremity function is a primary concern in osteopathic patient management.[72] Optimal joint mobility and balanced muscle and connective tissue function in the lower extremity are the foundation for weight-bearing functions of the entire body.[73] Manipulative interventions are often followed by additional postural interventions to optimize this important relationship to whole-body function. Standing anteroposterior and lateral postural films can be evaluated for sacral base unleveling associated with pelvic tilt and short leg syndromes.[74,75] Appropriate lift therapy can be implemented to reestablish the normal horizontal relationship of the sacral base to the lumbar spine.[76–78] Lumbopelvic instability of sagittal postural function may also require evaluation (i.e., for hyperlordosis syndromes) and treatment utilizing lifts, braces, belts, orthotics, ligament injections, and surgery if the patient is at high risk for neurologic compromise.[79–83] Additional consideration is given to the use of custom foot orthotics to optimize the mechanical relationships of the forefoot, hindfoot, and ankle.

Patient responses to osteopathic manipulation vary greatly, so frequency and duration of treatment are highly individualized.[84] Maintenance of optimal function is reinforced with a home exercise program that incorporates proprioceptive sensori motor retraining and stretching and strengthening to balance the functions of agonist and antagonist muscles and minimize substitution by synergistic muscles.[85] Additionally, patients are instructed in the proper biomechanics of sitting, standing, lifting, bending, reseating, reaching, sleeping, and breathing, as well as in the use of proper footwear.[86,87] Behavioral aspects of motivation, life-style habits, and psychoemotional stress are all important aspects of osteopathic management of the whole patient and should be carefully evaluated.[88,89]

CONCLUSION

The uniqueness of the osteopathic approach to evaluation and treatment of the athlete and lower extremity problems centers around the interrelationships between body regions and integrative whole-body function.[90] While relieving pain and restoring local function are important therapeutic goals, they are only part of the osteopathic approach to patient management. Osteopathic thinking considers the individual component parts in relationship to the whole person. Neuromuscular control mechanisms have central and peripheral relationships that relate lower extremity function to the rest of the body. Connective tissue serves an important role in transmitting and balancing mechanical and fluid forces necessary to carry out coordinated body functions. Integrative functions of the central and autonomic nervous systems and the respiratory and circulatory systems require optimal mobile function in their musculoskeletal relations. Psychoneuroimmunologic system interactions involve whole-body and local stress responses. They can be influenced by osteopathic manipulation and patient life-style management. Adequate provision for fulfilling physical, emotional, socioeconomic, and spiritual needs has a profound influence on the patient as a whole as well as on musculoskeletal performance. Enhancing these functions so that patients can excel in their personal and professional endeavors is the ultimate goal of osteopathic patient management.

REFERENCES

Introduction

1. Eisenberg DM, Kessler RC, Foster C et al: Unconventional medicine in the United States. N Engl J Med 328:246, 1993
2. Reilly DT: Research, homeopathy, and therapeutic consultation. Alternative Ther 1:65, 1995
3. Coulter HL: Divided legacy: a history of the schism. In Medical Thought: Vol. 4. Twentieth Century Medicine: The Bacteriological Era. North Atlantic Books, Berkeley, CA, 1995

Homeopathic Medicine

4. Hahnemann S: Essay on New Curative Principles. 1776
5. Bellavite P, Signorini A: Homeopathy: A Frontier of Medical Science. North Atlantic Books, Berkeley, CA, 1995
6. Gibson DM: Studies of Homeopathic Remedies. Beaconsfield Publishers Ltd., Bucks, England, 1987
7. HH Reckeweg: Materia Medica, Vols. 1 and 2. Aurelia-Verlag, Baden-Baden, 1989

Osteopathic Approach to the Athlete

8. Still AT: Philosophy of Osteopathy. p. 40. Author, Kirksville, M, 1899. (Reprinted by the Academy of Applied Osteopathy, Indianapolis, 1946)

9. Still AT: Philosophy and Mechanical Principles of Osteopathy. Author, Kansas City, 1902 (Reprinted by Osteopathic Enterprises, Kirksville, MO, 1986)

10. Northup GW: Osteopathic Medicine: An American Reformation. 2nd ed. American Osteopathic Association, Chicago, 1979

11. Trowbridge C: Andrew Taylor Still: 1828–1917. Thomas Jefferson University Press, Kirksville, MO, 1991

12. Buerger AA: Empirical Approaches to the Validation of Spinal Manipulation. Charles C Thomas, Springfield, IL, 1985

13. Buerger AA: Approaches to the Validation of Manipulation Therapy. Charles C Thomas, Springfield, IL, 1977

14. Gevitz N: The DO's: Osteopathic Medicine in America. Johns Hopkins University Press, Baltimore, 1982

15. MacDonald RS: An open controlled assessment of osteopathic manipulation in non-specific low back pain. Spine 15:364, 1990

16. Northup GW: Osteopathic Research Growth and Development. American Osteopathic Association, Chicago, 1987

17. Greenman PE (ed): Concepts and Mechanisms of Neuromuscular Functions. Springer-Verlag, Berlin, 1984

18. Johnston WL: Functional Methods: A Manual for Palpatory Skill and Development in Osteopathic Examination and Manipulation of Motor Function. American Academy of Osteopathy, Indianapolis, 1994

19. Northup GW: The Physiological Basis of Osteopathic Medicine. Postgraduate Institute of Osteopathic Medicine and Surgery, New York, 1970

20. Kuchera WA: Osteopathic Principles and Practice. 2nd ed. Grayden Press, Columbus, OH, 1994

21. Greenman PE: Models and mechanisms of osteopathic manipulative medicine. Osteopath Med News 4:1, 1987

22. Becker RF: The meaning of fascia and fascial continuity. Osteopath Ann 3:186, 1975

23. Cathie AG: Fascia of the body in relation to function and manipulative therapy. p. 74. In Yearbook of the Academy of Applied Osteopathy American Academy of Osteopathy, Indianapolis, 1960

24. Bandura A: Self efficacy mechanisms in physiological activiation and health promoting behavior. In Madden J IV (ed): Neurobiology of Learning, Emotion, and Affect. Raven, New York, 1991

25. Stanton DF: Chronic pain and the chronic pain syndrome: the usefulness of manipulation and behavioral interventions. Phys Med Rehabil Clin North Am 7:000, 1996

26. Gilliar WG: Neurologic basis of manual medicine. Phys Med Rehabil Clin North Am 7:693, 1966

27. Getting PA: Emerging principles governing the operation of neural networks. Annu Rev Neurosci 12:185, 1989

28. Korr IM (ed): Neurologic Mechanisms in Manipulative Therapy. Plenum Press, New York, 1978

29. Patterson MM: Eliza Burns Memorial Lecture, 1980: the spinal cord—active processor not passive transmitter. J Am Osteopath Assoc 80:210, 1980

30. Van Busker RL: Nociceptive reflexes in somatic dysfunction: a model. J Am Osteopath Assoc 90:791, 1990

31. Beal MC: Viscerosomatic reflexes: a review. J Am Osteopath Assoc 85:786, 1985

32. Patterson MM: The Central Connection: Somatovisceral/Viscerosomatic Interaction. American Academy of Osteopathy, Indianapolis, 1992

33. Willard FH: Nociception and the neuroendocrine immune connection. In Proceedings of the 1991 American Academy of Osteopathy International Symposium. University Classics Ltd, Athens, OH, 1991

34. Zink JG: Respiratory and circulatory care: the conceptual model. Osteopath Ann 5:108, 1977

35. Mochan E: Human regulatory adaptations in health and disease: a molecular perspective. p. 99. In Ward R (ed): Foundations for Osteopathic Medicine. Williams & Wilkins, Baltimore, 1997

36. Patterson MM: Neurophysiologic system: integration and disintegration. p. 137. In Ward R (ed): Foundations for Osteopathic Medicine. Williams & Wilkins, Baltimore, 1997

37. Portanova R: Endocrine system and body unity: osteopathic principles at a chemical level. p. 83. In Ward R (ed): Foundations for Osteopathic Medicine. Williams & Wilkins, Baltimore, 1997

38. Theobald RJ: Pharmacologic and osteopathic basic principles. p. 93. In Ward R (ed): Foundations for Osteopathic Medicine. Williams & Wilkins, Baltimore, 1997

39. Willard FH: Autonomic nervous system. p. 53. In Ward R (ed): Foundations for Osteopathic Medicine. Williams & Wilkins, Baltimore, 1997

40. Willard FH: Neuroendocrine, immune system, and homeostasis. p. 107. In Ward R (ed): Foundations for Osteopathic Medicine. Williams & Wilkins, Baltimore, 1997

41. Buzzell KA: The cost of human posture in locomotion. In The Physiological Basis of Osteopathic Medicine, The Postgraduate Institute of Osteopathic Medicine and Surgery, New York, 1970

42. Yelin E: The economic cost and social and psychological impact of musculoskeletal conditions. Arthritis Rheum 38:1351, 1995

43. Blood SD: Treatment of the sprained ankle. J Am Osteopath Assoc 790:680, 1980

44. Kuchera ML: Athletic functional demand and posture. J Am Osteopath Assoc 90:843, 1990

45. Peterson B: Postural Balance and Imbalance. American Academy of Osteopathy, Indianapolis, 1983

46. Bookhout MR: Exercise in somatic dysfunction. Phys Med Rehabil Clin North Am 7:845, 1996

47. Janda V: Muscle weakness and inhibition (pseudoparesis) in back pain syndrome. In Grieve G: Modern Manual Therapy of the Vertebral Column. Churchill Livingstone, Edinburgh, 1986

48. Janda V: Muscle, central nervous motor regulation and back problems. In Korr IM (ed): Neurological Mechanisms in Manipulative Therapy. Plenum Press, New York, 1977

49. Janda V: Treatment of chronic back pain. J Manual Med 6: 166, 1992

50. Johnston WL: Passive gross motion testing, part 1: its role in physical examination. J Am Osteopath Assoc 81:298, 1981

51. Johnston WL: Segmental definition, part 1: a focal point for diagnosis of somatic dysfunction. J Am Osteopath Assoc 88: 99, 1988

52. Bilkey W: Involvement of fascia in mechanical pain syndromes. J Manual Med 6:157, 1992

53. Hubbard RP: Mechanical behavior of connective tissue. p. 47. In Greenman PE (ed): Concepts and Mechanisms of Neuromuscular Functions. Springer-Verlag, New York, 1984

54. Viidik A: Interdependence between structure and function in collagenous tissues. p. 257. In Viidik A (ed): Biology of Collagen. Academic Press, New York, 1987

55. Woo S-L: Anatomy, biology, and biomechanics of tendon, ligament, and rotation. p. 45. In Simon SR (ed): Orthopedic Basic Science. American Academy of Orthopaedic Surgeons, 1994

56. Kuchera ML: Lower extremities. p. 623. In Ward R (ed): Foundations for Osteopathic Medicine. Williams & Wilkins, Baltimore, 1997

57. Vleeming A: Low back pain: the integrated function of the lumbar spine and sacroiliac joints. In Proceedings of the 2nd Interdisciplinary World Congress, San Diego, 1995

58. Giles LGF: Low back pain associated with leg length inequality. Spine 6:510, 1981

59. Hruby RJ: Pathophysiologic models in the selection of osteopathic manipulative techniques. J Osteopath Med 6:25, 1992

60. Lewitt K: Manipulative Therapy and Rehabilitation of the Motor System. 2nd ed. Oxford-Heinemann Ltd., London, 1991

61. Bowles CH: A functional orientation for technique. p. 177. In Page LE (ed): Yearbook of the Academy of Applied Osteopathy. American Academy of Osteopathy, Indianapolis, 1955

62. Bowles CH: Functional technique: a modern perspective. J Am Osteopath Assoc 80:326, 1981

63. Hoover HV: Fundamentals of technique. p. 25. In Yearbook of the Academy of Applied Osteopathy. Edward's Brothers Inc., Ann Arbor, MI, 1949

64. Johnston WL: Segmental definition, part 2: application of an indirect method in osteopathic manipulative treatment. J Am Osteopath Assoc 88:211, 1988

65. Johnston WL: Segmental definition, part 3: definitive basis for distinguishing somatic findings of visceral reflex origin. J Am Osteopath Assoc 88:347, 1988

66. Nei EA: Overview of techniques and system approaches to manipulation. Phys Med Rehabil Clin North Am 7:731, 1996

67. DiGiovanna EL: An Osteopathic Approach to Diagnosis and Treatment. JB Lippincott, Philadelphia, 1991

68. Jones LH: Spontaneous release by positioning. The DO 4: 109, 1964

69. Cantu RL: Myofascial Manipulation: Theory and Clinical Application. Aspen, Gaithersburg, MD, 1992

70. Lippincott HA: The osteopathic technique of William G. Southerland, DO. p. 1. In Northup DL (ed): Yearbook of the Academy of Applied Osteopathy. Edwards Brothers Inc., Ann Arbor, MI, 1949

71. Lippincott HA: Basic principles of osteopathic technique p. 45. In Yearbook of the Academy of Applied Osteopathy. Ewards Brothers Inc., Baqrnes MW (ed): Ann Arbor, MI, 1961

72. English WR: Manual medicine techniques used in the management of musculoskeletal somatic dysfunction of the lower extremity. Phys Med Rehabil Clin North Am 7:811, 1966

73. Cathie AG: Influence of the Lower Extremity upon the Structural Integrity of the Body. p. 157. American Academy of Osteopathy, Indianapolis, 1996

74. Kuchera ML: Postural considerations in coronal and horizontal planes. p. 983. In Ward R (ed): Foundations for Osteopathic Medicine. Williams & Wilkins, Baltimore, 1997

75. Willman MK: Radiographic technical aspects of the postural study. p. 1025. In Ward R (ed): Foundations for Osteopathic Medicine. Williams & Wilkins, Baltimore, 1997

76. Greenman PE: Lift therapy: use and abuse. J Am Osteopath Assoc 79:238, 1979

77. Hoffman KS: Effects of adding sacral base leveling to osteopathic manipulative treatment of back pain: a pilot study. J Am Osteopath Assoc 94:217, 1994

78. Irwin IE: Reduction of lumbar scoliosis by use of a heel lift to level the sacral base. J Am Osteopath Assoc 91:34, 1991

79. Dorman TA: Diagnosis and Injection Techniques in Orthopaedic Medicine. Williams & Wilkins, Baltimore, 1991

80. Kuchera ML: Gravitational stress, musculoligamentous strain and postural alignment. Spine: State of the Art Rev 9:463, 1995

81. Kuchera ML: Alteration of interpelvic spatial relationship utilizing an external pelvic orthosis in patients with low back pain. J Am Osteopath Assoc 92:1182, 1992

82. Kuchera ML: Postural considerations in the sagittal plane. p. 999. In Ward R (ed): Foundations for Osteopathic Medicine. Williams & Wilkins, Baltimore, 1997

83. Ongley NJ: A new approach to the treatment of chronic low back pain. Lancet 2:143, 1987

84. Kimberly PE: Formulating a prescription for osteopathic manipulative treatment. J Am Osteopath Assoc 75:486, 1976

85. Twomey LT: Supine exercise and spinal manipulation in the treatment of low back pain. Spine 20:615, 1995

86. Fisk JR: Back schools—past, present, and future. Clin Orthop 179:18, 1983

87. Triano JJ: Manipulative therapy vs. education programs in chronic low back pain. Spine 20:948, 1995

88. Roy R: The Social Context of the Chronic Pain Sufferer. University of Toronto Press, Toronto, 1992

89. Weiner H: Perturbing the Organism: The Biology of Stressful Experience. University of Chicago Press, Chicago, 1992

90. Prokop LL: The use of manipulation in sports medicine practice. Phys Med Rehabil Clin North Am 7:915, 1996

SUGGESTED READINGS

Homeopathic Medicine

Bianch-Ivo M: Geriatrics and Homotoxicology. Aurelia-Verlag, Baden-Baden, 1994 Cummings S, Ullman D: Everybody's Guide to Homeopathic Medicine. North Atlantic Press, Berkeley, CA, 1995

Subotnick SI: Sports and Exercise Injuries: Conventional, Homeopathic & Alternative Treatments. North Atlantic Press, Berkeley, CA, 1991

Osteopathic Approaches to the Athlete

Anderson R, Meeker WC, Wirick BE et al: A meta-analysis of clinical trials of spinal manipulation. J Manipulative Physiol Ther 15:181, 1992

Basmajian JV (ed): Rational Manual Therapies. Williams & Wilkins, Baltimore, 1993

Bourdillon JF: Spinal Manipulation. 5th ed. Butterworth-Heinemann, Oxford, 1992

Greenman PE: Principles of Manual Medicine. 2nd ed. Williams & Wilkins, Baltimore, 1996

LaBan MM: Manipulation: an objective analysis of the literature. Orthop Clin North Am 23:451, 1992

Mennell JM: Joint pain and back diagnosis and treatment using manipulative techniques. Aspen, Gaithersburg, MD, 1992

Mitchell FL: The Muscle Energy Manual. MET Press, East Lansing, MI, 1995

Vleeming A: Movement, the Pelvis, and Low Back Pain: An Interdisciplinary Approach. Churchill Livingstone, Edinburgh, in press

Ward R: Glossary of osteopathic terminology. Am Osteopath Assoc 80; 552, 1981

Ward R (ed): Foundations for Osteopathic Medicine. Williams & Wilkins, Baltimore, 1997

Sources for Further Information, Publications, or Courses on Homeopathic Medicine

American Holistic Medical Association
6932 Little River Turnpike
Annandale, VA 22003
(703) 642–5880

Biological Homeopathic Industries, Inc.
11600 Cochiti, S.E.
Albuquerque, NM 87123
(800) 621–7644

California State Homeopathic Medical Society
Richard Hiltner, M.D.
169 East El Robaar
Ojai, CA 93023
(805) 646–1495

Hahnemann College of Homeopathy
San Pablo Avenue
Albany, CA
(510) 524–3117

Homeopathy Educational Services
2124 Kittredge Street
Berkeley, CA 94704
(800) 359–9051

International Foundation for Homeopathy
2366 Eastwood Avenue
East Seattle, WA 98101
(206) 324–8230

National Center for Homeopathy
8012 North Fairfax Street, Suite 306
Alexandria, VA 22314
(703) 548–7790
Fax (703) 548–7792

National College of Homeopathic Medicine
11231 S.E. Market Street
Portland, OR 97126

Index

Note: Page numbers followed by f indicate figures; page numbers followed by t indicate tables.